Fundamental Skills and Concepts in Patient Care

Fundamental Skills and Concepts in Patient Care

SEVENTH EDITION

BARBARA KUHN TIMBY, RN,C, BSN, MA
Nursing Professor
Glen Oaks Community College
Centreville, Michigan

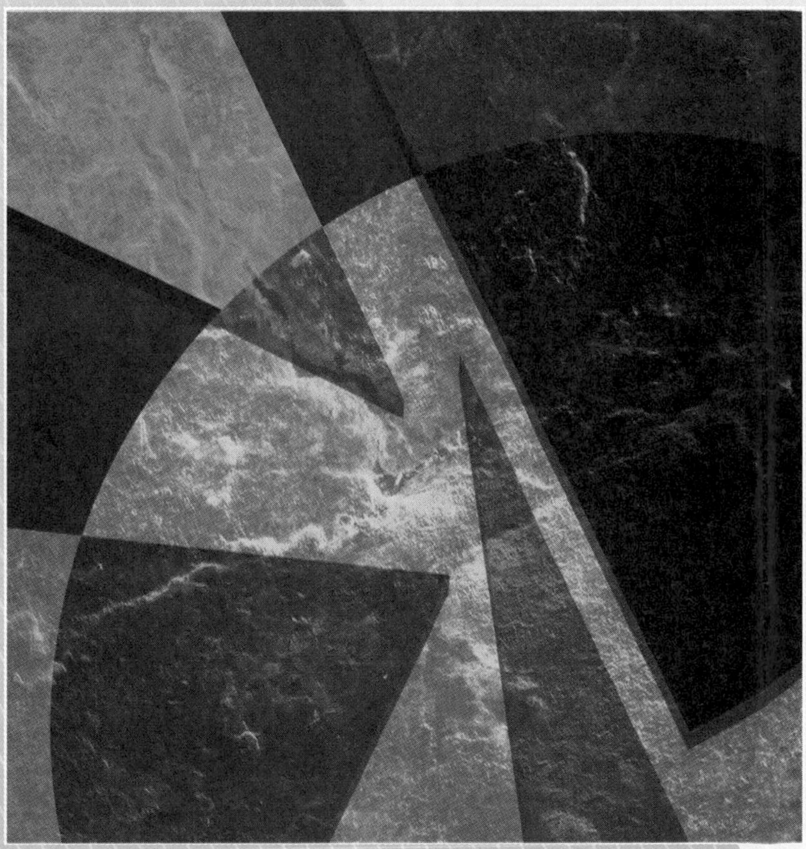

Lippincott
Philadelphia • New York • Baltimore

Acquisitions Editor: Ilze Rader
Managing Editor: Claudia Vaughn
Senior Project Editor: Tom Gibbons
Senior Production Manager: Helen Ewan
Senior Production Coordinator: Nannette Winski
Assistant Art Director: Doug Smock
Manufacturing Manager: William Alberti
Indexer: Ellen Brennan

7th Edition

Library of Congress Cataloging in Publications Data

Timby, Barbara Kuhn.
Fundamental skills and concepts in patient care / Barbara Kuhn Timby.—7th ed.
p. cm.
Includes bibliographical references and index.
ISBN 0-7817-1878-3 (paper: alk. paper)
1. Nursing. I. Title.
[DNLM: 1. Nursing Care. WY 100 T583f2000]
RT41.T54 2000
610.73—dc21 00-025008

Care has been taken to confirm the accuracy of the information presented and to describe generally accepted practices. However, the authors, editors, and publisher are not responsible for errors or omissions or for any consequences from application of the information in this book and make no warranty, express or implied, with respect to the contents of the publication.

The authors, editors and publisher have exerted every effort to ensure that drug selection and dosage set forth in this text are in accordance with current recommendations and practice at the time of publication. However, in view of ongoing research, changes in government regulations, and the constant flow of information relating to drug therapy and drug reactions, the reader is urged to check the package insert for each drug for any change in indications and dosage and for added warnings and precautions. This is particularly important when the recommended agent is a new or infrequently employed drug.

Some drugs and medical devices presented in this publication have Food and Drug Administration (FDA) clearance for limited use in restricted research settings. It is the responsibility of the health care provider to ascertain the FDA status of each drug or device planned for use in their clinical practice.

9 8 7 6 5 4 3 2 1

Contributor

Carol A. Miller, MSN, RN, C
Gerontological Clinical Nurse Specialist
Care & Counseling, Miller/Wetzler Associates
Clinical Faculty
Frances Payne Bolton School of Nursing
Case Western Reserve University
Nursing Consultant
Western Reserve Geriatric Education Center
Case Western Reserve University
Cleveland, Ohio

Reviewers

Karen L. Amsden, RN, BSN
Nursing Professor
Jefferson College
Hillsboro, Missouri

Virginia A. Armstrong, RN, PhD, PNP
Learning Solutions
DigitalThink, Inc.
San Francisco, California

Gail Barbich, RN, MSN
Practical Nursing Teacher
James Martin School at Swenson
Philadelphia, Pennsylvania

Elizabeth Cartieri
Sch. Training and Technology Center
Frackville, Pennsylvania

Annice D. Conaway, RN, MS
Department Head/Practical Nursing Program
J.F. Drake State Technical College
Huntsville, Alabama

Mary Ann Cosgarea, RN, BSN, BA
Nurse Administrator/Health Coordinator
Portage Lakes Career Center
W. Howard Nicol School of Practical Nursing
Green, Ohio

Melanie Daniel, RN, MSN
Nursing Instructor
Bevill State Community College
Sumiton, Alabama

Faith Chumchal Darilek, RN, BSN
Program Coordinator
Victoria College School of Vocational Nursing
Gonzales Campus
Gonzales, Texas

Marla J. De Jong, RN, MS, CCRN, CEN, Capt.
Critical Care Clinical Nurse Specialist
Keesler Medical Center
Keesler Air Force Base, Mississippi

Elizabeth M. Derouchie, RN, BSN, MEd
Vermont Technical College
Fanny Allen Memorial School for Practical Nursing
Colchester, Vermont

Rosanna Henry, RN, MSN
Nursing Instructor
U.P.M.C. Shadyside
School of Nursing
Pittsburgh, Pennsylvania

Phyllis Hime
Tennessee Technology Center
Morristown, Tennessee

Debra Mallory, RN, MS, NBA, CHt, CCS, CSW, NCBF
East Orange, New Jersey

Therese Solomon, RN, MSN
Assistant Professor
Westmoreland County Community College
Youngwood, Pennsylvania

Dawn Specht, RN, MSN, CEN, CCRN
Clinical Care Specialist
Critical Care/Neuroscience
Cooper Hospital
Camden, New Jersey

Kelly Stepp, RN, BSN
Greene County Vo-Tech
Waynesburg, Pennsylvania

Ann Stovall, RN, MSN
SCH Jasper Memorial Hospital
School of Vocational Nursing
Jasper, Texas

Mary Wallace, RN, BSE
Practical Nursing Director
North Arkansas College
Harrison, Arkansas

Preface

Fundamental Skills and Concepts in Patient Care is designed to assist beginning nursing students in acquiring a foundation of basic nursing theory and developing clinical skills. In addition, its content can serve as a ready reference for updating the skills of currently employed nurses or those returning to work after a period of inactive practice.

There are several underlying philosophical concepts in the text, such as:

- The human experience is a composite of physiologic, emotional, social and spiritual aspects that affect health and healing.
- Caring is the essence of nursing and is extended to every patient.
- Each patient is unique, and nursing care must be adapted to meet the individual needs of every person without compromising safety or achievement of desired outcomes.
- A supportive network of healthcare providers, family, and friends promotes health restoration and health promotion. Therefore, it is essential to include the patient's significant others in teaching, in formal discussions, and in the provision of services.
- Licensed nurses and student nurses are accountable for their actions and clinical decisions, and consequently each must be aware of legislation as it affects nursing practice.

The seventh edition of *Fundamental Skills and Concepts in Patient Care* has been carefully planned with three goals in mind. The first was to add new skills and concepts to provide an updated and comprehensive knowledge base for beginning nursing students. The second was to add new illustrations to enhance learning and promote visual appeal. The third was to design the book in ways that improve learning outcomes. Examples include:

- Providing a list of **Key Terms** in the chapter opening, printing the key term in bold when it is first used in the chapter, immediately following the key term with its definition in parentheses, and providing an alphabetized list of all key terms and definitions in the **Glossary** at the end of the text.
- Developing **Critical Thinking Exercises** that accompany each skill, as well as others at the end of the chapter, to help learners analyze and apply information rather than rely on memorization and rote performance.
- Including a list of **Suggested Readings** that directs students to information in the current literature that supplements the text in areas of particular topics.
- Supplying two **Appendices** that serve as helpful reference tools. The first includes a list and explanation of commonly used symbols and abbreviations. The second contains the most current list of nursing diagnoses accepted by the North American Nursing Diagnosis Association (NANDA).
- Organizing the content into **Units** that cluster chapters according to a common theme.
- Listing the titles of all units and chapters with their major topics and skills in the **Contents** section.
- Repeating the chapter contents and critical elements in a **Chapter Outline.**

This revision of *Fundamental Skills and Concepts in Patient Care* has been substantially revised in other ways in an effort to provide the beginning student with a contemporary framework for developing clinical skills. Chapters have been reorganized to provide more logical arrangement of content. For example, Chapter 17, Comfort, Rest, and Sleep, now includes skills for bedmaking that were previously located elsewhere. Chapter 19 is now entirely devoted to Pain Management.

There continues to be a strong focus on the **Nursing Process** in this edition. The concepts and paradigm for the nursing process appear in Chapter 2. The premise is that early familiarity with its components will reinforce its use in the **Skills** and sample **Nursing Care Plans** that appear throughout the text. Each skill chapter continues to have **Applicable Nursing Diagnoses** that correlate the types of problems recipients of the respective skills may have.

The **Skills** continue to be a strength of the seventh edition. They have been clustered together at the end of each chapter for ease of access. Moving their location from within the chapter to the end of the chapter helps avoid interrupting the narrative and distancing related **Tables** and **Displays** to locations where they previously seemed out of context. In addition, each illustration within the skills has been closely reviewed to ensure that it complies with **Standard Precautions,** infection control guidelines from the Centers for Disease Control and Prevention.

Because patient care extends beyond performing technical skills, this edition retains two recurring in-text displays, **Nursing Guidelines** and **Patient Teaching.** The Nursing Guidelines are mini-procedures, or directions for performing various kinds of nursing care or suggestions for managing patient care problems. The topics in the Patient Teaching sections help students prepare patients and their significant others for self-care and health maintenance.

Finally, the seventh edition continues to place a major emphasis on the geriatric population, who comprise the fastest-growing age group in America. Since they are most representative of the patients who nursing students care for, a recurrent display, **Focus on Older Adults,** is included in this edition. This section addresses unique characteristics and problems of aging adults as they pertain to the chapter content.

The seventh edition of *Fundamental Skills and Concepts in Patient Care* is accompanied by a complete teaching/learning package. To augment instruction, the **Instructor's Manual and Testbank** is three-hole-punched and the pages are perforated to allow the development of individual lesson plans. The Testbank portion contains over 700 NCLEX-style multiple-choice questions and rationales to assist faculty in developing and customizing their tests. To maximize learning, a **Study Guide,** which is also three-hole punched, includes chapter summaries, behavioral objectives, and a variety of learning exercises. **Performance Checklists,** which are perforated to facilitate removal and duplication, correlate with the skills in the text. They assist with faculty/student evaluation or student/peer evaluation in the clinical laboratory.

It is my belief that this text and its ancillary package will facilitate learning and produce safe, effective practitioners, capable of providing quality care for diverse patients in a variety of settings.

Barbara Kuhn Timby, RN, C, BSN, MA

Acknowledgments

Thanks go to the following people and the agencies for which they work for their help in preparing this book:

- Ilze Rader, Executive Editor, Nursing and Hospital Education, for guidance during manuscript preparation
- Mary Ann Foley, Development Editor, for polishing the manuscript and for always being there with kind words of encouragement
- Claudia Vaughn, Managing Editor, and Dale Thuesen, Editorial Assistant, for handling the details of manuscript compilation and tracking permissions, art, and photographs
- Tom Gibbons, Senior Production Editor, for editing manuscript and preparing it for publication
- Betsy Morgan, Director of the Learning Resources Center, Glen Oaks Community College, Centreville, Michigan, and her assistant, Judy Baumeister Fetch, for their assistance in literary searches of pertinent reference materials
- Administrators and personnel from The Community Health Center of Branch County, Coldwater, Michigan, and Three Rivers Area Hospital, Three Rivers, Michigan, for extending the use of their facilities for the purposes of updating photographs within the new edition
- Student nurses and their assigned patients, who agreed to be photographed during the course of nursing care
- Ken Timby, whose skills as a photographer have proved to be an invaluable asset to the revision of this and previous editions

Contents

SECTION II □ *Fundamental Nursing Skills* 115

UNIT IV

PERFORMING ASSESSMENT AND EVALUATION 117

UNIT V

ASSISTING WITH BASIC NEEDS 233

SECTION I

Fundamental Nursing Concepts

UNIT ONE

EXPLORING CONTEMPORARY NURSING

CHAPTER 1:
Nursing Foundations

CHAPTER 2:
Nursing Process

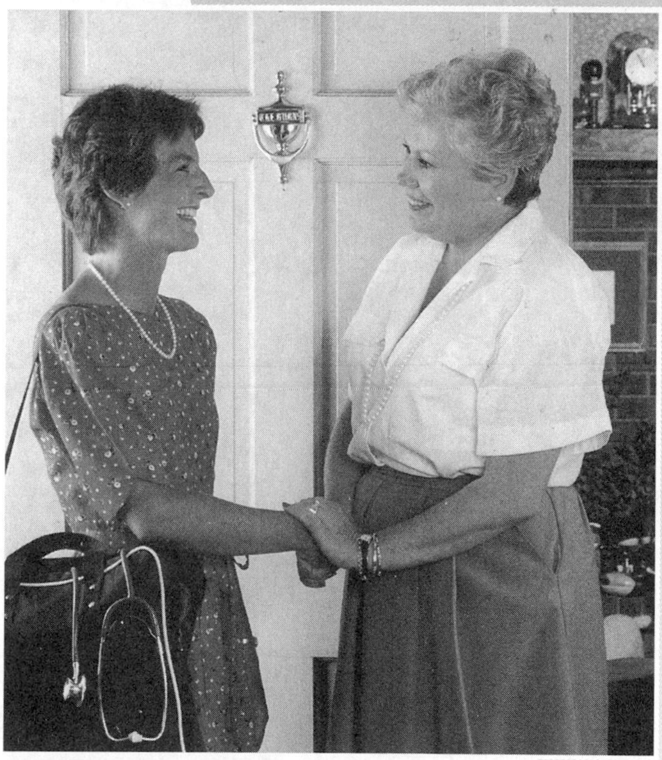

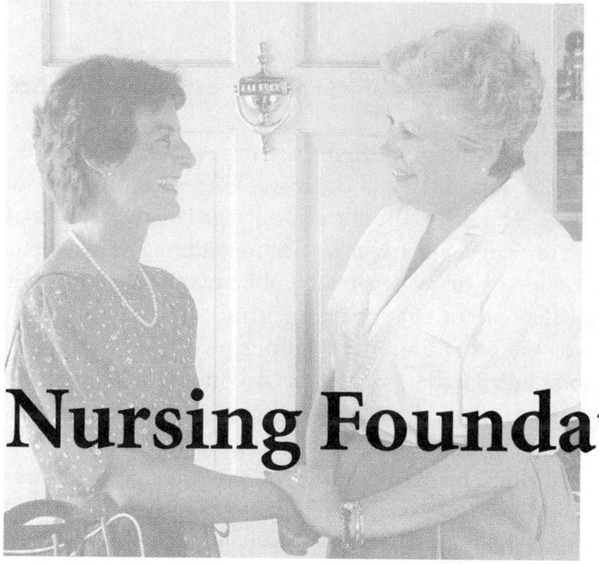

CHAPTER 1

Nursing Foundations

CHAPTER OUTLINE

Nursing Origins
The Nightingale Reformation
Establishing Nursing in the United States
Contemporary Nursing
The Educational Ladder
Continuing Education
Future Trends
Unique Nursing Skills

KEY TERMS

active listening
advanced practice
art
assessment skills
capitation
caring skills
clinical pathways
comforting skills
counseling skills
cross-trained
discharge planning
empathy
managed care practices
multicultural diversity
nursing skills
nursing theory
primary care
quality assurance
science
sympathy
theory

LEARNING OBJECTIVES

An understanding of the content within this chapter will be evidenced by the student's ability to:

- Name one historical event that lead to the demise of nursing in England before the time of Florence Nightingale.
- Identify four reforms for which Florence Nightingale is responsible.
- Describe at least five ways in which early U.S. training schools deviated from those established under the direction of Florence Nightingale.
- Name three ways that nurses used their skills in the early history of nursing in the United States.
- Explain how art, science, and nursing theory have been incorporated into contemporary nursing practice.
- Discuss the evolution that has occurred in definitions of nursing.
- List four types of educational programs that prepare students for beginning levels of nursing practice.
- Identify at least five factors that influence a person's choice of educational nursing program.
- State three reasons that support the need for continuing education in nursing.
- Name at least three current trends in health care and three trends in nursing.
- Describe four skills that all nurses use in clinical practice.

This chapter traces the historical development of nursing from its unorganized beginning to current practice. Ironically, nursing is returning to the community-based practice from which it originated.

Nursing Origins

Nursing is one of the youngest professions but one of the oldest arts. It evolved from the familial roles of nurturing and caretaking. Early responsibilities included assisting women during childbirth, suckling healthy newborns, and ministering to the ill, aged, and helpless within the household and surrounding community. Its hallmark was caring more than curing.

Eventually, the role of nursing expanded to include religious groups of nuns, priests, and brothers who combined their efforts to save souls with a commitment to care for the sick. Despite their zeal, they were overworked and overwhelmed due to their limited numbers, especially during periods when plagues and pestilence spread quickly among individuals in the community. Consequently, some convents and monasteries engaged conscientious penitent and disadvantaged lay people to assist with the burden of physical care.

Unfortunately, the character and quality of nursing care changed dramatically when religious groups in England were exiled to western Europe during the schism between King Henry VIII of England and the Catholic church. Thereafter, the management of parochial hospitals in England and the patients within them fell to the state. Hospitals became poorhouses, which some more accurately characterized as pesthouses.

The hospital labor force was recruited from the ranks of criminals, widows, and orphans. They repaid the Crown for their meager food and shelter by tending to the unfortunate sick. An example of the requirements for employment appears in Display 1-1. For the most part, nursing attendants were ignorant, uncouth, and apathetic to the needs of their charges. Without supervision, they rarely lived up to even their minimal job description. Infections, pressure sores, and malnutrition were a testimony to their neglect.

The Nightingale Reformation

In the midst of the deplorable health care conditions, Florence Nightingale, an Englishwoman born of wealthy parents, announced that she had been called by God to become a nurse. Despite her family's protests, she worked alongside nursing deaconesses, a Protestant order of women who cared for the sick, in Kaiserwerth, Germany.

After becoming suitably prepared through her nursing apprenticeship, Nightingale embarked on the next phase of her career. She worked at reforming and managing the care of women who were retired from the service of their affluent employers.

THE CRIMEAN WAR

While Nightingale was proving her ability to provide nursing care for the residents at the Institution for the Care of Sick Gentlewomen in Distressed Circumstances, England found itself allied with Turkey, France, and Sardinia in defending the Crimea, a peninsula on the north shore of the Black Sea (1854–1856).

The British soldiers suffered terribly, and their dire circumstances were made public by war correspondents at the front lines. The British public was outraged by the reports of the high rates of death and complications among its war casualties. Due to the widespread publicity, the government became the object of national criticism.

It was then that Florence Nightingale offered a strategic plan to Sidney Herbert, Secretary of War and an old family friend. She proposed that the sick and injured British soldiers at Scutari, a military barracks in Turkey, would fare better if cared for by a team of women she would train with nursing skills (Fig. 1-1). With Herbert's approval, Nightingale selected women whose reputations were beyond reproach. She intuitively realized that only individuals with devotion and idealism would be able to accept the discipline and hard work necessary for the task before them.

To the medical staff at Scutari, the arrival of a group of women implied that they were not capable of providing adequate care. Jealousy and rivalry caused the British medical officers to refuse any help from Nightingale and her 38 volunteers. When it became clear that the daily death rate, which averaged about 60%, would not subside, Nightingale's nurses were allowed to work. Under her supervision, the band of women cleaned up the filth and vermin and improved ventilation, nutrition, and sanitation. They staved off infection and gangrene and lowered the death rate to 1%.

Servicemen and their families alike were grateful; the country adored her. To show their appreciation, funds were donated

DISPLAY 1-1

Rules of Employment for Nursing Attendants—1789

- No dirt, rags, or bones may be thrown from the windows.
- Nurses are to punctually shift the bed and body linen of patients, viz., once in a fortnight (2 weeks), their shirts once in four days, their drawers and stockings once a week or oftener, if found necessary.
- All nurses who disobey orders, get drunk, neglect their patients, quarrel with men, shall be immediately discharged.

Goodnow M. Outlines of Nursing History. 5th ed. Philadelphia and London: WB Saunders, 1933, pp. 57–58.

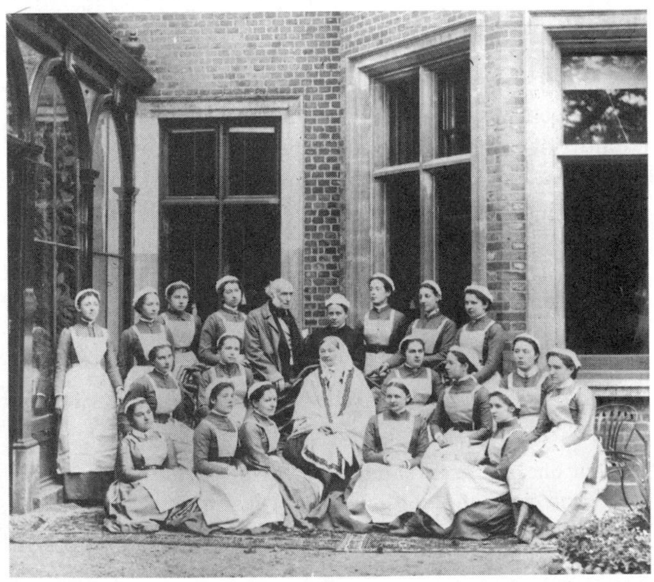

FIGURE 1–1. Florence Nightingale (*center*), her brother-in-law, Sir Harry Verney, and Miss Crossland, the nurse in charge of the Nightingale Training School at St. Thomas Hospital, with a class of student nurses. (Courtesy of The Florence Nightingale Museum Trust, London, England.)

to sustain the great work that Nightingale had begun. These funds were used to start the first Nightingale training school for nurses at St. Thomas Hospital in England. This school became the model for others in Europe and the United States.

NIGHTINGALE'S CONTRIBUTIONS

Nightingale changed the negative image of nursing to a positive one. She is credited with:

- Training people for the work they would perform
- Selecting only those with an upstanding character as potential nurses
- Improving sanitary conditions for patients
- Significantly reducing the death rate of British soldiers
- Providing classroom education and clinical teaching
- Advocating that nursing education should be a life-long process

Establishing Nursing in the United States

The Civil War came on the heels of the Nightingale reformation. Like England, the United States found itself involved in a war with no organized or substantial staff of trained nurses to care for its sick and wounded. The military had to rely on untrained corpsmen and civilian volunteers, often the mothers, wives, and sisters of soldiers.

The Union government appointed Dorothea Lynde Dix, a social worker who had proved her worth by reforming health conditions for the mentally ill, to select and organize women volunteers to care for the troops. In 1862, Dix followed Nightingale's advice and established the following selection criteria. Applicants were to be:

- Age 35 to 50
- Matronly and plain-looking
- Educated
- Neat, orderly, sober, and industrious, with a serious disposition

Applicants also had to submit two letters of recommendation attesting to their moral character, integrity, and capacity to care for the sick. Once selected, a volunteer nurse was to dress plainly in brown, gray, or black and had to agree to serve for at least 6 months (Donahue, 1985).

U.S. NURSING SCHOOLS

After the Civil War, attention turned to establishing training schools for nurses. Unfortunately, the United States deviated substantially from the Nightingale paradigm (Table 1-1). Whereas planned, consistent, formal education was the priority in Nightingale schools, the training of American nurses was more an unsubsidized apprenticeship.

TABLE 1–1. **Differences in Nightingale Schools and U.S. Training Schools**

Nightingale Schools	U.S. Training Schools
Training schools were affiliated with a few selective hospitals.	Any hospital, rural or urban, could establish a training school.
Training hospitals relied on a staff of employees to provide patient care.	Students staffed the hospital.
Costs for education were borne by the student or endowed from the Nightingale Trust Fund.	Students worked without pay in return for training—which more often than not consisted of performing housekeeping chores.
The training of nurses provided no financial advantages to the hospital.	Hospitals profited by eliminating the need to pay employees.
Class schedules were planned separate from practical experience.	No formal classes were held; training was an outcome of work.
There was a uniform core of curricular content.	The curriculum was unplanned and the content varied according to current cases.
Formal instruction was provided by a previously trained nurse with a focus on nursing care.	Instruction was usually informal, at the bedside, from the physician's perspective.
The number of clinical hours during training was restricted.	Students were expected to work 12 hours a day and live in or adjacent to the hospital in case they were unexpectedly needed.
At the end of the training period, graduates became paid employees or were hired to train other students.	At the end of training, students were discharged from the training hospital and new students took their places; most graduates sought private-duty positions.

Eventually, training schools became more organized and uniform in their curricula and the content taught. The training period lengthened from 6 months to 3 full years. Graduate nurses received a diploma attesting to their successful completion of training.

EXPANDING HORIZONS OF PRACTICE

Diplomas in hand, American nurses entered the 20th century by distinguishing themselves in caring for the sick and disadvantaged outside the walls of hospitals (Fig. 1-2). Nurses moved into the communities and established "settlement houses" where they lived and worked among the immigrant poor. Others provided midwifery services, especially in the rural hills of Appalachia. The success of their public health efforts in prenatal and obstetric care, teaching child care, and immunizing children is well documented.

Like other generations of nurses before them, they continued to volunteer during wars. Nurses offered their services to fight yellow fever, typhoid, malaria, and dysentery during the Spanish-American War. They replenished the nursing staff in military hospitals during World Wars I and II (Fig. 1-3). They worked side by side with physicians in Mobile Army Service Hospitals (MASH) during the Korean War, acquiring knowledge about trauma care that would later help to reduce the mortality rate of American soldiers in the Vietnam conflict. More recently, nurses answered the call during Operation Desert Storm. Whenever and wherever there is a need, nurses have put their own lives on the line.

Contemporary Nursing

COMBINING NURSING ART WITH SCIENCE

At first, the training of nurses consisted of learning the art of nursing. An **art** (ability to perform an act skillfully) was learned by watching and imitating the techniques performed

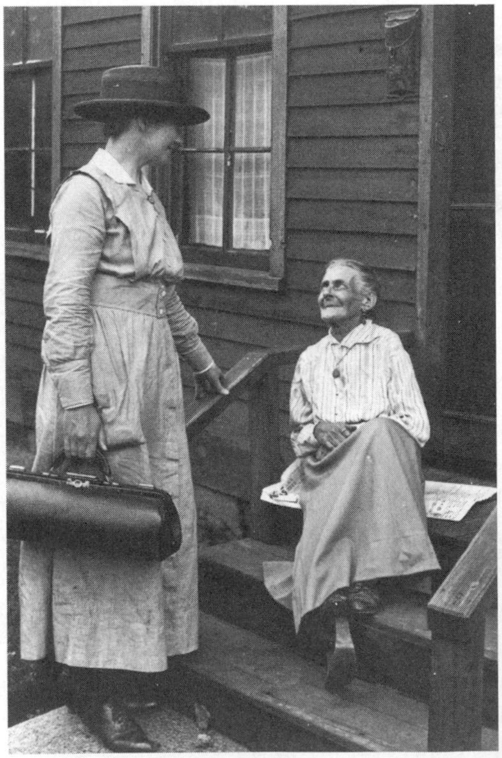

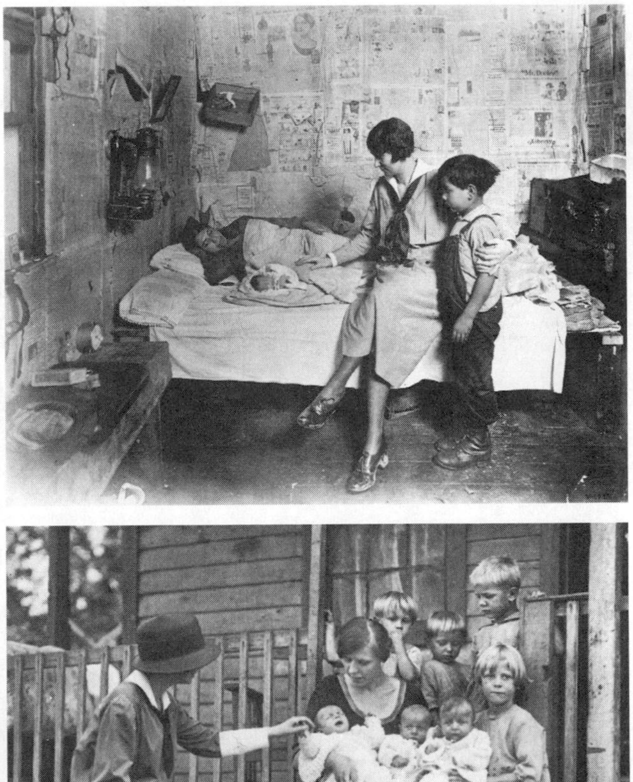

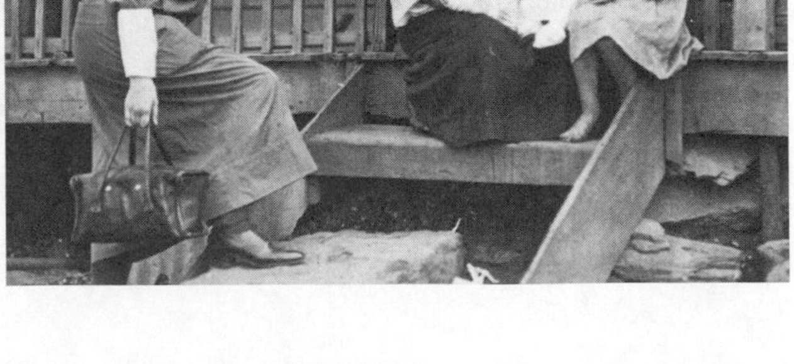

FIGURE 1–2. Community health nurses circa late 1800s to early 1900s. (Courtesy of Visiting Nurse Association, Inc. Detroit, MI.)

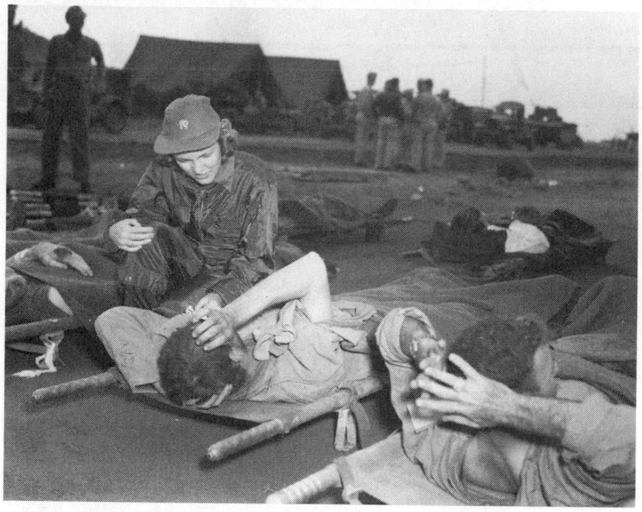

FIGURE 1–3. A military nurse comforts a soldier during World War II. (Courtesy of the National Archives, Washington, DC.)

by nurses with more experience. Nursing skills were passed on from mentor to student as a result of tradition.

Contemporary nursing practice has added another dimension: science. The English word "science" comes from the Latin word *scio,* which means, "I know." A **science** (body of knowledge unique to a particular subject) develops from observing and studying the relation of one phenomenon to another. By developing a unique body of scientific knowledge, it is now possible to predict which nursing interventions are most appropriate for producing desired outcomes.

INTEGRATING NURSING THEORY

The word **theory** (opinion, belief, or view that explains a process) comes from a Greek word that means vision. For example, a scientist may study the relation between sunlight and plants and derive a theory of photosynthesis that explains the process of how plants grow. Others who believe the theorist's view to be true may then apply the theory for their own practical use.

Nursing has undergone a similar scientific review. Nursing theorists, such as Florence Nightingale and others since, have examined the relationships among humans, health, the environment, and nursing. The outcome of the analysis becomes the basis for **nursing theory** (proposal on what is involved in the process called nursing). The theory is then adopted by a nursing program to serve as its conceptual framework or model for the school's philosophy, curriculum, and most importantly nursing approaches with patients. In similar fashion, psychologists have adopted Freud's psychoanalytic theory or Skinner's behavioral theory and used it as a model for their diagnostic and therapeutic interventions with clients.

Table 1-2 summarizes some nursing theories and discusses how each theory has been applied to nursing practice. These are only a few of the many theories that exist; additional information can be found in current nursing literature.

DEFINITIONS OF NURSING

In an effort to clarify for the public, and nurses themselves, just what nursing encompasses, various working definitions have been proposed. Nightingale is credited with the earliest modern definition: she defined nursing as "putting individuals in the best possible condition for nature to restore and preserve health."

Other definitions have been offered by nurses who have come to be recognized as authorities and therefore qualified spokespersons on the practice of nursing. One such authority is Virginia Henderson. Her definition, adopted by the International Council of Nurses, broadened the description of nursing to include health promotion, not just illness care. She stated in 1966:

> The unique function of the nurse is to assist the individual, sick or well, in the performance of those activities contributing to health or its recovery (or to a peaceful death) that he could perform unaided if he had the necessary strength, will or knowledge. And to do this in such a way as to help him gain independence as rapidly as possible.

Henderson proposed that nursing is more than carrying out medical orders. It involves a special relationship and service between the nurse and the patient (and his or her family). According to Henderson, the nurse acts as a temporary proxy, meeting the patient's health needs with knowledge and skills that neither the patient nor family members can provide.

The most recent definition of nursing comes from the American Nurses Association (ANA). In its 1980 report *Nursing: A Social Policy Statement,* nursing is defined as "the diagnosis and treatment of human responses to actual or potential health problems." The position of the ANA is that besides nursing's traditional dependent and interdependent functions, there is also an independent area of practice for using nursing skills. As the role of the nurse changes in the future, there will be further revisions to the definition of nursing and the scope of nursing practice.

The Educational Ladder

There are two basic educational options for those interested in pursuing a career in nursing: practical (vocational) nursing or one of several programs that prepare graduates for registered nursing. Each educational track provides the knowledge and skills for a particular entry level of practice. Some of the factors affecting the choice of a nursing program include:

- Career goals
- Geographic location of schools
- Costs involved
- Length of programs

TABLE 1–2. **Nursing Theories and Applications**

Theorist	Theory	Explanation
Florence Nightingale 1820–1910	**Environmental Theory**	
	Man	Individuals whose natural defenses are influenced by a healthful or unhealthful environment
	Health	A state in which the environment is optimal for the natural body processes to achieve reparative outcomes
	Environment	All the external conditions that are capable of preventing, suppressing, or contributing to disease or death
	Nursing	Putting the patient in the best condition for nature to act
	Synopsis of Theory	External conditions such as ventilation, light, odor, and cleanliness are capable of preventing, suppressing, or contributing to disease or death.
	Application to Nursing Practice	Nurses modify unhealthy aspects of the environment to put the patient in the best condition for nature to act.
Virginia Henderson 1897–1996	**Basic Needs Theory**	
	Man	Individuals with human needs that have meaning and value unique to each person
	Health	The ability to independently satisfy human needs composed of 14 basic physical, psychological, and social elements
	Environment	The setting in which an individual learns unique patterns for living
	Nursing	Temporarily assisting an individual who lacks the necessary strength, will, and knowledge to satisfy 1 or more of 14 basic needs
	Synopsis of Theory	Individuals have basic needs that are components of health. Their significance and value are unique to each person.
	Application to Nursing Practice	Nurses assist in performing those activities the patient would perform if he or she had strength, will, and knowledge.
Dorothea Orem 1914–	**Self-Care Theory**	
	Man	Individuals who use self-care to sustain life and health, recover from disease or injury, or cope with its effects
	Health	The result of practices that individuals have learned to carry out on their own behalf to maintain life and well-being
	Environment	External elements with which man interacts in his struggle to maintain self-care
	Nursing	A human service that assists individuals to progressively maximize their self-care potential
	Synopsis of Theory	Individuals learn behaviors that they perform on their own behalf to maintain life, health, and well-being.
	Application to Nursing Practice	Nurses assist patients with self-care to improve or maintain health.
Sister Callista Roy 1939–	**Adaptation Theory**	
	Man	Social, mental, spiritual, and physical beings who are affected by stimuli in the internal and external environment
	Health	The ability of an individual to adapt to changes in the environment
	Environment	Internal and external forces that are in a continuous state of change
	Nursing	A humanitarian art and expanding science that manipulates and modifies stimuli to promote and facilitate man's ability to adapt
	Synopsis of Theory	Man is a biopsychosocial being. A change in one component results in adaptive changes in the others.
	Application to Nursing Practice	Nurses assess biologic, psychological, and social factors interfering with health; alter the stimuli causing the maladaption; and evaluate the effectiveness of the action taken.

- Reputation and success of graduates
- Flexibility in course scheduling
- Opportunity for part-time versus full-time enrollment
- Ease of movement into the next level of education

PRACTICAL/VOCATIONAL NURSING

During World War II, many registered nurses enlisted in the military. This left civilian hospitals, clinics, schools, and other health care agencies with an acute shortage of trained nurses. To fill the void as expeditiously as possible, abbreviated programs in practical nursing were developed across the country to teach essential nursing skills. The goal was to prepare graduates to care for the health needs of well infants, children, and adults who were mildly or chronically ill or convalescing so that registered nurses could be used more effectively to care for acutely ill patients.

After the war, the need for practical nurses continued because many registered nurses opted for part-time employment or resigned to become full-time housewives. It became obvious that the role practical nurses were fulfilling in health care delivery would not be a temporary one. Consequently, leaders in practical nursing programs organized to form the National Association for Practical Nurse Education and Service, Inc. This group set about to standardize practical nurse education and to facilitate the licensure of graduates. By 1945, eight states had approved practical nurse programs (Mitchell & Grippando, 1997). In 1995, there were 1,107 practical nursing programs in the United States, with a reported enrollment of 57,906 students (Fig. 1-4).

Despite a slight recent decline in enrollment, the Bureau of Labor Statistics (1999) predicts:

> Job opportunities in the nursing profession are expected to rise faster than the norm over the next decade and will continue to make nursing an attractive career choice. . . . replacement due to attrition and retirement will provide numerous job openings.

Career centers, vocational schools, hospitals, independent agencies, and community colleges generally offer practical nursing programs. Clinical experience is arranged at local community hospitals, clinics, and nursing homes. The average length of a practical nursing program ranges from 1 year to 18 months, after which graduates are qualified to take their licensing examination. Because this is the shortest nursing preparatory program, it is considered by many to be the most economical. Licensed graduates provide direct health care for patients under the supervision of a registered nurse, physician, or dentist. To provide career mobility, many schools of practical nursing have developed "articulation agreements" to help their graduates enroll in another school that offers a path to registered nursing.

REGISTERED NURSING

Students can choose one of three paths to become a registered nurse: a hospital-based diploma program, a program that awards an associate degree in nursing, or a baccalaureate nursing program. All three meet the requirements for taking the national licensing examination (NCLEX-RN). A person licensed as a registered nurse may work directly at the bedside or supervise others in managing the care of groups of patients.

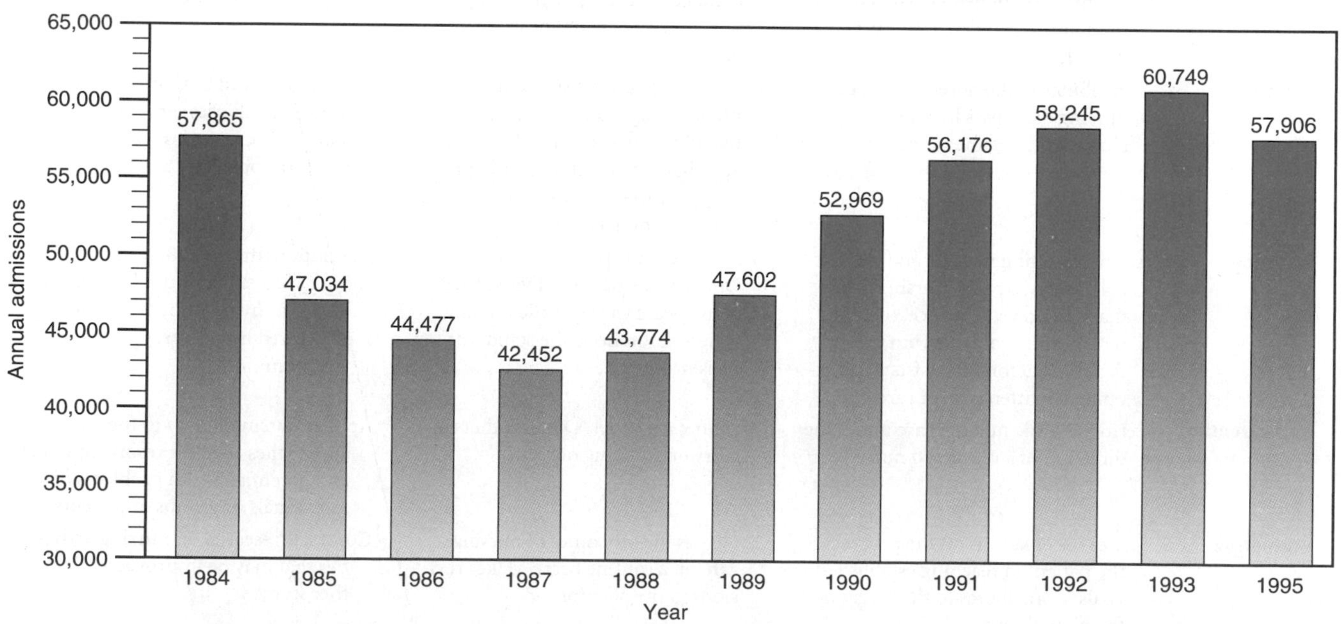

FIGURE 1–4. Trends in LPN/LVN enrollments 1984–1995. (National League for Nursing. Focus on Practical/Vocational Nursing, Vol. III, New York, 1997.)

Table 1-3 describes how educational programs prepare graduates to assume separate but coordinated types of responsibilities. However, when hiring new graduates, many employers do not differentiate between these educational programs, arguing that "a nurse is a nurse."

HOSPITAL-BASED DIPLOMA PROGRAMS

Diploma programs were the traditional route for nurses through the middle of this century. Their decline became obvious in the 1970s, and their numbers continue to dwindle (Fig. 1-5). The reason for their decline is twofold: first, there has been a movement to increase professionalism in nursing by encouraging education from colleges and universities, and second, hospitals can no longer financially subsidize schools of nursing.

Diploma nurses were, and are, well trained. Because of their vast clinical experience (compared with students from other types of programs), they are often characterized as more self-confident and more easily socialized into the role requirements of a graduate nurse.

A hospital-based diploma program is generally 3 years long. Many hospital schools of nursing collaborate with nearby colleges to provide basic science and humanities courses; these credits can be transferred if the graduate chooses to pursue an associate or baccalaureate degree at a later time.

ASSOCIATE DEGREE PROGRAMS

During World War II, hospital-based schools accelerated the education of some registered nursing students through the Cadet Nurse Corps because qualified nurses were being used for the war effort. Afterward, Mildred Montag, a doctoral nursing student, began to question whether it was necessary for students in a registered nursing program to spend 3 years acquiring a basic education. She believed that nursing education could be shortened to 2 years and relocated to vocational schools or junior or community colleges. The graduate from this type of program would acquire an associate degree in nursing, would be referred to as a technical nurse, and would not be expected to work in a management position.

This type of nursing preparation has proven extremely popular and now commands the highest enrollment among all registered nurse programs. Despite its condensed curriculum, graduates of associate degree programs have demonstrated a high level of competence in passing NCLEX-RN.

TABLE 1–3. **Levels of Responsibilities for the Nursing Process***

	Practical/Vocational Nurse	Associate Degree Nurse	Baccalaureate Nurse
Assessing	Gathers data by interviewing, observing, and performing a basic physical examination of people with common health problems with predictable outcomes.	Collects data from people with complex health problems with unpredictable outcomes, their family, medical records, and other health team members.	Identifies the information needed from individuals or groups to provide an appropriate nursing data base.
Diagnosing	Contributes to the development of nursing diagnoses by reporting abnormal assessment data.	Uses a classification list to write a nursing diagnostic statement, including the problem, its etiology, and signs and symptoms. Identifies problems that require collaboration with the physician.	Conducts clinical testing of approved nursing diagnoses. Proposes new diagnostic categories for consideration and approval.
Planning	Assists in setting realistic and measurable goals. Suggests nursing actions that can prevent, reduce, or eliminate health problems with predictable outcomes. Assists in developing a written plan of care.	Sets realistic, measurable goals. Develops a written individualized plan of care with specific nursing orders that reflects the standards for nursing practice.	Develops written standards for nursing practice. Plans care for healthy or sick individuals or groups in structured health care agencies or the community.
Implementing	Performs basic nursing care under the direction of a registered nurse.	Identifies priorities. Directs others to carry out nursing orders.	Applies nursing theory to the approaches used for resolving actual and potential health problems of individuals or groups of patients.
Evaluating	Shares observations on the progress of the patient in reaching established goals. Contributes to the revision of the plan of care.	Evaluates the outcomes of nursing care on a routine basis. Makes revisions in the plan for care.	Conducts research on nursing activities that may be improved with further study.

*Note that each more advanced practitioner can perform the responsibilities of those identified previously.

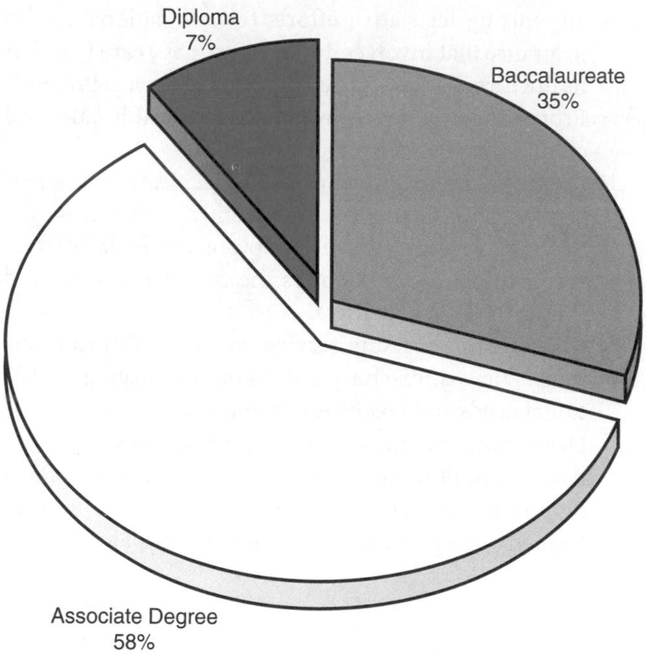

FIGURE 1–5. The distribution of basic RN programs. (National League for Nursing. Nursing Datasource, New York, 1997.)

BACCALAUREATE PROGRAMS

Although collegiate nursing programs were established at the beginning of the 20th century, until recently they have not attracted large numbers of students. Their popularity has been on the rise, perhaps because of the proposals by the ANA and the National League for Nursing to establish baccalaureate education as the entry level into nursing practice. The deadline for implementation of this goal, once set for 1985, has been postponed for three reasons:

- The date coincided with a national shortage of nurses.
- There was tremendous opposition from nondegreed nurses, who believed their titles and positions would be jeopardized.
- Employers feared that paying higher salaries to degreed personnel would escalate budgets beyond their financial limits.

Consequently, the adoption of a unified entry level into practice is still in limbo.

Although this is the longest and most expensive preparatory program, baccalaureate-prepared nurses have the greatest flexibility in qualifying for nursing positions, both staff and managerial. A nurse with a baccalaureate degree is usually preferred in areas such as public health, where there is a high degree of independent decision making.

Currently, many nondegreed nurses are returning to school to earn a baccalaureate degree. Articulation has been difficult for many due to problems transferring credits for the courses they took during their diploma or associate degree programs. To increase enrollment, some collegiate programs are offering nurses an opportunity to obtain credit by passing "challenge examinations." In addition, many colleges and universities are providing satellite or outreach programs to accommodate nurses who cannot go to school full-time or travel long distances.

GRADUATE NURSING PROGRAMS

Graduate nursing programs are available at both the master's and doctoral levels. Master's-prepared nurses fill roles as clinical specialists, nurse practitioners, administrators, and educators. Nurses with doctoral degrees conduct research, advise, administer, and instruct nurses pursuing undergraduate and graduate degrees. Although a graduate degree in nursing is preferred, some nurses pursue advanced education in fields outside nursing, such as business, leadership, and education, to enhance their nursing career.

Continuing Education

Continuing education in nursing is defined as any planned learning experience that takes place beyond the basic nursing program (ANA, 1974). Nightingale is credited with having said, "to stand still is to move backwards." The principle that learning is a life-long process still applies. Display 1-2 lists reasons why nurses, in particular, pursue continuing education. Several states now require nurses to show proof of continuing education to renew their nursing license.

Future Trends

Regardless of the educational preparation for nursing, nurses are becoming proactive in responding to the trends that are

DISPLAY 1-2

Rationale for Acquiring Continuing Education

- No basic program provides all the knowledge and skills needed for a lifetime career.
- Current advances in technology make previous practice obsolete.
- Assuming responsibility for self-learning demonstrates personal accountability.
- To ensure the public's confidence, nurses must demonstrate evidence of current competence.
- Practicing according to current nursing standards helps to ensure that care is legally safe.
- Renewal of state licensure is often contingent on evidence of continuing education.

affecting their role in health care (Table 1-4). Nurses are preparing for the 21st century by:

- Pursuing post-licensure education
- Training for **advanced practice** roles (nurse practitioner, nurse midwifery) to provide cost-effective health care in areas where there are inadequate numbers of primary care physicians
- Becoming **cross-trained** (ability to assume a nonnursing job position, depending on the census or levels of patient acuity on any given day). For example, nurses may be trained to provide respiratory treatments and obtain electrocardiograms, jobs previously performed by nonnursing health care workers.
- Learning more about **multicultural diversity** (unique characteristics of ethnic groups) as it affects health beliefs and values, food preferences, language and communication, and role relationships
- Supporting legislative efforts toward national health insurance that involves nurses in **primary care** (the first health care worker to assess a person with a health need)
- Promoting wellness through home health care and community-based programs
- Helping patients with chronic diseases learn techniques for living healthier and, consequently, longer lives
- Referring patients with health problems for early treatment; this practice requires the fewest resources and thus is the least expensive.
- Coordinating nursing services across health care settings—that is, **discharge planning** (managing transitional needs and ensuring continuity)
- Developing and implementing **clinical pathways** (standardized multidisciplinary plans for a specific diagnosis or procedure that identify aspects of care to be performed during a designated length of stay; Fig. 1-6)

TABLE 1–4. **Trends in Health Care and Nursing**

Health Care	Nursing
The most underserved health care populations include older adults, ethnic minorities, and the poor, who delay seeking early treatment because they cannot afford it.	Enrollments and numbers of graduates from LPN/LVN and RN educational programs are currently decreasing.
The number of uninsured has risen from 37 million in 1995 to 40 million.	More licensed nurses are earning master's and doctoral degrees.
Medicare and Medicaid benefits are being modified and reduced.	There may be a shortage of nurses in a variety of health care settings due to decreased enrollments, retirement, attrition, and cost-containment measures.
Chronic illness is the major health problem.	Hospital employment is decreasing.
Disease and injury prevention and health promotion are priorities.	There are higher patient-to-nurse ratios in employment settings.
Medicine tends to focus on high technology that improves outcomes for a select few.	There are more high-acuity patients in previously nonacute settings such as long-term and intermediate health care facilities.
Hospitals are downsizing and hiring unlicensed personnel to perform procedures once in the exclusive domain of licensed nurses for cost containment	Job opportunities have expanded to outpatient services, home health care, hospice programs, community health, and mental health agencies.
There are fewer primary care physicians in rural areas.	
Changes in reimbursement practices have created a shift in decision making from hospitals, nurses, and physicians to insurance companies.	
Health care costs continue to increase despite **managed care practices** (cost-containment strategies used to plan and coordinate a patient's care to avoid delays, unnecessary services, or overuse of expensive resources).	
Capitation (strategy for controlling health care costs by paying a fixed amount per member) encourages health providers to limit tests and services to increase profits.	
Hospitals, practitioners, and health insurance companies are being required to measure, monitor, and manage quality of care.	

- Participating in **quality assurance** (process of identifying and evaluating outcomes)

Unique Nursing Skills

Although the location for employment and the manner in which **nursing skills** (activities unique to the practice of nursing) are carried out differ according to educational preparation, all nurses share the same philosophical perspective. In keeping with the traditions of Nightingale, contemporary nursing practice continues to include assessment skills, caring skills, counseling skills, and comforting skills.

ASSESSMENT SKILLS

Before the nurse can determine what nursing care a person requires, he or she must determine the patient's needs and problems. This requires the use of **assessment skills** (acts that involve collecting data), which include interviewing, observing, and examining the patient and in some cases the patient's family (family is used loosely to refer to the people with whom the patient lives and associates). Although the patient and the family are the primary resources for information, the nurse also uses the patient's medical record and other health care workers as resources for obtaining facts. Assessment skills are discussed in more detail in Unit IV.

CARING SKILLS

Caring skills (nursing interventions that restore or maintain a person's health) may involve something as minimal as assisting with activities of daily living (ADLs). ADL is a term that refers to the acts that people do every day in the normal course of living, such as bathing, grooming, dressing, toileting, and eating. More and more, however, the role of the nurse is being extended to include the safe care of patients who require invasive or highly technical equipment. This textbook introduces the beginning nurse to the concepts and skills needed to provide care for patients whose disorders have fairly predictable outcomes. Once this foundation has been established, students may add to their initial knowledge base.

Traditionally, nurses have always been providers of physical care for people unable to meet their own health needs independently. But caring also involves the concern and attachment that results from the close relationship of one human being with another. Despite the close relationship that caring involves, the nurse ultimately wants patients to become self-reliant. The nurse who assumes too much care for patients, like the mother who continues to tie a child's shoes, often delays their independence.

COUNSELING SKILLS

A counselor is one who listens to a client's needs, responds with information based on his or her area of expertise, and facilitates the outcome that a client desires. Nurses implement **counseling skills** (interventions that include communicating with patients, actively listening to the exchange of information, offering pertinent health teaching, and providing emotional support) in nurse–patient relationships.

To understand the patient's perspective on a situation, the nurse uses therapeutic communication techniques to encourage verbal expression. Therapeutic and nontherapeutic communication techniques are discussed in Chapter 7. The interaction is facilitated by the use of **active listening** (demonstrating full attention to what is being said, hearing both the content being communicated and the unspoken message). Giving patients the opportunity to be heard helps them to organize their thoughts and evaluate their situation more realistically.

Once the patient's perspective is clear, the nurse provides pertinent health information without offering specific advice. By reserving personal opinions, nurses promote the right of every person to make his or her own decisions and choices on matters affecting health and illness care. The role of the nurse is to share information on potential alternatives, allow patients the freedom to choose, and support the decision that is made.

While giving care, the nurse finds many opportunities to teach patients how to promote healing processes, stay well, prevent illness, and carry out ADLs in the best possible way. People know much more about health and health care today, and they expect nurses to share accurate information with them.

Because patients do not always communicate their feelings to strangers, nurses use **empathy** (intuitive awareness of what the patient is experiencing) to perceive the patient's emotional state and need for support. This skill is different from **sympathy** (feeling as emotionally distraught as the patient). Empathy helps the nurse become effective in providing for the patient's needs while being compassionately detached.

COMFORTING SKILLS

Nightingale's presence and the light from her lamp communicated comfort to the frightened British soldiers. As a result of that heritage, contemporary nurses understand that illness often causes feelings of insecurity that may threaten the patient's or family's ability to cope; they may feel very vulnerable. It is then that the nurse uses **comforting skills** (interventions that provide stability and security during a health-related crisis) (Fig. 1-7). The nurse becomes the patient's guide, companion, and interpreter. This supportive relationship generally brings about trust and reduces fear and worry.

As a result of one woman's efforts, modern nursing was born. It has continued to mature and flourish ever since. The

text continued on page 18

DRG 209: (81.51)
Exp. LOS: 6 days
M.D.: ____________

RECOVERY PATHWAY TOTAL HIP

ADDRESSOGRAPH

(Recovery Pathways do not represent a standard of care. They are guidelines for consideration which may be modified according to the individual patient's need.)

	DATE: Pre-Admit	DAY OF WK: DATE: DAY 1 (OR Day)	DAY OF WK: DATE: DAY 2- 1st PostOp	DAY OF WK: DATE: DAY 3- 2nd PostOp	DAY OF WK: DATE: DAY 4- 3rd PostOp	DAY OF WK: DATE: DAY 5- 4th PostOp	DAY OF WK: DATE: DAY 6- 5th PostOp
Diagnostic Studies	Auto Blood Y N Pre-op Lab, EKG, CXR	X-ray Joint PACU Y N	CBC Y N PT/PTT (INR) Y N	CBC Y N ____________	____________	____________	____________
Treatments		- Waffle - Foley - TED Hose - in OR Y N - SCD in OR Y N - Drain Y N - IS	- TED Hose Y N - SCD Y N - Drain Y N - IS - Foley (consider D/C) Y N	⟶ - SCD Y N - IS (pt doing own) Y N - Drain D/C Y N - Foley D/C 0700 Y N	⟶ - SCD Y N - IS - Consider IV out Y N	⟶	⟶
Therapy PT (one time/day unless specified)	Pre-Op teaching Y N OT safety checklist	Total Hip protocol WB per M.D. (PT & OT) (Evaluation & Treatment) Y N	- Gait training 10-20' ____________ Y N - Total Hip precautions given Y N - OT - Precaution instruction Y N	- Gait training 20-25' as tol. ____ Y N - THR exercise x 10 rep with min Asst Y N - Understand total hip precautions Y N - Supine→sit w/__asst Y N - Sit→stand w/__asst Y N - OT: Pt participation as tol with LE dressing/bathing with equipment Y N	- Gait training 25-40' as tol ____ Y N - Transfer sit ⇆ stand minimal asst Y N - Exercise 10-15 reps Y N - Begin ↕ stairs Y N - OT: Transfer training - tub/ toilet/auto Y N	- Gait training 40-50' as tol ____ Y N - Transfer sit ⇆ stand Y N - in ⇆ OOB independently Y N - Exercise 15-20 reps Y N - ↕ stairs Y N - OT: Refining/ reviewing prior instruction with home safety, task simplification Y N	- Gait training 50-60' as tol_____ Y N - ↕steps independently YN - Independent with 15-20 reps of exercise Y N - Discharge Instructions
Multi-disciplinary Consults	SW Screen Medical Evaluation	Other MD consults			Consider Home Health Assessment Y N		
Medications	Physician preference	Antibiotics Analgesics	Antibiotics Analgesics	Antibiotics D/C Y N Analgesics (push po) Y N	Analgesics (po) Y N	Analgesics (po) Y N	Rx Written Analgesics
Nutrition	NPO after midnight	Clear liquids → DAT	Clear liquids → DAT	DAT GI function Y N	DAT	DAT	DAT

(continued)

	DATE: Pre-Admit	DAY OF WK: DATE: DAY 1 (OR Day)	DAY OF WK: DATE: DAY 2- 1st PostOp	DAY OF WK: DATE: DAY 3- 2nd PostOp	DAY OF WK: DATE: DAY 4- 3rd PostOp	DAY OF WK: DATE: DAY 5- 4th PostOp	DAY OF WK: DATE: DAY 6- 5th PostOp
Activity	Pre-Op Teaching	- BR w/position ▵ q2° - Maintain Abduction Y N - Dorsiplantar Flex q2° Y N - DB Y N - If early a.m. surgery - ↑ chair Y N	- Chair Y N - Dorsiplantar Flex q4° Y N - DB Y N	- Chair/Up in room, Hall as tol Y N - Dorsiplantar Flex q4° Y N - DB Y N	- Chair/up in room/hall Y N - Dorsiplantar Flex q4° Y N - DB Y N	- Chair/Up in room/Hall Independent Y N - Dorsiplantar Flex q4° Y N - DB Y N	- Chair/Up in room/Hall Independent Y N - Dorsiplantar flex q4° Y N - DB Y N
Teaching	- Video Education - Pain Mgmt - Lt supper/ suppository	- Reinforce pre-op education Y N - Hip Precautions Y N - Pain Scale (0-10) Y N	Continue to reinforce	Continue to reinforce: - Ted Hose Y N - Gait training/transfers Y N - Hip Precautions Y N	Continue to reinforce	- Coumadin (if going home on) Y N - Continue to reinforce	Discharge Instructions Follow-up appointments
Discharge Planning	Patient to bring pre-op instuctions with them	SS- meet with family - Develop initial plan Y N	SS - Monitor progress	- Assess rehab potential vs. ECF Y N	- Assess rehab potential vs. ECF Y N - Identify equipment needs (for home) Y N - Clarify plan with patient/ family Y N	- Assess rehab potential vs. ECF Y N - Order Equipment Y N - Clarify plan with patient/ family Y N - Coordinate discharge home (home health/ equipment needs) Y N	DC to home or ECF Home Health liaison to finalize HH involvement Y N
Expected Patient Outcomes	Patient states his responsibility/role in recovery Y N	Patient understands treatment rationale Y N	- Patient actively participates in care Y N - Verbalizes understanding of care Y N	- Verbalize hip precautions Y N	Verbalizes/ Demonstrates: - hip precautions Y N - discharge plans Y N - Discharge to Rehab Y N	- Patient/family demonstrates independence w/ADLs Y N Discharge to - ECF Y N - rehab Y N - Home Y N	Patient/family understands discharge instructions and is confident in ability to care for self. Y N - Discharge to home Y N

Signatures:

MR-

Rev. 3/1/94

FIGURE 1–6. Example of recovery pathway in managed care. (Courtesy of Elkhart General Hospital, Elkhart, IN.)

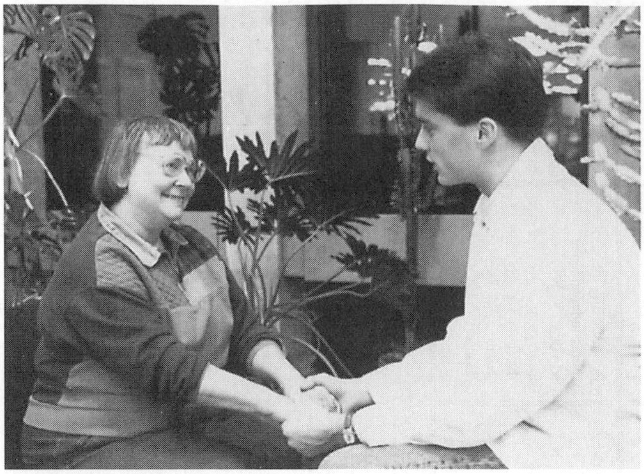

FIGURE 1–7. This nurse offers comfort and emotional support.

skills performed by Florence Nightingale on a very grand scale are repeated today during each and every nurse–patient relationship.

KEY CONCEPTS

- The art of nursing declined in England with the exile of Catholic religious orders back to Europe, forcing the government to assume responsibility for caring for the sick, aged, and infirm. Eventually, this care was delegated to untrained and for the most part uninterested people of questionable character.
- Florence Nightingale changed the image of nursing by training nurses to care for the sick, selecting only those with upstanding character as potential nurses, improving the sanitary conditions within patients' environments, significantly reducing the morbidity and mortality rates of British soldiers, providing formal nursing classes separate from clinical experience, and arguing that nursing education should be a life-long process.
- Training schools in the United States deviated from the pattern established by Nightingale. There were no criteria as to which hospitals were used for the training of nurses. Students staffed the hospitals without being paid. There was no uniformity in what was taught; students learned more by experience than by formal instruction. Nursing students were taught from a physician's perspective. Students were required to work and live at the beck and call of the hospital administrator, and after graduation students were left to seek employment elsewhere.
- Besides being employed within hospitals, early graduates of nursing programs met the health needs of the immigrant poor by living among them in settlement houses in the ghettos of large cities, by serving as midwives for rural women who lacked medical care, and by caring for sick and wounded soldiers.
- What started as an art, passing on the skills of nursing from one practitioner to another, was soon augmented by science, a unique body of knowledge making it possible to predict which nursing interventions would be most appropriate for producing desired outcomes. Most recently, nursing has become theory-based, which means that nursing scholars are proposing what the process of nursing encompasses by explaining the relationship between four essential components: humans, health, environment, and nursing.
- One of the earliest definitions of nursing outlined the scope of practice as caring for the sick. More recently, the definition has been refined, with the addition of the nurse's role in health promotion and independent practice.
- Those who wish to pursue a career in nursing may choose from a practical/vocational nursing program or a registered nursing program taught in a career center, hospital school, community or junior college, or university.
- The choice of nursing educational program depends on one's career goals, location of schools, costs involved, length of the program, reputation and success of graduates, flexibility in course scheduling, opportunities for part-time or full-time enrollment, and ease of articulation to the next level of education.
- Continuing education is necessary for contemporary nurses because it demonstrates personal accountability, promotes the public's trust, ensures competence in current nursing practice, and keeps the nurse abreast of how technology is affecting patient care.
- Several trends are affecting health care. Many people, such as older adults, minorities, and the poor, are not receiving adequate health care. The number of uninsured people is rising. Various cost-containment practices are in place that reduce a person's access to tests, treatment, and services.
- Some trends that are affecting nursing include reduced numbers of nursing students, increased ratios of patients to nurses in employment settings, and a higher acuity of patients in previously nonacute settings.
- Regardless of educational background, all nurses use assessment, caring, counseling, and comforting skills in clinical practice.

CRITICAL THINKING EXERCISES

- Describe the Nightingale reforms and explain which one you believe was most important.
- How would you define nursing?
- Do you think nursing in the 21st century will be better than it is currently, or worse? Support your opinion.

SELECTED READINGS

American Nurses Association. Standards for continuing education in nursing. Kansas City, 1974.

American Nurses Association. Nursing: a social policy statement. Kansas City, 1980.

Anderson R, Bennett PJ. Ask AONE's experts . . . about preparing for managed care. Nursing Management 1998;29(3):56.

Brewer CS. The history and future of nursing labor research in a cost-control environment. Research in Nursing & Health 1998;21(2):167–177.

Buerhaus PI. Is a nursing shortage on the way? Nursing 1998;28(8):34–35.

Bureau of Labor Statistics. Occupational outlook handbook. Washington DC, U.S. Dept. of Labor, 1999.

Donahue MP. The finest art. St. Louis, Mosby, 1985.

Henderson V. The nature of nursing. New York, Macmillan, 1966.

Houston CJ, Fox S. The changing health care market: implications for nursing education in the coming decade. Nursing Outlook 1998;46 (3):109–114.

Kurzen CR. Contemporary practical/vocational nursing. Philadelphia, Lippincott-Raven, 1997.

Mitchell PR, Grippando GM. Nursing perspectives and issues, 5th ed. Albany, Delmar, 1997.

National League for Nursing. Nursing datasource vol. III: focus on practical/vocational nursing. Sudbury, Jones and Bartlett, 1997.

National League for Nursing. Commission on a workforce for a restructured health care system, 1998. http://www:nln.org/

Nightingale F. Notes on nursing: what it is, and what it is not. London, Harrisson, 1859.

Ward SL. Caring and healing in the 21st century. American Journal of Maternal/Child Nursing 1998;23(4):210–215.

CHAPTER 2

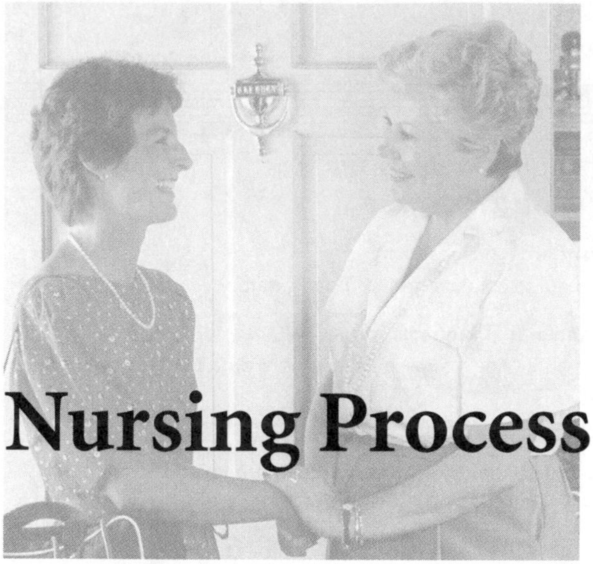

Nursing Process

CHAPTER OUTLINE

The Nursing Process
Assessment
Diagnosis
Planning
Implementation
Evaluation
Using the Nursing Process

☑ NURSING GUIDELINES

USING THE NURSING PROCESS

KEY TERMS

actual diagnosis	nursing process
assessment	objective data
collaborative problems	planning
critical thinking	possible diagnosis
data base assessment	potential diagnosis
diagnosis	short-term goals
evaluation	signs
focus assessment	standards for care
goal	subjective data
implementation	symptoms
long-term goals	syndrome diagnosis
nursing diagnosis	wellness diagnosis
nursing orders	

LEARNING OBJECTIVES

An understanding of the content within this chapter will be evidenced by the student's ability to:

- Define nursing process.
- List five steps in the nursing process.
- Describe six characteristics of the nursing process.
- Identify four sources for assessment data.
- Differentiate between a data base and focus assessment.
- Distinguish between a nursing diagnosis and a collaborative problem.
- List three parts of a nursing diagnostic statement.
- Describe the rationale for setting priorities.
- Discuss the circumstances when short-term and long-term goals are appropriate.
- Identify four ways for documenting a plan of care.
- Describe the information that is documented in reference to the plan of care.
- Discuss three outcomes that result from evaluation.

In the distant past, nursing practice involved actions that were based mostly on common sense and the examples set by older, more experienced nurses. The actual care of patients tended to be limited to the physician's medical orders. Although nurses today continue to work interdependently with other health care practitioners, they now plan and implement patient care more independently. In even stronger terms, nurses are held responsible and accountable for providing appropriate patient care that reflects currently accepted standards for nursing practice.

The Nursing Process

A *process* is a set of actions leading to a particular goal. The **nursing process** (an organized sequence of problem-solving steps: assessment, diagnosis, planning, implementation, and evaluation) is used to identify and manage health problems of patients (Fig. 2-1). It is the accepted standard for clinical practice established by the American Nurses Association (ANA) (Display 2-1). When nursing practice reflects the nursing process, patients receive quality care in minimal time with maximal efficiency.

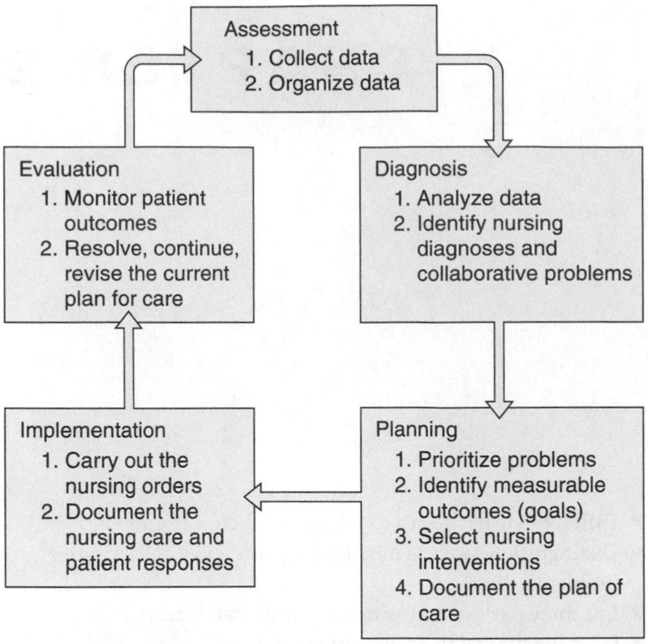

FIGURE 2–1. The steps in the nursing process.

DISPLAY 2–1

Standards of Clinical Nursing Practice

Standard I. Assessment

The nurse collects patient health data.

Standard II. Diagnosis

The nurse analyzes the assessment data in determining diagnoses.

Standard III. Outcome Identification

The nurse identifies expected outcomes individualized to the patient.

Standard IV. Planning

The nurse develops a plan of care that prescribes interventions to attain expected outcomes.

Standard V. Implementation

The nurse implements the interventions identified in the plan of care.

Standard VI. Evaluation

The nurse evaluates the patient's progress toward attainment of outcomes.

Reprinted with permission from Standards of Clinical Nursing Practice, 2nd ed, © 1998, American Nurses Association, Washington, D.C.

CHARACTERISTICS OF THE NURSING PROCESS

The nursing process has seven distinct characteristics. It is:

- *Within the legal scope of nursing.* The definitions of nursing in most state nurse practice acts describe nursing in terms of an independent problem-solving role that involves the diagnosis and treatment of human responses to actual or potential health problems.
- *Based on knowledge.* The ability to identify and resolve patient problems requires **critical thinking** (process of objective reasoning; analyzing facts to reach a valid conclusion). Critical thinking enables nurses to determine which problems necessitate collaboration with the physician and which ones fall within the independent domain of nursing. Critical thinking helps nurses select appropriate nursing interventions for achieving predictable outcomes.
- *Planned.* The steps of the nursing process are organized and systematic. One step leads to the next in an orderly fashion.
- *Patient-centered.* The nursing process makes it easier to formulate a comprehensive plan of care for each patient as a unique individual. Patients are expected, whenever possible, to be active participants in their care.
- *Goal-directed.* The nursing process involves a united effort between the patient and the nursing team to achieve desired outcomes.
- *Prioritized.* The nursing process provides a focused way to resolve the problems that represent the greatest threat to health.
- *Dynamic.* Because the health status of any patient is constantly changing, the nursing process acts like a continuous loop. Evaluation, the last step in the nursing process, involves data collection, beginning the process again.

Assessment

Assessment (the systematic collection of facts, or *data*) is the first step in the nursing process. Assessment begins with the nurse's first contact with a patient and is ongoing.

TYPES OF DATA

The data collected are either objective or subjective. **Objective data** (facts that are observable and measurable), such as the patient's blood pressure, are referred to as **signs** of a disorder. **Subjective data** (information that only the patient feels and can describe), such as pain, are called **symptoms** (Display 2-2).

DISPLAY 2-2

Examples of Objective and Subjective Data

Objective Data	Subjective Data
Weight	Pain
Temperature	Nausea
Skin color	Depression
Blood cell count	Fatigue
Vomiting	Anxiety
Bleeding	Loneliness

SOURCES FOR DATA

The primary source for information is the patient. Secondary sources include the patient's family, reports, test results, information in current and past medical records, and discussions with other health care workers.

TYPES OF ASSESSMENTS

There are two types of assessments: a data base assessment and a focus assessment (Table 2-1).

Data Base Assessment

A **data base assessment** (initial information about the patient's physical, emotional, social, and spiritual health) is lengthy and comprehensive. Data base information is obtained during the admission interview and physical examination (see Chap. 12). Hospitals generally provide a printed form to use as a guide (Fig. 2-2). Information obtained during a data base assessment serves as a reference for comparing all future data and provides the evidence used to identify the patient's initial problems.

Focus Assessment

A **focus assessment** (information that provides more details about specific problems) expands the original data base. For instance, if during the initial interview the nurse is informed that constipation is more often the rule than the exception for a patient, more questions follow. The nurse obtains data about the patient's dietary habits, level of activity, fluid intake, current medications, frequency of bowel elimination, and stool characteristics. The nurse may ask the patient to save a stool specimen for inspection.

Focus assessments are generally repeated frequently or on a scheduled basis to determine trends in a patient's condition and responses to therapeutic interventions. Performing postoperative surgical assessments (see Chap. 27), monitoring the patient's level of pain before and after administering medication, and checking the neurologic status of a patient with a head injury are examples of focus assessments that are frequently performed.

ORGANIZING DATA

Interpreting the data is easier if the information is organized. Organization involves grouping related information. For example, consider the following list of words: apple, wheels, orchard, pedals, tree, and handlebars. At first glance, they appear to be a jumble of terms. However, if asked to cluster the related terms, most would correctly group apple, tree, and orchard together, or wheels, pedals, and handlebars.

Nurses organize assessment data in much the same way. Using knowledge and past experiences, nurses group clusters

TABLE 2–1. **Comparison of Data Base and Focus Assessments**

Data Base Assessment	Focus Assessment
• Obtained on admission	• Compiled throughout subsequent care
• Consists of predetermined questions and systematic head-to-toe examination	• Unstructured questions and collection of physical assessments
• Performed once	• Repeated each shift or more often
• Suggests possible problems	• Rules out or confirms problems
• Findings are documented on an admission assessment form	• Findings are documented on a checklist or in progress notes
• Time-consuming; may take an hour or more	• Completed in a brief amount of time (about 15 minutes)
• Supplies a broad, comprehensive volume of data	• Limited amount of data is collected
• Provides breadth for future comparisons	• Adds depth to the initial data base
• Reflects the condition of the patient on entering the health care system	• Provides comparative trends for evaluating the patient's response to treatment

Community Health Center of Branch County

ADMISSION ASSESSMENT RECORD

RESPIRATION

[] PROBLEM [] POTENTIAL FOR REFERRAL	HISTORY OF: [] CHEST PAIN [] PNEUMONIA [] BRONCHITIS [] ASTHMA [] EMPHYSEMA
	SHORTNESS OF BREATH: [] YES [] NO [] WITH EXERCISE [] WITHOUT EXERCISE
	COUGH: [] YES [] NO [] PRODUCTIVE [] NON-PRODUCTIVE [] SPUTUM COLOR
	BREATH SOUNDS (DESCRIBE)
	RATE / RHYTHM / QUALITY: [] LABORED [] SHALLOW / SKIN COLOR: [] PINK [] PALE [] CYANOTIC
	ACCESSORY MUSCLES
	COMMENTS

CIRCULATION

[] PROBLEM [] POTENTIAL FOR REFERRAL	HISTORY OF: [] BLOOD CLOTS [] EDEMA [] ABNORMAL EKG [] NUMBNESS [] TINGLING [] POOR CIRCULATION [] FATIGUE [] HYPERTENSION
	APICAL RATE / APICAL RATE: [] REGULAR [] IRREGULAR / RHYTHM
	NECK VEIN DISTENSION: [] PRESENT [] ABSENT / NAIL BEDS: [] PINK [] PALE [] CYANOTIC
	PEDAL EDEMA: [] PRESENT [] ABSENT
	PEDAL PULSES: LEFT [] PRESENT [] WEAK [] ABSENT; RIGHT [] PRESENT [] WEAK [] ABSENT
	COMMENTS

NUTRITIONAL/METABOLIC

[] PROBLEM [] POTENTIAL FOR REFERRAL	HISTORY OF: [] DIABETES [] HYPOGLYCEMIA [] THYROID PROBLEMS / NUTRITIONAL STATUS: [] WELL NOURISHED [] EMACIATED [] OBESE
	MEALS PER DAY / DIET AT HOME / DIET PREFERENCE / LAST MEAL [] A.M. [] P.M. / RECENT WEIGHT CHANGES
	NUTRITIONAL DISTURBANCES: [] VOMITING [] NAUSEA [] ANOREXIA [] CHEWING PROBLEMS [] OTHER (DESCRIBE)
	JAUNDICE PRESENT: [] YES [] NO / DENTAL HYGIENE (DESCRIBE) / TEETH: [] OWN [] DENTURES / TONGUE CONDITION: [] DRY [] COATED [] MOIST [] SWOLLEN / ORAL MUCOSA: [] DRY [] MOIST / COLOR
	COMMENTS

ELIMINATION

[] PROBLEM [] POTENTIAL FOR REFERRAL	BOWEL HABITS, STOOLS PER DAY ______ / COLOR / [] SOFT FORMED [] DIARRHEA [] CONSTIPATED [] USE LAXATIVE / LAST BOWEL MOVEMENT
	BLADDER: [] DYSURIA [] URGENCY [] NOCTURIA [] CALCULI [] FREQUENCY [] HEMATURIA [] PROSTATE PROBLEM / BOWEL SOUNDS [] PRESENT [] ABSENT; OSTOMIES OR TUBES (DESCRIBE)
	ABDOMEN: [] TENDER [] SOFT [] FIRM [] DISTENDED [] NOT DISTENDED / URINARY DEVICES (DESCRIBE)
	COMMENTS

COGNITIVE/PERCEPTUAL

[] PROBLEM [] POTENTIAL FOR REFERRAL	HISTORY OF: [] SEIZURES [] FREQUENT [] INFREQUENT; [] HEADACHES [] FREQUENT [] INFREQUENT / LIMITATION OR RESTRICTION RELATED TO: [] HEARING - IMPAIRED [] YES [] NO; [] VISION - IMPAIRED [] YES [] NO
	LEVEL OF CONSCIOUSNESS: [] ALERT [] LETHARGIC [] CONFUSED [] LISTLESS [] RESPONDS TO PAIN [] UNRESPONSIVE
	ORIENTED TO: [] TIME [] PLACE [] PERSON / AFFECT: [] CALM [] WITHDRAWN [] APPREHENSIVE [] OTHER (DESCRIBE)
	BEHAVIOR: [] COOPERATIVE [] UNCOOPERATIVE / PUPILS: [] EQUAL [] REACTIVE [] OTHER (DESCRIBE)
	COMMUNICATION: [] SPEAKS ENGLISH [] ABLE TO READ [] ABLE TO WRITE [] COMMUNICATES ADEQUATELY
	AWARENESS: [] NO PROBLEM WITH MEMORY [] PROBLEM WITH MEMORY
	DISCOMFORT/PAIN: [] YES [] NO / WHERE / TYPE / PAIN MANAGEMENT / POTENTIAL RISK OF FALLS: [] YES [] NO
	COMMENTS

FIGURE 2–2. One page of a multipage admission assessment form is shown. (Courtesy of the Community Health Center of Branch County, Coldwater, MI.)

DISPLAY 2-3

Organization of Data

Assessment Findings

Lassitude; distended abdomen; dry, hard stool passed with difficulty; fever; weak cough; thick sputum

Related Clusters

Lassitude, fever
Weak cough, thick sputum
Distended abdomen; dry, hard stool passed with difficulty

of related data (Display 2-3). By organizing the data into small groups, the information is more easily analyzed and takes on more significance than when each fact is considered separately or when the group is examined as a whole.

Diagnosis

Diagnosis (identification of health-related problems) is the second step in the nursing process. Diagnosis is the result of analyzing the collected data and determining whether they suggest normal or abnormal findings.

NURSING DIAGNOSES

Nurses analyze data to identify one or more nursing diagnoses. A **nursing diagnosis** (health issue that can be prevented, reduced, resolved, or enhanced through independent nursing measures) is an exclusive nursing responsibility. Nursing diagnoses are categorized into five groups: actual, potential, possible, syndrome, and wellness diagnoses (Table 2-2).

TABLE 2-2. **Categories of Nursing Diagnoses**

Type	Explanation and Example
Actual diagnosis	A problem that currently exists *Impaired physical mobility related to pain as evidenced by limited range of motion, reluctance to move*
Potential diagnosis	A problem the patient is uniquely at risk for developing *Risk for fluid volume deficit related to persistent vomiting*
Possible diagnosis	A problem may be present, but requires more data collection to rule out or confirm its existence *Possible parental role conflict related to impending divorce*
Syndrome diagnosis	Cluster of problems that are present due to an event or situation (Carpenito, 1997) *Rape trauma syndrome* and *Disuse syndrome*
Wellness diagnosis	A health-related problem with which a healthy person obtains nursing assistance to maintain or perform at a higher level *Potential for enhanced breastfeeding*

The NANDA List

The ANA has designated the North American Nursing Diagnosis Association (NANDA) as the authoritative organization for developing and approving nursing diagnoses. NANDA is the clearinghouse for proposals suggesting diagnoses that fall within the independent domain of nursing practice. The proposals are reviewed for their appropriateness. While research is ongoing, they are incorporated into a list that is published for clinical use. The most recent index, which is revised every 2 years, is provided on the inside cover.

Although entries in the NANDA list change, most authorities believe that the language of approved diagnoses should be used whenever possible. When a patient's problem does not fit into any of the categories approved by NANDA, the nurse can use his or her own terminology when stating the nursing diagnosis.

DIAGNOSTIC STATEMENTS

A nursing diagnostic statement contains one to three parts:

1. Name of the health-related issue or problem as identified in the NANDA list
2. Etiology (its cause)
3. Signs and symptoms

The name of the nursing diagnosis is linked to the etiology with the phrase "related to," and the signs and symptoms are identified with the phrase "as manifested by" (Display 2-4).

Different types of diagnoses have different stems. Potential problems are prefaced with the term "*risk for,*" as in Risk for

DISPLAY 2-4

Parts of a Nursing Diagnostic Statement

1. Sleep pattern disturbance = problem
2. Related to excessive intake of coffee = etiology
3. As manifested by difficulty in falling asleep, feeling tired during the day, and irritability with others = signs and symptoms

impaired skin integrity related to inactivity. The word "*possible*" is used in a diagnostic statement to indicate uncertainty—for example, Possible sexual dysfunction related to anxiety. Wellness diagnoses are prefaced with the phrase "*Potential for enhanced.*"

Potential and possible nursing diagnoses do not include the third part of the statement. In potential nursing diagnoses, the signs or symptoms have not yet been manifested; in possible nursing diagnoses, the data are incomplete. However, the factors that place the patient at risk or make the nurse suspect such a diagnosis are identified in the nursing assessment documentation.

Syndrome diagnoses and wellness diagnoses are one-part statements; they are not linked with an etiology or signs and symptoms.

COLLABORATIVE PROBLEMS

Collaborative problems (physiologic complications whose treatment requires both nurse- and physician-prescribed interventions) represent an interdependent domain of nursing practice (Fig. 2-3). The nurse is specifically responsible and accountable for:

- Correlating medical diagnoses or medical treatment measures with the risk for unique complications
- Documenting the complications for which patients are at risk
- Making pertinent assessments to detect complications
- Reporting trends that suggest a complication is developing
- Managing the emerging problem with nurse- and physician-prescribed measures
- Evaluating the outcomes

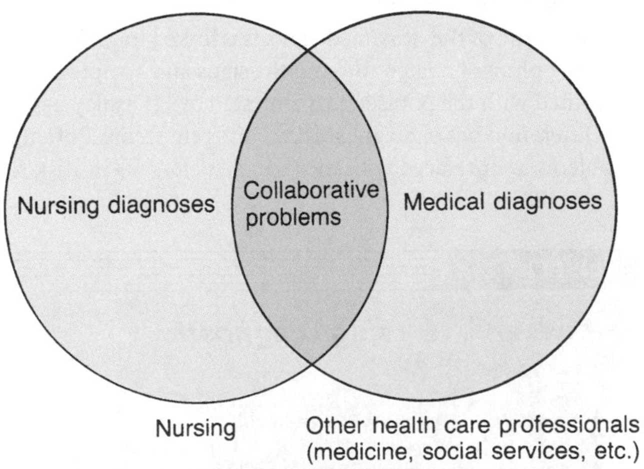

FIGURE 2–3. These two overlapping circles illustrate that the nurse independently treats nursing diagnoses. Doctors, other health professionals, and nurses work together on collaborative problems. (Carpenito LJ. Nursing diagnosis: application to clinical practice. 3rd ed, p 28. Philadelphia: JB Lippincott, 1989.)

Collaborative problems are identified on a patient's plan for care with the abbreviation PC, which stands for potential complication (Table 2-3). Because in a sense a collaborative problem requires the nurse to use diagnostic processes, some nursing leaders are proposing that the term "collaborative diagnosis" be used instead (Alfaro-LeFevre, 1998).

Planning

The third step in the nursing process is **planning** (process of prioritizing nursing diagnoses and collaborative problems, identifying measurable goals or outcomes, selecting appropriate interventions, and documenting the plan for care). Whenever possible, the patient is consulted when developing the plan and making revisions.

SETTING PRIORITIES

Not all of the patient's problems can be resolved during a typically short hospital stay. Therefore, it is important to determine which problems require the most immediate attention. This is done by setting priorities. Prioritization involves ranking from greatest to least importance.

There is more than one way to determine priorities. One method frequently used by nurses is to rank nursing diagnoses using Maslow's Hierarchy of Human Needs (see Chap. 4). Problems interfering with physiologic needs have priority over those affecting other levels of needs (Display 2-5). The ranking can change as problems are resolved or new problems develop.

ESTABLISHING GOALS

A **goal** (expected or desired outcome) helps the nursing team know whether the nursing care has been appropriate for managing the patient's nursing diagnoses and collaborative problems. Therefore, a written goal accompanies each one. Although the terms goal and outcome are sometimes used interchangeably, outcomes are generally more specific (Display 2-6). What is important is that the goal statement or outcome contains the criteria or objective evidence for verifying that the patient has improved. Depending on the agency, nurses may identify short-term goals, long-term goals, or both.

Short-Term Goals

Short-term goals (outcomes that can be met in a few days to a week) are used more often in acute care settings, because most hospital stays are no longer than a week. Short-term goals have the following characteristics (Display 2-7). They are:

TABLE 2-3. **Correlation of Collaborative Problems**

Medical Diagnosis or Medical Treatment	Possible Consequence	Collaborative Problem
Myocardial infarction (heart attack)	Abnormal heart rhythm	PC: Dysrhythmias
Heart failure	Fluid in the lungs	PC: Pulmonary edema
Severe burns	Serum moves into tissue, depleting blood volume	PC: Hypovolemic shock
HIV positive (infected with AIDS virus)	Decreased blood cells that fight infection	PC: Immunodeficiency
Gastric decompression (suctioning stomach fluid)	Removes acid and electrolytes	PC: Alkalosis PC: Electrolyte imbalance
Cardiac catheterization (inserting a catheter into the heart)	Arterial bleeding	PC: Hemorrhage

- *Developed from the problem portion of the diagnostic statement*
- *Patient-centered,* reflecting what will be accomplished from the patient's perspective, not the nurse's
- *Measurable,* identifying specific criteria that provide evidence that the goal has been reached
- *Realistic.* Setting unattainable goals is self-defeating and creates frustration.
- *Accompanied by a target date* for accomplishment, the predicted time when the goal will be met. Identifying a target date builds a time line for evaluation into the nursing process.

DISPLAY 2-5

Prioritizing Nursing Diagnoses

Human Need	Examples of Nursing Diagnoses
Physiologic	Altered nutrition: Less than body requirements Ineffective breathing pattern Pain Impaired swallowing Urinary retention
Safety and security	Risk for injury Impaired verbal communication Altered thought processes Anxiety Fear
Love and belonging	Social isolation Impaired social interactions Altered family processes Parental role conflict
Esteem and self-esteem	Body image disturbance Powerlessness Caregiver role strain Ineffective breastfeeding
Self-actualization	Altered growth and development Spiritual distress

Long-Term Goals

Long-term goals (desirable outcomes that take weeks or months to accomplish) are generally identified for patients who have chronic health problems that require extended care in a nursing home or who receive community health services or home health care. An example of a long-term goal for the patient with a cerebrovascular accident (stroke) is the return of full or partial function to a paralyzed limb. This goal is not likely to be achieved at the time of discharge. However, if short-term goals are achieved in the hospital, long-term goals are more likely to be achieved.

Goals for Collaborative Problems

Goals for collaborative problems are written from a nursing rather than from a patient perspective. They focus on what the nurse will monitor, report, record, or do to promote early detection and treatment (Alfaro-LeFevre, 1998).

The format for writing a nursing goal is, "The nurse will manage and minimize (identify complication) by (insert evidence of assessment, communication, and treatment activities)," or "(identify complication) will be managed and minimized by (evidence)." For example, if the nurse identifies gastrointestinal bleeding as a PC, the goal could be stated,

DISPLAY 2-6

Goals versus Outcomes

Goal

The patient will be well hydrated by 8/23.

Outcome

The patient will have adequate hydration as evidenced by an oral intake between 2,000–3,000 mL/24 hours and a urine output ± 500 mL of the intake amount by 8/23.

DISPLAY 2-7

Components of Short-Term Goals

Nursing Diagnostic Statement

Constipation related to decreased fluid intake, lack of dietary fiber, and lack of exercise as manifested by absence of a normal bowel movement for the past 3 days, abdominal cramping, and straining to pass stool.

Short-Term Goal

The patient will	*patient-centered*
have a bowel movement	identifies *measurable* criteria that reflect the *problem portion* of the diagnostic statement
in 2 days (specify date)	identifies a *target date* for achievement within a *realistic* time frame

"The nurse will examine emesis and stools for blood and report positive test findings, changes in vital signs, and decreased red blood cell counts to the physician" or "Gastrointestinal bleeding will be managed and minimized as evidenced by negative Hemoccult tests, red blood cell count greater than 2.5 million/dl, and vital signs within normal ranges."

SELECTING NURSING INTERVENTIONS

Planning the measures that will be used to accomplish identified goals involves critical thinking. Nursing interventions are directed at eliminating the etiologies. The selection of strategies is based on the knowledge that certain nursing actions produce a desired effect. Whatever interventions are planned, they must be safe, within the legal scope of nursing practice, and compatible with medical orders.

Initial interventions are generally limited to selected measures that have the potential for achieving success. Some interventions are held in reserve in case the goal is not accomplished.

DOCUMENTING THE PLAN OF CARE

The plan of care can be written by hand (Fig. 2-4), standardized, computer-generated, or based on an agency's written standards or clinical pathways. Whatever method is used, the Joint Commission on Accreditation of Healthcare Organizations (JCAHO) requires that every patient's medical record provide evidence of the planned nursing interventions for meeting the patient's needs (Carpenito, 1991).

Nursing orders (directions for a patient's care) identify the what, when, where, and how for performing nursing interventions. Nursing orders provide specific instructions so that all health team members understand exactly what to do for the patient (Display 2-8). Nursing orders are also signed to indicate accountability.

Standardized care plans are preprinted. Both computer-generated and standardized plans provide general suggestions for managing the nursing care of patients with a particular problem. It is up to the nurse to transform the generalized interventions into specific nursing orders and to eliminate whatever is inappropriate or unnecessary.

Agency-specific **standards for care** (policies that indicate which activities will be provided to ensure quality patient care) and clinical pathways (see Chap. 1) relieve the nurse from writing time-consuming plans. Both tools help nurses use their time efficiently and ensure consistent patient care.

COMMUNICATING THE PLAN

Consistency and continuity of care are needed to achieve goals. Therefore, the nurse shares the plan of care with nursing team members, the patient, and the patient's family. In some agencies, the patient signs the written care plan.

The plan of care is a permanent part of the patient's medical record. It is placed in the patient's chart, kept separately at the patient's bedside, or located in a temporary folder at the nurses' station for easy access. Wherever it is located, it is referred to daily by each nurse assigned to the patient, reviewed for appropriateness, and revised according to changes in the patient's condition.

Implementation

Implementation (carrying out the plan of care) is the fourth step in the nursing process. The nurse implements medical orders as well as nursing orders, which should complement each other. Implementing the plan involves the patient and one or more members of the health care team. A wide circle of care providers with assorted roles may be called on to participate, either directly or indirectly, in carrying out one patient's plan of care (Fig. 2-5).

DOCUMENTATION

The medical record is legal evidence that the plan of care has been more than just a paper trail. The information in the chart shows a correlation between the plan and the care that

Name: Mrs. Rita Williard Age: 68 Date of Admission: 11/10

Diagnosis on admission: CVA c̄ left-sided weakness

Nursing diagnosis: Impaired Physical Mobility, High Risk for Injury, Situational Low Self-esteem

Long-term goals: Independent mobility using walker or quad cane, record of personal safety, positive self-regard

DATE	PROBLEM	GOAL	TARGET DATE	NURSING ORDERS
11/10	1 Impaired Physical Mobility related to left sided weakness as manifested by decreased muscle strength in left leg and arm, slowed gait, dragging foot.	The patient will stand and pivot from bed to wheelchair or commode.	11/24	1) Passive ROM t.i.d. to left arm and leg 2) Physical therapy b.i.d. for practice at parallel bars 3) Apply left leg brace and sling to left arm when up 4) Assist to balance on right leg at bedside before and after physical therapy daily C. Meyer, RN
11/10	2 Risk for Injury related to motor deficit	The patient will transfer from bed to wheelchair without injury	12/1	1) Keep side rails up and trapeze over bed 2) Use shoe & nonskid sole on right foot (leg brace on left) before transfer 3) Dangle for 5 minutes before attempting to stand 4) Lock wheels on wheelchair before transfer 5) Obtain help of second assistant 6) Block left foot to avoid slipping during pivot 7) Place signal light on right side within reach at all times C. Meyer, RN
12/2	3 Situational Low Self-Esteem related to dependence on others as manifested by statements, I need as much help as a baby; I feel so useless; How embarrassing to be so dependent.	The patient will identify one or more examples of improved mobility and self-care	12/18	1.) Allow to express feelings without disagreeing or interrupting. 2.) Reinforce concept that the right side of body is unaffected. 3.) Help to set and accomplish one realistic goal daily. S. Moore, RN

FIGURE 2–4. Sample nursing care plan.

has been provided. In other words, the nurse's charting (see Chap. 9) reflects the written plan. Nurses are just as accountable for carrying out nursing orders as they are for physician's orders.

In addition to identifying the nursing interventions that have been provided, the record also describes the quantity and quality of the patient's response. Quoting the patient helps identify what is occurring from the patient's point of view and safeguards against making incorrect assumptions.

In short, appropriate documentation maintains open lines of communication among members of the health care team, ensures the continuing progress of the patient, complies with accreditation standards, and helps ensure reimbursement from government or private insurance companies.

DISPLAY 2-8

Nursing Orders

Nursing Order	Weakness	Improvement
Encourage fluids.	Lacks specificity Likely to be interpreted differently May result in inconsistent or less than-adequate care	Provide 100 mL of oral fluid every hour while awake.

Evaluation

Evaluation (process of determining whether a goal has been reached) is the fifth and final step in the nursing process. Although this is considered the last step, the entire process is an ongoing one. By analyzing the patient's response, evaluation helps to determine the effectiveness of nursing care (Display 2-9).

Before revising a plan of care, it is important to discuss any lack of progress with the patient. In this way, both the nurse and the patient can speculate on what activities need to be discontinued, added, or changed. Other health team members who are familiar with a particular patient or problems similar to those of the patient may offer their expertise as well. The evaluation of a patient's progress may be the subject of a nursing team conference. Some units even invite the patient and family to participate.

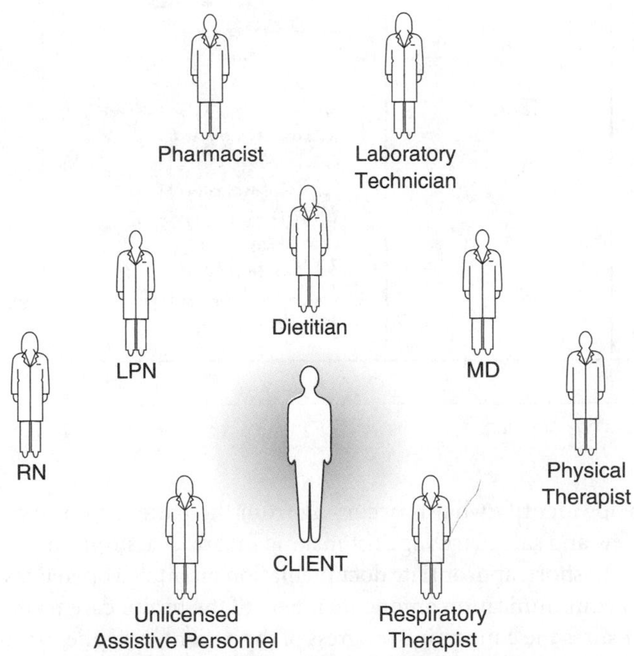

FIGURE 2–5. Members of the healthcare team.

Using the Nursing Process

Use of the nursing process is the standard for clinical nursing practice. Nurse practice acts hold nurses accountable for demonstrating all of these aspects when caring for patients. To do less implies negligence. More detailed discussions of the nursing process can be found in specialty texts and in some of the suggested readings at the end of this chapter. The guidelines that follow reiterate the sequence of steps in the nursing process.

Nursing Guidelines For

Using the Nursing Process

- Collect information about the patient.
  RATIONALE: Data collection is the basis for identifying problems.
- Organize the data.
  RATIONALE: Organizing related data simplifies the process of analysis.
- Analyze the data for what is normal and abnormal.
  RATIONALE: Abnormalities provide clues to the patient's problems.
- Identify actual, potential, possible, syndrome and wellness nursing diagnoses and collaborative problems.
  RATIONALE: Problem identification directs the nurse to select methods for maintaining or restoring the patient's health.
- Prioritize the problem list.
  RATIONALE: Setting priorities targets problems that require the most immediate attention.
- Set goals with specific criteria for evaluating whether the problems have been prevented, reduced, or resolved.
  RATIONALE: Goals predict the expected outcomes from nursing care.
- Select a limited number of appropriate nursing interventions.
  RATIONALE: The nurse uses scientific knowledge to determine which measures will be most effective in accomplishing the goals of care.

DISPLAY 2–9

Outcomes From Evaluation

Analysis	Reason	Action
Goals have been reached.	Plan was effective and implemented consistently.	Discontinue the nursing orders.
Some progress has been made.	Care has been inconsistent.	Check that nursing orders are clear and specific.
	Target date was too ambitious.	Continue care as planned; readjust target date.
	Patient's response has been less than expected.	Revise the plan by adding additional nursing interventions or more frequent implementation.
No progress has occurred.	Inaccurate initial diagnosis	Revise problem list; write new goals and nursing orders.
	New problems have occurred.	Add new problems, goals, and nursing orders.
	Unrealistic target date	Revise expected date for achievement.
	Ineffective nursing interventions	Add new nursing orders; discontinue ineffective measures; readjust target date.

☑ Give specific directions for nursing care.
RATIONALE: Specific directions promote consistency and continuity among care givers.

☑ Document the plan for care using whatever written format is acceptable.
RATIONALE: A written plan provides a means of communication and reference for the nursing team to follow.

☑ Discuss the plan with nursing team members, the patient, and family.
RATIONALE: Verbally sharing the plan ensures that everyone is informed and goal-directed.

☑ Put the plan into action.
RATIONALE: Work produces results.

☑ Observe the patient's responses.
RATIONALE: Evaluating outcomes is the basis for determining the effectiveness of the plan of care.

☑ Chart all nursing activities and the patient's responses.
RATIONALE: Documentation demonstrates that the planned care has been implemented and provides information about the patient's progress.

☑ Compare the patient's responses with the goal criteria.
RATIONALE: If the planned care is appropriate, there should be some measure of progress toward accomplishing goals.

☑ Discuss the progress, or lack of it, with the patient, family, and other nursing team members.
RATIONALE: Pooling resources may provide better alternatives when revising the plan of care.

☑ Change the plan in areas that are no longer appropriate.
RATIONALE: The nursing care plan changes according to the needs of the patient.

☑ Continue to implement and evaluate the revised plan of care.
RATIONALE: The nursing process is a continuous sequence of actions that is repeated until the goals have been met.

KEY CONCEPTS

- The nursing process is an organized sequence of steps used to identify health problems and manage patient care.
- The steps in the nursing process are assessment, diagnosis, planning, implementation, and evaluation.
- The nursing process is within the legal scope of nursing, based on unique knowledge, planned, patient-centered, goal-directed, prioritized, and dynamic.
- Resources for data include the patient, the patient's family, medical records, and other health care workers.
- A data base assessment provides a vast amount of information about a patient at the time of admission. Focus assessments, which are ongoing, expand the data base with additional information.
- A nursing diagnosis is a health problem that nurses can independently treat. A collaborative problem is a

physiologic complication that requires the skills and interventions of both nurses and physicians.

- A nursing diagnostic statement generally consists of three parts: the problem, the etiology for the problem, and the signs and symptoms or evidence for the problem.
- Because hospital stays are becoming very short, setting priorities for care helps to maximize efficiency in a minimal amount of time.
- Short-term goals are those the nurse expects to accomplish in a few days to a week when caring for patients in an acute care setting such as a hospital. Long-term goals may take weeks to months to accomplish. They are identified when caring for patients with chronic problems who are receiving nursing care in a long-term health facility or through community health agencies or home health care.
- The plan of care is documented by writing the problems, goals, and nursing orders by hand, individualizing a standardized or computer-generated care plan, or following an agency's written standards for care or clinical pathways.
- Implementation of the plan of care is demonstrated by correlating the written plan with the nurse's documentation in the medical record.
- When evaluating the patient's progress, nursing orders are discontinued if the goal has been met and the problem no longer exists. The care plan is revised if there has been progress but the goal remains unmet or if there has been no progress in reaching a desired outcome.

CRITICAL THINKING EXERCISES

- If an unconscious patient is brought to the nursing unit, how can a nurse gather data?
- There are three nursing diagnoses on a patient's plan of care: Ineffective breathing, Social isolation, and Anxiety. Which has the highest priority, and why?
- A nurse, while reviewing a patient's plan of care, notices that no progress has been made in accomplishing the goal by its projected target date. What actions are appropriate at this time?

SUGGESTED READINGS

Alfaro-LeFevre R. Applying nursing process: a step-by-step guide, 4th ed. Philadelphia, JB Lippincott, 1998.

Brooks JT. An analysis of nursing documentation as a reflection of actual nurse work. MedSurg Nursing 1998;7(4):189–198.

Brugh LA. Automated clinical pathways in the patient record: legal implications. Nursing Case Management 1998;3(3):131–137.

Carpenito LJ. Has JCAHO eliminated care plans? American Nurse 1991; 23(6):6.

Carpenito LJ. Nursing diagnosis: application to clinical practice, 7th ed. Philadelphia, JB Lippincott, 1997.

Daley JM, Mass M, McCloskey JC, Bulechek GM. A care planning tool that proves what we do. RN 1996;59(6):26–29.

Dozier AM. Professional standards: linking care, competence, and quality. Journal of Nursing Care Quality 1998;12(4):22–29.

Greenwald D. Nursing care plans: issues and solutions. Nursing Management 1996;27(3):33–40.

Quinn K. Protocols in practice. Navigating critical pathway selection. Nursing Case Management 1998;3(3):117–119.

UNIT TWO

INTEGRATING BASIC CONCEPTS

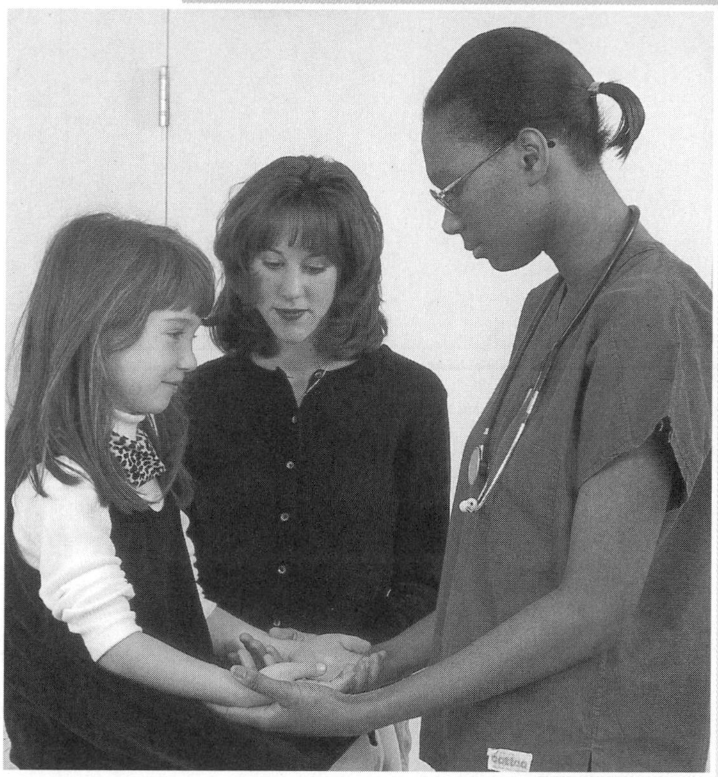

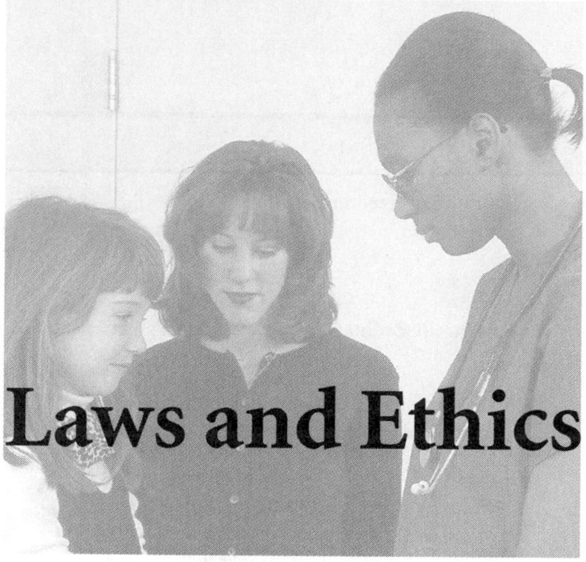

Laws and Ethics

CHAPTER 3

CHAPTER OUTLINE

Laws
Professional Liability
Ethics

KEY TERMS

administrative laws
advance directive
allocation of scarce resources
anecdotal record
assault
battery
board of nursing
civil laws
code of ethics
common law
confidentiality
criminal laws
defamation
defendant
deontology
ethical dilemma
ethics
false imprisonment
felony
Good Samaritan laws
incident report
intentional tort
invasion of privacy
laws
liability insurance
libel
malpractice
misdemeanor
negligence
nurse practice act
plaintiff
reciprocity
restraints
slander
statute of limitations
statutory laws
teleology
tort
truth telling
unintentional tort
whistle-blowing

LEARNING OBJECTIVES

An understanding of the content within this chapter will be evidenced by the student's ability to:

- Name six types of laws.
- Discuss the purpose of nurse practice acts and the role of the state board of nursing.
- Explain the difference between intentional and unintentional torts.
- Describe the difference between negligence and malpractice.
- Define the term ethics.
- Explain the purpose for a code of ethics.
- Describe two types of ethical theories.
- List five ethical issues that are common in nursing practice.

Laws, ethics, patient rights, and nursing duties affect nurses throughout their careers. This chapter introduces basic legal and ethical concepts and issues that affect the practice of nursing.

Laws

Laws (rules of conduct established and enforced by the government of a society) are intended to protect both the public as a whole and each person. There are six categories of laws: constitutional, statutory, administrative, common, criminal, and civil laws (Table 3-1).

CONSTITUTIONAL LAW

The founders of the United States wrote the country's first set of formal laws within the framework of the Constitution. The document, which has endured with few amendments, defines the division of power among three branches of government and the process of checks and balances, protecting the nation as a whole. It also identifies the rights and privileges to which all its citizens are entitled.

STATUTORY LAWS

Statutory laws (those enacted by federal, state, or local legislatures) are sometimes identified as public acts, codes, or ordinances. For example, the legislative branch of state govern-

TABLE 3–1. **Types of Laws**

Category	Purpose	Example
Constitutional	Protects fundamental rights and freedoms of U.S. citizens; defines the duties and limitations of the executive, legislative, and judicial branches of government	Bill of Rights, freedom of speech
Statutory	Identifies local, state, or federal rules that are necessary for the public's welfare	Public health ordinances, tax laws, nurse practice acts
Administrative	Develops regulations with which to carry out the mission of a public agency	Board of nursing in each state enacts and enforces rules as they relate to the nurse practice act
Common	Interprets legal issues based on previous court decisions in similar cases (legal precedents)	Tarrasoff *vs.* Board of Regents of University of California [1976] justifies breaching a mental patient's confidentiality when the identity of a potential criminal victim is revealed
Criminal	Determines the nature of criminal acts that endanger all of society	Identifies the differences in first-degree and second-degree murder, manslaughter, etc.
Civil	Determines the circumstances and manner in which an individual may be compensated for being the victim of another person's action or omission of an action	Dereliction of duty, negligence

ments assumes responsibility for enacting statutes that ensure that those who provide health care are competent. A **nurse practice act** (statute that legally defines the unique role of the nurse and differentiates it from that of other health care practitioners, such as physicians) is one example of a statutory law (Display 3-1). Although each state's nurse practice act is unique, all generally contain three elements:

- They define the scope of nursing practice.
- They establish the limits to that practice.
- They identify the titles that nurses may use, such as licensed practical nurse (LPN), licensed vocational nurse (LVN), or registered nurse (RN).

ADMINISTRATIVE LAWS

Administrative laws (legal provisions through which federal, state, and local agencies maintain self-regulation) affect the power to manage governmental agencies. Some administrative laws give federal and state governments the legal authority to ensure the health and safety of their citizens. The state board of nursing is an example of an administrative agency that enforces administrative law.

State Boards of Nursing

Each state's **board of nursing** (regulatory agency for managing the provisions of a state's nurse practice act) develops rules and regulations for the education and licensing of individuals who wish to practice as nurses within the state. The state board of nursing also is responsible for suspending and revoking licenses and reviewing applications asking for **reciprocity** (licensure based on evidence of having met licensing criteria in another state). A license in one state does not give

DISPLAY 3–1

Sample Nurse Practice Act

"Practical nurse" or "licensed practical nurse" means a person who is licensed as a practical nurse under this Act and practices practical nursing as defined in paragraph (j) of this Section. Only a practical nurse licensed under this Act is entitled to use the title "licensed practical nurse" and the abbreviation "L.P.N.". "Practical nursing" means the performance of nursing acts requiring the basic nursing knowledge, judgment, and skill acquired by means of completion of an approved practical nursing education program. Practical nursing includes assisting in the nursing process as delegated by and under the direction of a registered professional nurse. The practical nurse may work under the direction of a licensed physician, dentist, podiatrist, or other health care professional determined by the Department.

From: Nursing and Advanced Practice Nursing Act and Rules for the Administration of Nursing and Advanced Practice Nursing Act, 1999. Public Act 90-0818. Illinois Department of Professional Regulation. Amended by P.A. 90-0061, effective December 10, 1997; P.A. 90-0248, effective January 1, 1998; P.A. 90-0742, Section 17, effective August 13, 1998.

a person a right to automatic licensure in another. Reciprocity is important for nurses who live in one state and work in another, those who wish to practice in more than one state, or those who move from one state to another. However, reciprocity has been abused: in the past, a nurse whose license had been revoked as a punitive measure in one state could move to another and obtain a license there. However, legislation has been enacted to track incompetent practitioners. Since 1989, the names of licensed health care workers who are disciplined by hospitals, courts, licensing boards, professional associations, insurers, and peer review committees are submitted to a National Practitioner Data Bank, a computerized resource sponsored by the Office of Quality Assurance, a branch of the Department of Health and Human Services. The information is made available to licensing boards and health care facilities that hire nurses throughout the nation.

COMMON LAW

Common law (decisions based on prior cases of a similar nature) is based on a principle referred to as *stare decisis* ("let the decision stand") in which prior outcomes serve as a guideline for decisions in other jurisdictions that deal with comparable circumstances. Common law refers to litigation that falls outside the realm of constitutional, statutory, and administrative laws.

CRIMINAL LAWS

Criminal laws (penal codes that protect the safety of all citizens from persons who are a threat to the public good) are used to prosecute individuals who commit crimes. The state represents "the people" when prosecuting individuals accused of crimes. Crimes are either misdemeanors or felonies.

Shoplifting is an example of a **misdemeanor** (minor criminal offense). If the person is convicted, a small fine, a short period of incarceration, or both may be levied. The fine is paid to the state.

Murder is a **felony** (serious criminal offense), as are falsifying medical records, insurance fraud, and stealing narcotics. Conviction is punishable by a lengthy prison term or even execution. The state generally prohibits felons from obtaining an occupational license, and the state will revoke such a license if its holder is convicted of a felony.

CIVIL LAWS

Civil laws (statutes that protect the personal freedoms and rights of individuals) include the right to be left alone, freedom from threats of injury, freedom from offensive contact, and freedom from character attacks. Charges are brought by the **plaintiff** (person claiming injury) against the **defendant** (person charged with violating the law). The case is referred to as a **tort** (litigation in which one person asserts that an injury, which may be physical, emotional, or financial, occurred as a consequence of another person's actions or failure to act).

It does not take the same quality or quantity of evidence to be convicted in a civil lawsuit as in a criminal case. If found guilty of a tort, the defendant is required to pay the plaintiff restitution for damages. Torts are classified as intentional or unintentional.

Intentional Torts

Intentional torts (lawsuits in which a plaintiff charges that the defendant committed a deliberately aggressive act) include assault, battery, false imprisonment, invasion of privacy, and defamation.

Assault

Assault (act in which there is a threat or attempt to do bodily harm) may be in the form of physical intimidation, a remark, or a gesture. The plaintiff interprets the threat to mean that force may be forthcoming. A nurse may be accused of assault if he or she makes a verbal threat to restrain a patient unnecessarily—for example, to curtail the use of the signal light.

Battery

Battery (unauthorized physical contact) can include touching a person's body, clothing, chair, or bed. A charge of battery can be made even if the contact does not actually cause physical harm to the individual. The criterion is that the contact took place without the plaintiff's consent.

Sometimes nonconsensual physical contact can be justified. For example, health professionals can use physical force to subdue mentally ill individuals or those under the influence of alcohol or drugs if their actions endanger their own safety or that of others. However, documentation must show that the situation required the degree of restraint that was used. Excessive force is never appropriate when less would have been effective. When recording information about these types of situations, the nurse must describe the behavior and the response of the patient when lesser forms of restraint were used first.

To protect health care workers from being charged with battery, adult patients are asked to sign a general permission for care and treatment at the time of admission (Fig. 3-1) and additional written consent forms for tests, procedures, or surgery. Consent is obtained from a parent or guardian if the patient is a minor or is mentally retarded or mentally incompetent. In an emergency, consent can be implied. In other words, it is assumed that in life-threatening circumstances, if a patient were able to understand the risks, consent for treatment would be given.

THREE RIVERS AREA HOSPITAL
THREE RIVERS, MICHIGAN 49093

CONSENT FOR INPATIENT, OUTPATIENT, MEDICAL AND / OR SURGICAL TREATMENT

PATIENT'S NAME: ______________________________

DATE & TIME: ______________________________

I, the undersigned, knowing that I have a condition requiring hospital and medical treatment, do hereby voluntarily consent to such routine diagnostic procedures and hospital care by Dr. __________ __________, his assistants or his designees, including such hospital personnel as he deems necessary.

I am aware that the practice of medicine is not an exact science and I acknowledge that no guarantees have been made to me as to the results of said outpatient care which I have hereby authorized.

If applicable, I hereby authorize Three Rivers Area Hospital to retain, preserve, and use of scientific or teaching purposes, or otherwise dispose of, at their convenience, any specimens, tissues, parts or organs taken from my (or patient's) body, as a result of the procedure or procedures authorized above.

I understand that the physician is not an employee or agent of Three Rivers Area Hospital but that as a practicing physician in the State of Michigan, he is granted the privilege to utilize the facilities of care at this hospital.

This notice is to inform you that Michigan law allows this hospital to test your blood for the presence of antibodies which may indicate you have been exposed to HIV (AIDS). This test is permitted by Michigan law and may be done without your permission if any hospital personnel are exposed to blood and body fluids in the course of care for you. This is for your protection as well as for the course of care for you. This is for your protection as well as for the protection of the physicians, nurses and other associates of this hospital.

This form has been fully explained to me and I certify that I understand its contents.

______________________________ ______________
Patient's Signature Date

______________________________ ______________
Witness Date

If patient is unable to sign or is a minor, complete the following:
Patient is a minor, __________ years of age, and/or is unable to sign because:

____

______________________________ ______________
Signature (Closest Relative or Legal Guardian) Date

______________________________ ______________
Relationship to patient Witness

FIGURE 3–1. Consent for treatment form.

False Imprisonment

False imprisonment (interference with an individual's freedom to move about at will without legal authority to do so) can be alleged if a nurse detains a competent patient from leaving the hospital or other health care agency. If a patient wants to leave without being medically discharged, it is customary to have him or her sign a form indicating personal responsibility for leaving against medical advice (AMA) (Fig. 3-2). However, if the patient refuses to sign the paper, he or she cannot be barred from leaving.

Forced confinement is legal under two conditions: if there is a judicial restraining order (for example, a prisoner admitted for medical care) or if there is a court-ordered commitment (for example, a mentally ill person who is dangerous to himself or others).

The unnecessary or unprescribed restraint of an individual can lead to charges of false imprisonment, battery, or both. **Restraints** (devices or chemicals that restrict movement) include cloth limb restraints, bedrails, chairs with locking lap trays, and sedative drugs. These interventions are intended to subdue a patient's activity.

THREE RIVERS HOSPITAL
THREE RIVERS, MICHIGAN 49093

Release from Responsibility for Discharge

Date: ______________________ Time: ______________ A.M. / P.M.

PATIENT: ______________________________

This is to certify that I ______________________________, a patient in the ______________________________ Hospital am being discharged against the advice of the attending physician and the hospital administration. I acknowledge that I have been informed of the risk involved and hereby release the attending physician and the hospital from all responsibility for any ill effects which may result from such discharge.

Witnesses:

____
(Signature of Patient)

____

(To be signed by the legal representative in case of a minor or of a patient who is not mentally competent, otherwise by the patient.)

FIGURE 3–2. Release form for discharging oneself against medical advice.

The Nursing Home Reform Act of the Omnibus Budget Reconciliation Act (OBRA) passed in 1987 and implemented in 1990 states that residents in nursing homes have "the right to be free of, and the facility must ensure freedom from, any restraints imposed or psychoactive drug administered for purposes of discipline or convenience, and not required to treat the residents' medical symptoms." This is not to say that restraints cannot be used. However, they should be used as a last resort rather than the initial intervention. Their use must be justified and accompanied by informed consent from the patient or a responsible relative.

Before using restraints, the best legal advice is to try alternative measures for protecting wandering patients, reducing the potential for falls (see Chap. 18), and ensuring that patients do not jeopardize medical treatment by pulling out feeding tubes or other therapeutic devices. If less restrictive alternatives are unsuccessful, a medical order must be obtained before each and every instance in which restraints are used. In acute care hospitals, medical orders for restraints are renewed every 24 hours. Once restraints are applied, charting must indicate regular patient assessment, provisions for fluids and nourishment and bowel and bladder elimination, and attempts to release the patient from the restraints for a trial period to justify their continued use. Once the patient is no longer a danger to himself or herself or others, the restraints must be removed.

Invasion of Privacy

Civil law protects individuals from **invasion of privacy** (failure to leave individuals and their property alone). Some examples include trespassing, illegal search and seizure, wiretapping, and revealing personal information about someone, even if the information is true. Medical instances in which privacy laws are violated include photographing a patient without consent, revealing a patient's name in a public report, or allowing an unauthorized person to observe the patient's care. To ensure and protect patients' rights to privacy, medical records and information are kept confidential. Personal names and identities are concealed or obliterated in case studies or research. Privacy curtains are used during care, and permission is obtained if a nursing or medical student will be present as an observer during a procedure.

Defamation

Defamation (an act in which *untrue* information harms a person's reputation) is unlawful. Examples include **slander** (character attack that is uttered orally in the presence of others) and **libel** (damaging statement that is written and read by others). Injury is considered to occur because the derogatory remarks attack the character and good name of an individual. Therefore, nurses must avoid making negative comments about patients, physicians, or other coworkers.

Unintentional Torts

Unintentional torts (situations that result in an injury, although the person responsible did not mean to cause harm) involve allegations of negligence or malpractice.

Negligence

Negligence (harm that results because an individual did not act *reasonably*) implies that a person acted carelessly. In negligence cases, a jury decides whether any other prudent person would have acted differently than the defendant, given the same set of circumstances. For example, a person's car breaks down on the highway, and the driver pulls off to the side of the road, raises the hood, and activates the emergency flashing lights. If the disabled car is struck by another vehicle and the driver of the second car sues, the guilt or innocence of the driver of the disabled car hinges on whether the jury believes the driver's action was reasonable. *Reasonableness is based on the jury's opinion of what constitutes good common sense.*

Malpractice

Malpractice (professional negligence), which differs from simple negligence, holds professionals to a higher standard of accountability. Rather than being held accountable for acting as an ordinary, reasonable lay person, in a malpractice case the court determines whether a nurse or other health care worker acted in a manner comparable to that of his or her peers. Four elements must be proven to win a malpractice lawsuit: duty, breach of duty, causation, and injury (Display 3-2).

Because the jury may be unfamiliar with the scope of nursing practice, other resources may be presented in court to prove breach of duty. Some examples include the employing agency's standards for care, written policies and procedures, care plans or clinical pathways, and the testimony of expert witnesses.

The best protection from malpractice lawsuits is competent nursing. Competency is demonstrated by participating in continuing education programs, taking nursing courses at a college or university, and becoming certified. Defensive nursing practice also involves thorough and objective documentation (see Chap. 9).

One of the best methods for avoiding a lawsuit is to administer compassionate care. The "golden rule" of doing unto others as you would have them do unto you is a good principle to follow. Patients who perceive the nurse as caring and concerned tend to be satisfied with their care. These techniques communicate a caring attitude:

- Smiling
- Introducing yourself
- Calling the patient by the name he or she prefers
- Touching the patient appropriately to demonstrate concern
- Responding quickly to the call light
- Telling the patient how long you will be gone, if you need to leave the unit, informing the patient who will be caring for him or her in your absence, and informing him or her when you return
- Spending time with the patient other than performing required care
- Being a good listener
- Explaining everything so that the patient can understand it
- Being a good host or hostess—offering visitors extra chairs, letting them know where they can obtain snacks and beverages, and directing them to the restrooms and parking areas
- Accepting justifiable criticism without becoming defensive
- Saying "I'm sorry"

Patients can sense when a nurse wants to do a good job rather than just do a job. The relationship that develops is apt to reduce the potential for a lawsuit, even if harm occurs.

Professional Liability

All professionals, including nurses, are held responsible and accountable for providing safe, appropriate care. Because nurses have specialized knowledge and proximity to patients, they have a primary role in protecting patients from preventable or reversible complications.

The number of lawsuits involving nurses is increasing. Therefore, it is to every nurse's advantage to obtain liability insurance and to become familiar with legal mechanisms, such as Good Samaritan laws and statutes of limitations, that may prevent or relieve culpability, as well as with strategies for providing a sound legal defense, such as written incident reports and anecdotal records.

DISPLAY 3-2

Elements in a Malpractice Case

Duty

An obligation existed to provide care for the person who claims to have been injured or harmed

Breach of Duty

Failure to provide appropriate care, or the care that was provided was done so in a negligent manner—that is, in a manner that conflicts with how others with similar education would have acted given the same set of circumstances

Causation

The professional's action, or lack of it, caused the plaintiff harm.

Injury

Physical, psychological, or financial harm occurred.

LIABILITY INSURANCE

Liability insurance (a contract between an individual or corporation and a company who is willing to provide legal services and financial assistance when the policyholder is involved in a malpractice lawsuit) is a necessity for all nurses. Although many agencies that employ nurses have liability insurance with an umbrella clause that includes its employees, nurses should obtain their own personal liability insurance. The advantage is that the nurse involved in a lawsuit will have a separate attorney working on his or her sole behalf. Because the damages sought in malpractice lawsuits are so costly, the attorneys hired by the hospital are sometimes more committed to defending the hospital against liability and negative publicity, rather than defending an employed nurse whom they also are being paid to represent.

Student nurses are held accountable for their actions during clinical practice and should also carry liability insurance. Liability insurance is available through the National Federation for Licensed Practical Nurses, the National Student Nurses' Association, the American Nurses Association (ANA), and other private insurance companies.

REDUCING LIABILITY

It is unrealistic to think that lawsuits can be avoided completely, but there are some avenues that protect nurses and other health care workers from being sued or provide a foundation for a sound legal defense.

Good Samaritan Laws

Good Samaritan laws (legal immunity for passersby who provide emergency first aid to accident victims) have been enacted in most states. The legislation is based on the Biblical story of the person who gave aid to a beaten stranger along a roadside. Although laws of this nature are helpful, none of the Good Samaritan laws provides absolute exemption from prosecution in the event of an injury. Paramedics, ambulance personnel, physicians, and nurses who stop to provide assistance are still held to a higher standard of care because they supposedly have training above and beyond that of average lay persons.

Statute of Limitations

Each state establishes a **statute of limitations** (designated amount of time within which a person can file a lawsuit). The length of time varies from state to state and is generally calculated from when the incident occurred. However, when the injured party is a minor, the statute of limitations sometimes does not commence until the victim reaches adulthood. Once the time period expires, an injured party can no longer sue, even if his or her claim is legitimate.

Incident Reports

An **incident report** (written account of an unusual event involving a patient, employee, or visitor that has the potential for being injurious; Fig. 3-3) is kept separate from the medical record. Incident reports serve two purposes: to determine how hazardous situations can be prevented, and to serve as a reference in case of future litigation. Incident reports must include five important pieces of information:

- When the incident occurred
- Where it took place
- Who was involved
- What happened
- What actions were taken at the time

All witnesses are identified by name. Any pertinent statements made by the injured person, before or after the incident, are quoted. Accurate and detailed documentation can often help prove that the nurse acted reasonably or appropriately in the circumstances.

Anecdotal Records

An **anecdotal record** (personal, handwritten account of an incident) is not recorded on any official form, nor is it filed with administrative records. The information is retained by the nurse. The notation is safeguarded and may be used later to refresh the nurse's memory if a lawsuit develops. Anecdotal notes can be used in court on advice of an attorney.

MALPRACTICE LITIGATION

A successful outcome in a malpractice lawsuit depends on many variables, such as the physical evidence and the expertise of one's lawyer. However, the appearance, demeanor, and conduct of the nurse defendant inside and outside the courtroom can help or damage the case. The suggestions in Display 3-3 may be helpful if a nurse becomes involved in malpractice litigation.

Ethics

The word ethics comes from the Greek word *ethos,* meaning customs or modes of conduct. **Ethics** (moral or philosophical principles) direct actions as being either right or wrong. Various organizations, such as those representing nurses, have identified standards for ethical practice, known as a code of ethics, for members within their discipline.

CODES OF ETHICS

A **code of ethics** (a list of written statements describing ideal behavior) serves as a model for personal conduct. The National

THREE RIVERS AREA HOSPITAL INCIDENT REPORT
Confidential - DO NOT DUPLICATE
Forward to Risk Management within 48 hours

Addressograph

Identification Sex Age Incident Date Time Shift Department
__Inpatient __M ___ __/__/__ __:__ __1st
__Outpatient __F __2nd ________
__Visitor __3rd

Reason for hospitalization/presence on premises: ____________________

I. Location of Incident
__Patient Room #______
__Patient Bathroom
__Corridor
__Other ______________

II. Type of Incident
__Fall
__Medication
__Infusion
__Lost/Found
__Burn
__Treatment/Procedure
__Equipment
__Needle/Sponge Count
__Other__________

III. Description of Incident ____________________

IV. Nature of Incident

A. Falls:

Activity Order:	Pt. Condition Prior to:	Fall Involved:	Patient/Visitor was:
__Restraints	__Weak, unsteady	__Chair, W/C	__Lying
__Bedrest only	__Alert, oriented	__Stretcher	__Standing
__BRP	__Disoriented/confused	__Tub/Shower	__Getting on/off
__Up w/asst.	__Senile	__Toilet	__Sitting
__Up AD LIB	__Unconscious	__Floor Condition(below)	__Ambulating
	__Medicated/Sedated	__Bed	__Other________
	Med. Name ________	__Side Rails Up	________
	Last Dose ________	__Side Rails Down	________

B. Medications:

Incident Involved:
__Wrong Med, Tx, Procedure
__Wrong Patient
__Wrong Time
__Omission
__Incorrect Dose
__Incorrect Method of Administration

__Adverse Reaction
__Infiltration
__Other__________

Factors:
__Patient I.D. Not Checked
__Transcription
__Labeling
__Physician orders not clear
__Physician orders not checked
__Misread label/dose
__Charting
__Wrong Med from Pharmacy
__Defective equipment
__Communications
__Other__________

C. Other:
__Loss of Property
__Struck by object, equipment
__Equipment malfunction
__Anesthesia
__Patient ID
__Other__________

V. Nature of Injury (Injury sustained as a result of incident):
__Asphyxia, Strangulation, Inhalation
__Head Injury
__Contagious or infectious Disease Exposure
__Fracture or dislocation
__Viscera Injury
__Sprain or strain
__Contusion, Cut, Laceration
__Burn or Scald
__Chemical Burn
__No injury
__No apparent injury
__Other__________

VI. Action Taken:
Physician Notified __Yes __No
PT/Visitor seen by MD/T&EC __Yes __No
MD Name ____________ Time __:__
Physician's Findings: ____________________

Other follow up: __No __Yes - Specify ____________________

____________ __/__/__ ____________ __/__/__
Name of Person Reporting Date Department Director Date

____________ __/__/__ ____________ __/__/__
Supervisor Date Risk Management Date

8311-109

FIGURE 3–3. An incident report form.

DISPLAY 3-3

Legal Advice

1. Notify the claims agent of your professional liability insurance company.
2. Contact the National Nurses Claims Data Base through the American Nurses Association. This confidential service provides information that supports nurses involved in litigation.
3. Discuss the particulars of the case only with your attorney.
4. Tell your attorney everything.
5. Avoid giving public statements.
6. Reread the patient's record, incident sheet, and your anecdotal note before testifying.
7. Ask to reread information again in court if it will help to refresh your memory.
8. Dress conservatively, in a businesslike manner. Avoid excesses in makeup, hairstyle, or jewelry.
9. Look directly at whomever asks a question.
10. Speak in a modulated but audible voice that can be heard easily by the jury and others in the court.
11. Tell the truth.
12. Use language with which you are comfortable. Do not try to impress the court with legal or medical terms.
13. Say as little as possible in court under cross-examination.
14. Answer the prosecuting lawyer's questions with "Yes" or "No"; limit answers to only the questions that are asked.
15. If you do not know or cannot remember information, say so.
16. Wait to expand on information if asked by your defense attorney.
17. Remain calm, objective, and cooperative.

DISPLAY 3-4

Code for Nurses

1. The nurse provides services with respect for human dignity and the uniqueness of the client, unrestricted by considerations of social or economic status, personal attributes, or the nature of health problems.
2. The nurse safeguards the client's right to privacy by judiciously protecting information of a confidential nature.
3. The nurse acts to safeguard the client and the public when health care and safety are affected by incompetent, unethical, or illegal practice by any person.
4. The nurse assumes responsibility and accountability for individual nursing judgments and actions.
5. The nurse maintains competence in nursing.
6. The nurse exercises informed judgment and uses individual competency and qualifications as criteria in seeking consultation, accepting responsibilities, and delegating nursing activities.
7. The nurse participates in activities that contribute to the ongoing development of the profession's body of knowledge.
8. The nurse participates in the profession's efforts to implement and improve standards of nursing.
9. The nurse participates in the profession's efforts to establish and maintain conditions of employment conducive to high-quality nursing care.
10. The nurse participates in the profession's effort to protect the public from misinformation and misrepresentation and to maintain the integrity of nursing.
11. The nurse collaborates with members of the health professions and other citizens in promoting community and national efforts to meet the health needs of the public.

Reprinted with permission from Code for Nurses With Interpretive Statements. Kansas City, American Nurses Association, 1985.

Association for Practical Nurse Education and Services, the National Federation for Licensed Practical Nurses, and the International Council of Nurses are examples of organizations that have composed codes of ethics. Display 3-4 is a current code of ethics that was revised in 1985 by the ANA. Because of rapidly changing technology, no code of ethics is ever specific enough to provide guidelines for each and every dilemma that nurses may face.

SOLVING ETHICAL DILEMMAS

An **ethical dilemma** (choice between two undesirable alternatives) occurs when individual values and laws conflict. This is especially true in relation to health care. From time to time, nurses find themselves in situations that may be considered legal but are personally unethical—or ethical but illegal. For instance, abortion is legal, but some believe it is unethical. Assisted suicide is illegal (except in Oregon), but some believe it is ethical.

Using Ethical Theories

Nurses generally use one of two ethical problem-solving theories, either teleologic or deontologic principles, to guide them in solving ethical dilemmas.

Teleology (ethical theory based on final outcomes) is also known as *utilitarianism* because the ultimate ethical test for any decision is based on what is best for the greatest number of people. Therefore, the choice that benefits many people justifies the harm that may come to a few. A teleologist would argue that selective abortion (destroying some fetuses in a multiple pregnancy) is ethically correct because it is done to ensure the full-term birth of the remaining healthy fetuses. In other words, terminating the life of a fetus is justified in some situations but may not be justified in all cases. Ethical dilemmas are analyzed on a case-by-case basis.

Deontology (ethical study based on duty or moral obligations) proposes that the outcome is not the primary issue—rather, decisions must be based on the ultimate morality of the act itself. In other words, certain actions are always right or wrong regardless of extenuating circumstances. The deontologist would argue that destroying any fetus is wrong, whether it is done to save others or not, because killing is always immoral. The deontologist believes that health care providers have a moral duty to maintain and preserve life. Therefore, it is immoral for a nurse to assist with abortion, to assist a terminally ill person with suicide, or to support the execution of a convicted prisoner.

Additional Guidelines

It may not always be possible or practical to analyze ethical issues from a teleologic or deontologic point of view. The following additional guidelines may be helpful:

- Make sure that whatever is done is in the patient's best interest.
- Preserve and support the Patient's Bill of Rights (Display 3-5).
- Work cooperatively with the patient and other health practitioners.
- Follow written policies, codes of ethics, and laws.
- Follow your conscience.

Ethics Committees

Ethical decisions are complex, especially when they affect the lives of patients. Because making a judgment for another is a weighty responsibility, ethics committees have been established in many health agencies. Ethics committees are composed of professionals and nonprofessionals who represent a broad cross-section of people within the community with varying viewpoints. Their diversity encourages healthy debate about ethics issues. Ethics committees are best used in a policy-making capacity before any specific dilemma occurs. However, ethics committees are also called on to offer advice to protect a patient's best interests and to avoid legal battles.

COMMON ETHICS ISSUES

Several ethical issues recur in nursing practice. Some common examples include telling the truth, maintaining confidential-

DISPLAY 3-5

A Patient's Bill of Rights

1. The patient has the right to considerate and respectful care.
2. The patient has the right to and is encouraged to obtain from physicians and other direct caregivers relevant, current, and understandable information concerning diagnosis, treatment, and prognosis.
3. The patient has the right to make decisions about the plan of care prior to and during the course of treatment and to refuse a recommended treatment or plan of care to the extent permitted by law and hospital policy and to be informed of the medical consequences of this action.
4. The patient has the right to have an advance directive (such as a living will, health care proxy, or durable power of attorney for health care) concerning treatment or designating a surrogate decision maker with the expectation that the hospital will honor the intent of that directive to the extent permitted by law and hospital policy.
5. The patient has the right to every consideration of privacy. Case discussion, consultation, examination, and treatment should be conducted so as to protect each patient's privacy.
6. The patient has the right to expect that all communications and records pertaining to his or her care will be treated as confidential by the hospital, except in cases such as suspected abuse and public health hazards when reporting is permitted or required by law.
7. The patient has the right to review the records pertaining to his or her medical care and to have the information explained or interpreted as necessary, except when restricted by law.
8. The patient has the right to expect that, within its capacity and policies, a hospital will make reasonable response to the request of a patient for appropriate and medically indicated care and services. The hospital must provide evaluation, service, and/or referral as indicated by the urgency of the case.
9. The patient has the right to ask and be informed of the existence of business relationships among the hospital, educational institutions, other health care providers, or payers that may influence the patient's treatment and care.
10. The patient has the right to consent to or decline to participate in proposed research studies or human experimentation affecting care and treatment or requiring direct patient involvement, and to have those studies fully explained prior to consent.
11. The patient has the right to expect reasonable continuity of care when appropriate and to be informed by physicians and other caregivers of available and realistic patient care options when hospital care is no longer appropriate.
12. The patient has the right to be informed of hospital policies and practices that relate to patient care, treatment, and responsibilities. The patient has the right to be informed of available resources for resolving disputes, grievances, and conflicts. The patient has the right to be informed of the hospital's charges for services and available payment methods.

ity, withholding or withdrawing medical treatment, advocating for the most ethical allocation of scarce resources, and protecting vulnerable individuals from unsafe practices or practitioners.

Truth Telling

Truth telling (ethical principle proposing that all patients have the right to complete and accurate information) implies that physicians and nurses have a duty to tell patients the truth about matters concerning their health. Respect for this right is demonstrated by explaining to the patient the status of his or her health problem, benefits and risks of treatment, alternative forms of treatment, and consequences if the treatment is not administered.

It is the physician's duty to inform patients. Conflict occurs when the patient has not been given full information, when the facts have been misrepresented, or when the patient misunderstands the information. In some cases, physicians are reluctant to talk honestly with patients or the proposed treatment is presented in a biased manner. Often the nurse is forced to choose between remaining silent in allegiance to the physician or providing truthful information to the patient. Either action may have frustrating consequences.

Confidentiality

Confidentiality (safeguarding an individual's personal health information from public disclosure) is the foundation for developing trust. Health information that the patient confides must not be divulged to unauthorized individuals without the patient's written permission. Even giving medical information to a patient's health insurance company requires a signed release.

Consequently, nurses must use discretion when sharing information verbally so that it is not overheard indiscriminately. Now that vast amounts of information about patients are stored on computers, the duty to protect confidentiality extends to safeguarding written and electronic data.

Withholding and Withdrawing Treatment

Technology is often used to prolong life at all costs, beyond justifying its benefits. Decisions involving life and death may in some cases continue to circumvent patients, a clear violation of ethical principles. Legislation now makes it mandatory to discuss the issue of terminal care with patients. Since the Patient Self-Determination Act was approved by Congress in 1990, health care agencies that are reimbursed through Medicare must ask patients whether they have executed an **advance directive** (written statement identifying a competent person's wishes concerning terminal care). In some cases, the advance directive may legally appoint another individual to make a proxy decision on the patient's behalf (see Chap. 38).

Advance directives are not reserved for elderly adults; they can be completed by any competent adult. They are best composed before a health crisis develops. Therefore, nurses should inform all patients about their right to self-determination, encourage them to compose an advance directive, and support the decisions they make.

Allocation of Scarce Resources

Allocation of scarce resources (process of deciding how to distribute limited life-saving equipment or procedures among several who could benefit) is a difficult decision to make. In effect, it means that those who receive the resource will live and those who do not will die prematurely. One decision-making strategy is to take a "first come, first served" approach. Another approach is to project what would produce the most good for the most people, even though forecasting the future is humanly impossible.

Whistle-Blowing

Whistle-blowing (reporting incompetent or unethical practices), as the name implies, calls attention to an unsafe or potentially harmful situation. In most circumstances, it occurs in the institution where the reporting person is employed. For instance, a nurse may report another nurse or physician who cares for patients while under the influence of alcohol or a controlled substance.

Whenever a problem is identified, the first step is to report the situation to an immediate supervisor. If the supervisor takes no action, the nurse is faced with an ethical dilemma about what further steps to take. It may become necessary to go beyond the administrative hierarchy and make public revelations.

The decision to "blow the whistle" involves personal risks and may result in grave consequences such as character assassination, retribution in the form of crimes against one's person or property, negative evaluations, demotions, or isolation. Nevertheless, the ethical priority is protecting patients in general and the community at large.

KEY CONCEPTS

- There are six types of laws: constitutional, statutory, administrative, common, criminal, and civil.
- Administrative laws give federal and state governments the legal authority to ensure the health and safety of citizens.
- Criminal laws protect the public's welfare; civil laws protect personal freedoms and rights of individuals.

- Each state's nurse practice act defines the unique role of the nurse and differentiates it from that of other health care practitioners.
- Each state's board of nursing is the regulatory agency for managing its nurse practice act.
- Two categories of criminal acts are misdemeanors, which are minor offenses, and felonies, which are more serious.
- Violations of civil laws include intentional and unintentional torts. In an intentional tort, a private citizen sues another for a deliberately aggressive act. In an unintentional tort, the lawsuit charges that harm occurred due to a person's negligence even though no harm was intended.
- Negligence lawsuits allege that a person's actions, or lack thereof, caused harm. The defendant is held to a standard expected of any other reasonable person.
- In the case of malpractice, the plaintiff alleges that a professional's actions, or lack thereof, caused harm. The defendant is held to the standard expected of others with similar knowledge and education.
- In a malpractice case, the prosecution must prove that the defendant had a duty to carry out in relation to the plaintiff, that the defendant breached that duty, that the breach of duty was the direct cause for harm, and that injury occurred.
- Liability for malpractice may be limited or reduced by the use of Good Samaritan laws, expiration of the statute of limitations, a timely and well-written incident report, or a privately composed anecdotal record.
- Ethics refers to moral or philosophical principles that classify actions as right or wrong.
- A code of ethics is a written statement that describes ideal behavior for members of a particular discipline.
- There are two ethical theories: teleology and deontology. Teleology proposes that the best ethical decision is the one that will result in benefits for the majority of individuals. Deontology proposes that the basis for an ethical decision is simply whether the action is morally right or wrong.
- Some common ethical issues that nurses encounter in everyday practice include telling the truth, protecting patients' confidentiality, ensuring that patients' wishes for withholding and withdrawing treatment are followed, advocating for the nondiscriminatory allocation of scarce resources, and reporting incompetent or unethical practices.

CRITICAL THINKING EXERCISES

- What are the legal and ethical implications of working as a nurse while under the influence of an illegal controlled substance such as morphine?
- What actions might protect a nurse from being sued when a patient assigned to his or her care falls out of bed?
- Two patients need a liver transplant. What information would you want to know to determine which patient should receive the organ?
- Take a teleologist and a deontologist viewpoint in relation to assisted suicide, withholding nourishment from an infant who is severely retarded, or using animals for drug experiments.

SUGGESTED READINGS

American Hospital Association. A patient's bill of rights. Chicago, American Hospital Association, 1992.

American Nurses Association. Code for nurses, with interpretive statements. Kansas City, MO, ANA, 1985.

Ashley RC. Avoiding malpractice—beyond the scope of employment. Journal of Nursing Law 1997;4(4):45–50.

Badzek LA, Leslie NS, Corbo-Richert B. An ethical perspective. End-of-life decisions: are they honored? Journal of Nursing Law 1998;5(2):51–63.

Cypher DP. Healthcare rationing: issues and implications. Nursing Forum 1997;32(4):25–33.

Dunlap RK. Teaching advanced directives: the why, when, and how. Journal of Gerontological Nursing 1997;23(12):11–16.

Hall JK. Speak up! Killing, not caring. RN 1997;60(6):68.

Harrington N, Smith NE, Spratt WE. LPN to RN transitions. Philadelphia, Lippincott, 1996.

Kurzen CR. Contemporary practical/vocational nursing, 3d edition. Philadelphia, Lippincott, 1997.

Martin RH. Advanced directives: legal implications for nurses. Journal of Nursing Law 1997;4(2):7–15.

McCormack P. Quality of life and the right to die: an ethical dilemma. Journal of Advanced Nursing 1998;28(1):63–69.

Nursing and Advanced Practice Nursing Act and Rules for the Administration of Nursing and Advanced Practice Nursing Act. Public Act 90-0818, 1999. Illinois Dept. of Professional Regulation. http://www:state.il.us/dpr/who/ar/NURSE.htm

O'Boyle ME. Legal and ethical issues. Home Health Care Management & Practice 1997;9(6):1–83.

Trott MC. Legal issues for nurse managers. Nursing Management 1998; 29(6):38–42.

Yeo H. Informed consent in the neonatal unit: the ethical and legal rights of parents. Journal of Neonatal Nursing 1998;4(4):17–20.

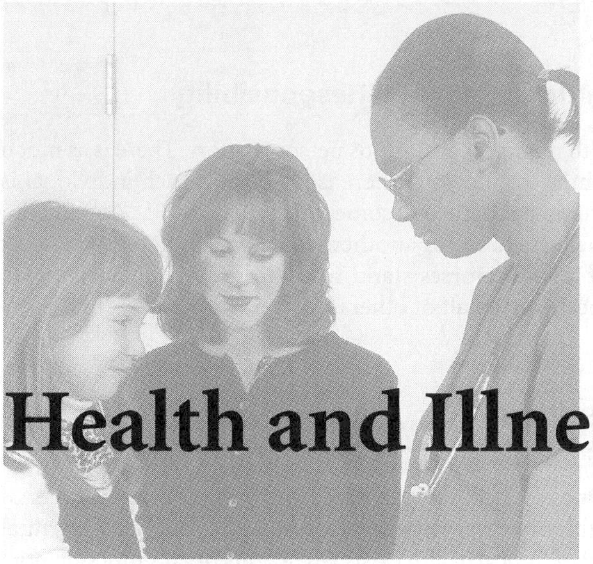

CHAPTER 4

Health and Illness

CHAPTER OUTLINE

Health
Wellness
Illness
Health Care System
National Health Goals
Nursing Team
Continuity of Health Care

KEY TERMS

acute illness
beliefs
case method
chronic illness
congenital disorder
continuity of care
exacerbation
extended care
functional nursing
health
health care system
hereditary condition
holism
human needs
idiopathic illness
illness
morbidity
mortality
nurse-managed care
nursing team
primary care
primary illness
primary nursing
remission
secondary care
secondary illness
sequelae
team nursing
terminal illness
tertiary care
values
wellness

LEARNING OBJECTIVES

An understanding of the content within this chapter will be evidenced by the student's ability to:

- Describe how the World Health Organization (WHO) defines health.
- Discuss the difference between values and beliefs.
- List three health beliefs that are common among Americans.
- Explain the concept of holism.
- Identify five levels of human needs.
- Define illness.
- Explain the meaning of terms used to describe illnesses, such as morbidity, mortality, acute, chronic, terminal, primary, secondary, remission, exacerbation, hereditary, congenital, and idiopathic.
- Differentiate between primary, secondary, tertiary, and extended care.
- Identify three national health goals targeted for the year 2000.
- Discuss five patterns for administering patient care.

Neither health nor illness is an absolute state; rather, there are fluctuations along a continuum throughout life (Fig. 4-1). Because it is impossible to be well and stay well forever, or to get well and remain well forever, nurses are committed to helping individuals prevent illness and restore or improve their health. These goals are accomplished by helping people live healthy lives, encouraging early diagnosis of disease, and implementing measures to prevent the complications of disorders that eventually develop.

Health

The World Health Organization (WHO) is globally committed to "Health for All." In the preamble to its constitution, WHO defines **health** as "a state of complete physical, mental, and social well-being, not merely the absence of disease or infirmity." However, how each person perceives and defines health varies. It is important to respect individual differences rather than impose standards that may be unrealistic for the person.

HEALTH VALUES AND BELIEFS

An individual's behaviors are outcomes of his or her values and belief system. **Values** (ideals that an individual feels

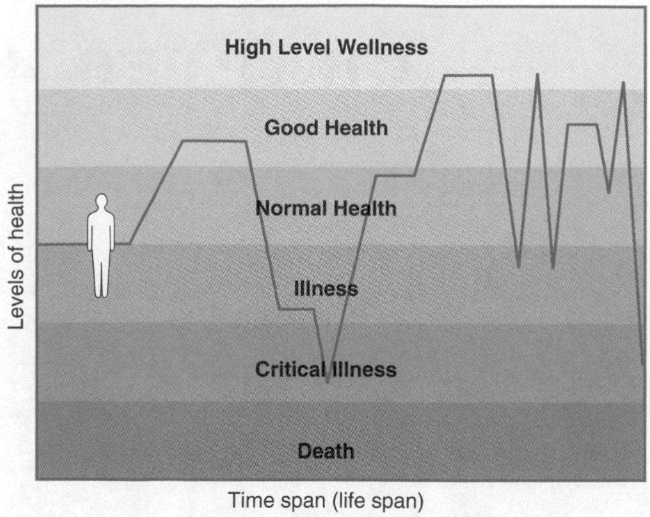

FIGURE 4–1. The health–illness continuum shows the different levels of health a person experiences over a lifetime.

are important) include knowledge, wealth, financial security, marital fidelity, and health, to name a few. **Beliefs** (concepts that individuals hold to be true), along with values, guide a person's actions. Both health values and beliefs demonstrate or affirm what is personally significant. When health is valued, actions are taken to preserve it. Most Americans believe health is a resource, a right, and a personal responsibility.

Health: A Limited Resource

A resource is a possession that is valuable because its supply is limited and there is no substitute. Given that definition, health is considered quite precious. People often say, "as long as you have your health, you have everything," and "health is wealth."

Health: A Right

The United States was established on the principle that everyone is equal and entitled to life, liberty, and the pursuit of happiness. If this premise is accepted, then it would seem that everyone, regardless of age, gender, ethnic origin, social position, or wealth, is entitled to equal services for sustaining health. Unfortunately, as will be discussed later, there are health disparities among various groups within the United States. These groups include the poor, older adults, and people with disabilities. However, efforts are underway to eliminate social barriers and to promote equal access to health care (see discussion of Healthy People 2010 later in this chapter).

If all are equally deserving of health, it follows that the nation in general and nurses in particular have a duty to protect and preserve the health of those who may be unable to assert this right for themselves.

Health: A Personal Responsibility

Health requires continuous personal effort. There is as much potential for illness as there is for health. Each individual is instrumental in the outcome. Pilch (1981) said, "No one can do wellness to or for another; you alone do it, but you don't do it alone." Nurses stand ready to provide assistance and advocate on behalf of others.

Wellness

Wellness (a full and balanced integration of all aspects of health) involves physical, emotional, social, and spiritual health. Physical health exists when body organs function normally. Emotional health results when one feels safe and copes effectively with the stressors of life. Social health is an outcome of feeling accepted and useful. Spiritual health is characterized as believing that one's life has purpose. The four components are collectively referred to as the concept of holism (Fig. 4-2).

HOLISM

Holism (the sum of physical, emotional, social, and spiritual health) determines how "whole" or well an individual feels. Any change in one component, positive or negative, automatically creates repercussions in the others. Take, for example, the person who has a heart attack. There is an obvious

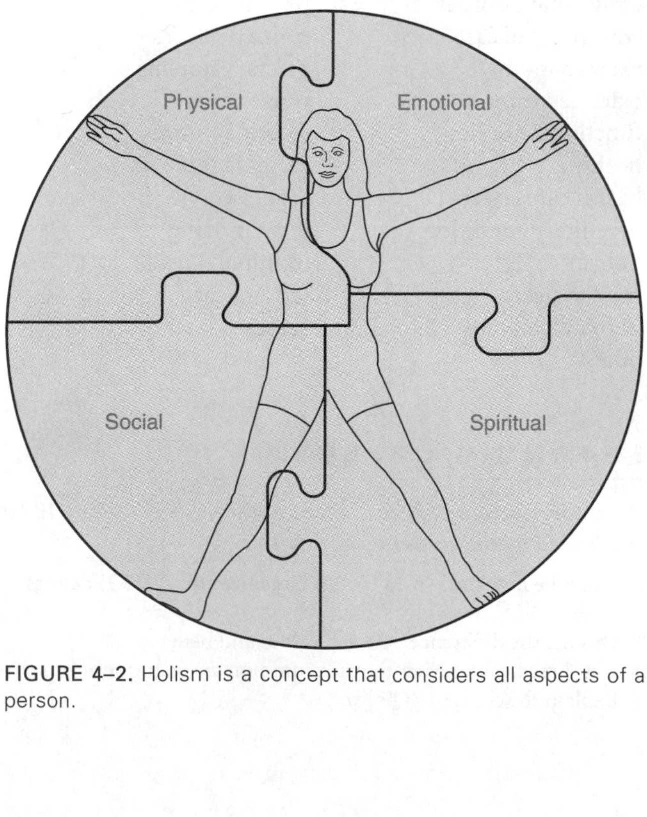

FIGURE 4–2. Holism is a concept that considers all aspects of a person.

and immediate impairment in the person's physical health. The emotional, social, and spiritual aspects of health also are affected by the psychological significance associated with the health change, the temporary or permanent alterations in social roles, and the philosophical issues that develop as the patient ponders the potential for death. Nurses, therefore, profess to be "holistic practitioners" because they are committed to restoring balance in each of the four spheres that affect health. The strategy for accomplishing this is generally based on a hierarchy of human needs.

Hierarchy of Human Needs

In the 1960s, Abraham Maslow, a psychologist, identified five levels of **human needs** (factors that motivate behavior). He grouped the needs in tiers, or a sequential hierarchy (Fig. 4-3), according to their significance: physiologic (first level), safety and security (second level), love and belonging (third level), esteem and self-esteem (fourth level), and self-actualization (fifth level).

The first-level physiologic needs are the most important. They are the activities, such as breathing and eating, that are necessary for sustaining life. Each higher level is less important to survival than the levels previous to it. Maslow believed that until physiologic needs are satisfied, humans could not or would not seek to fulfill other needs. However, by progressively satisfying needs at each subsequent level, individuals will realize their maximum potential for health and well-being. Nurses have adopted Maslow's hierarchy as a tool for setting priorities for patient care.

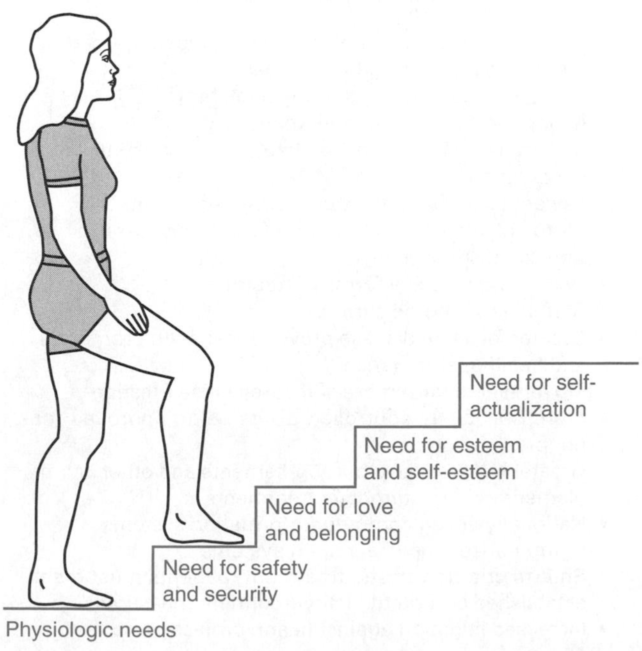

FIGURE 4–3. Maslow's hierarchy of human needs.

Illness

Illness (a state of discomfort) results when a person's health becomes impaired through disease, deterioration, or injury. Several terms—morbidity and mortality; acute, chronic, and terminal; primary and secondary; remission and exacerbation; hereditary, congenital, and idiopathic–are used when referring to illnesses.

MORBIDITY AND MORTALITY

Morbidity (incidence of a specific disease, disorder, or injury) refers to the rate or numbers of people affected. Federal statistics are compiled on the basis of age, gender, or per 1,000 people within the population. **Mortality** (incidence of deaths) denotes the number who died of a particular disease or condition. Table 4-1 lists the 10 leading causes of death among all Americans of all ages in 1997.

ACUTE, CHRONIC, AND TERMINAL ILLNESSES

An **acute illness** (one that comes on suddenly and lasts a short time) is one method for classifying a change in health. Influenza is an example of an acute illness. Many acute illnesses are cured. However, some lead to long-term problems due to their **sequelae** (singular: sequela; ill effects that result from permanent or progressive organ damage caused by a disease or its treatment).

Chronic illness (one that comes on slowly and lasts a long time) increases as individuals age. Arthritis, a joint disease, is an example of a chronic disease. Many older adults are living

TABLE 4–1. **U.S. Mortality Statistics, 1997**

Rank	Cause of Death	Number
1	Heart disease	2,322,421
2	Cancer	733,834
3	Cerebrovascular disease	544,278
4	Chronic lung disease	106,431
5	Accidents	93,874
	Motor vehicle (43,449)	
	All other (50,425)	
6	Pneumonia and influenza	82,579
7	Diabetes	61,559
8	AIDS	32,655
9	Suicide	30,862
10	Chronic liver disease	25,135

Reported in Monthly Vital Statistics Report, Vol. 46, No. 1, supp. 2, p. 32–33. Hyattsville, MD, National Center for Health Statistics, 1997.

with persistent health problems and disabilities because they survived acute illnesses that killed others years ago.

A **terminal illness** (one in which there is no potential for cure) is one that eventually is fatal. The terminal stage of an illness is one in which a person is approaching death.

PRIMARY AND SECONDARY ILLNESSES

A **primary illness** (one that develops independently of any other disease) is different than a **secondary illness** (disorder that develops from a pre-existing condition). For example, a pulmonary disease acquired from smoking is a primary illness. If pneumonia or heart failure occurs as a consequence of smoke-damaged lung tissue, it is considered a secondary problem. In essence, the primary condition predisposed the smoker, in this case, to the secondary condition.

REMISSION AND EXACERBATION

A **remission** (disappearance of signs and symptoms associated with a particular disease) is yet another term used in relation to illnesses. Although a remission resembles a cured state, the relief may be only temporary. The duration of a remission is unpredictable. An **exacerbation** (reactivation of a disorder, or one that reverts from a chronic to an acute state) can occur periodically in patients with long-standing diseases. Often, remissions and exacerbations are related to how well or poorly the immune system is functioning, the stressors the patient is facing, and the patient's overall health status (nutrition, sleep, hydration, and so on).

HEREDITARY, CONGENITAL, AND IDIOPATHIC ILLNESSES

A **hereditary condition** (disorder acquired from the genetic codes of one or both parents) may or may not produce symptoms immediately after birth. Cystic fibrosis, a lung disease, and Huntington's chorea, a neurologic disorder, are examples of inherited illnesses. The first is diagnosed soon after birth; the second is not manifested until adulthood.

Congenital disorders (those present at birth but which are the result of faulty embryonic development) cannot be genetically predicted. Maternal illness, such as rubella (German measles) or exposure to toxic chemicals or drugs, especially during the first 3 months of pregnancy, often predisposes the fetus to congenital disorders. Several decades ago, many pregnant women took the drug thalidomide and subsequently gave birth to infants with missing arms and legs. There is a great deal of concern about the role of alcohol in producing fetal alcohol syndrome, a permanent but preventable form of retardation, and the effects of exposure to other environmental toxins. Although the etiologies for some congenital disorders are well established, congenital disorders can occur randomly.

Treatment of an **idiopathic illness** (one whose cause is unexplained) focuses on relieving the signs and symptoms, because the etiology is unknown.

Health Care System

The **health care system** (network of available health services) involves agencies and institutions where individuals seek treatment for a health problem or assistance with maintaining or promoting their health.

The health care system, patients, and their diseases have drastically changed during the past 25 years (Display 4-1). Advances in technology and discoveries in science have created more elaborate methods of diagnosing and treating diseases, creating a need for more specialized care. What was once a system in which individuals would seek medical advice and treatment from one physician, clinic, or hospital has developed into a complex system for health care.

DISPLAY 4–1

Trends in Health and Health Care

- Increased older adult population
- Greater ethnically diverse groups
- More chronic, but preventable, illnesses
- Growing numbers of older adults with cognitive disorders such as Alzheimer's disease
- Higher incidence of drug-resistant infections
- Decreased incidence of and death rates from HIV infection with increased life expectancy associated with expensive drug therapy
- Expanding application of genetic engineering (treating diseases by altering genetic codes)
- Greater success in organ transplantation
- Major efforts at cost containment
- Continued rising costs of health care despite cost-containment measures
- Fewer insured and more underinsured citizens
- More outpatient or ambulatory (1-day stay) care
- Shorter hospital stays
- Use of less invasive forms of treatment
- Shift to more home care
- Greater focus on disease prevention, health promotion, and health maintenance
- Movement toward more self-care and self-testing
- More previously controlled drugs being approved for nonprescription use
- Greater interest in herbal supplements and other "complementary" or alternative treatments
- Nationally linked computer information systems
- Computerized medical record systems
- Shift to criterion-based treatment (patients must meet established criteria to justify treatment measures)
- Increased litigation against health professionals

HEALTH CARE SERVICES

Types of health care vary according to the needs of the patient. Patients may seek or be referred to resources that provide primary, secondary, tertiary, or extended care.

Primary Care

Primary care (health services provided by the first health care professional or agency an individual contacts) is usually provided by a family practice physician, nurse practitioner, or physician's assistant in an office or clinic. Cost-conscious health care reforms are likely to lead to the provision of primary care by advanced practice nurses.

Secondary Care

An example of **secondary care** (health services to which primary care givers refer patients for consultation and additional testing) is the referral of a patient to a cardiac catheterization laboratory.

Tertiary Care

Tertiary care (health services provided at hospitals or medical centers where complex technology and specialists are available) may require the patient to travel some distance from home. There is a growing trend to provide as many secondary and tertiary care services as possible on an outpatient basis or to require no more than 24 hours of inpatient care.

Extended Care

Extended care (services that meet the health needs of patients who no longer require acute hospital care) includes rehabilitation, skilled nursing care in a person's home or a nursing home, and hospice care for dying patients. Extended care is an important component of the health care system because it allows earlier discharge from secondary and tertiary care agencies and reduces the overall expense of health care.

National Health Goals

A national health-promotion effort during the past 20 years has identified goals and strategies for improving the nation's health by preventing major chronic illnesses, injuries, and infectious diseases by the year 2000 (Display 4-2). The campaign has been carried out with the combined expertise of the Public Health Service, each state's health department, national health organizations, the Institute of Medicine of the National Academy of Sciences, and selected individuals from the public at large. To meet these goals, health care workers are challenged to implement strategies to improve the overall health of individuals living in the United States.

In a midway review, some progress was noted (U.S. Department of Health and Human Services, 1997):

- A dramatic decline in the death rate from AIDS, from the leading cause of death among people age 25 to 44 to the second-leading cause of death in that age group. The reduction may be due in part to better combinations in drug therapy.
- A drop in the teenage birth rate by 12% since 1991
- Lower infant mortality rates, although death rates for African-American infants continue to be higher than those for whites (14.2 per 1,000 live births compared with 6.0 per 1,000 live births)
- Increased numbers of pregnant women receiving prenatal care: 82% received initial care in the first trimester
- Fewer suicides (4%) and homicides (11%) in 1996
- Life expectancy up from 75.8 years to 76.1 years

DISPLAY 4-2

National Health Promotion and Disease Prevention Objectives

Goals

- Increase the span of healthy life for Americans
- Reduce health care disparities among Americans
- Achieve access to preventive services for all Americans

Strategies

- Increase physical activity and fitness
- Improve nutrition
- Reduce tobacco, alcohol, and drug use
- Improve family planning
- Improve mental health and prevent mental disorders
- Reduce violent and abusive behavior
- Enhance educational and community-based programs
- Reduce unintentional injuries
- Improve occupational safety and health
- Improve environmental health
- Ensure food and drug safety
- Improve oral health
- Improve maternal and infant health
- Reduce heart disease and stroke
- Prevent and control cancer
- Reduce diabetes and chronic disabling conditions
- Prevent and control HIV (human immunodeficiency virus) infections
- Reduce sexually transmitted diseases
- Increase immunizations and prevent infectious diseases
- Expand access and use of clinical preventive services
- Improve surveillance and data systems.

Healthy People 2000, U.S. Department of Health and Human Services, 1990

Because of these preliminary successes in health promotion and disease prevention, new objectives and strategies have been defined for *Healthy People 2010.* Although the work is ongoing, preliminary goals and focus areas have been suggested (Fig. 4-4). The final framework will probably continue the emphasis on improving the quality of life, not just increasing life expectancy, with additional emphasis on community preventive services to reduce disparities in disadvantaged target populations.

Nursing Team

The goal of the **nursing team** (personnel who care for patients directly) is to help patients attain, maintain, or regain health (Fig. 4-5). The team may include several types of professionals as well as allied health care workers with special training, such as respiratory therapists, physical therapists, and technicians.

Nurses use their unique skills in the hospital as well as other employment areas. Because nurses have skills that assist the healthy, the dying, and all those in between, they work in a variety of settings, such as health maintenance organizations, physical fitness centers, diet clinics, public health departments, home health agencies, and hospices. Wherever nursing personnel work together, one of several patterns for managing patient care is used.

MANAGEMENT PATTERNS

There are five common management patterns: functional nursing, case method, team nursing, primary nursing, and nurse-managed care. Each has advantages and disadvantages. Students are likely to encounter one or all of these methods in their clinical experience.

Functional Nursing

One method used when providing patient care is **functional nursing** (pattern in which each nurse on a patient unit is assigned specific tasks). For example, one is assigned to give all the medications, another performs all the treatments (such as dressing changes), and another works at the desk transcribing physicians' orders and communicating with other nursing departments about patient care issues. This pattern is being used less often because its focus tends to be more on completing the task rather than caring for individual patients.

Case Method

The **case method** (pattern in which one nurse manages all the care a patient needs for a designated period of time) should not be confused with managed care, which is discussed later. The case method is most often used in home health and public health nursing.

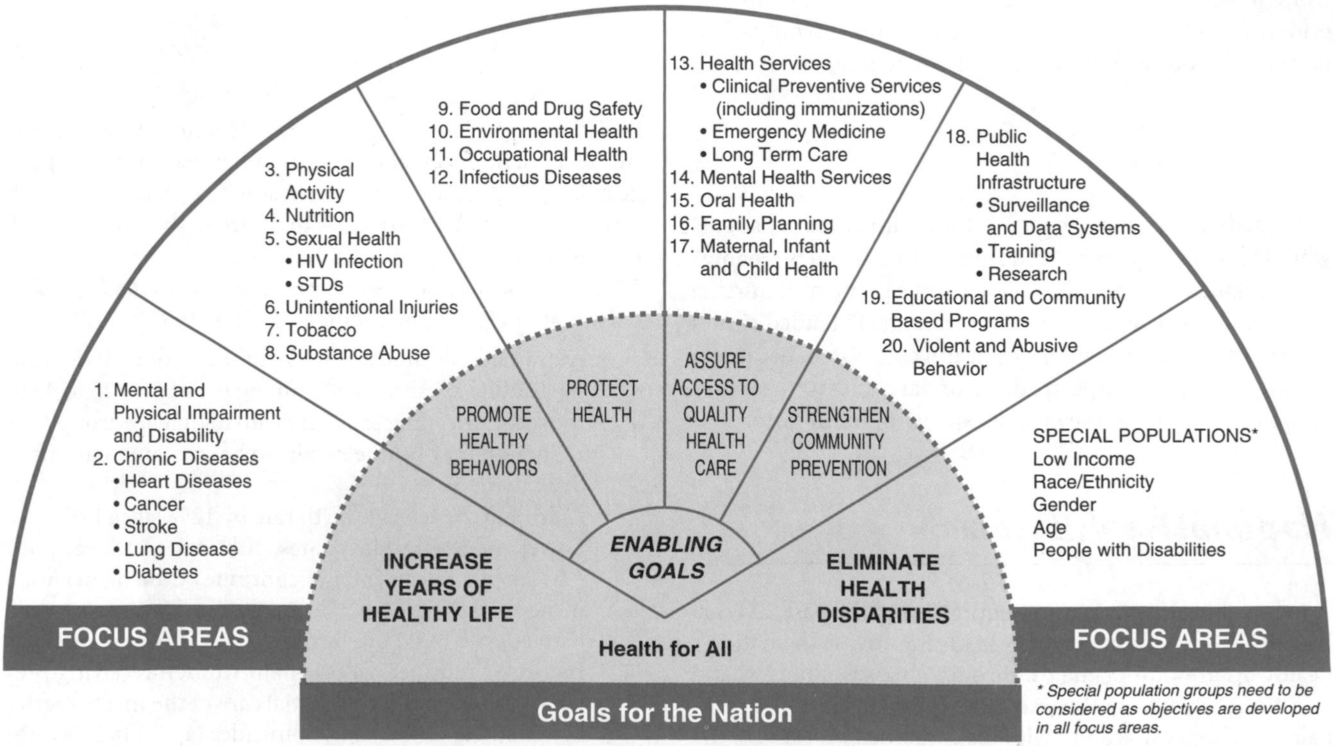
1. Mental and Physical Impairment and Disability
2. Chronic Diseases
• Heart Diseases
• Cancer
• Stroke
• Lung Disease
• Diabetes
3. Physical Activity
4. Nutrition
5. Sexual Health
• HIV Infection
• STDs
6. Unintentional Injuries
7. Tobacco
8. Substance Abuse
9. Food and Drug Safety
10. Environmental Health
11. Occupational Health
12. Infectious Diseases
13. Health Services
• Clinical Preventive Services (including immunizations)
• Emergency Medicine
• Long Term Care
14. Mental Health Services
15. Oral Health
16. Family Planning
17. Maternal, Infant and Child Health
18. Public Health Infrastructure
• Surveillance and Data Systems
• Training
• Research
19. Educational and Community Based Programs
20. Violent and Abusive Behavior
SPECIAL POPULATIONS*
Low Income
Race/Ethnicity
Gender
Age
People with Disabilities
PROMOTE HEALTHY BEHAVIORS
PROTECT HEALTH
ASSURE ACCESS TO QUALITY HEALTH CARE
STRENGTHEN COMMUNITY PREVENTION
ENABLING GOALS
INCREASE YEARS OF HEALTHY LIFE
ELIMINATE HEALTH DISPARITIES
Health for All
FOCUS AREAS
FOCUS AREAS
Goals for the Nation
* Special population groups need to be considered as objectives are developed in all focus areas.

FIGURE 4–4. Components of proposed *Healthy People 2010.*

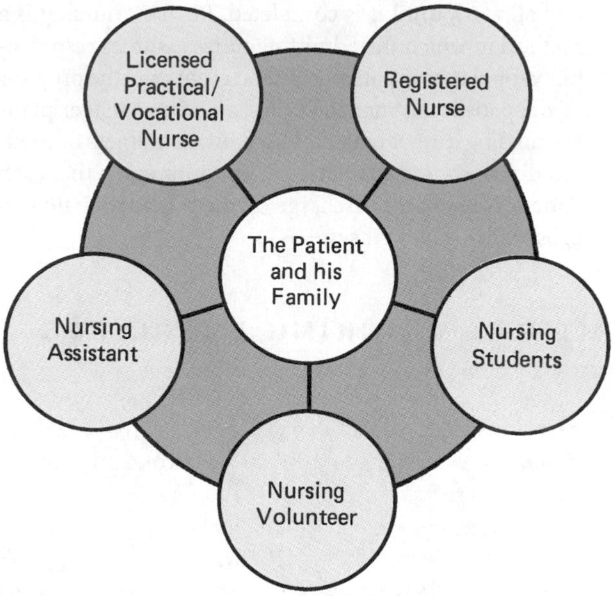

FIGURE 4–5. The nursing team.

Team Nursing

Team nursing (pattern in which nursing personnel divide the patients into groups and complete their care together) is organized and directed by a nurse called the team leader. The leader may assist with but usually supervises the care that other team members provide. All team members report the outcomes of their care to the team leader. The team leader is responsible for evaluating whether the goals of patient care are met.

Conferences are an important part of team nursing. They may cover a variety of subjects but are planned with certain goals in mind, such as determining the best approaches to each patient's health problems, increasing the team members' knowledge, and promoting a cooperative spirit among nursing personnel.

Primary Nursing

In **primary nursing** (pattern in which the admitting nurse assumes responsibility for planning patient care and evaluating the progress of the patient), the primary nurse may delegate the patient's care to someone else in his or her absence but is consulted when new problems develop or the plan of care requires modifications. The primary nurse remains responsible and accountable for specific patients until they are discharged.

Nurse-Managed Care

A new type of nursing-care delivery system is being implemented in several areas of the United States. It is called **nurse-managed care** (pattern in which a nurse manager plans the nursing care of patients based on their type of case or medical diagnosis) by some and case management by others. A clinical pathway typically is used in a managed care approach (see Chap. 1 for more information on managed care and an example of a clinical pathway).

This innovative system was developed in response to several problems affecting health care delivery today, such as the nursing shortage and the need to balance the costs of medical care with limited reimbursement systems. Nurse-managed care is similar to the principles used by successful businesses. In the business world, corporations pay executives to forecast trends and determine the best strategies for making profits. In nurse-managed care, a professional nurse acts as a case manager who evaluates whether predictable outcomes are met on a daily basis. By meeting the outcomes in a timely manner, the patient is ready for discharge by the time designated by prospective payment systems, if not before.

Pilot studies indicate that this approach ensures that standards of care are met with greater efficiency and cost savings. Hospitals who are adopting case-managed care report that they are operating within their budgets and decreasing their financial losses.

Continuity of Health Care

Continuity of care (maintenance of health care from one level of health to another and from one agency to another) ensures that the patient navigates the complicated health care system with a maximum of efficiency and a minimum of frustration. The goal is to avoid causing a patient, whether healthy or ill, to feel isolated, fragmented, or abandoned. All too often this occurs when one health practitioner fails to consult or communicate with others involved in the patient's care. Chapters 9 and 10 give examples of how nurses communicate among themselves and with personnel in other institutions to ensure that patient care is both continuous and goal-directed.

KEY CONCEPTS

- The World Health Organization (WHO) defines health as "a state of complete physical, mental, and social well-being and not merely the absence of disease or infirmity."
- Values are the ideals that an individual believes are honorable attributes. Beliefs are concepts that individuals hold to be true.
- Most Americans believe that health is a resource, a right, and a personal responsibility.
- How "whole" or well a person feels is the sum of his or her physical, emotional, social, and spiritual health, a concept referred to as holism. Any change in one component, positive or negative, automatically creates repercussions in the others.

- There are five levels of human needs: physiologic (first level), safety and security (second level), love and belonging (third level), esteem and self-esteem (fourth level), and self-actualization (fifth level). By satisfying needs at each subsequent level, individuals can realize their maximum potential for health and well-being.
- Illness is a state of discomfort that results when a person's health becomes impaired through disease, stress, or an accident or injury.
- Morbidity refers to the incidence of a specific disease, disorder, or injury. Mortality refers to the death rate from a specific condition.
- An acute illness is one that comes on suddenly and lasts a short time. A chronic illness is one that comes on slowly and lasts a long time. A terminal illness is one in which there is no potential for cure.
- A primary illness is one that developed independently of another disease. Any subsequent disorder that develops from a pre-existing condition is referred to as a secondary illness.
- Remission refers to the disappearance of the signs and symptoms associated with a particular disease. An exacerbation refers to the time when the disorder becomes reactivated or reverts from a chronic to an acute state.
- A hereditary condition is one acquired from the genetic codes of one or both parents. Congenital disorders are those that are present at birth but result from faulty embryonic development. An idiopathic illness whose cause is unexplained.
- Primary care refers to the services provided by the first health care professional or agency an individual contacts. Secondary care pertains to the services to which primary care givers refer patients for consultation and additional testing, such as a cardiac catheterization laboratory. Tertiary care takes place in a hospital where complex technology and specialists are available. Extended care involves meeting the health needs of patients who no longer require hospital care but who continue to need health services.
- Three national health goals have been set for the year 2000: to increase the span of healthy life for Americans, to reduce health care disparities among Americans, and to achieve access to preventive health services for all Americans. Because of positive outcomes, a second plan, known as *Healthy People 2010,* will be implemented.
- One of several patterns may be used when providing nursing care for patients. In functional nursing, each nurse on a unit is assigned specific tasks. The case method involves assigning one nurse to administer all the care a patient needs for a designated period of time. In team nursing, many nursing personnel divide the patient care, and all work until it is completed. Primary nursing is a method in which the admitting nurse assumes responsibility for planning patient care and evaluating the progress of the patient. In managed care, a nurse manager plans the nursing care of patients based on their illness or medical diagnosis and evaluates patient progress so that each patient is ready for discharge by the time designated by prospective payment systems.

CRITICAL THINKING EXERCISES

- A friend complains she has been having frequent bouts of indigestion. Explain how primary, secondary, and tertiary care might be involved in this person's care.
- If you were asked to participate in planning the goals and strategies for *Healthy People 2010,* what suggestions would you make to promote health and reduce chronic illness?
- Which pattern for managing patient care seems to be most advantageous for nurses? Which pattern might patients prefer? Give reasons for your selections.

SUGGESTED READINGS

Anderson KH, Valentine K. Establishing and sustaining a family nursing center for families with chronic illness: the Wisconsin experience. Journal of Family Nursing 1998;4(2):127–141.

Burtt K. Issues update. Nurses step to the forefront of elder care. American Journal of Nursing 1998;98(7):64–66.

Girvin J. Pointers to the future ... primary health care team. Nursing Management 1998;4(9):8–9.

Lambert S, Newton M, deMeneses M. Barriers to mammography in older low-income African American Women. Journal of Multicultural Nursing and Health 1998;4(2):6–19.

Maltby HJ, Robinson S. The role of baccalaureate nursing students in the matrix of health promotion. Journal of Community Health 1998;15(3):135–142.

Muscari ME. Adolescent health. Coping with chronic illness. American Journal of Nursing 1998;98(9):20–22.

National Center for Health Statistics. Monthly Vital Statistics Report, 46(1), Supp. 2, 32–33. Hyattsville, MD, U.S. Dept. of Health & Human Services, Centers for Disease Control & Prevention, 1997.

Office of Disease Prevention & Health Promotion. Healthy People Progress Reviews. Washington DC: Department of Health & Human Services, Public Health Service, 1997.

Pilch JJ. Your invitation to full life. Minneapolis, Winston Press, 1981.

Rubenstein LZ, Nahas R. Primary and secondary prevention strategies in the older adult. Geriatric Nursing 1998;19(1):11–28.

Rydholm L. Patient-focused care in parish nursing. Holistic Nursing Practice 1997;11(3):47–60.

Taylor P, Ferszt G. The nurse as patient advocate. Nursing 1998;28(8):70–71.

U.S. Department of Health and Human Services. Healthy People 2000: National health promotion and disease prevention objectives. Boston: Jones and Bartlett, 1992.

CHAPTER 5

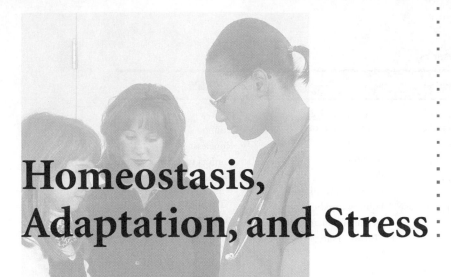

Homeostasis, Adaptation, and Stress

CHAPTER OUTLINE

Homeostasis
Physiologic Adaptation
Stress
Psychological Adaptation
Nursing Implications

KEY TERMS

adaptation
coping mechanisms
coping strategies
feedback loop
general adaptation syndrome
holism
homeostasis
neurotransmitters
stress
stressors

LEARNING OBJECTIVES

An understanding of the content within this chapter will be evidenced by the student's ability to:

- Explain homeostasis.
- List four categories stressors that affect homeostasis.
- Identify two beliefs that are based on the philosophic concept of holism.
- Explain the purpose underlying adaptation and identify two possible outcomes of unsuccessful adaptation.
- Trace the structures through which adaptive changes take place.
- Differentiate between sympathetic and parasympathetic adaptive responses.
- Define stress.
- List 10 factors that affect the stress response.
- Discuss the three stages of the general adaptation syndrome and the consequences that result.
- Name three levels of prevention that apply to the reduction or management of stress-related disorders.
- Explain how psychological adaptation occurs and give two possible outcomes that may result.
- List eight nursing activities that are helpful in the care of stress-prone patients.
- List four approaches for preventing, reducing, or eliminating a stress response.

Health is a tenuous state. To sustain it, the body continuously adapts to **stressors** (changes that have the potential for disturbing equilibrium). As long as the stressors are minor, the response is negligible and generally unnoticed. However, when a stressor is intense or when multiple stressors occur at the same time, the effort to restore balance may result in uncomfortable signs and symptoms many call "stress." If stress is prolonged, stress-related disorders and even death may occur. This chapter explores the nature of homeostasis, adaptive mechanisms for homeostatic regulation, the effect of stress, and nursing interventions that promote and restore health.

Homeostasis

Homeostasis (relatively stable state of physiologic equilibrium) literally means "staying the same." Although it sounds contradictory, staying the same requires constant physiologic activity. Constancy is maintained by making adjustments and readjustments in response to changes in the internal and external environment that foster disequilibrium.

HOLISM

Although homeostasis tends to be primarily associated with a person's physical status, it is also affected by emotional, social, and spiritual components. **Holism** (philosophic concept of interrelatedness) implies that multiple entities contribute to the *whole* of a person (see Chap. 4). Based on the principles of holism, stressors may be physiologic, psychological, social, or spiritual (Table 5-1).

TABLE 5–1. **Common Stressors**

Physiologic	Psychological	Social	Spiritual
Prematurity	Fear	Gender, racial, age discrimination	Guilt
Aging	Powerlessness	Isolation	Doubt
Injury	Jealousy	Abandonment	Hopelessness
Infection	Rivalry	Poverty	Conflict in values
Malnutrition	Bitterness	Conflict in relationships	Pressure to join, abandon, or change religions
Obesity	Hatred	Political instability	Religious discrimination
Surgery	Insecurity	Denial of human rights	
Pain		Threats to safety	
Fever		Illiteracy	
Fatigue		Infertility	
Pollution			

Holism leads to two commonly held beliefs: humans are directly influenced by both the mind and body, and the relationship between the mind and body has a potential for sustaining health as well as causing illness. Consequently, it is helpful to understand how the mind perceives information and makes adaptive responses.

Physiologic Adaptation

Adaptation (the manner in which an organism responds to change) requires the use of self-protective properties and mechanisms for regulating homeostasis. With physiologic adaptation, cells, tissues, and entire body systems become involved. The orchestration of homeostatic adaptive responses is mediated through neurotransmitters, which convey messages to coordinate the functions of the central nervous system, autonomic nervous system, and endocrine system.

CENTRAL NERVOUS SYSTEM

The central nervous system is composed of the brain and spinal cord. The brain is divided into the cortex and the structures that make up the subcortex (Fig. 5-1).

Cortex

The cortex is considered the higher functioning portion of the brain, allowing individuals to think abstractly, use and understand language, accumulate and store memories, and

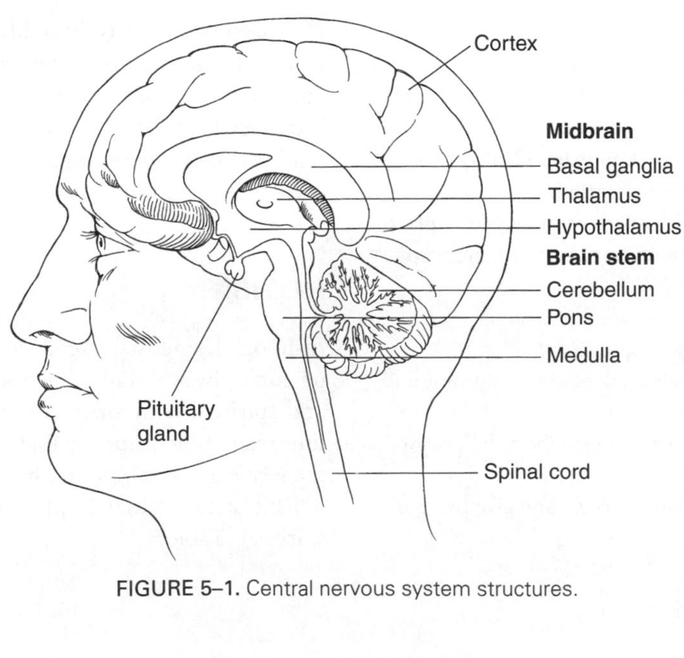

FIGURE 5–1. Central nervous system structures.

make decisions about the information it receives. The cortex also influences other primitive areas of the brain located in the subcortex.

Subcortex

The subcortex consists of the structures in the midbrain and brain stem. The midbrain, which lies between the cortex and the brain stem, includes the basal ganglia, thalamus, and hypothalamus. The brain stem, so named because it resembles a stalk, contains the cerebellum, medulla, and pons.

The subcortical structures are primarily responsible for regulating and maintaining physiologic activities that promote survival. These include the regulation of breathing, heart contraction, blood pressure, body temperature, sleeping, appetite, and a variety of other organ functions, including the stimulation and inhibition of hormone production.

Reticular Activating System (RAS)

The RAS, an area of the brain through which a network of nerves passes, is the communication link between the body and the mind. Information about a person's internal and external environment is funneled through the RAS to the cortex on both a conscious and an unconscious level (Fig. 5-2). The cortex processes the information and generates behavioral and physiologic responses through activation of the hypothalamus. The hypothalamus influences the autonomic nervous system and endocrine functions (Fig. 5-3).

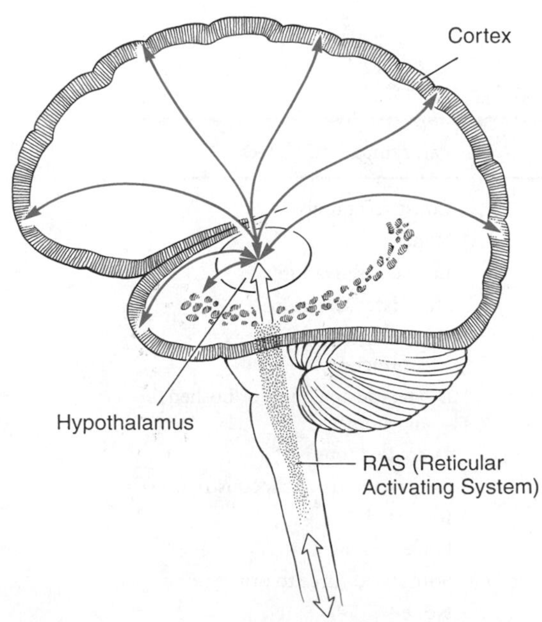

FIGURE 5–2. The reticular activating system is the link in the mind-body connection.

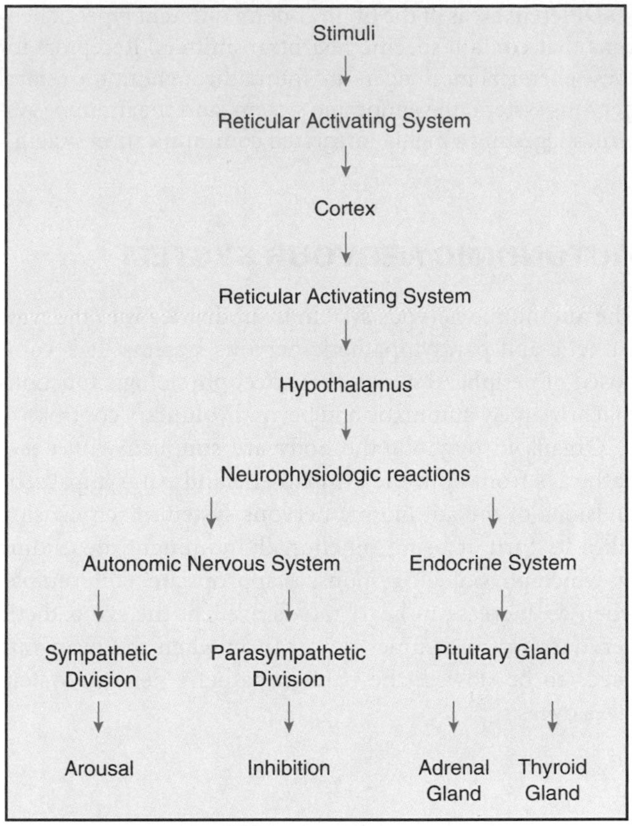

FIGURE 5–3. Homeostatic adaptive pathways.

NEUROTRANSMITTERS

Neurotransmitters (chemical messengers synthesized in the neurons) allow communication between neurons across the synaptic cleft, subsequently affecting thinking, behavior, and body function. When released, neurotransmitters temporarily bind to receptor sites on the postsynaptic neuron and transmit their information. Once this is accomplished, the neurotransmitter is broken down, recaptured for later use, or weakened.

Common neurotransmitters include serotonin, dopamine, norepinephrine, acetylcholine, and gamma-aminobutyric acid. Other chemical messengers, called neuropeptides, are actually a separate type of neurotransmitter. Neuropeptides include substance P, endorphins, enkephalins, and neurohormones.

Each neurotransmitter and neuropeptide exerts different effects. For example, serotonin stabilizes mood, induces sleep, and regulates temperature. Norepinephrine heightens arousal and raises energy level. Acetylcholine prepares the person for action and together with dopamine promotes movement. Gamma-aminobutyric acid inhibits the excitatory neurotransmitters, such as norepinephrine and dopamine. Substance P transmits the pain sensation, whereas endorphins and enkephalins interrupt the transmission of substance P and promote a sense of well-being.

Different areas of the brain contain different types of neurons that contain specific neurotransmitters. Receptors for these chemical messengers are found throughout the central nervous system, the endocrine system, and the immune system, suggesting a highly integrated communication system.

AUTONOMIC NERVOUS SYSTEM

The autonomic nervous system is subdivided into the sympathetic and parasympathetic nervous systems. It is composed of peripheral nerves that affect physiologic functions that are largely automatic and beyond voluntary control.

Organs throughout the body are supplied with nerve pathways from both the sympathetic and parasympathetic divisions of the autonomic nervous system. Each division takes its turn at being functionally dominant, depending on which physiologic response is appropriate. For example, when an increase in heart rate is needed, the sympathetic nervous system assumes dominance; when the heart rate needs to be slowed, the parasympathetic nervous system takes over.

Sympathetic Nervous System

When confronted with a situation that the mind perceives to be dangerous, the sympathetic nervous system prepares the body for fight or flight. It accelerates the physiologic functions that ensure survival through strength or a rapid escape. The individual becomes active, aroused, and emotionally charged.

Parasympathetic Nervous System

The parasympathetic nervous system tends to restore equilibrium after the danger is no longer apparent. It does so by inhibiting the physiologic stimulation created by its counterpart, the sympathetic nervous system. However, the parasympathetic nervous system does not produce an opposite reaction for every sympathetic effect (Table 5-2). This has led some to believe that the parasympathetic nervous system offers an alternate but equally effective mechanism for responding to threats from the internal or external environment.

For example, physiologic deceleration, produced by the parasympathetic nervous system, has been likened to the manner in which opossums and other animals "play dead" when they sense they are being stalked by predators. Simulating the appearance of death often causes the predator to leave the animal alone, thus saving its life. Therefore, it has been proposed that humans, too, may respond to stimuli they perceive as threatening by slowing their physiologic responses as well as by speeding them up (Nuernberger, 1981).

Thus, the autonomic nervous system provides the initial and immediate response to a perceived threat through either sympathetic or parasympathetic pathways. To sustain the response, the endocrine system becomes involved.

ENDOCRINE SYSTEM

The endocrine system is a group of glands, located throughout the body, that produce hormones (Fig. 5-4). Hormones are chemicals that are manufactured in one part of the body but whose actions have physiologic effects on target cells located elsewhere.

TABLE 5–2. **Sympathetic and Parasympathetic Effects**

Target Structure	Sympathetic Effect	Parasympathetic Effect
Iris of the eye	Dilates pupils	Constricts pupils
Sweat glands	Increases perspiration	None
Salivary glands	Inhibits salivation	Increases salivation
Digestive glands	Inhibits secretions	Stimulates secretions
Heart	Increases rate and force of contraction	Decreases rate and force of contraction
Blood vessels in skin	Constrict, causing pale appearance	Dilate, causing blush or flushed appearance
Skeletal muscles	Increased tone	Decreased tone
Bronchial muscles	Relaxed (bronchodilation)	Contracted (bronchoconstriction)
Digestive motility (peristalsis)	Decreased	Increased
Kidney	Decreased filtration	None
Bladder muscle (detrusor)	Inhibited (suppressed urination)	Stimulated (urge to urinate)
Liver	Release of glucose	None
Adrenal medulla	Stimulated	None

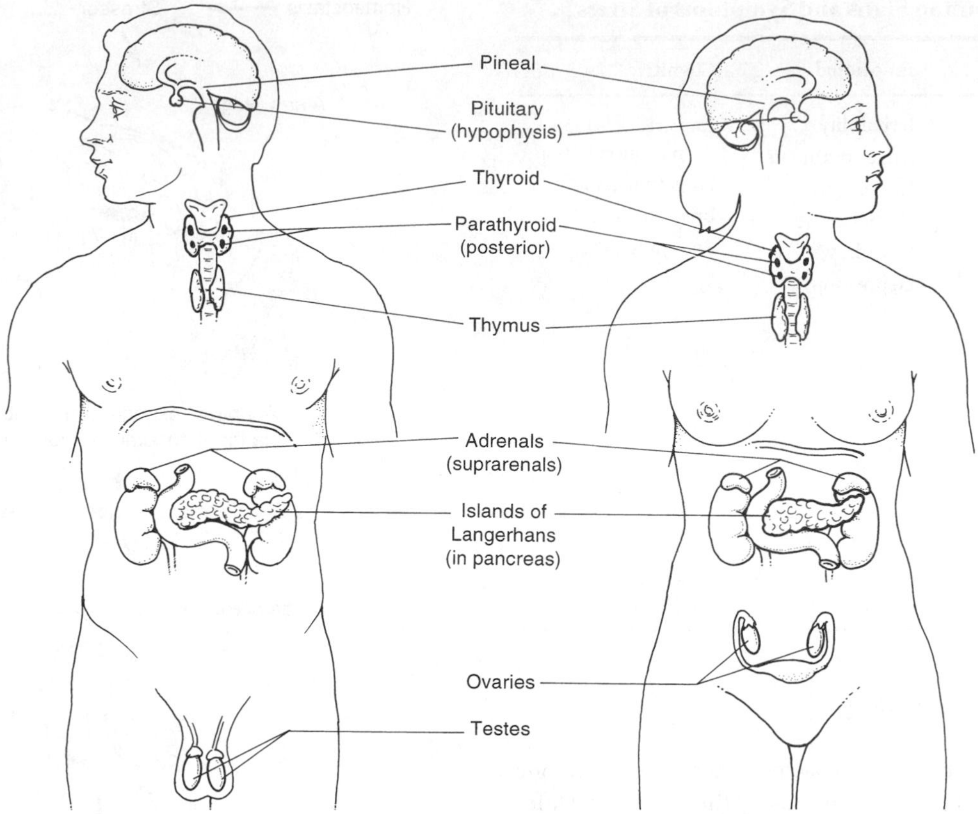

FIGURE 5–4. Endocrine glands. (Timby BK, Scherer JC, Smith NE: Introductory Medical-Surgical Nursing. 7th ed, p. 792. Philadelphia: Lippincott Williams and Wilkins, 1999.)

Neuroendocrine Control

The pituitary gland, located in the brain, is considered the master gland, producing hormones that influence other endocrine glands. The pituitary gland is connected to the hypothalamus, a subcortical structure, through both vascular connections and nerve endings. For pituitary function to occur, the cortex first stimulates the hypothalamus, which then activates the pituitary gland.

Feedback Loop

Hormone levels are controlled by a **feedback loop** (mechanism by which hormone production is turned off and on; Fig. 5-5). Feedback can be negative or positive. Most hormones are secreted in response to negative feedback; when levels decrease, the releasing gland is stimulated. In positive feedback the opposite occurs, keeping concentrations of hormones within a stable range at all times. Homeostasis is maintained when hormones are released as they are needed or inhibited when an adequate amount is present.

As long as the demands on the central nervous system, autonomic nervous system, and endocrine system are within the body's adaptive capacity, homeostasis is maintained. However, when the internal or external changes overwhelm homeostatic adaptation, stress results.

Stress

Stress (physiologic and behavioral reactions that occur in response to disequilibrium) results in physical, emotional, and cognitive changes (Table 5-3).

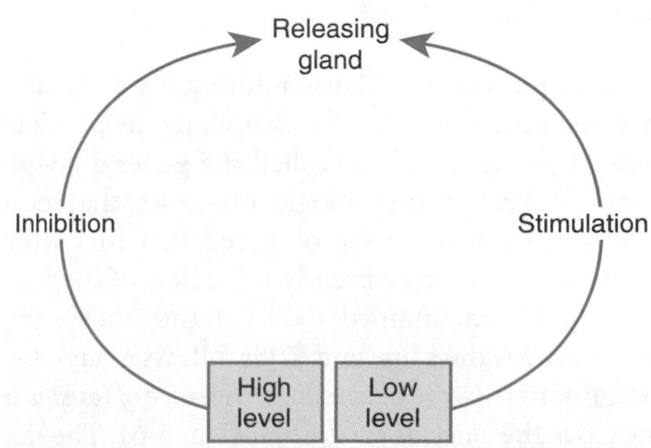

FIGURE 5–5. A feedback loop regulates hormone levels.

TABLE 5–3. **Common Signs and Symptoms of Stress**

Physical	Emotional	Cognitive
Rapid heart rate Rapid breathing Increased blood pressure Difficulty falling asleep, or excessive sleep Loss of appetite, or excessive eating Stiff muscles Hyperactivity or inactivity Dry mouth Constipation or diarrhea Lack of interest in sex	Irritability Angry outbursts Hypercritical Verbal abuse Withdrawal Depression	Impaired attention and concentration Forgetfulness Preoccupation Poor judgment

NATURE OF STRESS

Although humans have the capacity to adapt, not everyone responds to a similar stressor in exactly the same way. Differences may vary according to:

- The intensity of the stressor
- The number of stressors
- The duration of the stressor
- Physical health status
- Life experiences
- Coping strategies
- Social support
- Personal beliefs
- Attitudes
- Values

Because of unique differences, the outcomes may be adaptive or maladaptive, depending on each person's stress response.

STRESS RESPONSE

Hans Selye, a physician in Canada during the early 20th century, devoted much of his life to researching the physiology of the stress response, which he called the **general adaptation syndrome** (collective physiologic processes that occur in response to a stressor). Selye observed that this syndrome occurs repeatedly and consistently regardless of the nature of the stressor. He maintained that (1) the body's physical response is always the same and (2) it follows a one-, two-, or three-stage pattern—the *alarm stage*, the *stage of resistance*, and in some cases the *stage of exhaustion* (Fig. 5-6). The first two stages parallel the processes that occur in maintaining homeostasis. Therefore, brief stress responses generally result in adaptive outcomes and restoration of equilibrium. However, when the second stage, the stage of resistance, is prolonged, the process tends to become maladaptive and pathologic, leading to stress-related disorders and in some cases death.

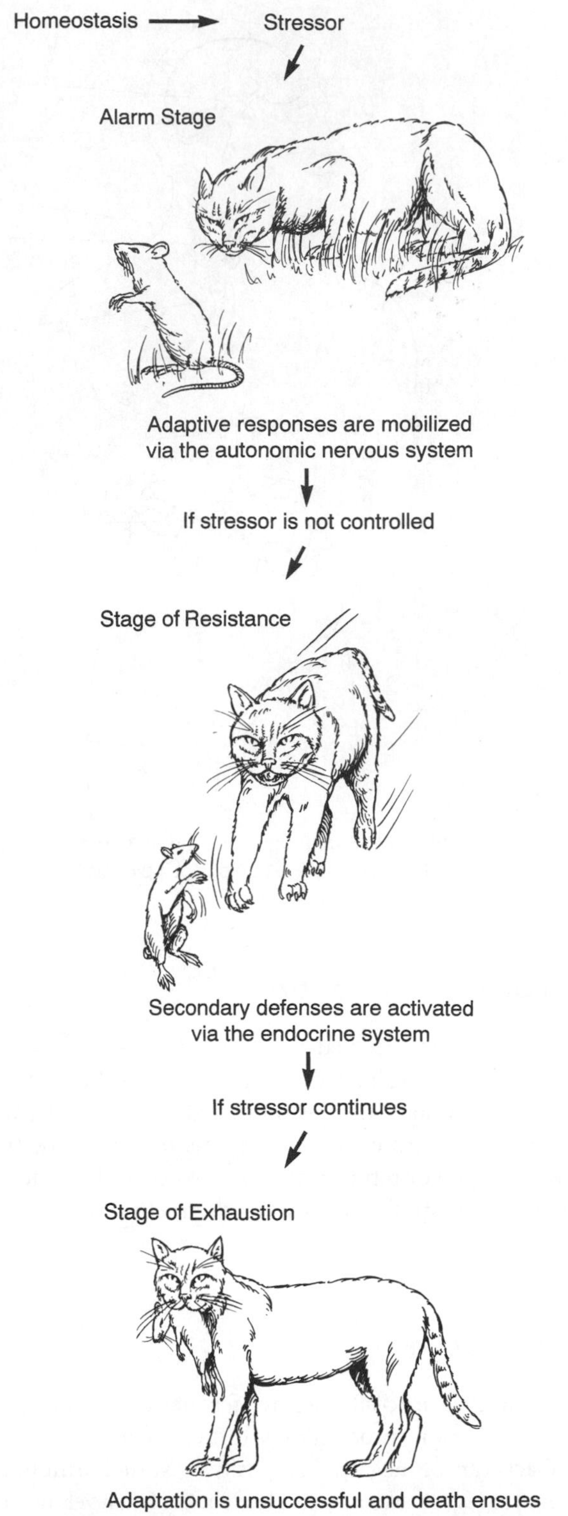

Homeostasis
Stressor
Alarm Stage
Adaptive responses are mobilized via the autonomic nervous system
If stressor is not controlled
Stage of Resistance
Secondary defenses are activated via the endocrine system
If stressor continues
Stage of Exhaustion
Adaptation is unsuccessful and death ensues

FIGURE 5–6. Stages of the general adaptation syndrome.

STRESS-RELATED DISORDERS

Stress-related disorders are diseases that result from prolonged stimulation of the autonomic nervous system and the endocrine system (Display 5-1). Many stress-related diseases involve allergic, inflammatory, or altered immune responses. They are characterized by physical conditions that cycle through asymptomatic periods (absence of the disorder) to episodes that often occur when the person is under stress. The brain–immune connection suggests that changes in body chemistry during periods of stress trigger the following: an autoimmune (self-attacking) response, like those associated with rheumatoid arthritis and other connective tissue disorders; failure to respond, as in immunosuppression; or a weakened immune response, which may be the case with infections and cancer. Consequently, psychological variables have the potential to influence the onset and progression of immune system-mediated diseases (Cohen and Herbert, 1996).

Holmes and Rahe (1967) developed a tool, the Social Readjustment Rating Scale, to predict a person's potential for developing a stress-related disorder. The rating scale is based on the number and significance of social stressors experienced in any 6-month period (Display 5-2). The risk for a stress-related disorder increases as the person's score rises. Although the dollar amounts in the mortgage-related items are outdated, being in debt is still a major stressor. Therefore, with only a minor adjustment, the assessment tool continues to have diagnostic value.

Preventive Approaches

By offering appropriate interventions to people with severe or accumulated stressors, stress-related illness can be prevented or minimized. Prevention takes place at three levels:

DISPLAY 5-1

Stress-Related Disorders

- Hypertension
- Headaches
- Gastritis
- Ulcerative colitis
- Asthma
- Rheumatoid arthritis
- Skin disorders
- Hyper/hypoinsulinism
- Hyper/hypothyroidism
- Depressive disorders
- Cancer
- Low back pain
- Irritable bowel syndrome
- Allergies
- Anxiety disorders
- Infertility
- Impotence
- Bruxism (tooth grinding)

- *Primary prevention* involves eliminating the potential for an illness before it occurs; for example, teaching principles of nutrition and methods for maintaining normal weight and blood pressure.
- *Secondary prevention* includes screening individuals for risk factors and providing a means for early diagnosis of disease; for example, regularly measuring the blood pressure of hypertension-prone individuals.
- *Tertiary prevention* minimizes the consequences of a disorder through aggressive rehabilitation or appropriate management of the disease; for example, frequently turning, positioning, and exercising stroke victims facilitates ambulation and the ability to perform activities of daily living.

Psychological Adaptation

Just as the physical body adapts to stressors, the psyche (mind) mounts other defenses as well. Sigmund Freud explained that humans unconsciously use defensive coping mechanisms to protect their ego, or reality base, from feeling less than adequate.

COPING MECHANISMS

Coping mechanisms (unconscious tactics used to protect the psyche) are listed in Table 5-4. These manipulations of reality act as psychological first aid, allowing people to avoid temporarily the emotional impact of a stressful situation. When used appropriately and in moderation, coping mechanisms enable individuals to maintain their mental equilibrium. An equally effective adaptive response involves implementing coping strategies.

COPING STRATEGIES

Coping strategies (stress reduction activities selected on a conscious level) help individuals deal with a stress-provoking event or situation. Examples of therapeutic coping strategies are:

- Seeking professional assistance in a crisis
- Using problem-solving techniques
- Demonstrating assertive behavior
- Practicing progressive relaxation
- Turning to a comforting other or higher power

Given the benefits of psychological adaptation, the person usually acquires insight, gains confidence to confront reality, and develops emotional maturity.

DISPLAY 5-2

The Social Readjustment Rating Scale

Rank	Life Event	LCU Value	Rank	Life Event	LCU Value
1	Death of spouse	100	23	Son or daughter leaving home	29
2	Divorce	73	24	Trouble with in-laws	29
3	Marital separation	65	25	Outstanding personal achievement	28
4	Jail term	63	26	Wife begins or stops work	26
5	Death of close family member	63	27	Begin or end school	26
6	Personal injury or illness	53	28	Change in living conditions	25
7	Marriage	50	29	Revision of personal habits	24
8	Fired at work	47	30	Trouble with boss	23
9	Marital reconciliation	45	31	Change in work hours or conditions	20
10	Retirement	45	32	Change in residence	20
11	Change in health of family member	44	33	Change in schools	20
12	Pregnancy	40	34	Change in recreation	19
13	Sex difficulties	39	35	Change in church activities	19
14	Gain of new family member	39	36	Change in social activities	18
15	Business readjustment	39	37	Mortgage or loan less than $10,000	17
16	Change in financial state	38	38	Change in sleeping habits	16
17	Death of close friend	37	39	Change in number of family get-togethers	15
18	Change to different line of work	36	40	Change in eating habits	15
19	Change in number of arguments with spouse	35	41	Vacation	13
20	Mortgage over $10,000	31	42	Christmas	12
21	Foreclosure of mortgage or loan	30	43	Minor violations of the law	11
22	Change in responsibilities at work	29			

Social events are ranked from most stressful to least stressful. Each event is assigned a life change unit (LCU) that correlates with the severity of the stressor. The sum of LCUs over the past 6 months is calculated. A score of less than 150 LCUs is considered low risk, a score between 150 to 199 is an indication of mild risk, moderate risk is associated with a score between 200 to 299, and a score over 300 places the person at major risk.

Holmes TH, Rahe RH. The Social Readjustment Rating Scale. Journal of Psychosomatic Research. August 1967;11:216.

MALADAPTIVE COPING

If coping mechanisms are overused or used over a long span of time, they may have a maladaptive effect, distorting reality to such an extent that the person fails to recognize and correct his or her weaknesses. Consequently, the person may avoid taking responsibility for solving personal psychosocial problems.

Maladaption also occurs when individuals elect to use nontherapeutic coping strategies, such as using mind- and mood-altering substances, sleeping excessively as an escape tactic, avoiding rather than dealing with conflict, and abandoning social interactions and activities. Negative coping strategies may provide immediate temporary relief from a stressor, but they eventually cause problems.

Nursing Implications

Nurses must be aware of potential stressors affecting patients because they add to the cumulative effect of other stressful life events. One research study ranked the stressors experienced by patients in a list modeled after the Social Readjustment Rating Scale (Display 5-3). By being aware of how an illness or hospital stay affects patients, nurses can be instrumental in supporting those who are especially vulnerable.

When a person is experiencing a stressor, nurses do one or several of the following:

- Identify the stressors.
- Assess the patient's response to stress.
- Eliminate or reduce the stressors.
- Prevent additional stressors from occurring.
- Promote the patient's physiologic adaptive responses.
- Support the patient's psychological coping strategies.
- Assist in maintaining a network of social support.
- Implement stress reduction and stress management techniques.

STRESS REDUCTION TECHNIQUES

Stress reduction techniques are methods that promote physiologic comfort and emotional well-being. Some general inter-

TABLE 5–4. **Coping Mechanisms**

Mechanism	Explanation	Example
Repression	Forgetting about the stressor	Wiping the experience of being sexually abused from conscious memory
Suppression	Purposely avoiding thinking about a stressor	Resolving to "sleep on a problem" or turn the problem over to a higher power like God
Denial	Rejecting information	Refusing to believe something like a life-threatening diagnosis
Rationalization	Relieving oneself of personal accountability by attributing responsibility to someone or something else	Blaming failure on a test to the manner in which the test was constructed
Displacement	Taking anger out on something or someone else who is less likely to retaliate	Kicking the wastebasket after being reprimanded by the boss
Regression	Behaving in a manner that is characteristic of a much younger age	Wanting to be bottle-fed like a newborn sibling
Projection	Attributing that which is unacceptable in oneself onto another	Accusing a person of another race of being prejudiced
Somatization	Manifesting emotional stress through a physical disorder	Developing diarrhea that conveniently excuses one from going to work
Compensation	Excelling at something to make up for a weakness of another kind	Becoming a motivational speaker although physically handicapped
Sublimation	Channeling one's energies into an acceptable alternative	Turning to sportscasting when an athletic career is not realistic
Reaction formation	Acting just the opposite of one's feelings	Being extremely nice to someone who is intensely disliked
Identification	Taking on the characteristics of another	Imitating the style of dress or speech of an actor or musician

ventions that are appropriate during the care of any patient include providing adequate explanations in understandable language, keeping the patient and family informed, demonstrating confidence and expertise when providing nursing care, remaining calm during crises, being available to the patient, responding promptly to the patient's signal for assistance, encouraging family interaction, advocating on behalf of the patient, and referring the patient and family to organizations or individuals that provide postdischarge assistance.

STRESS MANAGEMENT

People who are susceptible to intense stressors or who are likely to experience stressors over a long period may benefit from additional stress management approaches. Stress management refers to therapeutic activities that are used to reestablish balance between the sympathetic and parasympathetic nervous systems (Table 5-5). Techniques that counter sympathetic stimulation have a calming effect; stimulating tactics counterbalance parasympathetic dominance.

Physical and emotional responses to stress are also mediated by interventions that cause the release of endorphins or the manipulation of sensory stimuli.

Endorphins

Endorphins are natural body chemicals that produce effects similar to those of opiate drugs, such as morphine. In addition to decreasing the sensation of pain, these chemicals promote a sense of pleasantness, tranquillity, and well-being.

Endorphins are manufactured in the pituitary gland but are present in the blood and other tissues (Porth, 1998). Some believe that certain activities, such as massage, sustained aerobic exercise, and laughter, trigger the release of endorphins. Once released, endorphins attach themselves to receptor sites in the brain—perhaps in the limbic system, the center where emotions are experienced.

Sensory Manipulation

Sensory manipulation involves altering moods, feelings, and physiologic responses by stimulating pleasure centers in the brain using sensory stimuli. Research is being conducted on the stress-reducing effects of certain colors, full-spectrum lighting in the home and workplace, music, and specific aromas that conjure up pleasant associations, such as the smell of baking bread.

DISPLAY 5-3

Patient-Related Stressors

Thinking you might lose your sight
Thinking you might have cancer
Thinking you might lose a kidney or some other organ
Knowing you have a serious illness
Thinking you might lose your hearing
Not being told what your diagnosis is
Not knowing for sure what illness you have
Not getting pain medication when you need it
Not knowing the results or reasons for your treatments
Not getting relief from pain medications
Being fed through tubes
Missing your spouse
Not having your questions answered by the staff
Not having enough insurance to pay for your hospitalization
Not having your call light answered
Having a sudden hospitalization you weren't planning to have
Being hospitalized far from home
Knowing you have to have an operation
Not having family visit you
Feeling you are getting dependent on medications
Having nurses or doctors talk too fast or use words you can't understand
Having medications cause you discomfort
Thinking about losing income because of your illness
Having the staff be in too much of a hurry
Not knowing when to expect things will be done to you
Being put in the hospital because of an accident
Being cared for by an unfamiliar doctor
Not being able to call family or friends on the phone
Having to eat cold or tasteless food
Worrying about your spouse being away from you
Thinking you might have pain because of surgery or test procedures
Being in the hospital during holidays or special family occasions
Thinking your appearance might be changed after your hospitalization
Being in a room that is too cold or too hot
Not having friends visit you
Having a roommate who is unfriendly
Having to be assisted with a bedpan
Having a roommate who is seriously ill or cannot talk with you
Being aware of unusual smells around you
Having to stay in bed or the same room all day
Having a roommate who has too many visitors
Not being able to get newspapers, radio, or TV when you want them
Having to be assisted with bathing
Being awakened in the night by the nurse
Having strange machines around
Having to wear a hospital gown
Having to sleep in a strange bed
Having to eat at different times than you usually do
Having strangers sleep in the same room with you

The events in this list are arranged in order of their perceived significance as a stressor. The first event is the most stressful, and the rest follow in descending order.

TABLE 5–5. **Interventions for Stress Management**

Intervention	Explanation
Modeling	Promotes the ability to learn an adaptive response by exposing a person to someone who demonstrates a positive attitude or behavior
Progressive relaxation	Eases tense muscles by clearing the mind of stressful thoughts and focusing on consciously relaxing specific muscle groups
Imagery	Uses the mind to visualize calming, pleasurable, positive experiences
Biofeedback	Alters autonomic nervous system functions by responding to electronically displayed physiologic data
Yoga	Reduces physical and emotional tension through postural changes, muscular stretching, and focused concentration
Meditation and prayer	Reduces physiologic activation by placing one's trust in a higher power
Placebo effect	Alters a negative physiologic response through the power of suggestion

KEY CONCEPTS

- Homeostasis refers to a relatively stable state of physiologic equilibrium.
- Homeostasis is affected by physiologic, psychological, social, and spiritual stressors.
- The philosophic concept of holism leads to two commonly held beliefs: humans are directly influenced by both the mind and body, and the relationship between the mind and body has the potential for sustaining health as well as causing illness.
- Adaptation refers to the manner in which an organism responds to change. If done successfully, it is the key to maintaining and preserving homeostasis. Unsuccessful adaptation leads to illness and death.
- Adaptive changes occur through the cortex, which communicates with and through the reticular activating system, the hypothalamus, the autonomic nervous system, and the pituitary gland, along with other endocrine glands under its control.
- The sympathetic nervous system, a division of the autonomic nervous system, accelerates the physiologic func-

tions that ensure survival through strength or a rapid escape.

- The parasympathetic nervous system, a second division of the autonomic nervous system, inhibits physiologic stimulation, which restores homeostasis and provides an alternative mechanism for dealing with stressors.
- Stress involves the physiologic and behavioral reactions that occur when the body's equilibrium is disturbed.
- Individuals vary in their response to stressors, depending on the intensity of the stressor, the number of stressors being experienced at any given time, the duration of the stressor, and the individual's physical status, life experiences, coping strategies, social support system, and personal beliefs, attitudes, and values.
- The general adaptation syndrome, a physiologic stress response described by Hans Selye, consists of the alarm stage, the stage of resistance, and the stage of exhaustion. In most cases, the alarm stage and the stage of resistance lead to a restoration of homeostasis. However, when the stage of resistance is prolonged, adaptive resources are overwhelmed and the individual enters the stage of exhaustion, which is characterized by stress-related disorders and in some cases death.
- Stress-related disorders or their consequences are minimized at three levels. Primary prevention involves reducing the potential for a disorder. Secondary prevention involves public screening and early diagnosis. Tertiary prevention uses rehabilitation and aggressive management when a disorder develops.
- Psychological adaptation occurs through the use of coping mechanisms and coping strategies.
- The healthy use of coping mechanisms and coping strategies allows people to avoid temporarily the emotional impact of a stressful situation, permitting them to deal with reality eventually and gain emotional maturity.
- The unhealthy use of coping mechanisms tends to distort reality to such an extent that the person fails to see or correct his or her weaknesses. Nontherapeutic coping strategies provide temporary relief but eventually cause problems.
- The nursing care of patients under stress includes identifying stressors, assessing the patient's response to stressors, eliminating or reducing stressors, preventing additional stressors, promoting adaptive responses, supporting coping strategies, maintaining a patient's network of support, and implementing stress reduction and stress management techniques.
- Four methods for preventing, reducing, or eliminating a stress response include using stress reduction techniques, such as providing adequate explanations in understandable language; implementing stress management interventions, such as progressive relaxation; promoting the release of endorphins through massage, for example; and manipulating sensory stimuli, as might be done with aromatherapy.

CRITICAL THINKING EXERCISES

- Develop a list of stressors that are unique to students or student nurses, using the Social Readjustment Rating Scale and the list of patient-related stressors as models.
- Identify at least five interventions that are both realistic and helpful in reducing the stressors associated with being a student.
- Which stress management technique from among those in Table 5-5 is best? Explain the reasons for your choice.

SUGGESTED READINGS

Cohen S, Herbert T. Health psychology: psychological factors and physical disease from the perspective of human psychoneuroimmunology. Annual Review of Psychology 1996;47:113–142.

Davidhizar R, Gigar JN. Patients' use of denial: coping with the unacceptable. Nursing Standard 1998;12(43):44–46.

Freud S. The ego and the mechanisms of defense. London, Hogarth Press, 1937.

Holmes TH, Rahe RH. The social readjustment rating scale. Journal of Psychosomatic Research 1967;11(8):216.

Kauffman E, Harrison MB, Burke SO, Wong C. Family matters. Stress-point intervention for parents of children hospitalized with chronic conditions. Pediatric Nursing 1998;24(4):362–366.

Nuernberger P. Freedom from stress. Honesdale, PA, The Himalayan International Institute of Yoga Science and Philosophy, 1981.

O'Neill DP, Kenny EK. State of the science. Spirituality and chronic illness. Image: Journal of Nursing Scholarship 1998;30(3):275–280.

Pelletier-Hibbert M. Coping strategies used by nurses to deal with the care of organ donors and their families. Heart & Lung: Journal of Acute and Critical Care 1998;27(4):230–237.

Porth CM. Pathophysiology: concepts of altered health states, 5th ed. Philadelphia, Lippincott Williams & Wilkins, 1998.

Rimmer L. Client challenge. The clinical use of aromatherapy in the reduction of stress. Home Healthcare Nursing 1998;16(2):123–126.

Schiraldi GR, Spalding TW, Hofford CW. Expanding health educators' roles to meet critical needs in stress management and mental health. Journal of Health Education 1998;29(2):68–76.

Selye H. The stress of life. New York, McGraw-Hill, 1956.

Stetson B. Holistic health stress management program: nursing student and client health outcomes. Journal of Holistic Nursing 1997;15(2):143–157.

Topf M. Theoretical considerations for research on environmental stress and health. Image: Journal of Nursing Scholarship 1994;26(4):289–293.

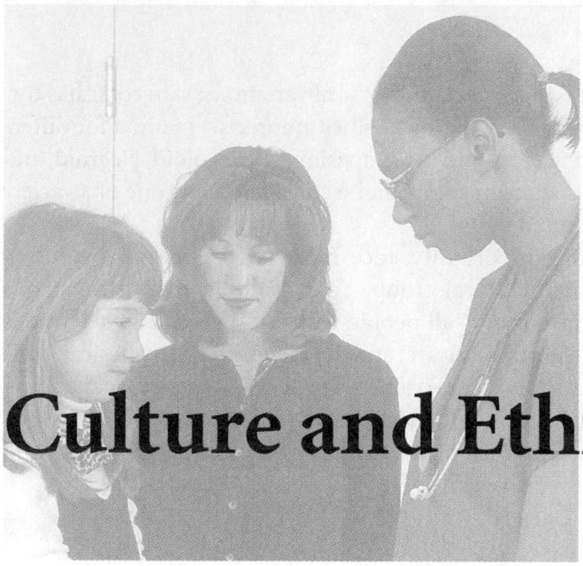

CHAPTER 6

Culture and Ethnicity

CHAPTER OUTLINE

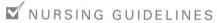

NURSING GUIDELINES

COMMUNICATING WITH NON-ENGLISH-SPEAKING PATIENTS

KEY TERMS

acultural nursing care	ethnicity
African Americans	ethnocentrism
Anglo-Americans	folk medicine
Asian Americans	Latinos
bilingual	Native Americans
cultural shock	race
culturally sensitive nursing care	stereotypes
culture	subcultures
	transcultural nursing

LEARNING OBJECTIVES

An understanding of the content within this chapter will be evidenced by the student's ability to:

- Differentiate between culture, race, and ethnicity.
- Discuss two factors that interfere with perceiving others who are dissimilar as individuals.
- Explain why the American culture is described as being Anglicized.
- List at least five characteristics of Anglo-American culture.
- Define the term subculture and list four major subcultures in the United States.
- List five ways in which individuals from subcultural groups differ from Anglo-Americans.
- Describe four characteristics of culturally sensitive care.
- List at least five ways of demonstrating cultural sensitivity.

Nurses have always cared for patients with differences of one kind or another. Patients vary according to their age, gender, race, health status, education, religion, occupation, and economic level. Culture, which is the focus of this chapter, is yet another characteristic that contributes to the diversity of patients.

Despite the fact that differences exist, the traditional tendency has been to treat patients as though there were none. Although equal treatment may be politically correct, many nurses now believe that ignoring differences contradicts what is in the best interest of patients. Consequently, there is a movement toward eliminating **acultural nursing care** (care that avoids concern for cultural differences) and promoting **culturally sensitive nursing care** (care that respects and is compatible with each patient's culture).

Culture

Culture (values, beliefs, and practices of a particular group; Giger and Davidhizar, 1995) incorporates the attitudes and customs that are learned by socialization with others. They are passed on from one generation to the next. The components of any cultural group include, but are not limited to, its language, communication style, traditions, religion, art, music, manner of dress, health beliefs, and health practices.

The United States has been described as a "melting pot" in which culturally diverse groups have become assimilated; however, that is not the case. Individuals from various cultural groups have settled, lived, and worked in the United States while continuing to sustain their particular identities (Table 6-1).

TABLE 6–1. **Culturally Diverse Groups Within the United States**

City or Region	Predominant Cultural Group
New England	Irish
Detroit, Buffalo, Chicago	Polish
Upper Midwest (Minnesota, North Dakota)	Scandinavians
Ohio and Pennsylvania	Amish
Washington state and Oregon	Southeast Asians (Laotian, Vietnamese)
New York (Spanish Harlem)	Puerto Rican
Miami (Little Cuba)	Cuban
San Francisco (Chinatown)	Chinese
Manhattan (Little Italy)	Italian
Louisiana	Cajan (French/Indian)
Southwest	Latin American/Native American
Hawaiian Islands	Pacific Islanders/Japanese/Chinese

Race

Cultural groups tend to share biologic and physiologic similarities as well. **Race** (biologic variations) is a term used to categorize people with genetically shared physical characteristics. Some examples include skin color, eye shape, and hair texture. Despite wide ranges in physical variations, skin color has traditionally been the chief, albeit imprecise, method for differentiating races into three divisions: Mongoloid, Negroid, and Caucasian. Skin color can be considered just one of a variety of inherited traits.

More importantly, race must not be equated with any particular cultural group. To do so leads to two erroneous assumptions: (1) all people with common physical features share the same culture, and (2) all people with physical similarities have cultural values, beliefs, and practices that are different from **Anglo-Americans** (individuals in the United States who trace their ancestry to the United Kingdom and Western European countries).

Ethnicity

Ethnicity (bond or kinship a person feels with his or her country of birth or place of ancestral origin) may exist regardless of whether a person has ever lived outside the United States. Pride in one's ethnicity is demonstrated by valuing certain physical characteristics, giving one's children ethnic names, wearing unique items of clothing, appreciating folk music and dance, and eating native dishes (Fig. 6-1).

Because cultural characteristics and ethnic pride represent the norm in a homogeneous group, they tend to go unnoticed.

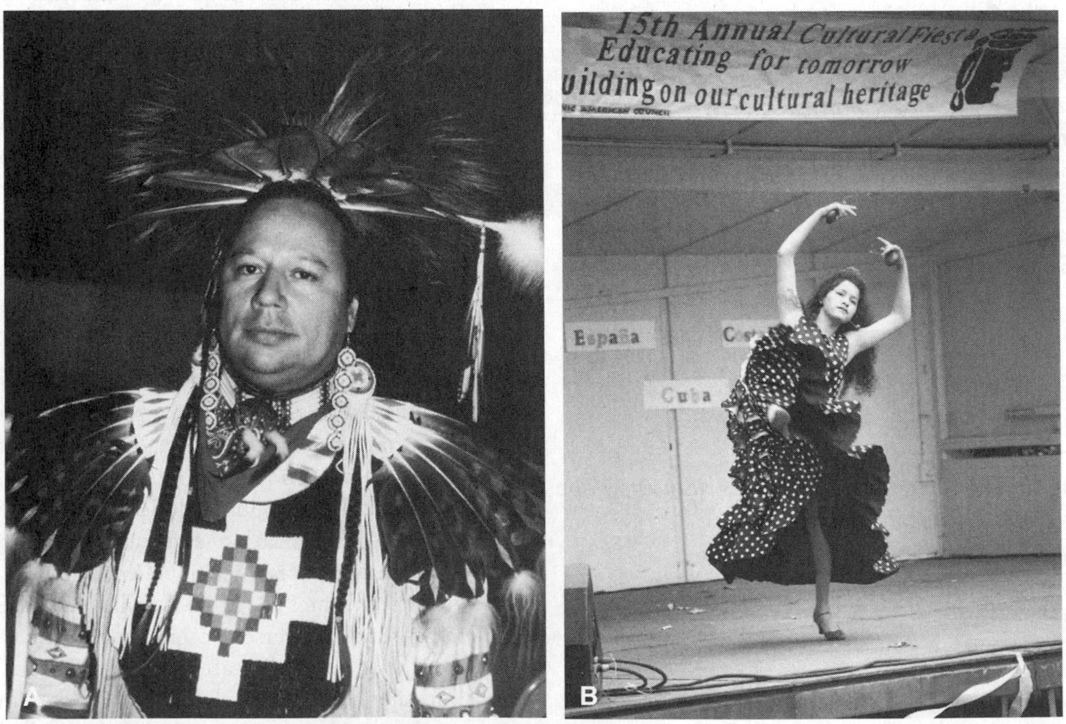

FIGURE 6–1. (*A*) A Native American in tribal dress during an Indian powwow. (*B*) Latin American ethnicity is celebrated at a festival that includes folk dancing and music. (Courtesy of Ken Timby.)

However, when two or more cultural groups mix, as they often do at the borders of various countries or through the process of immigration, their unique differences become more obvious. One or both groups may experience **cultural shock** (bewilderment over the behavior that is culturally atypical). Consequently, many ethnic groups have been victimized as a result of bigotry based on stereotypical assumptions and ethnocentrism.

STEREOTYPING

Stereotypes (fixed attitudes about *all* individuals who share a common characteristic) develop with regard to age, gender, race, sexual preference, or ethnicity. Because stereotypes are preconceived ideas that are usually unsupported by facts, they tend to be neither real nor accurate. In fact, they can be dangerous because they interfere with accepting others as unique individuals.

ETHNOCENTRISM

Ethnocentrism (belief that one's own ethnicity is superior to all others) also interferes with intercultural relationships. Ethnocentrism is manifested by treating anyone who is "different" as deviant and undesirable. This form of cultural intolerance was the basis for the Holocaust, during which the Nazis attempted to carry out genocide, the planned extinction of an entire ethnic group—European Jews. It continues to play a role in the ethnic rivalries between Bosnians and Serbs in Eastern Europe, Arabs and Jews in the Middle East, Tutsis and Huntas in West Africa, and wherever culturally diverse groups live in close proximity. Similar conflicts also occur among ethnic groups in the United States.

DISPLAY 6–1

Examples of American Cultural Characteristics

- English is the language of communication.
- The pronunciation or meaning of some words varies according to regions within the United States.
- The customary greeting is a handshake.
- A distance of 4 to 12 feet is customary when interacting with strangers or doing business (Giger and Davidhizar, 1995).
- In casual situations, it is acceptable for women as well as men to wear pants; blue jeans are a common mode of dress.
- Most Americans are Christians.
- Sunday is recognized as the Sabbath.
- Government is expected to remain separate from religion.
- Guilt or innocence for alleged crimes is decided by a jury of one's peers.
- Selection of a marriage partner is an individual's choice.
- Legally, men and women are equals.
- Marriage is monogamous (only one spouse); fidelity is expected.
- Divorce and subsequent remarriages are common.
- Parents are responsible for their minor children.
- Aging adults live separately from their children.
- Status is related to occupation, wealth, and education.
- Common beliefs are that everyone has the potential for success and that hard work leads to prosperity.
- Daily bathing and use of a deodorant are standard hygiene practices.
- Anglo-American women shave the hair from their legs and underarms; most men shave their faces daily.
- Health care is provided by licensed practitioners.
- Drugs and surgery are the traditional forms of medical treatment.
- Americans tend to value technology and equate it with quality.
- As a whole, Americans are time oriented, and therefore rigidly schedule their activities according to clock hours.
- Forks, knives, and spoons are used, except when eating "fast foods," for which using the fingers is appropriate.

Anglo-American Culture

The American culture can be described as *Anglicized*, or English-based, because it evolved primarily from its early English settlers. Display 6-1 provides an overview of some common characteristics of the American culture. However, to suggest that everyone who lives in America embraces the totality of its culture would be foolhardy.

AMERICAN SUBCULTURES

Although it is a gross oversimplification, there are four major **subcultures** (unique cultural groups that coexist within the dominant culture) in the United States. In addition to Anglo-Americans, there are African Americans, Latinos, Asian Americans, and Native Americans (Table 6-2).

The term **African Americans** (those whose ancestral origin is Africa) is used here in lieu of Black Americans to avoid any association based only on skin color. **Latinos** (those who trace their ethnic origin to South America) are sometimes referred to as *Hispanics* if they are of Spanish descent or *Chicanos* when speaking of people from Mexico. **Asian Americans** (those who come from China, Japan, Korea, the Philippines, Thailand, Indochina, and Vietnam) make up the third subculture. **Native Americans** (Indian nations found in North America, including the Eskimos and Aleuts) include approximately 1.5 million American Indians and Alaskan Natives belonging to 557 federally recognized tribes in the United States (Indian Health Services, 1998).

TABLE 6–2. **American Subcultural Groups***

Group	Representative Countries	Percent of American Population
African American	Africa, Haiti, Jamaica, West Indies, Dominican Republic	12.7
Latino	Mexico, Puerto Rico, Cuba, South and Central America	9
Asian American	China, Japan, Korea, Philippines, Thailand, Indochina, Vietnam, Pacific Islands	3
Native American	North American Indian nation and tribes, Eskimos, Aleuts	0.9

*As reported by the U.S. Census Bureau, 1994.

Although Anglo-American culture predominates in the United States, those who trace their ancestry to the United Kingdom and Western European countries are gradually becoming the minority. The Bureau of the Census predicts that by the middle of the 21st century, the majority of American citizens will be of African, Asian, Hispanic, or Arabic descent (Kavanaugh 1993). The population will become even more diverse, prompting the need for transcultural nursing.

Transcultural Nursing

Transcultural nursing (providing nursing care within the context of another's culture) is a term coined by Madeline Leininger in the 1970s. It incorporates:

- Assessments of a cultural nature
- Acceptance of each patient as an individual
- Knowledge of health problems that affect particular cultural groups
- Planning care within the patient's health belief system to achieve the best health outcomes

To provide culturally sensitive care, nurses must become skilled at managing language differences, understanding biologic and physiologic variations, promoting health teaching that will reduce prevalent diseases, and respecting alternative health beliefs or health practices.

Some forewarning about making generalizations is necessary, because after learning about differences among cultural groups, nurses may themselves fall into the trap of stereotyping. Assuming that all individuals who affiliate themselves with a particular group behave alike or hold the same beliefs is always incorrect. Diversity exists even within cultural groups.

CULTURAL ASSESSMENT

To provide culturally sensitive care, the nurse strives to gather data about the unique characteristics of patients. Pertinent data include:

- Language and communication style
- Hygiene practices, including feelings about modesty and accepting help from others
- Special clothing or ornamentation
- Religion and religious practices
- Rituals surrounding birth, passage from adolescence to adulthood, illness, and death
- Family and gender roles, including child-rearing practices and kinship with older adults
- Proper forms of greeting and showing respect
- Food habits and dietary restrictions
- Methods for making decisions
- Health beliefs and medical practices

Language

Because language is the primary way for sharing and gathering information, the inability to communicate is one of the biggest deterrents to providing culturally sensitive care. Foreign travelers and many residents in the United States do not speak English, or have learned it as their second language and do not speak it well. It is estimated that 13.8% of those who live in America speak a language other than English in their home (Perkins et al, 1998). Those who can communicate in English may still prefer to use their primary language, especially when under stress.

Equal Access

Federal law, specifically Title IV of the Civil Rights Act of 1994, states that individuals with limited English proficiency are entitled to the same health care and social services as those who speak English fluently. In other words, *all* patients have a right to unencumbered communication with a health provider. Using children as interpreters or requiring patients to provide their own interpreters is a civil rights violation. The Joint Commission on Accreditation of Healthcare Organizations requires that hospitals have a way of providing effective communication for each patient.

The use of untrained interpreters, volunteers, or family is not considered appropriate because it undermines confidentiality and privacy. It also violates family roles and boundaries. It increases the potential for modifying, condensing, omitting, or adding information or projecting the interpreter's own values during communication between the patient or the health care provider. To comply with the laws and accreditation requirements, health care agencies are strongly encouraged to train professional interpreters. A competent trained interpreter demonstrates the skills listed in Display 6-2.

DISPLAY 6–2

Characteristics of a Skilled Interpreter

- Learns the goals of the interaction
- Demonstrates courtesy and respect for the patient
- Explains his/her role to the patient
- Positions himself/herself to avoid disrupting direct communication between the health care worker and patient
- Has a good memory for what is said
- Converts the information in one language accurately into the other without commenting on the content
- Possesses knowledge of medical terminology and vocabulary
- Attempts to preserve the emphasis and emotions that are expressed by both persons
- Asks for clarification if verbalizations from either party are unclear
- Indicates instances where a cultural difference has the potential to impair communication
- Maintains confidentiality

Nurse–Patient Communication

If the nurse is not **bilingual** (able to speak a second language), an alternative method for communicating must be used.

Nursing Guidelines For

Communicating with Non-English-Speaking Patients

☑ Greet or say words and phrases in the patient's language, even if it is not possible to carry on a conversation.
RATIONALE: Using familiar words indicates a desire to communicate with the patient, even if the nurse lacks the expertise to do so.

☑ Refer to an English/foreign language dictionary, such as *Taber's Cyclopedic Medical Dictionary.*
RATIONALE: Some dictionaries provide a list of medical words and phrases that may help in obtaining pertinent information.

☑ Compile a looseleaf folder or file cards of medical words in one or more languages spoken by patients in the community, and place it where other reference books are located on the nursing unit.
RATIONALE: A home-made reference provides a readily available language resource for communicating with others in the local area.

☑ Request a trained interpreter. If that option is not possible, call ethnic organizations or church pastors to obtain a list of individuals who speak the patient's language and may be willing to act as translators in an emergency.
RATIONALE: Someone who is proficient at speaking the language is more effective in obtaining necessary information and explaining proposed treatments than someone who is relying on a rough translation.

☑ Contact an international telephone operator in a crisis, if there is no other option for communicating with a patient.
RATIONALE: International telephone operators are generally available 24 hours a day; however, their main responsibility is the job for which they were hired.

☑ When it is possible to choose from several interpreters, select one who is the same gender as the patient and approximately the same age.
RATIONALE: Some patients feel embarrassed to relate personal information to someone with whom they have little in common.

☑ Look at the patient, not the interpreter, when asking questions and listening for a response.
RATIONALE: Eye contact indicates that the patient is the primary focus of the interaction and helps the nurse interpret nonverbal clues.

☑ If the patient speaks some English, speak slowly, not loudly, using simple words and short sentences.
RATIONALE: Lengthy or complex sentences are barriers when communicating with someone who is not skilled in a second language.

☑ Avoid using technical terms, slang, or phrases with a double or colloquial meaning.
RATIONALE: The patient may not understand the spoken vernacular, especially if he or she learned English from a textbook rather than conversationally.

☑ Ask questions that can be answered by a yes or no.
RATIONALE: Direct questions avoid the need to provide an elaborate response in English.

☑ If the patient appears confused by a question, repeat it without changing the words.
RATIONALE: Rephrasing tends to compound the patient's confusion because it forces him or her to translate yet another group of unfamiliar words.

☑ Give the patient sufficient time to respond.
RATIONALE: The process of interpreting what has been said in English and then converting the response from the native language back into English requires extra time.

☑ Use nonverbal communication or pantomime.
RATIONALE: Body language is universal and tends to be communicated and interpreted quite accurately.

☑ Be patient.
RATIONALE: Anxiety is communicated interpersonally and tends to heighten frustration.

- ☑ Show the patient written English words.
  RATIONALE: Some non-English-speaking individuals can read better than they can understand spoken English.
- ☑ Work with the health agency's records committee to obtain consent forms, authorization for health insurance benefits, and copies of patient's rights that are written in languages other than English.
  RATIONALE: Legally, patients must understand what they are consenting to.
- ☑ Develop or obtain foreign translations describing common procedures, routine care, and health promotion. One resource is the *Patient Education Resource Center* in San Francisco, which provides publications in many languages on numerous health topics.
  RATIONALE: All patients are entitled to explanations and educational services.

Communication Styles

Even when individuals from different cultural groups speak the same language, the manner in which they do so may cause conflicts and miscommunication. What may be an accepted pattern during verbal interactions for one may be unusual, rude, or offensive to another. Therefore, understanding some unique cultural characteristics involving verbal and nonverbal aspects of communication may ease the transition toward culturally sensitive care.

Verbal Differences

General communication patterns can be found among the major American subcultures. The nurse should carefully observe or tactfully question the patient about communication styles and tailor the interview accordingly.

Native Americans tend to be private people and may be hesitant to share personal information with a stranger. Questioning may be interpreted as prying or meddling. The nurse should be patient when awaiting an answer and should listen carefully; impatience is considered disrespectful (Lipson et al, 1996). Navajos, currently the largest tribe of Native Americans, believe that no person has the right to speak for another and may refuse to comment on a family member's health problems.

Because Native Americans traditionally preserved their heritage through oral rather than written history, they may be skeptical of Anglo-American nurses who write down what they say. If possible, write notes after the interview rather than during it.

African Americans have good reason to mistrust the medical establishment, because they have been uninformed subjects in research projects in the past and have sometimes been treated as second-class citizens when seeking health care. The nurse must demonstrate professionalism by addressing patients by their last names and introducing himself or herself. Follow up thoroughly with requests. Respect the patient's privacy, and ask open-ended rather than direct questions until trust has been established. Because of their experiences as victims of discrimination, African Americans may be hesitant to give any more information than what is asked.

Latinos are characteristically more comfortable sitting close to the interviewer and letting the interaction unfold slowly. Many Latinos speak English but still have difficulty with medical terminology. They may be embarrassed to ask the interviewer to speak slowly, so the nurse must provide information and ask questions carefully. Latino men generally are protective and authoritarian regarding women and children. Men expect to be consulted in decisions concerning a family member.

Asian Americans may feel more comfortable more than an arm's length away from the interviewer. They tend to respond with brief or more factual answers with little elaboration, perhaps because traditionally they value simplicity, meditation, and introspection. Asian Americans may not openly disagree with authority figures, such as physicians and nurses, because of their respect for harmony. Their reticence can conceal a potential for noncompliance when a particular therapeutic regimen is unacceptable from their perspective.

Nonverbal Differences

Although it may be natural for Anglo-Americans to look directly at a person while speaking, it may offend Asian Americans or Native Americans, who are likely to believe that lingering eye contact is an invasion of privacy. Even the Anglo-American custom of a strong handshake can be interpreted as offensive by some Native Americans, who may be more comfortable with just a light passing of the hands.

Anglo-Americans in general express their feelings, both positive and negative. Asian Americans, however, tend to control their emotions and the expression of physical discomfort (Zborowski, 1952, 1969), especially when among people with whom they are unfamiliar. Similarly, Latino men may not demonstrate their feelings or readily discuss their symptoms because it may be interpreted as less than manly (Andrews and Boyle, 1995). The Latino cultural response can be attributed to *machismo,* a belief that virile men are physically strong and must deal with their emotions in private. Because this type of behavior is atypical from an Anglo-American perspective, nurses are more apt to overlook the emotional and physical needs of individuals from these cultural groups.

Biologic Variations

The biologic characteristics of primary importance to nurses are those that involve the skin and hair.

Skin Characteristics

The skin assessment techniques that are commonly taught are biased toward persons with white skins. To provide culturally sensitive care, nurses must modify their assessment techniques to obtain accurate data.

The best technique for observing baseline skin color in a dark-skinned person is to use natural or bright artificial light. Because the palms of the hands, the feet, and the abdomen contain the least amount of pigmentation and are less likely to have been tanned, they are often the best structures to inspect.

According to Giger and Davidhizar (1995), all skin, regardless of a person's ethnic origin, contains an underlying red tone. Its absence or a lighter appearance indicates pallor, a characteristic of anemia or inadequate oxygenation. The color of the lips and nailbeds, common sites for assessing cyanosis in whites, may be highly pigmented in other groups, and normal findings may be misinterpreted. The conjunctiva and oral mucous membranes are likely to provide more accurate data. The sclera or the hard palate, rather than the skin, is a better location for assessing jaundice. However, the sclera in some nonwhites may have a yellow cast due to carotene and fatty deposits; this should not be misconstrued as jaundice (Spector, 1996).

Rashes, bruising, and inflammation may not be as obvious among persons with darker skin. Palpating for variations in texture, warmth, and tenderness is a better assessment technique than inspection. Keloids (irregular, elevated thick scars) are common among dark-skinned persons (Fig. 6-2). Keloids are thought to form due to a genetic tendency to produce excessive amounts of transforming growth factor beta (TGFβ), a substance that promotes fibroblast proliferation during tissue repair.

Some nurses, when bathing a dark-skinned person, misinterpret the brown discoloration on a washcloth as a sign of poor hygiene. In reality, this is caused by the normal shedding of dead skin cells, which retain their pigmentation.

Hypo- and hyperpigmentation are conditions in which the skin is not a uniform color. Hypopigmentation may result when the skin becomes damaged. Regardless of ethnic origin, damaged skin characteristically manifests temporary redness, which then fades to a lighter hue; in dark-skinned patients, the effect is much more obvious. Vitiligo, a disease that affects whites as well as those with darker skin, produces irregular white patches on the skin due to the absence of melanin (Fig. 6-3). Other than hypopigmentation, there are no physical symptoms, but the cosmetic effects may create emotional distress. Patients concerned about the irregularity of their skin color may use a pigmented cream to disguise areas that are noticeable.

Mongolian spots, an example of hyperpigmentation, are dark-blue areas on the lower back of darkly pigmented infants and children (Fig. 6-4). They are rare among whites and tend to fade by the time a child is 5 years old. Mongolian spots can be mistaken as a sign of physical abuse or injury by nurses unfamiliar with ethnic differences. The two can be differentiated by pressing the pigmented area: Mongolian spots will not produce pain when pressure is applied.

Hair Characteristics

Hair color and texture are also biologic variants. Dark-skinned people usually have dark-brown or black hair. Hair texture, also an inherited characteristic, is the result of the amount of protein molecules within the hair. Variations range from straight to very curly hair. The curlier the hair, the more difficult it is to comb. In general, using a wide-toothed comb or pick, wetting the hair with water before combing, or applying a moisturizing cream makes hair grooming more manageable. Some patients with very curly hair prefer to arrange it in small, tightly braided sections.

Physiologic Variations

Three inherited enzymatic variations are prevalent among members of various subcultures in the United States: absence or insufficiency of the enzymes lactase, glucose-6-phosphate dehydrogenase (G-6-PD), and alcohol dehydrogenase (ADH).

Lactase Deficiency

Lactase is a digestive enzyme that converts lactose, the sugar in milk, into simpler sugars, glucose and galactose. A lactase

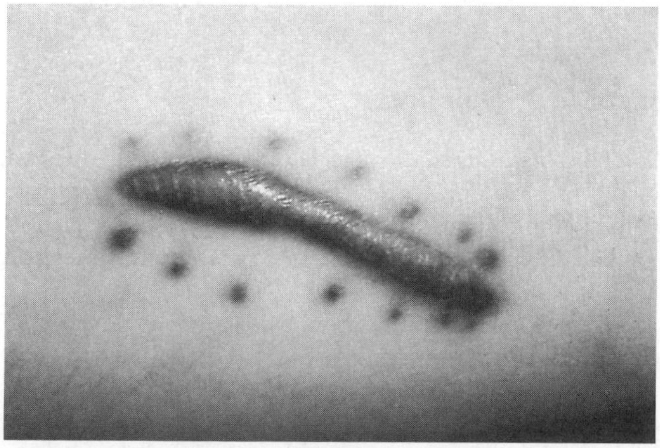

FIGURE 6–2. Keloids are raised, thick scars. (Jackson DB, Saunders R. Child Health Nursing: A Comprehensive Approach to the Care of Children and Their Families. Philadelphia, JB Lippincott, 1993)

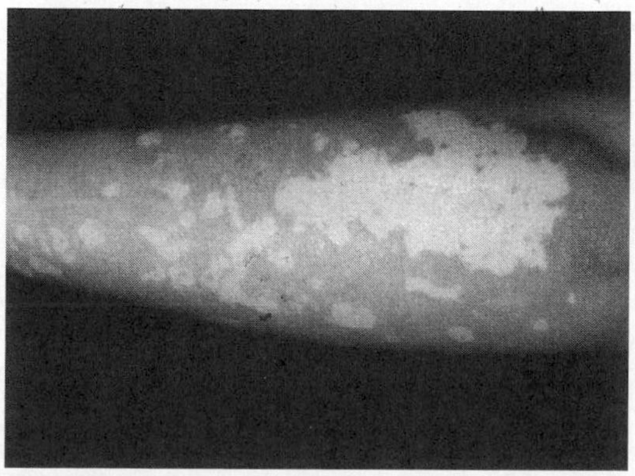

FIGURE 6–3. Vitiligo of forearm in a black patient. (Sauer GC, Hall JC. Manual of Skin Diseases, 7th ed. Philadelphia, Lippincott-Raven, 1996.)

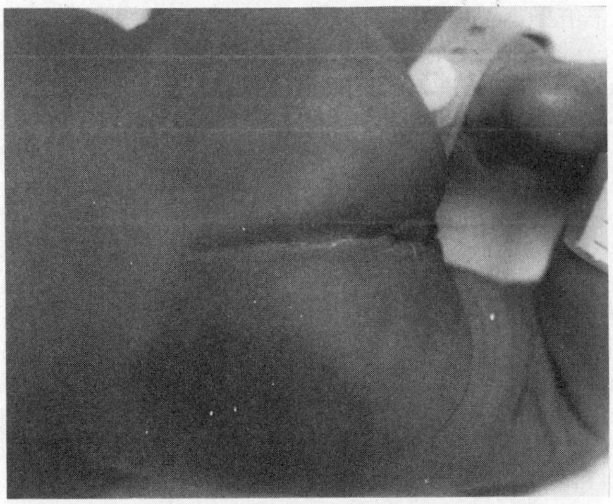

FIGURE 6-4. Mongolian spots are blue discolorations that are common in dark-skinned infants. (Courtesy of Ken Timby.)

deficiency causes an intolerance to dairy products. Without lactase, individuals have cramps, intestinal gas, and diarrhea approximately 30 minutes after ingesting milk or foods that contain milk. The symptoms may continue for 2 hours (Dudek, 1997). The discomfort may be prevented by eliminating or reducing sources of lactose in the diet. Liquid tube-feeding formulas and those used for bottle-fed infants can be prepared using milk substitutes.

Patient Teaching For

Reducing or Eliminating Lactose

Teach the patient or the family to do the following:

- Avoid milk, dairy products, and packaged foods that list dry milk solids or whey among their ingredients (for example, some breads, cereals, puddings, gravy mixes, caramels, and chocolate).
- Use nondairy creamers, which are lactose-free, instead of cream.
- Consume only small amounts of milk or dairy products at a time.
- Substitute milk that has been cultured with the *Acidophilus* organism, which changes lactose into lactic acid.
- Drink LactAid, a commercial product in which the lactose has been preconverted into other absorbable sugars.
- Use kosher foods, which are prepared without milk; they can be identified by the word *pareve* on the label.

Because milk is a good source of calcium, which is necessary for health, affected patients are taught to obtain calcium from other sources, such as green leafy vegetables, dates, prunes, canned sardines and salmon with bones, egg yolk, whole grains, dried peas and beans, and calcium supplements.

G-6-PD Deficiency

G-6-PD is an enzyme that helps red blood cells to metabolize glucose. African Americans and people from Mediterranean countries commonly lack this enzyme. The disorder is manifested in males, because the gene is sex-linked, but females can carry and transmit the faulty gene.

A G-6-PD deficiency makes red blood cells vulnerable during stress, when metabolic needs are increased. When this happens, red blood cells are destroyed at a much greater rate than in unaffected persons. If the production of new red blood cells cannot match the rate of destruction, anemia develops.

Because several drugs can precipitate the anemic process (Table 6-3), it is important for the nurse to intervene if these drugs, or those that depress red cell production, are prescribed for the ethnic patients who are at greatest risk. At the very least, the nurse must monitor susceptible patients and advocate for laboratory tests, such as red blood count and hemoglobin levels, that will indicate whether adverse effects are occurring.

ADH Deficiency

When alcohol is consumed, it is eventually broken down into acetic acid and carbon dioxide through a process of chemical reactions involving enzymes, one of which is ADH. Asian Americans and Native Americans often metabolize alcohol at a different rate because of physiologic variations in their enzyme system. The result is that affected individuals experience dramatic vascular effects, such as flushing and rapid heart rate, soon after consuming alcohol. In addition, middle metabolites of alcohol (those formed before acetic acid) remain unchanged for a prolonged period. Many scientists believe that the middle metabolites, such as acetaldehyde, are extremely toxic and subsequently play a primary role in causing organ damage. The rate of death from cirrhosis among Native Americans has been estimated to be at least four times that in the general population (National Clearinghouse for Alcohol and Drug Information, 1993).

Disease Prevalence

Several diseases, including sickle cell anemia, hypertension, diabetes, and stroke, occur with much greater frequency among ethnic subcultures than in the general population. The incidence of chronic illness affects morbidity differently as well (Table 6-4).

The incidence of some chronic diseases and their complications may be due in part to variations in social factors such as poverty. Minority cultural groups tend to be less affluent, and consequently their access to expensive health care is often limited. Without preventive health care, early detection, and treatment, higher death rates are bound to occur. The United

TABLE 6–3. **Drugs That Precipitate Glucose 6-Phosphate Dehydrogenase Anemia**

Drug Category	Example	Use
Quinine compounds	Primaquine phosphate	Prevention and treatment of malaria
Urocosurics	Probenecid (Benemid)	Treatment of gout
Sulfonamides	Sulfasalazine (Azulfidine)	Treatment of urinary infections

States has, therefore, committed itself to reducing the disparity in health care among all Americans (see Chap. 4).

With the knowledge that special populations are at higher risk for chronic diseases, culturally sensitive nurses focus heavily on health teaching, participate in community health screenings, and campaign for more equitable health services.

Health Beliefs and Practices

There are many differences in health beliefs among subcultures living in the United States. They are maintained due to strong ethnic influences. Health beliefs, in turn, affect health practices (Table 6-5).

Folk medicine (health practices unique to a particular group of people) has come to mean the methods of disease prevention or treatment that are outside the mainstream of conventional practice. These treatments are generally provided by lay rather than formally educated and licensed individuals. Besides culturally specific health practices, such as those sought from a *curandero* (Latino practitioner who is thought to have spiritual and medicinal powers), a *shaman* (holy man with curative powers), or an herbalist, many people in the United States also turn to alternative quasimedical therapy (Display 6-3). Alternative medicine attracts people for a variety of reasons: the expense of mainstream medical care, dissatisfaction with prior treatment or progress, or intimidation from the health care establishment.

Just because a health belief or practice is different does not make it wrong. Culturally sensitive nurses respect the patient's belief system and integrate scientifically based treatment along with folk and quasimedical practices.

CULTURALLY SENSITIVE NURSING

Accepting that Americans are multicultural is a first step toward transcultural nursing. The following recommendations are ways to demonstrate culturally sensitive nursing care:

- Learn to speak a second language.
- Use culturally sensitive techniques for improving interactions, such as sitting in the patient's comfort zone and making appropriate eye contact.

TABLE 6–4. **Leading Causes of Death Among U.S. Cultural Groups**

Rank	All Americans*	African Americans*	Latinos*	Native Americans†	Asian Americans‡
1	Heart disease	Heart disease	Heart disease	Heart disease	Heart disease
2	Cancer	Cancer	Cancer	Cancer	Cancer
3	Cerebrovascular disease	Cerebrovascular disease	Accidents	Accidents	Cerebrovascular disease
4	Chronic lung disease	HIV infection	Cerebrovascular disease	Diabetes	Accidents
5	Accidents	Accidents	HIV infection	Chronic liver disease	Pneumonia/influenza
6	Pneumonia/influenza	Diabetes	Diabetes	Cerebrovascular disease	Chronic lung disease
7	Diabetes	Homicide	Homicide	Pneumonia/influenza	Diabetes
8	HIV infection	Pneumonia/influenza	Pneumonia/influenza	Suicide	Suicide
9	Suicide	Chronic lung disease	Chronic liver disease	Homicide	Homicide
10	Chronic liver disease	Perinatal conditions	Chronic lung disease	Chronic lung disease	Congenital anomalies

* Leading causes of death, U.S. population, 1998, National Vital Statistics Report, Vol. 47, No. 9. National Center for Health Statistics (CDC)

† Leading causes of death for American Indians and Alaska Natives 1991–1993, Indian Service and National Center for Health Statistics (CDC)

‡ Monthly vital statistics report, vol. 46, No. 1 (5), National Center for Vital Statistics, CDC. August 14, 1997.

TABLE 6–5. **Common Health Beliefs and Practices**

Cultural Group	Health Belief	Health Practices
Anglo-Americans	Illness is caused by infectious microorganisms, organ degeneration, and unhealthy lifestyles.	Physicians are consulted for diagnosis and treatment; nurses provide physical care.
African Americans	Supernatural forces can cause disease and influence recovery.	Individual and group prayer is used to speed recovery.
Asian Americans	Health is the result of a balance between *yin* and *yang* energy; illness results when equilibrium is disturbed.	Acupuncture, acupressure, food, and herbs are used to restore balance.
Latinos	Illness and misfortune occur as a punishment from God, referred to as *castigo de Dios,* or they are caused by an imbalance of "hot" or "cold" forces within the body.	Prayer and penance are performed to receive forgiveness; the services of lay practitioners who are believed to possess spiritual healing power are used; foods that are "hot" or "cold" are consumed to restore balance.
Native Americans	Illness occurs when the harmony of nature (Mother Earth) is disturbed.	A *shaman,* or medicine man, who has both spiritual and healing power, is consulted to restore harmony.

- Become familiar with physical differences among ethnic groups.
- Perform physical assessments, especially of the skin, using techniques that will provide accurate data.
- Learn or ask patients about their cultural beliefs concerning health, illness, and techniques for healing.
- Consult the patient on ways to solve health problems.
- Never ridicule a cultural belief or practice, verbally or nonverbally.
- Integrate cultural practices that are helpful or harmless within the plan of care.
- Modify or gradually change practices that are unsafe.
- Avoid removing religious medals or clothes that hold symbolic meaning for the patient. If they must be removed, keep them safe and replace them as soon as possible.
- Provide food that is customarily eaten.
- Advocate that patients be routinely screened for diseases to which they are genetically or culturally prone.
- Facilitate rituals by the person the patient identifies as a healer within his or her belief system.
- Apologize if cultural traditions or beliefs are violated.

DISPLAY 6–3

Examples of Alternative Medical Therapy

- Homeopathy—Is based on the principle of similars; uses diluted herbal and medicinal substances that cause similar symptoms of a particular illness in healthy persons. Example: quinine is used to treat malaria because it causes chills, fever, and weakness (symptoms of malaria) when administered to healthy people.
- Naturopathy—Uses botanicals, nutrition, homeopathy, acupuncture, hydrotherapy, and manipulation to treat illness and restore a person to optimal balance.
- Chiropractic—Is based on the belief that illnesses and pain are the result of spinal malalignment; uses manipulations and adjustments of joint articulations, massage, and physiotherapy to correct dysfunction.
- Environmental medicine—Proposes that health, particularly in super-sensitive individuals, is affected by allergies to environmental substances in the home and workplace; advocates reduction in exposure to chemicals to control conditions that have been undiagnosed or misdiagnosed by mainstream physicians.

KEY CONCEPTS

- Culture refers to the values, beliefs, and practices of a particular group. Race refers to biologic variations. Ethnicity is the bond or kinship a person feels with his or her country of birth or place of ancestral origin.
- Two factors that interfere with perceiving others as individuals are stereotyping, which involves ascribing fixed beliefs about individuals based on some general characteristic, and ethnocentrism, the belief that one's own ethnicity is superior to all others.
- American culture is said to be Anglicized because many of the values, beliefs, and practices evolved from the early English settlers.
- Some examples of Anglo-American culture include speaking English; valuing work, time, and technology; holding parents responsible for the health care, behavior, and education of minor children; keeping government separate from religion; and seeking the assistance of licensed individuals when health care is necessary.
- A subculture is a unique cultural group that coexists within the dominant culture. There are four major subcultures living within the United States: African Americans, Latinos, Asian Americans, and Native Americans.

- Subcultural groups differ from Anglo-Americans in one or more of the following ways: language, communication style, biologic and physiologic variations, prevalence of diseases, and health beliefs and practices.
- There are four characteristics of culturally sensitive nursing care: data collection of a cultural nature, acceptance of each patient as an individual, knowledge of health problems that affect particular cultural groups, and planning care within the patient's health belief system to achieve the best health outcomes.
- Some ways that nurses can demonstrate cultural sensitivity include learning a second language, performing physical assessments and care according to the patient's unique biologic differences, consulting each patient as to his or her cultural preferences, arranging for modifications in diet and dress according to the patient's customs, and allowing patients to continue relying on cultural health practices (if they are not harmful).

CRITICAL THINKING EXERCISES

- During the Vietnam conflict, nurses cared for both American casualties and sick and wounded Vietnamese. Discuss how American nurses and their non-American patients may have experienced culture shock during this time.
- A nurse working for a home health agency is assigned to the home care of a non-English-speaking patient from Pakistan. Discuss how a culturally sensitive nurse might prepare for this patient's care.
- A pregnant Haitian woman explains to a nurse that she is wearing a chicken bone around her neck to protect her unborn child from birth defects. Discuss how it would be best to respond to this woman from a culturally sensitive perspective.

SUGGESTED READINGS

Andrews MM, Boyle JS. Transcultural concepts in nursing care, 2nd ed. Philadelphia, JB Lippincott, 1995.

Davidhizar R, Bechtel GA. Assessing the patient from a cultural perspective. Journal of Practical Nursing 1998;48(3):16–27.

Davidhizar R, Dowd SB, Bowen M. Global issues. The educational role of the surgical nurse with the multicultural patient and family. Today's Surgical Nurse 1998;20(4):20–24.

Doswell WM, Erlen JA. Multicultural issues and ethical concerns in the delivery of nursing care interventions. Nursing Clinics of North America 1998;33(2):353–361.

Dudek SG. Nutrition handbook for nursing practice, 3rd ed. Philadelphia, Lippincott-Raven, 1997.

Giger JN, Davidhizar RE. Transcultural nursing: assessment and Intervention, 2d ed. St. Louis, Mosby, 1995.

Indian Health Services, http://www.ihs.gov/, accessed June 1999.

Kavanaugh KH. Transcultural nursing: facing the challenges of advocacy and diversity/universality. Journal of Transcultural Nursing 1993;5:4–13.

Leininger M. Major directions for transcultural nursing: a journey into the 21st century. Journal of Transcultural Nursing 1996;7(2):28–31.

Lester N. Cultural competence: a nursing dialogue, part one. American Journal of Nursing 1998;98(8):26–34.

Lester N. Cultural competence: a nursing dialogue, part two. American Journal of Nursing 1998;98(9):36–43.

Lipson JG, Dibble SL, Minarik PA. Culture and nursing care: a nursing guide. San Francisco, UCSF Nursing Press, 1996.

National Clearinghouse for Alcohol and Drug Information. Prevalence of substance use among racial and ethnic subgroups in the United States, 1991–1993. Substance Abuse & Mental Health Services Administration, 1993.

Perkins J, Simon H, Cheng F, Olson K, Vera Y. Ensuring linguistic access in health care settings: legal rights and responsibilities. National Health Law Program, http://www.healthlaw.org/lingexecsumm.html, accessed 12/21/98.

Polaschek NR. Cultural safety: a new concept in nursing people of different ethnicities. Journal of Advanced Nursing 1998;27(3):452–457.

Rosenbaum JN. Leininger's theory of culture care diversity and universality: transcultural critique. Journal of Multicultural Nursing & Health 1997;3(3):24–36.

Spector RE. Cultural diversity in health and illness, 4th ed. East Norwalk: Appleton & Lange, 1996

Uema J. Insights on death and dying. Pain management: worlds apart. Nursing 1998;28(9):20–22.

U.S. Bureau of the Census. General population characteristics. Washington DC, U.S. Government Printing Office, 1994.

Wilson UM. Nursing care of American Indian patients. In MS Orgue, B Block, LSA Monrroy, eds. Ethnic nursing care: a multicultural approach. St. Louis, Mosby, 1983:271–295.

Wing DM. A comparison of traditional folk healing concepts with contemporary healing concepts. Journal of Community Health Nursing 1998;15(3):143–154.

Zborowski M. Cultural components in responses to pain. Journal of Social Issues 1952;8:16–30.

Zborowski M. People in pain. San Francisco, Jossey Bass, 1969.

UNIT THREE

FOSTERING COMMUNICATION

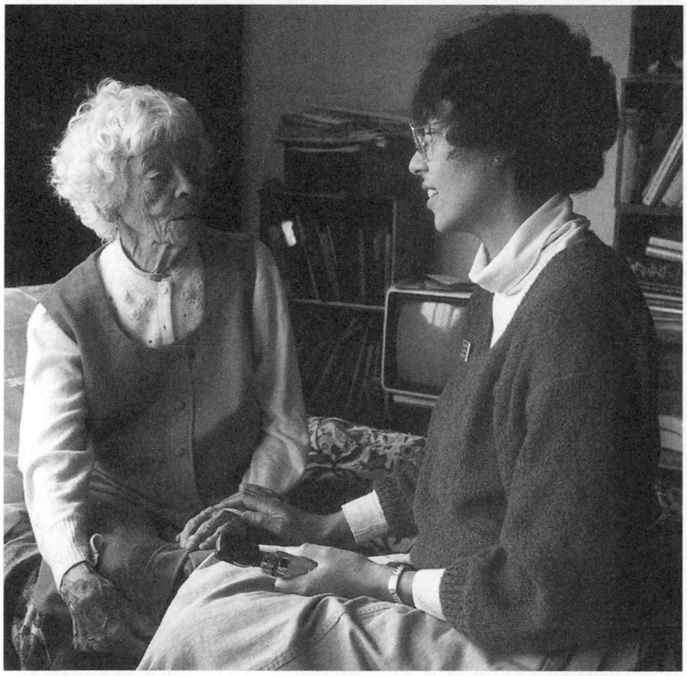

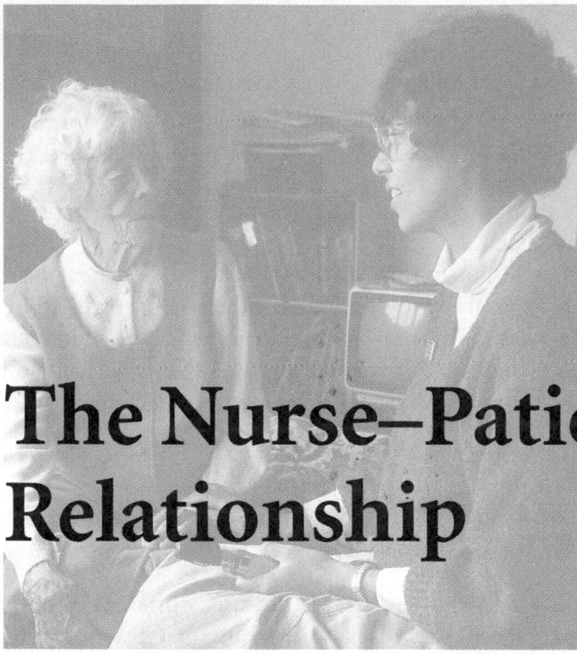

CHAPTER 7

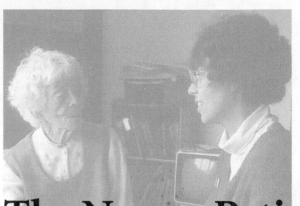

The Nurse–Patient Relationship

CHAPTER OUTLINE

KEY TERMS

affective touch
communication
intimate space
introductory phase
kinesics
nonverbal communication
paralanguage
personal space
proxemics
public space
relationship
silence
social space
task-related touch
terminating phase
therapeutic verbal communication
touch
verbal communication
working phase

LEARNING OBJECTIVES

An understanding of the content within this chapter will be evidenced by the student's ability to:

- Describe the current role expectations for patients.
- List at least five principles that form the basis of a nurse–patient relationship.
- Identify the three phases of a nurse–patient relationship.
- Differentiate between social communication and therapeutic verbal communication.
- Give five examples of therapeutic and nontherapeutic communication techniques.
- List at least five factors that affect oral communication.
- Describe the four forms of nonverbal communication.
- Differentiate task-related touch from affective touch.
- List at least five situations in which affective touch may be appropriate.

Nurses provide services, or skills, that assist individuals, called patients or clients, to resolve health problems that are beyond their own capabilities or to cope with those that will not improve. There are several differences between the services that nurses provide and those provided by other caring people (Display 7-1).

An intangible factor that helps place nurses in high regard is the relationship that develops between nurses and patients. One of the primary keys to establishing and maintaining a positive nurse–patient relationship is the manner and style of a nurse's communication.

The Nurse–Patient Relationship

A **relationship** (association between two people) is established between the nurse and patient when nursing services are provided. The nurse–patient relationship could also be called a therapeutic relationship, because the desired outcome of the association is almost always one of moving toward a goal of restored health. A therapeutic relationship differs from a social relationship. A therapeutic relationship is patient-centered, with a focus on goal achievement. It is also time-limited: the relationship ends when the goals are achieved.

The relationship between nurses and patients has gradually changed. In the past, patients were expected to play a passive role, allow others to make decisions for them, and submit to treatments without question or protest. Nurses now encourage and expect persons for whom they care to become actively involved, to communicate, to question, to assist in planning their care, and to retain as much independence as possible (Display 7-2).

DISPLAY 7-1

Differentiating Caring Acts From Nursing Acts

Caring Acts	Nursing Acts
Prompted by observing a person in distress	Prompted by a concern for the well-being of everyone
Motivated by sympathy	Motivated by altruism
Spontaneous	Planned
Goal is to relieve crisis	Goal is to promote self-reliance
Outcomes are short-term	Outcomes are long-term
Assume major responsibility for resolving the person's problem	Expect mutual cooperation in resolving health problems
Experience-based	Knowledge-based
Modeled on a personal moral code	Modeled on a formal code of ethics
Guided by common sense	Legally defined
Accountability based on acting reasonably prudent	Accountability based on meeting professional standards

UNDERLYING PRINCIPLES

A therapeutic nurse–patient relationship is more likely to develop when the nurse:

- Treats each patient as a unique person
- Respects the patient's feelings
- Strives to promote the patient's physical, emotional, social, and spiritual well-being
- Encourages the patient to participate in problem solving and decision making
- Accepts that a patient has the potential for growth and change
- Communicates using terms and language the patient understands
- Uses the nursing process to individualize the patient's care
- Incorporates people to whom the patient turns to for support, such as family and friends, when providing care
- Implements health care techniques that are compatible with the patient's value system and cultural heritage

DISPLAY 7-2

Responsibilities Within the Nurse–Patient Relationship

Nursing Responsibilities	Patient Responsibilities
Possess current knowledge	Identify current problem
Be aware of unique age-related differences	Describe desired outcomes
Perform technical skills safely	Answer questions honestly
Be committed to patient care	Provide accurate historical and subjective data
Be available and courteous	Participate to fullest extent possible
Allow participation in decisions	Be open and flexible to alternatives
Remain objective	Comply with the plan for care
Advocate on the patient's behalf	Keep appointments for follow-up care
Provide explanations in language that is easily understood	
Promote independence	

PHASES OF THE NURSE–PATIENT RELATIONSHIP

Nurse–patient relationships are ordinarily brief. They begin when people seek services that will maintain or restore health, or prevent disease. They end when patients can achieve their health-related goals independently. This type of relationship is generally described as having three phases: the introductory phase, the working phase, and the terminating phase.

Introductory Phase

The relationship between the patient and the nurse begins with the **introductory phase** (period of getting acquainted). Each person usually brings preconceived ideas about the other to the initial interaction. These assumptions are eventually either confirmed or dismissed.

The patient initiates the relationship by identifying one or more health problems for which help is being sought. It is important for the nurse to demonstrate courtesy, active listening, empathy, competency, and appropriate communication skills to ensure that the relationship begins positively.

Working Phase

The **working phase** involves mutually planning the patient's care and putting the plan into action. Both the nurse and the patient participate. Each shares in performing those tasks that will lead to the desired outcomes identified by the patient. During the working phase, the nurse tries not to retard the patient's independence: doing too much can be as harmful as doing too little.

Terminating Phase

The nurse–patient relationship is self-limiting. The **terminating phase** occurs when there is mutual agreement that the patient's immediate health problems have improved. The nurse uses a caring attitude and compassion in facilitating the patient's transition of care to other health care services or independent living.

BARRIERS TO A THERAPEUTIC RELATIONSHIP

It is impossible to develop positive relationships with every patient; Display 7-3 lists examples of behaviors that are likely to interfere. The best approach is to treat patients in the manner one would like to be treated.

DISPLAY 7-3

Barriers to a Nurse–Patient Relationship

- Appearing unkempt: long hair that dangles on or over the patient during care, offensive body or breath odor, wrinkled or soiled uniform, dirty shoes
- Failing to identify oneself verbally and with a name tag
- Mispronouncing or avoiding the patient's name
- Using the patient's first name without permission
- Showing disinterest in the patient's personal history and life experiences
- Sharing personal or work-related problems with the patient or with staff in the presence of the patient
- Using crude or distasteful language
- Revealing confidential information or gossip about other patients, staff, or people known in common
- Focusing on nursing tasks rather than the patient's responses
- Being inattentive to the patient's requests (such as for food, pain relief, assistance with toileting, bathing)
- Abandoning the patient at stressful or emotional times
- Failing to keep promises, such as consulting with the physician about a current need or request
- Going on a break or to lunch without keeping the patient informed and identifying who has been delegated for the patient's care during the temporary absence

Communication

Communication (exchange of information) involves both sending and receiving messages between two or more people, followed by feedback indicating that the information was understood or requires further clarification (Fig. 7-1).

Communication takes place simultaneously on a verbal and nonverbal level. Because no relationship can exist without verbal and nonverbal communication, nurses must develop skills that enhance their therapeutic interactions with patients.

VERBAL COMMUNICATION

Verbal communication (communication that uses words) includes speaking, reading, and writing. Verbal communication is used by both the nurse and patient to gather facts. It is also used to instruct, clarify, and exchange ideas.

The ability to communicate orally or in writing is affected by:

- Attention and concentration
- Language compatibility
- Verbal skills
- Hearing and visual acuity
- Motor functions involving the throat, tongue, and teeth
- Sensory distractions

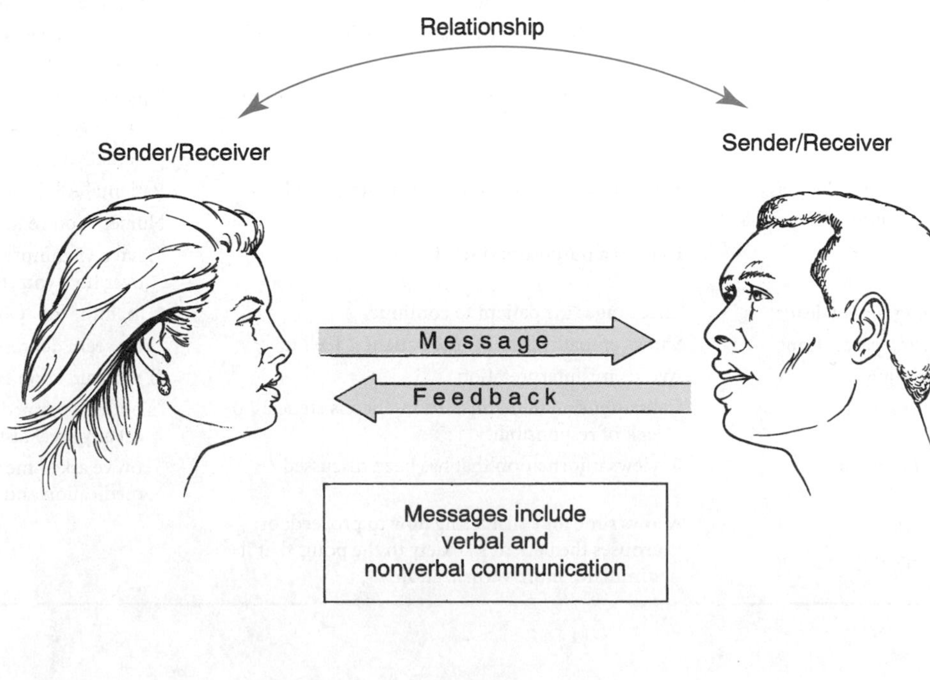

FIGURE 7–1. Communication is a two-way process between a sender and a receiver.

- Interpersonal attitudes
- Literacy
- Cultural similarities

The nurse promotes the factors that enhance the communication of verbal content and controls or eliminates those that interfere with the accurate perception of expressed ideas.

THERAPEUTIC VERBAL COMMUNICATION

Communication can take place on a social or therapeutic level. Social communication is superficial; it includes common courtesies and exchanges about general topics. **Therapeutic verbal communication** (using words and gestures to accomplish a particular objective) is extremely important, especially when the nurse is exploring problems with the patient or encouraging the expression of feelings. Techniques that the nurse may find helpful are described in Table 7-1.

The nurse must never assume that a quiet, uncommunicative patient has no problems or understands everything. It is never appropriate to probe and pry; rather, it may be advantageous to wait and be patient. It is not unusual for reticent patients to share their feelings and concerns after they decide the nurse is sincere and trustworthy.

Vocal, emotional patients must also be handled delicately. For instance, when patients are angry or crying, the best nursing approach is to allow them to express their emotions. Allowing patients to display their feelings without fear of retaliation or censure contributes to a therapeutic relationship.

Although nurses often have the best intentions of interacting therapeutically with patients, some fall into traps that block or hinder verbal communication. Table 7-2 lists common examples of nontherapeutic communication.

LISTENING

Listening is as important during communication as speaking. Giving attention to what patients say provides a stimulus for meaningful interaction. It is important to avoid giving signals that indicate boredom, impatience, or the pretense of listening. For example, looking out a window or interrupting is a sign of disinterest. When communicating with most Americans, it is best to position oneself at the person's level and make frequent eye contact (Fig. 7-2). Refer to Chapter 6 for cultural exceptions. Nodding and making comments such as, "Yes, I see," encourages the patient to continue and shows full involvement in what is being said.

TABLE 7–1. **Therapeutic Verbal Communication Techniques**

Technique	Use	Example
Broad openings	Relieves tension before getting to the real purpose of the interaction	"Wonderful weather we're having."
Giving information	Provides facts	"Your surgery is scheduled at noon."
Direct questioning	Acquires specific information	"Do you have any allergies?"
Open-ended questioning	Encourages the patient to elaborate	"How are you feeling?"
Reflecting	Confirms that the conversation is being followed	Patient: "I haven't been sleeping well." Nurse: "You haven't been sleeping well."
Paraphrasing	Restates what the patient has said to demonstrate listening	Patient: "After every meal, I feel like I will throw up." Nurse: "Eating makes you nauseous, but you don't actually vomit."
Verbalizing what has been implied	Shares how a statement has been interpreted	Patient: "All the nurses are so busy." Nurse: "You're feeling that you shouldn't ask for help."
Structuring	Defines a purpose and sets limits	"I have 15 minutes. If your pain is relieved, I could go over how your test will be done."
Giving general leads	Encourages the patient to continue	"Uh, huh," or "Go on."
Sharing perceptions	Shows empathy for how the patient is feeling	"You seem depressed."
Clarifying	Avoids misinterpretation	"I'm afraid I don't quite understand what you're asking."
Confronting	Calls attention to manipulation, inconsistencies, or lack of responsibility	"You're concerned about your weight loss, but you didn't eat any breakfast."
Summarizing	Reviews information that has been discussed	"You've asked me to check on increasing your pain medication and getting your diet changed."
Silence	Allows time for considering how to proceed; or, arouses the patient's anxiety to the point that it stimulates more verbalization	

TABLE 7–2. **Nontherapeutic Communication Techniques**

Technique and Consequence	Example	Improvement
Giving False Reassurance		
Trivializes the unique feelings of the patient and discourages further discussion	"You've got nothing to worry about. Everything will work out just fine."	"Tell me about your specific concerns."
Using Clichés		
Provides worthless advice and curtails exploring alternatives	"Keep a stiff upper lip."	"It must be difficult for you right now."
Giving Approval or Disapproval		
Holds the patient to a rigid standard; implies that future deviation may lead to subsequent rejection or disfavor	"I'm glad you're exercising so regularly."	"Are you having any difficulty fitting regular exercise into your schedule?"
	"You should be testing your blood sugar each morning."	"Let's explore some ways that will help you test your blood sugar each morning."
Agreeing		
Does not allow the patient flexibility to change his or her mind	"You're right about needing surgery immediately."	"Having surgery immediately is one possibility. What others have you considered?"
Disagreeing		
Intimidates the patient; makes the patient feel foolish or inadequate	"That's not true! Where did you get an idea like that?"	"Maybe I can help clarify that for you."
Demanding an Explanation		
Puts the patient on the defensive; the patient may be tempted to make up an excuse rather than risk disapproval for an honest answer	"Why didn't you keep your appointment last week?"	"I see you couldn't keep your appointment last week."
Giving Advice		
Discourages independent problem solving and decision making; provides a biased view that may prejudice the patient's choice	"If I were you, I'd try drug therapy before having surgery."	"Share with me the advantages and disadvantages of your options as you see them."
Defending		
Indicates such a strong allegiance that any disagreement to the contrary is not acceptable	"Ms. Johnson is my best nursing assistant. She wouldn't have let your light go unanswered that long."	"I'm sorry you had to wait so long."
Belittling		
Disregards how the patient is responding as an individual	"Lots of people learn to give themselves insulin."	"You're finding it especially difficult to stick yourself with a needle."
Patronizing		
Treats the patient in a condescending manner as less than capable of making an independent decision	"Are *we* ready for *our* bath yet?"	"Would you like your bath now, or should I check with you later?"
Changing the Subject		
Alters the direction of the discussion to a topic that is safer or more comfortable	Patient: "I'm so scared that a mammogram will show I have cancer."	
	Nurse: "Tell me more about your family."	"It is a serious disease. What concerns you the most?"

SILENCE

Silence (intentionally withholding verbal commentary) plays an important role in communication. At first glance, it may seem contradictory to include silence as a form of verbal communication. However, one of its uses is to encourage the patient to participate in verbal discussions. Other therapeutic uses for silence include relieving a patient's anxiety just by providing a personal presence and providing a brief period of time during which patients can process information or respond to a question.

Patients may use silence to camouflage their fears or to express contentment. Silence also is used for introspection when we need to explore feelings or when we pray. Interrupting someone who is deep in concentration disturbs the thinking process. A common obstacle to effective communi-

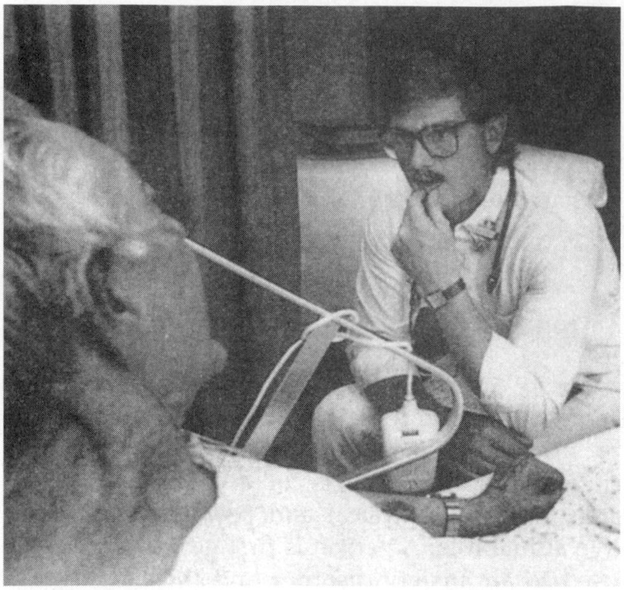

FIGURE 7–2. Appropriate positioning, space, eye contact, and attention promote therapeutic communication. (Courtesy of Susan Weaver, Bay Health Systems.)

cation is ignoring the importance of silence and talking excessively.

NONVERBAL COMMUNICATION

Nonverbal communication (exchange of information without using words) involves what is *not* said. The manner in which verbal information is conveyed affects its meaning. A person has less control over nonverbal than verbal communication. Words can be chosen with care, but a facial expression is harder to control. As a result, messages are often communicated more accurately through nonverbal communication.

People communicate nonverbally through techniques described as kinesics, paralanguage, proxemics, and touch.

Kinesics

Kinesics (body language) includes nonverbal techniques such as facial expressions, posture, gestures, and body movements. Some add that clothing style and accessories such as jewelry also affect the context of communication.

Paralanguage

Paralanguage (vocal sounds that are not actually words) also communicates a message. Some examples include drawing in a deep breath to indicate surprise, clucking the tongue to indicate disappointment, and whistling to get someone's attention. Vocal inflections, volume, pitch, and rate of speech also add another dimension to communication. Crying, laughing, and moaning are additional forms of paralanguage.

Proxemics

Proxemics (use and relationship of space to communication) varies among people from different cultural backgrounds. Generally, there are four zones that are observed in interactions between Americans (Hall, 1959, 1963, 1966): **intimate space** (within 6 inches), **personal space** (6 inches to 4 feet), **social space** (4 to 12 feet), and **public space** (more than 12 feet; Table 7-3).

Most Americans comfortably tolerate strangers in a 2- to 3-foot area. Venturing closer may cause some to feel anxious. Understanding the patient's comfort zone helps the nurse know how spatial relations affect nonverbal communication.

Closeness is common in nursing because of the many times nurses and patients are in direct physical contact. Therefore, physical nearness and touching within intimate and personal spaces can be misinterpreted by some as having sexual connotations. Approaches that may prevent such misunderstanding include explaining beforehand how a nursing procedure will be performed, ensuring that the patient is properly draped, and asking that another staff person of the patient's gender be present during an examination or procedure.

Touch

Touch (tactile stimulus produced by making personal contact with another person or object) occurs frequently in nurse–patient relationships. While caring for patients, touch

TABLE 7–3. **Communication Zones**

Zone	Distance	Purpose
Intimate space	Within 6 inches	• Lovemaking • Confiding secrets • Sharing confidential information
Personal space	6 inches to 4 feet	• Interviewing • Physical assessment • Therapeutic interventions involving touch • Private conversations • Teaching one-on-one
Social space	4 to 12 feet	• Group interactions • Lecturing • Conversations that are not intended to be private
Public space	12 or more feet	• Giving speeches • Gatherings of strangers

can be task-oriented, affective, or both (Burnside, 1988; Brady and Nesbitt, 1991). **Task-oriented touch** involves the personal contact that is required when performing nursing procedures (Fig. 7-3). **Affective touch** is used to demonstrate concern or affection (Fig. 7-4).

Affective touch has different meanings to different people, depending on their upbringing and their cultural background. Because nursing care involves a high degree of touching, the nurse must be sensitive to how it is perceived. Most people respond positively to being touched, but there may be a great deal of variation among individuals. Therefore, affective touching must be used cautiously, even though its intention is to communicate caring and support. In general, affective touch is therapeutic when a patient is:

- Lonely
- Uncomfortable
- Near death
- Anxious, insecure, or frightened
- Disoriented
- Disfigured
- Semiconscious or comatose
- Visually impaired
- Sensory deprived

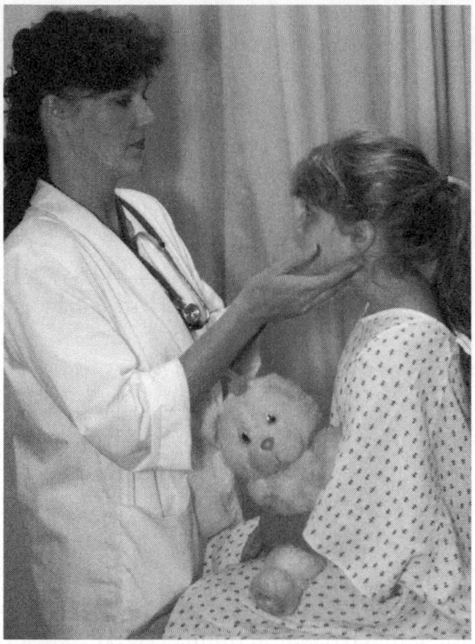

FIGURE 7–3. Examining a patient involves task-oriented touch. (Courtesy of Ken Timby.)

FOCUS ON OLDER ADULTS

- Begin initial contacts with an exchange of names and, if appropriate, a handshake.
- Before calling a person by his or her first name, obtain permission or wait until being invited to use a more familiar form of address, which is reserved for family and close friends in some cultures.
- Never treat older adults as if they are children; avoid using any terms that are demeaning or connote childlike or infantile behavior or actions, for example, remarks such as "He acts just like a baby," and references to incontinence products as diapers.
- Use touch purposefully as a primary method of nonverbal communication and to reinforce verbal messages; recognize that touch as a form of communication is usually more important to older adults than to younger adults.
- Sit in a face-to-face position, provide good lighting while avoiding background glare, and eliminate as much background noise as possible.
- Promote as much control over decisions and choices as possible. Dependence is often difficult to accept; independence maintains self-esteem and dignity.
- Allow older adults to pace their own care and maintain as much independence as possible, even when this requires more time.
- Encourage reminiscing; ask about past events and relationships that are associated with positive experiences and feelings. Giving older adults an opportunity to talk about earlier times in their lives reinforces their value and unique identity.
- Be aware of subtle verbal messages that convey bias or inequality; for example, calling white men "Mister" but men of color by their first names.
- Avoid addressing older adults in familiar terms such as "Dear," "Grandma," or "Pop," unless the older adult suggests it.

KEY CONCEPTS

- Patients are expected to be actively involved in their care, to communicate, to ask questions, to assist in planning their care, and above all to retain as much independence as possible
- Some principles underlying a therapeutic nurse–patient relationship include treating each patient as a unique person; respecting the patient's feelings; striving to promote the patient's physical, emotional, social, and spiritual well-being; encouraging the patient to participate

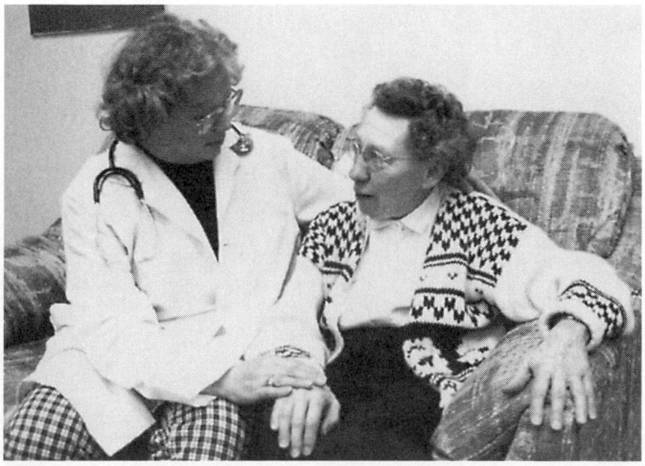

FIGURE 7–4. This nurse uses affective touch as she talks with her homebound patient. (Courtesy of Ken Timby.)

in problem solving and decision making; and accepting that a patient has the potential for growth and change.

- A nurse–patient relationship usually encompasses three phases: the introductory phase, the working phase, and the termination phase.
- Communication involves sending and receiving messages between two or more people, followed by feedback indicating that the information was understood or requires further clarification. Therapeutic communication refers to using words and gestures to accomplish a particular objective.
- Examples of therapeutic verbal communication techniques include questioning, reflecting, paraphrasing, sharing perceptions, and clarifying. Examples of nontherapeutic communication techniques include giving false reassurance, using clichés, giving approval or disapproval, demanding an explanation, and giving advice.
- Some factors that may affect oral communication include language compatibility; verbal skills; hearing and visual acuity; motor functions involving the throat, tongue, and teeth; sensory distractions; and interpersonal attitudes.
- There are four forms of nonverbal communication: kinesics (body language), paralanguage (vocal sounds), proxemics (how space is used in communication), and touch.
- Task-related touch involves the personal contact that is required when performing nursing procedures. Affective touch is used to demonstrate concern or affection.
- There are many situations in which affective touch is appropriate. Some include when caring for patients who are lonely, uncomfortable, near death, or anxious and those with sensory deprivation.

CRITICAL THINKING EXERCISES

- Because nursing is a service-oriented profession, what specific services might a person expect from a nurse that would be different from those expected in a relationship with a physician?
- It has been observed that older adults are not touched with the same frequency as patients in other age groups. Discuss reasons for this.

SELECTED READINGS

Advice prn: nurse/patient relationship: grist for gossip. Nursing 1998; 28(1):12.

Alavi C, Cattoni J. Good nurse, bad nurse. Journal of Advanced Nursing 1995;21:344–349.

Ausdenmoore MM. A touching moment ... healing touch. Nursing 1998;28(4):32–36.

Bischko D. Tips, tools, and techniques. The art of nursing: the client-nurse relationship as a therapeutic tool. Nursing Case Management 1998;3(4):148–150.

Brady BA, Nesbitt SN. Using the right touch. Nursing 1991;21(5):46–47.

Burnside I. Nursing and the aged, 3rd ed. St. Louis, Mosby, 1988.

Davidhizar R, Giger JN. When touch is not the best approach. Journal of Clinical Nursing 1997;6(3):203–206.

Hall ET. The silent language. New York, Fawcett, 1959.

Hall ET. A system for the notation of proxemic behavior. American Anthropologist 1963;65(3):1003–1026.

Hall ET. The hidden dimension. New York, Doubleday, 1966.

Hoffman MJ. Therapeutic touch is back. Caring 1998;17(4):26–30.

Lomax B. Learning to understand a patient's silence. Nursing Times 1997;93(17):48–49.

Meehan TC. Therapeutic touch as a nursing intervention. Journal of Advanced Nursing 1998;28(1):117–125.

Sears M. Relationship. Using therapeutic communication to connect with others. Home Healthcare Nurse 1998;14(8):614–617.

Shafer P. When a client develops an attraction: successful resolution versus boundary violation. Journal of Psychiatric and Mental Health Nursing 1997;4(3):203–211.

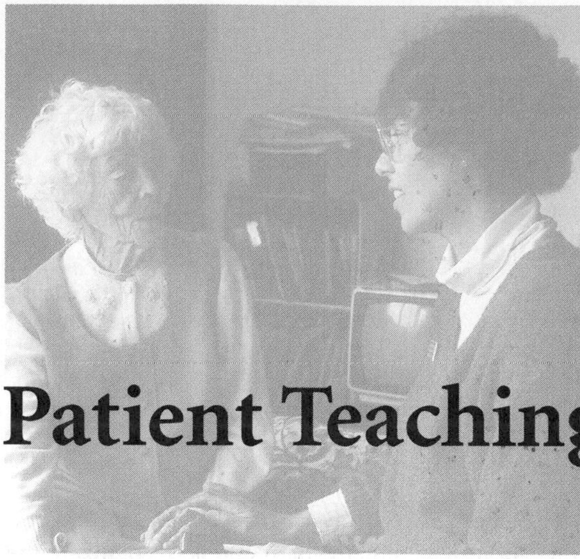

CHAPTER 8

Patient Teaching

CHAPTER OUTLINE

Patient Teaching
Assessing the Learner
Informal and Formal Teaching

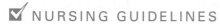

☑ NURSING GUIDELINES

TEACHING PATIENTS WITH SENSORY IMPAIRMENTS
TEACHING ADULT PATIENTS

KEY TERMS

affective domain
androgogy
cognitive domain
functionally illiterate
gerogogy
illiterate
literacy
pedagogy
psychomotor domain

LEARNING OBJECTIVES

An understanding of the content within this chapter will be evidenced by the student's ability to:

- Describe the three domains of learning styles.
- Discuss three age-related categories of learners.
- Discuss at least five characteristics that are unique to older adult learners.
- Identify at least four factors that are assessed before teaching patients.

One of the most important nursing uses for communication is patient teaching. Health teaching promotes the patient's independent ability to meet his or her own health needs. An old proverb that reinforces how education promotes self-care says, "Give a man a fish and he will eat for a day; teach a man to fish and he will eat for a lifetime."

Patient Teaching

Health teaching is no longer an optional nursing activity. State nurse practice acts require it, and it is a criteria for accreditation by the Joint Commission on Accreditation of Healthcare Organizations. Patient teaching is likewise addressed in the American Nurses Association's *Social Policy Statement* (Display 8-1).

If teaching standards are not met, nurses are at risk for being sued if discharged patients are readmitted or harmed because they were uninformed or failed to understand the information that was taught. The best proof of compliance with teaching standards is to include in the patient's medical record who was taught, what was taught, the method of teaching, and the evidence that learning took place. Teaching generally includes combinations from the following subject areas:

- Self-administration of medications
- Directions and practice in using equipment for self-care
- Dietary instructions
- Rehabilitation program
- Available community resources
- Plan for medical follow-up
- Signs of complications and actions to take

Limited hospitalization time demands that nurses begin teaching as soon as possible after admission rather than waiting until discharge.

Assessing the Learner

To implement effective teaching, the nurse must determine the patient's:

- Preferred learning style
- Age and developmental level
- Capacity to learn

DISPLAY 8-1

Social Policy Statement Regarding Teaching

The nature of the (nurse–patient) relationship therefore allows the nurse to assist people effectively, whether giving physical care, providing emotional support, *engaging in health teaching or counseling,* or assisting recovery or a peaceful death.

Excerpted and reprinted with permission from American Nurses Association. Social policy statement. Washington DC, ANA, 1995:10.

- Motivation
- Learning readiness
- Learning needs

LEARNING STYLES

A style of learning refers to the manner in which a person prefers to acquire knowledge. Learning styles include three general domains: cognitive, affective, and psychomotor. The **cognitive domain** (style of processing information by listening or reading facts and descriptions) is illustrated in Figure 8-1. The **affective domain** (learning by appealing to a person's feelings, beliefs, or values) and the **psychomotor domain** (learning by doing) are the other two components of the triad. Display 8-2 lists some activities that are associated with each of the learning domains.

One way to determine the patient's preferred learning style is to ask a question such as, "When you learned to add fractions, what helped you most: hearing the teacher's explanation or reading about it in a mathematics book, recognizing the value of the exercise, or actually working sample problems?"

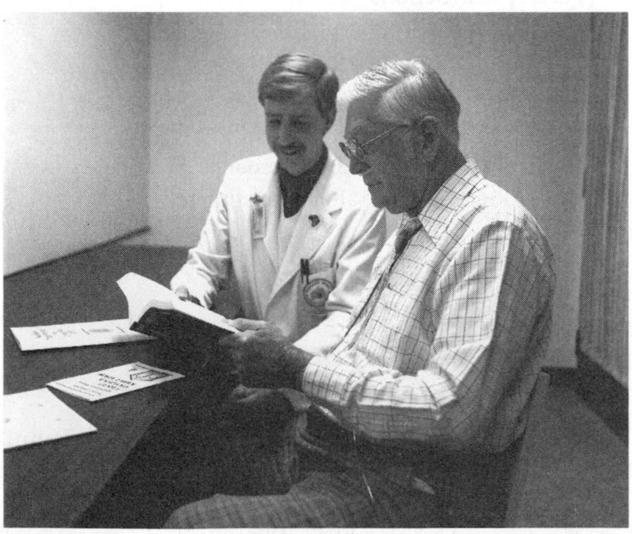

FIGURE 8–1. The nurse uses pamphlets and a book, which appeal to this patient who prefers the cognitive domain of learning. (Courtesy of McLaren Regional Medical Center, Flint, MI.)

DISPLAY 8-2

Activities that Promote Learning

Cognitive Domain	Psychomotor Domain	Affective Domain
Listing	Assembling	Advocating
Identifying	Changing	Supporting
Locating	Emptying	Accepting
Labeling	Filling	Promoting
Summarizing	Adding	Refusing
Selecting	Removing	Defending

Although most favor one domain, learning tends to be optimized by presenting information through a combination of teaching approaches. This is evidenced by the fact that "learners retain 10% of what they read, 20% of what they hear, 30% of what they see, 50% of what they see and hear, 70% of what they teach/talk, and 90% of what they talk/do" (Heinrich et al., 1992; Rega, 1993).

AGE AND DEVELOPMENTAL DIFFERENCES

Educators emphasize that learning takes place differently depending on a person's age and developmental level. Experts agree that teaching tends to be more effective when it is designed to accommodate unique age-related differences. Recently a distinction has been made between learners at the early and later ends of the adult spectrum. Currently there are three major categories:

- **Pedagogy** (science of teaching children or those who have comparable cognitive ability)
- **Androgogy** (principles of teaching adult learners)
- **Gerogogy** (techniques that enhance learning among older adults)

Nurses and anyone else who provides instruction must be aware of the learning characteristics of children, adult, and older adult learners (Table 8-1). Although most patients with health problems are in their geriatric years, nurse educators are advised to prepare themselves for teaching young adults who belong to "Generation X" as they age. Generation Xers are those born between 1961 and 1981; they have been greatly affected by technology and imposed independence as a consequence of growing up in a single-parent household or one in which both parents worked. In general, Generation Xers have the following learning characteristics:

- They are technologically literate, having grown up with computers.

TABLE 8–1. **Age-Related Differences Among Learners***

Pedagogic Learners	Androgogic Learners	Gerogogic Learners
Physically immature	Physically mature	Undergoing degenerative changes
Lack experience	Building experience	Vast experience
Compulsory learners	Voluntary learners	Crisis learners
Passive	Active	Passive/active
Need direction and supervision	Self-directed and independent	Need structure and encouragement
Motivated to learn by potential rewards or punishment	Seek knowledge for its own sake or personal interest	Motivated by a personal need or goal
Learning is subject-centered	Learning is problem-centered	Learning is self-centered
Short attention span	Longer attention span	Attention affected by low energy level, fatigue, and anxiety
Convergent thinkers (uni-directional; *eg*, see one application for new information)	Divergent thinkers (process multiple applications for new information)	Practical thinkers (process new information as it applies to a unique personal problem)
Need immediate feedback	Can postpone feedback	Respond to frequent feedback
Rote learning	Analytical learning	Experiential learning
Short-term retention	Long-term retention	Short-term unless reinforced by immediate use
Task-oriented	Goal-oriented	Outcome-oriented
Think concretely	Think abstractly	Concrete/abstract
Respond to competition	Respond to collaboration	Respond to family encouragement

*Each learner is unique and may demonstrate characteristics associated with other age groups.

- They crave stimulation and a quick response time.
- They expect immediate answers and feedback.
- They become bored with memorizing information and doing repetitious tasks.
- They like a variety of instructional methods from which they can choose.
- They respond best when they find the information to be relevant.

CAPACITY TO LEARN

For the person to receive, remember, analyze, and apply new information, a certain amount of intellectual ability must exist. Illiteracy, sensory deficits, cultural differences, a shortened attention span, and lack of motivation and readiness require special adaptations when implementing health teaching.

Literacy

It is essential to determine a patient's level of **literacy** (ability to read and write) before developing a teaching plan. Approximately 21% of American adults are **illiterate** (unable to read or write) (Davis et al., 1998). An additional 27% are considered **functionally illiterate** (possess minimal literacy skills), which means they can sign their name and can perform simple mathematical tasks (such as making change), and read at or below a ninth-grade level. Functional illiteracy may be the consequence of a learning disability, not a below-average intellectual capacity.

Because many illiterate or functionally illiterate people are not apt to volunteer this information, literacy may be difficult to assess. Those who are illiterate and functionally illiterate usually develop elaborate mechanisms to disguise or compensate for their learning deficits. To protect the patient's self-esteem, the nurse can ask, "How do you learn best?" and plan accordingly. Some approaches that are useful when teaching patients who are illiterate or functionally illiterate include:

- Using verbal and visual modes for instruction
- Repeating directions several times in the same sequence so the patient can memorize the information
- Providing pictures, diagrams, or audiotapes for future review

Sensory Deficits

The abilities to see and hear are essential to almost every learning situation. Older adults tend to have visual and auditory deficits, although such deficits are not exclusive to this population. Some techniques for teaching patients with sensory impairment follow.

Nursing Guidelines For

Teaching Patients with Sensory Impairments

- ☑ Make sure the patient with visual impairment is wearing prescription eyeglasses, and the hearing-impaired patient is wearing a hearing aid, if available.
  RATIONALE: Visual and auditory aids maximize the ability to perceive sensory stimuli.

For the visually impaired patient:

- ☑ Speak in a normal tone of voice.
  RATIONALE: A visually impaired patient is not necessarily hearing-impaired. Increasing volume does not compensate for reduced vision.
- ☑ Use at least a 75-to 100-watt light source, preferably in a lamp that shines over the patient's shoulder.
  RATIONALE: Ceiling lights tend to diffuse light rather than concentrate it on a small area where the patient needs to focus.
- ☑ Avoid standing in front of a window through which bright sunlight is shining.
  RATIONALE: It is difficult to look into bright light.
- ☑ Provide a magnifying glass for reading.
  RATIONALE: Magnification enlarges standard or small print to a size that is comfortable to read.
- ☑ Obtain pamphlets in large size (12- to 16-point) print and serif lettering, which has horizontal lines at the bottom and top of each letter (Fig. 8-2).
  RATIONALE: Letters and words are usually more distinct when they are set in large print with a type style that promotes visual discrimination.
- ☑ Avoid using materials printed on glossy paper.
  RATIONALE: Glossy paper reflects light, causing a glare that makes reading uncomfortable.
- ☑ Select black print on white paper.
  RATIONALE: Black print on white provides maximum contrast and makes the letters more legible.

For the hearing-impaired patient:

- ☑ Use a magic slate, chalk board, flash cards, and writing pads to communicate.
  RATIONALE: Writing can be substituted for verbal instructions.
- ☑ Lower the voice pitch.
  RATIONALE: Hearing loss is generally in the higher-pitch ranges.
- ☑ Try to select words that do not begin with "f," "s," "k," and "sh."
  RATIONALE: These letters are formed with high-pitched sounds and are therefore difficult for the hearing-impaired person to discriminate.
- ☑ Rephrase rather than repeat when the patient does not understand.
  RATIONALE: Rephrasing may provide additional visual or auditory clues to facilitate the patient's understanding.
- ☑ Insert a stethoscope into the patient's ears and speak into the bell with a low voice.
  RATIONALE: The stethoscope acts as a primitive hearing aid. It directs sounds directly to the ears and reduces background noise.

12 pt. Times

Aa Bb Cc Dd Ee Ff Gg Hh Ii Jj Kk Ll
Oo Pp Qq Rr Ss Tt Uu Vv Ww Xx Yy

14 pt. Times

Aa Bb Cc Dd Ee Ff Gg Hh Ii Jj Kk
Oo Pp Qq Rr Ss Tt Uu Vv Ww Xx

16 pt. Times

Aa Bb Cc Dd Ee Ff
Oo Pp Qq Rr Ss Tt

FIGURE 8–2. Selecting printed materials with 12- to 16-point size type, black print on white paper, and serif lettering helps to improve visual clarity.

Cultural Differences

Because teaching and learning involve language, the nurse must modify teaching approaches if the patient cannot speak English or if English is a second language (see Chap. 6, Nursing Guidelines for Communicating with Non–English-Speaking Patients). Language barriers do not justify omitting health teaching. In most cases, if neither the nurse nor the patient speaks a compatible language, a translator is used.

Attention and Concentration

The patient's attention and concentration affect the duration, delivery, and teaching methods that are employed. Some approaches that are helpful include the following:

- Observe the patient, and implement health teaching when he or she is most alert and comfortable.
- Keep the teaching session short.
- Use the patient's name frequently throughout the instructional period; this refocuses his or her attention.
- Show enthusiasm, which is likely to be communicated to the patient.
- Use colorful materials, gestures, and variety to stimulate the patient.
- Involve the patient in an active way.
- Vary the tone and pitch of voice to stimulate the patient aurally.

MOTIVATION

Optimal learning takes place when a person has a purpose for acquiring new information. The relevance for learning is also an individual variable. The desire for learning may be to satisfy intellectual curiosity, restore independence, prevent complications, or facilitate discharge and return to the comfort of home. Less desirable reasons for learning are to please others and to avoid criticism.

LEARNING READINESS

When the capacity and motivation for learning exist, the final component, learning readiness, is determined. Readiness refers to the patient's physical and psychological well-being. A person who is in pain, is too warm or cold, is having difficulty breathing, or is depressed or fearful, for example, is not in the best condition for learning to take place. In these situations, it is best to restore comfort and then attend to teaching.

LEARNING NEEDS

The best teaching and learning takes place when they are individualized. To be most efficient and personalized, the nurse needs to gather pertinent information from the patient. Second-guessing what the patient wants and needs to know often leads to wasted time and effort.

The following are questions the nurse can ask to assess the patient's learning needs:

- What does being healthy mean to you?
- What things in your life interfere with being healthy?
- What don't you understand as fully as you would like to?
- What activities do you need help with?
- What do you hope to accomplish before being discharged?
- How can we help you at this time?

Informal and Formal Teaching

Informal teaching is unplanned and occurs spontaneously at the bedside. Formal teaching requires a plan. Without a plan, teaching becomes haphazard. The potential for reaching goals, providing adequate information, and ensuring the patient's comprehension are jeopardized unless there is some organization of time and content. Potential teaching needs are generally identified at the time of the patient's admission, but they may be amended as the patient's care and treatment progress.

A student nurse may work with a staff nurse or instructor in developing a teaching plan. Usually one or more nurses carry out certain specific parts of a teaching plan (Fig. 8-3). This is the most desirable approach so that a patient is not overwhelmed with processing volumes of new information or learning skills that are difficult for a novice to perform.

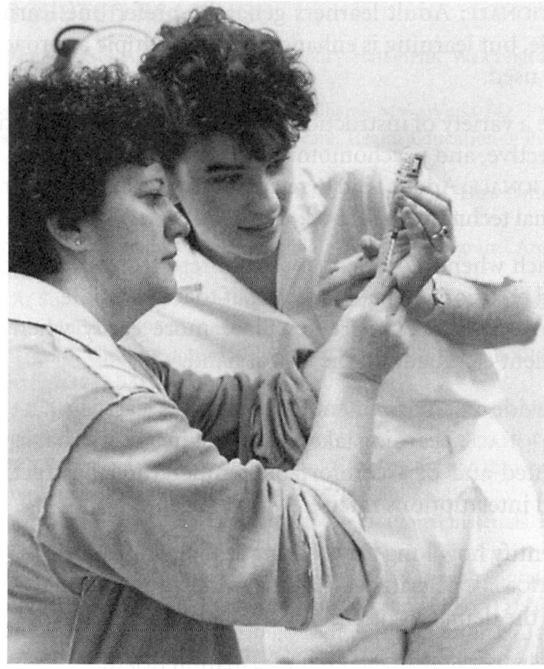

FIGURE 8–3. Diabetic teaching is performed at the bedside. The nurse promotes multisensory stimulation by giving the patient verbal explanations and encouraging her to look at and hold the insulin bottle and syringe. (Courtesy of Ken Timby.)

The nursing guidelines that follow serve as a model when an adult patient needs teaching.

Nursing Guidelines For

Teaching Adult Patients

☑ Find out what the patient wants to know.
RATIONALE: Learning is facilitated when there is personal interest.

☑ Determine what the patient should know if he or she is to remain healthy.
RATIONALE: Patients are not always aware of what information is vital to maintain their health and safety.

☑ Collaborate with the patient on content, goals, and a realistic time for accomplishing the task.
RATIONALE: Adult learners tend to prefer collaboration and active involvement in the learning process.

☑ Develop a written plan that builds from simple to complex, familiar to unfamiliar, normal to abnormal.
RATIONALE: Adult learners learn best by applying information from their present level of knowledge or past experiences.

☑ Divide the information into manageable amounts.
RATIONALE: Too much information at one time tends to overwhelm learners.

☑ Select teaching methods and resources that are compatible with the patient's preferred style for learning.

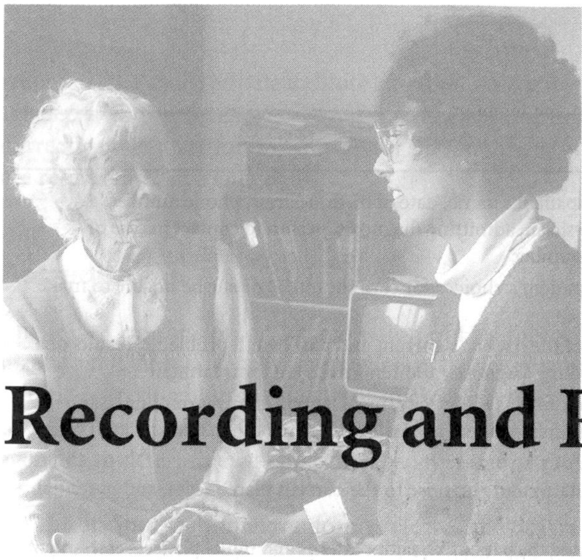

CHAPTER 9

Recording and Reporting

CHAPTER OUTLINE

Medical Records
Methods of Charting
Documenting Information
Communication for Continuity and Collaboration

☑ NURSING GUIDELINES

MAKING ENTRIES IN A PATIENT'S RECORD

KEY TERMS

auditors
change of shift report
chart
charting
charting by exception
checklist
computerized charting
continuous quality improvement
documenting
flow sheet
focus charting
Kardex
medical records
military time
narrative charting
nursing care plan
PIE charting
problem-oriented records
quality assurance
recording
rounds
SOAP charting
source-oriented records
traditional time
total quality improvement

LEARNING OBJECTIVES

An understanding of the content within this chapter will be evidenced by the student's ability to:

- Identify seven uses for medical records.
- List six components that are generally found in any patient's medical record.
- Differentiate between source-oriented and problem-oriented records.
- Identify six methods of charting.
- List four aspects of documentation that are required in the medical records of all patients cared for in acute care settings.
- Discuss why it is important to use only approved abbreviations when charting.
- Explain how to convert traditional time to military time.
- List at least 10 guidelines that apply to charting.
- Identify four written forms used for communicating information about patients.
- List five ways that health care workers exchange patient information, other than by reading the medical record.

Nurses must communicate information clearly, concisely, and accurately, both in writing and when speaking. This chapter describes various written and spoken forms of communication and nursing responsibilities for record-keeping and reporting.

Medical Records

Medical records (written collection of information about a person's health problems, the care provided by health practitioners, and the progress of the patient) are also referred to as health records or patient records. Medical records contain many different printed forms (Table 9-1). The collection of forms is placed in a **chart** (binder or folder that enables the orderly collection, storage, and safekeeping of a person's medical records). The paper forms in the chart may be color-coded or separated by tabbed sheets. All personnel involved in a patient's health care contribute to the medical record by **charting, recording,** or **documenting** (process of writing information) on the health agency's forms.

USES

Besides serving as a permanent health record, a chart provides a means for sharing information among health care workers, thus ensuring patient safety and continuity of care. From

PATIENT ACCESS TO RECORDS

Historically, patients were not allowed to see their medical records, but today health agencies are more flexible on this issue. The Patient's Bill of Rights (see Chap. 3) states that patients have a right to read their medical records. Consequently, many institutions have written policies that describe the guidelines by which patients can have access to their own medical records. Policies range from complete, unrestricted access on the patient's written request to arranging access to their record in the presence of the patient's physician or the hospital administrator. Nurses must follow whatever policies have been established.

TYPES OF PATIENT RECORDS

Although health records in most agencies contain similar information, the record is generally organized in one of two ways. Health care agencies may adopt either a source-oriented or a problem-oriented format.

Source-Oriented Records

The traditional type of patient record is **source-oriented records** (records organized according to the source of documented information). This type of record contains separate forms on which physicians, nurses, dietitians, physical therapists, and so on make written entries about their own specific activities in relation to the patient's care.

One of the criticisms of source-oriented records is that it is difficult to demonstrate that there is a unified, cooperative approach for resolving the patient's problems among caregivers. More often than not, the fragmented documentation gives the impression that each professional is working independently of the others.

Problem-Oriented Records

A second type of patient record is **problem-oriented records** (records organized according to the patient's health problems). In contrast to source-oriented records, which contain numerous locations for information, problem-oriented records contain four major components: the data base, the problem list, the plan of care, and progress notes (Table 9-2). The information is compiled and arranged to emphasize goal-directed care, to promote recording of pertinent information, and to facilitate communication among health care professionals.

TABLE 9–2. **Common Components of a Problem-Oriented Record**

Component	Description
Data base	Contains initial health information
Problem list	Consists of a numeric list of the patient's health problems
Plan of care	Identifies methods for solving each identified health problem
Progress notes	Describes the patient's responses to what has been done and revisions to the initial plan

Methods of Charting

A variety of styles are used to record information on the patient's record. Examples include narrative notes, SOAP charting, focus charting, PIE charting, charting by exception, and computerized charting.

NARRATIVE CHARTING

Narrative charting (style of documentation generally used in source-oriented records) involves writing information about the patient and patient care in chronologic order. There is no established format for narrative notations; the content resembles a log or journal (Fig. 9-1).

Narrative charting is time-consuming to write and read. The caregiver must sort through the lengthy notation for specific information that correlates the patient's problems with care and progress. Depending on the skill of the person writing the entries, pertinent documentation may be omitted or insignificant information included.

SOAP CHARTING

SOAP charting (documentation style more likely to be used in a problem-oriented record) acquired its name from the four essential components included in a progress note:

- S = subjective data
- O = objective data
- A = analysis of the data
- P = plan for care

Some agencies have expanded the SOAP format to SOAPIE or SOAPIER (I = interventions, E = evaluation, R = revision to the plan of care) (Table 9-3).

Any of the variations in the SOAP format tends to keep the documentation focused on pertinent information. SOAP charting also helps to demonstrate interdisciplinary cooperation, because everyone involved in the care of a patient makes entries in the same location in the chart.

FOCUS CHARTING

Focus charting (modified form of SOAP charting) uses the word *focus* rather than problem, because some believe that the word *problem* carries negative connotations. A focus can be the patient's current or changed behavior, significant events in the patient's care, or even a NANDA nursing diagnosis category. Instead of making entries using the SOAP format, a DAR model is used (D = data, A = action, R = response) (Fig. 9-2). DAR notations tends to reflect the steps in the nursing process.

Three Rivers Area Hospital
214 SPRING STREET
THREE RIVERS, MICHIGAN 49093

NURSING NOTES

ROOM NO.________
NAME________
DOCTOR________

Date Time	NURSES REMARKS	Signature
1330	States "I'm having chest pain. It's like an elephant is sitting on me."	—— B. Zook, RN
1340	BP $^{150}/_{90}$, P-122 and irregular. Skin is pale and moist. O_2 started at 5L/min. —— Nitroglycerin $\bar{i}$ tab. administered sublingually.	—— B. Zook, RN.
1350	Dr. Johnson notified of the change in condition. EKG ordered. 1000 cc 5% D/W started IV $\bar{c}$ #20 gauge angiocath in (L) arm. IV running at 20 gtts/minute.	—— B. Zook, RN.
1410	EKG obtained. BP $^{142}/_{84}$ P-110 and still irregular, skin pink but moist. No relief from Nitroglycerin. States "It's still pretty bad."	B. Zook, RN.
1420	Morphine 10 mg. administered sub-q for chest pain and anxiety.	—— B. Zook, RN
1430	Transferred to CCU per bed. Clothing, dentures, and eye-glasses accompanied transfer.	—— B. Zook RN
1440	Family notified of transfer.	— B. Zook, RN

FIGURE 9–1. Sample of narrative charting. (Courtesy of Three Rivers Area Hospital, Three Rivers, MI.)

PIE CHARTING

PIE charting (method of recording the patient's progress under the headings of problem, intervention, and evaluation) is similar to the SOAPIE format. The PIE style of documentation prompts the nurse to address specific content in a charted progress note.

When the PIE method is used, assessments are documented on a separate form and the patient's problems are given a corresponding number. The number is subsequently used in the progress notes when referring to the interventions and the patient's responses (Fig. 9-3).

CHARTING BY EXCEPTION

Charting by exception (documentation method in which only abnormal assessment findings or care that deviates from

Washington Hospital Center

Requested by — Page – 1

RoutneNurseCare

DATE (1999) / TIME	6/18 2200	6/19 0400	1300	6/20 2200	6/21 0200	2000	2310
Bath Care	Complt	None	Partl	Complt	Partl	Complt	None
Oral Care	q4h	q8h	q4h	q2h	q4h	q4h	q4h
Skin Care	Yes	Yes	Yes	Yes	Yes	Yes	Yes
Freq. Turned	q2h	q2h	q2h	q2h	q2h	q2h	q2h
ROMq4	Ys-Act	No	Ys-Act	Ys-Pas	Ys-Pas	Ys-Pas	
Decubitus care	None	None	None			None	None
Foly/Texs Care	Yes	Yes	Yes	Yes	Yes	Yes	Yes
Line Dressing	Ok	Ok	Ok	None	None	Ok	Ok
IV tubing	Ok	Ok	Chnged	Ok	Chnged	Chnged	Chnged
HeprinLk Flush	None	None		Yes	None		None
OOB	Assist	Bedrst	Assist			Assist	Bedrst
OOB-hrs	>1hr		>2hr			>1hr	
Slept-hrs	1–4hr	>4hr	1–4hr			<1hr	>4hr
Nares Care	q8h	q8h		q8h	q8h	q8h	q8h
ET/Trach Care	q8h	q8h	q8h	q8h	q8h	q4h	q8h
Chest PT	q6h	q6h		q6h	q6h	q6h	q6h
Restr.check q2		Yes	None				
Pulse check q8	Palp	Palp	Palp	Palp	Palp	Palp	Palp
NG/Dobpatentq4	Yes	Yes	Yes	Yes	Yes	Yes	Yes
BowelSounds q8	Normal	Normal	Normal	Normal	Normal	Normal	Normal
Wound Dressing						Ok	
Daily Wght (kg)			66.1	65.5			
Alrmlmitchk q4	Yes	Yes	Yes	Yes	Yes	Yes	Yes
Stop cock chk					No	Yes	
CXR done			No	No	No		Yes
12 Lead EKG			No	No	No		
Pt.Clasificati	B	B	B	B	B	B	B

Critical Care Data RoutneNurseCare	Date: 6/22/99	Patient : Hosp. No.: Location : 4G08

FIGURE 9–5. Sample of computerized charting.

on a 24-hour clock), which uses a different four-digit number for each hour and minute of the day (Fig. 9-6 and Table 9-5). The first two digits indicate the hour within the 24-hour period; the last two digits indicate the minutes.

The use of military time avoids confusion, because no number is ever duplicated, and the labels A.M., P.M., midnight, and noon are not needed. Military time begins at midnight (2400 or 0000). One minute after midnight is 0001. A zero is placed before the hours of one through nine in the morning; for example, 0700 refers to 7 A.M. and is stated as "oh seven hundred." After noon, 12 is added to each hour; therefore, 1 P.M. is 1300. Minutes are given as 1 to 59.

DISPLAY 9–2

Content of Nursing Documentation

Nurses are usually responsible for documenting:

- Assessment data*
- Patient care needs
- Routine care, such as hygiene measures
- Safety precautions that have been used
- Nursing interventions described in the care plan
- Medical treatments prescribed by the physician
- Outcomes of treatment and nursing interventions
- Patient activity
- Medication administration
- Percentage of food consumed at each meal
- Visits or consults by physicians or other health professionals
- Reasons for contacting the physician and the outcome of the communication
- Transportation to other departments, like the radiography department, for specialized care or diagnostic tests, and time of return
- Patient teaching and discharge instructions
- Referrals to other health care agencies

**In acute care settings, a registered nurse is required by JCAHO to document the admission nursing assessment findings and develop the initial plan of care. Some aspects of the initial data collection may be delegated to the practical or vocational nurse.*

Nursing Guidelines For

Making Entries in a Patient's Record

☑ Make sure the patient's name is identified on the form.
RATIONALE: If a sheet of paper becomes separated from the chart, proper identification ensures that it will be reinserted into the appropriate record.

☑ Use a pen to make entries; use the color of ink indicated by agency policy.
RATIONALE: Ink is permanent. Black ink photocopies better than other colors.

☑ Write or print information so it can be read easily.
RATIONALE: The entry loses its value for exchanging information if it is unreadable. Illegible entries become questionable in a court of law.

☑ Record the date and time of each entry.
RATIONALE: Legal issues often involve when events took place.

☑ Make entries as promptly as possible after performing a procedure or obtaining assessment data.
RATIONALE: The potential for inaccuracies or omissions increases when documentation is delayed.

☑ Fill all the space on each line of the form; draw a line through any blank space on an unfilled line.
RATIONALE: Filling space reduces the possibility that someone else will add information to what appears to be the original documentation.

☑ Never chart nursing activities before they have been performed.
RATIONALE: Making early entries can cause legal problems, especially if the patient's condition suddenly changes.

☑ Follow agency policy for the interval between entries.
RATIONALE: Frequent charting indicates that the patient has been observed and attended to at reasonable periods of time.

☑ Indicate the current time when charting a late entry (documentation of information that occurred earlier but was accidentally omitted), and identify the time that the omitted entry took place.
RATIONALE: Correlating time with actual events promotes logic and order when evaluating the patient's progress.

☑ Delete articles (a, an, the).
RATIONALE: Extra words add length to the entry.

☑ Do not state the patient's name; do not use *pt.* as an abbreviation.
RATIONALE: It is understood that all the entries refer to the patient identified on the chart form.

☑ Use only agency-approved abbreviations and symbols.
RATIONALE: Using approved abbreviations promotes consistent interpretation.

☑ Never use ditto marks.
RATIONALE: Even if information is repetitious, it must be documented separately.

☑ Identify actual or approximate sizes when describing assessment data rather than using relative descriptions such as large, moderate, or small.
RATIONALE: Nonspecific measurements are subject to wide interpretation and are therefore less accurate and informative.

☑ Draw a line through a mistake rather than scribbling through or in any other way obscuring the original words. Put the word *error* followed by a date and initials next to the entry, and immediately enter the corrected information. Some agencies specify that the nurse must indicate the nature of the error (for example, "wrong medical record").
RATIONALE: Correcting an error must be done in such a way that all words can be clearly read. Obliterated words can cast suspicion that the record was tampered with to conceal damaging information. A jury seeing the word *error* without any explanation might assume that the nurse made an error in care rather than documentation.

☑ Document information clearly and accurately, without any subjective interpretation. Quote the patient, if a statement is pertinent.
RATIONALE: The chart is a record of facts, not opinions.

TABLE 9–4. **Commonly Used Abbreviations**

Abbreviation	Meaning	Abbreviation	Meaning
abd.	abdomen	OB	obstetrics
a.c.	before meals	OD	right eye
ad lib	as desired	OOB	out of bed
AMA	against medical advice	OR	operating room
amt.	amount	OS	left eye
approx.	approximately	OU	both eyes
b.i.d.	twice a day	per	by or through
BM	bowel movement	P	pulse
BP	blood pressure	p.c.	after meals
bpm	beats per minute	p.o.	by mouth
BRP	bathroom privileges	postop.	postoperative
$\bar{c}$	with	preop.	preoperative
C	centigrade	pt.	patient
cc	cubic centimeter	PT	physical therapy
CCU	coronary care unit	q	every
c/o	complains of	q.d.	every day
dc	discontinue	q.i.d.	four times a day
ED	emergency department	q.o.d.	every other day
et	and	q.s.	quantity sufficient
H_2O	water	R, Rt, or R	right
HS	hour of sleep, bedtime	R	respirations
I & O	intake and output	$\bar{s}$	without
IM	intramuscular	ss	one half
IV	intravenous	SS	soap suds
kg	kilogram	stat	immediately
L, Lt, or L	left	t.i.d.	three times a day
L	liter	TPR	temperature, pulse, respirations
lb	pound	UA	urinalysis
NKA	no known allergies	via	by way of
NPO	nothing by mouth	WC	wheelchair
NSS	normal saline solution	WNL	within normal limits
O_2	oxygen	Wt.	weight

- ☑ Avoid phrases such as "appears to be" or "seems to be."
  RATIONALE: Phrases implying uncertainty suggest that the nurse lacks reasonable knowledge.

- ☑ Record adverse reactions; include the measures used to manage them.
  RATIONALE: Documentation may be necessary to demonstrate that the nurse acted reasonably and that the care was not substandard.

- ☑ Identify the specific information that is taught and the evidence of the patient's learning.
  RATIONALE: Ensures continuity in preparing the patient for discharge.

- ☑ Sign each entry with a first initial, last name, and title.
  RATIONALE: The signature demonstrates accountability for what has been written.

Communication for Continuity and Collaboration

Although the record serves as an ongoing source of information about the patient's status, other methods of communication are used to promote continuity of care and collabora-

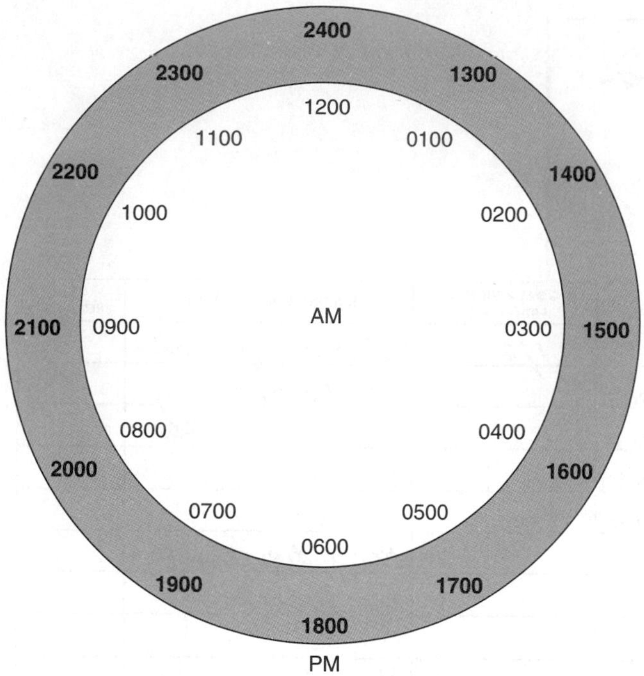

FIGURE 9–6. Military time is based on a 24-hour numbering system.

tion among the health care personnel involved in the patient's care. These methods are in written or verbal form.

WRITTEN FORMS OF COMMUNICATION

Other written forms of communication include the nursing care plan, the nursing Kardex, checklists, and flow sheets.

Nursing Care Plans

A **nursing care plan** (written list of the patient's problems, goals, and nursing orders for patient care) promotes the prevention, reduction, or resolution of health problems. The principles and style for writing a diagnostic statement, goals, and nursing orders are described in Chapter 2.

Present JCAHO standards require that the record show evidence of a plan of care; however, the plan of care does not need to be identified separately. Standards IM.7 through IM.7.2 state: "Nursing care data related to patient assessments, nursing diagnoses or patient needs, nursing interventions, and patient outcomes are permanently integrated into the clinical information system" (that is, the medical record). Nevertheless, many agencies require a separate nursing care plan as a means of demonstrating compliance with the JCAHO standards. The plan of care is revised as the patient's condition changes.

Most nursing care plans are handwritten on a form developed by the agency (Fig. 9-7). Some agencies use preprinted care plans, computer-generated care plans, standards of care, or clinical pathways or cite the plan of care within progress notes.

Because the nursing care plan is part of the permanent record and thus is a legal document, it is compiled and maintained following documentation principles. All entries and revisions are dated. The written components are clear, concise, and legible. Information is never obliterated. Only approved abbreviations are used. Each addition or revision to the plan is signed.

TABLE 9–5. **Military Time Conversions**

Traditional Time	Military Time
Midnight	0000 or 2400
12:01 A.M.	0001
1:30 A.M.	0130
Noon	1200
1:00 P.M.	1300
3:15 P.M.	1515
7:59 P.M.	1959
10:47 P.M.	2247

Nursing Kardex

The nursing **Kardex** (quick reference for current information about the patient and the patient's care) is shown in Figure 9-8. The Kardex forms for all patients are kept in a folder that allows caregivers to flip from one to another. The Kardex is used to:

- Locate patients by name and room number
- Identify each patient's physician and medical diagnosis
- Serve as a reference for a change of shift report
- Serve as a guide for making nursing assignments
- Provide a rapid resource for current medical orders on each patient
- Check quickly on a patient's type of diet
- Alert nursing personnel to a patient's scheduled tests or test preparations
- Inform staff of a patient's current level of activity
- Identify comfort or assistive measures a patient may require
- Provide a tool for estimating the personnel-to-patient ratio for a nursing unit

The information in the Kardex changes frequently, sometimes even several times in one day. The Kardex form is not a part of the permanent record. Therefore, information can be written in pencil or erased.

DISCHARGE GOALS:

Pt will be discharged home with approximated incision, pain within tolerable level, normal vital signs, voiding well, able to eat sufficient food, clear lungs, and active bowel sounds

DIRECTIONS: Each entry must be signed with nurse's name and title.

DATE	PATIENT PROBLEM/NURSING DIAGNOSIS	GOAL/EXPECTED OUTCOMES	GOAL REVIEWED WITH PT./S.O.	NURSING ORDER/ACTIONS	DATE RESOLVED
1/7	Risk for infection related to impaired skin integrity 2° to surgical incision	Pt. will remain free of infection as evidenced by absence of redness, swelling, drainage from wound and afebrile for length of stay	1/7	1. Observe appropriate handwashing before and after patient care. 2. Keep dressing dry and intact. 3. Provide aseptic wound care. D. Miller, LPN	
1/7	Risk for ineffective breathing pattern related to abdominal incisional pain	Pt.'s respiratory rate will remain within normal limits (16-20/min) for length of stay.	1/7	1. Give analgesic for pain rated 75 on a scale of 1-10 2. Instruct to splint incision when turning and deep breathing. D. Miller, LPN	

FIGURE 9–7. Sample nursing care plan.

Checklists

A **checklist** (form of documentation in which the nurse indicates with a check mark or initials that routine care has been performed) is an alternative to writing a narrative note. Checklists are used primarily to avoid documenting types of care that are regularly repeated, such as bathing and mouth care. This charting technique is especially helpful when the care is similar each day and the patient's condition does not differ much for extended periods of time.

Flow Sheets

A **flow sheet** (form of documentation that contains sections for recording frequently repeated assessment data) enables nurses to evaluate trends, because similar information is located on one form. Some provide room for recording numbers or brief descriptions.

INTERPERSONAL COMMUNICATION

Besides using written resources such as the chart as a means for exchanging information, communication also takes place during personal interactions among health professionals (Fig. 9-9). Some examples are:

- Change of shift reports
- Patient care assignments
- Team conferences
- Rounds
- Telephone calls

BATH:
_____ Complete
_____ Partial
_____ Self
_____ Tub
_____ Shower

ACTIVITY:
_____ Bed Rest
_____ BRP only
_____ Dangle
_____ Ambulate
_____ Change pos.
_____ Up as tol.

HYGIENE:
_____ Dentures
_____ Oral Care
_____ Special
____

DIET:
_____ NPO
_____ Hold Brkfst
_____ Feed
_____ Liquid
_____ Soft
_____ General
_____ Special

FLUIDS:
_____ I & O
_____ Restrict to:
____
_____ Increase to:
____
_____ IV

VITAL SIGNS:
_____ TPR
_____ BP

BOWEL/BLADDER:
_____ Catheter
_____ Commode
_____ Incontinent
_____ Ostomy
Type: __________

SAFETY MEASURES:
_____ Siderails
_____ Restraints
Jacket: _____
Wrist: _____
Ankles: _____
Constant: _____
When OOB: _____
Night only _____
_____ Supervise Smoking
_____ Other (list)
____

PHYSICAL TRAITS:
_____ Left handed
_____ Right handed
_____ Paraplegic
_____ Hemiplegic
L __ R __
_____ Blind
L __ R __
_____ Deaf
L __ R __
_____ Speech Imp.
_____ Other (list)
____

ALLERGIES (in red) If none, so state:
____
____
____

DIAGNOSIS: OPERATION: DATE: RELIGION:

ROOM: NAME: AGE: DOCTOR:

FIGURE 9–8. Sample of a Kardex form. (Courtesy of Fairview Medical Care Facility, Centreville, MI.)

Change of Shift Report

A **change of shift report** (discussion between a nursing spokesperson from the shift that is ending and personnel coming on duty; Fig. 9-10) includes a summary of each patient's condition and current status of care (Display 9-3).

To maximize the efficiency of change of shift reports, nurses should do the following:

- Be prompt, so that the report can start and end on time.
- Come prepared with a pen and paper or clipboard.
- Avoid socializing during reporting sessions.
- Take notes.

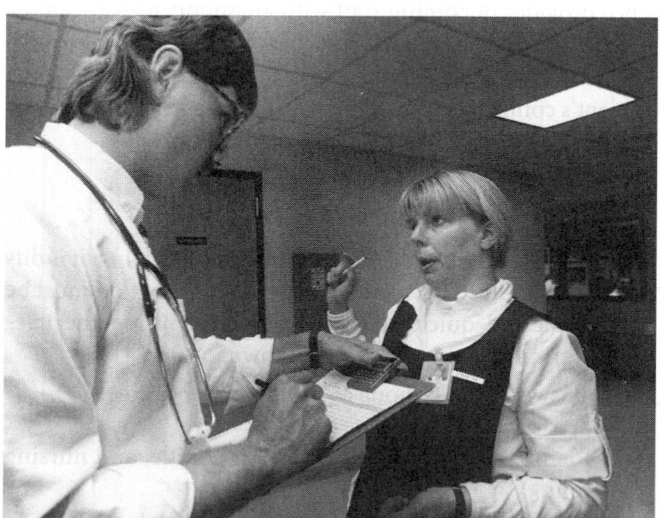

FIGURE 9–9. A staff nurse discusses patient care with a student nurse. (Courtesy of Suzanne Weaver/Bay Health Systems.)

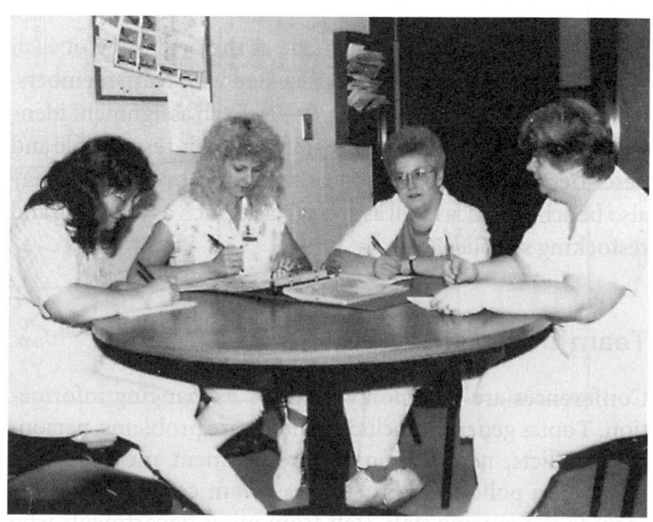

FIGURE 9–10. Nurses begin their shift by receiving a report on their patients.

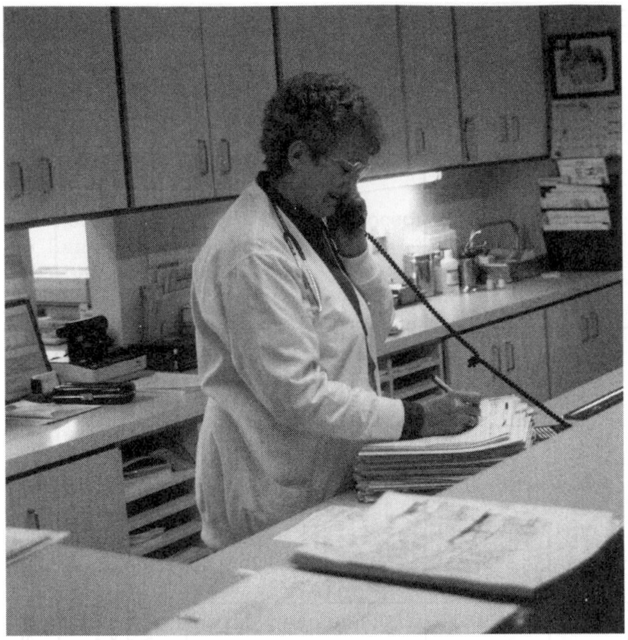

FIGURE 9–13. A nurse reports information to the physician and other departments involved in patient care. (Courtesy of Ken Timby.)

- Spell the patient's name if there is any chance of confusion.
- Converse in a courteous and business-like manner.
- Repeat information to ensure it has been heard accurately.

When notifying a physician about a change in a patient's condition, document in the patient's record the information reported and the instructions received. If the nurse believes that the physician has not responded in a safe manner to the information given, the nursing supervisor or the head of the medical department is notified.

KEY CONCEPTS

- Medical records are used as a permanent account of a person's health problems, care, and progress; for sharing information among health care personnel; as a resource for investigating the quality of care in an institution; to acquire and maintain JCAHO accreditation; to obtain reimbursement for billed services and products; for conducting research; and as legal evidence in malpractice cases.
- Medical records generally contain an information sheet about the patient, medical information, a plan of care, nursing documentation, medication administration records, and laboratory and diagnostic test results.
- Health care agencies may organize the information in the medical record using a source-oriented format or a problem-oriented format. Source-oriented records categorize the information according to the source reporting the information; problem-oriented records are organized according to the patient's health problems, regardless of who is doing the documentation.
- Information may be documented in the medical record using one of the following methods: narrative charting, SOAP charting, focus charting, PIE charting, charting by exception, and computerized charting.
- Regardless of the charting style, all documentation in an acute health care agency includes ongoing assessment data, a plan of care, a record of the care provided, and the outcomes of the implemented care.
- Only agency-approved abbreviations are used when documenting information to promote clarity in communication among health professionals and to ensure accurate interpretation of the documented information if the chart is subpoenaed as legal evidence.
- Military time is based on a 24-hour clock. Each time is indicated using a different four-digit number. After noon, the time is identified by adding 12 to each hour.
- Some principles of charting include the following: ensure that the documentation form identifies the patient; use a pen; print or write legibly; record the time of each entry; fill all the space on a line; use only approved abbreviations; describe information objectively, providing precise measurements when possible; avoid obliterating information; and sign each entry by name and title.
- Written forms of communication other than the medical record include the nursing care plan, nursing Kardex, checklists, and flow sheets.
- Besides the written record, information may be exchanged among the health care team during change of shift reports, patient care assignments, team conferences, rounds, and telephone calls.

CRITICAL THINKING EXERCISES

- Which method of charting described in this chapter is best? Support your opinion with several reasons.
- Explain the consequences that might occur if a nurse's documentation contained illegible writing, unapproved abbreviations, and misspelled words. How would you help the nurse improve his or her documentation?

SUGGESTED READINGS

Black J. Charting chuckles. Nursing 1997;27(12):53.

Brooks JT. An analysis of nursing documentation as a reflection of actual nurse work. MedSurg Nursing 1998;7(4):189.

Calfee BE. Charting tips. Making calls to the physician. Nursing 1998; 28(10):17.

Calfee BE. Legally speaking: Charting with tact. Journal of Practical Nursing 1997;47(3):21.

Cirone NR. Correcting charting errors. Nursing 1998;28(4):65.

Cirone NR. Handling late entries. Nursing 1998;28(7):17.

Cirone NR. Taking orders by phone? Nursing 1998;28(8):56.
Cornelius N. Professional practice. 10 rules to good charting. Care Connection 1998;13(3):7.
DeMarzo D. Charting by exception. Caring 1997;16(3):36.
Documentation: Nix creative charting. Nursing 1997;27(10):14.
Eggland ET. Documenting psychiatric and behavioral outcomes. Nursing 1997;27(4):25.
How to document objectively. Nursing 1997;27(7):17.
Joint Commission on Accreditation of Healthcare Organizations. Comprehensive accreditation manual for hospitals. Oak Terrace, IL: JCAHO, 1998.
Mattox DB. Documentation: Keep it simple. Home Health Focus 1996; 3(6):44.
McLean P. The significance of good charting. Canadian Nurse 1997; 93(10):47.
Minda S, Brundage DJ. Time differences in handwritten and computer documentation of nursing assessment. Computers in Nursing 1994;12(6):277.
Ormsby J. My greatest challenge: Communication and documentation must be accurate and detailed. Home Health Focus 1997;4(3):24.
Pabst MK, Scherubel JC, Minnick AF. The impact of computerized documentation on nurses' use of time. Computers in Nursing 1996;14(1):25.
Sullivan GH. Be cautious when updating charts at a later date. RN 1998; 61(7):60.
Tammelleo AD. Charting by exception: There are perils. RN 1994;57(10):71.
Ten rules for good charting. (1998) Nursing 28(5):27.
Wolverton MK, Scheider K, Burke LJ, Murphy J. In defense of charting by exception. RN 1995;58(3):6.

SECTION II

Fundamental Nursing Skills

UNIT FOUR

PERFORMING ASSESSMENT AND EVALUATION

CHAPTER 10:
Admission, Discharge, Transfer, and Referrals

CHAPTER 11:
Vital Signs

CHAPTER 12:
Physical Assessment

CHAPTER 13:
Special Examinations and Tests

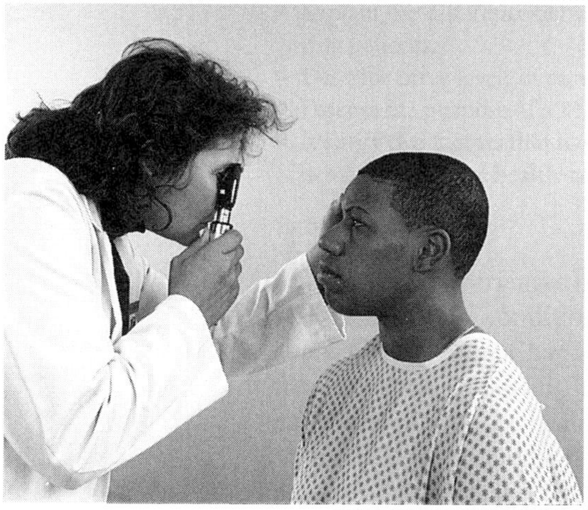

2. Collection of billing information by the admitting department of the health care agency
3. Completion of the agency's admission procedure by nursing personnel
4. Documentation of the patient's medical history and findings of a physical examination
5. Initial medical orders for treatment

The various types of admissions are listed in Table 10-1.

MEDICAL AUTHORIZATION

Before patients are admitted, a physician determines that their condition requires special tests, technical care, or treatment that cannot be provided other than in a hospital or other health care agency. Some patients are scheduled for nonurgent care, such as certain types of surgery, when there is a date and time that is mutually agreeable. However, most patients are seen just before their admission by a primary care or emergency room physician. The physician advises both the patient and nursing staff to proceed with the admission process.

THE ADMITTING DEPARTMENT

In the admitting department, clerical personnel begin to gather information from the prospective patient or a family member. The medical record is initiated with the data obtained at this time. A form is prepared with the patient's address, place of employment, insurance company and policy numbers, and other personal data. This information is used primarily by the hospital's business office for record keeping and future billing.

Patients who are extremely unstable or in severe discomfort may bypass the admitting department and be transported directly to the nursing unit. Someone from the family is eventually directed to the admitting department on the patient's behalf, or personnel are sent to the patient's bedside to obtain needed information.

Generally the admissions clerk prepares an identification bracelet for the patient. The identification bracelet contains the patient's name and identification number, the name of the patient's physician, and the patient's room number. The bracelet is applied by someone in the admitting department or by the admitting nurse (Fig. 10-1). For the patient's safety, the bracelet must remain on throughout his or her stay. Other than asking a patient's name, the bracelet is the single most important method for identifying the patient. If the identification bracelet is missing or has been removed, the nurse is responsible for replacing it as soon as possible.

Once the preliminary data have been collected, the nursing unit is notified and the patient is escorted to the location where he or she will receive care. The form initiated in the admitting department is delivered to the nursing unit along with a plastic card, called an adressograph plate. The card is used to identify all future pages within the patient's medical record.

NURSING ADMISSION ACTIVITIES

Preparing the Patient's Room

When the nurse is informed by the admissions department that the patient is about to be escorted to the unit, the room is checked to ensure it is clean and stocked with basic equipment for initial care (Display 10-1). Personal care items such as soap, skin lotion, toothbrush, toothpaste, razor, paper tissues, and denture containers are provided later for patients who do not have them. The nurse places oxygen administration equipment, a stand for supporting intravenous fluids, or anything else that facilitates initial treatment.

Welcoming the Patient

One of the most important steps in the admission process is to make the patient feel welcome. Therefore, on arrival, the nurse greets the patient warmly with a smile and a handshake (Fig. 10-2). The admitting nurse wears a name tag, introduces

TABLE 10–1. **Types of Admissions**

Type	Explanation	Example
Inpatient	Length of stay generally more than 24 hours	Acute pneumonia
Planned (nonurgent)	Scheduled in advance	Elective or required major surgery
Emergency admission	Unplanned; stabilized in emergency department and transferred to nursing care unit	Unrelieved chest pain, major trauma
Direct admission	Unplanned; emergency department bypassed	Acute condition such as prolonged vomiting or diarrhea
Outpatient	Length of stay less than 24 hours; possible return on a regular basis for continued care or treatment	Minor surgery, cancer therapy, physical therapy
Observational	Monitoring required; need for inpatient admission determined within 23 hours	Head injury, unstable vital signs, premature or early labor

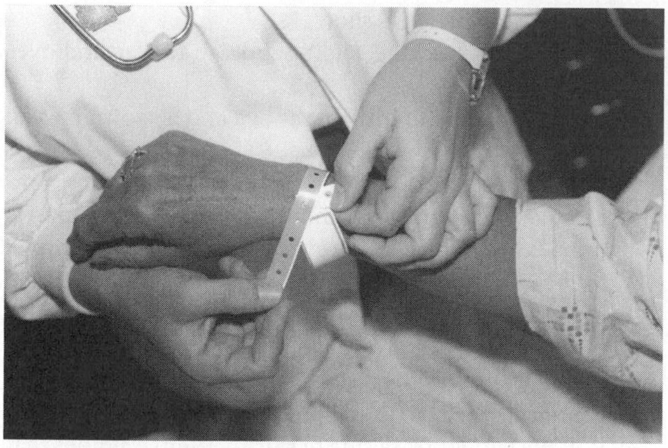

FIGURE 10–1. Applying an identification bracelet. (Courtesy of Ken Timby.)

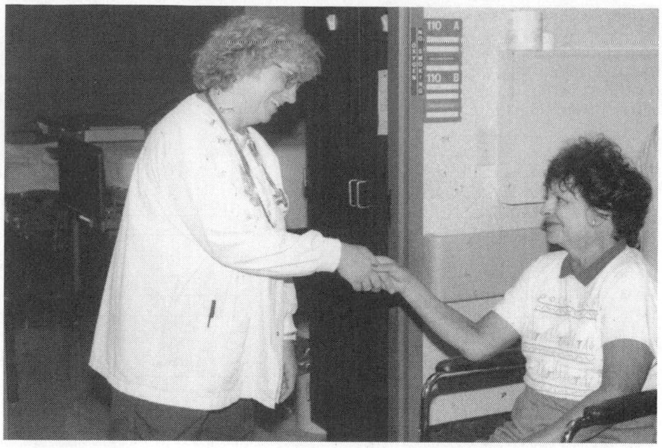

FIGURE 10–2. Greeting a new patient. (Courtesy of Ken Timby.)

himself or herself, and also introduces patients who will share a room. Being treated courteously and in a friendly manner helps put the patient at ease. If the patient feels unexpected or unwanted, he or she is likely to have a poor, and lasting, first impression of the unit.

Orienting the Patient

Orientation (helping a person become familiar with a new environment) facilitates comfort and adaptation. When orienting a patient, the nurse describes:

- The location of the nursing station, toilet, shower or bathing area, and lounge available to the patient and visitors
- Where clothing and personal items can be stored
- How to call for nursing assistance from the bed and bathroom
- How to adjust the hospital bed
- How to regulate the room lights
- How to use the telephone and any policy about diverting incoming calls to the nursing station during the night
- How to operate the television
- The daily routine, such as meal times
- When the doctor usually visits
- When surgery is scheduled
- When laboratory or diagnostic tests are performed

Some hospitals provide booklets with general information about the agency, such as the gift shop hours, newspaper deliveries, and the location of the chapel or the name of the chaplain. However, such booklets should never take the place of the nurse's individualized explanations.

DISPLAY 10–1

Basic Room Supplies

Each bedside stand is generally stocked with:

- Wash basin
- Soap dish
- Emesis basin
- Water carafe
- Bedpan and urinal

Safeguarding Valuables and Clothing

Certain items, such as prescription and nonprescription medications, valuable jewelry, and large sums of money, should be given to family members to take home. If this is not possible, *the agency's policies must be carefully observed.* Some institutions provide outpatients with a locker where they can store their personal effects. Others allow inpatients to place their valuables in the hospital's safe temporarily. A notation is made in the medical record identifying the type of valuables and the manner in which they were safeguarded. It is best to be as descriptive as possible. For example, rather than indicating that a ring was placed in the safe, it is better to describe the type of metal and stones in the ring.

Losing a patient's personal items can have serious legal implications for both the nurse and the health care agency. The patient may sue, claiming the belongings were lost or stolen because they were handled carelessly. Therefore, it is best to have a second nurse, supervisor, or security person present when assuming responsibility for safeguarding valuables.

One method for avoiding discrepancies between the items that were entrusted to the nurse and those that are eventually returned is to make an inventory (Fig. 10-3). The nurse and the patient both sign the inventory. One copy is given to the patient, and another is attached to the chart. When items are added or returned, the list is revised and the patient signs the new inventory. Problems with theft or loss may occur if items are brought in without subsequent documentation.

(Please check articles of clothing with patient and describe.)

Dress 1 - BLUE & WHITE	Pants
Slip 1 - WHITE (½ SLIP)	Shirt
Bra 1 - WHITE	Undershirt
Panties 1 - WHITE	Undershorts
Hose	Socks
Girdle	Tie
Slippers 1 - PINK	Shoes 1 - WHITE
Nightgown 1 - BLUE, 1 - PINK	Pajamas
Suit	Robe
Sweater	Coat
Slacks	Truss
Blouse	Backsupport
Shorts	Belt
Skirt	Hat

Other items not listed:

Check valuables below and describe if necessary:

Watch

Medals

Earrings

Rings - Type & Number 1 - YELLOW METAL, PLAIN BAND

Other Jewelry

Dentures - Yes ✓ No ___ Prosthesis - Yes ___ No ✓

Contact Lenses - Yes ___ No ✓ Glasses - Yes ✓ No ___

Removed - Yes ___ No ___ Hearing Aid - Yes ___ No ✓

Wallet ✓ Color RED With Pt. ✓ In Safe ___ To Family or Friend ___

Purse ✓ Color WHITE With Pt. ✓ In Safe ___ To Family or Friend ___

Cash $25.00 With Pt. ___ In Safe ✓ To Family or Friend ___

Checks/Check Book ___ With Pt. ___ In Safe ___ To Family or Friend ___

The above list is correct:

Patient's signature Helen Jones Witness Nancy Smith, L.P.N.

Clothing taken home by

Relationship

Witness

Received by on Nursing Unit

FIGURE 10–3. Inventory of the patient's personal belongings.

Patient-owned equipment, such as a walker or wheelchair, should be identified with a large label that is easily read. Labeling personal equipment helps prevent it from being confused with hospital property. Most agencies have facilities in the patient's room for storing street clothing.

Because eyeglasses and dentures are removed from time to time, they may be lost or broken. Generally, the health care agency is responsible for replacing these items if they are accidentally damaged or lost through the negligence of staff.

Helping the Patient Undress

To facilitate a physical examination, the patient must undress. If the patient cannot undress without the nurse's help, the nurse should do the following:

- Provide privacy.
- Have the patient sit on the edge of the bed, which has already been lowered.
- Remove the patient's shoes.
- Gather each stocking, sliding it down the leg and over the foot.
- Help the patient to turn on the bed and lie down if weak or tired.
- Release fasteners, such as zippers and buttons, and remove the item of clothing in whatever manner is most comfortable and least disturbing. For example, fold or gather a garment and work it up and over the body. Have the patient lift the hips to slide clothes up or down.
- Lift the patient's head so garments can be guided over the head.
- Roll the patient from side to side to remove clothes that fasten up the front or back.
- Cover the patient with a bath blanket after removing the outer clothing, or put a hospital gown on the patient. Explain that hospital gowns fasten in the back.

Compiling the Nursing Data Base

At the time of admission, the nurse begins assessing the patient and collecting information for the data base (see Chap. 2). Although the registered nurse is responsible for the admission assessment, some aspects may be delegated to the practical nurse or other ancillary staff. Physical assessment skills, which include taking vital signs, are discussed in more depth in Chapters 11 and 12.

Skill 10-1 describes the basic steps in admitting a patient. Additions or modifications to the procedure depend largely on the patient's condition and agency policies. Once the admission assessment is performed, the nurse identifies the patient's problems and develops the initial plan for nursing care. The physician is notified once the admission procedure is completed.

MEDICAL ADMISSION RESPONSIBILITIES

The patient's physician provides medical orders for medications and other treatments, laboratory and diagnostic tests, activity, and diet. The physician also must obtain a medical history and perform a physical examination within 24 hours of admission. This task, likewise, can be delegated to some other member of the medical team such as a medical student, intern, or resident.

The medical history and physical examination generally includes the following information: identifying data, chief complaint, history of present illness, personal history, past health history, family history, review of body systems, and conclusions (Display 10-2). If the physician is unsure of the actual medical diagnosis, the term *rule out,* or the abbreviation *R/O,* is used to indicate that the condition is suspected, but addi-

DISPLAY 10–2

Components of a Medical History and Physical Examination

Identifying Data
- Age, gender, marital status
- General appearance
- Circumstances surrounding physician involvement
- Reliability of patient as historian
- Others providing information about the patient's history

Chief Complaint
- Reason for seeking care (from patient's perspective)

Present Illness
- Chronologic description of onset, frequency, and duration of current signs and symptoms
- Outcomes of earlier attempts at self-treatment and medical treatment

Personal History
- Occupation
- Highest level of education
- Religious affiliation
- Residence
- Country of origin
- Primary language
- Military service
- Foreign travel or residence (date, location, length)

Past Health History
- Childhood disease summary
- Physical injuries
- Major illnesses and surgeries
- Previous hospitalizations (medical or psychiatric)
- Drug history
- Alcohol and tobacco use
- Allergy history

Family History
- Health problems in immediate family members (living and deceased)
- Longevity and cause of death among deceased blood relatives (especially parents and grandparents)

Review of Body Systems
- Results of physical examination

Conclusions
- Primary diagnosis (from chief complaint and physical examination)
- Secondary diagnoses reflecting stable or pre-existing conditions possibly affecting patient's treatment

tional diagnostic data must be obtained before it can be confirmed.

COMMON RESPONSES TO ADMISSION

Nurses and physicians must remember that no matter how many times they have admitted patients, it is a unique and emotionally traumatic experience for the patient. Leaving the security of home and entering the unfamiliar environment of a health care facility compounds the stress of physical illness and contributes to emotional and social distress.

Although the specific responses to admission are unique to each patient, some common reactions include anxiety, loneliness, decreased privacy, and loss of identity. In addition, the nurse may identify one or more of the following nursing diagnoses that develop as a consequence of admission:

- Anxiety
- Fear
- Decisional conflict
- Self-esteem disturbance
- Powerlessness
- Social isolation
- Risk for ineffective management of therapeutic regimen: individual

Anxiety

Anxiety is an uncomfortable feeling caused by insecurity. It has been defined by the North American Nursing Diagnosis Association (1998) as "a vague, uneasy feeling of discomfort accompanied by an autonomic response; the source is often nonspecific or unknown to the individual."

Many adults do not manifest their anxiety in obvious ways. Observant nurses may note that adults appear sad or worried, are restless, have a reduced appetite, and have trouble sleeping (see Chap. 5). Because adults have a greater capacity to process information than children, it is helpful to acknowledge their uneasiness and to provide explanations and instructions before any new experience occurs. The nursing care plan in this chapter provides an example of how the nursing process is used when planning the care of a patient with anxiety.

Loneliness

Loneliness occurs when a patient cannot interact with family and friends. Although nurses can never replace the people who are significant to a patient, they act as temporary surrogates and should make frequent contact with the patient. To help combat loneliness, many hospitals and nursing homes have adopted liberal visiting hours. Age restrictions are also being lifted to allow more contact between children and their sick relatives.

Decreased Privacy

Privacy is at a premium in most health care agencies. Few patients have a room to themselves; in fact, most patients have little more than a few feet they can consider their personal space. Patients often share a room with a stranger, room doors are open most of the time, and many people pass by at all hours of the day and night; all of these compromise privacy.

To compensate, nurses should demonstrate respect for and ensure the protection of each patient's right to privacy. Patients must always be protected from the view of others when personal care is given. If a patient's door is closed or the curtains are pulled, the nurse should knock or ask permission to enter. If there is a place in the health care agency where patients can find solitude, such as a chapel or reading room, the information is included in the admission orientation.

Loss of Identity

Becoming an inpatient may temporarily deprive the person of his or her personal identity. For example, when patients are required to wear hospital gowns, they tend to look somewhat the same. Consequently, patients may be treated in an impersonal manner—simply as a face or a warm body with no name. This attitude makes patients feel like they are receiving care, but without caring.

Therefore, nurses should learn and use the patient's name. First names are used only if the patient requests it. Patients also are encouraged to display family pictures or other small personal objects that reaffirm their unique life and personality. In long-term care facilities, many patients are urged to dress in their own clothing and are invited to furnish their rooms with personal items from home.

The Discharge Process

Regardless of where patients are admitted and for whatever reason, the goal is to keep the admission as brief as possible and to discharge patients back to their homes as soon as possible. **Discharge** (termination of care from a health care agency) generally consists of obtaining a written medical order for discharge, completing discharge instructions, notifying the business office, helping the patient leave the agency, writing a summary of the patient's condition at discharge, and requesting that the room be cleaned.

OBTAINING AUTHORIZATION FOR MEDICAL DISCHARGE

The physician determines when the patient is well enough to be discharged. Generally, the physician waits to write the medical order until after examining the patient. Before leaving the nursing unit, the physician writes the discharge order, provides written prescriptions for the patient, and indicates when and where a follow-up appointment should take place.

Leaving Against Medical Advice

Leaving against medical advice (AMA) is a term that applies to situations in which the patient leaves before the physician authorizes the discharge. Many times the situation arises because the patient is unhappy with some aspect of care. In some cases, the nurse may negotiate a compromise or persuade the patient to delay taking such action. In the meantime, the nurse informs the physician and nursing supervisor of the patient's wish to leave.

If the patient is determined to leave, the nurse asks him or her to sign a special form (see Chap. 3). This signed form releases the physician and agency from future responsibility for any complications that may occur. If the patient refuses to sign, he or she cannot be prevented from leaving. The fact that the form was presented and subsequently refused is, however, noted in the patient's medical record.

PROVIDING DISCHARGE INSTRUCTIONS

Planning for discharge actually begins when patients are admitted. Shortly after admission, the nurse identifies the anticipated knowledge, skills, and community resources that each patient will need to maintain a safe level of self-care. One discharge planning technique involves using the acronym METHOD as a guide (Table 10-2). The actual teaching identified in the discharge plan is provided periodically throughout the patient's stay and documented in the patient's record (see Chap. 8).

Before the patient leaves, the nurse reviews the teaching that has been provided, gives the patient prescriptions to have filled, and advises the patient to make an office appointment for the date specified by the physician. A written summary of discharge instructions is provided. The patient signs one sheet and a carbon copy is attached to the patient's medical record.

NOTIFYING THE BUSINESS OFFICE

Before the patient leaves the agency, the business office is notified. At that time, clerical personnel verify that all insurance information is complete and that the patient has signed a consent form authorizing the release of medical information to the

TABLE 10–2. **The METHOD Discharge Planning Guide**

Topic	Nursing Activity	Example
M—Medications	Instruct the patient about drugs that will be self-administered.	Insulin
E—Environment	Explore how the home environment can be modified to ensure the patient's safety.	Remove scatter rugs
T—Treatments	Demonstrate how to perform skills involved in self-care and provide opportunities for returning the demonstration.	Dressing changes
H—Health teaching	Identify information that is necessary for maintaining or improving health.	Signs and symptoms of complications
O—Outpatient referral	Explain what community services are available that may ease the patient's transition to independent living.	Physical therapy
D—Diet	Arrange for the dietitian to provide verbal and written instructions on modifying or restricting certain foods or suggestions for altering their methods of preparation.	Low-fat diet

insurance carrier. If records are incomplete or if the patient has no health insurance, the patient must make arrangements for future financial payments before being discharged.

DISCHARGING A PATIENT

When all the preliminary business is completed, the nurse helps the patient gather his or her belongings, plan for transportation, and actually leave the agency.

Gathering Belongings

If necessary, the nurse helps the patient repack his or her personal items. The inventory of valuables is used to ensure that nothing has been lost or forgotten. Because most hospitals dispose of the plastic supplies (basin, bedpan, urinal, and so forth), the nurse can offer them to the patient; otherwise they are discarded in the soiled utility room. A wheeled cart is helpful to transport the patient's belongings.

Arranging Transportation

The nurse should inform patients about the agency's "checkout time"—the time before which they can avoid being charged for another full day. In most cases, the patient contacts a family member or friend for assistance with transportation. If no transportation is available, the patient may use public transportation or an ambulance to get home. Van transportation may be available for older adults through the local Commission on Aging, but 24-hour advance notification is usually needed.

Escorting the Patient

When the patient is ready, he or she is taken to the door in a wheelchair or allowed to walk there with assistance. The patient may choose to have discharge prescriptions filled at the hospital's pharmacy before leaving. Generally the nurse remains with the patient until he or she is safely inside a vehicle or waiting in the lobby for a ride.

Skill 10-2 provides a step-by-step description of the discharge process.

WRITING A DISCHARGE SUMMARY

Once the patient has left, the nurse documents the discharge activities (see Skill 10-2).

TERMINAL CLEANING

Except in unusual circumstances, housekeeping personnel prepare the patient unit for the next admission. The bed is stripped of linen and cleaned with a disinfectant, and the bedside cabinet is restocked with basic equipment. The admitting department is then notified that the unit is ready. This prevents a patient from being assigned to a room that still requires cleaning.

Patient Transfer

A **transfer** (discharging a patient from one unit or agency and admitting him or her to another without going home in the interim) may take place when a patient's condition changes for better or worse. Generally, a transfer has some advantage for the patient. It may facilitate more specialized care in a life-threatening situation (Fig. 10-4), or it may reduce health care costs. Many hospitals are creating **stepdown units** or **progressive care units** (units for patients who were once in critical condition but have recovered sufficiently to require less intensive nursing care).

TRANSFER ACTIVITIES

Transferring a patient to a different nursing unit is less complex than transferring him or her to another agency.

TABLE 10–3. **Discharge Outcomes of Hospitalized Older Adults**

Age Range (years)	Discharged Home	Referred to Home Care Programs	Transferred to Nursing Homes	Discharged to Rehabilitation Facilities
65–74	85.7%	6.7%	3.9%	1.1%
75 and older	69.2%	12.3%	15.9%	1.5%

(Densen PM. Tracing the elderly through the health care system: An update. Rockville MD, Agency for Health Care Policy and Research, U.S. Department of Health and Human Services, January 1991.)

skilled care. Some older adults have private insurance policies that assist with Medicare copayments. If that is not the case, or if patients continue to require skilled care beyond 100 days, they must bear the cost personally until they are considered indigent. Once patients have exhausted their own financial resources and those of their spouse, they may apply to the state for Medicaid or its equivalent.

Intermediate Care Facilities

A nursing home may also be licensed as an **intermediate care facility** (agency that provides health-related care and services to people who because of their mental or physical condition require institutional care, but not 24-hour nursing care). Patients who require intermediate care may need supervision because they tend to wander or are confused. They need nursing care for assistance with oral medications, bathing, dressing, toileting, and mobility.

Medicare does not provide reimbursement for intermediate care. The costs are assumed by the patient or through state welfare programs, such as Medicaid, for impoverished residents. Some nursing homes do not accept Medicaid patients because the fees for reimbursement are fixed by the state at much lower amounts than Medicare and private insurance provide.

Basic Care Facilities

A third type of nursing home is a **basic care facility** (agency that provides extended custodial care). The emphasis is on providing shelter, food, and laundry services in a group setting. These patients assume much of the responsibility for their own activities of daily living, such as hygiene and dressing, preparing for sleep, and joining others for meals.

Intermediate and basic care may be provided at a skilled nursing facility, but usually in separate wings.

Determining the Level of Care

The level of care is determined at admission. Each patient is assessed using a standard form developed by the Health Care Financing Association called a *Minimum Data Set for Nursing Home Resident Assessment and Care Screening.* By federal law, the Minimum Data Set (MDS) is repeated at 3-month intervals, or whenever a patient's condition changes. The MDS requires assessment of:

- Cognitive patterns
- Communication/hearing patterns
- Vision patterns
- Physical functioning and structural problems
- Continence patterns in the last 14 days
- Psychosocial well-being
- Mood and behavior patterns
- Activity pursuit patterns
- Disease diagnoses
- Health conditions
- Oral/nutritional status
- Oral/dental status
- Skin condition
- Medication use
- Special treatments and procedures

Problems identified on the MDS are then reflected in the nursing care plan.

Selecting a Nursing Home

When the need arises, family members are often ill prepared for selecting a nursing home. Brochures on choosing a nursing home are available from the American Association of Retired Persons, the Commission on Aging, and each state's public health and welfare departments. The following guidelines are important.

Patient Teaching For

Selecting a Nursing Home

Teach the patient or family to do the following:

- Find out the levels of care (skilled, intermediate, or basic) the nursing home is licensed to provide.

- Review inspection reports on each home. This information is available on a fee-per-page basis from the state's public health department.
- Ask others in the community, including the family physician, for recommendations.
- Visit nursing homes with, and again without, an appointment. Go at least once during a meal time.
- Note the appearance of residents and the manner in which staff respond to their needs.
- Observe the cleanliness of the surroundings and the presence of any unpleasant odors.
- Request brochures that identify medical care, nursing services, rehabilitation therapy, social services, activities programs, religious observances, and residents' rights and privileges.
- Clarify charges and billing procedures.
- Analyze whether the overall impression of the home is positive or negative.

Patient Referral

A **referral** (process of sending someone to another person or agency for special services) is made to a private practitioner or a community agency. Table 10-4 lists some common community services to which persons with declining health, physical disabilities, or special needs are referred.

Thinking about a referral is part of good discharge planning. For example, a nurse or the agency's discharge planner may help refer patients for home health care. Because planning, coordinating, and communicating take time, referrals are initiated as soon as possible once the need is identified. Early planning helps ensure **continuity of care** (uninterrupted patient care despite the change in caregivers), thus avoiding any loss of progress that has been made.

HOME HEALTH CARE

Home health care (health care provided in the home by an employee of a home health agency; Fig. 10-6) may be provided by public agencies (regional, state, or federal, such as the public health department) or private agencies.

The number of patients who receive home health care continues to rise. This growth is, in part, an outcome of the limitations imposed by Medicare and insurance companies on the number of hospital and nursing home days for which care is reimbursed. Another factor is the growing number of older adults in the population who are chronically ill and in need of assistance.

According to *Profile of Older Americans: 1998* (Duncker and Greenberg, 1998), more than half of those older than 65 reported having at least one disability; about one third were severely disabled. In contrast, for persons age 15 to 64, fewer than 20% had a disability, and only 8% were severely disabled. In the older adult population, 14% had difficulty with basic activities of daily living such as bathing, dressing, eating, and getting around the house; 21% had difficulty with activities such as preparing meals, shopping, doing housework, managing money, using the phone, and taking medications.

Home care nursing services help shorten the time spent recovering in the hospital, prevent admissions to extended care facilities, and reduce the number of readmissions to acute care facilities. Display 10-3 identifies the responsibilities assumed by home health nurses who provide community-based care.

TABLE 10–4. **Common Community Services**

Organization	Service
Commission on Aging	Assists older adults with transportation to medical appointments, outpatient therapy, and community meal sites
Hospice	Supports the family and terminally ill patients who choose to stay at home
Visiting Nurses' Association	Offers intermittent nursing care to home-bound patients
Meals on Wheels	Provides one or two hot meals per day, delivered either at home or at a community meal site
Homemaker Services	Sends adults to the home to assist in shopping, meal preparation, and light housekeeping
Home health aides	Assist with bathing, hygiene, and medications
Adult protective services	Makes social, legal, and accounting services available to incompetent adults who may be victimized by others
Respite care	Provides short-term, temporary relief to full-time caregivers of homebound patients
Older Americans' Ombudsman	Investigates and resolves complaints made by, or on behalf of, nursing home residents; at least one full-time ombudsman is mandated for each state

CRITICAL THINKING EXERCISES

- Discuss how the admission of a child might be different from that of an adult.
- Describe the similarities and differences between an admission to a hospital and one to a nursing home.
- Besides being ready for a new patient and greeting the patient warmly, what other factors might help to make a good first impression on patients?

SUGGESTED READINGS

Bean P, Waldron K. Readmission study leads to continuum of care. Nursing Management 1995;26(9):65–68.

Chest pain: admit, send home, or something else? Patient Focused Care 1997;5(11):126–129.

Duncker A, Greenberg S. Profile of older Americans: 1998. Washington DC: American Association of Retired Persons and Administration on Aging, U.S. Department of Health & Human Services, Program Resources Department; *www.aoa:dhhs.gov/aoa/stats/profile/default/html*

Dunn D. Preoperative assessment criteria and patient teaching for ambulatory surgery patients. Journal of Perianesthesia Nursing 1998;13(5): 274–291.

Green K, Lydon S. Continuing care extra: the continuum of patient care. American Journal of Nursing 1998;98(10):16BBB–16DDD.

Joint Commission on the Accreditation of Healthcare Organizations. Comprehensive accreditation manual for hospitals. Oak Terrace, IL: JCAHO, 1998.

Jones B. Nutrition: taking the tube home. Nursing Times 1998;94(33):67–68.

Kammer CH. Stress and coping of family members responsible for nursing home placement. Research in Nursing & Health 1994;17(2):89–98.

Kernaghan SG. Program profile: hospitals, nursing homes design uniform patient transfer. Continuum: An Interdisciplinary Journal on Continuity of Care 1996;16(2):19–21.

Miller CA. Nursing care of older adults, 3d ed. Philadelphia, Lippincott Williams & Wilkins, 1999.

North American Nursing Diagnosis Association. NANDA nursing diagnoses: definitions and classification, 1999–2000. Philadelphia, NANDA, 1999.

Pesce L. Evaluating nursing intensity: it's time to transfer the patient. Nursing Management 1995;26(2):36–39.

Spear H. Anxiety. 1996;RN 59:40–45.

Steefel L. Making the switch to home care. Nursing Spectrum 1998;10A(6): 4–5.

Stewart S, Voss DW. A study of unplanned readmissions to a coronary care unit. Heart & Lung 1997;26(3):196–203.

Walker J, Brooksby A, McInerny J, Taylor A. Patient perceptions of hospital care: building confidence, faith and trust. Journal of Nursing Management 1998;6(4):193–200.

Weber MW. Neonates making the transition from intensive care to home care. Caring 1998;17(5):26–29.

SKILL 10-1

ADMITTING A PATIENT

Suggested Action	Reason for Action
Assessment	
Obtain the name, admitting diagnosis, and condition of the patient and the room to which the patient has been assigned.	Provides preliminary data from which to plan the activities that may be involved in admitting the patient
Check the appearance of the room and presence of basic supplies.	Demonstrates concern for cleanliness, order, and patient convenience
Planning	
Assemble equipment that will be needed: admission assessment form, thermometer, blood pressure cuff (if not wall-mounted), stethoscope, scale, urine specimen container.	Enhances organization and efficient time management
Obtain special equipment, such as an IV pole or oxygen, that may be needed, according to the needs of the patient.	Facilitates immediate care of the patient without causing unnecessary delay or discomfort
Arrange the height of the bed to coordinate with the expected mode of arrival.	Reduces the physical effort in moving from a wheelchair or stretcher to the bed
Fold the top linen to the bottom of the bed if the patient will be immediately confined to bed.	Reduces obstacles that may interfere with the patient's comfort and ease of transfer

continued

SKILL 10-1

ADMITTING A PATIENT *Continued*

Suggested Action	Reason for Action
Implementation	
Greet the patient by name and demonstrate a friendly smile; extend a hand as a symbol of welcome.	Promotes feelings of friendliness and personal regard to help reduce initial anxiety
Introduce yourself to the patient and those who have accompanied the patient.	Establishes the nurse–patient relationship on a personal basis
Observe the patient for signs of acute distress.	Determines if the admission process requires modification
Attend to urgent needs for comfort and breathing.	Demonstrates concern for the patient's well-being
Introduce the patient to his or her roommate, if there is one, and anyone else who enters the room.	Promotes a sense of familiarity to relieve social awkwardness; demonstrates concern for the patient's emotional comfort
Offer the patient a chair unless the patient requires immediate bed rest.	Demonstrates concern for the patient's physical comfort
Check the patient's identification bracelet.	Enhances safety by accurately identifying the patient
Orient the patient to the physical environment of the room and the nursing unit.	Aids in adapting to unfamiliar surroundings
Demonstrate how to use the equipment in the room such as the adjustments for the bed, how to signal for a nurse, use of the telephone and television.	Promotes comfort and self-reliance; ensures safety
Explain the general routines and schedules that are followed for visiting hours, meals, and care.	Reduces uncertainty about when to expect activities
Explain the need to examine the patient and ask personal health questions.	Prepares the patient for what will follow next
Ask whether the patient would like family members to leave or remain.	Promotes a sense of control over decisions and outcomes
Make provisions for privacy.	Demonstrates respect for the patient's dignity
Request that the patient undress and don a patient gown; assist as necessary.	Facilitates physical assessment
Ask the patient about the need to urinate at the present time, and obtain a urine specimen if ordered.	Shows concern for the patient's immediate comfort; facilitates physical assessment of the abdomen
Weigh the patient before helping him or her into bed.	Avoids disturbing the patient once settled in bed
Assist the patient to a comfortable position in bed.	Shows concern for the patient's comfort; facilitates the examination
Take care of the patient's clothing and valuables according to agency policy.	Provides safeguards for the patient's possessions
Ask the patient to identify allergies to food, drugs, or other substances and to describe the type of symptoms that accompany a typical allergic reaction.	Aids in preventing the potential for an allergic reaction during care; prepares staff for the manner in which the patient reacts to the allergen
Wash hands thoroughly.	Reduces the direct transmission of microorganisms from the nurse's hands to the patient
Obtain the patient's temperature, pulse, respiratory rate, and blood pressure.	Contributes to the initial data base assessment
Place the signal cord where it can be conveniently reached.	Reduces the potential for accidents by ensuring that the patient can make his or her needs known

continued

SKILL 10-1

ADMITTING A PATIENT *Continued*

Suggested Action	Reason for Action
Make sure the bed is in low position, and follow agency policy about raising the side rails on the bed.	Promotes safety. Side rails are considered a form of physical restraint; their use may require written permission from the patient.
Remove the urine specimen, if obtained at this time, attach a laboratory request form, and place it in the refrigerator or take it to the laboratory.	Ensures proper identification of the specimen, specifies the test to be performed, and prevents changes that may affect test results
Wash hands thoroughly.	Removes microorganisms acquired from contact with the patient or the urine specimen
Report the progress of the patient's admission to the registered nurse, who may perform the nursing interview and physical assessment or delegate components at this time.	Complies with JCAHO standards; the entire admission assessment must be completed within 24 hours; parts of the assessment may be performed at periodic intervals
Inform family or friends that they may resume visiting when the nursing activities are completed.	Facilitates the patient's network of support

Evaluation

- Patient is comfortable and oriented to room and routines.
- Safety measures are implemented.
- Data base assessments are initiated.
- Status and progress are communicated to nursing team.

Document

- Date and time of admission
- Age and gender of patient
- Overall appearance
- Mode of arrival to unit
- Room number
- Initial vital signs and weight
- List of allergies, if any; quote the patient's description of a typical reaction; or indicate if the patient has no allergies by using the abbreviation NKA (no known allergies) or whatever abbreviation is acceptable
- Disposition of urine specimen
- Present condition of patient.

SAMPLE DOCUMENTATION

Date and Time 68-year-old female admitted to Room 258 by wheelchair from admitting dept. with moderate dyspnea. O_2 running at 2 L per nasal cannula. Weighs 173 lbs. on bed scale wearing only a patient gown. T 98.4°, P 92, R 32, BP 146/68 in R arm while sitting up. Unable to void at the present time. Allergic to penicillin, which causes "hives and difficulty breathing." In high Fowler's position at this time with a respiratory rate of 24 at rest.

________________________ SIGNATURE/TITLE

continued

SKILL 10-1

ADMITTING A PATIENT *Continued*

CRITICAL THINKING

- What aspects of an admission could be delegated to a nursing assistant? What are the responsibilities of the nurse who has delegated a task?
- What actions might you take if a family member or a significant other chooses to remain with the patient after he or she has been escorted to a room on the nursing unit?
- What information is important to provide to the family of a new patient?
- What are some emotional responses that the family of a new patient might be experiencing?

SKILL 10-2

DISCHARGING A PATIENT

Suggested Action	Reason for Action
Assessment	
Determine that a medical order has been written.	Provides authorization for discharging the patient
Check for written prescriptions and other medical discharge instructions.	Enables the patient to continue self-care
Note if there are any new medical orders that must be carried out before the patient's discharge.	Ensures that the patient will leave in the best possible condition
Review the nursing discharge plan.	Determines if more health teaching is needed or if the instructions have been completed
Planning*	
Discuss the patient's time frame for leaving the hospital.	Helps in coordinating nursing activities within the patient's schedule
Coordinate the discharge with the home health care agency, hospice organization, or company supplying oxygen or other medical equipment.	Facilitates continuity of care
Determine the patient's mode of transportation.	Clarifies if the services of a cab company or other resource may be needed
*Notify the business office of the patient's impending discharge.	Allows time for the clerical department to review the patient's billing information and determine the necessity for further actions
*Inform the housekeeping department that the patient will be leaving.	Alerts cleaning staff that the patient unit will need terminal cleaning
*Cancel any meals that the patient will miss after discharge.	Avoids wasting food
*Notify the pharmacy of the approximate time of discharge.	Eliminates wasted drugs
Plan to provide hygiene and medical treatments early.	Prevents delays in the patient's departure
Implementation	
Wash hands.	Reduces transmission of microorganisms
Provide for hygiene but omit changing the bed linen.	Eliminates unnecessary work

* Starred activities may be delegated to a clerk.

continued

SKILL 10-2

DISCHARGING A PATIENT *Continued*

Suggested Action	Reason for Action
Complete medical treatment and nursing interventions according to the plan for care.	Promotes continuation of nursing care
Help the patient dress in street clothing.	Demonstrates concern for the patient's appearance
Review discharge instructions and complete health teaching.	Promotes safe self-care
Have the patient sign the discharge instruction sheet and paraphrase the information it contains.	Validates that the patient has understood instructions for maintaining health
Assist the patient with packing personal items; if appropriate, have the patient sign the clothing inventory or valuables list.	Reduces claims that personal items were lost or stolen; signing a clothing inventory or valuables list is more likely to apply when a patient is discharged from a nursing home or rehabilitation center
Obtain a cart for the patient's belongings.	Eases the work of transporting multiple or heavy items
Assist the patient into a wheelchair when transportation is available.	Reduces the potential for a fall if the patient is weak or unsteady
Stop, if necessary, at the business office.	Complies with billing procedures
Escort the patient to the waiting vehicle.	Promotes safety while still in the hospital
Return any forms from the business office.	Confirms that the patient has left the hospital
Replace the wheelchair in its proper location on the nursing unit.	Makes equipment available for others to use
Wash hands.	Reduces the transmission of microorganisms
Complete a discharge summary in the medical record.	Closes the medical record for this admission

Evaluation

- Health condition is stable (if being transferred in unstable condition, is accompanied by qualified personnel who have the knowledge and skills to intervene in emergencies).
- Patient is able to paraphrase discharge instructions accurately.
- Business office indicates that billing records are in order.
- Patient experiences no injuries during transport from room to vehicle.

Document

- Date and time of discharge
- Condition at time of discharge
- Summary of discharge instructions
- Mode of transportation
- Identity of person(s) who accompanied patient

SAMPLE DOCUMENTATION

Date and Time No fever or wound tenderness at this time. Sutures removed. Abdominal incision intact. No dressing applied. Given prescription for Keflex. Able to repeat how many capsules to administer per dose, the appropriate times for administration, and possible side effects. Repeated signs and symptoms of infection and the need to report them immediately. Instructed to shower as usual and temporarily avoid lifting objects over 10 lbs. Informed to make follow-up appointment in 1 week with physician as indicated on discharge instruction sheet. Given patient's copy of written discharge instructions. Escorted to business office in wheelchair accompanied by spouse. Assisted into private car without any unusual events.

__________________________________ SIGNATURE/TITLE

continued

SKILL 10-2

DISCHARGING A PATIENT *Continued*

CRITICAL THINKING

- What information is important to obtain from the patient to ensure a safe transition to self-management after discharge?
- If the patient cannot assume independent self-management at the time of discharge, what alternatives are possible?

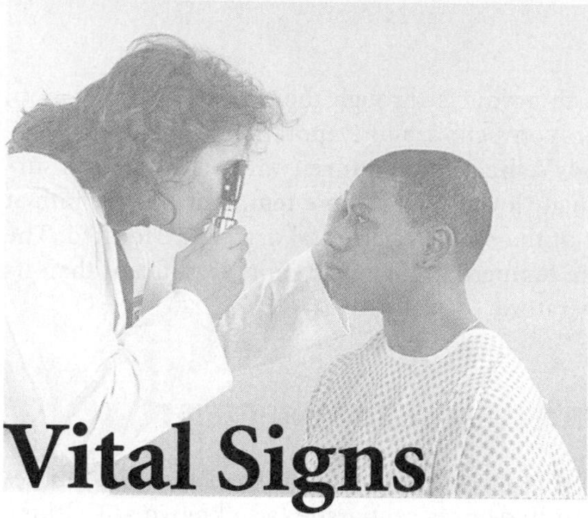

CHAPTER 11

Vital Signs

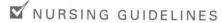

CHAPTER OUTLINE

Body Temperature
Pulse
Respiration
Blood Pressure
Documenting Vital Signs
Nursing Implications

NURSING GUIDELINES

PATIENTS WITH A FEVER
PATIENTS WITH A SUBNORMAL TEMPERATURE
ASSESSING POSTURAL HYPOTENSION

SKILLS

SKILL 11-1: ASSESSING BODY TEMPERATURE
SKILL 11-2: ASSESSING THE RADIAL PULSE
SKILL 11-3: ASSESSING THE RESPIRATORY RATE
SKILL 11-4: ASSESSING BLOOD PRESSURE

NURSING CARE PLAN

HYPERTHERMIA

KEY TERMS

afebrile
afterload
antipyretics
apical heart rate
apical-radial rate
apnea
arrhythmia
auscultatory gap
automated monitoring devices
bradypnea
blood pressure
bradycardia
cardiac output
centigrade scale
cerumen
clinical thermometers
core temperature
diastolic pressure
Doppler stethoscope
drawdown effect
dyspnea
dysrhythmia
Fahrenheit scale
febrile
fever
frenulum
hypertension
hyperthermia
hyperventilation
hypotension
hypothalamus
hypothermia
hypoventilation
Korotkoff sounds
metabolic rate
offsets
orthopnea
orthostatic hypotension
palpitation
postural hypotension
preload
pulse
pulse deficit
pulse pressure
pulse rate
pulse rhythm
pulse volume
pyrexia
respiration
respiratory rate
set point
shell temperature
speculum
sphygmomanometer
stertorous breathing
stethoscope
stridor
systolic pressure
tachycardia
tachypnea
temperature translation
thermistor
training effect
ventilation
vital signs
whitecoat hypertension

LEARNING OBJECTIVES

An understanding of the content within this chapter will be evidenced by the student's ability to:

- List four physiologic components that are measured when assessing vital signs.
- Differentiate between shell and core body temperature.
- Identify the two scales that are used to measure temperature.
- Explain how to convert from one temperature scale to the other.
- List four temperature assessment sites, and indicate the site that is considered the closest to core temperature.
- Name four types of clinical thermometers.
- Discuss the difference between a fever and hyperthermia.
- Name the four phases of a fever.
- List at least four signs or symptoms that accompany a fever.
- Give two reasons for using an infrared tympanic thermometer when the body temperature is subnormal.

- List at least four signs and symptoms that accompany a subnormal body temperature.
- Identify three characteristics that are noted when assessing a patient's pulse.
- Name the most commonly used site for pulse assessment and three other assessment techniques that may be used.
- Explain the difference between respiration and ventilation.
- Name and explain at least four terms used to describe abnormal breathing characteristics.
- Discuss the physiologic data that can be inferred from a blood pressure assessment.
- Explain the difference between systolic and diastolic blood pressure.
- Name three pieces of equipment for assessing blood pressure.
- Describe the five phases of Korotkoff sounds.
- Identify three alternative techniques for assessing blood pressure.

Vital signs (body temperature, pulse rate, respiratory rate, and blood pressure) are objective data that indicate how well or poorly the body is functioning. Vital signs are very sensitive to alterations in physiology; therefore, they are measured at regular intervals to monitor a patient's health status (Display 11-1). This chapter describes how to assess each component of the vital signs and explains what the measurements indicate.

Body Temperature

Body temperature refers to the warmth of the human body. Body heat is produced primarily by exercise and the metabolism of food. Heat is lost from the skin, the lungs, and the body's waste products through the processes of radiation, conduction, convection, and evaporation (Table 11-1).

The body's **shell temperature** (warmth at the skin surface) is usually lower than its **core temperature** (warmth at the center of the body) where vital organs are located. The body's core temperature is much more significant than its shell temperature.

DISPLAY 11–1

Recommendations for Measuring Vital Signs

Vital signs are taken:

- On admission, when obtaining data base assessments
- According to written medical orders
- Once per day when a patient is stable
- At least every 4 hours when one or more vital signs is abnormal
- Every 5 to 15 minutes when a patient is unstable or at risk for rapid physiologic changes, such as after surgery
- Whenever a patient's condition appears to have changed
- A second time, or at more frequent intervals, when there is a significant difference from the previous measurement
- When a patient reports feeling unusual
- Before, during, and after a blood transfusion
- Before administering medications that affect any of the vital signs, and afterward to monitor the drug's effect

TEMPERATURE MEASUREMENT

Temperature is measured either in degrees Fahrenheit, abbreviated °F, or in degrees centigrade (also known as Celsius), abbreviated °C. Both scales measure ranges in temperature from the point at which water freezes and boils.

The **Fahrenheit scale** (scale that uses 32°F as the temperature at which water freezes and 212°F as the point at which it boils) is generally used in the United States to measure and report body temperature. The **centigrade scale** (scale that uses 0°C as the temperature at which water freezes and 100°C as the point at which it boils) is used more often in scientific research and in countries where the metric system is used. Nurses are required to use both scales from time to time and must be able to convert between the two measurements (Display 11-2).

NORMAL BODY TEMPERATURE

In normal, healthy adults, shell temperature generally ranges from 96.6° to 99.3°F or 35.8° to 37.4°C (Porth, 1999). Core body temperature, according to Severine and McKenzie (1997), ranges from 96.9° to 100.4°F (36° to 38°C).

If a patient's temperature is above or below normal, the nurse should report the temperature, reassess at frequent intervals, and implement nursing and medical interventions for restoring normal body temperature as appropriate.

TABLE 11–1. **Mechanisms of Heat Loss**

Method	Description	Example
Radiation	Transfer of heat into the air space of the environment	Body heat warms the air within a sleeping bag.
Conduction	Transfer of heat through contact with a solid substance	Heat from the hands warms an iced drink.
Convection	Transfer of heat by moving it through air, gas, or liquid currents	Warmed air escapes during exhalation from the lungs.
Evaporation	Transfer of heat by changing fluid to a vapor (moisture-filled air)	Warm body fluid in the form of perspiration leaves the skin as a vapor.

DISPLAY 11-2

Temperature Conversion Formulas

To convert Fahrenheit to centigrade, use the formula:

$$°C = \frac{(°F - 32)}{1.8}$$

Example: Step 1: 98.6°F − 32 = 66.6
Step 2: 66.6 ÷ 1.8 = 37°C

To convert centigrade to Fahrenheit, use the formula:

$$°F = (°C \times 1.8) + 32$$

Example: Step 1: 15°C × 1.8 = 27
Step 2: 27 + 32 = 59°F

Temperature Regulation

The **hypothalamus** (structure within the brain) acts as the center for temperature regulation. When functioning appropriately, it maintains the core temperature **set point** (optimal body temperature) within 1°C by responding to slight changes in skin surface and blood temperatures (Fig. 11-1).

Temperatures higher than 105.8°F (41°C) or lower than 93.2°F (34°C) indicate that the hypothalamic regulatory center is impaired. According to Porth (1998), the chance of survival tends to diminish when body temperatures exceed 110°F (43.3°C) or fall below 84°F (28.8°C).

Factors Affecting Body Temperature

Age

Infants and older adults have more difficulty maintaining normal body temperature. Both have limited body fat, which would otherwise provide insulation and prevent heat loss. Their ability to shiver and perspire may also be inadequate, putting them at risk for abnormally low or high body temperatures.

Newborns and young infants tend to experience temperature fluctuations because they have a **metabolic rate** (use of calories for sustaining body functions) twice that of adults. Older adults are compromised by impaired circulation, which interferes with losing or retaining heat through the dilation or constriction of blood vessels near the skin.

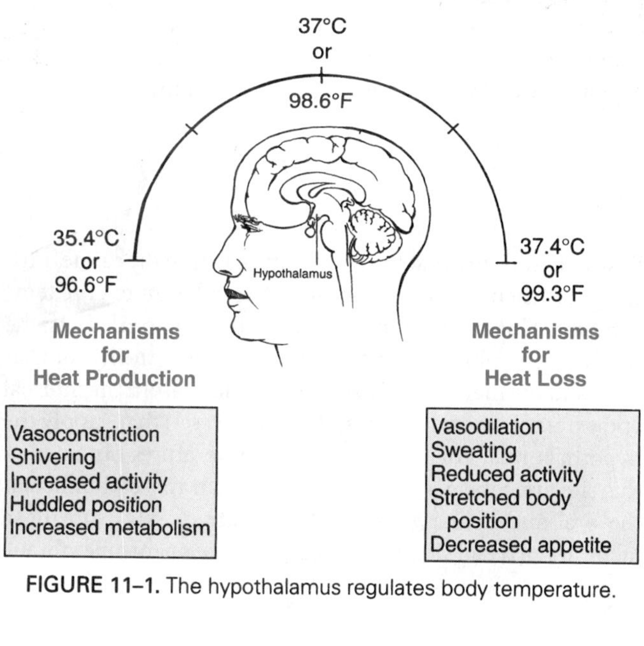

FIGURE 11–1. The hypothalamus regulates body temperature.

Gender

Women of childbearing age have a slight rise in body temperature when ovulating. This is probably due to hormonal changes, affecting metabolism or tissue injury and repair after an ovum (egg) is released. The change in body temperature is so small that most women are unaware of it unless they are monitoring their temperature on a daily basis.

Exercise and Activity

Both exercise and activity involve muscle contraction, which produces body heat. To provide energy, the metabolic rate is also increased, leading to the combustion of calories. This combination increases heat production, which raises the body temperature if compensatory cooling mechanisms are inadequate or impaired.

Circadian Rhythm

Circadian rhythms are physiologic changes, such as fluctuations in body temperature and other vital signs, that occur in 24-hour cycles. Body temperature fluctuates 0.5° to 2.0°F (0.28° to 1.1°C) during a 24-hour period. It tends to be lowest from midnight to dawn and highest in the late afternoon to early evening. People who routinely work at night and sleep during the day have temperature fluctuations that cycle in reverse.

Emotions

Emotions affect the metabolic rate by triggering hormonal changes through the sympathetic and parasympathetic pathways of the autonomic nervous system (see Chap. 5). People who tend to be consistently anxious and nervous are likely to have higher-than-average body temperatures. Conversely, people who are apathetic and depressed are prone to have body temperatures in the lower ranges of normal.

Illness or Injury

Diseases, disorders, or injuries that affect the function of the hypothalamus or mechanisms for heat production and loss alter body temperature, sometimes dramatically. Some examples include tissue injury, infections and inflammatory disorders, fluid loss, injury to the skin, impaired circulation, and head injury.

Drugs

Drugs affect body temperature by increasing or decreasing the metabolic rate and energy requirements. Some drugs, such as aspirin and acetaminophen, directly lower body temperature by acting on the hypothalamus itself. However, in the absence of a fever, their use will not lower body temperature to subnormal levels.

ASSESSMENT SITES

Body temperature can be assessed at a variety of locations. The most practical assessment sites are the mouth, rectum, axilla, and ear (tympanic membrane). These areas are anatomically close to superficial arteries containing warm blood, or they are enclosed areas where heat loss is minimal, or both.

Temperature measurements vary slightly depending on the assessment site (Table 11-2). To evaluate trends in body temperature, the nurse documents the assessment site as O for oral, R for rectal, AX for axillary, and T for tympanic ear membrane and takes the temperature by the same route each time.

Oral Site

The oral site, or mouth, is a convenient assessment site. It generally measures 0.8° to 1.0°F (0.5° to 0.6°C) below core temperature. The area under the tongue is in direct proximity to the sublingual artery. As long as the patient keeps the mouth closed and breathes at a normal rate, the tissue remains at a fairly consistent temperature. Poor placement of the thermometer or premature removal can result in measurements that are off by as much as 1.5°F (0.9°C).

The oral site is contraindicated for patients who are uncooperative, very young, unconscious, or prone to seizures, those who have had oral surgery, mouth breathers, and those who continue to talk during temperature assessment. To ensure accuracy, oral temperature assessment is delayed for at least 30 minutes after the patient has been chewing gum, has smoked a cigarette, or has consumed hot or cold food or beverages.

TABLE 11–2. **Equivalent Mercury Thermometer Measurements According to Site**

Assessment Site	Fahrenheit	Centigrade
Oral	98.6°	37°
Rectal equivalent	99.6°	37.5°
Axillary equivalent	97.6°	36.4°

Rectal Site

The rectum is considered one of the most accurate sites for assessing body temperature. It differs only about 0.2°F (0.1°C) from core temperature. However, rapid fluctuations in temperature may not be identified for as long as an hour because the area retains heat longer than other sites. In addition, it is an embarrassing and emotionally traumatic site for patients who are alert. Further, the presence of stool in the rectum, improper placement of the thermometer, and premature removal affect the accuracy of rectal temperature assessment.

Axillary Site

The axilla, or underarm, is an alternative site for assessing body temperature. Temperature measurements from this site are generally 1°F (0.6°C) lower than those obtained at the oral site and reflect shell rather than core temperature (except in newborns). Because infants can be injured internally with thermometers and because they lose heat through their skin at a greater rate than other age groups, the axilla and the groin are preferred sites for temperature assessment in this age group.

The axillary site has several advantages for all age groups. It is readily accessible in most instances. It is safe. There is less potential for spreading microorganisms than with the oral and rectal sites, and it is less disturbing psychologically than the rectal site. However, this route requires the longest assessment time (8 to 11 minutes), and temperature assessment may be inaccurate if the patient has poor circulation or has recently bathed the area or rubbed it with a towel.

The Ear

Research indicates that the temperature within the ear near the tympanic membrane has the closest correlation to core temperature. This conclusion is based on two anatomic facts: the tympanic membrane is just 1.4″ (3.8 cm) from the hypothalamus, and the membrane is warmed by blood from the internal and external carotid arteries, the same vessels that supply the hypothalamus. For these reasons, temperatures obtained at this site are considered more reliable than those obtained at the oral and axillary sites and correlate closely with those taken at the rectal site. Also, because the tympanic membrane is fairly deep within the head, it is less affected by warm or cool air temperatures.

THERMOMETERS

There are several types of **clinical thermometers** (instruments used to measure body temperature), among them glass, electronic, chemical, and infrared thermometers (Table 11-3).

Glass Thermometers

A glass thermometer, which is calibrated in either the Fahrenheit or centigrade scale, has two parts—the bulb and the stem (Fig. 11-2). The bulb is either long and slender or more bluntly rounded. The long slender bulb provides a larger surface for contact with tissues and is therefore preferred for taking oral temperatures. The more rounded bulb is less fragile and more appropriate for rectal placement. The stem is a long tube that contains liquid mercury. When mercury is heated, it expands and moves up through the stem. The stem is calibrated in whole degrees and tenths of degrees. The highest point to which the mercury rises is read as the body temperature. Temperatures are recorded in tenths, such as 97.8°F.

Glass mercury thermometers have largely been replaced in health care agencies by electronic and infrared thermometers, but they are still widely used by patients at home. Because glass thermometers are not disposable, nurses must teach patients and their family members how to use and clean them.

TABLE 11–3. **Types of Clinical Thermometer**

Type	Advantages	Disadvantages
Glass	Inexpensive Small Portable Widely available	Breakable Difficult to read Cleaning necessary before use by another patient Unable to sterilize using heat Time-consuming to use Accuracy affected by eating, drinking, smoking, talking, mouth breathing, stool in the rectum, vasoconstriction of skin and mucous membranes Porous; possible inaccuracy from mercury evaporation High risk for injury if broken during use Environmental pollution from mercury, if not properly disposed
Electronic	Faster than glass Accurate No sterilization or disinfection needed Easy to use	Expensive Recharging necessary Probe needs to be held by patient or nurse Interference with simultaneously taking the patient's pulse while holding the probe with one hand and the unit in the other
Infrared (tympanic)	Fastest Convenient Closest approximation of core temperature Least invasive Accuracy unaffected by eating, drinking, or breathing Most sanitary No sterilization or disinfection required	Expensive Battery recharging necessary Accuracy affected by improper placement and probe size Actual ear and core temperature ranges are slightly different from oral, rectal, and axillary sites Tip requires cleaning with a paper tissue or alcohol swab Extreme hot or cold environmental temperatures affecting electronics
Chemical	Inexpensive Safe; nonbreakable Sanitary Temperature registers in approximately 45 seconds No cleaning or disinfection necessary Easily used by untrained individuals	Measurements vary at different body sites depending on blood flow and room temperature

Patient Teaching For
Cleaning Glass Thermometers

Teach the patient or the family to do the following:

- Don gloves if there is the potential for contact with blood or stool, as may be the case with rectal assessment.
- Hold the thermometer at the tip of the stem and keep the bulb in a downward position, away from your hand.
- Wipe the soiled thermometer toward the bulb with a clean, soft tissue using a firm twisting motion.
- Wash the thermometer with soap or detergent solution, again using friction.
- Rinse the thermometer under cold running water.
- Dry the thermometer with a soft towel.
- Soak the thermometer in 70% to 90% isopropyl alcohol or a 1:10 solution of household bleach (1 part bleach to 10 parts water).
- Rinse the thermometer after disinfecting it.
- Store the thermometer in a clean, dry container.

Electronic Thermometers

An electronic thermometer (Fig. 11-3) uses a temperature-sensitive probe covered with a disposable sheath. The probe is attached by a coiled wire to a display unit. Electronic thermometers are portable. They are recharged when not in use.

Electronic thermometers generally have two types of probes: one for oral or axillary use and another for rectal use. Some types offer the option of providing the measurement in Fahrenheit or centigrade.

There is no established length of time for probe placement. The electronic unit senses when the temperature ceases to change and emits a beep. The signal, which usually sounds in 30 to 60 seconds, alerts the nurse to remove the probe and read the displayed measurement.

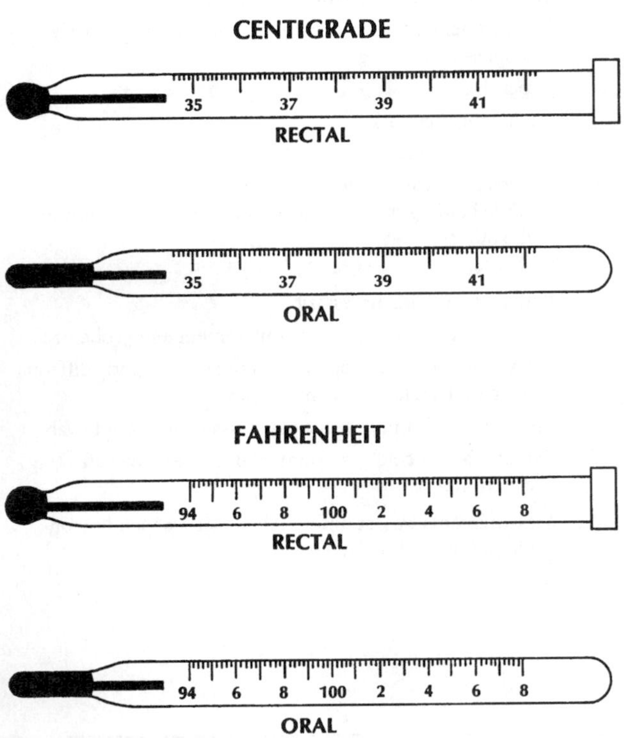

FIGURE 11–2. Glass mercury thermometers.

Infrared (Tympanic) Thermometers

Infrared tympanic thermometers are the newest type of electronic equipment for assessing body temperature. The device consists of a hand-held covered probe that is inserted into the ear canal (Fig. 11-4); its base charging unit is sometimes referred to as its cradle.

The probe contains an infrared sensor that detects the warmth radiating from the tympanic membrane (eardrum) and converts the heat into a temperature measurement in 2 to 5 seconds. The potential for transferring microorganisms from one patient to another is reduced because the probe cover is changed after each use, and because the ear does not contain mucous membrane and its accompanying secretions.

Despite the advantages of these thermometers, some reports (Severine and McKenzie, 1997) have found that infrared thermometers produce inaccurate measurements if:

- The ear canal is not straightened appropriately.
- The probe is too large for the ear canal (a problem with infants and small children).
- The sensor is directed at the ear canal rather than directly at the tympanic membrane.
- There is impacted **cerumen** (ear wax), a common problem among older adults.
- The **drawdown effect** (cooling of the ear when it comes in contact with the probe) occurs.

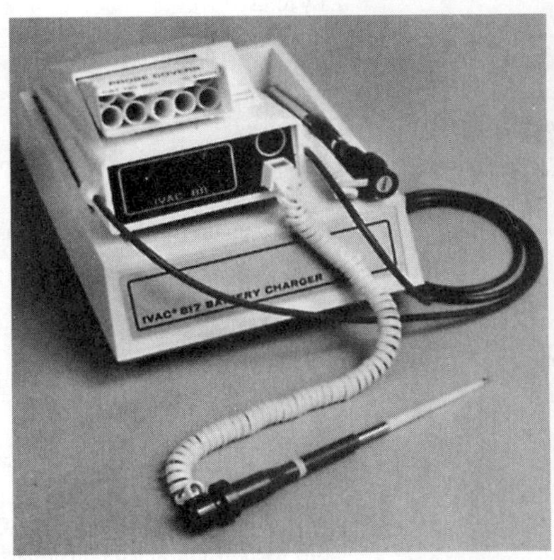

FIGURE 11–3. Electronic thermometer. (Courtesy of the IVAC Corporation, San Diego, CA.)

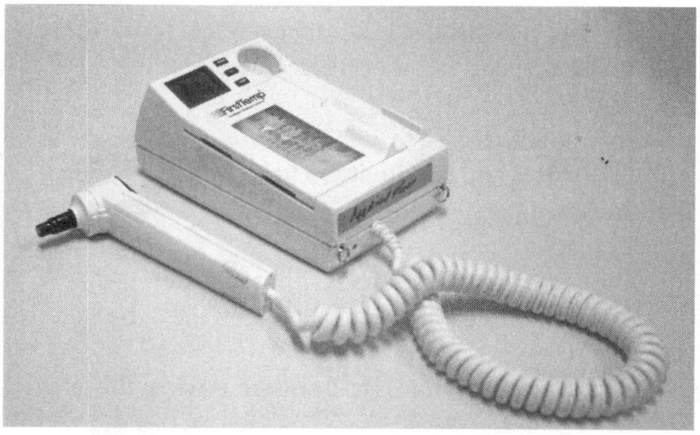

FIGURE 11–4. Infrared tympanic thermometer.

The first use of a tympanic thermometer after recharging is not always as accurate as a second reading. Another criticism of tympanic temperature measurement is that currently there is no standard for actual ear or core temperatures. At present, tympanic thermometers use internally calculated **offsets** (predictive mathematical conversions) for oral and rectal temperatures. These offsets vary from manufacturer to manufacturer.

Chemical Thermometers

Various types of chemical thermometers are available. One example is a paper or plastic strip with chemically treated dots (Fig. 11-5). The temperature is determined by noting how many dots change color after the strip is held in the mouth. Chemical dot thermometers are discarded after one use. They are used for assessing the temperature of patients who require isolation precautions for infectious diseases. Their use eliminates the need to clean a multiuse thermometer, such as an electronic or infrared one. Some physician's offices also use chemical dot thermometers because they are disposable.

A second type of chemical thermometer is made of a heat-sensitive tape or patch that is applied to the abdomen or forehead (Fig. 11-6). The tape or patch changes color according to the body temperature. Heat-sensitive tapes and patches can be reused several times before being thrown away.

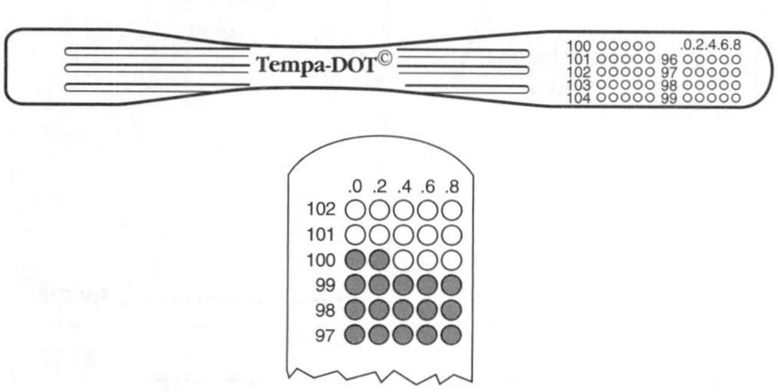

FIGURE 11–5. Chemical thermometer.

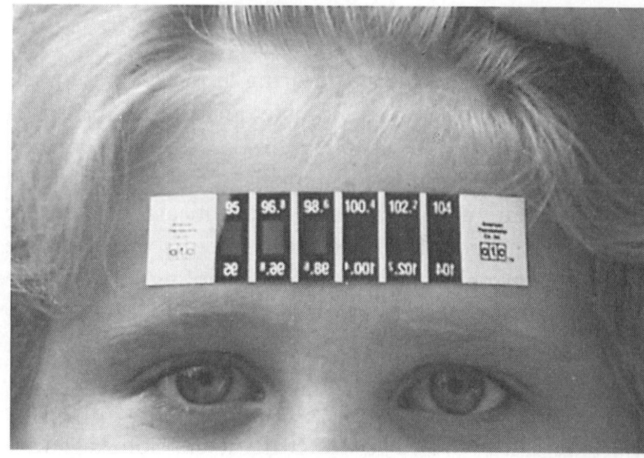

FIGURE 11–6. Disposable chemical thermometer with heat-sensitive liquid crystals.

Automated Monitoring Devices

Some agencies use **automated monitoring devices** (equipment that allows for the simultaneous collection of multiple vital sign data). They may measure the temperature, blood pressure, and pulse (Fig. 11-7) as well as other information such as heart rhythm and pulse oximetry. Some models can store and display the trends in vital signs.

Most automated monitors are portable and can be moved from room to room or remain at one patient's bedside. Their chief advantage is that they save time and money. Agencies have found that the use of automated monitors allows some potentially unstable patients to be cared for on a general medical-surgical unit rather than in the more expensive intensive care unit. To ensure reliable data, the accuracy of automated devices needs to be cross-checked with manual devices from time to time.

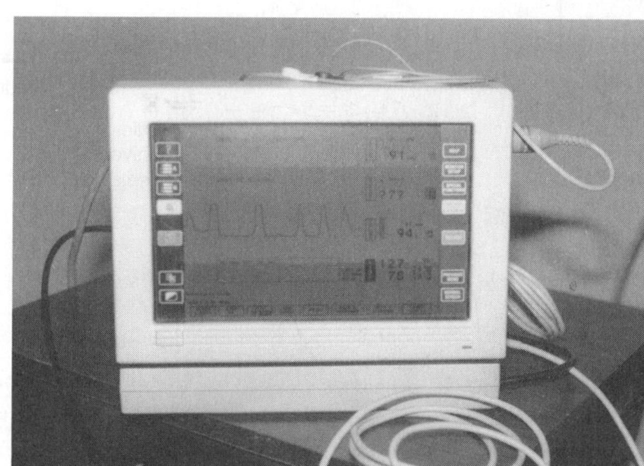

FIGURE 11–7. An automated monitoring device. (Courtesy of Ken Timby.)

Continuous Monitoring Devices

Continuous temperature monitoring devices are used primarily in critical care areas. Body temperature is measured using probes within the esophagus of anesthetized patients or by means of a **thermistor** (temperature sensor) attached to a pulmonary artery catheter. These measurements are generally required when caring for patients with extreme hypo- or hyperthermia. Warming or cooling blankets are usually used at the same time (see Chap. 28). The assessment aids in evaluating the effectiveness of these treatment devices.

Skill 11-1 describes how to assess body temperature using electronic, infrared, and glass thermometers. Some agencies also use automated and continuous monitoring devices.

ELEVATED BODY TEMPERATURE

A **fever** (body temperature that exceeds 99.3°F [37.4°C]) is a common indication of illness. **Pyrexia** (Greek word for fire) is a term used to describe a warmer-than-normal set point. A person with a fever is said to be **febrile** (condition in which the temperature is elevated) as opposed to **afebrile** (absence of a fever).

Hyperthermia (excessively high core temperature) describes a state in which the temperature usually exceeds 105.8°F (40.6°C). At this level, the person is at extremely high risk for brain damage or death from complications associated with increased metabolic demands.

The following are common signs and symptoms associated with a fever:

- Pinkish, red (flushed) skin that is warm to the touch
- Restlessness or, in others, excessive sleepiness
- Irritability
- Poor appetite
- Glassy eyes and sensitivity to light
- Increased perspiration
- Headache
- Above-normal pulse and respiratory rates
- Disorientation and confusion (when the temperature is high)
- Convulsions in infants and children (when the temperature is high)
- Fever blisters about the nose or lips in patients who harbor the herpes simplex virus.

Phases of a Fever

A fever generally progresses through four distinct phases:

1. *Prodromal phase:* the patient has nonspecific symptoms just before the temperature rises
2. *Onset* or *invasion phase:* obvious mechanisms for increasing body temperature develop
3. *Stationary phase:* the fever is sustained
4. *Resolution* or *defervescence phase:* the temperature returns to normal (Fig. 11-8.)

If the fever suddenly drops to normal, it is referred to as a resolution by crisis. If it gradually descends, it is a resolution lysis.

Fevers and the manner in which they subside take a variety of courses. Common variations in fever patterns are described in Table 11-4.

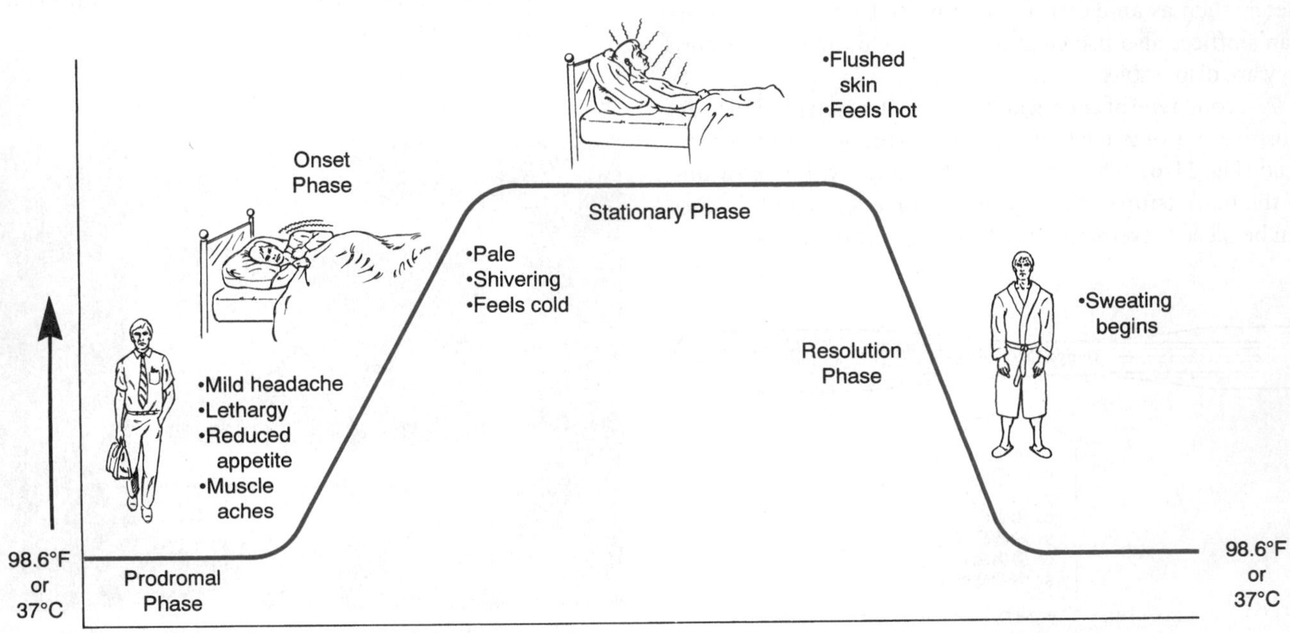

FIGURE 11–8. Phases of a fever and physiologic changes.

TABLE 11–4. **Variations in Fever Patterns**

	Type of Fever	Description
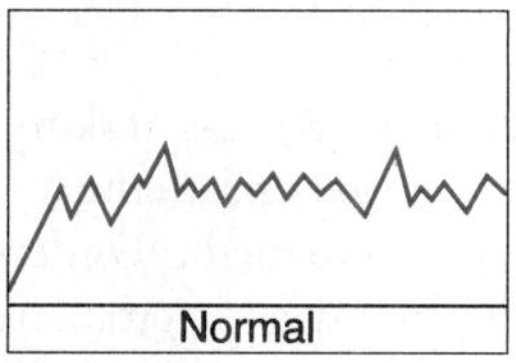	Sustained fever	Remains elevated with little fluctuation
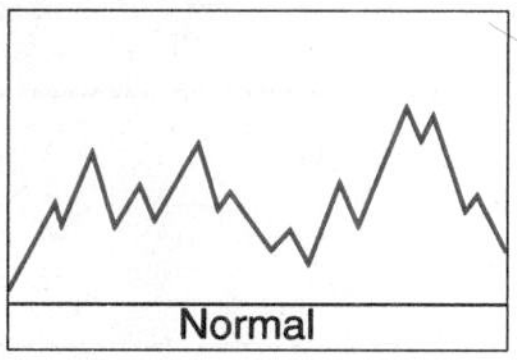	Remittent fever	Fluctuates several degrees, but never reaches normal between fluctuations
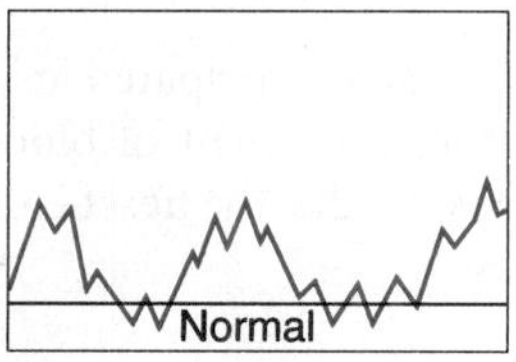	Intermittent fever	Cycles frequently between periods of normal or subnormal temperatures and spikes of fever
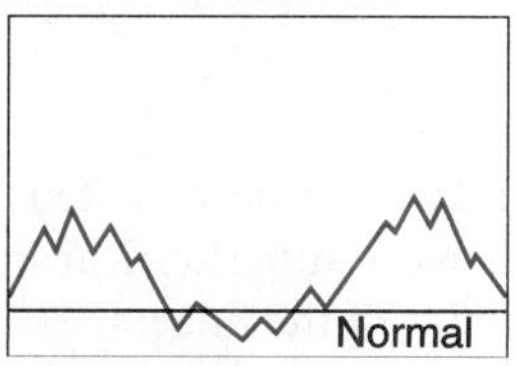	Relapsing fever	Reoccurs after a brief but sustained period during which the temperature has been normal

Nursing Management

A fever is considered an important body defense for destroying infectious microorganisms. Therefore, as long as the fever remains below 102°F (38.9°C) and the person does not have a chronic medical condition, providing fluids or rest may be all that is necessary. **Antipyretics** (drugs that reduce fever) such as aspirin or acetaminophen are helpful when the temperature is 102° to 104°F (38.9° to 40°C). Physical cooling measures are used for temperatures between 104° and 105.8°F (40° to 40.6°C). If the temperature is higher than 105.8°F (40.6°C), or if a high temperature is unchanged after a sufficient response time with conventional interventions, more aggressive treatment is warranted.

Nursing Guidelines For

Patients with a Fever

☑ Cover patients when shivering is evident.
RATIONALE: Prevents heat loss and assists the hypothalamus in reaching a higher set point.

☑ Keep patients in a warm but not hot environment.
RATIONALE: Provides comfort while the body adapts to the new set point.

☑ Remove blankets or heavy clothing once shivering subsides.
RATIONALE: Facilitates heat loss from radiation and convection and maintains body temperature within the new set point.

☑ Limit activity.
RATIONALE: Reduces heat production.

☑ Provide liberal amounts of oral fluids.
RATIONALE: Replaces fluid loss due to perspiration and increased metabolism.

☑ Provide light but high-calorie nourishment.
RATIONALE: Compensates for increased metabolic rate, delayed gastric emptying, and decreased intestinal motility (Letizia and Janusek, 1994).

☑ Administer antipyretics according to medical orders. Aspirin is contraindicated for use in children with fevers because it is associated with Reye's syndrome.
RATIONALE: Blocks the set point elevation in the hypothalamus.

☑ Apply cool cloths or an ice bag to the forehead, behind the neck, and between the axillary and inguinal skin folds.
RATIONALE: Cools blood that flows near the peripheral skin surface.

☑ Promote room ventilation.
RATIONALE: Disperses heat via air currents.

☑ Keep the humidity level low.
RATIONALE: Facilitates evaporation.

☑ Apply tepid water to the skin, as in a sponge bath, 30 minutes after administering an antipyretic.
RATIONALE: Increases heat loss through evaporation after allowing the set point to be lowered.

☑ Discontinue physical cooling measures if the patient begins to shiver.
RATIONALE: Shivering raises body heat and defeats the purpose of the sponge bath.

☑ Apply an electronically regulated cooling pad beneath the patient as directed by a physician (see Chap. 28).
RATIONALE: Cools blood as it circulates through the skin.

SUBNORMAL BODY TEMPERATURE

There are several ranges of **hypothermia** (core body temperature less than 95°F [35°C]). A person is considered *mildly hypothermic* at temperatures of 95° to 93.2°F (35° to 34°C), *moderately hypothermic* at 93° to 86°F (33.8° to 30°C), and *severely hypothermic* at below 86°F (30°C).

Cold body temperatures are best measured with a tympanic thermometer for two reasons. First, other clinical thermometers do not have the capacity to measure temperatures in hypothermic ranges. Second, the blood flow in the mouth, rectum, or axilla is generally so reduced that measurements taken from these sites are inaccurate.

The following are common signs and symptoms associated with hypothermia:

- Shivering until body temperature is extremely low
- Pale, cool skin
- Puffiness of skin
- Impaired muscle coordination
- Listlessness
- Slow pulse and respiratory rates
- Irregular heart rhythm
- Decreased ability to think coherently and use good judgment
- Diminished ability to feel pain or other sensations

In some illnesses, such as hypothyroidism and starvation, the patient typically has a subnormal temperature. Therefore, the nurse must assess patients just as closely when the body temperature falls below normal ranges as when it is elevated.

Death usually occurs in severely hypothermic patients. However, patients have been known to live even with very low temperatures, as in near-drownings in cold water and exposure in extremely cold environments. This phenomenon has led to the saying among paramedics and emergency department personnel that "patients aren't dead until they're warm and dead."

Nursing Management

Various supportive measures may be implemented when patients have subnormal body temperatures.

Nursing Guidelines For

Patients with a Subnormal Temperature

☑ Raise the room temperature.
RATIONALE: Warms the surface of the body.

☑ Remove wet clothing.
RATIONALE: Reduces heat loss.

☑ Apply layers of dry clothing and loosely woven blankets.
RATIONALE: Traps body heat next to the skin.

☑ Warm blankets and clothing in a warming oven or microwave if the body temperature is quite low.
RATIONALE: Raises the temperature of woven fabrics above ambient (room) temperature.

☑ Position the patient so that the arms are next to the chest and the legs are tucked toward the abdomen.
RATIONALE: Prevents heat loss.

☑ Cover the head with a cap or towel.
RATIONALE: Reduces heat loss from exposed body areas.

☑ Provide warm fluids.
RATIONALE: Conducts heat to internal organs.

☑ Massage the skin unless it has been frostbitten.
RATIONALE: Produces mechanical friction, which produces warmth.

☑ Apply bags filled with warm water between areas of skin folds, or place an electronic warming pad beneath the back and hips (see Chap. 28), according to medical orders.
RATIONALE: Transfers heat to the blood as it circulates through the skin.

Pulse

The **pulse** (wavelike sensation that can be palpated in a peripheral artery) is produced by the movement of blood during the heart's contraction. In most adults, the heart contracts 60 to 100 times a minute at rest.

PULSE RATE

The **pulse rate** (number of peripheral pulsations palpated in a minute) is counted by compressing a superficial artery against an underlying bone with the tips of the fingers.

Rapid Pulse Rate

The pulse rate of adults is considered rapid if it exceeds 100 beats per minute (bpm) at rest. **Tachycardia** (heart rate between 100 and 150 bpm) is a fast heart rate, but heart and pulse rates can exceed 150 beats per minute. Rapid contraction, if sustained, tends to overwork the heart and may not oxygenate cells adequately because the heart has such little time between contractions to fill with blood.

The term **palpitation** (awareness of one's own heart contraction without having to feel the pulse) can accompany tachycardia. Patients with a rapid pulse rate are monitored closely, and the results are reported and recorded according to agency policy.

Slow Pulse Rate

The pulse rate of adults is considered slower than normal if it falls below 60 beats per minute. **Bradycardia** (heart rate less than 60 bpm) is less common than tachycardia; it merits prompt reporting and continued monitoring.

Factors Affecting Pulse and Heart Rates

Any factors that affect the rate of heart contraction also cause a comparable effect in the pulse rate. Because one is dependent on the other, the pulse rate can never be faster than the actual heart rate per minute. Heart and pulse rates may vary depending on the following:

- *Age.* Some common rates are listed in Table 11-5.
- *Circadian rhythm.* Rates tend to be lower in the morning and increase later in the day.
- *Gender.* Men average approximately 60 to 65 beats per minute at rest; the average rate for women is about 7 or 8 beats per minute faster.
- *Body build.* Tall, slender persons usually have slower heart and pulse rates than short, stout persons.
- *Exercise and activity.* Rates increase with exercise and activity and decrease with rest. However, with regular aerobic exercise, a **training effect** (the heart rate and consequently the pulse rate become consistently lower than average) occurs. This effect develops because the heart muscle becomes efficient at supplying body cells with a sufficient volume of oxygenated blood with fewer beats. Those who are physically fit exhibit slower pulse rates even during exercise.
- *Stress and emotions.* Stimulation of the sympathetic nervous system and emotions such as anger, fear, and excitement increase heart and pulse rates. Pain, which is stressful (especially when it is moderate to severe), can trigger faster rates.
- *Body temperature.* For every one degree of Fahrenheit elevation, the heart and pulse rate increase 10 bpm. A one-degree increase in centigrade measurement causes a 15-bpm increase (Porth, 1999). With a fall in body temperature, an opposite effect occurs.
- *Blood volume.* Excessive blood loss causes the heart and pulse rates to increase. With decreased red blood cells or inadequate hemoglobin to distribute oxygen to cells, the heart rate accelerates in an effort to keep cells adequately supplied.
- *Drugs.* Certain drugs can slow or speed the rate of heart contraction. Digitalis preparations and sedatives typically slow the heart rate. Caffeine, nicotine, cocaine, thyroid replacement hormones, and adrenalin increase heart contractions and subsequently the pulse rate.

TABLE 11–5. **Normal Pulse Rates per Minute at Various Ages**

Age	Approximate Range	Approximate Average
Newborn	120–160	140
1–12 months	80–140	120
1–2 years	80–130	110
3–6 years	75–120	100
7–12 years	75–110	95
Adolescence	60–100	80
Adulthood	60–100	80

PULSE RHYTHM

The **pulse rhythm** (pattern of the pulsations and the pauses between them) is normally regular. That is, the beats and the pauses occur similarly throughout the time the pulse is palpated.

An **arrhythmia** or **dysrhythmia** (irregular pattern of heartbeats), with a consequently irregular pulse rhythm, is reported promptly. Some types of arrhythmias indicate potentially life-threatening cardiac dysfunctions that may warrant more sophisticated monitoring and treatment. Details about arrhythmias and their causes can be found in textbooks that discuss cardiac disorders.

PULSE VOLUME

Pulse volume (quality of the pulsations that are felt) is usually related to the amount of blood pumped with each heartbeat, or the force of the heart's contraction. A normal pulse is described as feeling *strong* when it can be felt with mild pressure over the artery. A *feeble, weak,* or *thready pulse* describes a pulse that is difficult to feel or, once felt, is easily obliterated with slight pressure. A rapid, thready pulse is usually a serious sign and is reported promptly. A *bounding* or *full pulse* produces a pronounced pulsation that does not easily disappear with pressure.

Another way to describe the volume or quality of the pulse is with corresponding numbers (Table 11-6). When documenting pulse volume, the nurse should follow agency policy about using descriptive terms or a numbering system.

ASSESSMENT SITES

The arteries used for pulse assessment lie close to the skin. Most, but not all, are named for the bone over which they are located (Fig. 11-9). These pulse sites are collectively called *peripheral pulses* because they are distant from the heart. Of all the peripheral pulses, the radial artery, located on the inner (thumb) side of the wrist, is the site most often used for pulse assessment.

Three alternative assessment techniques can be used in lieu of, or in addition to, assessment of a peripheral pulse. These techniques include counting the apical heart rate, obtaining an apical-radial rate, and using a Doppler ultrasound device over a peripheral artery.

Apical Heart Rate

The **apical heart rate** (number of ventricular contractions per minute) is considered more accurate than the radial pulse for two reasons. First, the sound of each heartbeat is obvious and distinct. Second, sometimes the heart contraction is not strong enough to be felt at a peripheral pulse site. However,

TABLE 11–6. **Identifying Pulse Volume**

Number	Definition	Description
0	Absent pulse	No pulsation is felt despite extreme pressure.
1+	Thready pulse	Pulsation is not easily felt; slight pressure causes it to disappear.
2+	Weak pulse	Stronger than a thready pulse; light pressure causes it to disappear.
3+	Normal pulse	Pulsation is easily felt; moderate pressure causes it to disappear.
4+	Bounding pulse	The pulsation is strong and does not disappear with moderate pressure.

counting the apical rate is not as convenient as a radial pulse assessment. An apical heart rate is generally assessed when the peripheral pulse is irregular or difficult to palpate due to a rapid rate or thready quality, or when it is necessary to obtain an actual heart rate.

The apical heart rate is counted by listening at the chest with a stethoscope or by feeling the pulsations in the chest at an area called the *point of maximum impulse* for 1 full minute. As the name suggests, the heartbeats are best heard, or felt, at the apex, or lower tip, of the heart. The apex in a healthy adult is slightly below the left nipple, in line with the middle of the clavicle (Fig. 11-10).

When assessing the apical heart rate by listening to the chest—which is generally the more accurate technique—the nurse listens for the "lub/dub" sound. The lub sound is louder if the stethoscope has been correctly applied. These two sounds equal one pulsation at a peripheral pulse site. The apical heart rate is counted for 1 full minute, and the rhythm is also evaluated.

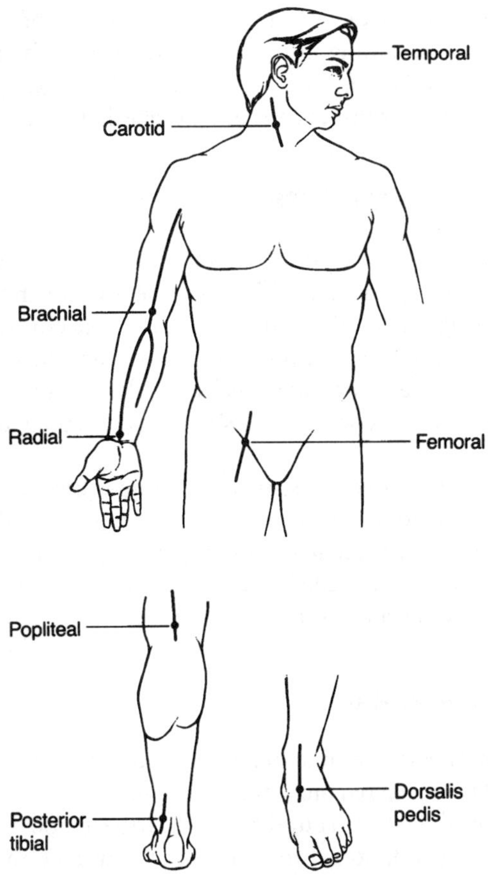

FIGURE 11-9. Peripheral pulse sites.

Apical-Radial Rate

The **apical-radial rate** (number of sounds heard at the heart's apex and the rate of the radial pulse during the same period) is counted by separate nurses at the same time using one watch or clock (Fig. 11-11). The apical and radial rates should be the same, but in some patients they are not. The **pulse deficit** (difference between the apical and radial pulse rates) is noted. If a significant pulse deficit is present—and the rates have been counted accurately—the findings are reported promptly and documented in the patient's medical record.

Doppler Ultrasound Device

A Doppler ultrasound device is an electronic instrument that detects the movement of blood through peripheral blood vessels and converts the movement to a sound. This instrument is most helpful when slight pressure occludes pulsations or arterial blood flow is severely compromised.

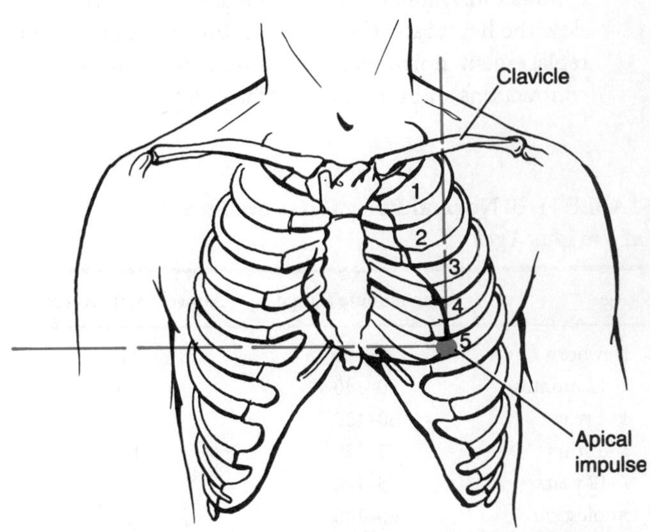

FIGURE 11-10. The apical heart rate is assessed to the left of the sternum at the interspace below the fifth rib in midline with the clavicle.

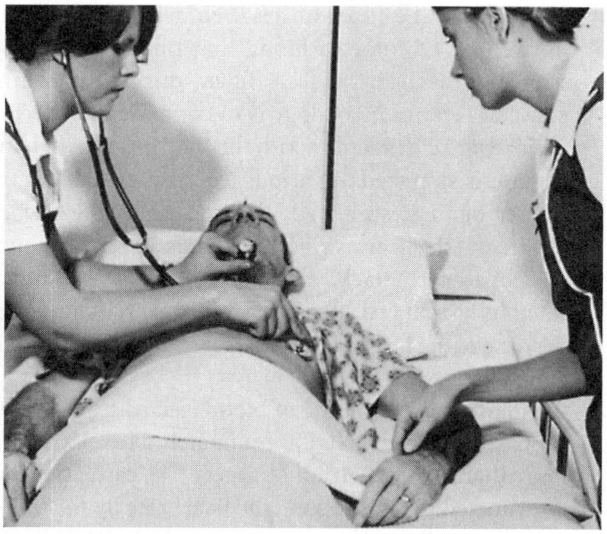

FIGURE 11–11. One nurse counts the radial pulse while the other counts the apical rate.

When the device is used, conductive gel is applied over the arterial site and the probe is moved at an angle over the skin until a pulsating sound is heard (Fig. 11-12). The pulsating sounds are counted, much like the palpated pulsations. The nurse documents the assessment site and the rate, followed by the abbreviation D to indicate it was obtained using a Doppler device.

Skill 11-2 describes how to assess the rate, rhythm, and volume of the pulse at the radial artery.

Respiration

Respiration (exchange of oxygen and carbon dioxide), when it occurs between the alveolar and capillary membranes, is called *external respiration.* The process of exchanging oxygen and carbon dioxide between the blood and body cells is called *internal respiration* or *tissue respiration.*

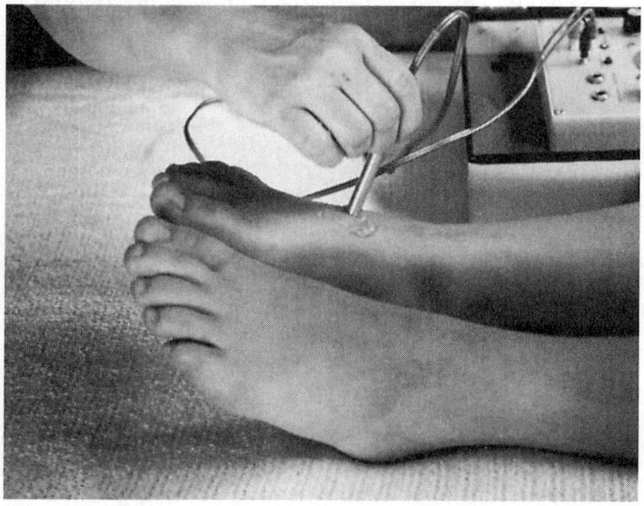

FIGURE 11–12. Using a Doppler ultrasound device.

Ventilation (movement of air in and out of the chest) involves *inhalation* or *inspiration* (breathing in) and *exhalation* or *expiration* (breathing out). Ventilation is controlled by the medulla, the respiratory center in the brain. The medulla is sensitive to the amount of carbon dioxide in the blood and adapts the rate of ventilations accordingly. Breathing can be voluntarily controlled to a certain extent.

RESPIRATORY RATE

The **respiratory rate** (number of ventilations per minute) varies considerably in healthy people, but normal ranges have been established (Table 11-7). Factors that influence the pulse rate generally also affect the respiratory rate. The faster the pulse rate, the faster the respiratory rate, and vice versa. The ratio of one respiration to approximately four or five heartbeats is fairly consistent in normal people.

Rapid Respiratory Rate

Resting respiratory rates that exceed the standards for a patient's age are considered abnormal. **Tachypnea** (rapid respiratory rate) often accompanies an elevated temperature or diseases that affect the cardiac and respiratory systems.

Slow Respiratory Rates

Bradypnea (slower-than-normal respiratory rate at rest) can occur as a result of medications—for instance, morphine sulfate slows the respiratory rate. Slow respirations may also be observed in patients with neurologic disorders or those experiencing hypothermia.

BREATHING PATTERNS AND ABNORMAL CHARACTERISTICS

Various breathing patterns and abnormal characteristics may be identified when assessing respiratory rates. *Cheyne-Stokes*

TABLE 11–7. **Normal Respiratory Rates at Various Ages**

Age	Average Range
Newborn	30–80
Early childhood	20–40
Late childhood	15–25
Adulthood	
Men	14–18
Women	16–20

respiration refers to a breathing pattern in which there is a gradual increase in the depth of respirations followed by a gradual decrease, and then a period when breathing stops briefly before resuming again. Cheyne-Stokes respiration is a serious sign that may occur as death approaches.

Hyperventilation (rapid or deep breathing, or both) and **hypoventilation** (diminished breathing) affect the volume of air entering and leaving the lungs. Changes in ventilation may occur in patients with airway obstruction or pulmonary or neuromuscular diseases.

Dyspnea (difficult or labored breathing) is almost always accompanied by a rapid respiratory rate as patients work to improve the efficiency of their breathing. Patients with dyspnea usually appear anxious and worried. The nostrils flare (widen) as the patient fights to fill the lungs with air. Abdominal and neck muscles may be used to assist other muscles in breathing. When observing the patient, the nurse should note how much and what type of activity brings on dyspnea. For example, walking to the bathroom may bring on dyspnea in a patient, but sitting in a chair may not.

Orthopnea (breathing that is facilitated by sitting up or standing) occurs in patients with dyspnea who find it easier to breathe in this manner. The sitting or standing position causes organs in the abdominal cavity to fall away from the diaphragm with gravity. This gives more room for the lungs to expand within the chest cavity, allowing the person to take in more air with each breath.

Apnea (absence of breathing) is a life-threatening situation if it lasts more than 4 to 6 minutes. Prolonged apnea leads to brain damage or death. Brief periods of apnea lower the oxygen levels in the blood and can trigger serious abnormal cardiac rhythms (see Chap. 20 for more on sleep apnea).

Terms such as **stertorous breathing** (noisy ventilation) and **stridor** (harsh, high-pitched sound heard on inspiration when there is laryngeal obstruction) are used to describe sounds that accompany breathing. Infants and young children with croup often have stridor when breathing.

The nurse uses a stethoscope to listen to the sounds of air moving through the chest. The technique and the characteristics of lung sounds are described in Chapter 12.

Skill 11-3 lists techniques to use when counting the respiratory rate.

Blood Pressure

Blood pressure (force exerted by blood within the arteries) is created and affected by several physiologic variables:

- Circulating blood volume, which averages 4.5 to 5.5 L in adult women and 5.0 to 6.0 L in adult men. Lower-than-normal volumes decrease blood pressure; excess blood volume increases it.
- Contractility of the heart, which is influenced by the stretch of cardiac muscle fibers. Based on *Starling's law of the heart,* the force of heart contraction is related to **preload** (volume of blood that fills the heart and stretches the heart muscle fibers during its resting phase). A common analogy is to compare the effect of preload and contractility with the snap of a rubber band when it is stretched to various lengths—the longer the rubber band is stretched, the greater it snaps when released. If the heart is scarred from tissue damage, such as after a heart attack, stretching is impaired and contractility is reduced. Regular aerobic exercise increases the tone of the heart muscle, making it an efficient muscular pump.
- **Cardiac output** (volume of blood ejected from the left ventricle per minute) is approximately 5 to 6 L (slightly more than a gallon) in adults at rest. The cardiac output is estimated by multiplying the heart rate by the stroke volume (amount of blood that leaves the heart with each contraction). The average stroke volume in adults is 70 ml. With exercise, the cardiac output can increase as much as five times the resting volume. Bradycardia can severely reduce cardiac output and thus blood pressure.
- Blood viscosity (thickness) creates a resisting force when the heart contracts. The resistance compromises stroke volume and cardiac output. Blood thickens when there are more cells and proteins in proportion to water in plasma. Circulating viscous blood also tires the heart and weakens its ability to contract.
- Peripheral resistance, which is referred to as **afterload** (force against which the heart pumps when ejecting blood), is increased when the valves of the heart and arterioles (small subdivisions of arteries) are narrowed or calcified. Afterload is decreased when arteries dilate.

In healthy people, the arterial walls are elastic and easily stretch and recoil to accommodate the changing volume of circulating blood. Measuring the blood pressure helps to assess the efficiency of the circulatory system. Blood pressure measurements reflect (1) the ability of the arteries to stretch, (2) the volume of circulating blood, and (3) the amount of resistance the heart must overcome when it pumps blood.

FACTORS AFFECTING BLOOD PRESSURE

Besides the physiologic variables that create blood pressure, other factors cause temporary or permanent alterations. They include:

- *Age.* Blood pressure tends to rise with age due to *arteriosclerosis,* a process in which arteries lose their elasticity and become more rigid, and *atherosclerosis,* a process in which the arteries become narrowed with fat deposits. The rate at which these conditions occur depends on heredity and lifestyle habits such as diet and exercise.

- *Circadian rhythm.* Blood pressure tends to be lowest after midnight, begins rising at approximately 4 or 5 A.M., and peaks during late morning or early afternoon.
- *Gender.* Women tend to have lower blood pressure than men of the same age.
- *Exercise and activity.* Blood pressure rises during exercise and activity, when the heart pumps a greater volume of blood. Regular exercise, however, helps to maintain the blood pressure within normal levels.
- *Emotions and pain.* Strong emotional experiences and pain tend to cause blood pressure to rise from sympathetic nervous system stimulation.
- *Miscellaneous factors.* As a rule, a person has a lower blood pressure when lying down than when sitting or standing, although the difference in most people is insignificant. Blood pressure also seems to rise somewhat when the urinary bladder is full, when the legs are crossed, or when the person is cold. Drugs that stimulate the heart such as nicotine, caffeine, and cocaine also tend to constrict the arteries and raise blood pressure.

PRESSURE MEASUREMENTS

When the blood pressure is assessed, both systolic and diastolic pressure measurements are obtained. **Systolic pressure** (pressure within the arterial system when the heart contracts) is higher than **diastolic pressure** (pressure within the arterial system when the heart relaxes and fills with blood).

Blood pressure measurement is expressed as a fraction. The numerator is the systolic pressure and the denominator is the diastolic pressure. The pressure is expressed in millimeters of mercury, abbreviated mm Hg. Thus, a recording of 140/80 means the systolic blood pressure was measured at 140 mm Hg and the diastolic blood pressure was measured at 80 mm Hg.

The **pulse pressure** (difference between systolic and diastolic blood pressure measurements) is computed by subtracting the smaller figure from the larger. For example, when the blood pressure is 126/88 mm Hg, the pulse pressure is 38. A pulse pressure between 30 and 50 is considered to be in a normal range, with 40 being a healthy average.

Studies of healthy persons show that blood pressure can fluctuate within a wide range and still be normal. Because individual differences can be considerable, it is important to analyze the usual ranges and patterns of blood pressure measurements for each person. A rise or fall of 20 to 30 mm Hg in the usual pressure is significant, even if it is well within the generally accepted range for normal.

ASSESSMENT SITES

The blood pressure is most often assessed over the brachial artery at the inner aspect of the elbow area. Exceptions for using one or both arms include situations in which a patient has had one or both breasts removed and when a patient has had vascular surgery to permit dialysis treatments for kidney failure. If the arms are missing or the site is inaccessible or inappropriate for use, the blood pressure is measured over the popliteal artery behind the knee. It also is possible to use the lower arm and radial artery for assessing the blood pressure if needed. Documentation of the site is essential.

EQUIPMENT FOR MEASURING BLOOD PRESSURE

Blood pressure is measured with a stethoscope, an inflatable cuff, and a **sphygmomanometer** (a device for measuring blood pressure).

Sphygmomanometer

A sphygmomanometer contains a manometer, a gauge for measuring the pressure of a gas or liquid. Most manometers have either a mercury or aneroid gauge (Fig. 11-13). Some sphygmomanometers are portable; others are wall-mounted. There are also electronic sphygmomanometers patients can use to monitor their blood pressure at home.

Mercury Gauge Manometer

A mercury gauge manometer contains liquid mercury within a column that is calibrated in millimeters. To ensure an accurate measurement, the mercury must be even with the zero at the base of the calibrated column when not in use. It also must be positioned vertically, with the gauge at eye level. Positioning

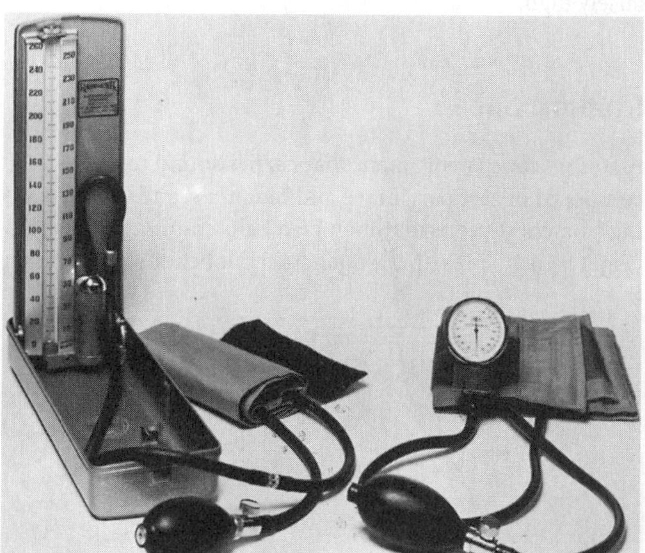

FIGURE 11–13. Mercury gauge manometer (*left*) and aneroid gauge (*right*).

the gauge in this manner allows the nurse to observe the column of mercury, the top of which appears slightly curved, more accurately (Fig. 11-14).

Aneroid Manometer

An aneroid manometer contains a gauge with a needle that moves about a dial that is calibrated in millimeters. The needle must be positioned initially at zero to ensure an accurate recording.

There are advantages and disadvantages to using a mercury, aneroid, or electronic sphygmomanometer (Table 11-8). However, any type, provided it is working properly and is used correctly, can measure blood pressure accurately. The readings obtained with one type are comparable to those obtained with the others.

Inflatable Cuff

The cuff of a sphygmomanometer contains an inflatable bladder to which two tubes are attached. One is connected to the manometer, which registers the pressure. The other is attached to a bulb, which is used to inflate the bladder with air. A screw valve on the bulb allows the nurse to fill and empty the bladder. As the air escapes, the pressure is measured.

Cuffs come in a variety of sizes. The nurse must select a cuff with an appropriate bladder size for the body proportions of each patient. A common guide (Fig. 11-15) is to use a cuff whose bladder width is at least 40% and whose length is 80% to 100% of midlimb circumference (National Heart, Lung, and Blood Institute, 1997). If the cuff is too wide, the blood pressure reading will be falsely low. If the cuff is too narrow, the blood pressure reading will be falsely high.

Stethoscope

A **stethoscope** (instrument that carries sound to the ears) is composed of eartips, a brace and binaurals, and tubing leading to a chest piece that may be a bell, diaphragm, or both (Fig. 11-16). The eartips are generally rubber or plastic. When

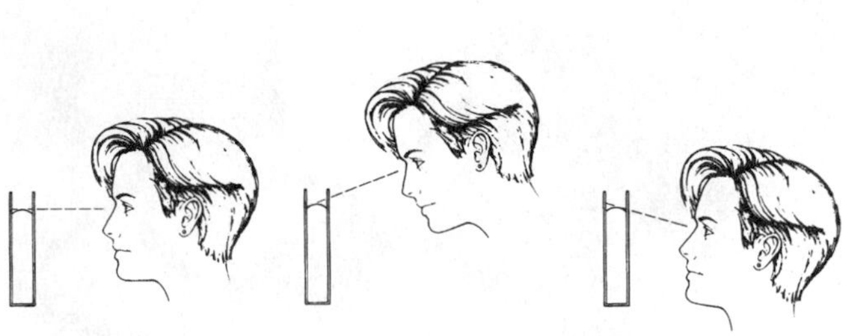

FIGURE 11–14. To avoid inaccurate interpretation of a mercury gauge manometer, it is read at eye level.

the stethoscope is used, the eartips are positioned downward and forward within the ears to produce the best sound perception. If stethoscopes are used by various people, the eartips are cleaned between uses with alcohol pads. Personal stethoscopes also need periodic cleaning to keep the eartips free of cerumen and dirt.

The brace and binaurals are generally made of metal. They connect the eartips to the tubing and chest piece. The brace prevents the tubing from kinking and distorting the sound. Stethoscope tubing is rubber or plastic. The best length for good sound conduction is about 20″ (50 cm).

The bell, or cup-shaped chest piece, is used for detecting low-pitched sounds such as those produced in blood vessels. The diaphragm, or disk-shaped chest piece, detects high-pitched sounds, such as those in the lungs, heart, or abdomen. If the diaphragm becomes cracked, it must be replaced. When the bell is used, care is taken to position it lightly over the anatomic area, because pressure flattens the skin and creates the same effect as a diaphragm.

MEASURING BLOOD PRESSURE

The first time the blood pressure is measured, it is assessed in each arm. The blood pressure measurements should not vary more than 5 to 10 mm Hg between the two unless pathology (disease) is present. Some agencies include a blood pressure assessment of the patient in lying, sitting, and standing positions for the initial data base. Several variables can result in inaccurate blood pressure measurements (Table 11-9).

Korotkoff Sounds

Most blood pressure recordings are obtained indirectly. That is, they are determined by applying a blood pressure cuff, briefly occluding arterial blood flow, and listening for **Korotkoff sounds** (sounds that result from the vibrations of blood within the arterial wall or changes in blood flow). The blood pressure measurements are determined by correlating the phases of Korotkoff sounds with the numbers on the gauge of the sphygmomanometer. If Korotkoff sounds are difficult to hear, they can be intensified in one of two ways:

- Have the patient elevate the arm before and during inflation of the cuff, and then lower the arm after it is fully inflated.
- Have the patient open and close the fist after the cuff has been inflated.

Korotkoff sounds have five unique phases (Fig. 11-17).

Phase I begins with the first faint but clear tapping sound that follows a period of silence as pressure is released from the cuff. When the first sound occurs, it corresponds to the peak pressure in the arterial system during heart contraction, or the systolic pressure measurement. It is recorded as the first number in the fraction.

TABLE 11–8. **Comparisons of Sphygmomanometer Equipment**

Type	Advantages	Disadvantages
Mercury	Easy to read Consistent Accurate Considered the standard for assessing blood pressures No readjustment required	Bulky Breakable glass column Hazardous if mercury spills Flat surface during use necessary Essential for gauge to be read at eye level Stethoscope and accurate hearing needed
Aneroid	Inexpensive Easy to carry and store Ability to read gauge from any position	Delicate Periodic checking against a mercury sphygmomanometer necessary for accuracy Gauge possibly clumsy to attach to cuff Stethoscope and accurate hearing necessary Calibration check and readjustment recommended yearly Manufacturer repair required
Electronic	Digital display of measurement No stethoscope required Accurate for people with hearing loss Facilitation of BP measurement of newborns and infants in whom auscultation (listening with a stethoscope) is difficult	Expensive Batteries necessary Accuracy can be influenced by body movements and improper cuff application Calibration check and readjustment recommended yearly Manufacturer repair needed

(Adapted from Blood pressure: buying and caring for home equipment. American Heart Association, 1999.)

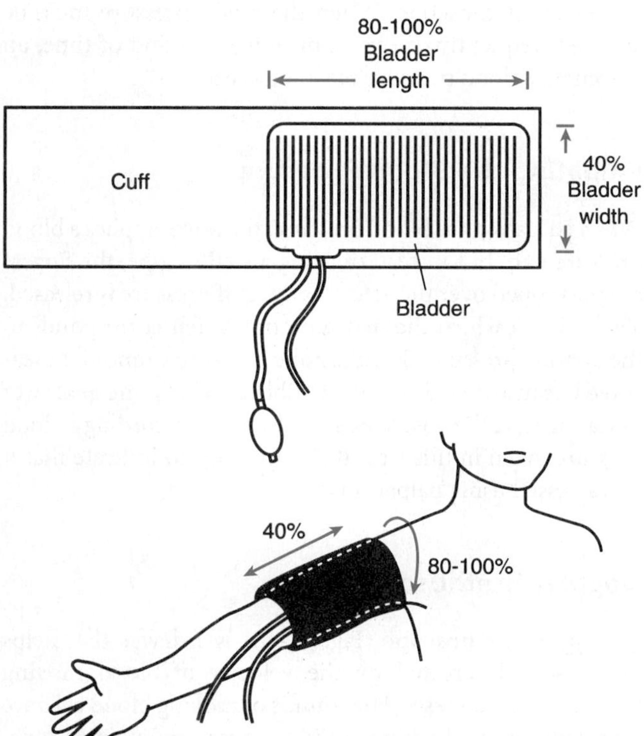

FIGURE 11–15. To determine the appropriate size of blood pressure cuff, the width of the bladder should be 40% of the mid-arm circumference and the length should be at least 80%.

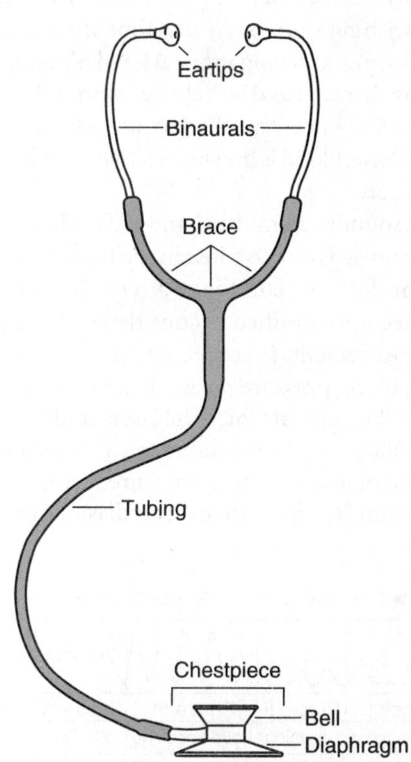

FIGURE 11–16. Parts of a stethoscope.

TABLE 11–9. **Common Causes of Blood Pressure Assessment Errors**

Cause	Effect	Correction
Inaccurate manometer calibration	Falsely high or low readings	Recalibrate, repair, or replace gauge.
Loosely applied cuff	High reading	Wrap snugly with equal pressure about extremity.
Cuff too small for extremity	High reading	Select appropriate size.
Cuff too large for extremity	Low reading	Select appropriate size.
Cuff applied over clothing	Creates noises or interferes with sound perception	Remove arm from sleeve or have patient don a gown.
Tubing that leaks	Rapid loss of pressure	Replace or repair.
Improper positioning of eartips	Poor sound conduction	Reposition and retake blood pressure.
Impaired hearing	Altered sound perception	Use an alternative assessment technique or equipment.
Loud environmental noise	Interferes with sound perception	Reduce noise and reassess.
Impaired vision	Inaccurate observation of gauge	Correct vision; reposition gauge within adequate range.
Rapid cuff deflation	Inaccurate observation of gauge	Reassess and deflate at 2 to 3 mm Hg/second.

The first sound, which is heard for at least two consecutive beats, may be missed if the cuff pressure is not pumped high enough initially. Palpating for the disappearance of a distal pulse when inflating the cuff helps to ensure that the cuff pressure is above arterial pressure.

Phase I sounds may briefly disappear before they become re-established, especially in patients with blood pressures that are above normal. An **auscultatory gap** (period during which sound disappears) can span a range of as much as 40 mm Hg. Failure to identify the first sound preceding an auscultatory gap results in an inaccurate blood pressure measurement.

Phase II is characterized by a change from the tapping sounds to swishing sounds. At this time the diameter of the artery is widening, allowing more arterial blood flow.

Phase III is characterized by a change to sounds that are loud and distinct. They are described as crisp knocking sounds. During this phase, blood is flowing relatively freely through the artery once more.

Phase IV sounds are muffled and have a blowing quality. The sound change is due to a loss in the transmission of pressure from the deflating cuff to the artery. The point at which the sound becomes muffled is considered the first diastolic pressure measurement. It is generally preferred when documenting the blood pressure measurements in children.

Phase V is the point at which the last sound is heard, or the second diastolic pressure measurement. This is considered the best reflection of adult diastolic pressure, because phase IV is often 7 to 10 mm Hg higher than direct diastolic pressure measurements. When recording adult blood pressure measurements, the pressures at phase I and phase V are used.

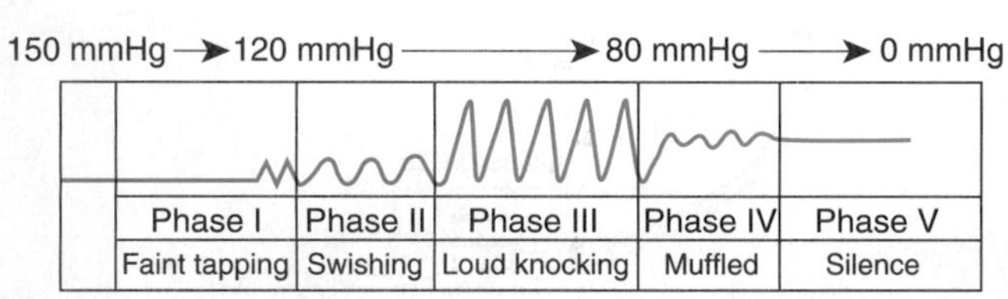

FIGURE 11–17. Characteristics of Korotkoff sounds.

ALTERNATIVE ASSESSMENT TECHNIQUES

When it is difficult to hear Korotkoff sounds in the usual manner, no matter how conscientious the effort to augment them, the blood pressure is assessed by palpation or by using a Doppler stethoscope. When the blood pressure must be assessed frequently or over a prolonged period of time, an automated blood pressure machine is used.

Palpating the Blood Pressure

When palpating the blood pressure, the nurse applies a blood pressure cuff, but instead of using a stethoscope, the fingers are positioned over the artery as the cuff pressure is released. The point at which the first pulsation is felt corresponds to the systolic pressure. The diastolic pressure cannot be measured because there is no perceptible change in the quality of pulsations like there is in the sounds. When recording a blood pressure taken in this way, it is important to indicate that it was assessed using palpation.

Doppler Stethoscope

A **Doppler stethoscope** (Fig. 11-18) is a device that helps detect sounds created by the velocity of blood moving through a blood vessel. The sounds of moving blood cells are reflected toward the ultrasound receiver, producing a tone. The nurse notes the pressure at which the sound occurs. The onset of sound represents the peak pressure of arterial blood flow. A description of how the Doppler is used was given ear-

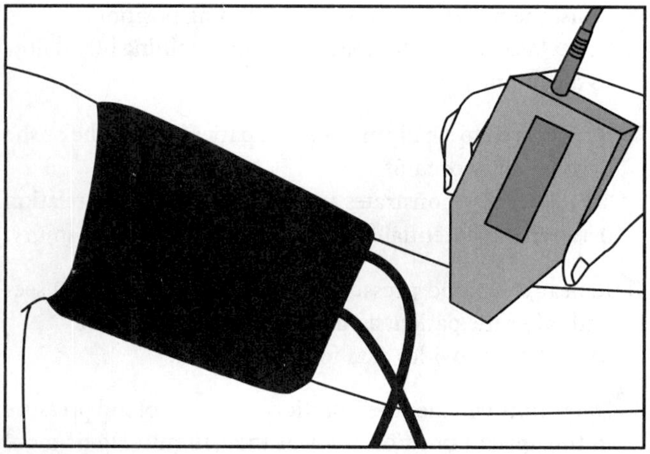

FIGURE 11–18. A Doppler stethoscope is used when Korotkoff sounds are difficult to hear.

lier in this chapter. When documenting the pressure measurement, a D is used to indicate that it was obtained with a Doppler.

Automatic Blood Pressure Monitoring

An automatic blood pressure monitoring device consists of a blood pressure cuff attached to a microprocessing unit. Such devices are used to diagnose unusual fluctuations in blood pressure that cannot be identified during single or sporadic monitoring. When used, the device records the patient's blood pressure every 10 to 30 minutes or as needed throughout a 24-hour period. The data are stored in the microprocessor's memory. Measurements are printed or transferred by hand to a flow sheet for vital signs. A portable model that is supported either at the shoulder or waist is worn by outpatients to help diagnose conditions in which the blood pressure is altered.

Directions for standard blood pressure measurement are given in Skill 11-4.

ABNORMAL BLOOD PRESSURE MEASUREMENTS

Blood pressures above or below normal ranges may indicate significant health problems.

High Blood Pressure

Hypertension (high blood pressure) exists when the systolic pressure, diastolic pressure, or both is sustained above normal levels for the person's age. The Joint National Committee on Detection, Evaluation, and Treatment of High Blood Pressure (1997) considers a systolic pressure of 140 mm Hg or greater in adults 18 years or older, and a diastolic pressure of 90 mm Hg or greater, to be abnormally high (Table 11-10).

TABLE 11–10. **Classification of Adult Blood Pressure Measurements**

Category*	Systolic (mm Hg)		Diastolic (mm Hg)
Optimal†	<120	and	<80
Normal	<130	and	<85
High-normal	130–139	or	85–89
Hypertension‡			
Stage 1	140–159	or	90–99
Stage 2	160–179	or	100–109
Stage 3	≥180	or	≥110

* Not taking antihypertensive drugs and not acutely ill. When systolic and diastolic blood pressures fall into different categories, the higher category should be selected to classify the individual's blood pressure status. For example, 160/92 mm Hg should be classified as stage 2 hypertension, and 174/120 mm Hg should be classified as stage 3 hypertension. Isolated systolic hypertension is defined as SBP of 140 mm Hg or greater and DBP below 90 mm Hg and staged appropriately (e.g., 170/82 mm Hg is defined as stage 2 isolated systolic hypertension). In addition to classifying stages of hypertension on the basis of average blood pressure levels, clinicians should specify presence or absence of target organ disease and additional risk factors. This specificity is important for risk classification and treatment.

† Optimal blood pressure with respect to cardiovascular risk is below 120/80 mm Hg. However, unusually low readings should be evaluated for clinical significance.

‡ Based on the average or two or more readings taken at each of two or more visits after an initial screening.

(Classification terms and measurements from the 1997 Joint National Committee Report on Detection, Evaluation, and Treatment of High Blood Pressure.)

An occasional elevation in blood pressure does not necessarily mean a person has hypertension. It does mean that the blood pressure should be monitored at various intervals, depending on the significance of the pressure measurements (Table 11-11). This is especially important to determine whether the elevated blood pressure is a sustained phenomenon or is due to **whitecoat hypertension** (condition in which the blood pressure is elevated when taken by a health care worker but is normal at other times).

Hypertensive blood pressure measurements are often associated with:

- Anxiety
- Obesity
- Vascular diseases
- Stroke
- Heart failure
- Kidney diseases

Low Blood Pressure

Hypotension (low blood pressure) exists when the blood pressure measurements are below the normal systolic values for the person's age. Having a consistently low pressure, 96/60 mm Hg for example, seems to cause no harm. In fact, low blood pres-

TABLE 11–11. **Recommendations for Follow-Up Based on Initial Set of Blood Pressure Measurements**

Initial Blood Pressure (mm Hg)*		
Systolic	*Diastolic*	Follow-Up Recommended†
<130	<85	Recheck in 2 years.
130–139	85–89	Recheck in 1 year.‡
140–159	90–99	Confirm within 2 months.‡
160–179	100–109	Evaluate or refer to source of care within 1 month.
≥180	≥110	Evaluate or refer to source of care immediately or within 1 week, depending on clinical situation.

* If systolic and diastolic categories are different, follow recommendations for shorter follow-up (e.g., patient with 160/86 mm Hg should be evaluated or referred to source of care within 1 month).

† Modify the scheduling of follow-up according to reliable information about past blood pressure measurements, other cardiovascular risk factors, or target organ disease.

‡ Provide advice about lifestyle modifications.

(From the sixth report of the Joint National Committee for the Detection, Evaluation, and Treatment of High Blood Pressure, National Heart, Lung, and Blood Institute, National Institutes of Health, 1997).

sure is usually associated with efficient functioning of the heart and blood vessels. However, persons with low blood pressure should continue to be monitored to evaluate its significance. Low blood pressure measurements may be an indication of shock, hemorrhage, or side effects from drugs.

Postural Hypotension

Postural or **orthostatic hypotension** (sudden but temporary drop in blood pressure when rising from a reclining position) is most common in those with circulatory problems, those who are dehydrated, or those who take diuretics or other drugs that lower the blood pressure. A consequence of a sudden drop in blood pressure is dizziness and fainting. Patients who are in high-risk categories or who become symptomatic during care are assessed for postural hypotension using the following nursing guidelines.

Nursing Guidelines For
Assessing Postural Hypotension

☑ Have the patient lie down for at least 3 minutes.
RATIONALE: Allows time for the blood pressure to stabilize.

☑ Take the patient's blood pressure and pulse.
RATIONALE: Establishes a baseline for comparison.

☑ Assist the patient to a sitting or standing position.
RATIONALE: Stimulates reflexes for maintaining blood flow to the brain.

☑ Be prepared to steady or assist the patient should he or she become dizzy or faint.
RATIONALE: Demonstrates an understanding of the relation between the potential for hypotension and risk for injury.

☑ Repeat the blood pressure and pulse assessment 30 seconds after the patient assumes an upright position.
RATIONALE: Provides data for comparison.

☑ Determine whether the systolic or diastolic blood pressure in the upright position is lower than 10 mm Hg or more from the reclining blood pressure and the heart rate increases 10% or more (Bickley and Hoekelman, 1998).
RATIONALE: Validates that the patient is experiencing postural hypotension.

Documenting Vital Signs

Once vital sign measurements are obtained, they are documented in the medical record so that patterns and trends can be analyzed (Fig. 11-19) The data, along with any other subjective or objective information, may also be entered elsewhere in the patient's record, such as in the narrative nursing notes.

Nursing Implications

Vital sign assessment is part of every patient's care and forms the basis for identifying problems. Based on the analysis of assessment data, the nurse may identify one or more of the following nursing diagnoses:

- Hyperthermia
- Hypothermia
- Ineffective thermoregulation
- Decreased cardiac output
- Risk for injury
- Ineffective breathing pattern

The nursing care plan in this chapter describes approaches that are used for a patient with Hyperthermia. Hyperthermia is defined in the NANDA taxonomy (1999) as "a state in which an individual's body temperature is elevated above normal range." If the alteration is so severe that it requires medical interventions, it is considered a collaborative problem.

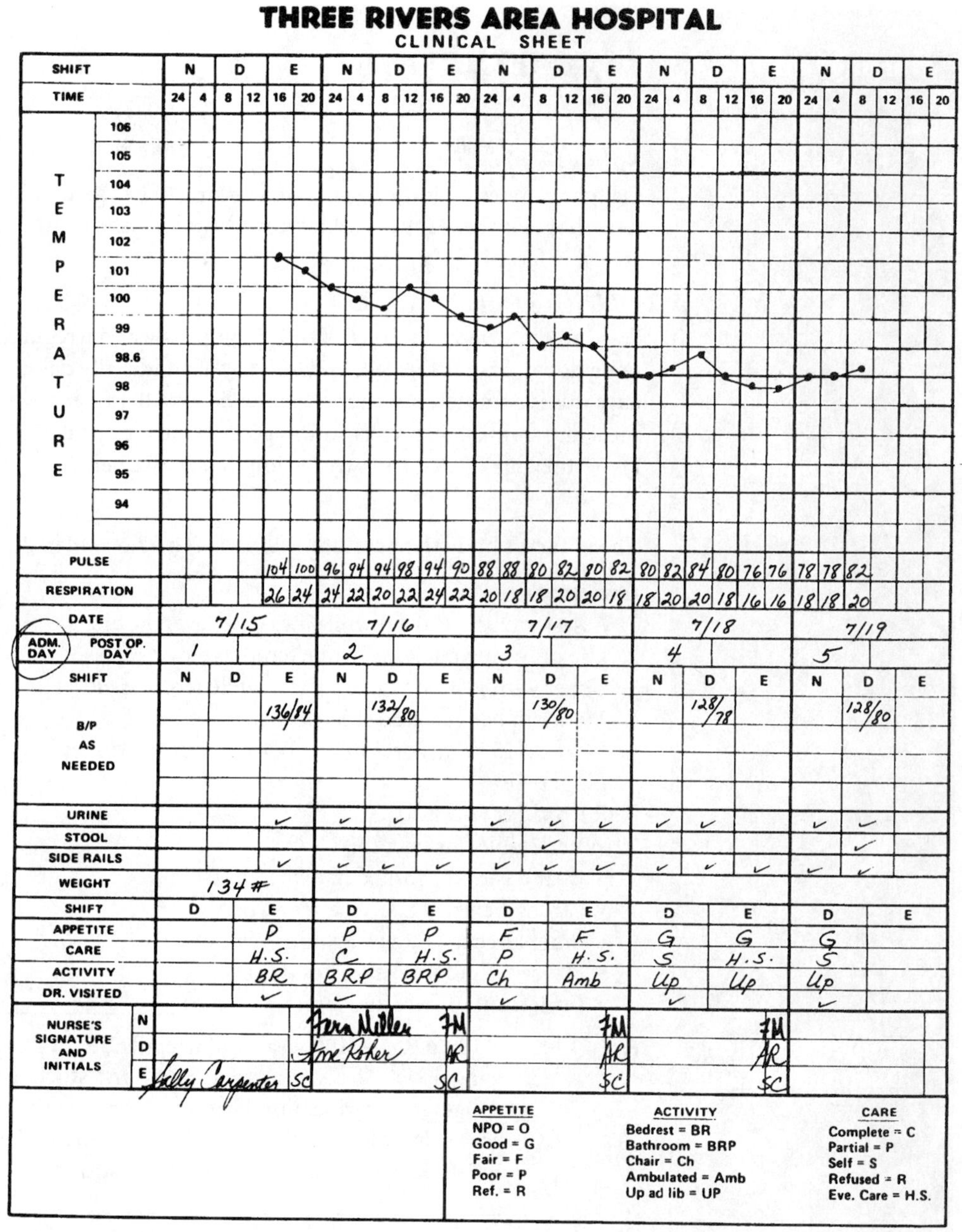

FIGURE 11–19. Graphic recording of vital signs.

KEY CONCEPTS

- Vital signs include temperature, pulse, respirations, and blood pressure.
- Shell temperature is the degree of warmth at the skin surface; core temperature is the degree of warmth near the center of the body, where vital organs are located.
- Temperature is measured using the centigrade or Fahrenheit scale.
- The mouth, rectum, axilla, and ear are common sites for assessing body temperature; the temperature of the tympanic membrane in the ear is the closest approximation of core temperature.
- Glass mercury, electronic, infrared, and chemical thermometers are used to assess body temperature.
- A fever exists when a patient has a body temperature that exceeds 99.3°F (37.4°C), hyperthermia, on the other hand, is a life-threatening condition characterized by a body temperature that exceeds 105.8°F (40.6°C).
- A fever generally has four phases: prodromal, onset or invasion, stationary, and resolution or defervescence.
- A fever is accompanied by chills, flushed skin, irritability, and headache, as well as several other signs and symptoms.
- An infrared tympanic thermometer is the best assessment tool for measuring subnormal temperatures because glass and electronic thermometers cannot measure temperatures in hypothermic ranges, and the

Nursing Care Plan

Hyperthermia

Assessment

Subjective Data

Daughter states, "Mother insists on working in her garden in this heat. Luckily the neighbors saw her faint, or who knows how long she would have lain there." Patient states, "I feel dizzy."

Objective Data

76-year-old woman. T 102.6 (O), P 104 thready and irregular, R 28, BP 106/52 in R arm lying down. Skin is flushed, hot, and dry. Can identify daughter by name and relationship. Says this is summer, but cannot name the month or year. Knows she is in the hospital. Last meal and fluid consumed 6 hours ago. Not currently taking any type of medication.

Diagnosis

Hyperthermia related to overexertion in hot weather

Plan

Goal

The patient's body temperature will return to 98.6 ± 1° in 24 hours (1600 on 8/7).

Orders: 8/6

1. Assess vital signs $\bar{q}$ 4 h while awake on even hours.
2. Use only hospital gown while temp. is elevated.
3. Cover with just one cotton sheet while temp. is elevated.
4. Maintain bed rest and side-rails.
5. Provide 1500 mL oral intake before bedtime. Likes lemonade, apple juice, and ginger ale.
6. Record I & O
7. When stable, instruct to:
   - wear a wide-brimmed hat when outside
   - garden before 9 A.M. or after 7 P.M.
   - limit sun exposure to 30 min
   - increase fluid intake on hot days
   - sit in front of fan after coming inside. ________________ S. EVANS, RN

Implementation (Documentation)

8/6 1800 T 100.4 (O), P 100 weak and irregular, R 20 $\bar{s}$ effort. BP 108/60 R arm while lying down. Dress, undergarments, and stockings removed and given to daughter. Wearing hospital gown covered with top sheet. Bed is in low position with side-rails up. Feels "dizzy" when head is elevated. BP 104/60 R arm lying; BP 90/50 3 minutes after assuming a sitting position. Bed rest maintained.
________________ A. WHITE, LPN

Evaluation (Documentation)

2000 T 100 (O), P 96 full but irregular, R 20. BP 110/64 R arm lying down. Skin is pink, dry, and cool. Drinking liquids. Urinating comparable amounts. Urine has changed from dark yellow to light yellow. Can identify current year correctly. No further dizziness experienced. Teaching postponed at this time.
________________ A. WHITE, LPN

blood flow in the mouth, rectum, and axilla is generally so low that measurements taken from these sites are inaccurate.

- Subnormal temperatures are accompanied by shivering, pale skin, listlessness, and impaired muscle coordination, as well as several other signs and symptoms.
- A pulse assessment includes the rate per minute, rhythm, and volume.
- The radial artery is the most common pulse assessment site; however, similar data may be obtained by assessing the apical heart rate or the apical-radial rate, or by using a Doppler ultrasound device.
- Respiration refers to the exchange of oxygen and carbon dioxide. Ventilation is the movement of air in and out of the chest. The rate of ventilations is assessed when obtaining vital signs.

FOCUS ON OLDER ADULTS

- Because older adults tend to have a lower "normal" body temperature, knowing an older person's baseline body temperature is important when assessing for an elevated body temperature.
- Some older adults have a delayed and diminished febrile response to illnesses. Careful assessment is essential to identify temperature elevations.
- Older adults are more susceptible to hypothermia and heat-related conditions. Environmental factors, such as extreme heat and cold conditions and inadequately heated or cooled living environments, pose additional risk factors for developing hypothermia and heat-related illnesses.
- To avoid "white coat hypertension" (i.e., elevated blood pressure readings associated with clinical settings), older adults are encouraged to use validated self-monitoring devices or obtain blood pressure readings at community settings where they feel more comfortable (Joint National Committee on Prevention, Detection, Evaluation, and Treatment of High Blood Pressure and the National High Blood Pressure Education Program Coordinating Committee, 1997).
- Blood pressure is assessed in each arm when collecting baseline assessment and documenting subsequent trends. Also, older adults need to have their blood pressure assessed while lying and sitting to detect the possibility of postural hypotension.
- Older adults are more susceptible to arrhythmias and to postural and postprandial (a drop in blood pressure of 20 mm Hg within 1 hour of eating a meal) hypotension.
- Some older adults have a wide pulse pressure because of a rising systolic pressure exceeding the rate of diastolic elevation, and they have a higher incidence of hypertension.
- The same criteria defining normal and abnormal (or high) blood pressure are used for older adults.
- Manifestations of cardiovascular disease typically are more subtle and variable in older adults.
- Older adults generally have more profound responses to cardiovascular medications than younger adults.

- Some of the abnormal breathing characteristics that may be noted are tachypnea (rapid breathing), bradypnea (slow breathing), dyspnea (labored breathing), and apnea (absence of breathing).
- Blood pressure measurements reflect the ability of the arteries to stretch, the volume of circulating blood, and the amount of resistance the heart must overcome when it pumps blood.
- Systolic pressure is the pressure within the arterial system when the heart contracts. Diastolic pressure is the pressure within the arterial system when the heart relaxes and fills with blood.
- A stethoscope, inflatable cuff, and sphygmomanometer are usually required for measuring blood pressure.
- During blood pressure assessment, five distinct sounds, called Korotkoff sounds, are heard. Phase I is characterized by faint tapping sounds; in phase II, the sounds are swishing; in phase III, the sounds are loud and crisp; in phase IV, the sound becomes suddenly muffled; and in phase V there is one last sound, followed by silence.
- Besides mercury and aneroid manometers, blood pressure may be measured with an electronic sphygmomanometer, which provides a digital display of the pressure measurements.
- The blood pressure also can be measured by palpating the brachial pulse while releasing the air from the cuff bladder or by using a Doppler stethoscope or an automated blood pressure machine.

CRITICAL THINKING EXERCISES

- If a neighbor with no medical experience asks how to tell if her child, age 4, has a fever, what advice would you give?
- An 80-year-old patient explains that as an economy measure, she keeps her thermostat set at 65°F. What health information would be appropriate, considering this woman's age?
- While participating in a community health assessment, you discover a person with a blood pressure that measures 190/110. What actions would be appropriate at this time?

SUGGESTED READINGS

Vital signs: a cuff in time. Nursing 1997;27(2):12–13.

American Heart Association. Blood pressure: buying and caring for home equipment. Dallas, American Heart Association, 1999.

Bayne CG. Technology assessment: are we monitoring the right parameters? Nursing Management 1997;28(5):74–76.

Bickley LS, Hoekelman RA. Bates' guide to physical examination and history taking, 7th ed. Philadelphia, Lippincott-Raven, 1998.

Erikson RS, Meyer LT. Accuracy of infrared ear thermometry and other temperature methods in adults. American Journal of Critical Care 1994;3(1): 40–54.

Erikson RS, Meyer LT, Woo TM. Accuracy of chemical dot thermometers in critically ill adults and young children. Image: Journal of Nursing Scholarship 1996;18(1):23–28.

Holtzclaw BJ. Monitoring body temperature. AACN Clinical Issues in Critical Care Nursing 1993;4(1):44–55.

Joint National Committee on Prevention, Detection, Evaluation, and Treatment of High Blood Pressure and the National High Blood Pressure Education Program Coordinating Committee. The sixth report of the Joint National Committee on Prevention, Detection, Evaluation, and Treatment of High Blood Pressure. Archives of Internal Medicine 1997; 157:2413–2446.

Letizia M, Janusek L. The self-defense mechanism of fever. MedSurg Nursing 1994;3(10):373–377.

Murphy L, et al. Managing vital signs monitoring problems. Nursing 1996; 26(11):32gg–32ii.

North American Nursing Diagnosis Association. NANDA nursing diagnoses: definitions and classification, 1999–2000. Philadelphia, NANDA, 1999.

Porth CM. Pathophysiology: concepts of altered health states, 5th ed. Philadelphia, Lippincott Williams & Wilkins, 1999.

Schumacher SB. Monitoring vital signs to identify postoperative complications. MedSurg Nursing 1995;4(2):142–145.

Severine JE, McKenzie NE. Advances in temperature monitoring: a far cry from shake and take. Nursing 1997;27(5):1–16.

SKILL 11-1

ASSESSING BODY TEMPERATURE

Suggested Action	Reason for Action
Assessment	
Determine when and how frequently to monitor the patient's temperature (refer to Display 11-1), and the type of thermometer that has been previously used.	Demonstrates accountability for making timely and appropriate assessments; ensures consistency in technique for gathering data
Review the data collected in previously recorded temperature measurements.	Aids in identifying trends and analyzing significant patterns
If using an oral glass or electronic thermometer:	
Observe the patient's ability to support a thermometer within the mouth and breathe adequately through the nose with the mouth closed.	Shows consideration for accuracy because thermal energy is transferred from the oral cavity to the thermometer probe; escape of heat invalidates the measurement
Read the patient's history for any reference to recent seizures or a seizure disorder.	Shows consideration for safety and identifies possible contraindication for oral site
Determine if the patient consumed any hot or cold substances or smoked a cigarette within the past 30 minutes.	Shows consideration for accuracy because the temperature in the oral cavity can be temporarily altered from substances recently placed within the mouth.
Planning	
Arrange to take the patient's temperature as near to the scheduled routine as possible.	Ensures consistency and accuracy
Gather supplies, including a thermometer, watch, and probe cover or disposable sleeve if needed. Include lubricant, paper tissues, and gloves if using the rectal site or other route if there is a potential for contact with body secretions.	Promotes efficiency, accuracy, and safety
(The use of gloves is determined on an individual basis. The virus that causes AIDS has not been shown to be transmitted through contact with oral secretions unless they contain blood; thorough handwashing is always appropriate after any patient contact.)	
Implementation	
Introduce yourself to the patient if this has not been done during earlier contact.	Demonstrates responsibility and accountability
Explain the procedure to the patient.	Reduces apprehension and promotes cooperation
Wash your hands.	Reduces the spread of microorganisms
ELECTRONIC THERMOMETER	
Implementation	
Remove the electronic unit from the charging base.	Promotes portability
Select the oral or rectal probe depending on the intended site for assessment.	Ensures appropriate use
Insert the probe into a disposable cover until it locks into place (see Fig. A).	Protects the probe from contamination with secretions that contain microorganisms

continued

SKILL 11–1

ASSESSING BODY TEMPERATURE *Continued*

Suggested Action | **Reason for Action**

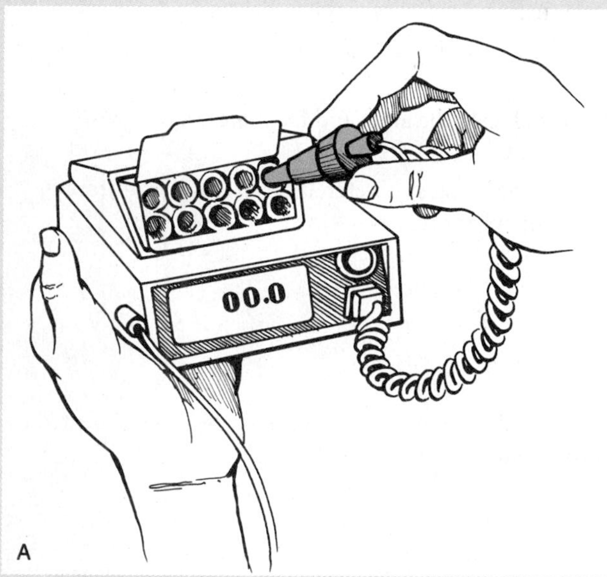

Inserting the probe into a disposable cover.

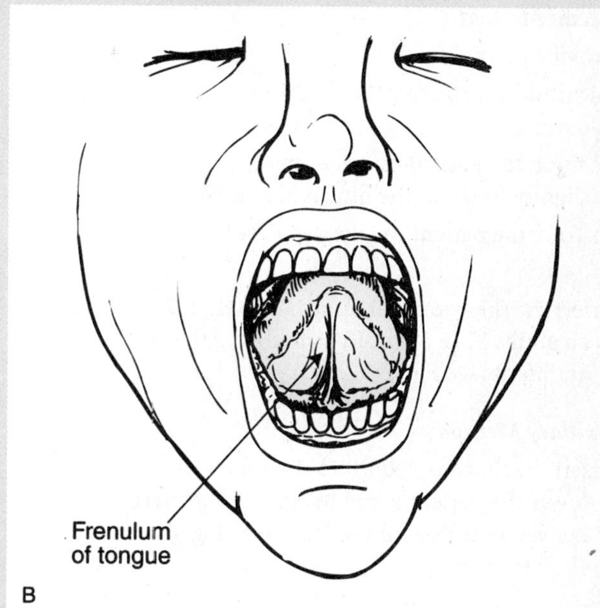

Location for oral temperature assessment.

Oral Method

Place the covered probe beneath the tongue to the right or left of the **frenulum** (structure that attaches the underneath surface of the tongue to the fleshy portion of the mouth (see Fig. B).

Locates the probe near the sublingual artery to ensure correct location

Hold probe in place (see Fig. C).

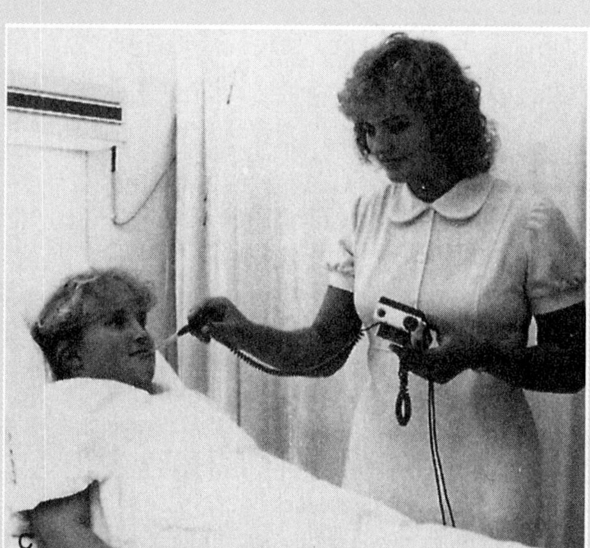

Maintaining the probe in position. (Courtesy of Ken Timby.)

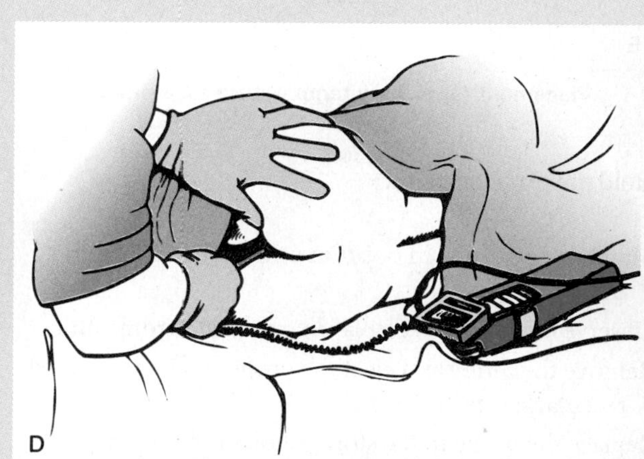

Rectal thermometer insertion.

continued

SKILL 11-1

ASSESSING BODY TEMPERATURE *Continued*

Suggested Action	Reason for Action
Rectal Method	
Provide privacy.	Demonstrates respect for the patient's dignity
Lubricate approximately 1″ (2.5 cm) of the rectal probe cover.	Promotes comfort and ease of insertion
Position the patient on his or her side with the upper leg slightly flexed at the hip and knee (Sims' position).	Helps to locate the anus and facilitate probe insertion
Instruct the patient to take deep breaths.	Relaxes the rectal sphincter and reduces discomfort during insertion
Insert the thermometer approximately 1.5″ (3.8 cm) in an adult, 1″ (2.5 cm) in a child, and 0.5″ (1.25 cm) in an infant (see Fig. D).	
Axillary Method	
Insert the thermometer into the center of the axilla and lower the patient's arm to enclose the thermometer between the two folds of skin (see Fig. E).	Confines the tip of the thermometer so it is unaffected by room air

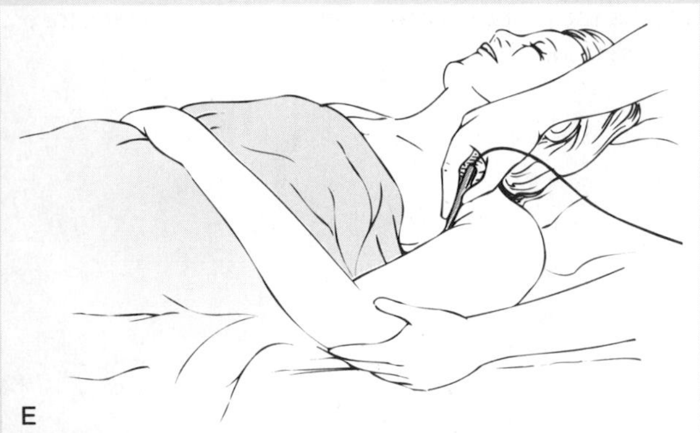

E

Placement for axillary temperature assessment.

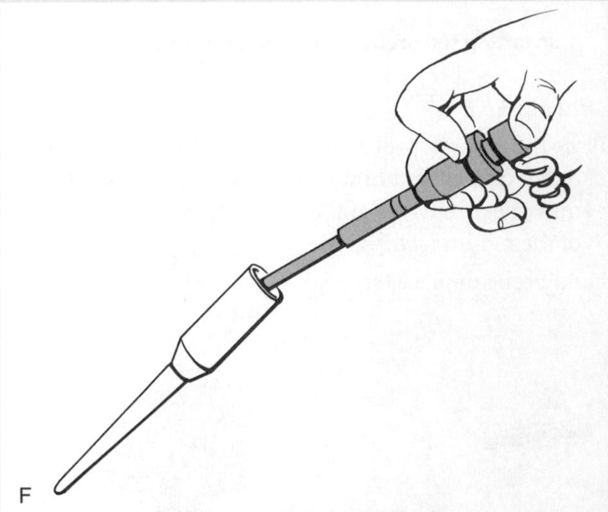

F

Releasing the probe cover.

Suggested Action	Reason for Action
Hold the probe in place.	Supports the probe so it does not drift away from its intended location; ensures valid data collection
Maintain the probe in position until an audible sound occurs.	Signals when the sensed temperature remains constant
Observe the numbers displayed on the electronic unit.	Indicates temperature measurement
Remove the probe and eject the probe cover into a lined receptacle (see Fig. F).	Confines contaminated objects to an area for proper disposal without direct contact
Replace the probe in the storage holder within the electronic unit.	Prevents damage to the probe attachment

continued

SKILL 11-1

ASSESSING BODY TEMPERATURE *Continued*

Suggested Action	Reason for Action
Wipe lubricant and any stool from around the patient's rectum.	Demonstrates concern for the patient's comfort
Remove and discard gloves, if worn; wash your hands.	Reduces the transmission of microorganisms
Return the electronic unit to its charging base.	Facilitates reuse
Record assessment measurement on the graphic sheet or flowsheet, or in the narrative nursing notes.	Provides documentation for future comparisons
Verbally report elevated or subnormal temperatures.	Alerts others to monitor the patient closely and make changes in the plan for care

INFRARED TYMPANIC THERMOMETER

Implementation

Suggested Action	Reason for Action
Remove the thermometer component from its holding cradle (see Fig. G).	Facilitates insertion of the tympanic **speculum** (funnel-shaped instrument used to widen and support an opening in the body)

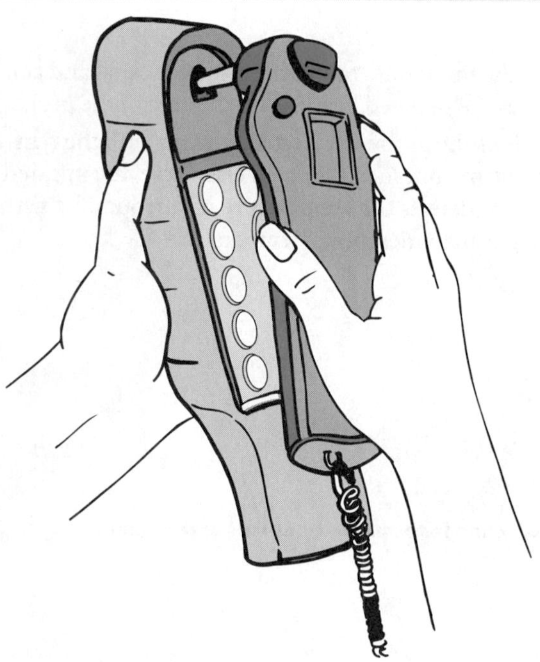

G

Tympanic thermometer and cradle.

Suggested Action	Reason for Action
Inspect the tip of the thermometer for damage and the lens for cleanliness.	Promotes safety and hygiene
Replace a cracked or broken tip; clean the lens with a dry wipe or lint-free swab moistened with a small amount of isopropyl alcohol, and then wipe to remove the alcohol film.	Ensures accurate data collection
Wait 30 minutes after cleaning with alcohol.	Allows the thermometer to readjust after the cooling effect created by alcohol evaporation.

continued

SKILL 11-1

ASSESSING BODY TEMPERATURE *Continued*

Suggested Action	Reason for Action
Cover the speculum with a disposable cover until it locks in place.	Maintains cleanliness of the tip
Press the mode button to select the choice of **temperature translation** (conversion of tympanic temperature into an oral, rectal, or core temperature).	Adjusts the tympanic measurement, norms for which have not been established, into more common frames of reference. The rectal equivalent is recommended for children who are 3 years old or less.
Depress the mode button for several seconds to select either Fahrenheit or centigrade.	Eliminates need to calculate conversion measurements by hand
Hold the probe in your dominant hand.	Improves motor skill and coordination
Position the patient with the head turned 90°, exposing the same ear as the hand holding the probe.	Promotes proper probe placement; if the right hand is holding the probe, the right ear is assessed
Wait for a "Ready" message to be displayed.	Indicates the offset has been programmed
Pull the external ear of adults up and back by grasping the external ear at its midpoint with your nondominant hand; for children 6 years old or less, pull the ear down and back.	Straightens the ear canal
Insert the probe into the ear, advancing it with a gentle back-and-forth motion until it seals the ear canal.	Seats the tip of the probe within the ear canal and confines the radiated heat within the area of the probe
Point the tip of the probe in an imaginary line between the sideburn hair and the eyebrow on the opposite side of the face (see Fig. H).	Positions the probe in direct alignment with the tympanic membrane; if pointed elsewhere, the infrared sensor detects the temperature of surrounding tissue rather than membrane temperature

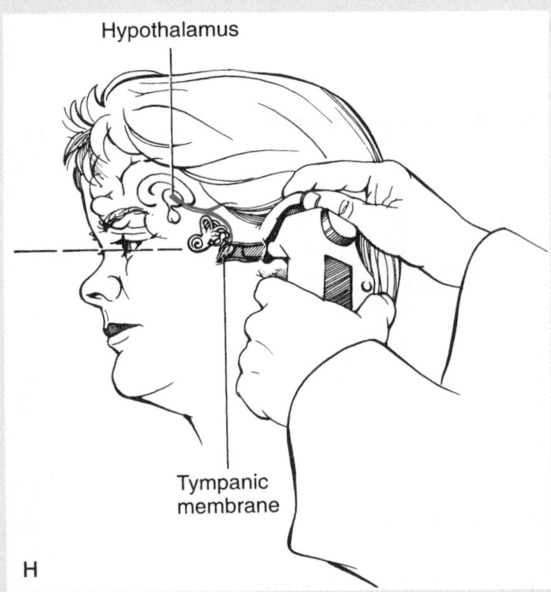

Placement of probe for accurate tympanic assessment.

Suggested Action	Reason for Action
Press the button that activates the thermometer as soon as the probe is in position.	Initiates electronic sensing; for some models, this action must be done within 25 seconds of having removed the thermometer from its holding cradle
Keep the probe within the ear until the thermometer emits a sound or flashing light.	Indicates that the procedure is complete

continued

SKILL 11-1

ASSESSING BODY TEMPERATURE *Continued*

Suggested Action	Reason for Action
Repeat the procedure after waiting 2 minutes if this is the first use of the tympanic thermometer since it was recharged.	Ensures accuracy with a second assessment
Read the temperature, remove the thermometer from the ear, and release the probe cover into a lined receptacle.	Controls the transmission of microorganisms
Return the thermometer to its charging cradle.	Ensures that the thermometer is charged when needed again

GLASS THERMOMETER

Implementation

Oral Method

Suggested Action	Reason for Action
Grasp the thermometer at the stem and shake it with a snapping motion from the wrist until the mercury is well within the bulb.	Makes room for the mercury to expand and rise when exposed to heat
Place the bulb of the thermometer under the patient's tongue (see Fig. I).	Locates the bulb near the sublingual artery

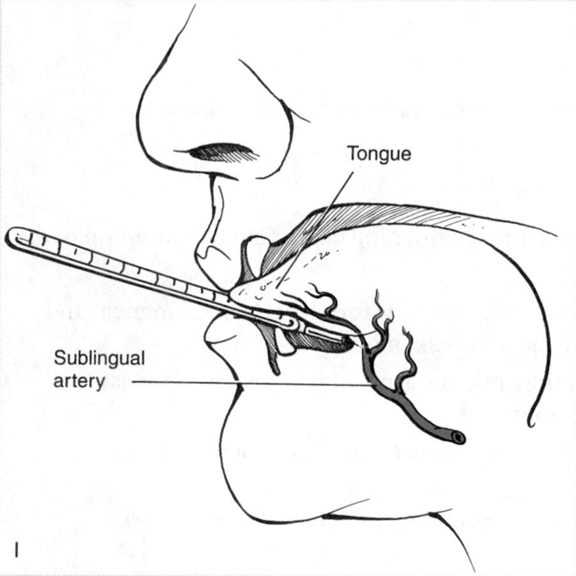

Assessing oral temperature using a glass thermometer.

Suggested Action	Reason for Action
Leave the thermometer in place at least 3 minutes if the patient is not feverish, or 5 minutes if the temperature has been borderline or elevated above normal in previous measurements.	Ensures adequate time for the thermometer to reach the maximum measurement
Remove the thermometer and wipe it toward the bulb with a tissue, using a firm twisting motion.	Removes mucus, making it easier to see the numerical markings
Read the thermometer by holding it horizontally at eye level and rotating it until the column of mercury can be seen (see Fig. J).	Places the mercury and calibrations in a position where they can be read most accurately

continued

SKILL 11-1

ASSESSING BODY TEMPERATURE *Continued*

Suggested Action	Reason for Action
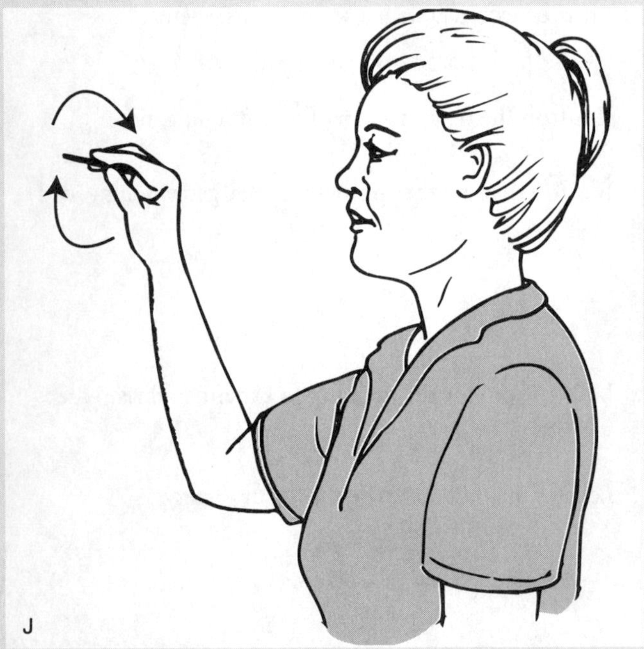	**Reading a glass mercury thermometer.**
Follow agency policy for cleaning and disinfecting the thermometer; wash your hands.	Reduces the transmission of microorganisms

Rectal Method

Refer to description of rectal method using an electronic thermometer for positioning the patient and insertion of the thermometer.

Suggested Action	Reason for Action
Hold the thermometer in place for at least 2 minutes, or as specified by agency policy.	Allows sufficient time for accurate measurement and reduces the risk of injury
Remove the thermometer and place it on a paper tissue.	Confines microorganisms to a source that is easily disposed of
Wipe lubricant and any stool from around the patient's rectum.	Demonstrates concern for the patient's comfort
Wipe lubricant, mucus, and stool from the thermometer.	Facilitates examination of the calibrated marks
Read the thermometer, place it on a clean tissue, and remove gloves.	Ensures that the thermometer can be transported without actually touching it
Wash your hands.	Reduces the transmission of microorganisms
Restore the patient to a therapeutic position or one of comfort and lower the bed.	Ensures comfort and safety
Enclose the thermometer within the tissue and transport it to the appropriate area for cleaning and disinfection	Reduces the transmission of microorganisms
Document the recorded measurement and specify that it was obtained rectally.	Facilitates analysis and future comparisons

continued

SKILL 11-1

ASSESSING BODY TEMPERATURE *Continued*

Evaluation

- Thermometer remained inserted the appropriate length of time.
- Level of temperature is consistent with accompanying signs and symptoms.
- Thermometer and surrounding tissue remain intact.

Document

- Date and time
- Degree of heat to the nearest tenth
- Temperature scale
- Site of assessment
- Accompanying signs and symptoms
- To whom abnormal information was reported, and outcome of the interaction

SAMPLE DOCUMENTATION

Date and Time T 102.4°F (O). States, "I feel cold and my throat hurts." Pharynx looks beefy red. Reported to Dr. Washington. New orders for throat culture. ____________________ SIGNATURE/TITLE

CRITICAL THINKING

- Discuss the site and type of thermometer that is appropriate to use when assessing the temperature of the following patients:
  A 78-year-old patient in a coma
  A 55-year-old patient whose nose is packed with gauze to control a nosebleed
  A 40-year-old patient who has had her gallbladder removed
  An 18-month-old infant who has been vomiting
  A 2-year-old who actively avoids any contact with the nurse
- If a patient's temperature is elevated at the morning assessment, when and how often would you reassess the patient's temperature?
- If a nursing assistant reported that a patient, who has been running a fever for the past 24 hours, now has a temperature of 96.2°F, what actions are appropriate to take?

SKILL 11-2

ASSESSING THE RADIAL PULSE

Suggested Action	Reason for Action
Assessment	
Determine when and how frequently to monitor the patient's pulse (refer to Display 11-1).	Demonstrates accountability for making timely and appropriate assessments
Review the data collected in previous assessments of the pulse or abnormalities in other vital signs.	Aids in identifying trends and analyzing significant patterns
Read the patient's history for any reference to cardiac or vascular disorders.	Demonstrates an understanding of factors that may affect the pulse rate
Review the list of prescribed drugs for any that may have cardiac effects.	Helps in analyzing the results of assessment findings
Planning	
Arrange to take the patient's pulse as near to the scheduled routine as possible.	Ensures consistency and accuracy
Make sure a watch or wall clock with a second hand is available.	Ensures accurate timing when counting pulsations
Plan to assess the patient's pulse after a 5-minute period of inactivity.	Reflects the characteristics of the pulse at rest rather than data that may be influenced by activity
Plan to use the right or left radial pulse site, unless it is inaccessible or difficult to palpate.	Provides consistency in evaluating data
Implementation	
Introduce yourself to the patient, if this has not been done during earlier contact.	Demonstrates responsibility and accountability
Explain the procedure to the patient.	Reduces apprehension and promotes cooperation
Raise the height of the bed.	Reduces musculoskeletal strain
Wash your hands.	Reduces the spread of microorganisms
Help the patient to a position of comfort.	Avoids influencing the pulse rate due to stress or pain
Rest or support the patient's forearm with the wrist extended.	Provides access to the radial artery and places the arm in a relaxed position

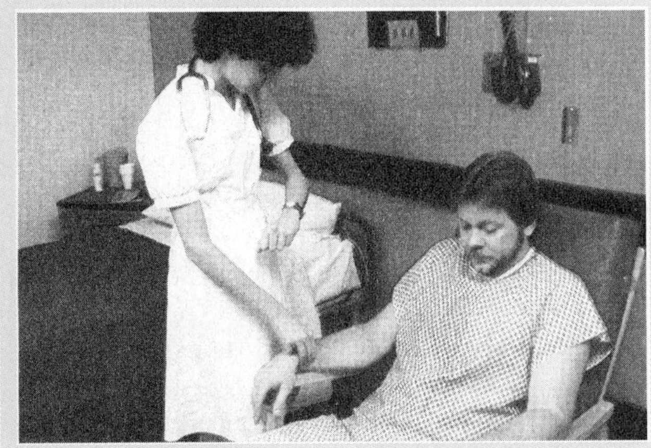

The pulse is supported during pulse assessment.

continued

SKILL 11-2

ASSESSING THE RADIAL PULSE *Continued*

Suggested Action	**Reason for Action**
Press the first, second, and third fingertips toward the radius while feeling for a recurrent pulsation.	Ensures accuracy, because the nurse may feel his or her own pulse if the thumb is used; light palpation should not obliterate the pulse.

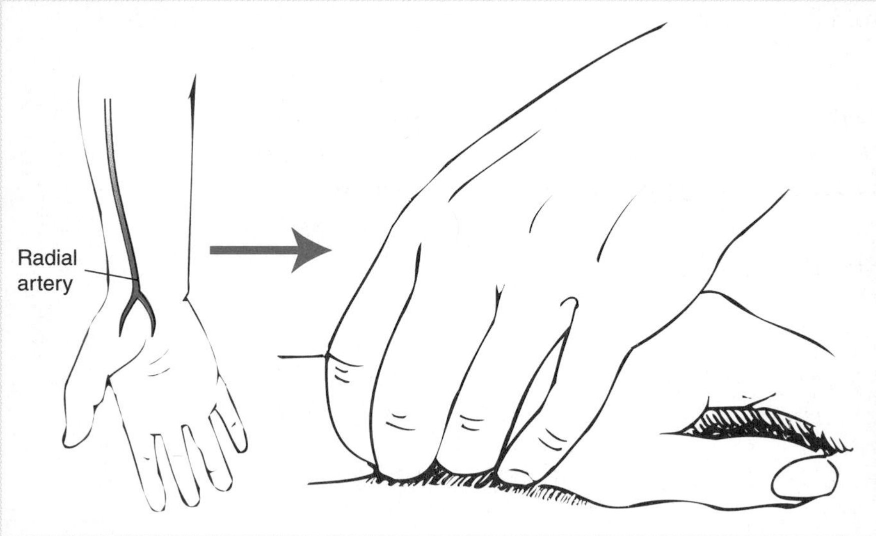

Locating the radial pulse.

Suggested Action	**Reason for Action**
Palpate the rhythm and volume of the pulse once it is located.	Provides comprehensive assessment data
Note the position of the second hand on the clock or watch.	Identifies the point at which the assessment begins
Count the number of pulsations for 15 or 30 seconds and multiply the number by 4 or 2, respectively. If the pulse is irregular, count for a full minute.	Provides pulse rate data. A regular pulse rate should not vary whether it is counted for a full minute or some portion thereof, whereas the rate of an irregular pulse may be significantly inaccurate if assessed for less than a full minute.
Write down the pulse rate.	Ensures accurate documentation
Restore the patient to a therapeutic position or one that provides comfort, and lower the bed.	Demonstrates responsibility for patient care, safety, and comfort
Record assessed measurement on the graphic sheet or flow sheet, or in the narrative nursing notes.	Provides documentation for future comparisons
Verbally report rapid or slow pulse rates.	Alerts others to monitor the patient closely and make changes in the plan for care

Evaluation

- Pulse rate remained palpable throughout the period of assessment.
- Pulse rate is consistent with the patient's condition.

Document

- Date and time
- Assessment site

continued

SKILL 11-2

ASSESSING THE RADIAL PULSE *Continued*

- Rate of pulsations per minute, pulse volume, and rhythm
- Accompanying signs and symptoms if appropriate
- To whom abnormal information was reported and outcome of the interaction

SAMPLE DOCUMENTATION

Date and Time Radial pulse 88 bpm, full, and regular. ______________________ SIGNATURE/TITLE

CRITICAL THINKING

- If a patient's arms are inaccessible, perhaps because both are in plaster casts, list at least two alternative sites for assessing the pulse rate and characteristics.
- If you find it difficult to assess a peripheral pulse accurately, discuss possible actions you could take.
- Discuss factors that can affect pulse assessment if the patient is an infant, a toddler (2 years old), or an older adult.

SKILL 11-3

ASSESSING THE RESPIRATORY RATE

Suggested Action	Reason for Action
Assessment	
Determine when and how frequently to monitor the patient's respiratory rate (refer to Display 11-1).	Demonstrates accountability for making timely and appropriate assessments
Review the data collected in previous assessments of the respiratory rate and other vital signs.	Aids in identifying trends and analyzing significant patterns
Read the patient's history for any reference to respiratory, cardiac, or neurologic disorders.	Demonstrates an understanding of factors that may affect the respiratory rate
Review the list of prescribed drugs for any that may have respiratory or neurologic effects.	Helps in analyzing the results of assessment findings
Planning	
Arrange to count the patient's respiratory rate as close to the scheduled routine as possible.	Ensures consistency and accuracy
Make sure a watch or wall clock with a second hand is available.	Ensures accurate timing
Plan to assess the patient's respiratory rate after a 5-minute period of inactivity.	Reflects the characteristics of respirations at rest rather than under the influence of activity

continued

SKILL 11-3

ASSESSING THE RESPIRATORY RATE *Continued*

Suggested Action	Reason for Action
Implementation	
Introduce yourself to the patient, if this has not been done during earlier contact.	Demonstrates responsibility and accountability
Explain the procedure to the patient.	Reduces apprehension and promotes cooperation
Raise the height of the bed.	Reduces musculoskeletal strain
Wash your hands.	Reduces the spread of microorganisms
Help the patient to a sitting or lying position.	Facilitates the ability to observe breathing
Note the position of the second hand on the clock or watch.	Identifies the point at which the assessment begins
Choose a time when the patient is unaware of being watched; it may be helpful to count the respiratory rate while appearing to count the pulse or while the patient is holding a thermometer in the mouth.	Discourages conscious control of breathing or talking during the time that the rate of breathing is being assessed
Observe the rise and fall of the patient's chest for a full minute, if breathing is unusual. If breathing appears noiseless and effortless, count the ventilations for a fractional portion of a minute and then multiply to calculate the rate.	Determines the respiratory rate per minute
Write down the respiratory rate.	Ensures accurate documentation
Restore the patient to a therapeutic position or one that provides comfort, and lower the bed	Demonstrates responsibility for patient care, safety, and comfort
Record assessed measurement on the graphic sheet or flow sheet, or in the narrative nursing notes.	Provides documentation for future comparisons
Verbally report rapid or slow respiratory rates or any other unusual characteristics.	Alerts others to monitor the patient closely and make changes in the plan for care

Evaluation

- Respiratory rate is counted for an appropriate amount of time.
- Respiratory rate is consistent with the patient's condition.

Document

- Date and time
- Rate per minute
- Accompanying signs and symptoms if appropriate
- To whom abnormal information was reported and outcome of the interaction

SAMPLE DOCUMENTATION

Date and Time Respiratory rate of 20/min at rest. Breathing is noiseless and effortless.

______________________________ SIGNATURE/TITLE

CRITICAL THINKING

- Discuss additional data to investigate if a patient had a respiratory rate less than 12 per minute or over 28 per minute.
- What action would you take if a patient had bradypnea or tachypnea?

SKILL 11-4

ASSESSING BLOOD PRESSURE

Suggested Action	Reason for Action
Assessment	
Determine when and how frequently to monitor the patient's blood pressure (refer to Display 11-1).	Demonstrates accountability for making timely and appropriate assessments
Review the data collected in previous assessments.	Aids in identifying trends and analyzing significant patterns
Determine in which arm and in what position previous assessments were made.	Ensures consistency when evaluating data
Read the patient's history for any reference to cardiac or vascular disorders.	Demonstrates an understanding of factors that may affect the blood pressure
Review the list of prescribed drugs for any that may have cardiovascular effects.	Helps in analyzing the results of assessment findings
Planning	
Gather the necessary supplies: blood pressure cuff, sphygmomanometer, and stethoscope.	Promotes efficient time management. A mercury sphygmomanometer is preferred, but a recently calibrated aneroid or a validated electronic device can be used.
Select a cuff that is an appropriate size for the patient.	Ensures valid assessment findings
Arrange to take the patient's blood pressure as near to the scheduled routine as possible.	Ensures consistency
Plan to assess the blood pressure after at least 5 minutes of inactivity, unless it is an emergency situation.	Reflects the blood pressure under resting conditions
Wait 30 minutes from the time the patient has ingested caffeine or used tobacco.	Avoids obtaining a higher-than-usual measurement due to arterial constriction
Plan to use the right or left arm unless inaccessible	Provides consistency in evaluating data
Implementation	
Introduce yourself to the patient, if this has not been done during earlier contact.	Demonstrates responsibility and accountability
Explain the procedure to the patient.	Reduces apprehension and promotes cooperation
Raise the height of the bed.	Reduces musculoskeletal strain
Wash your hands.	Reduces the spread of microorganisms
Help the patient to a sitting position or one of comfort.	Relaxes the patient and reduces elevation in blood pressure due to stress or discomfort
Support the patient's forearm at the level of the heart with palm of the hand upward.	Ensures collecting accurate data and facilitates locating the brachial artery
Expose the inner aspect of the elbow by removing clothing or loosely rolling up a sleeve.	Facilitates application of the blood pressure cuff and optimum sound perception
Center the cuff bladder so that the lower edge is about 1″ to 2″ (2.5 to 5 cm) above the inner aspect of the elbow (see Fig. A).	Places the cuff in the best position for occluding the blood flow through the brachial artery
Wrap the cuff snugly and uniformly about the circumference of the arm.	Ensures the application of even pressure during inflation
Position the mercury manometer on an even surface at eye level; make sure the aneroid gauge can be clearly seen.	Prevents errors when observing the gauge

continued

SKILL 11-4

ASSESSING BLOOD PRESSURE *Continued*

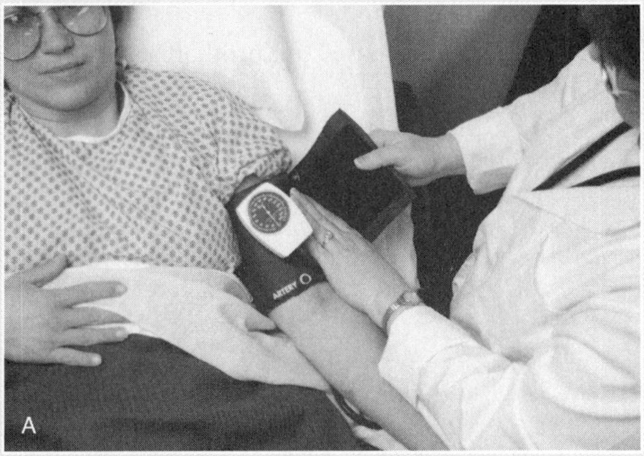

Applying the blood pressure cuff. (Courtesy of Ken Timby.)

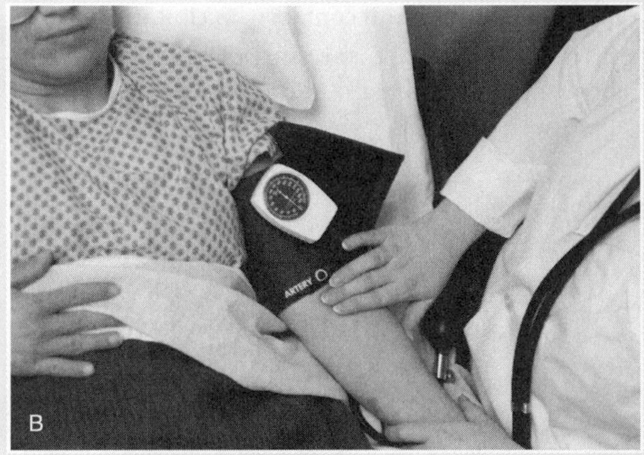

Palpating the brachial artery. (Courtesy of Ken Timby.)

Suggested Action	Reason for Action
Palpate the brachial pulse (see Fig. B).	Determines the most accurate location for assessment and hearing Korotkoff sounds
Tighten the screw valve on the bulb (see Fig. C).	Prevents loss of pumped air
Compress the bulb until the pulsation within the artery stops.	Provides an estimation of systolic pressure
Deflate the cuff and wait 15 to 30 seconds.	Allows the return of normal blood flow
Place the eartips of the stethoscope within the ears, and position the bell of the stethoscope lightly over the location of the brachial artery (see Fig. D). The diaphragm may be used, but it is not the preferred option.	Ensures accurate assessment

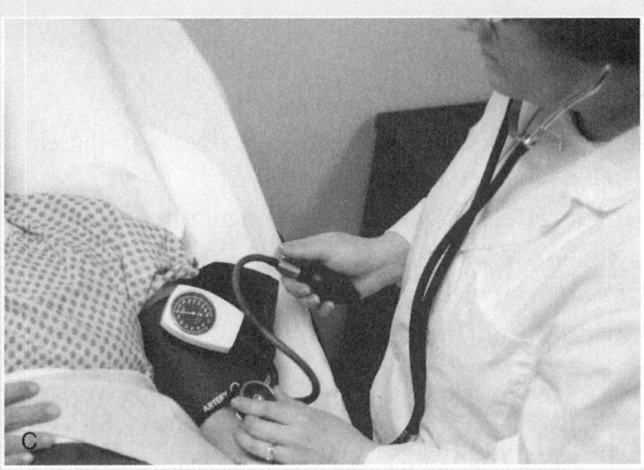

Tightening the screw valve. (Courtesy of Ken Timby.)

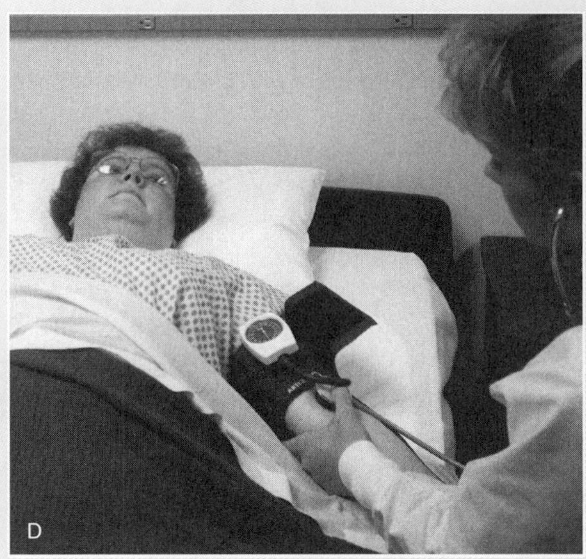

Placing the stethoscope. (Courtesy of Ken Timby.)

continued

SKILL 11-4

ASSESSING BLOOD PRESSURE *Continued*

Suggested Action	Reason for Action
Keep the tubing free from contact with clothing.	Reduces sound distortion
Pump the cuff bladder to a pressure that is 30 mm Hg above the point where the pulse previously disappeared (see Fig. E).	Facilitates identifying phase I of Korotkoff sounds

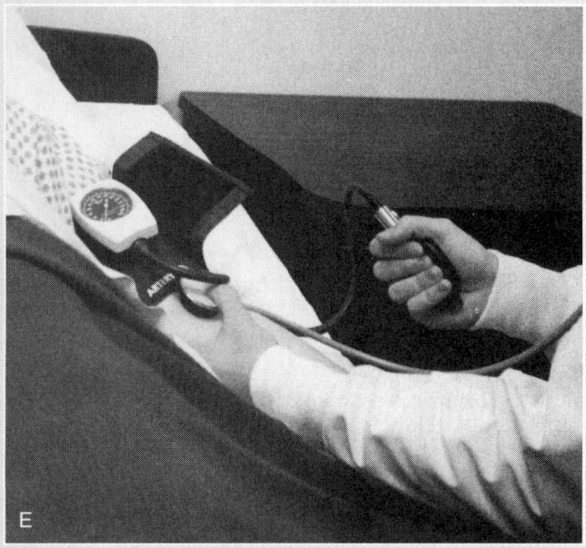

Pumping the bulb. (Courtesy of Ken Timby.)

Suggested Action	Reason for Action
Loosen the screw on the valve.	Releases air from the cuff bladder
Control the release of air at a rate of approximately 2 to 3 mm Hg per second.	Ensures accurate assessment between the time when a sound is perceived and the numbers are noted on the gauge
Listen for the onset and changes in Korotkoff sounds.	Aids in determining the systolic and diastolic pressure
Read the manometer gauge to the closest even number when phase I, IV, or V is noted.	Follows recommended standards for children or adults
Release the air quickly when there has been silence for at least 10 mm Hg.	Indicates phase V is complete
Write down the blood pressure measurements.	Ensures accurate documentation
Repeat the assessment after waiting at least 1 minute if unsure of the pressure measurements.	Allows time for the arterial pressure to return to baseline before another assessment
Restore the patient to a therapeutic position or one that provides comfort, and lower the bed.	Demonstrates responsibility for patient care, safety, and comfort
Wash hands.	Reduces the spread of microorganisms
Record assessed measurement on the graphic sheet or flow sheet, or in the narrative nursing notes.	Provides documentation for future comparisons
Verbally report elevated or low blood pressure measurements.	Alerts others to monitor the patient closely and make changes in the plan for care

continued

SKILL 11-4

ASSESSING BLOOD PRESSURE *Continued*

Evaluation

- Korotkoff sounds are heard clearly.
- Blood pressure is consistent with the patient's condition.

Document

- Date and time
- Systolic and diastolic pressure measurements
- Assessment site
- Position of the patient
- Accompanying signs and symptoms if appropriate
- To whom abnormal information was reported, and outcome of the interaction

SAMPLE DOCUMENTATION

Date and Time BP 136/72 in R arm while in sitting position. ______________________ SIGNATURE/TITLE

CRITICAL THINKING EXERCISES

- Discuss modifications in the blood pressure assessment procedure for the following situations:
  - The patient has intravenous fluid infusing in one arm and has had a mastectomy on the other side.
  - A patient's condition becomes unstable and requires blood pressure measurement approximately every 5 minutes.
  - The patient's Korotkoff sounds are very faint, and the measurements could be inaccurate.

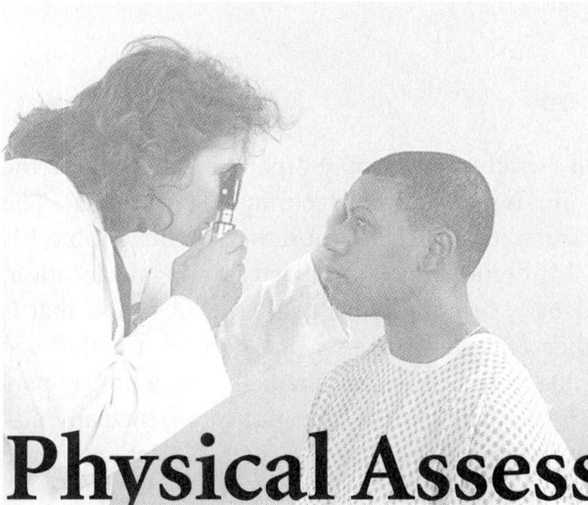

Physical Assessment

CHAPTER 12

CHAPTER OUTLINE

NURSING GUIDELINES

OBTAINING WEIGHT AND HEIGHT
ASSESSING PUPILLARY RESPONSE
PERFORMING A VOICE TEST FOR HEARING ACUITY
ASSESSING LUNG SOUNDS
ASSESSING SENSORY SKIN PERCEPTION
ASSESSING BOWEL SOUNDS

SKILLS

SKILL 12-1: PERFORMING A PHYSICAL ASSESSMENT

NURSING CARE PLAN

HEALTH SEEKING BEHAVIORS

KEY TERMS

accommodation
audiometry
auscultation
body systems approach
capillary refill time
cerumen
consensual response
drape
edema
extraocular movements
head-to-toe approach
hearing acuity
inspection
Jaeger chart
mental status assessment
palpation
percussion
physical assessment
Rinne test
smelling acuity
Snellen eye chart
turgor
visual acuity
visual field examination
Weber test

LEARNING OBJECTIVES

An understanding of the content within this chapter will be evidenced by the student's ability to:

- List four purposes for a physical assessment.
- Name four assessment techniques.
- List at least five items that are needed when performing a basic physical assessment.
- Discuss at least three criteria for an appropriate assessment environment.
- Identify at least five assessments that can be obtained during the initial survey of patients.
- State two reasons for draping patients.
- Explain the difference between a head-to-toe approach to physical assessment and a body systems approach.
- List six areas into which the body may be divided for organizing data collection.
- Identify two types of self-examinations that nurses should teach their adult patients.

The first step in the nursing process is assessment, or gathering information. **Physical assessment** (systematic examination of body structures) is one method for gathering health data.

This chapter describes how to perform a physical assessment from a generalist's or beginning nurse's point of view, and identifies common assessment findings. Advanced physical assessment skills are learned through additional education and experience or by consulting specialty texts.

Overview of Physical Assessment

Physical assessment is performed on every patient to gather objective data. This is accomplished with the use of different techniques and equipment. Although the environment may vary, it should be one that is conducive to patient privacy and comfort and ensures accurate data collection.

PURPOSES

The overall goal of a physical assessment is to gather objective data about a patient. To achieve this goal, patients are thoroughly examined on admission, briefly at the beginning of each shift, and any time their condition changes. The purposes of assessment are as follows:

- To evaluate the patient's current physical condition
- To detect early signs of developing health problems
- To establish a baseline for future comparisons
- To evaluate responses to medical and nursing interventions

TECHNIQUES

There are four basic physical assessment techniques: inspection, percussion, palpation, and auscultation.

Inspection

Inspection (purposeful observation) is the most frequently used assessment technique. It involves examining particular parts of the body, looking for specific normal and abnormal characteristics (Fig. 12-1*A*). With advanced instruction, some nurses learn to use special examination instruments to inspect parts of the body, such as the interior of the eyes, that are potentially inaccessible to ordinary vision and inspection techniques.

Percussion

Percussion (striking or tapping a part of the body) is the least-used nursing assessment technique (Fig. 12-1B). The fingertips are used to produce vibratory sounds (Table 12-1). The quality of the sound aids in determining the location, size, and density of underlying structures. A sound that is different than expected suggests that there is a pathologic change in the area being examined. If percussion is performed correctly, the patient does not experience any discomfort. Pain could indicate the presence of a disease process or tissue injury.

Palpation

Palpation (lightly touching the body or applying pressure) is a third assessment technique. *Light palpation* involves the use of the fingertips, the back of the hand, or the palm of the hand (Fig. 12-2). Light palpation is best used when feeling the surface of the skin, structures that lie just beneath the skin, the pulsation from peripheral arteries, and vibrations in the chest. *Deep palpation* is performed by depressing tissue approximately 1″ (2.5 cm) with the forefingers of one or both hands.

Palpation provides information about:

- The size, shape, consistency, and mobility of normal tissue and unusual masses
- The symmetry or asymmetry of bilateral (both sides of the body) structures, such as the lobes of the thyroid gland
- The temperature and moisture of the skin
- The presence of tenderness
- Unusual vibrations

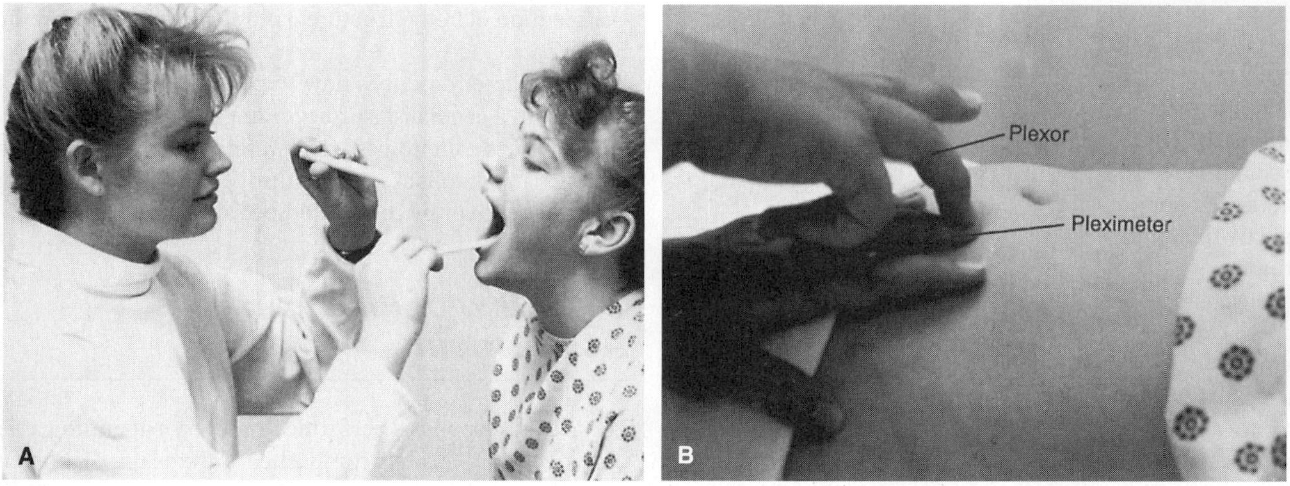

FIGURE 12–1. *(A)* Inspection. *(B)* Percussion. (Courtesy of Ken Timby.)

TABLE 12–1. **Percussion Sounds**

Sound	Intensity	Descriptive Term	Common Locations
Muted	Soft	Flat	Muscle, bone
Thud	Soft to moderate	Dull	Liver, full bladder, tumorous mass
Empty	Moderate to loud	Resonant	Normal lung
Cavernous	Loud	Tympanic	Intestine filled with air
Booming	Very loud	Hyperresonant	Barrel-shaped chest overinflated with trapped air due to chronic lung disease

Auscultation

Auscultation (listening to body sounds) is a frequently used assessment technique. The heart, lungs, and abdomen are the structures that are most often assessed by auscultation. A stethoscope is required for hearing soft sounds (Fig. 12-3), but in some cases loud sounds, such as those associated with hyperactivity in the intestinal tract, are audible with gross hearing.

The technique of auscultation must be practiced repeatedly on a variety of healthy and ill people to gain proficiency with the equipment and experience in interpreting data. To ensure that assessment findings are accurate, noise in the environment is eliminated or reduced as much as possible.

EQUIPMENT

The items generally needed for a basic physical assessment are listed in Display 12-1. Additional examination equipment is used by more advanced practitioners.

ENVIRONMENT

Patients are assessed in a special examination room or at the bedside. Regardless of the assessment location, the area should have:

- Easy access to a restroom
- A door or curtain that ensures privacy
- Adequate warmth for patient comfort
- A padded, adjustable table or bed
- Sufficient room for moving to either side of the patient
- Adequate lighting
- Facilities for handwashing
- A clean counter or surface for placing examination equipment
- A lined receptacle for soiled articles

Performing a Physical Assessment

Basic activities involved in a physical assessment include gathering general data, draping and positioning the patient, select-

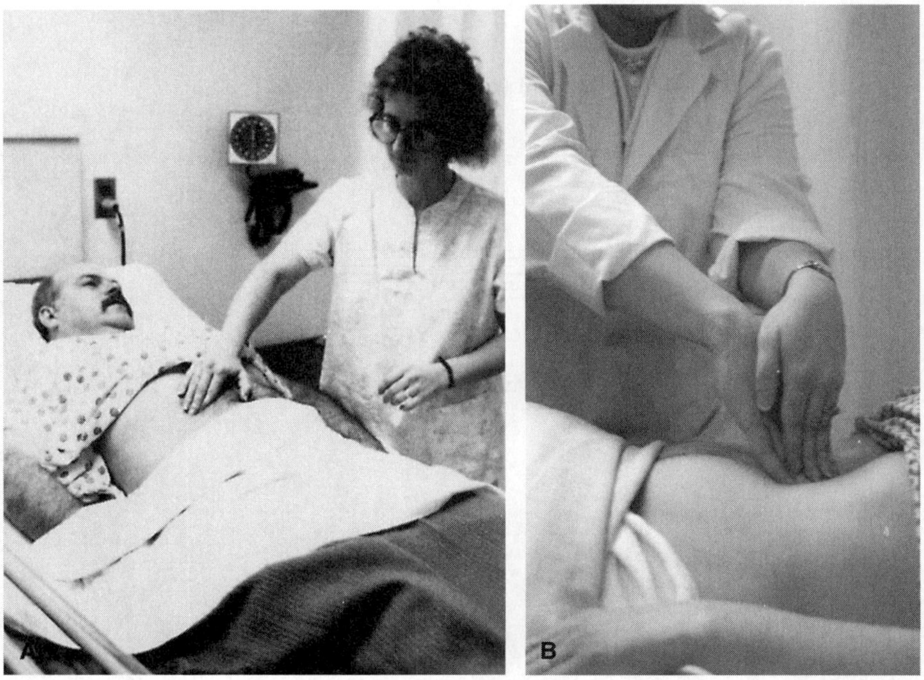

FIGURE 12–2. Palpation techniques. (*A*) Light palpation. (*B*) Deep palpation. (Courtesy of Ken Timby.)

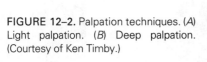

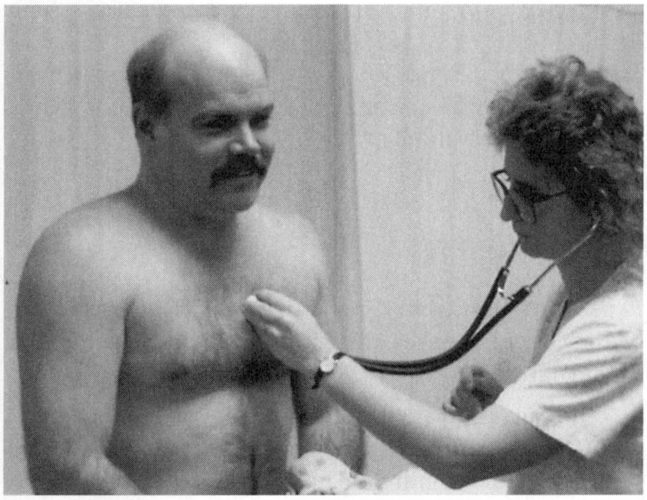

FIGURE 12–3. Auscultation. (Courtesy of Ken Timby.)

ing a systematic approach for collecting data, and examining the patient.

GENERAL DATA

A great deal of general data is obtained during the nurse's first contact with the patient. At this time the nurse develops an overall appraisal of the patient's general condition. By observing and interacting with the patient before the actual physical examination, the nurse notes the patient's:

- Physical appearance in relation to clothing and hygiene
- Level of consciousness
- Body size
- Posture
- Gait and coordinated movement (or lack of it)
- Use of ambulatory aids
- Mood and emotional tone

DISPLAY 12–1

Physical Assessment Equipment

For a basic physical assessment, the nurse needs:

- Gloves
- Patient gown
- Cloth or paper drapes
- Scale
- Stethoscope
- Sphygmomanometer
- Thermometer
- Pen light or flashlight
- Tongue blade
- Assessment form and pen

Some preliminary data, such as measuring the vital signs (see Chap. 11) and obtaining the patient's weight and height, are gathered at this time.

WEIGHT AND HEIGHT

The patient's weight and height are documented because they provide more reliable data than the nurse's subjective assessment of body size. The recorded measurements are extremely important in assessing trends in future weight loss or gain. For hospitalized patients, weight and height also are used to calculate dosages of some drugs. In most cases, adult patients and older children are weighed and measured using a standing scale (Fig. 12-4).

Nursing Guidelines For

Obtaining Weight and Height

☑ Check to see that the scale is calibrated at zero.
RATIONALE: Ensures accuracy.

☑ Ask or assist the patient to remove all but a minimum of clothing. Shoes should be removed.
RATIONALE: Facilitates measuring body weight.

☑ Place a paper towel on the scale before the patient stands on it in bare feet.
RATIONALE: Helps reduce contact with microorganisms present on equipment that is used by other people.

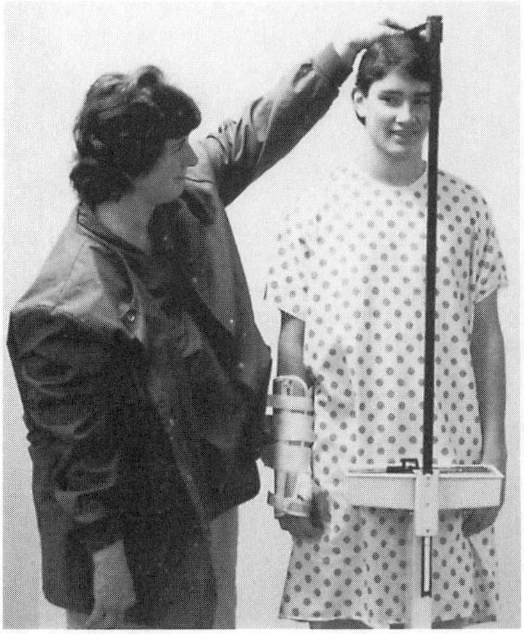

FIGURE 12–4. Assessment of height and weight. (Courtesy of Ken Timby.)

☑ Assist the patient onto the scale.
RATIONALE: Prevents injury should the patient become dizzy or unstable.

☑ Position the heavier weight in a calibrated groove of the scale arm.
RATIONALE: Provides a rough approximation of the gross body weight.

☑ Move the lighter weight across the calibrations for individual pounds and ounces until the bar balances in the center of the scale.
RATIONALE: Correlates with the actual weight.

☑ Read the weight and write it down.
RATIONALE: Ensures accurate documentation.

☑ Raise the measuring bar well above the patient's head.
RATIONALE: Provides room for positioning the patient without injury.

☑ Ask the patient to stand straight and look forward.
RATIONALE: Facilitates measuring height.

☑ Lower the measuring bar until it lightly touches the top of the patient's head.
RATIONALE: Correlates with actual height.

☑ Note the height and write it down.
RATIONALE: Ensures accurate documentation.

Medically unstable patients, those who are grossly obese, or those who cannot stand are weighed with an electronic bed or chair scale (Fig. 12-5). Electronic scales, which are battery-powered, can weigh persons who are 400 to 500 lbs (181 to 227 kg) while avoiding the potential for a patient fall or injury to the nurse. Several models store the weight of the patient in memory. The weight can be automatically recalled until another patient is weighed. The electronic scales are portable and can be transported from storage to a patient room when needed.

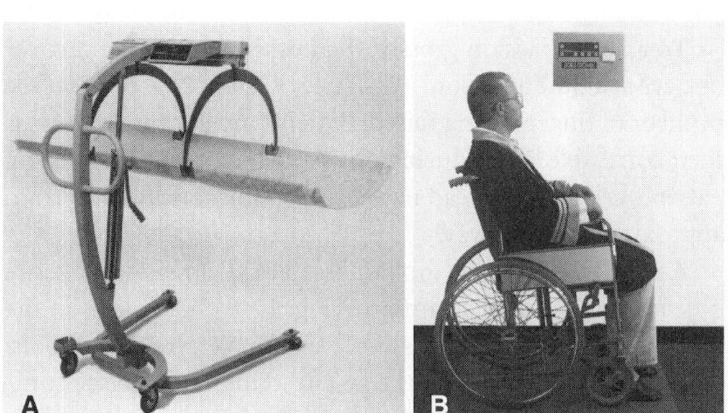

FIGURE 12–5. (*A*) Bed-sling scale. (*B*) Chair scale. (Courtesy of Scale-Tronix, Inc., White Plains, NY.)

DRAPING AND POSITIONING

Because patients are assessed while naked (or wearing only a loose patient gown), they generally appreciate being covered with a **drape** (sheet of soft cloth or paper). A drape provides more modesty than warmth.

The examination usually begins with the patient in a standing or sitting position (Fig. 12-6). Some components of the physical assessment require the patient to recline and turn from side to side. Specific positions for special examinations are described and illustrated in Chapters 13 and 23.

APPROACHES FOR DATA COLLECTION

Once the patient is draped and positioned, further data collection is facilitated by following a systematic, organized pattern. Two common approaches for data collection are the head-to-toe approach and the body systems approach.

Head-to-Toe Approach

A **head-to-toe approach** (gathering data from the top of the body to the feet) has three advantages:

1. It prevents overlooking some aspect of data collection.
2. It reduces the number of position changes required of the patient.

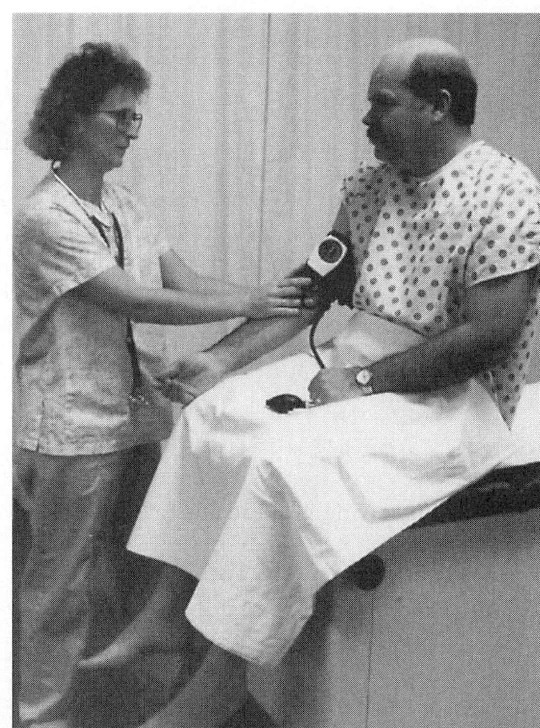

FIGURE 12–6. Patient is prepared for examination. (Courtesy of Ken Timby.)

3. It generally takes less time, because the nurse is not constantly moving about the patient in what may appear to be a haphazard manner.

Body Systems Approach

A **body systems approach** (data collection according to the functional systems of the body) involves examining the structures in each system separately. For example, the skin, mucous membranes, nails, and hair are assessed because they are all components of the integumentary system. When the cardiovascular system is assessed, the nurse palpates peripheral pulses, listens to heart sounds, and so on. One advantage of collecting data in this manner is that the assessment findings tend to be clustered, making problems more easily identifiable. Disadvantages are that the nurse examines portions of the body several times before completing the assessment, and the patient may become fatigued by frequent position changes during the examination.

Regardless of the approach used for data collection, the objective is to obtain essentially the same basic data. Consequently, each nurse develops his or her own order and sequence for examining patients, or an assessment form is used as a guide. Nurses should conduct the assessment consistently each time to avoid omitting essential information.

The procedure for performing a physical assessment is described in Skill 12-1. Specific assessment techniques, their purpose, and the data they provide are described later in the chapter.

Data Collection

When collecting data, the body may be divided into six general areas: the head and neck, the chest, the extremities, the abdomen, the genitalia, and the anus and rectum. The discussion that follows identifies the structures that are commonly assessed, specific assessment techniques, and common assessment findings.

HEAD AND NECK

The assessments involving the head and neck involve several body systems.

Head

At the patient's head, the nurse begins assessing the patient's mental status, the symmetry of craniofacial structures (eyes, ears, nose, mouth) and their function. The skin, oral and nasal mucous membranes, hair, and scalp also are assessed.

Mental Status Assessment

A **mental status assessment** (technique for determining the level of a patient's cognitive functioning) helps determine a patient's attention and concentration, memory, and ability to think abstractly. For most patients, documenting that they are alert and oriented is all that is necessary. However, more objective assessment data are important when caring for the following patients:

- Previously unconscious patients
- Patients who were recently resuscitated
- Patients with periods of confusion
- Head injury victims
- Patients who took an overdose of drugs
- Patients with a history of chronic alcoholism
- Patients with psychiatric diagnoses

A common assessment tool is the Mini-Mental State Examination (Display 12-2). After performing a mental status assessment, it is important to document the patient's score or objectively describe his or her performance, even if it was accurate. The assessment is performed daily to detect an improvement or worsening of mental status.

Eyes

Probably one of the most obvious assessments, when examining the head, is the appearance of the eyes. The eyes are generally of similar size and distance from the center of the face. Each iris is the same color, the sclerae (plural of sclera) appear white, the corneas are clear, and eyelashes are present along the margins of each eye. Structures within the eye are examined by more advanced practitioners with an instrument called an *ophthalmoscope* (Fig. 12-7). After gross inspection, functions such as visual acuity, pupil size and response, and ocular movement are assessed.

Visual acuity (ability to see both far and near) is not assessed in every patient who is hospitalized. However, it is always appropriate to ask whether the patient wears glasses or contact lenses, has a false eye, or considers himself or herself blind.

To assess far vision grossly, the nurse has the patient cover one eye at a time and from a distance of about 20 feet count the number of fingers being raised. Patients are permitted to wear their corrective lenses during this assessment. For close vision, patients are asked to read newsprint (if they are literate) from approximately 14″ away.

A **Snellen eye chart** (tool for assessing far vision) is a more objective assessment technique (Fig. 12-8). Each line on the chart is printed in progressively smaller letters or symbols. Patients are asked to read the smallest line they can see comfortably from a distance of 20 feet both with and without their corrective lenses. The patient's vision is then compared with norms.

DISPLAY 12-2

Mini-Mental State Examination

Maximum Score	
	Orientation
5	What is the (year) (season) (date) (day) (month)?
5	Where are we (state) (county) (city) (hospital) (floor)?
	Registration
3	Name three objects: One second to say each. Then ask subject all three after you have said them. Give one point for each correct answer. Repeat them until subject learns all three. Count trials and record number.
	Attention and Calculation
5	Begin with 100 and count backwards by 7 (stop after five answers). Alternatively, spell "world" backwards.
	Recall
3	Ask for the three objects repeated above. Give one point for each correct answer.
	Language
2	Show a pencil and a watch and ask subject to name them.
1	Repeat the following: "No 'if's,' 'and's,' or 'but's.'"
3	A three-stage command, "Take a paper in your right hand; fold it in half and put it on the floor."
1	Read and obey the following: (show subject the written item). CLOSE YOUR EYES
1	Write a sentence.
1	Copy a design (complex polygon as in Bender-Gestalt).
30	Total score possible
<20	Suggests significant cognitive impairment

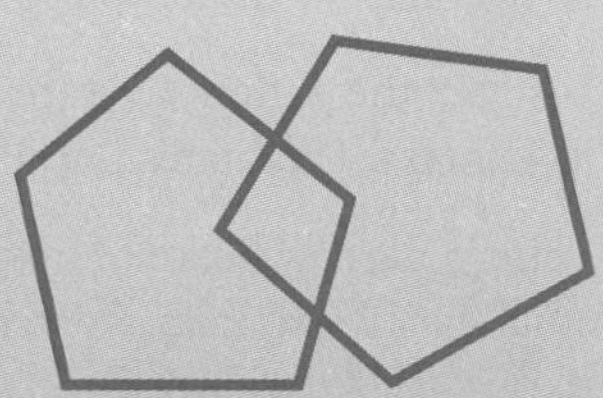

Folstein MF, Folstein S, McHugh PR. Mini-mental state: a practical method for grading the cognitive state of patients for the clinician. Journal of Psychiatric Research 1975; 12:189–198, with permission from Pergamon Press Ltd. Headington Hill Hall, Oxford OX3 OBW, UK.)

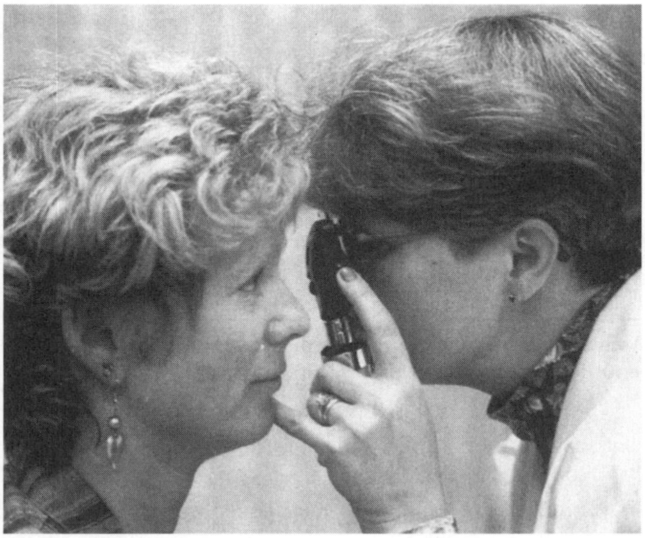

FIGURE 12–7. An ophthalmoscopic examination. (Courtesy of Ken Timby.)

Normal vision is the ability to read printed letters seen by most people without prescription lenses at a distance of 20 feet. This number is written as a fraction: 20/20. If, at 20 feet from the chart, a person sees only the first line—one that can be seen by persons with normal vision from 200 feet away—the patient's visual acuity is recorded as 20/200. Near vision is tested using a **Jaeger chart** (visual assessment tool with small print).

The size of each pupil is estimated in millimeters under normal light conditions (Fig. 12-9). Normal pupils are round and equal in size. There is also a **consensual response** (brisk, equal, and simultaneous constriction of both pupils when one eye and then the other is stimulated with light) (Fig. 12-10*A*). In addition, the pupils are assessed for **accommodation** (ability to constrict when looking at a near object and dilate when looking at an object in the distance) (Fig. 12-10*B*). Normal findings are documented using the abbreviation *PERRLA: P*upils *E*qually *R*ound and *R*eact to *L*ight and *A*ccommodation.

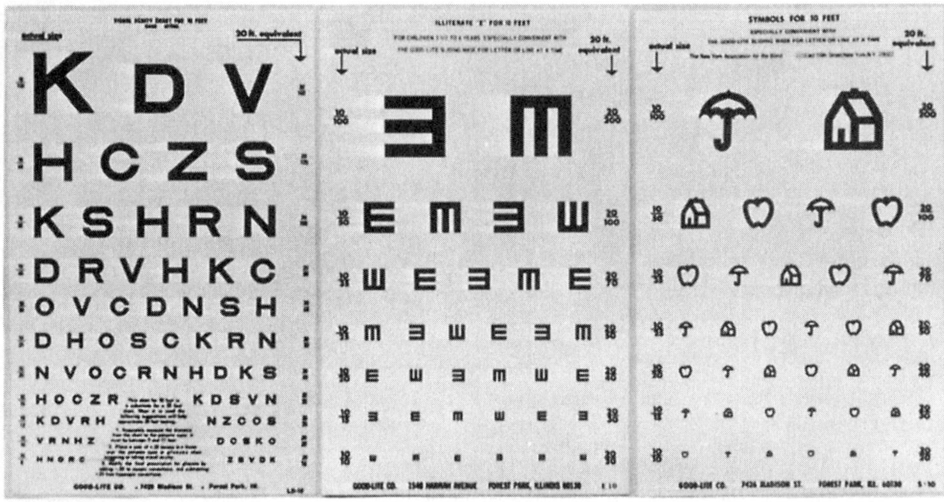

FIGURE 12–8. Three examples of Snellen eye charts. (Courtesy of Ken Timby.)

Nursing Guidelines For
Assessing Pupillary Response

☑ Dim the lights in the examination area.
RATIONALE: Facilitates pupil dilation.

☑ Instruct the patient to stare straight ahead.
RATIONALE: Facilitates pupil dilation.

☑ Bring a narrow beam of light, like that from a pen light or small flashlight, from the temple toward the eye.
RATIONALE: Provides a direct stimulus for pupil constriction.

☑ Observe the pupil of the stimulated eye as well as the unstimulated pupil. The response should be the same.
RATIONALE: Indicates status of brain function.

☑ Repeat the assessment by directly stimulating the opposite eye.
RATIONALE: Provides comparative data.

☑ Ask the patient to look at a finger or object approximately 4″ (10 cm) from his or her face.
RATIONALE: Produces a situation in which the pupils should get smaller.

☑ Tell the patient to look from the near object to another that is more distant.
RATIONALE: Produces a situation in which the pupils should get larger.

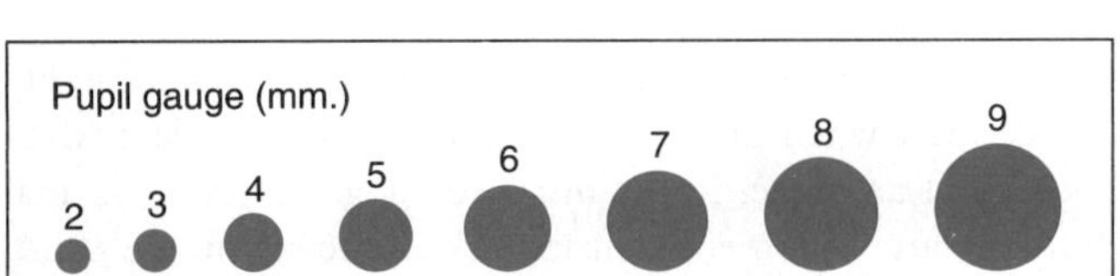

FIGURE 12–9. Pupil size assessment guide.

Extraocular movements (eye movements controlled by several pairs of eye muscles) are also observed. The patient is asked to focus on and track the nurse's finger or some other object as it is moved in each of six positions (Fig. 12-10C). During the assessment, both eyes should move in a coordinated manner. Absence of movement in one or the other eye may indicate cranial nerve damage; irregular or uncoordinated movement may suggest other neurologic pathology.

A **visual field examination** (assessment of peripheral vision and continuity in the visual field) is performed grossly by the nurse, or it can be tested with more sophisticated ophthalmic equipment. The nurse stands directly in front of the patient, and each covers an eye. The patient is instructed to look straight ahead and indicate when a light or the nurse's finger is seen as it is brought from several sectors of the periphery toward the center. If the patient's and the nurse's visual fields are normal, they will see the object at the same time. Certain eye and neurologic disorders are associated with changes in the visual field.

Ears

During a physical assessment, the external ears are examined by inspection and palpation. More advanced practitioners use an instrument called an *otoscope* to examine the tympanic membrane, or eardrum.

A gross examination of the ear is performed by:

- Observing the appearance of the ears. Both should be similar in size, shape, and location.
- Moving the skin behind and in front of the ears as well as the underlying cartilage to determine whether there is any tenderness
- Shining a pen light or other light source within each ear to illuminate the ear canal.

To obtain optimal visualization, the curved ear canal is straightened as much as possible. For children, this is done by

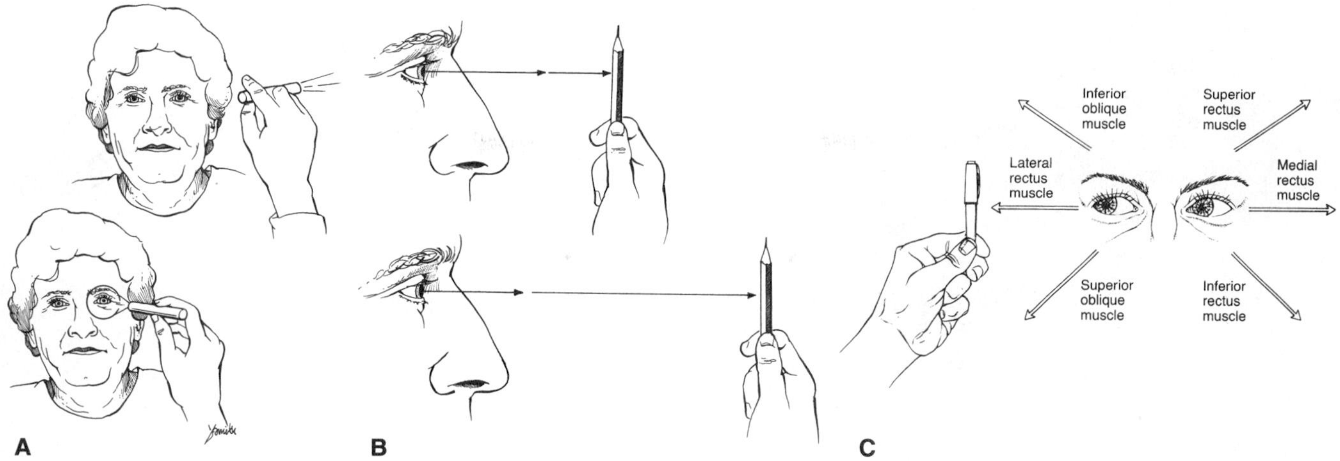

FIGURE 12–10. (*A*) Testing pupil response to light. (*B*) Testing accommodation. (*C*) Assessing extraocular movements.

pulling the ear down and back; for an adult, the ear is pulled up and back (Fig. 12-11). **Cerumen** (yellowish-brown, waxy secretion produced by glands within the ear) is a common finding. Any other type of drainage is abnormal, and its characteristics are described and reported.

If the patient relies on a hearing aid for amplifying sound, that information is noted on the assessment form. The nurse may discover changes in **hearing acuity** (ability to hear and discriminate sound) by performing a voice test or the Weber or Rinne test.

Nursing Guidelines For

Performing a Voice Test for Hearing Acuity

- ☑ Stand approximately 2 feet behind and to the side of the patient.
  RATIONALE: Simulates the distance between most people during social interaction and prevents the patient from observing visual cues.

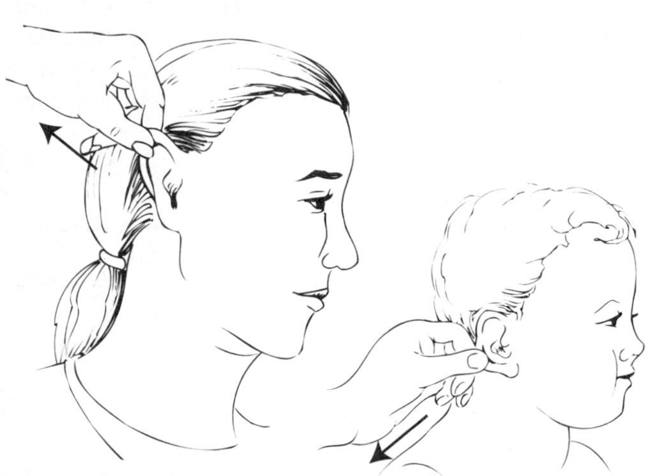

FIGURE 12–11. Technique for straightening the ear canal of an adult and child.

- ☑ Instruct the patient to cover the ear on the opposite side (Fig. 12-12).
  RATIONALE: Facilitates sound conduction to the tested ear only.
- ☑ Whisper a color, number, or name into the uncovered ear.
  RATIONALE: Delivers a high-pitched sound, the most common type of hearing loss, toward the tested ear.
- ☑ Instruct the patient to repeat the whispered word.
  RATIONALE: Reveals the ability to discriminate sound.
- ☑ Continue the same pattern using several more words; increase the volume from a soft to medium to loud whisper or spoken voice if the patient's response is inaccurate.
  RATIONALE: Provides more reliable data.
- ☑ Repeat the test on the opposite ear.
  RATIONALE: Provides separate assessment findings for each ear.

The Weber and Rinne tests help to determine whether patients have impaired hearing due to sensory nerve damage or disorders that interfere with sound conduction through the ear.

The **Weber test** (assessment technique for determining equality or disparity of bone-conducted sound) is performed by striking a tuning fork on the nurse's palm and placing the vibrating stem in the center of the head (Fig. 12-13). The patient is asked whether the sound is heard equally in both ears. This indicates a normal finding, or that the hearing in both ears is equally diminished. Hearing the sound louder in one ear is a sign of unequal hearing (hearing loss greater in one ear).

The **Rinne test** (assessment technique for comparing air versus bone conduction of sound) is also performed with a tuning fork. The tuning fork is first struck, and the stem is placed on the mastoid area behind the ear (Fig. 12-14). This tests for bone conduction of sound waves in the tested ear. The patient reports when the sound stops. The tines of the still-vibrating tuning fork are then moved near the ear canal. The

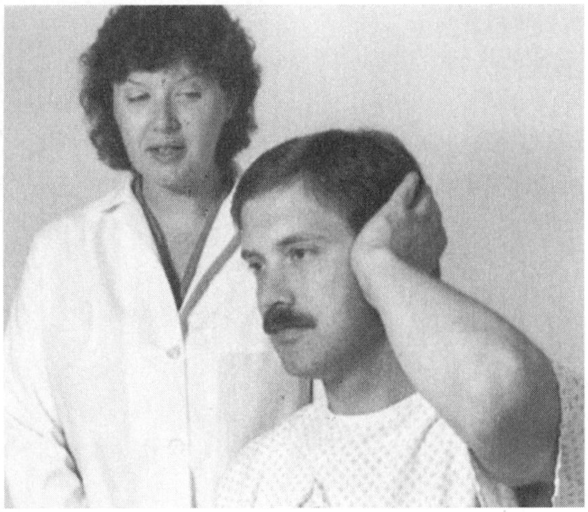

FIGURE 12–12. Voice test.

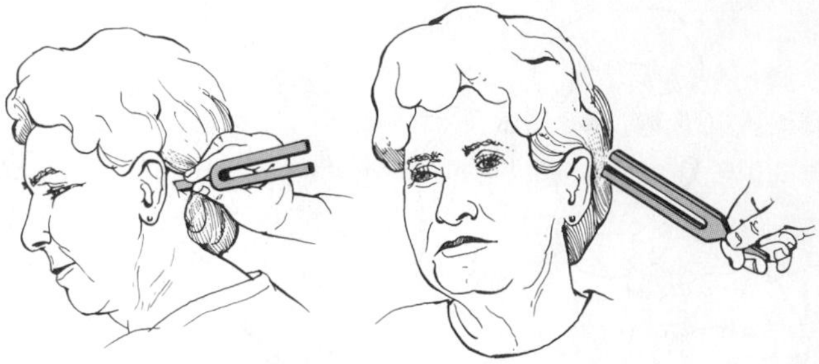

FIGURE 12–14. Rinne test.

patient is asked whether sound is perceived. This tests air conduction of sound in the tested ear. Both ears are assessed separately. Normally, sound is heard longer by air conduction. If the patient does not continue to hear sound when the tuning fork is beside the ear, it indicates a problem with the ear structures that collect and transmit sound through the ear.

Audiometry (measurement of hearing acuity at various sound frequencies) is a sophisticated test to identify a person's range of hearing. An audiometric test is performed by an *audiologist,* a professional trained to test hearing with standardized instruments. When audiometric hearing tests are used, exact pitch and volume deficits are measured. Hearing is measured in decibels (intensity of sound)—the greater the intensity of sound, the more impaired the hearing (Table 12-2).

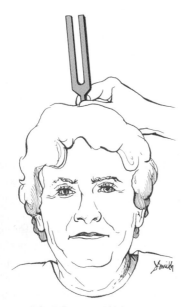

FIGURE 12–13. Weber test.

Nose

The nose and nasal passages are inspected by having the patient assume a "sniffing" position. The septum (tissue that divides the nose in half) should be in midline, causing the nasal passages to be equal in size. Deeper inspection is facilitated by pressing at the tip of the nose. Air should move fairly quietly through the nose during breathing. Normal mucous membrane within the nose is pink, moist, and free of obvious drainage. The presence of a deviated septum, lesions or growths, flaring of the nostrils, or unusual drainage is documented in the assessment findings.

Smelling acuity (ability to smell and identify odors) is not commonly performed unless there is some reason to suspect that it is impaired. To test a patient's smelling acuity:

1. Have the patient occlude one nostril and close his or her eyes.
2. Place substances with strong odors, such as lemon, vanilla extract, coffee, peppermint, or alcohol, one at a time, beneath the patent (open) nostril.
3. Ask the patient to inhale and identify the substance.

Mouth and Oral Mucous Membranes

The mouth is surrounded by the lips and contains the tongue and teeth. These structures are inspected by having the patient open his or her mouth widely. The tongue is normally in midline when it protrudes. The presence of dentures, missing or malpositioned teeth, or a partial plate is documented. Sometimes unusual breath odors are diagnos-

TABLE 12–2. **Hearing Acuity Levels**

Hearing Level	Decibel Range
Normal	0–25 dB
Mildly impaired	26–30 dB
Moderately impaired	31–55 dB
Moderately to severely impaired	56–70 dB
Severely impaired	71–90 dB
Profoundly impaired	91 dB or greater

tic. For example, the odor of alcohol or acetone suggests additional health problems.

Normal oral mucous membranes are pink and intact. They are kept moist by salivary glands located below the tongue. When the patient smiles, purses the lips as though preparing to whistle, or shows the teeth, the lips should look the same.

The tongue contains many taste buds that detect particular taste characteristics (Fig. 12-15). Although assessing taste is rarely done, it is facilitated by placing substances on the tongue and asking the patient to identify them with the eyes closed. To ensure valid results, the patient is encouraged to sip water between assessments.

Facial Skin

Characteristics of the facial skin are noted while assessing the head. Although skin assessment begins in this area, it continues as other areas of the body are examined. Regardless of where the skin is examined, it should be smooth, unbroken, of uniform color according to the patient's ethnic or racial origin, warm, and resilient. It should feel neither wet nor dry. Variations in skin color that are diagnostic are listed in Table 12-3.

While examining the skin, the nurse may detect one or more alterations in its integrity:

- A *wound* is a break in the skin.
- An *ulcer* is an open crater-like area.
- An *abrasion* is an area that has been rubbed away by friction.
- A *laceration* is a torn, jagged wound.
- A *fissure* is a crack in the skin, especially in or near mucous membranes.
- A *scar* is a mark left by the healing of a wound or lesion.

Other common skin lesions and their characteristics are described in Table 12-4. Additional skin assessments are described in later discussions about assessments in other areas of the body.

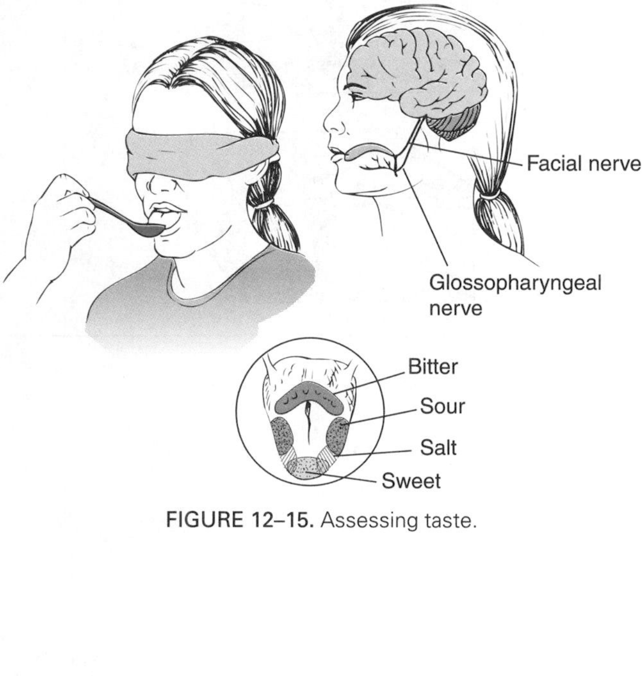

FIGURE 12–15. Assessing taste.

TABLE 12–3. **Common Skin Color Variations**

Color	Term	Possible Causes
Pale, regardless of race	Pallor	Anemia, blood loss
Red	Erythema	Superficial burns, local inflammation, carbon monoxide poisoning
Pink	Flushed	Fever, hypertension
Purple	Ecchymosis	Trauma to soft tissue
Blue	Cyanosis	Low tissue oxygenation
Yellow	Jaundice	Liver or kidney disease, destruction of red blood cells
Brown	Tan	Ethnic variation, sun exposure, pregnancy, Addison's disease

Hair

The assessment of the hair includes scalp hair, eyebrows, and eyelashes. The color, texture, and distribution (presence or absence in unusual locations for gender or age) are noted. The hair is also inspected for debris, such as blood in a patient with head trauma, nits (eggs from a lice infestation), or scales from scalp lesions. As the physical assessment progresses, the characteristics of body hair are also observed.

Scalp

The scalp is assessed by separating the hair at random areas and inspecting the skin. The nurse looks for signs indicating that the scalp is smooth, intact, and free of lesions. While examining the scalp, the nurse also palpates the skull for any unusual contour.

Neck

The neck supports the head in midline. The patient should be able to bend the head forward, backward, and to either side, as well as rotate it in a 180° arc. The trachea, or windpipe, should appear in the center of the neck. The pulsations in the carotid arteries (see Chap. 11) are visible and easily palpated. There should be no unusual bulges or fullness in the neck. Some nurses lightly palpate the lymph nodes in the neck area or assess for an enlarged thyroid gland.

CHEST AND SPINE

The chest is a cavity surrounded by the ribs and the vertebrae. It is the area where the heart and lungs are located. The nurse observes the shape of the chest and how it moves during breathing, notes the curved appearance of the spine, and assesses skin turgor, the breasts, heart sounds, and lung sounds.

TABLE 12–4. **Common Skin Lesions**

Type of Lesion	Description	Example	Illustration
Macule	Flat, round, colored, nonpalpable area	Freckles	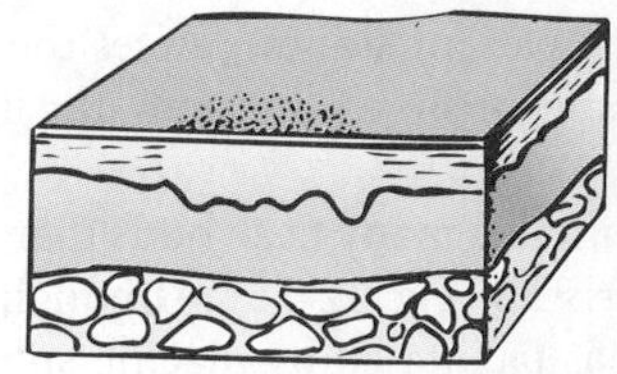
Papule	Elevated, palpable, solid	Wart	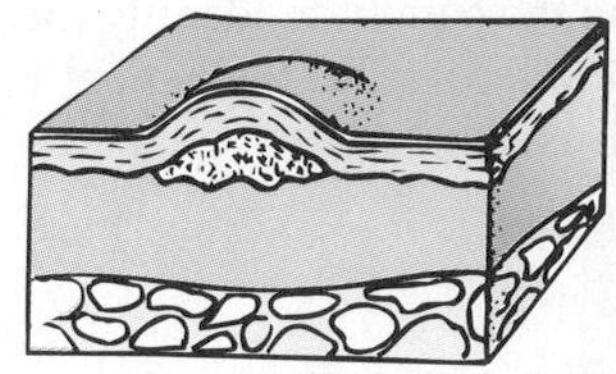
Vesicle	Elevated, round, filled with serum	Blister	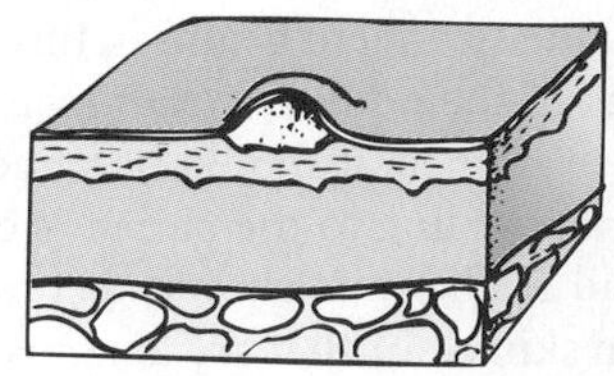
Wheal	Elevated, irregular border, no free fluid	Hives	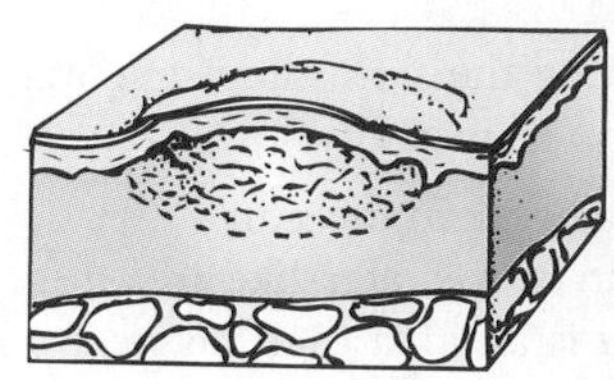
Pustule	Elevated, raised border, filled with pus	Boil	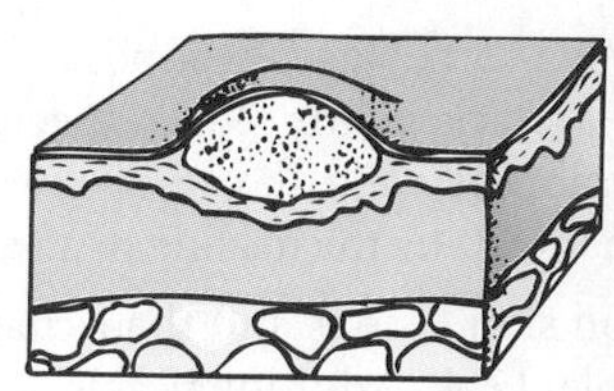
Nodule	Elevated, solid mass, deeper and firmer than papule	Enlarged lymph node	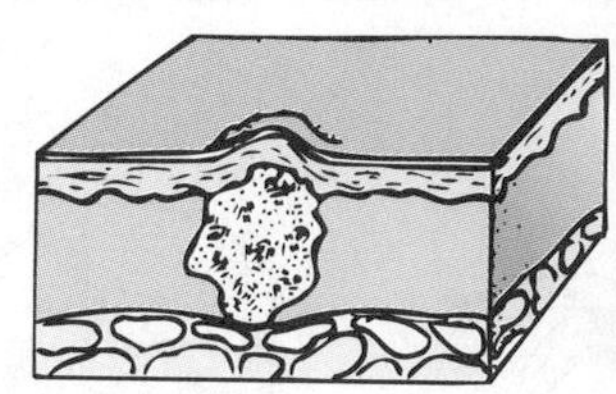
Cyst	Encapsulated, round fluid-filled or solid mass beneath the skin	Tissue growth	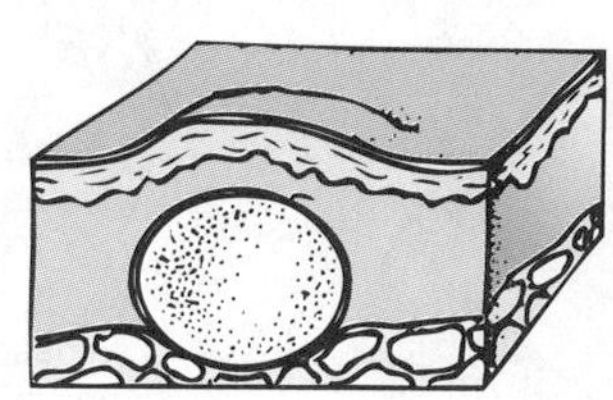

Turgor (resiliency of the skin) is a combination of the elastic quality of the skin and the pressure exerted on it by fluid within the tissue. To assess skin turgor, the skin is grasped between the thumb and fingers in an attempt to lift it from the underlying tissue. The area over the chest is a good assessment location because the skin in other areas tends to become loose with age. When the tissue is released, it should immediately return to its original position. Prolonged tenting indicates dehydration.

Chest Shape and Movement

In the normal adult, the lateral dimension of the chest is approximately twice the anterior-posterior dimension. Various musculoskeletal abnormalities, cardiac or respiratory diseases, or trauma cause changes in chest shape (Fig. 12-16). With normal breathing, the chest expands equally on both sides. To assess chest expansion:

- Place the thumbs side by side over the posterior vertebrae at about the level of the 10th rib (Fig. 12-17).
- As the patient inhales, note how far the thumbs separate; normally the distance is 1″ to 2″ (3 to 5 cm).

Spine

The spine, or column of vertebrae, appears in midline with gentle concave and convex curves when viewed from the side. The shoulders are at equal height. Some common deviations may be noted (Fig. 12-18). *Lordosis* is a condition in which the natural lumbar curve of the spine is exaggerated. *Kyphosis* causes an increased curve in the thoracic area. *Scoliosis* is a pronounced lateral curvature of the spine.

Breasts

Although abnormalities such as tumors occur in both women and men, they are more common in women. Usually more advanced practitioners examine a patient's breasts, but because breast tumors are common and early diagnosis carries a better prognosis, all nurses have a responsibility for teaching women how to examine their breasts on a routine basis.

Patient Teaching for
Self-Breast Examination

Teach the patient to do the following:

- Examine the breasts monthly about a week after a menstrual period, or on a specific date post-menopause.
- Begin the examination in the shower.
- Use the right hand to examine the left breast and the left hand to examine the right breast.
- Place the hand on the side that will be examined behind the head.
- Glide the flat portion of the fingers over all aspects of each breast in a circular fashion.
- Determine whether there are any lumps, hard knots, or thickened areas.
- Next, stand in front of a mirror.
- Look at both breasts with the arms relaxed at the side, with the hands pressing on the hips, and with the hands elevated above the head.
- Look for dimpling in the skin or retraction of either nipple.
- Lie down for the remainder of the examination.
- Put a pillow or folded towel under the shoulder on the side where the first breast will be examined; reverse the pillow before examining the second breast.

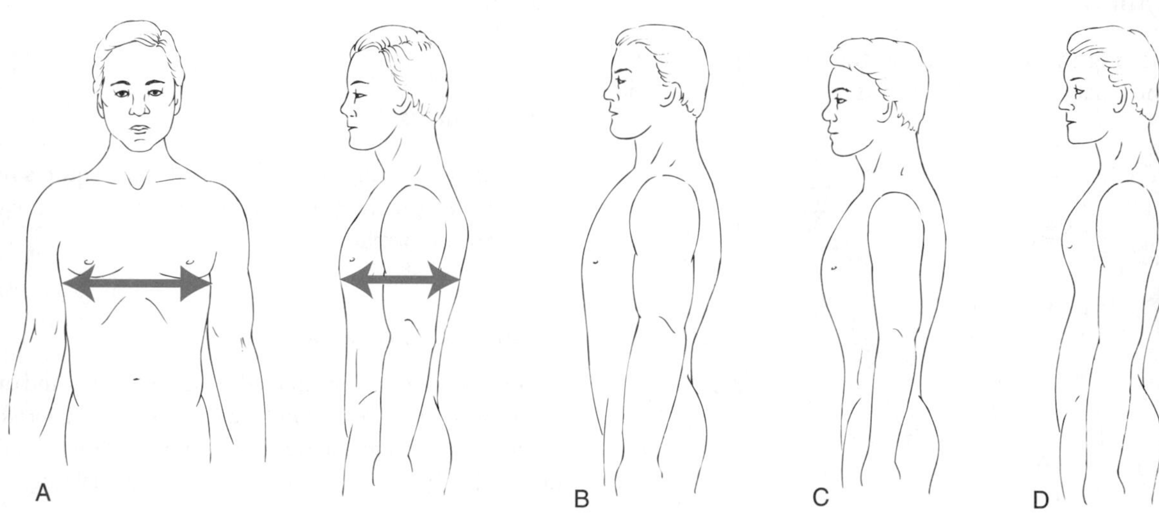

FIGURE 12–16. (*A*) Normal chest size and shape; anterolateral dimension is twice the anteroposterior dimension. (*B*) Barrel chest. (*C*) Pigeon chest. (*D*) Funnel chest.

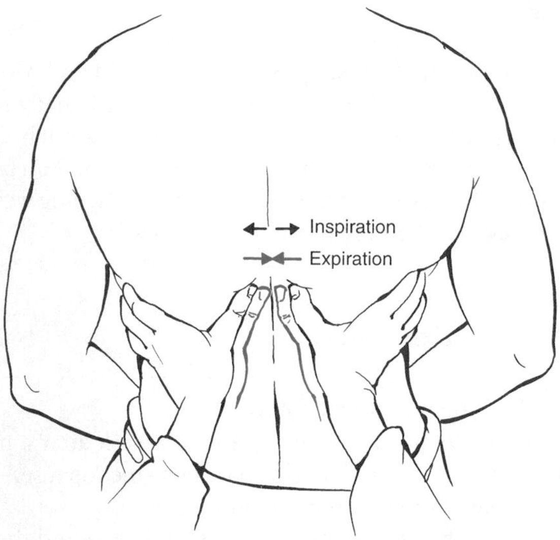

FIGURE 12–17. Assessing chest excursion.

- Again, place the arm behind the head.
- Press the flat surface of the fingers in small circular motions from the outer margin of the breast toward the nipple, or as in spokes in a wheel (Fig. 12-19).
- Feel upward toward the axilla of each arm.
- Complete at least three revolutions about the breast.
- Squeeze the nipple gently between the thumb and index finger to determine whether there is any clear or bloody discharge.
- Repeat the examination on the opposite breast and axilla.
- Report any unusual findings or changes to a physician.
- Self-breast examination is combined with additional examinations to ensure early diagnosis and treatment of cancerous tumors (Table 12-5).

Heart Sounds

When assessing the anterior chest, the nurse listens to the heart sounds that presumably are caused by the closing of the atrial and ventricular heart valves. A beginning nurse may limit the assessment to the apical area (see the section on apical heart rate in Chap. 11), but with experience nurses can expand their assessment skills to include auscultation at the aortic, pulmonic, tricuspid, and mitral areas (Fig. 12-20).

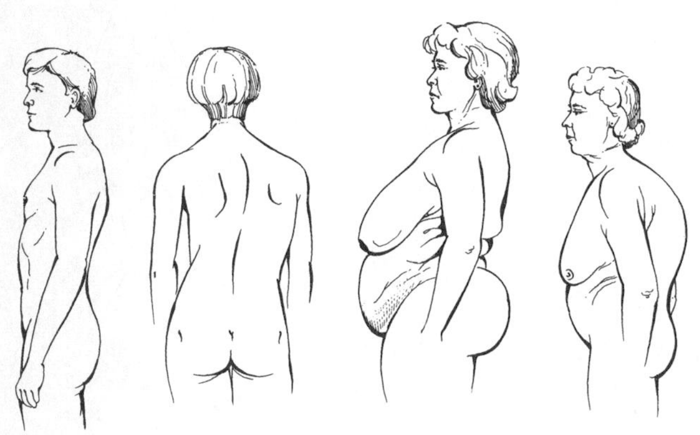

FIGURE 12–18. Variations in spinal curves: (*A*) normal, (*B*) scoliosis, (*C*) lordosis, and (*D*) kyphosis.

Normal Heart Sounds

There are two normal heart sounds, S_1 and S_2. S_1, the first heart sound, correlates with the "lub" sound and is louder at the apex or mitral area when the diaphragm of a stethoscope is used. Although the second heart sound, S_2 or the "dub" sound, can be heard in the mitral area, it is louder over the aortic area.

Sometimes there is tiny slurring, or *splitting,* of one or both sounds that lasts just a fraction of a second longer. It may sound like "lubba-dub" or "lub-dubba." Split sounds are generally attributed to the fact that the valves between the atria (or the ventricles) do not always close in exact unison. Splitting, if heard at all, is generally noted with the stethoscope at point P or T on the chest.

Abnormal Heart Sounds

The nurse may hear two additional sounds, S_3 and S_4, when auscultating the chest. An S_3 is normal in children but abnormal in most adults. An S_3 appears after the S_2 sound. It sounds like "lub-dub-**dub**" or the cadence of sounds in "Ken-tuck-**y.**" A third sound is much more pronounced than a split second sound. The S_4 is heard just before the S_1. It may sound more like "**lub**-lub-dub" or the syllables in "**Ten**-ne-ssee."

Identifying abnormal heart sounds—S_3, S_4, heart murmurs, clicks, and rubs—is a skill that is generally mastered after the nurse becomes proficient at distinguishing between S_1 and S_2. The beginning nurse should consult with an experienced nurse or the physician if there is any unusual characteristic in the S_1 and S_2 heart sounds.

Lung Sounds

Listening to the lungs is another skill that requires frequent and repeated practice, because some sounds are normal and others are abnormal.

Normal Lung Sounds

Normal lung sounds are created by air moving in and out of air passageways, which vary in location and size. Therefore, the sounds vary in pitch and duration depending on the area being auscultated (Fig. 12-21). There are four normal lung sounds:

- *Tracheal sounds* are loud and coarse. They are equal in length during inspiration and expiration and are separated by a brief pause in between.

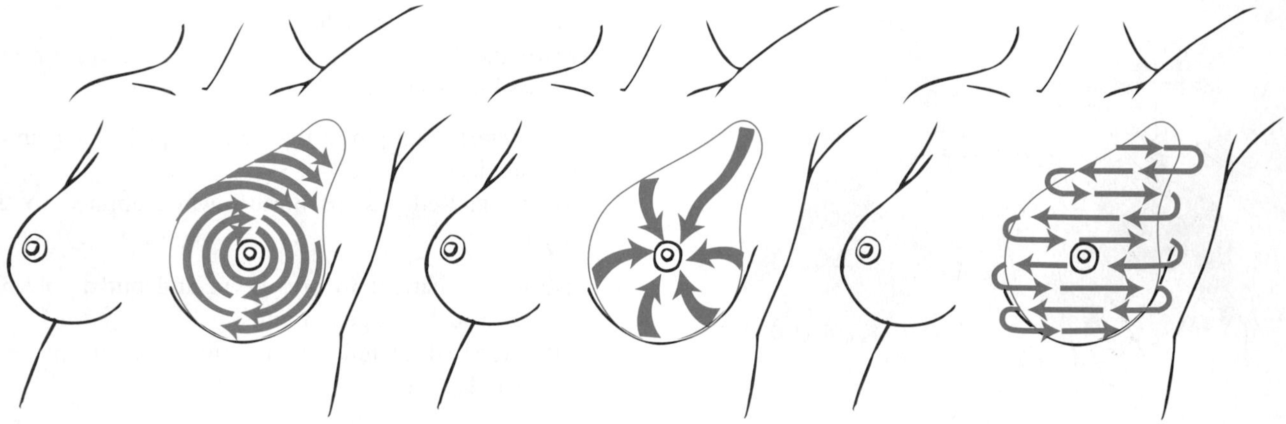

FIGURE 12–19. Patterns for palpating the breast when performing self breast examination.

- *Bronchial sounds,* heard over the upper part of the sternum, are harsh and loud. They are shorter on inspiration than expiration, with a pause between the two.
- *Bronchovesicular sounds* are heard on either side of the central chest or back. They are medium-range sounds that are equal in length during inspiration and expiration, with no noticeable pause.
- *Vesicular sounds* are located in the periphery of all the lung fields. Their soft, rustling quality is longer on inspiration than expiration, with no pause in between.

Abnormal Lung Sounds

Abnormal lung sounds, known as *adventitious sounds,* are those heard in addition to normal lung sounds. Most adventitious sounds are created by air moving through secretions or narrowed airways. Adventitious sounds are divided into four categories:

- *Crackles,* formerly called *rales,* are intermittent, high-pitched, popping sounds heard in distant areas of the lungs, primarily during inspiration. They resemble the sound of crisped rice cereal when milk is added. The sound is attributed to the opening of partially collapsed alveoli (terminal air sacs) or the movement of air over minute amounts of fluid in the periphery of the lungs during deep inspiration.
- *Gurgles,* formerly called *rhonchi,* are low-pitched, continuous, bubbling sounds heard in larger airways. They are more prominent during expiration. Some describe gurgles as sounding like wet snoring. Gurgles may clear with deep breathing or coughing.
- *Wheezes* are whistling or squeaking sounds caused by air moving through a narrowed passage. They can be heard anywhere throughout the chest during inspiration or expiration. Sometimes wheezes are audible without a stethoscope. Coughing and deep breathing do not usually alter a wheeze; if fact, if wheezing suddenly stops, it may mean that the air passage is totally occluded.
- *Rubs* are grating, or leathery, sounds caused by two dry pleural surfaces moving over one another.

Whenever adventitious sounds are heard, the nurse also assesses the characteristics of any cough that is present and the appearance of raised sputum.

TABLE 12–5. **Breast Examination Guidelines**

Technique	Age	Frequency
Self-examination	≥20 years	Once per month
Clinical examination	20–40 years	Every 3 years
by a nurse or physician	>40 years	Every year
Mammography	40 years	First examination
	>40 years	Every year

(Source: American Cancer Society, 1998.)

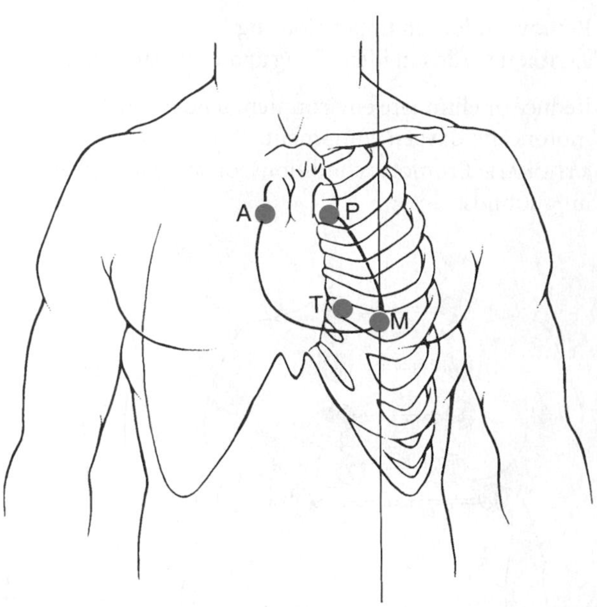

FIGURE 12–20. Locations for assessing heart sounds: M = mitral area, T = tricuspid area, P = pulmonic area, A = aortic area.

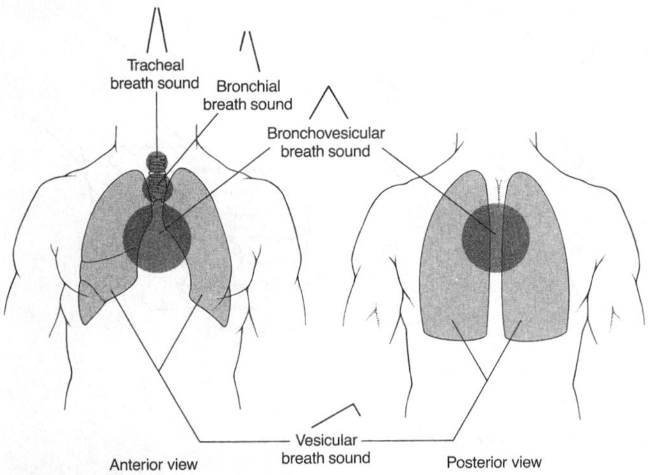

FIGURE 12–21. Locations of normal lung sounds. The symbols indicate the ratio of time they may be heard during inspiration and expiration, as well as the presence or absence of pauses between the two.

Nursing Guidelines For

Assessing Lung Sounds

- ☑ Wash your hands.
  RATIONALE: Reduces the spread of infection.
- ☑ Provide privacy.
  RATIONALE: Demonstrates concern for patient modesty.
- ☑ Raise the bed to a comfortable position for you.
  RATIONALE: Reduces strain on the musculoskeletal system.
- ☑ Assist the patient to a sitting position, if possible.
  RATIONALE: Facilitates auscultating the anterior, posterior, and lateral aspects of the chest with minimal exertion by the patient.
- ☑ Remove or loosen upper clothing.
  RATIONALE: Aids in identifying anatomic landmarks.
- ☑ Reduce or eliminate environmental noise, such as suction motors and oxygen equipment.
  RATIONALE: Promotes conditions for accurately identifying lung sounds.
- ☑ Ask the patient not to talk.
  RATIONALE: Talking interferes with concentration and distorts lung sounds.
- ☑ Warm the diaphragm of the stethoscope in the palm of your hand.
  RATIONALE: Reduces discomfort when applied to the chest.
- ☑ Instruct the patient to breathe in and out deeply but slowly, through an open mouth.
  RATIONALE: Reduces noise from air turbulence and prevents hyperventilation.
- ☑ Apply the chest piece to the upper back, but avoid placement over the scapulae or ribs.
  RATIONALE: Facilitates hearing sounds in the upper and lower lobes and reduces competing sounds from the heart.
- ☑ Listen for one complete ventilation (inspiration and expiration) at each area that is auscultated.
  RATIONALE: Ensures hearing characteristics during each phase of ventilation.
- ☑ If body hair causes noise, wet it or press harder with the chest piece.
  RATIONALE: Reduces sound distortion.
- ☑ Move the diaphragm from side to side from the apices (top) to the bases (bottom) of the lungs (Fig. 12-22)
  RATIONALE: Aids comparison of the sounds.
- ☑ Auscultate the lateral and anterior chest in a similar fashion.
  RATIONALE: Ensures a comprehensive assessment.
- ☑ Ask the patient to cough or breath deeply if crackles or gurgles are heard.
  RATIONALE: Helps to clear the air passages and open the alveoli.
- ☑ Reapply clothing and lower the bed.
  RATIONALE: Restores comfort and safety.
- ☑ Wash your hands.
  RATIONALE: Reduces the spread of microorganisms.

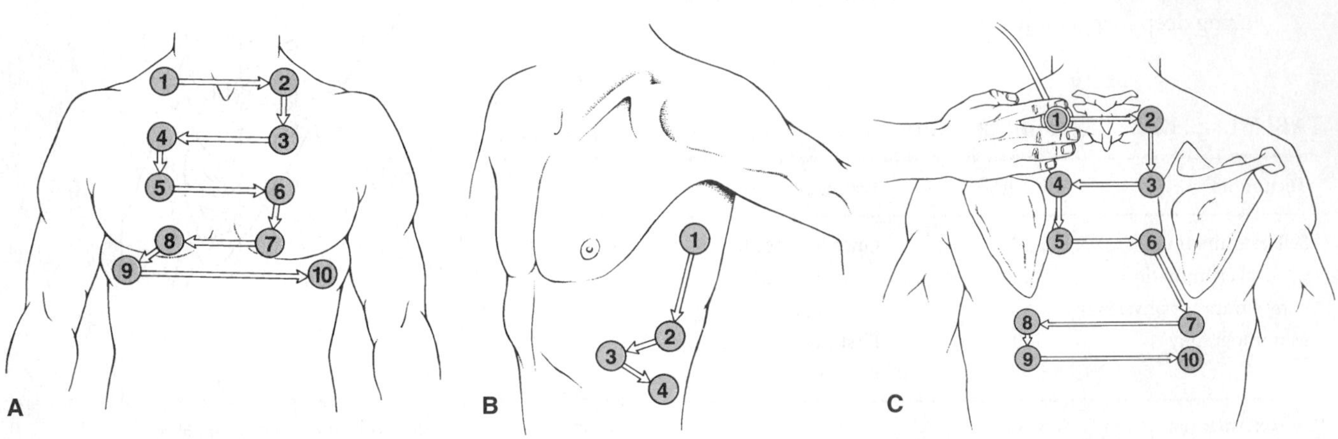

FIGURE 12–22. Auscultation sequence. (*A*) Anterior. (*B*) Lateral. (*C*) Posterior.

☑ Record assessment findings.
RATIONALE: Documents data that can be used for future comparisons.

☑ Repeat lung sound assessments according to agency policy or the patient's condition.
RATIONALE: Demonstrates responsibility, accountability, and good clinical judgment.

EXTREMITIES

The nurse notes the alignment, mobility, and strength of the extremities and compares their size. The nurse also feels the skin temperature, notes the characteristics of the nails and times the capillary refill, palpates local peripheral pulses (see Chap. 11), checks for edema, and may test the perception of skin sensations. Advanced practitioners assess deep tendon reflexes with a *reflex hammer*.

Muscle Strength

All four extremities are assessed separately to determine muscle strength. The patient is asked to grasp, squeeze, and release the nurse's fingers. As the nurse pulls and pushes on the forearm and upper arm, the patient is instructed to resist. To test the strength in the lower extremities, the nurse has the patient push and pull his or her foot against a resisting hand (Fig. 12-23).

Finger and Toe Nails

Changes in the shape and thickness of the finger and toe nails are often signs of chronic cardiopulmonary disease (Fig. 12-24) or fungal infections. Any unusual characteristics of the nails or tissue surrounding it are documented.

Capillary refill time (amount of time it takes blood to resume flowing in the base of the nail beds) is normally less than 3 seconds after the nail bed is compressed and released. To assess capillary refill time:

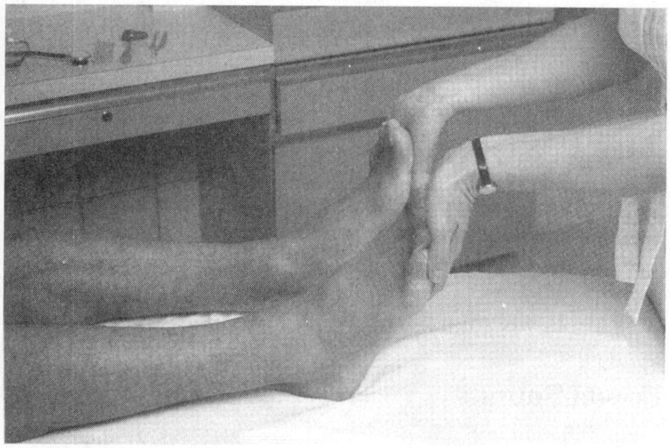

FIGURE 12–23. Assessing muscle strength of lower extremities. (From Rosdahl CB. Textbook of basic nursing, 7th ed. Philadelphia, Lippincott Williams & Wilkins, 1999).

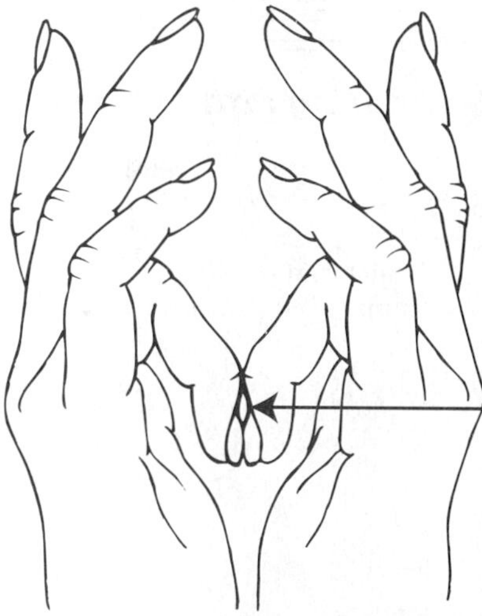

FIGURE 12–24. Technique for assessing clubbed fingernails. A diamond-shape space between the nails of the ring fingers is normal.

1. Observe the color in the nail bed.
2. Depress the nail bed, displacing capillary blood.
3. Release the pressure.
4. Note how many seconds it takes for the preassessment color to reappear. Watching a clock would interfere with an accurate assessment, so count, "one-one thousand, two-one thousand, three-one thousand" to estimate the time in seconds.

Edema

Edema (excessive amount of fluid within tissue) is a sign of abnormal fluid distribution. Patients with cardiovascular, liver, and kidney dysfunction are prone to develop edema. Subtle indications of edema include weight gain, tight rings, and patterns in the skin after socks or shoes have been removed. To determine the presence and extent of edema, the nurse presses a thumb or finger into the tissue. If an indentation remains (*pitting edema*), the nurse attempts to quantify its severity (Display 12-3).

Skin Sensation

During a comprehensive rather than a basic assessment, the ability of the patient to differentiate between light touch, warmth, cold, sharp, dull, and vibration is tested.

Nursing Guidelines For
Assessing Sensory Skin Perception

☑ Gather a cotton ball, a safety pin or pointed object, a small container of warm water and one of ice water, and a tuning fork.
RATIONALE: Provides a variety of test resources.

DISPLAY 12–3

Criteria for Estimating Pitting Edema

1+ Pitting Edema
- Slight indentation (2 mm)
- Normal contours
- Associated with interstitial fluid volume 30% above normal

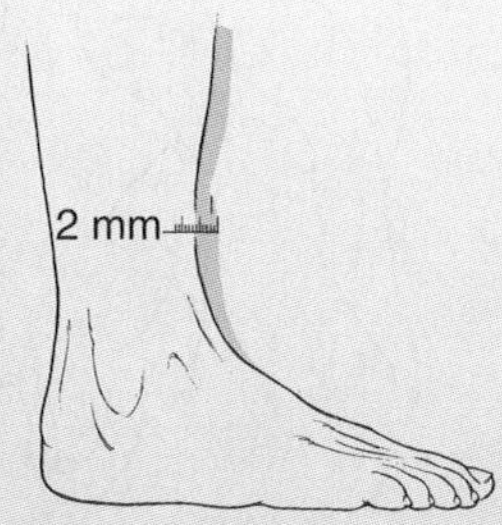

2+ Pitting Edema
- Deeper pit after pressing (4 mm)
- Lasts longer than 1+
- Fairly normal contour

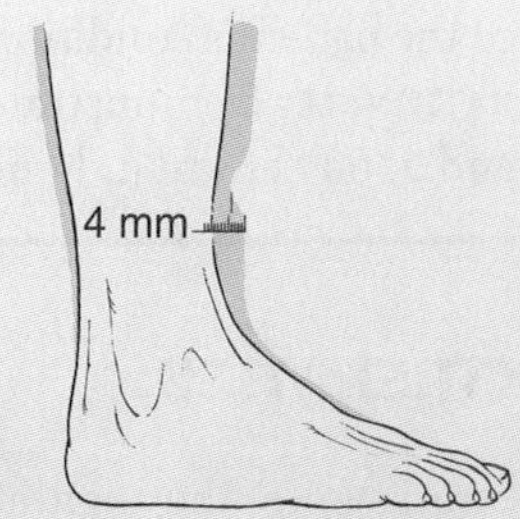

3+ Pitting Edema
- Deep pit (6 mm)
- Remains several seconds after pressing
- Skin swelling obvious by general inspection

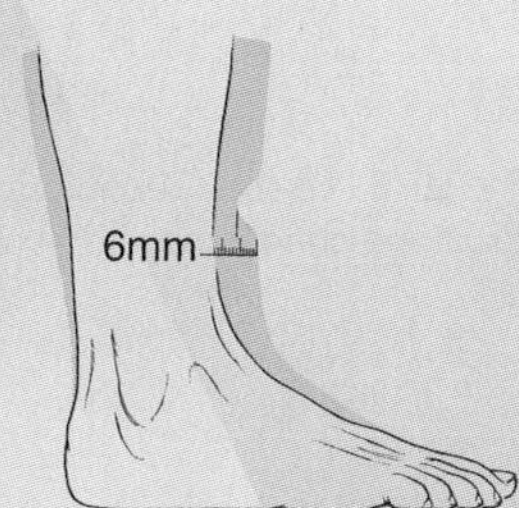

4+ Pitting Edema
- Deep pit (8 mm)
- Remains for a prolonged time after pressing, possibly minutes
- Frank swelling

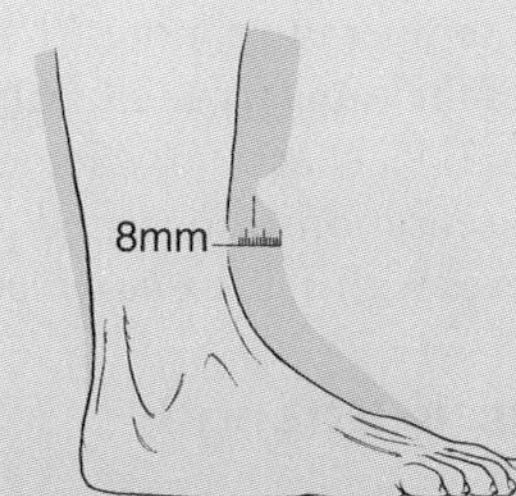

5+ Brawny Edema
- Fluid can no longer be displaced secondary to excessive interstitial fluid accumulation
- No pitting
- Tissue palpates as firm or hard
- Skin surface shiny, warm moist

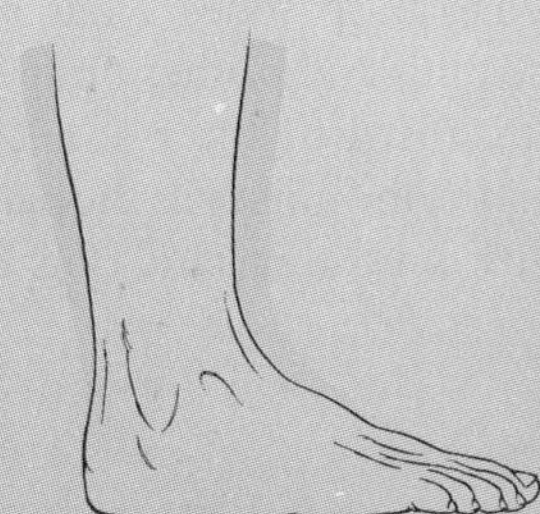

☑ Instruct the patient to shut both eyes.
RATIONALE: Reduces the potential for gathering invalid data.

☑ Explain that the skin will be touched at various places and on both sides of the body with test objects, and that he or she will be asked to identify the location and the characteristic of the sensation.
RATIONALE: Identifies the method of the test and how the patient is expected to respond.

☑ Touch the patient in a random pattern with the test objects.
RATIONALE: Avoids the potential for correct guessing.

☑ Use both the pointed end and the curved end of a safety pin to determine whether the patient can discriminate between sharp and dull. Take care not to puncture the skin.
RATIONALE: Prevents injury.

☑ Stroke the skin with the cotton ball and touch areas with the warm and cold containers.
RATIONALE: Assesses the ability to identify fine touch and differences in temperatures.

☑ Strike a tuning fork and place the stem against bony areas such as the wrists and along the length of the shins.
RATIONALE: Tests the ability to sense vibration.

ABDOMEN

Most of the gastrointestinal and accessory organs for digestion lie within the abdomen. The bladder, if distended, may rise into the abdomen.

For assessment, the abdomen is divided into four quadrants (Fig. 12-25). *The abdomen is always inspected and then auscultated—in that sequence—before using palpation or percussion techniques.* Touching or manipulating the abdomen can alter bowel sounds, producing invalid findings.

Bowel Sounds

Bowel sounds are produced by the wavelike muscular contractions of the large and small intestine that move fluid and

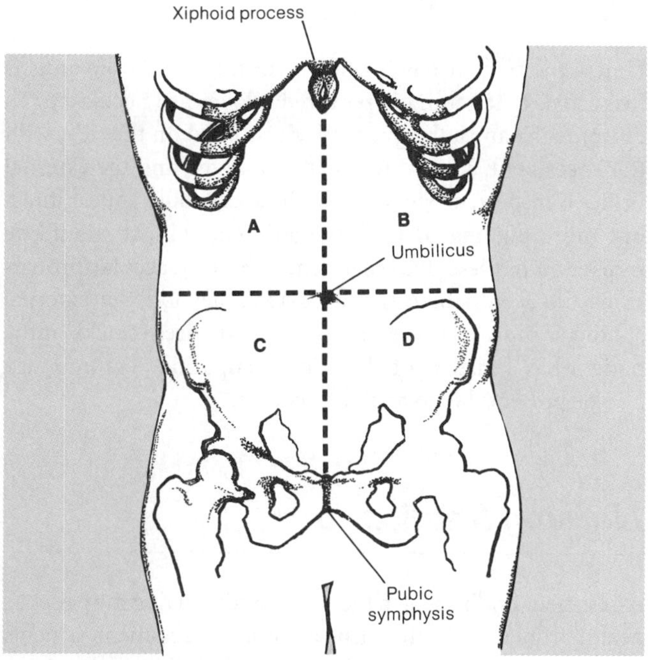

FIGURE 12-25. Four abdominal quadrants. (*A*) Right upper quadrant (RUQ), (*B*) left upper quadrant (LUQ), (*C*) right lower quadrant (RLQ), and (*D*) left lower quadrant (LLQ).

intestinal contents toward the rectum. Bowel sounds are routinely assessed on admission and once per shift.

Normal bowel sounds resemble clicks or gurgles and occur 5 to 34 times a minute (Bickley and Hoekelman, 1998). They are more frequent after the person eats. Bowel sounds are described as *hyperactive* if they are frequent, *hypoactive* if they occur after long intervals of silence, and *absent* if no sound is heard for 2 to 5 minutes. Occasionally, the nurse also detects the sound of blood pulsating through the abdominal aorta.

Nursing Guidelines For

Assessing Bowel Sounds

☑ Have the patient recline.
RATIONALE: Provides access to the abdomen.

☑ Reduce noise.
RATIONALE: Facilitates accurate assessment.

☑ Warm the diaphragm of the stethoscope.
RATIONALE: Promotes comfort.

☑ Place the diaphragm lightly in the lower right quadrant and listen for clicks or gurgles. Listening in this area usually provides adequate data, but most nurses move the chest piece over all four quadrants. If no sounds are heard initially, listen in that area for 2 to 5 minutes.
RATIONALE: Follows the anatomic areas of the upper to lower bowel.

☑ Document the frequency and character of the bowel sounds.
RATIONALE: Provides data for problem identification and future comparisons.

☑ Once auscultation is performed, the nurse notes the softness or firmness of the abdomen and feels for palpable masses (Display 12-4).

Abdominal Girth

If the abdomen appears unusually enlarged, the nurse measures the girth, or circumference, daily by placing a tape measure around the largest diameter of the abdomen. To ensure that the measurements are taken from the same location during subsequent assessments, the nurse makes guide marks on the skin using indelible pen (Fig. 12-26).

THE GENITALIA

In most cases, the genitalia are only inspected. If contact with genital structures or secretions is required, the nurse dons gloves. To eliminate the possibility of being falsely accused of sexual impropriety, it is a good practice to ask someone of the patient's gender to be present when the genitalia are touched.

During inspection, the condition of the skin and the distribution and any unusual characteristics of pubic hair are noted (lice may also infest pubic hair). A physician or nurse with advanced skills examines females internally with an

DISPLAY 12-4

Characteristics of Palpated Masses

Characteristic	*Description*
Mobility	Fixed—does not move Mobile—can be moved with palpation
Shape	Round—resembles a ball Tubular—is elongated Ovoid—resembles an egg Irregular—has no definite shape
Consistency	Edematous—leaves indentation when palpated Nodular—feels bumpy to touch Granular—feels gritty to touch Spongy—feels soft to touch Hard—feels firm to touch
Size	Measured in centimeters (1 cm = approximately ½")
Tenderness	Amount of discomfort when palpated—none, slight, moderate, or severe

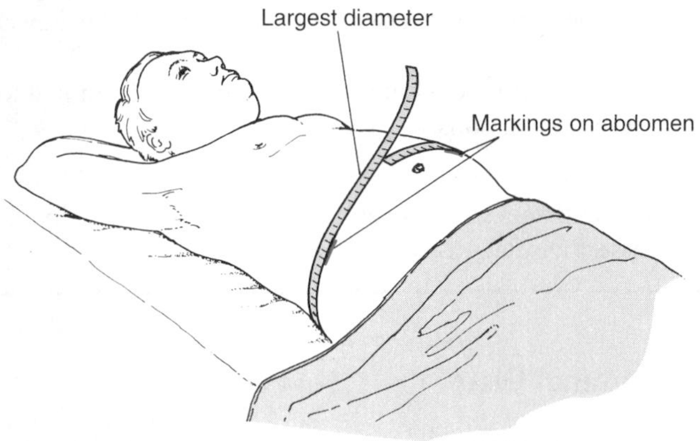

FIGURE 12–26. Measuring abdominal girth.

instrument called a *speculum* (see Chap. 13); in men, the prostate gland is palpated during a rectal examination.

The nurse observes whether males are circumcised and whether the scrotum appears to be of normal size. Whenever possible, men are instructed how to self-examine their testicles.

PATIENT TEACHING FOR *Testicular Self-Examination*

Teach the patient to do the following:

- Examine the testes monthly at a time when the testicles are warm and positioned loosely within the scrotum, like when bathing or showering.
- Elevate the penis with one hand.
- Gently roll each testicle within the scrotum between the thumb and the index finger.
- Feel each testicle vertically and horizontally (Fig. 12-27).
- Check for any unusual lumps; cancerous lumps are more often located on the upper and outer sides of the testes.
- Continue palpation, following the spermatic cord from the testicle to where it ascends into the abdomen.
- Report any unusual findings to a physician as soon as possible; an early diagnosis carries a better prognosis.

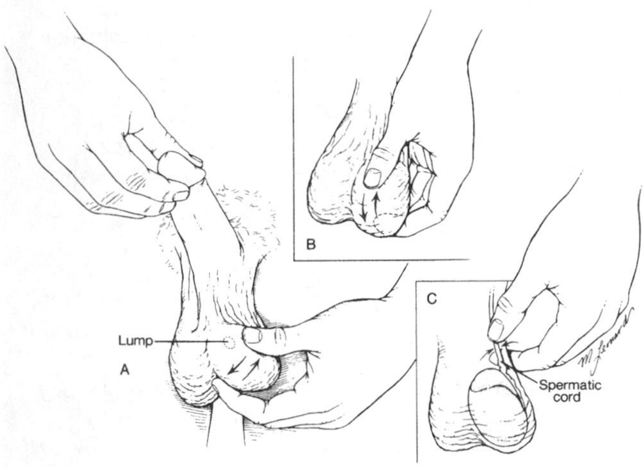

FIGURE 12–27. Testicular self-examination. (*A*) Horizontal palpation. (*B*) Vertical palpation. (*C*) Palpation of spermatic cord.

ANUS AND RECTUM

Unless the patient has specific symptoms, only the anus is inspected. If touching is required, gloves are necessary. To examine the anus, the patient is positioned on the side, with the knees bent. The buttocks are separated and the external orifice is inspected (Fig. 12-28). The area should appear intact but more pigmented than the adjacent skin; it should be moist and hairless. External hemorrhoids (saccular protrusions filled with blood) may extend beyond the external sphincter muscle. There may be rectal fissures (cracks) if the patient has a history of chronic constipation. Trauma may also be present due to anal intercourse.

Nursing Implications

Assessment findings form the basis for identifying the patient's health problems. Often during a physical assessment, patients reveal situations that caused their health to fail, or they indicate a desire for more health information. The following are some nursing diagnoses that may be outcomes after a physical assessment:

- Altered health maintenance
- Ineffective management of therapeutic regimen
- Knowledge deficit
- Noncompliance
- Health-seeking behaviors

The accompanying nursing care plan is an example of how the nursing process is used when a patient has the nursing diagnosis of Health-seeking behaviors, defined in the NANDA taxonomy (1999) as "a state in which an individual in stable health is actively seeking ways to alter personal health habits and/or the environment in order to move toward a higher level of health."

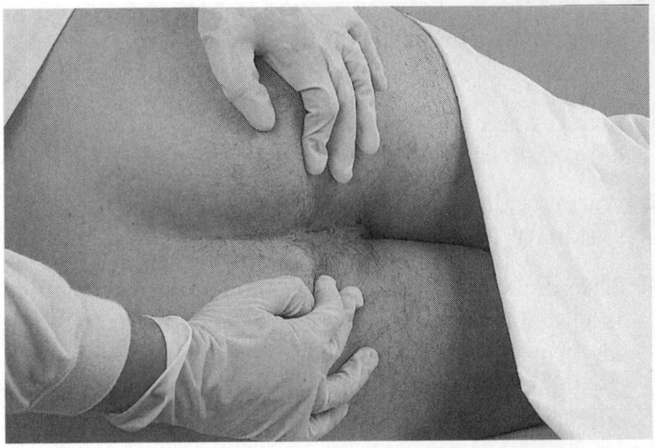

FIGURE 12–28. Inspection of the anus. (From Rosdahl CB. Textbook of basic nursing, 7th ed. Philadelphia, Lippincott Williams & Wilkins, 1999.)

Nursing Care Plan

Health-Seeking Behaviors

Assessment

Subjective Data

States, "I've been having sex with a lot of women. None of them have gotten pregnant and I haven't caught any diseases as far as I know. But, I don't want to take chances anymore."

Objective Data

19-year-old man scheduled for inguinal hernia repair as an outpatient in 3 days. Circumcised penis with bilaterally descended testicles. Slight bulge in R inguinal area. No discharge from penis. Has vaginal sex at least four times a week. Currently has three sexual partners. Requests information on safer sex practices and use of condoms.

Diagnosis

Health Seeking Behaviors: Preventing sexually transmitted diseases and pregnancy.

Plan

Goal

The patient will identify safer sex practices by 10/13 and use them during future sexual activities.

Orders: 10/10

1. Give assorted pamphlets and free condoms from Reproductive Control Clinic.
2. Emphasize the following safer sex practices:
   - Reduce sexual partners to one noninfected, faithful person.
   - Use a latex condom and nonoxynol-9 spermicide either over the tip of the condom or as a vaginal application.
   - Remove the condom-covered penis from the vagina before the penis becomes limp.
   - Do not have sexual contact again unless another condom is applied.
   - If a condom breaks or leaks, urinate immediately and wash the penis with soap and water.

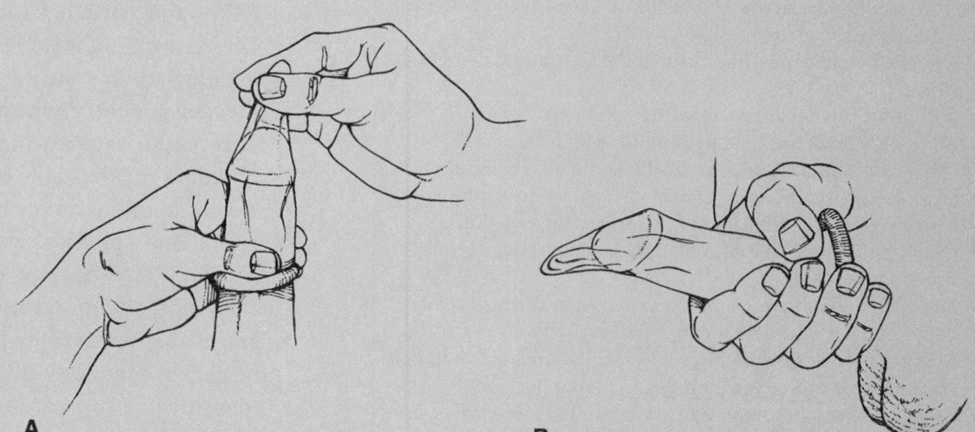

(*A*) To apply, roll the condom completely over the erect penis while pinching the space at the condom tip. (*B*) Hold the condom at the base of the penis during its removal from the vagina.

3. Give schedule of Reproductive Control Clinic hours ______________ B. VELASQUEZ, RN

Implementation (Documentation)

10/10 1300 Given the following pamphlets: "Choices" and "Understanding Safer Sex." Identified pages with illustrations for applying condoms. Given sample package of condoms. Clinic hours written on cover of pamphlets. Will discuss reading and use of condoms on return admission.
______________________________ B. VELASQUEZ, RN

continued

Nursing Care Plan ***Health-Seeking Behaviors*** *Continued*

Evaluation (Documentation)	10/13 0630 Says he has read sex information pamphlets given during preadmission exam. Used one sample condom s̄ problems. Asked, "What can my girlfriend do if the condom breaks?" Advised immediate insertion of an applicator filled with foam spermicide. To reduce risks of sexually transmitted diseases, a female sex partner should urinate and also wash well with soap and water. Told to avoid douching as this may push infectious organisms higher into the uterus or Fallopian tubes. Plans to buy more condoms. Says, "They're a lot cheaper than babies." ____________ B. VELASQUEZ, RN

FOCUS ON OLDER ADULTS

- The skin of older adults is usually dry, thin, and wrinkled.
- Non-pathologic skin lesions common in older adults include: lentigines (pale to dark brown macules), actinic keratosis (red, yellow, brown, or flesh-colored papules or plaques), and seborrheic keratosis (brown or black papules or plaques).
- A loss in height of 3/4 inch to 1 3/4 inches (2 to 4 cm) per decade is a normal consequence of osteoporosis, (bone demineralization) in older adults.
- Hair becomes grayer and thinner with increased age.
- Older adults experience a reduction in sweat gland activity, predisposing them to dry skin.
- A gradual decline in tactile sensitivity begins around the age of 20 years.
- Loss of subcutaneous fat causes the skin to sag.
- All sensory functions tend to diminish with increasing age.
- Older adults need referrals for further evaluation of vision and hearing impairments since they can benefit from hearing aids, corrective lenses, and medical and surgical interventions.
- Older adults often have difficulty hearing high-pitched consonants, such as "f," "s," "sh," "th," and "ch."
- Direct, non-glare lighting improves older adults' visual ability.
- Older adults have a weaker cough and gag reflex.
- Menstruation is rare after age 50 years. Vaginal bleeding or spotting often indicates a pathologic condition.
- Female breasts become flat and pendulous due to postmenopausal loss of estrogen.
- The incidence of cancer increases with age. The risk for breast cancer rises after menopause.
- The vaginal mucous membrane becomes dryer with age, leading to discomfort during intercourse.
- Older men usually retain their ability to produce sperm. However, the time needed to achieve an erection increases.
- The prostate gland tends to enlarge as men age, predisposing them to urinary retention and infection.
- Bladder capacity in both men and women diminishes with increased age.
- Muscular strength and joint flexibility decrease with age.

KEY CONCEPTS

- Physical assessments are performed to evaluate the patient's current physical condition, to detect early signs of developing health problems, to establish a data base for future comparisons, and to evaluate responses to medical and nursing interventions.
- There are four physical assessment techniques: inspection, percussion, palpation, and auscultation.
- Before performing a physical assessment, the nurse needs gloves, a patient gown, a cloth or paper drape, stethoscope, pen light, and tongue blade, as well as other assessment instruments for taking vital signs and weighing and measuring the patient.
- The assessment environment should be close to a restroom, private, warm, and adequately lighted. There should be an adjustable examination table or bed.
- During an initial survey of a patient, the nurse observes the patient's physical appearance, level of consciousness, body size, posture, gait, movement, use of ambulatory aids, and mood and emotional tone.
- Drapes are used during a physical examination to protect the patient's modesty and provide warmth.
- There are two approaches for data collection. The head-to-toe approach involves gathering data from the top of the body, working toward the feet. The systems approach organizes data collection according to the functional systems of the body.
- The body may be divided into six general components when organizing data collection: the head and neck, the chest, the extremities, the abdomen, the genitalia, and the anus and rectum.
- Whenever an opportunity arises, adult patients are taught how to perform breast and testicular self-examinations.

CRITICAL THINKING EXERCISES

- A patient reports that he has not had a bowel movement for 3 days, which is an unusual pattern for him. Discuss the physical assessments that are important to perform at this time.
- A nurse has documented that a patient has maculopapular skin lesions over her body. Describe how these would appear.
- You hear a patient coughing at frequent intervals. What physical assessments are appropriate?
- You are listening with a stethoscope at approximately the midchest, below the nipple line, of a male patient. Describe the characteristics of lung sounds normally heard in this location.

SUGGESTED READINGS

Adair JC. Is it Alzheimer's? Hospital Practice 1998;33(8):35–53.

American Cancer Society. Prevention and detection guidelines. Guidelines for cancer-related checkup. Atlanta, American Cancer Society, 1998. *www.cancer.org/guide/guidchec.html*

Arnold GJ, Neiheisel MB. A comprehensive approach to evaluating nipple discharge. Nurse Practitioner: American Journal of Primary Health Care 1997;22(7):96–111.

Baum NH. The testicular self-exam—30 seconds that can save your life. Hospital Medicine 1996;32(4):49–50.

Bickley LS, Hoekelman RA. Bates' guide to physical examination and history taking, 7th ed. Philadelphia, Lippincott-Raven, 1998.

Gallegos SJ, Michalee DL. Orthopedic essentials. Neurologic assessment of the orthopaedic patient. Orthopaedic Nursing 1996;15(5):23–29.

Geyer N, Naude S. Continuing education—clinical. Assessment of the musculoskeletal system. Nursing News 1996;20(9):41–45.

Kirton CA. Physical assessment. Assessing for ascites. Nursing 1996;26(4):53.

Koshti-Richman A. The role of nurses in promoting testicular self-examination. Nursing Times 1996;92(33):40–41.

Langan JC. Abdominal assessment in the home: from A to Zzz. Home Healthcare Nurse 1998;16(1):50–58.

Li JTC, Sheeler RD. The asthma physical exam: what's valuable, what's not? Journal of Respiratory Diseases 1996;17(9):735–738.

Ludwig LM. Cardiovascular assessment for home healthcare nurses, part I: initial cardiovascular assessment. Home Healthcare Nurse 1998;16(7): 450–456.

North American Nursing Diagnosis Association. NANDA nursing diagnoses: definitions and classification, 1999–2000. Philadelphia, NANDA, 1999.

O'Hanlon-Nichols T. Basic assessment series: the adult cardiovascular system. American Journal of Nursing 1997;97(12):34–40.

Peters J, Watts J. Accurate assessment of skin conditions—stop, look and listen. Practice Nurse 1998;15(9):525–530.

Underwood PW. Vital signs. Breast cancer awareness begins with you. American Journal of Nursing 1998;98(10):80.

Young T. Skin assessment and unusual presentations. Community Nurse 1997;3(5):33–36.

SKILL 12–1

PERFORMING A PHYSICAL ASSESSMENT

Suggested Action	Reason for Action
Assessment:	
Identify the patient.	Ensures that the assessment will be performed on the correct individual
Determine the age, gender, and race of the patient.	Forms the basis for planning techniques for physical assessment
Observe the patient's state of alertness and ability to move about.	Aids in determining the best location for the assessment and whether assistance will be required
Ask the patient's opinion about his or her health status and any current or recent signs and symptoms.	Helps focus attention during the assessment on particular structures and their functions
Planning	
Give the patient a specimen container, if a urine sample is needed.	Takes advantage of an opportunity when the patient's bladder contains urine
Have the patient empty his or her bladder before undressing.	Facilitates the examination and reduces discomfort
Pull the curtain or close the door and give the patient a drape or gown to put on after undressing.	Prepares the patient for accurate assessment and ensures privacy
Gather assessment equipment and supplies (see Display 12–1 for basic necessities).	Promotes organization and efficient time management
Decide whether to examine the patient using a head-to-toe or body systems approach.	Establishes the plan for assessment and ensures that the data will be gathered in a comprehensive manner

continued

SKILL 12-1

PERFORMING A PHYSICAL ASSESSMENT *Continued*

Suggested Action	Reason for Action
Implementation	
Explain how the assessment will be conducted.	May reduce anxiety
Explain that all information will be kept confidential among those involved in the patient's care.	Encourages the patient to be honest and open in identifying health problems
Wash your hands thoroughly and preferably in the presence of the patient.	Provides reassurance that the nurse is clean and conscientious about controlling the spread of microorganisms
Warm your hands before touching the patient.	Demonstrates concern for the patient's comfort
Obtain the patient's height, weight, and vital signs.	Contributes to the general survey of the patient
Assist the patient to sit at the bottom of the examination table.	Facilitates examination of the upper body without requiring the patient to change positions
Modify the patient's position if the examination is being conducted in locations other than an examination room.	Demonstrates adaptability
Explain each assessment technique before it is performed.	Reduces anxiety
Try to avoid tiring the patient, and apologize if the patient experiences discomfort.	Demonstrates concern for the patient's comfort
Help the patient to resume sitting after the examination.	Places the patient in the best position for communicating
Wash your hands once again.	Shows responsibility for controlling the spread of microorganisms
Review pertinent findings, both normal and abnormal, without making medical interpretations.	Demonstrates compliance with the patient's right to information
Offer the patient an opportunity to ask questions.	Encourages active participation in learning and decision making
Begin organizing assessment findings outside the examination room while the patient dresses or dons a bathrobe.	Ensures privacy
Help the patient leave the examination room.	Demonstrates courtesy and concern for the patient's safety
Dispose of soiled equipment, restore cleanliness and order to the examination room, and restock used supplies.	Shows consideration for the next person who uses the examination room

Evaluation

- All aspects of the assessment have been carried out.
- Comprehensive data have been collected.
- The patient remained safe, warm, and comfortable.
- The patient's questions or concerns have been addressed.

Document

- Date and time
- Normal and abnormal findings
- Any unexpected outcomes that occurred during the procedure, and the nursing actions that were taken
- To whom abnormal findings were verbally reported and outcome of the interaction

continued

SKILL 12-1

PERFORMING A PHYSICAL ASSESSMENT *Continued*

SAMPLE DOCUMENTATION

Date and Time 67-year-old man transported from bed to examination room per wheelchair for physical assessment. Able to cooperate without distress. Refer to assessment form for examination findings. ______________________________ SIGNATURE/TITLE

CRITICAL THINKING

- You have been asked to assess two new patients. One arrived by wheelchair and has been walking about the nursing unit. The other was transported by ambulance, has intravenous fluid infusing, and is receiving oxygen.
  - Which patient would you assess first? Why?
  - What differences might you use in the physical assessment of each of these two patients?

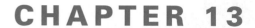

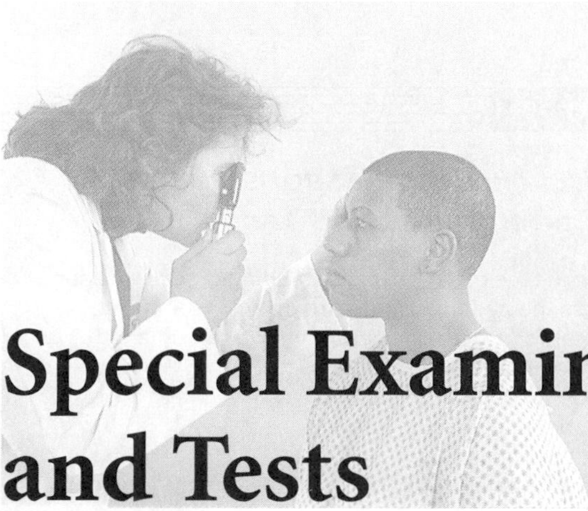

Special Examinations and Tests

CHAPTER 13

CHAPTER OUTLINE

Examinations and Tests
Common Diagnostic Examinations
Diagnostic Tests
Nursing Implications

NURSING GUIDELINES

ASSISTING WITH A PARACENTESIS
ASSISTING WITH A LUMBAR PUNCTURE
COLLECTING A SPECIMEN FOR A THROAT CULTURE

SKILLS

SKILL 13-1: ASSISTING WITH A PELVIC EXAMINATION
SKILL 13-2: ASSISTING WITH A SIGMOIDOSCOPY
SKILL 13-3: USING A GLUCOMETER

NURSING CARE PLAN

DECISIONAL CONFLICT

KEY TERMS

cold spot
computed tomography
contrast medium
culture
diagnostic examination
dorsal recumbent position
echography
electrocardiography
electroencephalography
electromyography
endoscopy
fluoroscopy
glucometer
gram staining
hot spot
knee–chest position
laboratory test
lithotomy position
lumbar puncture
magnetic resonance imaging
modified standing position
nuclear medicine department
Pap (Papanicolaou) test
paracentesis
pelvic examination
positron emission tomography
radiography
radionuclides
roentgenography
Sims' position
specimens
speculum
spinal tap
transducer
ultrasonography

LEARNING OBJECTIVES

An understanding of the content within this chapter will be evidenced by the student's ability to:

- Differentiate between an examination and a test.
- List 10 general nursing responsibilities that relate to assisting with special examinations and tests.
- Name five positions commonly used during tests or examinations.
- Explain what is involved in a pelvic examination and Pap smear.
- List six categories of tests or examinations that are commonly performed.
- Identify four word endings and their meanings that provide clues as to how tests or examinations are performed.
- Explain the following procedures: sigmoidoscopy, paracentesis, lumbar puncture, throat culture, and measurement of capillary blood glucose.
- Discuss at least three factors that are considered when examinations and tests are performed on older adults.

In addition to obtaining a health history and performing a physical assessment, the nurse gains additional assessment data by evaluating the results of special examinations and tests. This chapter gives an overview of some common diagnostic examinations and tests and the related nursing responsibilities. Tests involving the collection of urine and stool specimens are discussed in Chapters 30 and 31, respectively.

Examinations and Tests

A **diagnostic examination** (procedure that involves physical inspection of body structures and evidence of their functions) is facilitated by the use of technical equipment and techniques such as:

- Radiography (x-rays)
- Endoscopy (optical scopes)
- Radionuclide imaging (radioactive chemicals)
- Ultrasonography (high-frequency sound waves)
- Electrical graphic recordings

By learning root words and suffixes (word endings), which are primarily of Latin and Greek origin, it is possible to decipher many unfamiliar names of diagnostic examinations or tests (Table 13-1).

A **laboratory test** (procedure that involves the examination of body fluids or specimens) involves comparing the components of a collected specimen with normal findings. An examination may or may not include the collection of specimens.

GENERAL NURSING RESPONSIBILITIES

When patients undergo diagnostic examinations and tests, nurses have specific responsibilities before, during, and after the procedure (Display 13-1).

Preprocedural Care

Before a procedure begins, the nurse determines whether the patient understands the purpose of and the activities involved in the examination or test and agrees to proceed with it. Once consent is obtained, the patient is prepared, equipment and supplies are obtained, and the examination area is prepared.

DISPLAY 13–1

General Nursing Responsibilities for Examinations and Tests

- Determine the patient's understanding of the procedure.
- Witness the patient's signature on a consent form.
- Teach or follow test preparation requirements.
- Obtain equipment and supplies.
- Arrange the examination area.
- Position and drape the patient.
- Assist the examiner.
- Provide the patient with physical and emotional support.
- Care for specimens.
- Record and report appropriate information.

Clarifying Explanations

In some cases, a signed consent form is required before examinations or tests are performed. To be legally sound, consent must contain three elements: *capacity, comprehension,* and *voluntariness* (Display 13-2).

Although physicians are responsible for giving patients sufficient information to obtain their informed consent, not all patients fully understand the information. Some are too anxious to process details, others feel too insecure to ask questions, and still others express additional concerns after the physician has left. Often the nurse must repeat, simplify, clarify, or expand the original explanation.

There are no exact rules for clarifying explanations. In general, it is best to find out how much of the physician's explanation the patient understands, and to use the patient's questions as a guide for providing further information. Nurses should follow the suggestions for teaching and providing emotional support given in Chapter 8.

TABLE 13–1. **Deciphering Diagnostic Terms**

Suffix	Meaning	Examples	Description
-graphy	To record	Angiography	Test that records an image of blood vessels
-gram	An image	Angiogram	The actual image recorded during angiography
-scopy	To see	Sigmoidoscopy	Test in which the lower intestine is inspected
-scope	Examination instrument	Sigmoidoscope	A tube with a light and lens for looking within the lower intestine
-centesis	To puncture	Thoracentesis	Procedure in which a needle is used to puncture the thorax and withdraw fluid
-metry	To measure	Pelvimetry	Procedure in which the pelvis is measured
-meter	Instrument for obtaining measurements	Glucometer	Instrument for measuring glucose

DISPLAY 13–2

Elements of Informed Consent

Capacity	Indicates that the patient has the ability to make a rational decision; if not, a spouse, parent, or legal guardian must do so.
Comprehension	Indicates that the patient understands the physician's explanation of the risks, benefits, and alternatives that are available.*
Voluntariness	Indicates that the patient is acting on his or her own free will without coercion or threat of intimidation.

**Capacity and comprehension may be temporarily affected by sedative drugs or the effects of anesthesia.*

Preparing Patients

Some examinations and tests require special preparation of the patient, such as withholding food and fluids or modifying the diet. Because test preparation requirements vary from one health care agency to another, the nurse refers to written protocols in the agency's manual rather than relying on memory.

Once the specific requirements for a test are known, the nurse provides directions to the patient, nursing staff, and other hospital departments, such as the dietary department, that are affected by the test. Everyone who is involved must cooperate so that the test is conducted accurately. If the test preparations are not carried out correctly, the information is reported promptly, because the procedure may need to be canceled and rescheduled.

Because many tests and examinations are being done on an outpatient basis, the nurse must understand the patient's responsibilities and instruct him or her accordingly.

Patient Teaching Before

Special Examinations or Tests

Teach the outpatient or the family to do the following:

- Call (specify the number) if any test preparation instructions are not clearly understood or cannot be followed.
- Refrain from eating anything for at least 8 hours before a test or examination that requires a fasting state.
- Follow all dietary specifications for eating or omitting certain foods exactly as directed.
- Check with the physician about taking or readjusting the time schedule for taking prescribed medications on the day of the test or examination.
- Bathe or shower as usual on the day of the test or examination.
- Dress casually and in layers so that items of clothing can be removed or added to maintain comfort in the test environment.
- Ask a friend or family member to provide transportation to and from the site if there is a potential for drowsiness, lingering pain, or weakness after the procedure.
- Arrive at least a half hour before the test is scheduled.
- Identify yourself at the information or appointment desk when you arrive.
- Bring information to verify insurance or Medicare coverage.

Regardless of the type of examination or test, the nurse helps the patient change into an examination gown, applies an identification bracelet, takes vital signs, and suggests that he or she empties the bladder. The nurse continues to monitor the condition of waiting patients, who can experience adverse effects due to fatigue, delayed food consumption, or medical symptoms.

Obtaining Equipment and Supplies

If an examination or test is performed at the bedside or in an examination room on the nursing unit, equipment and supplies are obtained ahead of time. Nurses are relieved of this responsibility if the examination or test is carried out in other locations or when a special technician performs the procedure.

Some items the nurse needs are in prepackaged kits that are kept in a clean utility room (Fig. 13-1) or obtained from a central supply department. If packaged kits are used, the nurse checks the list of contents to determine what, if any,

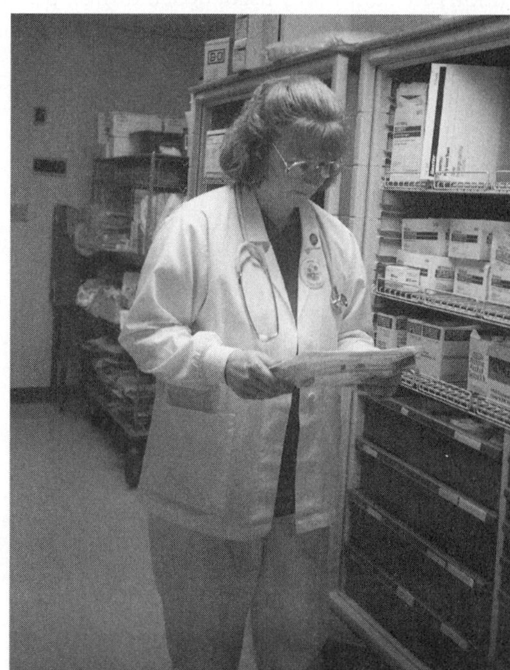

FIGURE 13–1. Obtaining equipment from the supply room. (Courtesy of Ken Timby.)

additional items are needed. Clean gloves, goggles, masks, and gowns are provided to prevent direct contact with blood or body secretions (see the section on standard precautions in Chap. 22).

ARRANGING THE EXAMINATION AREA

If the procedure is performed at the bedside, the nurse removes unnecessary articles from the area and provides privacy. Many nursing units contain an examination room that is clean, well-lighted, and stocked with frequently used equipment. The examination table is covered with sheets or paper dispensed from a roll. A lined receptacle is nearby for disposing of soiled items.

Equipment and supplies are arranged for easy access by the examiner (Fig. 13-2). Sterile items remain wrapped or covered until just before their use. Instruments that require electric power, batteries, or lights are checked before the examiner arrives so that nonfunctioning equipment can be replaced.

Procedural Responsibilities

During the examination or test, the nurse positions and drapes the patient, provides the examiner with technical assistance, and supports the patient physically and emotionally.

Positioning and Draping

Five positions are commonly used, depending on the type of examination, condition of the patient, and preference of the examiner. They include the dorsal recumbent position, Sims' or left lateral position, lithotomy position, knee–chest or genupectoral position, and modified standing position (Table 13-2).

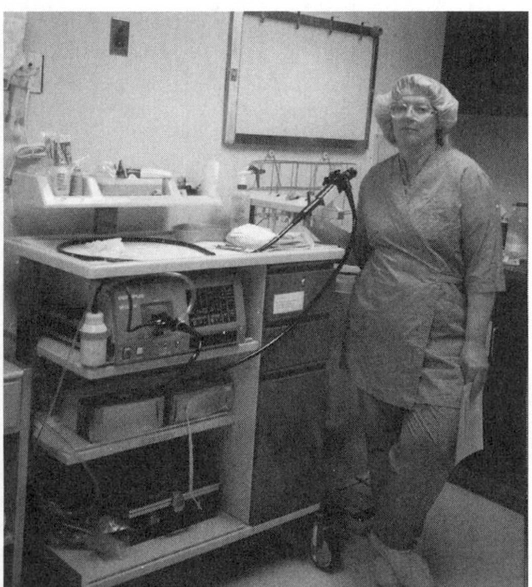

FIGURE 13–2. An endoscopic examination room. (Courtesy of Ken Timby.)

The **dorsal recumbent position** (reclining position with the knees bent, hips rotated outward, and feet flat) is commonly used for a variety of examinations. A bath blanket is used to drape the patient. A disposable pad is placed under the buttocks to absorb drainage.

The **lithotomy position** (reclining position with the feet in metal supports called *stirrups*) is used to facilitate gynecologic (female reproductive), urologic, and sometimes rectal examinations. A drape is used to cover the exposed perineum and legs.

Sims' position (position in which the patient is lying on the left side with the chest leaning forward, the right knee bent toward the head, the right arm forward, and the left arm extended behind the body) has indications similar to those for the lithotomy position. It is an alternative gynecologic or urologic position when a patient cannot abduct the hips (move the legs outward from midline) due to restricted joint movement (for instance, when the patient has arthritis). This position also provides access to the anus and rectum when the patient requires rectal administration of medication or instillation of enema solution.

The **knee–chest position** (position in which the patient rests on the knees and chest) is also called a *genupectoral position.* The head is turned to one side and is supported on a small pillow. A pillow is also placed under the chest for added comfort. The arms are above the head or bent at the elbows so they rest alongside the patient's head. A drape is placed so that the patient's back, buttocks, and thighs are covered. This is a very difficult position for most patients—especially older adults—to assume for any length of time. Therefore, the nurse should wait to position the patient in this manner until just before the examination. Some examination tables have movable sections that facilitate maintaining this position without much patient effort.

A **modified standing position** (position in which the upper half of the body is leaning forward) is used primarily when the prostate gland is examined. For comfort and safety, the draped patient stands in front of the examination table and leans forward from the waist.

Assisting the Examiner

The nurse must be familiar with the examination equipment and the order in which it is used. Instruments and equipment are placed on the side of the examiner's dominant hand, if possible. If not, the nurse anticipates what is needed during the procedure and hands one item at a time to the examiner.

If the skin and underlying tissue require local anesthesia, the nurse holds a container of the medication as the physician withdraws some of its contents (Fig. 13-3). The nurse always checks the drug name and concentration on the label

TABLE 13–2. **Indications for Common Examination Positions**

Position	Uses
A. Dorsal recumbent position 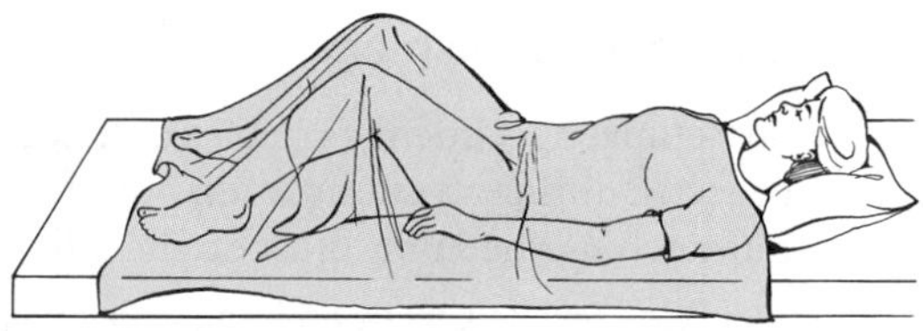	• External genitalia inspection • Vaginal examination • Rectal examination • Urinary catheter insertion
B. Lithotomy position 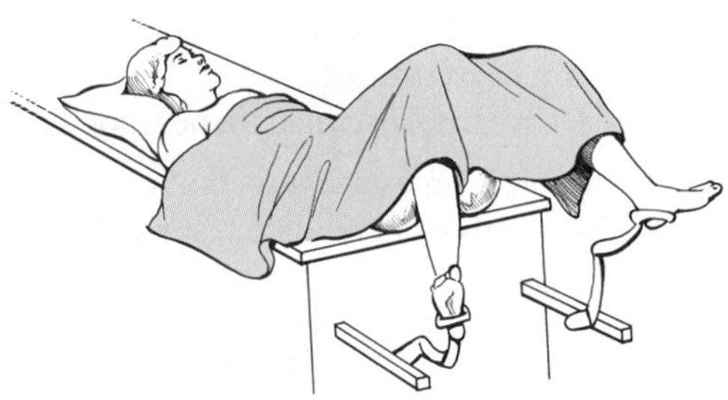	• Internal pelvic examination (female) • Obstetric delivery • Cystoscopic (bladder) examination • Rectal examination
C. Sims' position 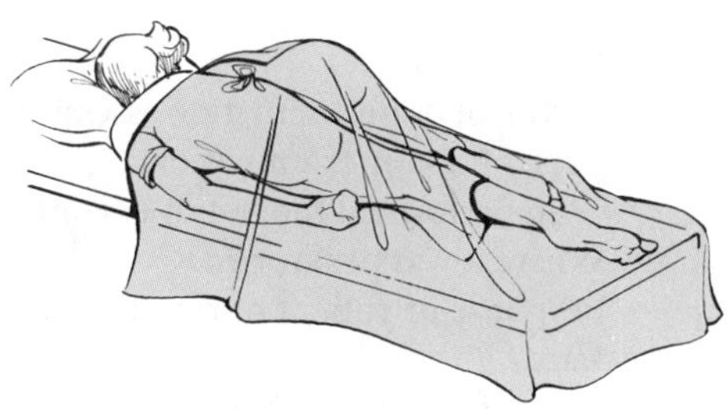	• Rectal examination • Vaginal examination • Rectal temperature assessment • Suppository insertion • Enema administration
D. Knee–chest position 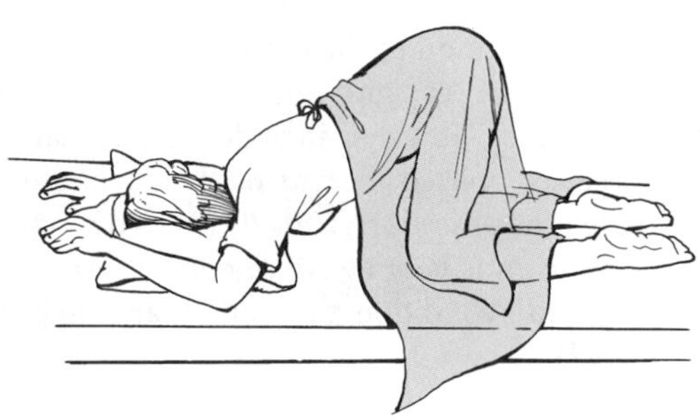	• Rectal and lower intestinal examinations • Prostate gland examination
E. Modified standing position 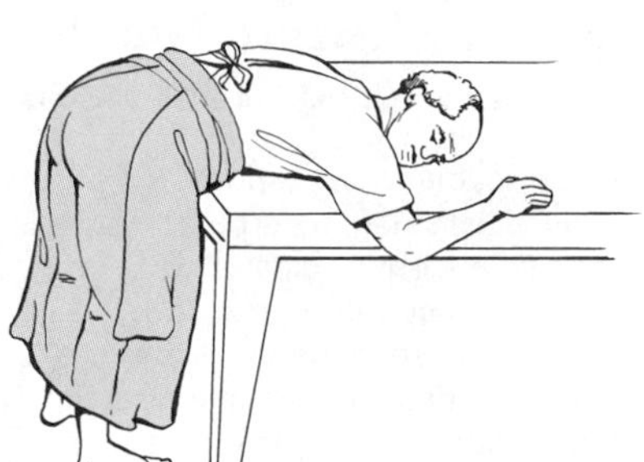	• Prostate gland examination

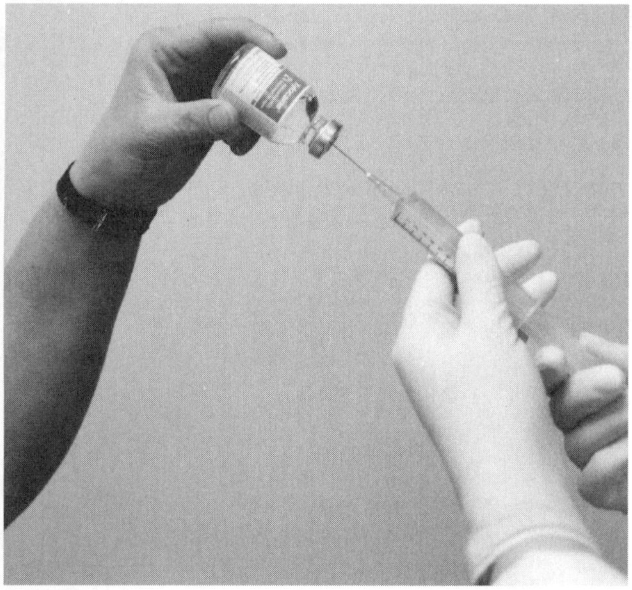

FIGURE 13–3. Holding local anesthetic with the label clearly visible to the physician. (Courtesy of Ken Timby.)

carefully. A second method for ensuring that the correct drug is used is to hold the container so that the examiner can read the label.

If the nurse is responsible for performing the test or examination, all equipment and supplies are obtained so that the patient is not left alone. If assistance or additional equipment is required, the nurse summons help with a telephone or call light within the examination room.

Providing Physical and Emotional Support

Throughout any examination or test, the nurse continuously observes the patient's physical and emotional reactions and responds accordingly. For example, comfort measures are in order if the patient is cold or in pain. Holding the patient's hand and offering words of encouragement help the patient endure temporary discomfort. The nurse's assessments of the patient are communicated to the examiner, who may shorten or modify the examination in some manner.

Postprocedural Care

After examinations and tests are completed, the nurse attends to the patient's comfort and safety, cares for specimens, and records and reports pertinent data.

Attending to the Patient

First, the patient is helped to a position of comfort. Vital signs are rechecked to verify that the patient's condition is stable. The patient is cleaned of any substances that caused soiling. Hospitalized patients are offered a clean gown; outpatients are directed to dress in their own clothing. When it is safe to do so, patients are escorted to their rooms or to the discharge area, and instructions for follow-up care are provided.

Caring for Specimens

Sometimes **specimens** (samples of tissue or body fluids) are collected during an examination or test. To ensure their accurate analysis, the nurse must do the following:

- Collect the specimen in an appropriate container.
- Label the specimen container with correct information.
- Attach the proper laboratory request form.
- Ensure that the specimen does not decompose before it can be examined.
- Deliver the specimen to the laboratory as soon as possible.

Display 13-3 lists factors that often interfere with accurate examinations or invalidate test results.

Recording and Reporting Data

Certain information needs to be documented whenever a patient undergoes a special examination or test. General information includes the following:

- Date and time
- Pertinent pre-examination assessments and preparation
- Type of test or examination
- Who performed the test or examination
- Where it was performed
- Response of patient during the examination and afterward
- Type of specimen obtained, if any
- Appearance, size, or volume of specimen
- Where the specimen was taken.

In addition to the written account of the examination, the nurse reports significant information to other nursing team members. This may include the fact that the examination has been completed, the patient's reactions during and immediately after the procedure, and any delayed reactions. When the nursing team is kept aware of current events and changes in the patient's condition, the plan of care can be revised and kept up to date.

DISPLAY 13–3

Common Factors That Invalidate Examination or Test Results

- Incorrect diet preparation
- Failure to remain fasting
- Insufficient bowel cleansing
- Drug interactions
- Inadequate specimen volume
- Failure to deliver specimen in a timely manner
- Incorrect or missing test requisition

Common Diagnostic Examinations

Many types of diagnostic examinations are commonly performed to assess and evaluate patients. Some of the more common are discussed in this section. Additional information can be found in laboratory and test manuals and courses in which specific diseases are studied; beginning nurses will also gain experiences with these examinations in the clinical setting.

PELVIC EXAMINATION

A **pelvic examination** (physical inspection of the vagina and cervix, with palpation of the uterus and ovaries) is usually performed by a physician, a physician's assistant, or a nurse practitioner. A specimen of cervical secretions is often collected for a **Pap (Papanicolaou) test** (screening test that detects abnormal cervical cells, the status of reproductive hormone activity, or the presence of normal or infectious microorganisms within the uterus or vagina; Table 13-3).

The American College of Obstetricians and Gynecologists (1995) recommends that women receive their first Pap test at age 18 or sooner if they are sexually active. Thereafter, the test should be performed every year for 3 years, and then every 3 years if the three previous Pap tests were normal—or at the discretion of the physician. Women in high-risk categories, such as those who are HIV-positive, those with sexually transmitted diseases, or those whose mothers took diethylstilbestrol (DES) during pregnancy require yearly screening.

TABLE 13–3. **Pap Test Results**

Test Component	Interpretation
Cellular Examination	
Class I	Negative; no abnormal cells
Class II	Unusual, but not cancerous
Class III	Suggestive of cancer, but not definite
Class IV	Strongly suggestive of cancer
Class V	Definitely cancerous
Hormonal Effects (on a 6-point scale)	
1	Marked estrogen effect
2	Moderate estrogen effect
3	Slight estrogen effect
4	Absent estrogen effect
5	Compatible with pregnancy
6	Too bloody, inflamed, or scanty to analyze
Identifiable Microorganisms (on a 5-point scale)	
1	Normal microorganisms
2	Scanty or absent microorganisms
3	*Trichomonas vaginalis* (protozoan organism)
4	*Candida* (yeastlike fungus)
5	Other or mixed collection of microorganisms

(Adapted from Fischbach F. A manual of laboratory and diagnostic tests, 5th ed. Philadelphia: Lippincott, 1996.)

Related Nursing Responsibilities

Skill 13-1 identifies the nursing responsibilities involved in assisting with a pelvic examination and collecting cervical secretions for a Pap test.

RADIOGRAPHY

Radiography or **roentgenography** (general term for procedures that use roentgen rays, or x-rays) produces images of body structures. The actual film image is technically called a *roentgenogram,* but it is commonly known as an x-ray. Roentgen rays produce electromagnetic energy that passes through body structures, leaving an image of dense tissue on special film. Table 13-4 lists common radiographic examinations and the indications for their use.

X-rays cannot be seen or felt, but the energy is absorbed by cells. Repeated exposure to x-rays, even at small doses, or a single exposure to a high dose causes cell damage that can

TABLE 13–4. **Common Radiographic Examinations**

Examination	Examples of Indications for Use
Chest x-ray (anterior, posterior, lateral views)	Detects pneumonia, broken ribs, lung tumors
Upper gastrointestinal x-ray (upper GI or barium swallow)	Aids in diagnosis of ulcers, gastrointestinal tumors, narrowing of the esophagus
Lower gastrointestinal x-ray (lower GI or barium enema)	Helps in diagnosis of polyps or tumors of the bowel, intestinal obstruction, and structural changes within the intestine
Cholecystography (x-ray of the gallbladder and ducts)	Facilitates determining the presence of gallstones and obstruction in the flow of bile
Intravenous pyelography (IVP)	Helps identify urinary malformations, tumors, stones, cysts, and obstructions in the kidneys and ureters
Retrograde pyelography	Same as for IVP, but the contrast medium is instilled through a urinary catheter
Angiography (x-ray of blood vessels)	Determines the location where and the extent to which blood vessels have narrowed, or evaluates improvement after treatment
Myelography (x-ray of spinal canal)	Detects spinal tumors, ruptured intervertebral disks, and bony changes in the vertebrae

lead to cancerous cell changes. Consequently, there is a tendency to be cautious about the number of x-ray studies that are taken. X-ray studies should not be taken during pregnancy if at all possible, because a developing fetus is at greater risk for cellular damage from x-rays.

Magnetic resonance imaging (MRI; technique for producing an image by using atoms subjected to a strong electromagnetic field) is a diagnostic alternative that does not involve exposure to the type of radiation produced with roentgenography (Fig. 13-4). However, because metal devices on or within the body are affected, patients with metal implants, pacemakers, or staples cannot undergo this type of diagnostic imaging.

Contrast Medium

A **contrast medium** (substance that adds density to a body organ or cavity, such as barium sulfate or iodine) makes hollow body areas appear more distinct when imaged on x-ray film. Some people are sensitive to substances used in contrast media and have an immediate allergic reaction to them.

Contrast media are administered orally or rectally or injected. **Fluoroscopy** (form of radiography in which an image is displayed in real time) is used to observe the movement of contrast media—for example, as it is being swallowed or injected.

Computed tomography (CT scan; form of roentgenography that shows planes of tissue) and some other types of x-ray examinations use contrast media. The CT contrast medium makes it possible to identify differences in tissue density when x-ray images are obtained from various angles and levels in the body (Fig. 13-5).

Related Nursing Responsibilities

For the patient undergoing radiographic examination, nursing responsibilities include the following:

- Assess vital signs before the examination to provide a baseline and to help detect changes in the patient's condition during or after the procedure.
- Remove any metal items, such as a religious medal, or clothing that contains metal, such as the hooks and eyes on a bra. Metal produces a dense image that may be confused with a tissue abnormality.
- Request a lead apron or collar to shield a fetus or vulnerable parts of the body during x-rays (Fig. 13-6).
- If the radiographic study involves administration of a contrast medium, ask the patient about allergies, especially to seafood or iodine, or previous adverse reactions during a diagnostic examination. A reaction can range from mild nausea and vomiting to shock and death.
- Know where emergency equipment and drugs are located in case there is an unexpected allergic reaction to contrast medium.
- To avoid interference with subsequent visual imaging, schedule procedures requiring iodine before those that use barium.

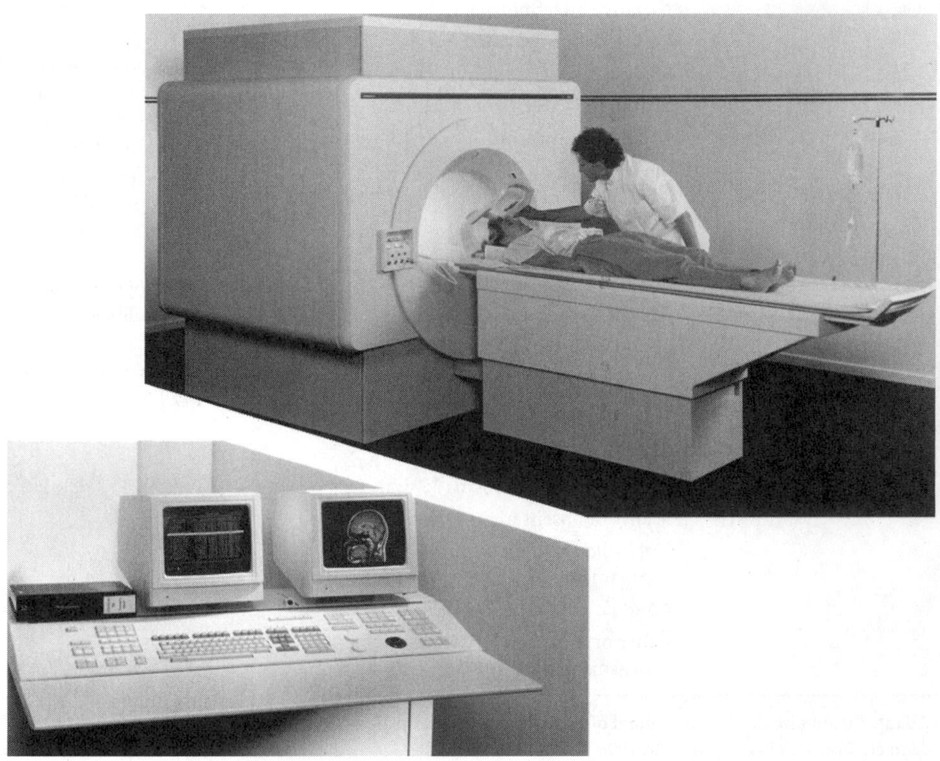

FIGURE 13–4. Magnetic resonance imaging. (Courtesy of Kalamazoo Neuro-Imaging Center, Inc., Kalamazoo, MI.)

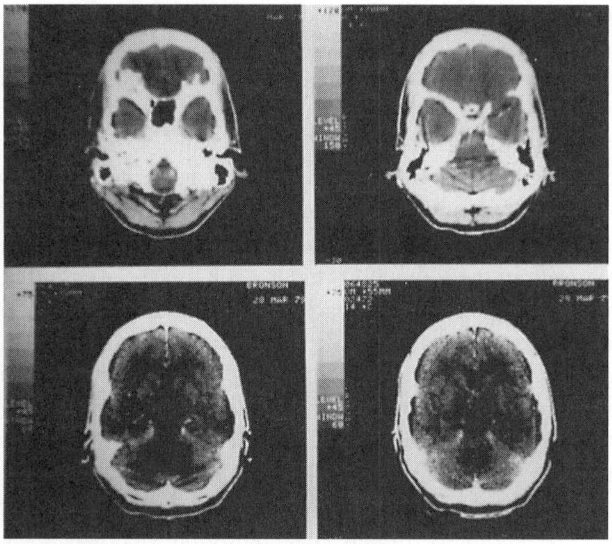

FIGURE 13–5. Cross-sections of cranial CT scan. (Courtesy of Ken Timby.)

- To promote urinary excretion, encourage the patient to drink a large amount of fluid after an examination involving iodine.
- Check on bowel elimination and stool characteristics for at least 2 days after barium contrast medium is administered. Barium retention can lead to constipation and bowel obstruction. Report absence of bowel elimination beyond 2 days. Administration of a prescribed laxative is often necessary.

ENDOSCOPIC EXAMINATIONS

Endoscopy (visual examination of internal structures) is performed using optical scopes. Endoscopes have a lighted

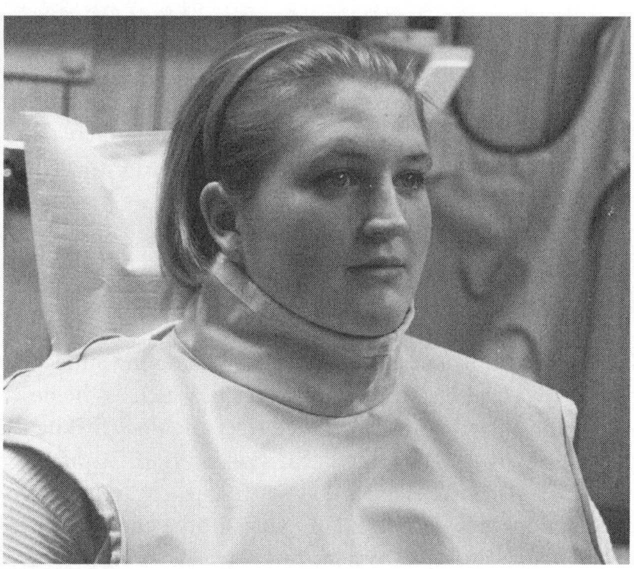

FIGURE 13–6. Lead thyroid collar and apron. (Courtesy of Ken Timby.)

mirror-lens system attached to a tube and are quite flexible so they can be advanced through curved structures.

Endoscopic examinations are named primarily for the structure that is being examined (Display 13-4). In addition to allowing the examiner to inspect the appearance of a structure, endoscopes also have attachments that permit various forms of treatment or the collection of specimens for microscopic analysis. Endoscopic examinations that produce discomfort or anxiety are performed under a light, short-acting form of anesthesia sometimes referred to as *conscious sedation.*

Endoscopic examinations are being performed more and more on an outpatient basis and in the physician's office. They are an economical alternative to invasive tests and procedures that previously required surgery.

Related Nursing Responsibilities

For the patient undergoing endoscopy, nursing responsibilities include the following:

- To prevent aspiration, withhold food and fluids for at least 6 hours before any procedure in which an endoscope is inserted into the upper airway or upper gastrointestinal tract.
- If conscious sedation is used, monitor the patient's vital signs, breathing, oxygen saturation (using pulse oximetry; see Chap. 20), and cardiac rhythm. Have oxygen and resuscitation equipment readily available.
- If topical anesthesia is used to facilitate the passage of an endoscope into the airway or upper gastrointestinal tract, withhold food or fluids for at least 2 hours after the procedure and until swallow, cough, and gag reflexes are present.
- Relieve a sore throat with ice chips, fluids, or gargles when it is safe to do so.
- Confirm that bowel preparation using laxatives and enemas has been completed before endoscopic procedures of the lower intestine.
- Report difficulty in arousing a patient or the presence of sharp pain, fever, unusual bleeding, nausea, vomiting,

DISPLAY 13–4

Examples of Endoscopic Examinations

- *Bronchoscopy*—inspection of the bronchi
- *Gastroscopy*—inspection of the stomach
- *Colonoscopy*—inspection of the colon
- *Esophagogastroduodenoscopy* (EGD)—inspection of the esophagus, stomach, and duodenum
- *Laparoscopy*—inspection of the abdominal cavity
- *Cystoscopy*—inspection of the urinary bladder

or difficulty with urination after any endoscopic examination.
- Skill 13-2 describes the nurse's role when assisting with a sigmoidoscopy.

RADIONUCLIDE IMAGING

Radionuclides (elements whose molecular structures are altered to produce radiation) are identified by a number followed by the chemical symbol, such as ^{131}I (radioactive iodine) and ^{99}Tc (radioactive technetium). When radionuclides are instilled in the body, usually by the intravenous route, they are absorbed by particular tissues or organs. With the use of a scanning device that detects radiation, an image of the size, shape, and concentration of the radionuclide is obtained. The terms **hot spot** (area where the radionuclide is intensely concentrated) and **cold spot** (area with little if any radionuclide concentration) refer to the amount of tissue absorption. **Positron emission tomography** (PET) combines the technology of radionuclide scanning with the layered analysis of tomography.

Radionuclide imaging offers two advantages over standard radiography: it visualizes areas within organs and tissue that are not possible with standard x-rays, and it involves less exposure to radiation than with roentgenography. However, tests using radionuclides are contraindicated for women who are pregnant or breast-feeding: the energy that is released is harmful to the rapidly growing cells of an infant or fetus.

Related Nursing Responsibilities

For the patient undergoing radionuclide imaging, nursing responsibilities include the following:

- If the patient is a woman, ask about her menstrual and obstetric history. Notify the **nuclear medicine department** (unit responsible for radionuclide imaging) if the patient is pregnant or breast-feeding.
- Ask about the allergy history, because iodine is commonly used in radionuclide examinations.
- Assist the patient to put on a gown, robe, and slippers. Make sure the patient has no internal metal devices or external metal objects, because these interfere with the diagnostic findings.
- Obtain an accurate weight, because the dose of radionuclide is calculated according to weight.
- Inform the patient that he or she will be radioactive for a brief period (usually less than 24 hours), but body fluids, such as urine, stool, and emesis, can be safely flushed away.
- Instruct premenopausal women to use effective birth control for the short period during which radiation continues to be present.

ULTRASONOGRAPHY

Ultrasonography (soft tissue examination that uses sound waves in ranges beyond human hearing) is also known as **echography**. During ultrasonography, which is similar to the echo location used by bats and dolphins and sonar devices on submarines, sound is projected through the body's surface from a hand-held probe called a **transducer.** The sound waves cause vibrations within body tissues, and images are produced as the waves are reflected back toward the machine. The reflected sound waves are converted into a visual image called an *ultrasonogram, sonogram,* or *echogram,* which can be viewed in real time on a monitor and recorded for future analysis. Doppler ultrasound, discussed in Chapters 11 and 12, is a variation of this type of technology.

Ultrasound examinations are used to visualize breast, abdominal, and pelvic organs; male reproductive organs; structures in the head and neck; the heart and valves; and the structures within the eyes. Air-filled structures, such as the lung or intestine, and extremely dense tissue, such as bones, do not image well. This type of examination is used in obstetrics to determine fetal size, the presence of more than one fetus, and the location of the placenta. The gender of the fetus can sometimes be determined by the outline of fetal anatomy in the late stages of pregnancy. Because ultrasound examinations do not involve radiation or contrast media, they are an extremely safe diagnostic tool.

Related Nursing Responsibilities

For the patient undergoing ultrasonography, nursing responsibilities include the following:

- Schedule abdominal and pelvic ultrasonography before any examinations that use barium for best visualization.
- Instruct patients undergoing abdominal ultrasonography to drink five to six full glasses of fluid approximately 1 to 2 hours before the test. They should not urinate until after the test is completed to ensure a full bladder.
- Explain that acoustic gel is applied over the area where the transducer is placed.

ELECTRICAL GRAPHIC RECORDINGS

Diagnostic information is obtained by using machines that record electrical impulses from structures such as the heart, brain, and skeletal muscles. These tests are identified by the prefix "electro-," as in **electrocardiography** (ECG or EKG; examination of the electrical activity in the heart), **electroencephalography** (EEG; examination of the energy emitted by the brain), and **electromyography** (EMG; examination of the energy produced by stimulated muscles).

To detect the electrical activity, wires called *electrodes* are attached to the skin (or muscle in the case of an EMG). They transmit the electrical activity to a machine that converts it into a series of waveforms (Fig. 13-7). Except for an awareness of the presence of the electrodes, the patient undergoing an ECG or EEG usually does not experience any other sensations. Occasionally there is slight discomfort during an EMG.

Related Nursing Responsibilities

For the patient undergoing an ECG, nursing responsibilities include the following:

- Attach the adhesive tabs to the skin where the electrode wires will be fastened. Clip hair in the area to reduce discomfort when the patches are removed.
- Avoid attaching the adhesive tabs over bones, scars, or breast tissue.

For the patient undergoing an ECG, nursing responsibilities include the following:

- Instruct the patient to shampoo the hair the evening before the procedure to facilitate firm attachment of the electrodes. The hair is shampooed after the test to remove adhesive from the scalp.
- Withhold coffee, tea, and cola beverages for 8 hours before the procedure. Consult with the physician about withholding scheduled medications, especially those that affect neurologic activity.

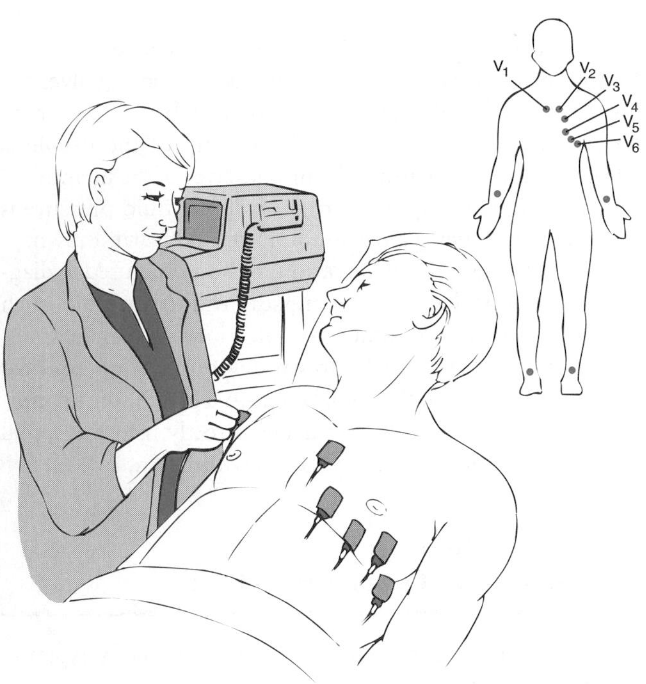

FIGURE 13–7. The nurse attaches electrodes to the patient's chest and limbs prior to an ECG.

- If a sleep-deprived EEG is scheduled, instruct the patient that he or she must stay awake after midnight before the examination.

For the patient undergoing an ECG, nursing responsibilities include the following:

- Tell the patient he or she will be instructed to contract and relax certain muscles during the examination.
- Explain that electrical current is applied to muscles during an EMG, but the sensation is not usually painful. Also, a muscle electrode is inserted with a small-gauge needle in 10 or more locations, but the experience is painless unless it touches a terminal nerve in the area.

Diagnostic Tests

Specimens, such as blood, urine, stool, sputum, intestinal secretions, spinal fluid, and drainage from wounds or infected tissue, are collected by nurses, laboratory personnel, and physicians. Tests on collected specimens are repeated at intervals to monitor the progress of patients. Students should refer to laboratory manuals to learn the purpose of specific tests and the nursing responsibilities that are involved.

Several examples of specimen collection are discussed in future chapters, where they are more pertinent. Nursing responsibilities for assisting with a paracentesis and a lumbar puncture, collecting a specimen for a throat culture, and measuring capillary blood glucose follow.

ASSISTING WITH A PARACENTESIS

A **paracentesis** (procedure for withdrawing fluid from the abdominal cavity) is always performed by a physician, with the assistance of a nurse. A paracentesis is most commonly done to relieve abdominal pressure and improve breathing, which generally becomes labored when fluid crowds the lungs. Sometimes 1 quart or more of fluid is removed. A specimen of the fluid may be sent to the laboratory for microscopic examination.

Nursing Guidelines For
Assisting with a Paracentesis

☑ Explain the procedure or clarify the physician's explanation to the patient.
RATIONALE: Prepares the patient for an unfamiliar experience, or promotes a clearer understanding.

☑ Ensure that the consent form has been signed, if needed.
RATIONALE: Provides legal protection.

☑ Measure and record the patient's weight, blood pressure, and respiratory rate, and measure the abdominal girth at its widest point with a tape measure.
RATIONALE: Serves as a basis for postprocedural comparisons.

☑ Obtain a prepackaged paracentesis kit, along with a vial of local anesthetic.
RATIONALE: Promotes efficient time management.

☑ Make sure that extra gloves, gown, mask, and goggles are available.
RATIONALE: Offers protection from contact with microorganisms, such as HIV, that may be present in blood or other body fluids.

☑ Encourage the patient to empty the bladder just before the procedure.
RATIONALE: Prevents accidental puncture of the bladder.

☑ Place the patient in a sitting position.
RATIONALE: Pools abdominal fluid in the lower areas of the abdomen and displaces the intestines posteriorly.

☑ Hold the container of local anesthetic so the physician can withdraw a sufficient amount.
RATIONALE: Prevents contaminating the physician's sterile gloves.

☑ Offer patient support as an area of the abdomen is anesthetized and then pierced with an instrument called a *trocar* and a hollow sheath called a *cannula* is inserted (Fig. 13-8).
RATIONALE: Relieves anxiety through empathetic concern.

☑ Reassess the patient periodically after cannula insertion; expect that the blood pressure and respiratory rate may decrease.
RATIONALE: Indicates the response of the patient.

☑ Place a Band-Aid or small dressing over the puncture site after the cannula is withdrawn.
RATIONALE: Acts as a barrier to microorganisms and absorbs drainage.

☑ Assist the patient to a position of comfort.
RATIONALE: Demonstrates concern for the patient's welfare.

☑ Measure the volume of fluid withdrawn.
RATIONALE: Contributes to accurate assessment of fluid volume.

☑ Label the specimen, if ordered, and send it to the laboratory with the appropriate requisition form.
RATIONALE: Facilitates appropriate analysis.

☑ Document pertinent information, such as the appearance and volume of the fluid, patient assessments, and disposition of the specimen.
RATIONALE: Adds essential data to the patient's medical record.

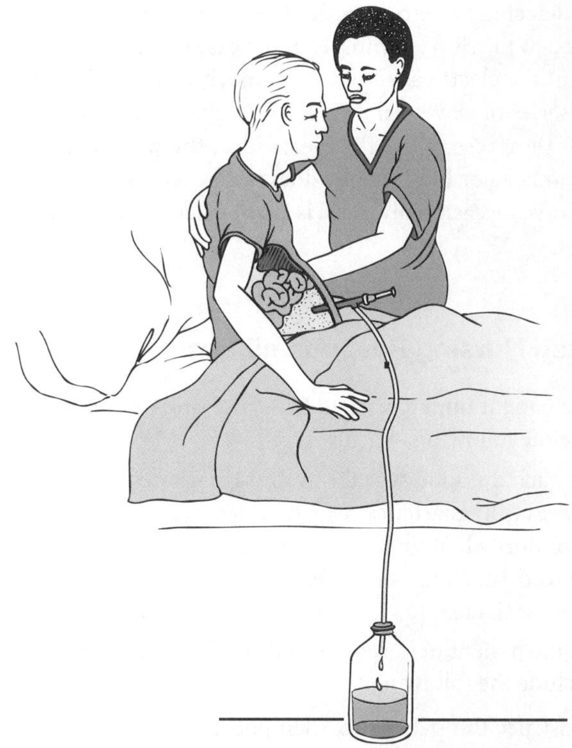

FIGURE 13–8. The nurse offers support during an abdominal paracentesis.

ASSISTING WITH A LUMBAR PUNCTURE

The physician requires nursing assistance when performing a **lumbar puncture** or **spinal tap** (procedure that involves the insertion of a needle between lumbar vertebrae in the spine but below the spinal cord itself). The tip of the needle is advanced until it is beneath the middle layer of the membrane that surrounds the spinal cord. The spinal fluid pressure is measured, and then a small amount of fluid is withdrawn.

This test is performed for various reasons. It is used to diagnose conditions that raise the pressure within the brain, such as brain or spinal cord tumors, or infections such as meningitis. Spinal fluid also is withdrawn before instilling contrast medium for x-rays of the spinal column. Finally, some conditions are treated by instilling drugs directly into the spinal fluid after a similar amount has been withdrawn.

Nursing Guidelines For
Assisting with a Lumbar Puncture

☑ Explain the procedure or clarify the physician's explanation to the patient.
RATIONALE: Prepares the patient for an unfamiliar experience, or promotes a clearer understanding.

☑ Ensure that the consent form has been signed, if needed.
RATIONALE: Provides legal protection.

☑ Perform a basic neurologic examination, including pupil size and response and muscle strength and sensation in all four extremities.
RATIONALE: Provides a baseline for future comparisons.

☑ Encourage the patient to empty the bladder.
RATIONALE: Promotes comfort during the procedure.

☑ Administer a sedative drug if ordered.
RATIONALE: Reduces anxiety.

☑ Obtain a prepackaged lumbar puncture kit, along with a vial of local anesthetic.
RATIONALE: Promotes efficient time management.

☑ Make sure that extra gloves, gown, mask, and goggles are available.
RATIONALE: Offers protection from contact with microorganisms, such as HIV, that may be present in blood or other body fluids.

☑ Place the patient on his or her side with the knees and neck acutely flexed (Fig. 13-9). or in a sitting position, bent from the hips.
RATIONALE: Separates the bony vertebrae.

☑ Instruct the patient that once the needle has been inserted, movement must be avoided.
RATIONALE: Prevents injury.

☑ Hold the container of local anesthetic so the physician can withdraw a sufficient amount.
RATIONALE: Prevents contaminating the physician's sterile gloves.

☑ Stabilize the patient's position at the neck and knees.
RATIONALE: Reinforces the need to remain motionless.

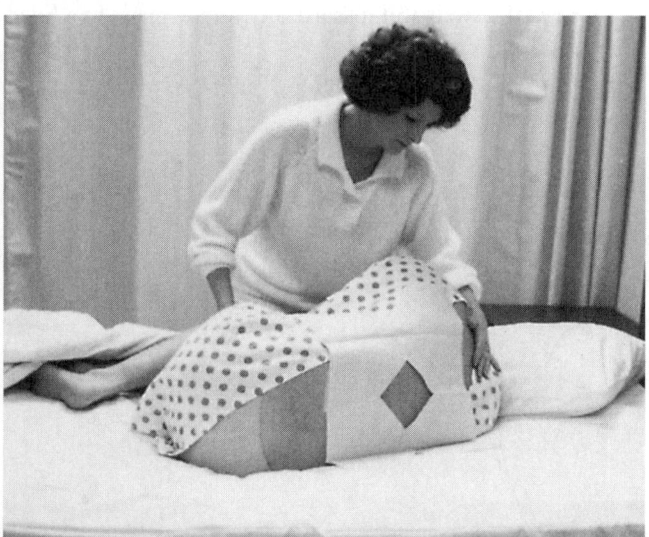

FIGURE 13–9. Positioning for lumbar puncture. (Courtesy of Ken Timby.)

☑ Support the patient emotionally as the skin is injected with local anesthesia and the needle is inserted.
RATIONALE: Relieves anxiety through empathetic concern.

☑ Tell the patient that it is not unusual to feel pressure or a shooting pain down the leg.
RATIONALE: Prepares the patient for expected sensations.

☑ Perform *Queckenstedt's test,* if asked, by compressing each jugular vein separately for approximately 10 seconds while the pressure is being measured.
RATIONALE: Indicates that an obstruction in spinal fluid is present if the pressure remains unchanged, rises slightly, or takes longer than 20 seconds to return to baseline.

☑ Observe that the physician fills three separate numbered containers with 5 to 10 mL in their appropriate sequence if laboratory analysis is desired.
RATIONALE: Suggests that if blood is present but in decreasing amounts in the third container, its source is most likely the trauma of the procedure rather than central nervous system pathology.

☑ Place a Band-Aid or small dressing over the puncture site after the needle has been withdrawn.
RATIONALE: Acts as a barrier to microorganisms and absorbs drainage.

☑ Position the patient flat on the back or abdomen; instruct the patient to remain flat and roll from side to side for the next 6 to 12 hours.
RATIONALE: Reduces the potential for a severe headache.

☑ Reassess the patient's neurologic status like before the procedure. Check the puncture site for bleeding or clear drainage.
RATIONALE: Provides comparative data for evaluating changes in the patient's condition.

☑ Offer oral fluids frequently.
RATIONALE: Helps in restoring the volume of spinal fluid.

☑ Label the specimens, if ordered, and send them to the laboratory with the appropriate requisition form.
RATIONALE: Facilitates appropriate analysis.

☑ Document pertinent information, such as the appearance of the fluid, patient assessments, and disposition of the specimen.
RATIONALE: Adds essential data to the patient's medical record.

COLLECTING A SPECIMEN FOR A THROAT CULTURE

A **culture** (incubation of microorganisms) is performed by collecting body fluid or substance suspected of containing infectious microorganisms, growing the living microorganisms in a nutritive substance, and examining their characteristics with a microscope. Cultures are commonly performed on urine, blood, stool, wound drainage, and throat secretions.

To identify and treat the cause of a throat infection (commonly a streptococcal bacteria), the nurse obtains a specimen from the throat. An abbreviated test that takes approximately 10 minutes is performed on throat specimens in many doctors' offices or student health clinics. A rapid preliminary diagnosis is made so that appropriate treatment can be initiated immediately. If the quick test is negative, a follow-up specimen is obtained and sent to the laboratory for culturing. Conclusive results of a bacterial culture generally requires 24 to 72 hours for sufficient microbial growth to take place.

Once bacteria grow within the nutritive medium, they are identified microscopically by their shape and by the color they acquire when stained with special dyes. **Gram staining** (process of adding a dye to a microscopic specimen) is named for the Danish physician who developed the technique. The gram stain helps determine whether a bacteria is gram-positive or gram-negative. *Gram-positive bacteria* appear violet after staining. Those that repel the violet dye but appear red, the color of a counterstain, are called *gram-negative bacteria* (Fischbach, 1996). Streptococci are round, grow in chains, and are gram-positive.

Once the presence of a microorganism is determined and it is identified, the most appropriate treatment can be provided. A throat culture is most often performed on young children, who are susceptible to complications from upper respiratory infections and infection of the tonsils. However, adults who tend to harbor infectious microorganisms in their pharynx are also tested. A culture may be repeated after a course of treatment to determine its effectiveness.

Nursing Guidelines For

Collecting a Specimen for a Throat Culture

☑ Check with the physician about proceeding with the throat culture if the patient is taking antibiotic drugs.
RATIONALE: Antibiotics affect the results of the test.

☑ Delay collecting a specimen if an antiseptic gargle has recently been used.
RATIONALE: Affects the diagnostic value of the test.

☑ Explain the purpose of and technique for obtaining the culture.
RATIONALE: Reduces anxiety and promotes cooperation.

☑ Collect supplies: sterile culture swab, glass slide, tongue blade, gloves, mask if the patient is coughing, paper tissues, and an emesis basin if the patient gags.
RATIONALE: Facilitates organization and efficient time management.

☑ Have the patient sit where there is optimum light.
RATIONALE: Enhances inspection of the throat anatomy.

☑ Don gloves and a mask, if necessary.
RATIONALE: Reduces the potential for transferring microorganisms.

☑ Loosen the cap on the tube in which the swab is located.
RATIONALE: Facilitates hand dexterity.

☑ Tell the patient to open the mouth wide, stick out the tongue, and tilt the head back.
RATIONALE: Promotes access to the back of the throat.

☑ Depress the middle of the tongue with a tongue blade in your nondominant hand (Fig. 13-10).
RATIONALE: Opens the pathway for the swab.

☑ Rub and twist the tip of the swab about the tonsil areas and the back of the throat without touching the lips, teeth, or tongue.
RATIONALE: Transfers microorganisms from the inflamed tissue to the swab.

☑ Be prepared for gagging.
RATIONALE: Stroking the back of the throat stimulates the gag reflex.

☑ Remove the swab and discard the tongue blade in a lined receptacle.
RATIONALE: Controls the spread of microorganisms.

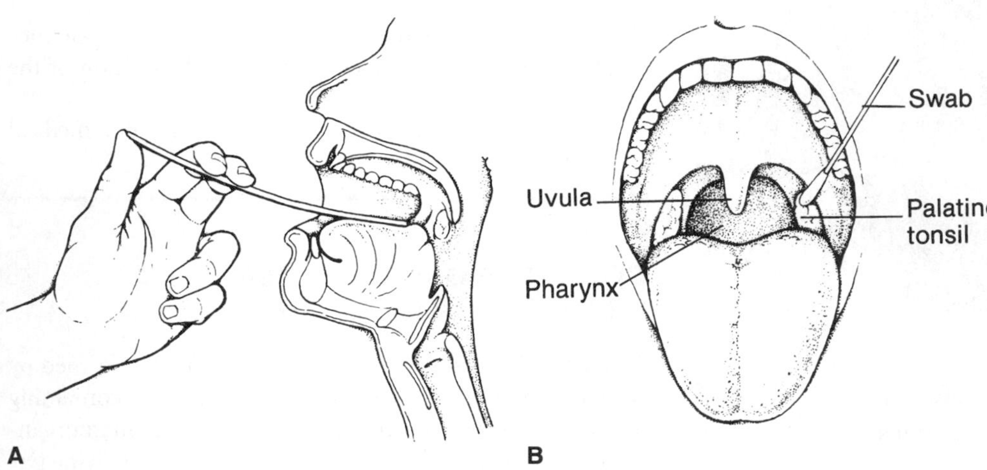

FIGURE 13–10. Throat culture. (*A*) Depressing the tongue. (*B*) Obtaining a specimen.

☑ Spread the secretions on the swab across the glass slide.
RATIONALE: Prepares a specimen for quick staining and microscopic examination.

☑ Replace the swab securely within the tube, taking care not to touch the outside of the container.
RATIONALE: Avoids collecting unrelated microorganisms and provides containment for the collected specimen.

☑ Crush the packet in the bottom of the tube.
RATIONALE: Releases nourishing fluid to promote growth of bacteria.

☑ Remove gloves, discard them in a lined receptacle, and wash your hands.
RATIONALE: Reduces the transmission of microorganisms.

☑ Label the culture tube with the patient's name, the date and time, and the source of the specimen.
RATIONALE: Provides laboratory personnel with essential information.

☑ Attend to staining and examination of the prepared glass slide, if appropriate.
RATIONALE: Provides tentative identification of streptococcal bacteria.

☑ Deliver the sealed culture tube to the laboratory, or refrigerate it if there will be a delay of longer than 1 hour.
RATIONALE: Ensures that the microorganisms will grow when transferred to other culture media.

MEASURING CAPILLARY BLOOD GLUCOSE

Glucose is the type of sugar present in blood as a result of eating carbohydrates. A certain amount is always present to keep cells supplied with a source of instant energy. The amount of blood sugar in a nonfasting state is generally 80 to 120 mg/dl (milligrams per deciliter). Normal blood levels are maintained by the body's production of glucagon and insulin, hormones that regulate glucose metabolism.

Persons with diabetes have an impaired ability to produce insulin and have difficulty regulating blood sugar levels. They control their disease with diet, exercise, and in some cases medications. Persons with diabetes may experience low or high blood sugar levels, both of which can have life-threatening consequences. Therefore, many diabetics measure their own capillary blood sugar levels rather than having venous blood drawn for laboratory analysis.

A **glucometer** (instrument that measures the amount of glucose in capillary blood) operates by assessing the amount of light that is reflected through a chemical test strip (Fig. 13-11). Based on the amount of measured sugar in the blood, diabetic patients adjust their intake of food or medication.

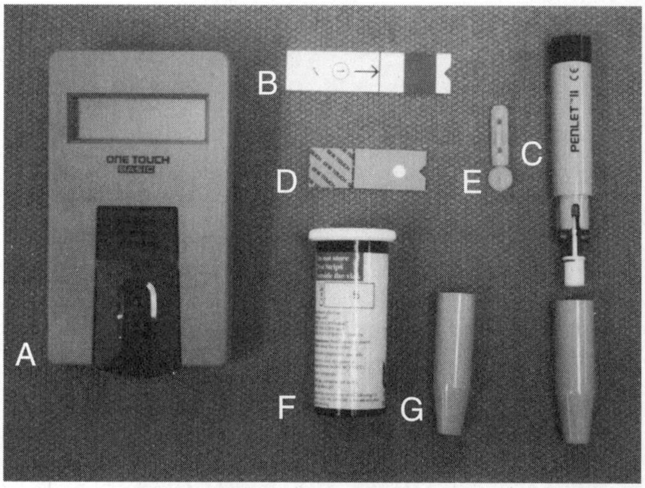

FIGURE 13–11. Equipment used to perform capillary blood glucose testing: (*A*) glucometer and test strip holder, (*B*) check strip, (*C*) lancet holder, (*D*) test strip, (*E*) lancet, (*F*) container of test strips, and (*G*) lancet cover. (Courtesy of Ken Timby.)

Because diabetes is such a common disorder, nurses are frequently called on to teach newly diagnosed diabetic patients how to test their own blood sugar levels. Nurses measure blood sugar levels for diabetic patients who are hospitalized or are being cared for in long-term care institutions.

There are several important points to remember about measuring blood glucose:

1. Several types of glucometers are available, and the manufacturer's instructions must be followed for accurate use.
2. The blood sugar is usually measured about a half-hour before eating and before bedtime to determine what are likely to be the lowest levels of glucose. This allows time for increasing or decreasing the consumption of food or administering additional prescribed insulin (see Chap. 34), referred to as *coverage.*
3. Measuring blood glucose involves a risk for contact with blood. Because blood may contain infectious viruses, gloves are *always* worn when performing this test. Researchers are working on developing noninvasive devices that will not require piercing the skin with a lancet, but such devices are not available at present.

Skill 13-3 presents the steps involved in using a One Touch glucometer.

Nursing Implications

Most patients who undergo special examinations and tests have emotional needs from the stress of a potential diagnosis or the anxiety created by undergoing something unfamiliar.

The following are some nursing diagnoses that may be identified during pre- and postprocedural stages of examinations and tests:

- Anxiety
- Fear
- Impaired adjustment
- Decisional conflict
- Health-seeking behavior
- Powerlessness
- Spiritual distress

The accompanying nursing care plan illustrates the nursing process as it relates to the nursing diagnosis of Decisional conflict, defined in the NANDA taxonomy (1999) as "the state of uncertainty about the course of action to be taken when choice among competing actions involves risk, loss, or challenge to personal life values."

Nursing Care Plan

Decisional Conflict

Assessment

Subjective Data

States, "I don't know what to do now that the amniocentesis shows that my baby will have cystic fibrosis. I know I can have an abortion, but I'm not sure I want to do that. I remember what it was like when my brother who had cystic fibrosis was always sick and then died. Why did this have to happen to me? I don't feel that any decision is possible right now."

Objective Data

28-year-old married woman who is 20 weeks pregnant. Date of last menstrual period: 7/2. Fetal heart rate is 140 in left lower quadrant. Says she has felt fetal movement. Had a younger brother who died at age 5 from cystic fibrosis. Sits with rigid posture almost immobile except wringing hands. Very little eye contact during interaction.

Diagnosis

Decisional Conflict related to birthing options of fetus with genetic disorder detected by amniocentesis.

Plan

Goal

The patient will make an informed choice concerning the outcome of the current pregnancy by the return office visit on 11/10.

Orders: 11/5

1. Ask to compose a written list of advantages and disadvantages to possible choices before return appointment on 11/10.
2. Encourage to discuss options with husband and other significant persons.
3. Offer referrals to the Cystic Fibrosis Foundation, pro-choice and right-to-life groups.
4. Support patient's decision even if it is contrary to one's personal choice.

F. BROWN, RN

Implementation (Documentation)

11/5 1415 Shared that this decision is difficult—other women dealing with these same circumstances have felt similarly. Reinforced that the choice is hers to make and also confident that she can make the one that is best for her. Asked to list any and all advantages and disadvantages in writing to help clarify options. Offered referral to supportive agencies. Asked for and was given the phone number of the Cystic Fibrosis Foundation. Encouraged to come with husband for sharing questions and concerns.

F. BROWN, RN

Evaluation (Documentation)

11/10 1300 Returned for office conference with husband. Contacted Cystic Fibrosis Foundation and attended a support group of parents. List of advantages and disadvantages completed by both patient and husband. Stated, "The treatment of cystic fibrosis seems to have improved in the 20 years since my brother died. We talked it over and even if we had a normal baby, there's the risk it would die while we are alive. The people at the CF meeting made us feel like we're not alone." Scheduled next prenatal visit for 12/15

F. BROWN, RN

FOCUS ON OLDER ADULTS

- Values for laboratory test results are often determined by using averaged statistics from younger adult age groups. Therefore, unless age-specific norms are available, results for older adults are subject to misinterpretation.
- When interpreting blood test results, the medications the older adult takes are reviewed and evaluated as to their potential effects on laboratory values.
- Knowing the usual range of laboratory results for older adults who have chronic conditions is important. The disorder or its treatment can cause abnormal test findings that may be considered normal or acceptable for the older adult.
- Older adults, especially those who are medically frail, may not be able to tolerate the withholding of food or fluids for long periods before tests or examinations. Assessing urinary output, blood pressure, and mental status provides data on how well an older adult is tolerating a fasting state.
- When older adults must abstain from food or fluid before a test or examination, administration of their prescribed medications with a small amount of water may be allowed, based on consultation with the physician.
- Older adults are more susceptible to dehydration. The resulting concentration of blood can cause false elevations of laboratory blood tests.
- Some older adults become exhausted by preparations for gastrointestinal examinations that require the use of laxatives and enemas.
- Providing a bedside commode and hands-on assistance is helpful for older adults, especially those with impaired mobility, when they are undergoing preparation for gastrointestinal examinations.
- A bed alarm that sounds when a patient gets out of bed or a chair is a safety measure for older adults who require assistance with toileting but are unreliable in requesting help.
- Because frail older adults fatigue easily, tests and examinations are coordinated with diagnostic personnel to eliminate long periods of fasting or waiting in uncomfortable environments.
- Older adults are likely to need additional clothing, slippers, and extra covers to keep them warm in waiting rooms and examination areas.
- After a diagnostic examination, older adults are offered food and fluid and a period of rest before resuming physically taxing activities.
- When working with an older adult who is cognitively compromised (e.g., dementia), a family member or responsible caregiver is instructed about test preparations. The caregiver or family member is included in the procedure as much as possible.

KEY CONCEPTS

- An examination is a procedure that involves the physical inspection of body structures and evidence of their functions. A test involves the examination of body fluids or specimens.
- Whenever patients undergo special examinations and tests, the nurse is generally responsible for determining the patient's understanding of the procedure, checking that the consent form is signed, following test preparation requirements or teaching outpatients how to prepare themselves, obtaining equipment and supplies, arranging the examination area, positioning and draping patients, assisting the examiner, providing patients with physical and emotional support, caring for specimens, and recording and reporting significant information.
- There are five common examination positions: dorsal recumbent, Sims', lithotomy, knee–chest, and modified standing.
- A pelvic examination involves the inspection and palpation of the vagina and adjacent organs. This examination often includes the collection of secretions for a Pap test to identify the presence of abnormal cells, levels of hormone activity, or identity of infectious microorganisms.
- Tests and examinations commonly involve the use of x-rays, endoscopes, radioactive substances, sound waves, and electrical activity.
- When determining how particular tests are performed, it is helpful to understand four word endings: *-graphy,* as in angiography, means to record an image; *-scopy,* as in bronchoscopy, means to look through a lensed instrument; *-centesis,* as in amniocentesis, means to puncture; and *-metry,* as in pelvimetry, means to measure with an instrument.
- Nurses are often called on to assist with sigmoidoscopy (inspecting the rectum and sigmoid section of the lower intestine with an endoscope), paracentesis (puncturing the skin and withdrawing fluid from the abdominal cavity), and lumbar puncture (inserting a needle between lumbar vertebrae in the spine but below the spinal cord itself), to collect a throat culture specimen, and to measure capillary blood glucose levels using a glucometer.
- When the patient undergoing special examinations and tests is an older adult, the nurse faces special challenges, such as preventing fatigue and dehydration, maintaining or adjusting current drug therapy, and avoiding misinterpretation of laboratory test results that are based on norms for younger adults.

CRITICAL THINKING EXERCISES

- Discuss how the procedure for a sigmoidoscopy or another test or examination may differ if it is performed on an outpatient basis rather than when the patient is an inpatient.
- How might diminished mentation (capacity to understand), reduced strength and stamina, and pain affect the performance of a diagnostic examination or test?

SUGGESTED READINGS

American College of Obstetricians and Gynecologists. Recommendations on frequency of Pap test screening, No. 152. Washington DC, ACOG, March 1995.

Butler RN. Type 2 diabetes: patient education and home blood glucose monitoring. Geriatrics 1998;53(5):60–67.

Clark BA. A new approach to assessment and documentation of conscious sedation during endoscopic examinations. Gastroenterology Nursing 1998;21(1):59–63.

Colodny CS. Procedures for your practice. Paracentesis and peritoneal lavage. Patient Care 1995;29(13):137–145.
Dumesic DA. Pelvic examination: what to focus on in menopausal women. Consultant 1996;36(1):39–46.
Fatchett J II. Basic abdominal sonography: procedural overview. Journal of Diagnostic Medical Sonography 1997;13(5):24S–28S.
Fischbach F. A manual of laboratory & diagnostic tests, 5th ed. Philadelphia: Lippincott, 1996.
Franges EZ. Lumbar punctures: helping a "sticky" procedure go smoothly. Nursing 1996;26(3):48–50.
Higgins C. Screening for cervical cancer. Nursing Times 1997;93(20):50–51.
Hill JM, Newton JL. Contrast echo: your role at the bedside. RN 1998;61(10): 32–36.
Klonoff DC. Noninvasive blood glucose monitoring. Diabetes Care 1997; 20(3): 433–437.
Kumar D. PET scanning. American Journal of Nursing 1998;98(7):16G–16H.
Leino-Kilpi H, Nyrhinen T, Katajisto J. Patients' rights in laboratory examinations: do they realize? Nursing Ethics 1997;4(6):451–464.
Lederman RJ. Geriatrics advisor. Lumbar puncture: essential steps to a safe and valid procedure. Geriatrics 1996;51(6):51–58.
McCarthy V. Patient education review. The first pelvic examination. Journal of Pediatric Health Care 1997;11(5):247–249.
Muram D, Aiken MM, Strong C. Children's refusal of gynecologic examinations for suspected child abuse. Journal of Clinical Ethics 1997;8(2):158–164.
North American Nursing Diagnosis Association. NANDA nursing diagnoses: definitions and classification, 1999–2000. Philadelphia, NANDA, 1999.
Panting A. Preparing patients for endoscopy. Nursing Times 1998;94(27):60.
Patient guide: what to expect with flexible sigmoidoscopy. Hospital Medicine 1995;31(8):39–40.
Strimke CL. Test your ECG monitoring IQ. Nursing 1997;27(6):32cc6–32cc9.
Wright DL. Improving the geriatric radiography experience. Seminars in Radiologic Technology 1998;6(2):46–77.

SKILL 13-1

ASSISTING WITH A PELVIC EXAMINATION

Suggested Action	Reason for Action
Assessment	
Determine the identity of the patient on whom the examination will be performed.	Prevents errors
Determine whether a Pap test is needed.	Indicates the need for additional equipment and supplies
Find out whether the patient has had a pelvic examination before.	Provides a basis for teaching
Ask whether the patient is currently menstruating or had intercourse within the last 48 hours.	Interferes with microscopic examination of collected specimens. Blood, mucus, and pus are three substances that obscure and distort cells, making it difficult to determine whether they are atypical. The examiner may wish to delay obtaining a specimen.
Inquire whether the patient has douched in the last 24 hours.	Suggests a need to reschedule the Pap smear, because an adequate sample of cells and secretions may not be available.
Ask the patient's age, the date of the last menstrual period, the number of pregnancies and live births, and a description of symptoms, such as bleeding or drainage, itching, or pain.	Provides data to determine the possibility of pregnancy, to compare cellular specimens with hormonal activity, and to provide clues as to possible pathology and the need for additional tests
Determine whether and what type of birth control is being used, if the patient is premenopausal. For oral contraceptives, identify the name of the drug and dosage.	Correlates the influence of prescribed hormones on cellular specimens
Ask menopausal women if they are taking estrogen replacement, including the brand name and dosage.	Correlates the influence of prescribed hormones on cellular specimens
Observe for impaired strength or joint limitation.	Suggests the need to modify the examination position
Planning	
Explain the procedure and give the patient an opportunity to ask questions.	Tends to reduce anxiety
Provide an examination gown and direct the patient to empty her bladder.	Facilitates palpation of the uterus and ovaries

continued

SKILL 13-1

ASSISTING WITH A PELVIC EXAMINATION *Continued*

Suggested Action	Reason for Action
Place a **speculum** (a metal or a disposable plastic instrument for widening the vagina; see Fig. A), gloves, examination light, lubricant, and the following materials for the Pap smear: long soft applicators and spatula (see Fig. B) and at least three glass slides, a chemical fixative, and a container for holding the slides, on the counter or on a tray in the examination room.	Promotes efficient time management. Metal specula (plural of speculum) are reused after sterilization. Select an appropriate size according to the individual patient.

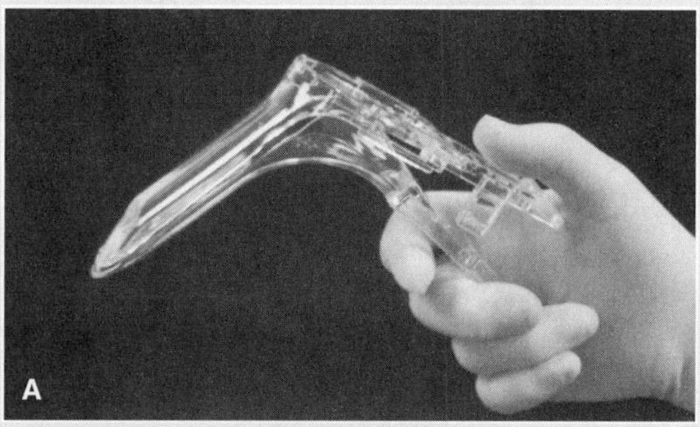

Vaginal speculum. (Courtesy of Ken Timby)

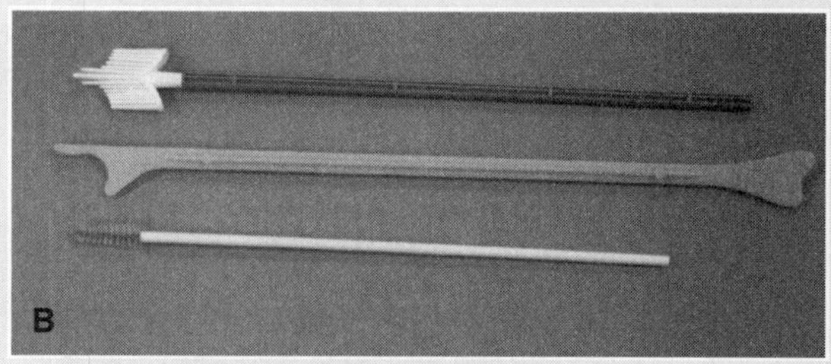

Applicators and spatula for obtaining cervical and vaginal specimens. (Courtesy of Ken Timby)

Suggested Action	Reason for Action
(A new technique of specimen preservation, approved by the Food and Drug Administration, eliminates using slides; instead, it involves rinsing the collection tool within a liquid transport medium.)	
Mark one slide with an E for endocervical, another with a C for cervical, and the last with a V for vaginal.	Identifies the location from which the specimens are taken; *endocervical* means inside the cervix. The cervix is the lower portion of the uterus, or womb.
Arrange for a female nurse to be with the patient during the examination, especially if the examiner is a man.	Reduces the potential for claims of sexual impropriety
Plan to assist with the collection of the vaginal and cervical secretions for the Pap test before the examiner proceeds to palpate the internal organs.	Prevents lubricant used during palpation from interfering with microscopic examination of the specimens
Implementation	
Place the patient in a lithotomy position; use an alternative position, such as Sims' or dorsal recumbent, if the patient is disabled.	Provides access to the vagina
Cover the patient with a cotton or paper drape.	Maintains modesty and privacy
Introduce the examiner to the patient if the two are strangers.	Tends to reduce anxiety
Fold back the drape just before the examination begins.	Exposes the genitalia while minimizing patient exposure
Direct the examination light from behind the examiner's shoulder toward the vaginal opening.	Illuminates the area, facilitating inspection

continued

SKILL 13-1

ASSISTING WITH A PELVIC EXAMINATION *Continued*

Suggested Action	Reason for Action
Wet the speculum with warm water; if a Pap smear will not be obtained, apply water-soluble lubricant to the speculum blades.	Eases insertion and provides comfort during insertion
Prepare the patient to expect the momentary insertion of the speculum. Explain that a loud click will be heard as it is locked in place.	Tends to reduce anxiety and aids in relaxation
Hand the examiner a soft-tipped applicator, spatula, and brush applicator in that order.	Facilitates collection of secretions for the Pap smear
Hold the slide marked E so the examiner can roll or slide the specimen across the slide; follow a similar pattern as the second and third samples are collected from the cervix and vagina (see Fig. C).	Deposits intact cells and secretions according to their source; excessive manipulation of the cells while being obtained or applied to the slide can make normal cells look like atypical cells.

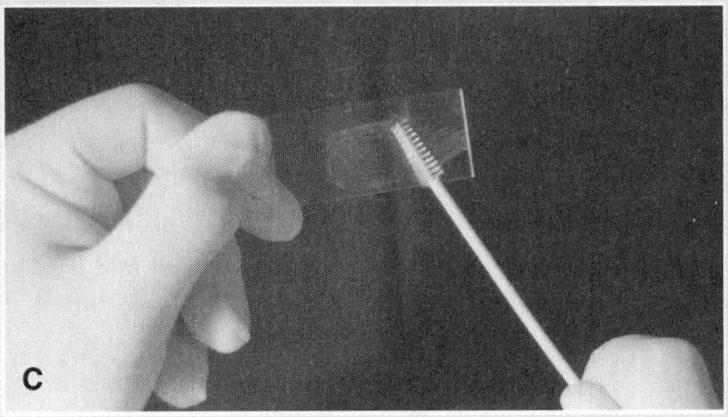

Transferring secretions to a glass slide. (Courtesy of Ken Timby)

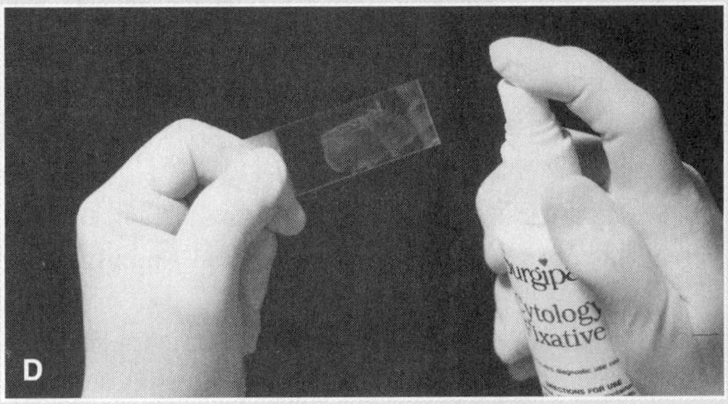

Preserving specimen. (Courtesy of Ken Timby)

Suggested Action	Reason for Action
Position the lined receptacle so the examiner can dispose of the collection device and the speculum after use.	Controls the spread of microorganisms
Place each slide in a chemical fixative solution or spray it with a similar chemical (see Fig. D).	Preserves the integrity of the specimens; delay in applying a fixative leads to air drying, enlargement of cells, and loss of details in the nucleus; making it difficult to determine whether the cells are atypical.
If using the new preservation technique, immerse the sampling device in the container of solution, cap it, and discard the tool.	Disperses the cells and breaks up blood, mucus, and nondiagnostic debris
Lubricate the gloved fingers of the examiner's dominant hand and prepare the patient for an internal examination of the vagina (and in some cases the rectum as well).	Reduces friction; keeps the patient informed of the progress of the examination
Don gloves and clean the skin of lubricant when the examination is completed; then remove the gloves.	Prevents the transmission of microorganisms; promotes comfort and hygiene
Wash hands.	Reduces the number of microorganisms on the hands
Lower both feet simultaneously from the stirrups, and assist the patient to sit up.	Reduces strain on abdominal and back muscles
Assist the patient from the room after she has dressed.	Maintains patient safety

continued

SKILL 13-1

ASSISTING WITH A PELVIC EXAMINATION *Continued*

Evaluation

- Patient demonstrated understanding of the purpose for the examination.
- Patient assumed and was maintained in a satisfactory position for examination.
- Patient privacy, comfort, and safety were maintained.
- Specimens were collected, identified, and preserved.

Document

- Date and time
- Pertinent preassessment data, if any
- Type of examination, including any specimens collected
- Examiner and/or location
- Condition of the patient afterward
- Disposition of specimens

SAMPLE DOCUMENTATION

Date and Time Taken to examination room by wheelchair for pelvic examination by Dr. Wood. Able to assume lithotomy position without difficulty. Smears of endocervical, cervical, and vaginal specimens obtained and sent to lab. Returned to room by wheelchair and assisted into bed. ______________________ SIGNATURE, TITLE

CRITICAL THINKING

- How might the pelvic examination be different if the person being examined is a rape victim or a child who has been sexually abused?
- Discuss factors during a pelvic examination and collection of a specimen that can lead to an inaccurate interpretation of the Pap test findings.
- Discuss reasons why many women ignore regular, routine pelvic examinations and Pap tests, despite the fact that they are the best methods for detection, treatment, and cure of early reproductive cancer.
- What are some strategies nurses can use to promote regular, routine pelvic examinations?

SKILL 13-2

ASSISTING WITH A SIGMOIDOSCOPY

Suggested Action	Reason for Action
Assessment	
Identify the patient on whom the examination will be performed.	Prevents errors
Check for a signed consent form.	Provides legal protection
Ask the patient to describe the procedure.	Indicates the accuracy of the patient's understanding and provides an opportunity to clarify the explanation

continued

SKILL 13-2

ASSISTING WITH A SIGMOIDOSCOPY *Continued*

Suggested Action	Reason for Action
Inquire about the patient's current symptoms and family history of significant diseases.	Provides information about the purpose for performing the procedure and an opportunity for reinforcing the need for future regular sigmoidoscopic examinations
Ask for a description of the patient's dietary and fluid intake and bowel cleansing protocol and results.	Indicates whether the patient complied with proper preparation for the procedure
Assess the patient's vital signs and obtain other physical assessments according to agency policy, such as weight or bowel sounds.	Provides a baseline for future comparisons
Ask for an allergy history and a list of medications being taken.	Influences drugs that may be prescribed and alerts staff to other medical problems
Planning	
Direct the patient to undress, don an examination gown, and use the restroom.	Facilitates the examination and gives the patient an opportunity to empty the bowel and bladder again
Prepare for the examination by placing a sigmoidoscope, gloves, gown, mask, goggles, lubricant, suction machine, and containers for biopsied tissue in the examination room.	Promotes efficient time management

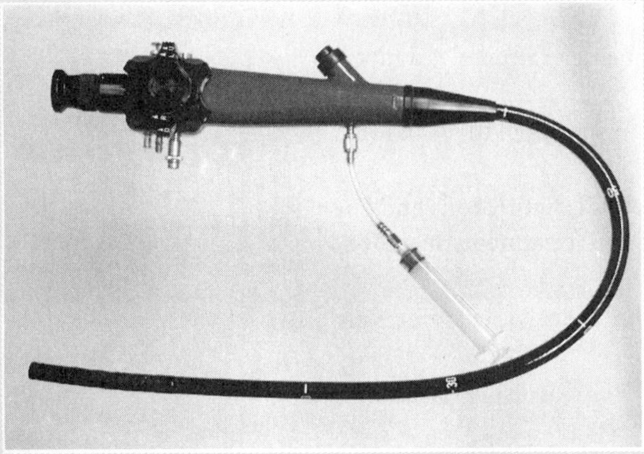

Flexible sigmoidoscope. (Courtesy of Ken Timby.)

Suggested Action	Reason for Action
Check that the light at the end of the sigmoidoscope and the suction equipment are operational	Avoids delay, inconvenience, and discomfort once the examination is in progress
Implementation	
Help the patient to assume a Sims' position, if a flexible sigmoidoscope will be used, or a knee–chest position, if a rigid sigmoidoscope is used.	Facilitates passage of the scope; an endoscopic table may be used in lieu of a self-maintained knee–chest position
Cover the patient with a cotton or paper drape.	Maintains modesty and privacy
Introduce the examiner to the patient if the two are strangers.	Tends to reduce anxiety
Lubricate the examiner's gloved fingers.	Reduces discomfort when the fingers are used to dilate the anal and rectal sphincters.

continued

SKILL 13–2

ASSISTING WITH A SIGMOIDOSCOPY *Continued*

Suggested Action	Reason for Action
Prepare the patient for the introduction of the examiner's fingers, followed by the insertion of the sigmoidoscope.	Tends to reduce anxiety by keeping the patient informed of each step and the progress that is being made
Acknowledge any discomfort that the patient may be experiencing and explain that the discomfort should be short-lived.	Indicates that the nurse empathizes with the patient's distress
Inform the patient if, and before, suction is used, air is introduced, or a sample of tissue is obtained.	Prepares the patient for unexpected sensations or temporary increase in discomfort
Open specimen container, cover the specimen with preservative, and recap the container.	Prevents loss and decomposition of the specimen
Inform the patient when the scope will be withdrawn.	Keeps the patient informed of progress
Don gloves and clean the skin of lubricant and stool after the examination is completed; then remove the gloves.	Prevents the transmission of microorganisms; promotes comfort and hygiene
Wash hands.	Reduces the number of microorganisms
Assist the patient from the room to an area where his or her clothing is located, or provide a clean gown.	Maintains patient safety and dignity
Explain that there may be slight abdominal discomfort until the instilled air has been expelled and that some rectal bleeding may be observed if a biopsy was taken.	Provides anticipatory health teaching
Stress that if severe pain occurs or bleeding is excessive, the physician should be notified.	Identifies significant data to be reported
Advise that food and fluids may be consumed as desired.	Clarifies dietary guidelines
Clean the sigmoidoscope and any other soiled equipment according to agency and infection control guidelines.	Prevents the transmission of microorganisms
Restore order and cleanliness to the examination room; restock supplies.	Prepares the room for future use
Complete laboratory requisition form, label specimen, and take both to the lab for analysis.	Facilitates microscopic examination

Evaluation

- Patient demonstrated understanding of the purpose for the examination.
- Appropriate dietary and bowel preparations were carried out.
- Patient assumed required position.
- Comfort and safety were maintained.
- Postprocedural instructions were given.
- Specimen was preserved, identified, and delivered appropriately.

Document

- Date and time
- Pertinent preassessment data, if any
- Type of examination and specimens collected, if any
- Examiner and/or location
- Condition of the patient afterward
- Instructions provided
- Disposition of specimen

continued

SKILL 13-2

ASSISTING WITH A SIGMOIDOSCOPY *Continued*

SAMPLE DOCUMENTATION

Date and Time Arrived ambulatory for routine sigmoidoscopic examination. No current symptoms, no known allergies. Takes Tenormin for hypertension. Last dose was @0700. BP 142/90 in right arm while sitting. T 98.2 P 90. R 22. Bowel sounds active in all four quadrants. Has eaten lightly this morning and self-administered two enemas last night with good results and one this morning with very little stool expelled. Placed in Sims' position for examination. Biopsy omitted. Instructed to resume eating and taking fluid as desired. Explained that gas pains are possible and that walking about will help, but to notify Dr. Ross if the discomfort is prolonged or severe. Discharged ambulatory accompanied by wife.

________________________ SIGNATURE, TITLE

CRITICAL THINKING

- Identify one reason why it is important for individuals to have an initial sigmoidoscopy after the age of 50 and every 3 to 5 years thereafter.
- How can nurses promote routine cancer screening procedures?

SKILL 13-3

USING A GLUCOMETER

Suggested Action	Reason for Action
Assessment	
Identify the patient on whom the examination will be performed.	Prevents errors
Find out whether the patient has ever had the blood sugar measured with a glucometer, or whether the patient has any questions.	Provides a basis for teaching
Review the previous blood sugar measurements and the trends that may be obvious.	Helps evaluate the reliability of the assessed measurement when it is obtained
Check to see whether insulin coverage has been ordered if the glucose levels are higher than normal.	Aids in quickly reducing high levels of blood glucose
Verify that the glucometer has been checked with a control strip within the last 24 hours.	Confirms that the machine is operating properly
Check the date on the container of test strips; discard if the date has expired.	Determines if the test strips are still appropriate for use. Discard unused test strips stored in a vial 4 months after they are opened.
Observe the code number on the container of test strips and compare it with the code number programmed into the glucometer (see Fig. A).	Ensures accuracy. Code numbers range from 1 to 16; if the numbers do not match, the meter number is changed.
Inspect the patient's fingers and thumb for a nontraumatized area; also inspect the earlobes, an acceptable alternative.	Avoids secondary trauma

continued

SKILL 13-3

USING A GLUCOMETER *Continued*

Suggested Action	Reason for Action
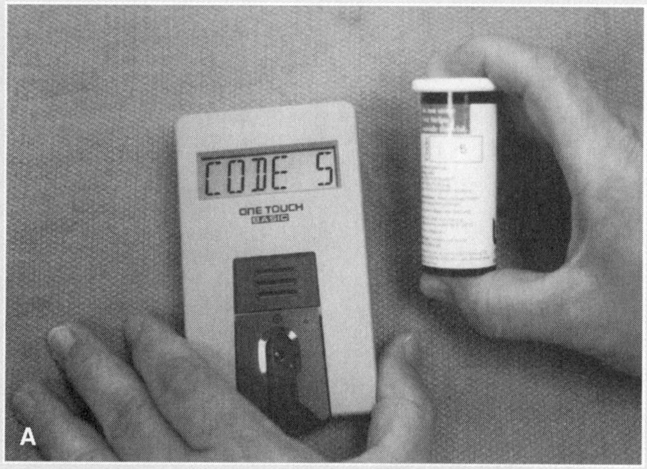	**Comparing code number on test strip bottle to glucometer code number. (Courtesy of Ken Timby.)**
Planning	
Test the machine's calibration with a control strip or solution supplied by the manufacturer, if it has not been done in 24 hours.	Verifies the machine's accuracy
Arrange care so that the test is performed about a half-hour before a meal and at bedtime.	Ensures consistency in obtaining data and facilitates detection of trends
Collect the necessary equipment and supplies: glucometer, lancets, lancet holder, test strips, and gloves.	Promotes efficient time management
Implementation	
Have the patient wash the hands with soap and warm water and towel dry.	Reduces the number of microorganisms on the skin; warmth dilates the capillaries and increases blood flow. Swabbing with alcohol is not necessary and can alter the results if not totally evaporated.
Turn on the machine; observe the last blood glucose reading, current test strip code, and the message "Insert strip."	Prepares the machine for testing the blood sample. The machine retains the last glucose measurement in its memory.
Place the notched end of one test strip into the holder with the test spot up (see Fig. B).	Locates the strip in position for the application of blood
Assemble the lancet within the spring-loaded lancet holder, and twist to remove the lancet cover.	Loads and holds the lancet in place
Place the cap of the holder over the lancet and pull the barrel until it clicks (see Fig. C).	Covers the sharp tip of the lancet; cocks the holder for a rapid thrust into the skin
Don clean gloves after washing your hands.	Provides a barrier against contact with blood
Select a nontraumatized side of a finger or thumb, avoiding the central pads (see Fig. D).	Avoids puncturing an area where there are sensitive nerve endings
Apply the cap covering the lancet firmly to the side of the finger and press the release button.	Thrusts the lancet into the skin
Release lancet and holder.	Opens a path for blood

continued

SKILL 13-3

USING A GLUCOMETER *Continued*

Suggested Action	Reason for Action

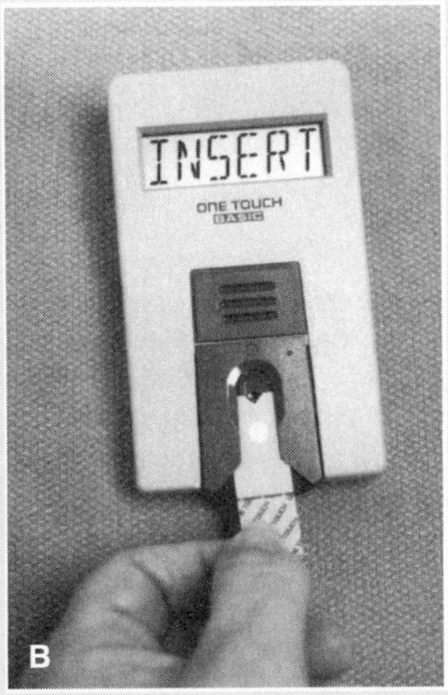

Insertion of test strip. (Courtesy of Ken Timby.)

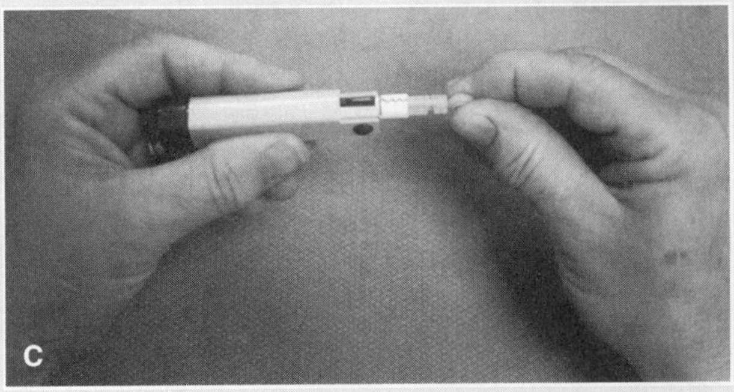

Lancet insertion. (Courtesy of Ken Timby.)

Suggested Action	Reason for Action
Hold the finger or thumb so that a large hanging drop of blood forms.	Uses gravity to aid in collecting blood
Touch the hanging drop of blood to the test spot on the strip, making sure that the spot is completely covered and stays wet during the test (see Fig. E).	Saturates the test spot to ensure accurate test results
Listen for the meter to beep, followed by series of beeps 45 seconds later.	Activates the timing mechanism

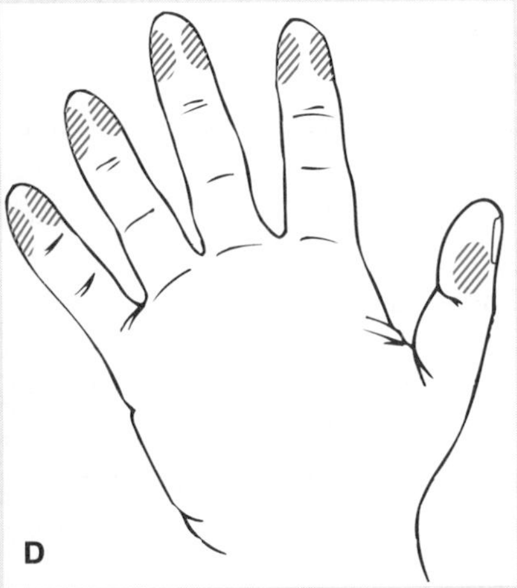

Appropriate puncture sites.

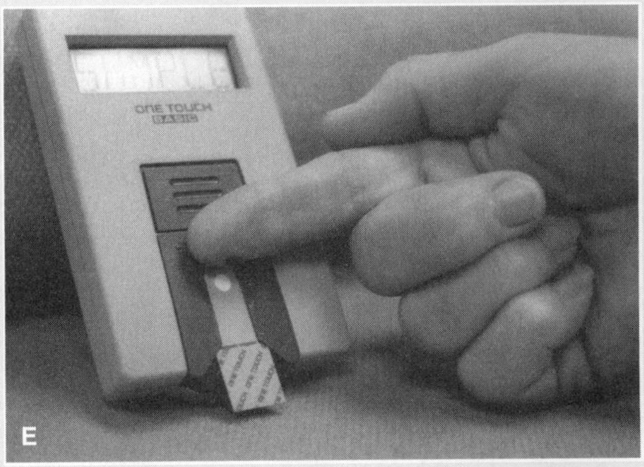

One large drop of blood is placed in the center of the test strip. (Courtesy of Ken Timby.)

continued

SKILL 13-3

USING A GLUCOMETER *Continued*

Suggested Action	Reason for Action
Read the display on the meter after the series of beeps.	Identifies the patient's blood sugar
Turn the machine off.	Extends the life of the battery
Offer the patient a Band-Aid or paper tissue.	Absorbs blood and controls bleeding
Pull back on the barrel to release the lancet.	Prevents potential for a needlestick injury
Dispose of the lancet in a puncture-resistant container.	Prevents injury and transmission of blood-borne infectious microorganisms
Clean the window of the glucometer and the hole of the test strip holder with a cotton swab or damp cloth to remove dirt, blood, or lint once a week or more often if needed.	Keeps the equipment free of debris, which can impair light detection
Remove gloves and immediately wash your hands.	Reduces the number of microorganisms
Remove the equipment from the bedside if it does not belong to the patient.	Facilitates the use of equipment that may be needed for other patients
Store the test strips in a cool dry place at 37° to 85°F (1.7° to 30°C).	Prevents decomposition due to heat and humidity
Record the glucose measurement in the patient's record.	Documents essential data
Report the blood sugar level to the nurse in charge.	Communicates information for making treatment decisions

Evaluation

- Patient demonstrates understanding of the purpose for the examination.
- Adequate amount of blood is obtained.
- Results are consistent with the patient's present condition, previous trends, and concurrent treatment.
- Additional treatment is provided depending on glucose measurement.

Document

- Date and time
- Pertinent preassessment data, if any
- Results obtained when using the glucometer. In most agencies, the test data are recorded on a diabetic flow sheet rather than being charted in narrative nursing notes.
- Treatment provided based on abnormal test results

SAMPLE DOCUMENTATION

Date and Time Blood sugar 210 mg per glucometer. 5 units of Humulin R insulin given subcutaneously as coverage. ________________________________ SIGNATURE, TITLE

CRITICAL THINKING

- Discuss a plan for ensuring that glucometer equipment is checked with a control strip or solution on a regular basis.
- Research nursing actions that are appropriate if the blood sugar measurement is significantly low (<60 mg/dl) or significantly high (>120 mg/dl).
- Besides the patient, who else should learn how to use a glucometer? Explain the reason for your answer.

UNIT FIVE

ASSISTING WITH BASIC NEEDS

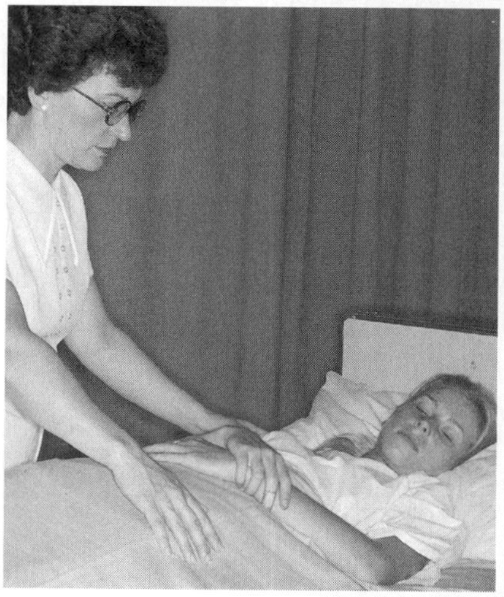

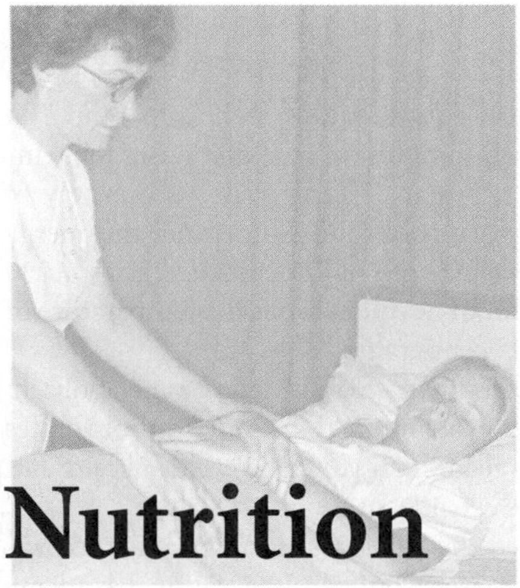

CHAPTER 14

Nutrition

CHAPTER OUTLINE

Overview of Nutrition
Nutritional Status Assessment
Management of Problems Interfering with Nutrition
Management of Patient Nutrition

NURSING GUIDELINES

OVERCOMING SIMPLE ANOREXIA
RELIEVING NAUSEA
MANAGING THE CARE OF A VOMITING PATIENT
PREVENTING AND RELIEVING STOMACH GAS

SKILLS

SKILL 14-1: SERVING AND REMOVING MEAL TRAYS
SKILL 14-2: FEEDING A PATIENT

NURSING CARE PLAN

IMPAIRED SWALLOWING

KEY TERMS

anorexia
anthropometric data
body-mass index
cachexia
calorie
carbohydrates
cellulose
complete proteins
diet history
dysphagia
emaciation
emesis
eructation
essential amino acids
fat
fat-soluble vitamins
flatus
food pyramid
incomplete proteins
kilocalorie
lipoproteins
malnutrition
megadoses
metabolic rate
midarm circumference
minerals
nausea
nonessential amino acids
nutrition
obesity
projectile vomiting
protein
protein complementation
regurgitation
retching
saturated fats
unsaturated fats
vegans
vegetarians
vitamins
vomiting
vomitus
water-soluble vitamins

LEARNING OBJECTIVES

An understanding of the content within this chapter will be evidenced by the student's ability to:

- Define the terms *nutrition* and *malnutrition.*
- List six components of basic nutrition.
- List at least five factors that influence nutritional needs.
- Discuss the purpose and components of the food pyramid.
- Describe three facts that are available on nutritional labels.
- Explain protein complementation.
- Identify four objective assessments for determining a person's nutritional status.
- Discuss the purpose of a diet history.
- List five common problems that can be identified from a nutritional assessment.
- Plan nursing interventions for resolving problems caused by or affected by nutrition.
- List seven common hospital diets.
- Discuss four nursing responsibilities for meeting the nutritional needs of patients.
- Identify three facts the nurse must know about a patient's diet.
- Describe and demonstrate techniques for feeding patients.
- Explain how to meet the nutritional needs of patients with visual impairment or dementia.
- Discuss at least three unique aspects of nutrition that apply to older adults.

Nutrition (the process by which the body uses food) is a basic need. **Malnutrition** (a condition resulting from a lack of proper nutrients in the diet) is common in poor, developing countries but also occurs among some groups in the United

States. Some examples of Americans who tend to have inadequate nutrition are:

- Elderly people who are socially isolated and live on fixed incomes
- Children of economically deprived parents
- Pregnant teenagers
- People with substance abuse problems such as alcoholism

More and more data support the fact that the quality of one's nutrition influences one's health and well-being. Therapeutic diets have been a standard technique in the treatment of diseases. Now, there is emphasis on improving nutrition to prevent disease. Healthy people in general are becoming selective about the quantity and quality of their daily food consumption. Consequently, nurses advise others about what and how much to eat, discourage food fads and unsafe dieting, and manage the care of patients whose ability to eat, digest, absorb, or eliminate food is impaired.

Overview of Nutrition

HUMAN NUTRITIONAL NEEDS

All humans have the same basic nutritional needs for health. Through the scientific study of nutrition, standards have been determined for the recommended daily amounts of:

- Calories
- Proteins, carbohydrates, and fats, which provide the calories for energy and substances needed for growth and repair of body structures
- Vitamins and minerals, which are essential for regulating and maintaining physiologic processes necessary for health but do not supply calories

Water, which is also necessary for life, is discussed in Chapter 15.

Although standards have been established for the types and amounts of dietary components needed to sustain health, individual nutritional needs are influenced by and may require adjustment according to:

- Age
- Weight and height
- Growth periods
- Activity
- Health status

Calories

Food is the source of energy for humans. Some nutrients produce more energy than others. By using a calorimeter, a device for measuring heat, the nutrients in food are burned in a laboratory and then analyzed to quantify their energy value.

The energy, or heat equivalent, of food is measured in calories. A **calorie** (cal) (amount of heat that raises the temperature of 1 gram of water 1° centigrade) is one way of expressing the energy value of food. Sometimes the energy equivalent of food is expressed in **kilocalories** (kcal) (1000 calories, or the amount of heat that raises the temperature of 1 kilogram of water 1° centigrade).

When proteins, carbohydrates, and fats are metabolized, they produce energy. Proteins yield 4 kcal/g, carbohydrates yield 4 kcal/g, and fats yield 9 kcal/g. Alcohol yields 7 kcal/g, but it is not considered an essential nutrient.

Average adults need 2000 to 3000 calories per day, according to the National Research Council of the National Academy of Science. However, unless the caloric intake includes adequate sources of proteins, carbohydrates, and fats, the person may be marginally nourished or malnourished. In other words, consuming 3000 calories of chocolate, exclusive of any other food, is not adequate to sustain a healthy state! Fortunately, most foods contain an assortment of nutrients, vitamins, and minerals.

Proteins

Protein (nutrient composed of *amino acids*, chemical compounds made up of nitrogen, carbon, hydrogen, and oxygen) is a component of every living cell. Amino acids are responsible for building and repairing cells. Twenty-two amino acids have been identified. Nine of the 22 are referred to as **essential amino acids** (protein components that must be obtained from food because they cannot be synthesized by the body). **Nonessential amino acids** (protein components manufactured within the body) is a misleading term: "nonessential" refers to the fact that these amino acids are not dependent on dietary intake, not that they are unnecessary for health.

Proteins are used primarily to build, maintain, and repair body tissue. The body spares protein for energy use as long as calories are available from carbohydrates and fats.

Dietary proteins come from animal and plant food sources. Good sources of protein include milk, meat, fish, poultry, eggs, legumes (peas, beans, peanuts), nuts, and components of grains. Animal sources are referred to as **complete proteins** (contain all the essential amino acids); plant sources are called **incomplete proteins** (contain only some of the essential amino acids). **Protein complementation** (combining plant sources of protein) helps the person acquire all the essential amino acids from nonanimal sources (Fig. 14-1). Protein complementation is discussed later in relation to vegetarian diets.

Carbohydrates

Carbohydrates (nutrients that contain molecules of carbon, hydrogen, and oxygen) are generally found in plant food

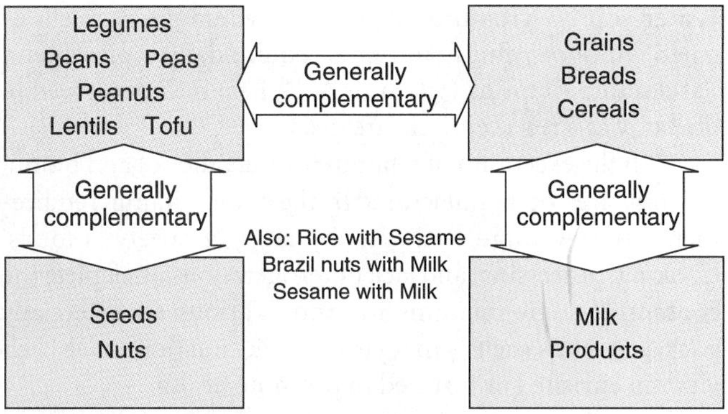

FIGURE 14–1. Complementary protein guide for meatless meals.

sources. They are classified according to the number of sugar, or saccharide, units they contain. Carbohydrates are subdivided into sugars, such as *monosaccharides* and *disaccharides,* and starches, called *polysaccharides.*

Carbohydrates, which make up the chief component of most diets, are used primarily as a source for quick energy. In addition to providing calories, carbohydrates contain **cellulose** (undigestible fiber in the stems, skins, and leaves of fruits and vegetables) that forms intestinal bulk. Fiber is important for promoting bowel elimination.

Sources of carbohydrates include cereals and grains, such as rice, wheat and wheat germ, oats, barley, corn and corn meal; fruits and vegetables; and sweeteners. Display 14-1 lists terms on food labels that identify ingredients that are, in essence, sugar. Foods that contain sugar as a major ingredient tend to supply calories but few if any other nutrients.

Fats

Fats (nutrients that contain molecules composed of glycerol and fatty acids called *glycerides*) are known collectively as *lipids.* Depending on the number of fatty acids that make up the fat molecule, fats are referred to as mono-, di-, or triglycerides.

DISPLAY 14–1

Label Ingredients that Represent Sugar

- Sucrose (table sugar)
- Fructose
- Glucose (dextrose)
- Brown sugar
- Corn sweetener
- Corn syrup
- Fruit juice concentrate
- Honey
- Invert sugar
- Lactose
- Maltose
- Molasses
- Raw sugar
- Syrup

Fats are a concentrated source of energy, supplying more than twice the calories per gram than either proteins or carbohydrates. Although fats are high in calories, they should not be eliminated from the diet. Fats provide energy and are necessary for many chemical reactions in the body. Fat is necessary for the absorption of some vitamins. Fats also add flavor to food, and because they leave the stomach slowly, they promote a feeling of having satisfied appetite and hunger.

Because fats are insoluble in water, they are carried throughout the bloodstream within molecules of protein referred to as **lipoproteins** (combination of fats and proteins). Lipoproteins vary in the proportion of protein to fat (Table 14-1). The more protein the molecule contains, the higher its density. The ratio of low-density lipoprotein (LDL), which contains substantial amounts of cholesterol, to high-density lipoprotein (HDL) is significant in predicting the risk for cardiovascular disease.

Saturated fats (lipids that contain as much hydrogen as their molecular structure can hold) are generally solid. Most saturated fats are found in animal sources. **Unsaturated fats** (lipids that are missing some hydrogen) more often have the composition of liquid oil. Unsaturated fats are found more often in plant sources such as corn. The following foods are rich in fat: beef and pork; butter, margarine, and vegetable oils; egg yolk; whole milk and cheese; peanut butter; salad dressings; avocados; chocolate; and nuts.

In general, Americans eat more fats than people in most other countries. The relation of fat consumption and obesity to disorders such as heart disease, hypertension, diabetes, and some types of cancer is becoming well documented. In an effort to improve the health of the nation, the Department of Health and Human Resources is continuing its national health initiative, *Healthy People 2010: National Health Promotion and Disease Prevention* (1999). Among its goals, the government is advocating that at least 50% of people aged 2 and older will consume no more than 30% of their daily calories from fat; of that, less than 10% will be saturated fat.

TABLE 14–1. **Classification of Lipoproteins**

Type of Lipoprotein	Function	Recommended Blood Level*
Very low density (VLDL)	Delivers triglycerides to cells; becomes a major source of LDL	Not usually reported
Low density (LDL)	Transports cholesterol to cells and tissues	<130 mg/dl
High density (HDL)	Mobilizes cholesterol from tissues; transfers cholesterol to the liver for eventual excretion	30–85 mg/dl

* Values must be adjusted for age and gender.

Minerals

Minerals (noncaloric substances in food that are essential to all cells) play a role in the regulation of many of the body's chemical processes, such as blood clotting and the conduction of nerve impulses. Table 14-2 lists some of the major and trace minerals of the body, their chief functions, and common dietary sources. As a national policy, specified amounts of certain minerals and vitamins are added to some processed foods. For example, enriched flour and bread contain thiamine, riboflavin, niacin, and iron to replace what is lost when the grain is milled into flour. *Fortified foods* have been enhanced by the addition of extra amounts of nutritional substances that are present in the food naturally.

Vitamins

Vitamins (chemical substances that are necessary in minute amounts for normal growth, maintenance of health, and functioning of the body; Table 14-3) were originally named as letters in the alphabet. Numbers were subsequently added to some letters as more were identified. Chemical names are now replacing the letter–number system of identification. **Water-soluble vitamins** (B complex, vitamin C) are eliminated with body fluids and thus require daily replacement. **Fat-soluble vitamins** (vitamins A, D, E, and K) are stored in the body as a reserve for future needs.

With the exception of vitamin K (menadione) and biotin, vitamins are not manufactured by the body. Vitamin requirements, however, are easily met by eating a variety of foods. Cooking, processing, and lack of refrigeration can deplete the content of some vitamins in food. Various commercially packaged foods such as margarine, milk, and flour have been vitamin enriched or fortified to promote health.

Generally, vitamin and mineral supplements are not necessary as long as a person eats a well-balanced diet. Consuming **megadoses** (amounts exceeding those considered adequate for health) can be dangerous. Some athletes and people with terminal diseases follow unconventional diets and take large doses of nutritional supplements. Athletes are motivated by a desire to alter their muscle mass, strength, and endurance; people with terminal diseases may do so in a desperate attempt to be cured. Although various deficiency diseases develop from inadequate nutrition, there is no conclusive evidence at this time that consuming excessive amounts of nutrients, vitamins, or minerals is a safe substitute for healthy eating or a singular established treatment for disease.

TABLE 14–2. **Common Dietary Minerals**

Mineral	Chief Functions	Common Dietary Sources
Sodium	Maintenance of water and electrolyte balance	Table salt Processed meat
Potassium	Maintenance of electrolyte balance Neuromuscular activity Enzyme reactions	Bananas Oranges Potatoes
Chloride	Maintenance of fluid and electrolyte balance	Table salt Processed meat
Calcium	Formation of teeth and bones Neuromuscular activity Blood coagulation Cell wall permeability	Milk Milk products
Phosphorus	Buffering action Formation of bones and teeth	Eggs Meat Milk
Iodine	Regulation of body metabolism Promotion of normal growth	Seafood Iodized salt
Iron	Component of hemoglobin Assistance in cellular oxidation	Liver Egg yolk Meat
Magnesium	Neuromuscular activity Activation of enzymes Formation of teeth and bones	Whole grains Milk Meat
Zinc	Constituent of enzymes and insulin	Seafood Liver

TABLE 14–3. **Vitamins**

Vitamin	Chief Functions	Common Dietary Sources
A (Retinol) Not destroyed by ordinary cooking temperatures	Growth of body cells Promotion of vision, healthy hair and skin, and integrity of epithelial membranes Prevention of xerophthalmia, a condition characterized by chronic conjunctivitis	Animal fats: butter, cheese, cream, egg yolk, whole milk Fish liver oil and liver Green leafy and yellow fruits and vegetables
B_1 (Thiamine) Not readily destroyed by ordinary cooking temperatures	Carbohydrate metabolism Functioning of nervous system Normal digestion Prevention of beriberi, a condition characterized by neuritis	Fish Lean meat and poultry Glandular organs Milk Whole-grain cereals Peas, beans, and peanuts
B_2 (Riboflavin) Not destroyed by heat except in presence of alkali	Formation of certain enzymes Normal growth Light adaptation in the eyes	Eggs Green leafy vegetables Lean meat Milk Whole grains Dried yeast
B_3 (Niacin)	Carbohydrate, fat, and protein metabolism Enzyme component Prevention of appetite loss Prevention of pellagra, a condition characterized by cutaneous, gastrointestinal, neurologic, and mental symptoms	Lean meat and liver Fish Peas, beans Whole-grain cereals Peanuts Yeast Eggs Liver
B_6 (Pyridoxine) Destroyed by heat, sunlight, and air	Healthy gums and teeth Red blood cell formation Carbohydrate, fat, and protein metabolism	Whole-grain cereals and wheat germ Vegetables Yeast Meat Bananas Blackstrap molasses
B_9 (Folic acid)	Protein metabolism Red blood cell formation Normal intestinal tract functioning	Green leafy vegetables Glandular organs Yeast
B_{12} (Cyanocobalamin)	Protein metabolism Red blood cell formation Healthy nervous system tissues Prevention of pernicious anemia, a condition characterized by decreased red blood cells	Liver and kidney Dairy products Lean meat Milk Saltwater fish and oysters
C (Ascorbic acid) Readily destroyed by cooking temperatures	Healthy bones, teeth, and gums Formation of blood vessels and capillary walls Proper tissue and bone healing Facilitation of iron and folic acid absorption Prevention of scurvy, a condition characterized by bleeding and abnormal bone and teeth formation	Citrus fruits and juices Tomatoes Berries Cabbage Green vegetables Potatoes
D (Calciferol) Relatively stable with refrigeration	Absorption of calcium and phosphorus Prevention of rickets, a condition characterized by weak bones	Fish liver oils, salmon, tuna Milk Egg yolk Butter Liver Oysters Formed in the skin by exposure to sunlight
E (Alpha-tocopherol) Heat-stable in absence of oxygen	Red blood cell formation Protection of essential fatty acids Important for normal reproduction in experimental animals (i.e., rats)	Green leafy vegetables Wheat germ oil Margarine Brown rice

continued

TABLE 14–3. **Vitamins** *Continued*

Vitamin	Chief Functions	Common Dietary Sources
Pantothenic acid	Metabolism	Liver Egg yolk Milk
H (Biotin) Heat-sensitive	Enzyme activity Metabolism of carbohydrates, fats, and proteins	Egg yolk Green vegetables Milk Liver and kidney Yeast
K (Menadione)	Production of prothrombin	Liver Eggs Green leafy vegetables Synthesized in the gastrointestinal tract by bacteria

NUTRITIONAL STANDARDS

Recently, several national efforts have taken place to educate the public about nutrition and to promote healthy or informed choices when purchasing food (Display 14-2). One strategy that is being used to achieve the objectives of *Healthy People 2010* is the use of the U.S. Department of Agriculture's food pyramid. Others include requiring simpler labels about nutrition on processed and packaged foods and establishing standard definitions for the terms used on food labels.

The Food Pyramid

The **food pyramid** (guide for promoting the healthy intake of food) is a helpful tool (Fig. 14-2). By using the simple pyramid design, average people can easily learn what foods and how much to consume on a daily basis. The number of servings from each category is ranked from most (bottom of the pyramid) to least (top of the pyramid). By following the pyramid's guidelines, Americans can achieve the dietary recommendations set by the U.S. Department of Health and Human Services and the U.S. Department of Agriculture for promoting health and preventing chronic disease (Display 14-3).

The number of servings needs to be modified in certain circumstances. Children, adolescents, pregnant women, and breastfeeding mothers require more servings per day of certain food groups, particularly the milk group.

Nutritional Labeling

Nutritional information has appeared on food labels since 1974. Today, all packages of fresh meat and poultry must provide printed disease prevention guidelines. There have also been major changes in the way nutritional information is provided on approximately 90% of processed and packaged food labels (Fig. 14-3). The labels continue to identify the amounts of each nutrient per serving, but the serving sizes are now identified in household measurements rather than in metric amounts. However, to interpret the information accurately, consumers must become familiar with some new or revised terms. For example, daily value (DV) is a term that replaces the previously used term, the recommended daily amount (RDA). DVs are calculated in percentages based on standards set for total fat, saturated fat, cholesterol, sodium, carbohydrate, and fiber in a 2000-calorie diet. The standards are:

- Total fat, 65 g
- Saturated fat, ≤20 g
- Cholesterol, 300 mg
- Sodium, <2400 mg
- Total carbohydrate, 300 g
- Dietary fiber, 25 g

People consuming diets of more than or less than 2000 calories must adjust the percentage of DVs; this may prove difficult for the average consumer.

An expanded table showing the DV equivalents for both a 2000- and a 2500-calorie diet appears on some food labels. Because the requirements for vitamins and minerals are not dependent on calories, those amounts apply to all consumers.

The federal Nutrition Labeling and Education Act requires companies to comply with standard definitions if they use health-related claims, such as "low-fat," on their labels (Display 14-4).

Nutritional Patterns and Practices

Eating Habits

Most eating habits are learned early in life. The kind of food that is consumed and a person's eating patterns are affected by cultural (Fig. 14-4), economic, emotional, and social variables. Some factors include:

DISPLAY 14-2

Proposed National Nutritional Objectives for 2010

- Reduce coronary heart disease deaths to no more than 100 per 100,000 people.
- Reverse the rise in cancer deaths to achieve a rate of no more than 130 per 100,000 people.
- Reduce overweight to a prevalence of no more than 20% among people aged 20 and older and no more than 15% among adolescents aged 12–19.
- Reduce growth retardation among low-income children aged 5 and younger to less than 10%.
- Reduce dietary fat intake to an average of 30% of calories among people aged 2 and older, and increase to at least 50% the number who consume less than 10% of calories from saturated fat.
- Increase complex carbohydrate and fiber-containing foods in diets of people aged 2 and older to an average of five or more daily servings for vegetables (including legumes) and fruits, and to an average of six or more daily servings for grain products.
- Increase to at least 50% the proportion of overweight people aged 12 and older who have adopted sound dietary practices combined with regular physical activity to attain an appropriate body weight.
- Increase calcium intake so at least 50% of people aged 11–24 and 50% of pregnant and lactating women consume an average of three or more daily servings of foods rich in calcium, and at least 75% of children aged 2–10 and 50% of people aged 25 and older consume an average of two or more servings daily.
- Decrease salt and sodium intake so at least 65% of home meal preparers prepare foods without adding salt, at least 80% of people avoid using salt at the table, and at least 40% of adults regularly purchase foods modified or lower in sodium.
- Reduce iron deficiency to less than 3% among children aged 1–4 and among women of child-bearing age.
- Increase to at least 75% the proportion of mothers who breast-feed their babies in the early postpartum period and to at least 50% the proportion who continue breast-feeding until their infants are 5–6 months old.
- Increase to at least 75% the proportion of parents and caregivers who use feeding practices that prevent "baby bottle tooth decay."
- Increase to at least 85% the proportion of people aged 18 and older who use food labels to make nutritious food selections.
- Achieve useful and informative nutrition labeling for virtually all processed foods and at least 40% of ready-to-eat carry-away foods.
- Increase to at least 5,000 brand items the availability of processed food products that are reduced in fat and saturated fat.
- Increase to at least 90% the proportion of school lunch, breakfast, and child care food services with menus that are consistent with the nutrition principles in the Dietary Guidelines for Americans.
- Increase to at least 80% the receipt of home food services by people aged 65 and older who have difficulty preparing their own meals or are otherwise in need of home-delivered meals.
- Increase to at least 75% the proportion of the nation's schools that provide nutrition education from preschool to 12th grade, preferably as part of comprehensive school health education.
- Increase to at least 50% the proportion of worksites with 50 or more employees that offer nutrition education and/or weight-management programs for employees.
- Increase to at least 75% the proportion of primary care providers who provide nutrition assessment and counseling and/or referral to qualified nutritionists or dietitians.
- Reduce the prevalence of blood cholesterol levels of 240 mg/dl or greater to no more than 20% among adults.
- Increase to at least 50% the proportion of people with high blood pressure whose blood pressure is under control.
- Reduce the mean serum cholesterol level among adults to no more than 200 mg/dl.

(Office of Disease Prevention and Health Promotion, U.S. Department of Health and Human Services. The 1995 midcourse revisions of Healthy People 2000 initiative. March 22, 1999.)

- Food preferences acquired during childhood
- Established patterns for meals
- Attitudes about nutrition
- Knowledge of nutrition
- Income level
- Time available for food preparation
- Number of people in the household
- Access to food markets
- Use of food for comfort, celebration, or symbolic reward
- Satisfaction or dissatisfaction with body weight
- Religious beliefs

Vegetarianism

Vegetarians (persons who restrict their consumption of animal food sources) modify their diets for religious and personal reasons. Vegetarianism is practiced in various forms, from **vegans** (persons who rely exclusively on plant sources for protein) to semivegetarians, who exclude only red meat.

Vegetarians, as a whole, have a lower incidence of colorectal cancer and fewer problems with obesity and diseases that are associated with a high-fat diet. However, a vegan diet, unless skillfully planned, can be inadequate in complete protein, calcium, riboflavin, vitamins B_{12} and D, and iron. Thus, teaching the vegan about protein complementation is necessary.

Patient Teaching For

Vegetarians

Teach the patient or the family to do the following:

- Plan menus a day or week at a time.
- Eat a wide variety of foods.
- Use complementary plant proteins.

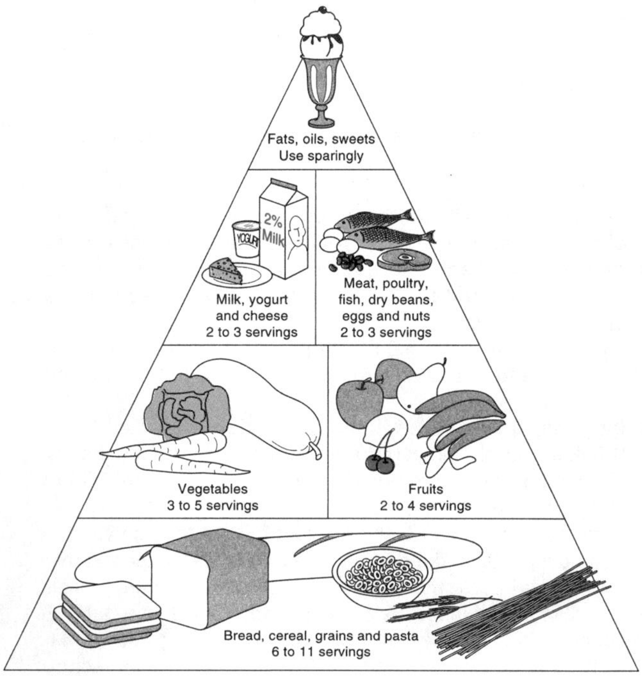

FIGURE 14–2. The food pyramid.

- Include dried fruit, molasses, and dried peas for iron.
- Enhance the absorption of iron by including a good source of vitamin C, such as orange juice, at each meal.
- Use whole grains and enriched flour, rather than refined, to obtain riboflavin.
- Add brewer's yeast, a source of B vitamins, to the dough of baked goods.
- Take a calcium supplement that supplies at least 800 mg (preferably 1200 mg) per day.
- Use soybean milk fortified with vitamin B_{12}, or consult with a physician concerning replacement therapy of at least 2 mcg/day.
- Select good sources of calcium, such as broccoli, collard and mustard greens, kale, and tofu.
- Breast-feed infants, if possible.

DISPLAY 14–3

Dietary Guidelines for Americans

- Balance the food you eat with physical activity. Maintain or improve your weight.
- Eat a variety of foods.
- Choose a diet with plenty of grain products, vegetables, and fruits.
- Choose a diet low in fat, saturated fat, and cholesterol.
- Choose a diet moderate in salt and sodium.
- Choose a diet moderate in sugars.
- If you drink alcoholic beverages, do so in moderation.

(U.S. Department of Agriculture and U.S. Department of Health and Human Services. Nutrition and your health: dietary guidelines for Americans, 4th ed. 1995.)

Nutrition Facts
Serving Size 1/2 of package (21g)
Servings Per Container 2

Amount Per Serving	
Calories 70	Calories from Fat 20
	% Daily Value*
Total Fat 2.5g	4%
Saturated Fat 1.5g	6%
Cholesterol Less than 5mg	1%
Sodium 940mg	39%
Total Carbohydrate 12g	4%
Dietary Fiber 1g	6%
Sugars 4g	
Protein 2g	
Vitamin A 0% •	Vitamin C 0%
Calcium 6% •	Iron 2%

* Percent Daily Values are based on 2,000 calorie diet. Your daily values may be higher or lower depending on your calorie needs:

	Calories:	2,000	2,500
Total Fat	Less than	65g	80g
Sat Fat	Less than	20g	25g
Cholesterol	Less than	300mg	300mg
Sodium	Less than	2,400mg	2,400mg
Total carbohydrate		300g	375g
Dietary Fiber		25g	30g

Calories per gram:
Fat 9 • Carbohydrate 4 • Protein 4

FIGURE 14–3. Sample label with nutritional information.

DISPLAY 14–4

Regulations for Labeling Terms

Calorie-free: <5 calories
Low calorie: ≤40 calories
Reduced calorie: at least 25% fewer calories than standard product
Light or "lite": ⅓ fewer calories or 50% less fat than regular product
Fat-free: <0.5 g fat; example: skim milk
Low fat: ≤3 g of fat; example: 1% milk
Reduced fat: at least 25% less fat than regular product; example: 2% milk
Cholesterol-free: <2 mg cholesterol and ≤2 g saturated fat
Low cholesterol: ≤20 mg cholesterol and ≤2 g saturated fat
Sugar-free: <0.5 g sugar
Fruit drink/beverage: <100% fruit juice
Imitation: new food that resembles a traditional food and contains less protein or less of any essential vitamin or mineral than the traditional food; example: imitation cheese

Figures are per serving.
(Food and Drug Administration. Better life for special diets. Pub. #98-2291. Washington DC: FDA, 1998. www.fda/gov/fdac/foodlabel/special.html, accessed 7/99.)

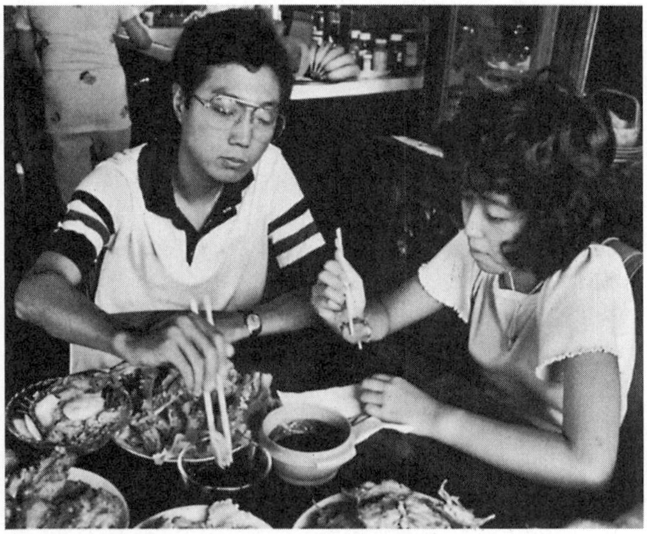

FIGURE 14–4. Cultural influences affect eating habits.

- Consider taking cod liver oil as a source of vitamin D.
- Purchase meat analogs, products with the taste and appearance of meat, poultry, or fish that are made from textured vegetable protein, in health food stores.
- Contact a Seventh-Day Adventist church, whose members practice vegetarianism, for information on sources for meatless products and food preparation classes.

Nutritional Status Assessment

Because eating is a basic need, nurses must identify any current or potential problems associated with nutrition. Subjective information can be obtained by asking focused questions in a diet history; objective data can be gathered using physical assessment techniques.

SUBJECTIVE DATA

A **diet history** (assessment technique for obtaining facts about an individual's eating habits and factors that affect nutrition) adds to the data base of nutrition information. Common components in a diet history include:

- Level of appetite
- Weight loss or gain of 10 lbs in the past 6 months
- Number of meals eaten per day
- Foods eaten in the previous 24 hours, in approximate household measurements
- Time when meals are generally eaten
- Frequency with which meals are eaten alone
- Food likes, dislikes, allergies, intolerances, and cultural beliefs about food
- Amount of alcohol consumed on a daily or weekly basis
- Vitamin or mineral supplements taken on a routine basis
- Any problems with eating, digestion, or elimination
- Special diets that have been medically prescribed or self-imposed
- Use of over-the-counter drugs such as antacids or laxatives
- Food supplements or restrictions, and the reason for them
- Desire to improve nutritional intake or to gain or lose weight

A comprehensive assessment also includes current and past medical conditions and surgical procedures.

OBJECTIVE DATA

The body is composed of water, fat, bone, and muscle. The nurse uses physical assessment techniques to determine how a person's body measurements or anthropometric data reflect his or her nutritional status.

Anthropometric Data

Anthropometric data (measurements that pertain to body size and composition) are obtained by measuring the patient's height and weight, calculating body-mass index, and measuring midarm circumference and triceps skinfold thickness. More sophisticated tests, such as bioelectrical impedance analysis, which calculates lean body mass, body fat, and total body water based on changes in conduction of an applied electrical current, are used at eating disorder clinics or fitness centers.

Obtaining the patient's height and weight is generally sufficient anthropometric data unless a severe nutritional problem is suspected or long-term therapy is anticipated. An actual weight, rather than the patient's estimate, is essential. A standing, chair, or bed scale is used depending on the patient's condition. The date and time, the type of scale, and the clothing worn by the patient are recorded. It is important to duplicate all of these factors when taking subsequent weights for comparison. The patient's height is measured without shoes and clothes. A gross assessment tool using weight and height is shown in Figure 14-5.

Body-mass index (BMI; numeric data used to compare a person's size in relation to established norms for the adult population) is calculated using height and weight (Display 14-5).

The **midarm circumference** (measurement for determining skeletal muscle mass) is one technique that, when combined with other body measurements, helps to assess a person's nutritional status. This measurement is based on the assumption that muscle is usually located in anatomic areas such as the biceps. When measuring the midarm circumference:

- Use the nondominant arm.
- Find the midpoint of the upper arm between the shoulder and elbow.
- Mark the midarm location.

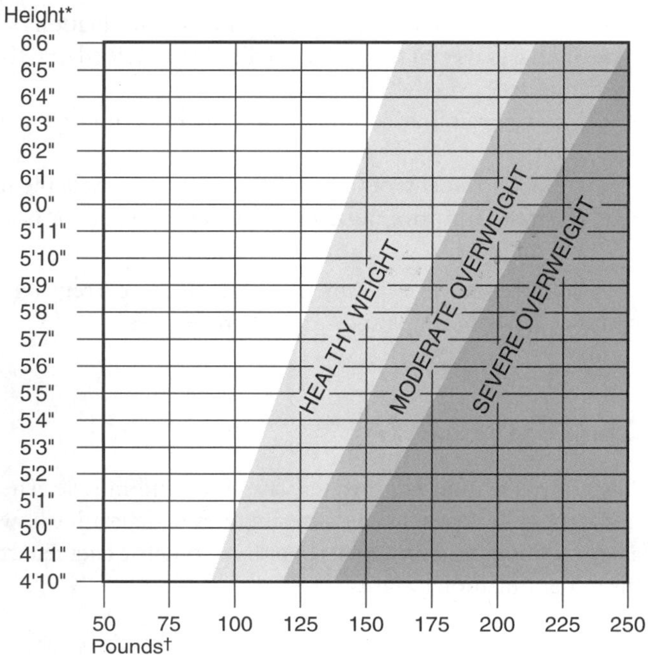

* Without shoes.

† Without clothes. The higher weights apply to people with more muscle and bone, such as many men.

Source: Report of the Dietary Guidelines Advisory Committee on the Dietary Guidelines for Americans, 1995, pages 23-24.

FIGURE 14–5. Tool for determining weight status.

DISPLAY 14–5

Body-Mass Index Formula, Calculation , and Interpretation

Formula

$$BMI = \frac{\text{weight in kg}}{\text{height in m}^2}$$

Calculation

1. Divide pounds by 2.2 = kilograms (kg).
2. Divide height in inches by 39.4 = meters (m).
3. Square the answer in step 2 by multiplying the number times itself.
4. Divide weight in kg by m².

Interpretation

Classification	BMI (kg/m²)
Underweight	<18.5
Normal	18.5 to 24.9
Overweight	25.0 to 29.9
Obesity (Class I)	30.0 to 34.9
(Class II)	35.0 to 39.9
Extreme Obesity (Class III)	≥40

(Adapted from WHO. Preventing and managing the global epidemic of obesity. Geneva, WHO, June 1997. In NIH. Clinical guidelines on the identification, evaluation, and treatment of overweight and obesity in adults. Pub. # 98-4083. Washington DC, NIH, September 1998.)

- Position the arm loosely at the patient's side.
- Encircle the arm with a tape measure at the marked position.
- Record the circumference in centimeters.

The thickness of the skinfold at the triceps or subscapular areas is generally obtained to aid in estimating the amount of subcutaneous fat deposits (Fig. 14-6). The skinfold thickness measurement relates to total body fat. To measure the triceps skinfold thickness:

- Use the same arm as for the midarm circumference measurement.
- Grasp and pull the skin separate from the muscle at the previously marked location.
- Place the calipers about the skinfold.
- Record the measurement in millimeters.

To calculate how much of the midarm circumference is actual muscle (midarm muscle circumference), multiply the triceps skinfold measurement by 0.314.

To interpret the significance of the midarm circumference measurement and the triceps skinfold thickness, the measurements are compared with averages provided in standardized charts (Table 14-4). Skinfold thickness norms do not exist for adults over age 75. The circumference of the abdomen may be a more accurate anthropometric measurement for older adults, but standardized norms have not been established.

Physical Assessment

In addition to the anthropometric data, the nurse assesses the following:

- General appearance
- Integrity of the mouth

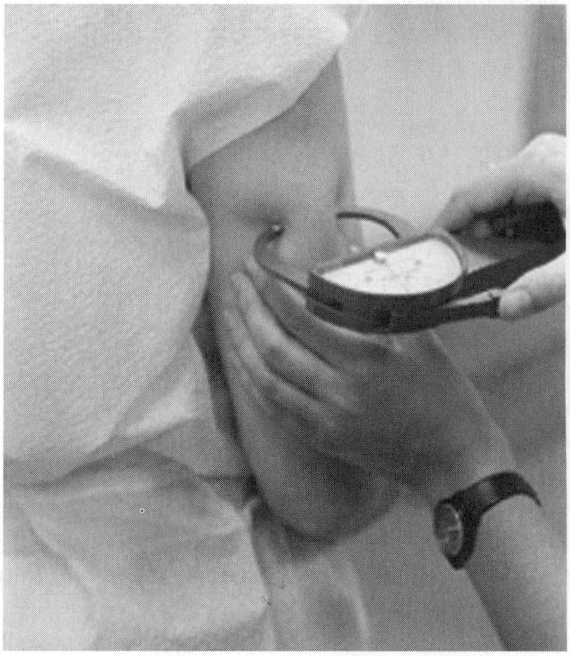

FIGURE 14–6. Measuring triceps skin-fold thickness with calipers. (Courtesy of Ken Timby.)

TABLE 14–4. **Anthropometric Measurements for Adults**

Measurement	Gender	Normal Range*
Midarm circumference	Male	29.3–17.6 cm
	Female	28.5–17.1 cm
Midarm muscle circumference	Male	25.3–15.2 cm
	Female	23.2–13.9 cm
Triceps skin fold	Male	12.5–7.3 mm
	Female	16.5–9.9 mm

* If measurements are below the lowest range for normal, nutritional support may be indicated. (Adapted from Jelliffe DB. The assessment of the nutritional status of the community. World Health Organization Monograph No. 53. Geneva, World Health Organization, 1986.)

- Condition of the teeth
- Ability to chew and swallow
- Gag reflex
- Characteristics of skin and hair
- Joint flexibility
- Hand strength
- Attention and concentration

Laboratory Data

Laboratory tests used in nutritional assessment include a complete blood count (CBC), especially the hemoglobin, hematocrit, and number of lymphocytes; serum albumin and transferrin levels, which indicate protein status; and cholesterol, triglyceride, and lipoprotein levels, which may reflect a need to adjust the amount of fat the patient eats.

Management of Problems Interfering with Nutrition

Based on the assessment data, the nurse may identify one or more of the following nursing diagnoses:

- Altered nutrition: less than body requirements
- Altered nutrition: more than body requirements
- Knowledge deficit: nutrition
- Self-care deficit: feeding
- Impaired swallowing
- Risk for aspiration

If a nutritional problem is beyond the scope of independent nursing practice, the nurse consults with the physician. If the problem can be resolved through independent nursing measures, the nurse may proceed by collaborating with the dietitian, selecting appropriate nursing interventions, and continuing to monitor the patient to evaluate the effectiveness of the nursing care plan.

The accompanying nursing care plan is an example of how the nurse manages the care of a patient who has a nursing diagnosis of Impaired swallowing. This diagnostic category is defined in the NANDA taxonomy (1999) as "abnormal functioning of the swallowing mechanism associated with deficits in oral, pharyngeal, or esophageal structure or function."

Nursing guidelines follow for managing the care of patients with other problems associated with nutrition and eating.

OBESITY

If a person wants to lose weight, the nurse must determine whether he or she actually needs to do so. A desire to lose weight may be based on wanting to resemble an unrealistic ideal. **Obesity** (condition in which a person's BMI exceeds $30/m^2$ or the triceps skinfold measurement exceeds 15 mm) indicates a need for healthy weight-reduction techniques. Research (Rexrode et al., 1998) has found that excess abdominal fat—a waist circumference over 40″ in men and over 35″ in women–is a greater health risk than fatty hips or thighs. Having a greater proportion of abdominal fat is associated with a higher incidence of heart and vascular disease, hypertension, and diabetes mellitus. Severely obese people are medically evaluated to determine whether there are physical etiologies for the disorder or health risks associated with a weight-loss program.

To lose 1 lb, the person must reduce his or her caloric intake by 3500 calories. Thus, decreasing one's intake of food by 500 calories per day will produce a 1-lb weight loss per week. By omitting 1000 calories per day, the person will lose 2 lbs per week. Generally, a sustained loss of 1 to 2 lb per week is a healthy goal. Patients trying to lose weight should be advised about healthy eating and about the hazards of unsupervised weight-loss techniques such as fasting, fad diets, or diet drugs.

Patient Teaching For

Promoting Weight Loss

Teach the patient or the family to do the following:

- When using the food pyramid, follow the requirements for a 2000-calorie diet.
- Limit the number of servings to the amounts suggested by the food pyramid:
  Grains—one slice of bread, 1 oz of cereal, or a half-cup of cooked pasta, rice, or cereal
  Vegetables—1 cup of raw leafy vegetables, a half-cup of other raw or cooked vegetables, or three-fourths of a cup of vegetable juice
  Fruits—one medium apple, banana, or orange; a half-cup of chopped, cooked, or canned fruit; or three-fourths of a cup of fruit juice
  Dairy—1 cup of milk or yogurt, 1.5 oz of natural cheese, or 2 oz of processed cheese

Meat—2 to 3 oz of cooked lean meat, poultry, or fish. A half-cup of cooked dry beans, one egg, 2 tablespoons of peanut butter, or one-third of a cup of nuts are the equivalent of 1 oz of meat.

- Use fats, oils, and sugar sparingly.
- Eliminate junk food (contributes calories but not much nutrition) and alcoholic beverages.
- Eat small but more frequent meals rather than three large meals per day. Any nutrients not used from large meals are stored as fat.
- Sit at the table to eat. Do not read or do other tasks while eating; distraction often fools the brain into thinking that food has not been consumed.
- Increase fiber in the diet from fresh fruits, vegetables, and whole grains. Fiber is not digested and may provide a full feeling without large numbers of calories.
- Participate in some regular, active form of exercise. Exercise raises the **metabolic rate** (speed at which calories are used) while suppressing the appetite. Information on activity and exercise is located in Chapter 23.

EMACIATION

Progressive or prolonged weight loss with a BMI of less than $16/m^2$ can have serious consequences. **Emaciation** (excessive leanness) and **cachexia** (general wasting away of body tissue) are consistent with severe malnourishment. States of severe malnourishment require collaboration with a physician, who will prescribe measures to ensure adequate nourishment, such as gastric or enteral tube feedings and parenteral nutrition (see Chap. 29).

Independent nursing interventions, including patient teaching, are appropriate for people who are approximately 10 lb below their ideal body weight. To gain 1 lb, a person must consume 3500 calories more than their metabolic needs. This is best done gradually.

Patient Teaching For

Promoting Weight Gain

Teach the patient or the family to do the following:

- Eat a variety of foods from the food pyramid, but increase the number of servings or serving sizes.
- Eat small amounts frequently.
- Eat with others.
- Snack on high-calorie but nutritious foods such as hard cheese, milkshakes, and nuts.
- Disguise extra calories by fortifying foods with powdered milk, gravies, or sauces.
- Garnish food with cubed or grated cheese, diced meat, nuts, or raisins.
- Rest after eating.

ANOREXIA

Anorexia (loss of appetite) is associated with multiple factors: illness, altered taste and smell, oral problems, and tension and depression. Simple anorexia is generally a short-lived symptom that requires no medical or nursing intervention. Anorexia nervosa, a psychobiologic disorder, is associated with a 20% to 25% loss in previously stable body weight. No matter what the etiology, the nurse never ignores that a patient is not eating. If food is uneaten, the nurse assesses for physiologic, emotional, cultural, or social etiologies that may be contributing factors.

Nursing Guidelines For

Overcoming Simple Anorexia

- ☑ Cater to the patient's food preferences.
  RATIONALE: More food is likely to be consumed if the patient selects it.
- ☑ Serve nutrient-dense foods (foods loaded with calories).
  RATIONALE: Nutrient-dense foods may compensate for a low intake of food.
- ☑ Offer small servings of food at frequent intervals.
  RATIONALE: Eating small amounts frequently may result in a cumulative intake that is within acceptable nutritional levels.
- ☑ Ensure that the patient is rested before meal time.
  RATIONALE: Lack of energy may overpower the desire to eat.
- ☑ Provide an opportunity for oral hygiene before meals.
  RATIONALE: Mouth care stimulates salivation and potentiates the pleasure from eating.
- ☑ Help the patient to a sitting position.
  RATIONALE: Seeing food stimulates the appetite center, and sitting also promotes access to the food.
- ☑ Arrange for the patient to eat with others.
  RATIONALE: Because eating is a social activity, the patient may eat more when seated with a group.
- ☑ Serve food attractively.
  RATIONALE: The visual presentation of food affects appetite stimulation in the brain.
- ☑ Suggest adding spices and herbs to foods.
  RATIONALE: Intensifying flavors and aromas may stimulate a desire to eat; however, it may have the opposite effect as well. When experimenting, add new seasonings to small amounts of food.
- ☑ Serve foods at their appropriate temperature.
  RATIONALE: More food may be eaten if hot foods are hot and cold foods are cold.

☑ Serve cool, bland foods to patients with mouth irritation.
RATIONALE: Hot or spicy foods intensify the irritation of oral structures.

NAUSEA

Nausea (feeling that usually precedes vomiting) is produced when gastrointestinal sensations, sensory data, and drug effects stimulate a portion of the medulla that contains the vomiting center.

Nausea may be associated with feeling faint or weak. Often, dizziness, perspiration, skin pallor, a rapid pulse rate, and a headache are present. The physician is consulted when nursing measures like the ones that follow are unsuccessful for overcoming nausea. Prescribed medications may be necessary.

Nursing Guidelines For

Relieving Nausea

☑ Check to see whether something as simple as an annoying odor or sight is contributing to nausea.
RATIONALE: Offensive sensory data can stimulate the vomiting center in the brain.

☑ Have the patient take deep breaths.
RATIONALE: Distraction can overcome nausea by directing conscious attention away from the unpleasant sensation.

☑ Avoid abrupt movements, and limit activities.
RATIONALE: Moving about may shift gastrointestinal structures and their contents, intensifying stimulation to the vomiting center.

☑ Limit the intake of food and fluid temporarily until signs of nausea subside.
RATIONALE: Distention of the stomach is a common trigger of the vomiting center.

☑ Avoid making negative comments about food.
RATIONALE: Verbal comments create visual images that may stimulate the vomiting center.

Once nausea is relieved, resuming fluid intake and nourishment becomes a priority. This process is started gradually. Sips of clear fluids are offered first. If fluids are tolerated, soft, bland foods are added in small amounts.

VOMITING

Vomiting (loss of stomach contents through the mouth) commonly accompanies nausea. **Emesis** or **vomitus** (substance that is vomited) is readily visible. **Retching** (act of vomiting without producing vomitus) may occur if the stomach is empty. **Regurgitation** (bringing stomach contents to the throat and mouth without the effort of vomiting) occurs commonly among infants after eating.

Projectile vomiting (vomiting that occurs with great force) is associated with certain disease conditions, such as increased pressure in the brain or gastrointestinal bleeding. Nausea may be present, but it often is not.

Nursing Guidelines For

Managing the Care of a Vomiting Patient

☑ Temporarily limit the intake of food.
RATIONALE: Adding contents to an already upset stomach may prolong episodes of vomiting.

☑ Lean the patient's head forward over a container or the toilet.
RATIONALE: Tilting the chin toward the chest reduces the possibility that vomitus will enter the lungs.

☑ Adjust the light, sound, ventilation, and temperature to a comfortable level.
RATIONALE: Reducing sensory stimulation may reduce the urge to vomit.

☑ Apply a cool washcloth to the forehead or back of the neck.
RATIONALE: Vomiting may be accompanied by an increase in perspiration and a clammy feeling to the skin.

☑ Rinse the mouth, offer mouthwash, or provide mouth care as soon as possible after vomiting.
RATIONALE: Gastric acid is harmful to the enamel of teeth. Emesis usually produces an unpleasant aftertaste.

☑ Turn a vomiting patient who is unconscious or weak onto the abdomen or side.
RATIONALE: Gravity helps emesis drain from the mouth rather than remaining in the throat, where it may be aspirated into the lungs.

☑ Use a suction machine to clear vomitus from the mouth and throat of a weak or unconscious patient.
RATIONALE: Suctioning pulls fluid from the oral cavity and airway, thus preventing choking and aspiration (see Chap. 36).

☑ Provide firm support with the hands or a pillow to the abdominal incision if the patient has had abdominal surgery. An abdominal binder may also help support the incision (see Chap 28).
RATIONALE: Strong muscle contractions may pull on stitches and increase pain and discomfort.

☑ Remove the container of emesis from the bedside as soon as possible. Provide ventilation to remove any lingering odors.
RATIONALE: The appearance and odor of vomitus may stimulate more vomiting.

The nurse describes the emesis in the patient's medical record. If possible, the amount of emesis is measured and the volume is recorded. Documentation includes the amount, color, appearance, and any unusual odor, such as the odor of fecal material or alcohol. If the characteristics of the emesis are unusual, a specimen is saved for the physician to examine. If there are any doubts about whether to discard or save the emesis, it is best to check with a more experienced nurse.

The physician is always consulted when vomiting is prolonged. It may be necessary to administer prescribed medications to relieve it.

STOMACH GAS

Air in the stomach is primarily a result of swallowing air. It becomes a problem only when it accumulates. **Eructation** (belching) is a discharge of gas from the stomach through the mouth. **Flatus** (gas that is formed in the intestine and released from the rectum) occurs when eructation does not occur. Nursing guidelines for relieving intestinal gas are discussed in Chapter 31.

Nursing Guidelines For

Preventing and Relieving Stomach Gas

☑ Suggest that patients chew food with the mouth closed.
RATIONALE: Laughing and talking while eating increase the amount of swallowed air.

☑ Advise against using a straw.
RATIONALE: Each swallow of liquid also contains the air in the straw.

☑ Advise against chewing gum and smoking cigarettes.
RATIONALE: Chewing gum increases salivation and results in swallowing both secretions and air. A portion of inhaled cigarette smoke may actually be swallowed.

☑ Limit or restrict foods that contain large volumes of air, such as soufflés, yeast breads, and carbonated beverages.
RATIONALE: Swallowing air trapped within food and drinking beverages that contain dissolved gas distend the stomach.

☑ Recommend that when under stress, the patient should avoid eating.
RATIONALE: Emotions delay stomach emptying. Any gas that is present is prevented from being distributed to the intestine.

☑ Propose walking about if uncomfortable.
RATIONALE: Activity helps gas rise to its highest point in the stomach, making belching easier.

☑ Consult with the physician about the use of medications that relieve gas accumulation. Instruct patients who purchase over-the-counter drugs to follow label directions for their use.
RATIONALE: Drugs containing simethicone tend to aid in the elimination of gas by reducing the surface tension of the gas bubbles trapped in the gastrointestinal tract. Simethicone is an ingredient in several nonprescription antacid products.

Management of Patient Nutrition

COMMON HOSPITAL DIETS

Some common hospital diets include:

- Regular or general: allows unrestricted food selections
- Light or convalescent: differs from regular diet in preparation; typically omits fried, fatty, gas-forming, and raw foods and rich pastries
- Soft: contains foods soft in texture; is usually low in residue and readily digestible; contains few or no spices or condiments; provides fewer fruits, vegetables, or meats than a light diet
- Mechanical soft: resembles a light diet but used for patients with chewing difficulties; provides cooked fruits and vegetables and ground meats
- Full liquid: contains fruit and vegetable juices, creamed or blended soups, milk, ices, ice cream, gelatin, junket, custards, and cooked cereals
- Clear liquid: consists of water, clear broth, clear fruit juices, plain gelatin, tea, and coffee; may or may not include carbonated beverages
- Special therapeutic: consists of foods prepared to meet special needs, such as low in sodium, fat, or fiber

Most inpatient agencies have a dietitian who plans the meals and a centralized food service that prepares patient meals.

Nurses are generally responsible for ordering and canceling diets for patients, serving and collecting meal trays, helping patients eat, and recording the percentage of food that is eaten. Nurses must know the type of diet prescribed for each patient, the purpose for the diet, and its characteristics. Care is taken that patients receive the correct diet and restricted foods are withheld.

MEAL TRAYS

Meals are usually served at the bedside, but some hospitals have cafeterias for ambulatory patients. Nursing homes generally have a dining room where patients eat in small groups. Nurses and dietary personnel work together to ensure that patients receive food at mealtimes and that the trays are collected afterward. The nursing responsibilities for serving and removing trays are identified in Skill 14-1.

FEEDING ASSISTANCE

Some patients need help with eating. Skill 14-2 provides suggested actions for feeding patients who can bite, sip, chew, and swallow but cannot cut food or use utensils for eating. Suggestions for helping patients with **dysphagia** (difficulty swallowing) and those who are blind or have both eyes patched, and for promoting self-feeding by those with dementia (impairment of intellectual functioning) follow.

Feeding the Patient with Dysphagia

The following techniques can be used when caring for patients who have difficulty chewing and swallowing food:

- Always have equipment for oral and pharyngeal suctioning at the bedside (see Chap. 36).
- If the patient has a tracheostomy tube or endotracheal tube, make sure the cuff is inflated (see Chap. 36).
- Place the patient in a sitting position.
- Provide oral hygiene to moisten the mouth.
- Initially, avoid dry foods, such as crackers, and sticky foods, such as bananas.
- Request semisolid foods with some texture, such as oatmeal, poached eggs, and mashed potatoes; they are easier to swallow than liquids and watery puréed food.
- Add commercial thickeners to change liquids to a semisolid consistency.
- Offer amounts of a quarter- to a half-teaspoon.
- Observe for swallowing.
- Ask the patient to speak; if the patient's voice sounds normal, not wet and gurgly, the food is most likely in the esophagus. If not, have the patient swallow several more times and cough to clear the airway, or suction the pharynx.
- Check the mouth for pockets of food that remain unswallowed before offering more.
- Keep the patient in a sitting position for at least a half-hour after eating to avoid pulmonary complications should regurgitation or vomiting occur.

Feeding the Visually Impaired Patient

When caring for patients who are temporarily or permanently sightless:

- Place a thick towel across the patient's chest and over the lap.
- If the patient can eat independently, consider using dishes with rims or bowls to prevent spilling.
- Arrange as much as possible to have finger foods (foods that may be eaten with the hands) prepared for the patient.
- Describe the food and indicate where it is located on the tray.
- Guide the patient's hand to reinforce the location of food and utensils.
- Prepare the food by opening cartons, cutting bite-size pieces, adding salt and pepper, buttering bread, and pouring coffee.
- Use the analogy of a clock when describing where food may be found on the plate. For example, "The potatoes are at 3 o'clock."
- If the patient needs to be fed, tell him or her what kind of food is being offered with each mouthful.
- Devise a system by which the patient can indicate when he or she is ready for more food or beverage, such as asking or raising a finger.
- Do not rush the patient; eating should be done at a leisurely pace.

Assisting the Patient with Dementia

Dementia refers to the deterioration of previous intellectual capacity. It is a common problem among those with neurologic conditions such as Alzheimer's disease. These patients often can retain their ability to carry out activities of daily living, such as self-feeding, by keeping their attention and concentration and repeating actions over and over. Therefore, the following are useful nursing actions:

- Have the same staff person help the patient, if possible, to develop a rapport with the patient and promote continuity of care.
- Be consistent with the time and place for eating.
- Reduce or eliminate distractions within the environment to promote concentration on the task at hand.
- Place the food tray close to the patient, not the staff person, to communicate visually and spatially that the food is to be eaten by the patient.
- Remove wrappers, containers, and food covers to reduce confusion.
- Pour milk from the carton into a glass so it is easily recognizable.
- Encourage the patient's participation by offering finger foods and utensils to stimulate awareness and memory.
- Ensure that the patient can see at least one other person who is also eating. This serves as a model for the desired behavior.
- Guide the hand with food to the patient's mouth.
- Reinforce a desired response by praising, touching, and smiling at the patient.
- Remain with the patient. Do not begin feeding, leave, and then return, because this interrupts the patient's attention and concentration.

Nursing Care Plan

Impaired Swallowing

Assessment

Subjective Data

States, "I'm losing weight. I've almost given up trying to eat. I get more on me than in me since my stroke."

Objective Data

67-year-old woman recovering from a cerebrovascular accident (CVA). Gag reflex is present on stimulating the throat with a cotton-tipped swab. Produces an audible cough on request. Food lodges in pockets of left cheek. Drools from left side of mouth when attempting to swallow.

Diagnosis

Impaired swallowing related to neuromuscular impairment

Plan

Goal

The patient will demonstrate swallowing techniques that result in an empty mouth and maintenance of present weight of 110 lb by 2/5.

Orders: 2/1

1. Weigh every day on standing scale at 0730 wearing slippers, patient gown, and cotton robe.
2. Maintain suction machine, suction catheter, and oxygen per mask at the bedside in case of choking.
3. Seat in a high-backed chair for meals.
4. Cover chest with towel.
5. Open sealed food containers.
6. Sit with patient and remain throughout meals.
7. Remind to place food on the unaffected (right) side of the mouth.
8. Instruct to take small portions of food with each bite and chew well before attempting to swallow.
9. Repeat the following instructions for swallowing:
   - Work the food to the back of mouth.
   - Lift tongue up to the roof of mouth.
   - Close lips tightly.
   - Lower chin toward chest.
   - Swallow once and repeat.
10. Give patient a hand mirror for inspecting the mouth.
11. Have patient use a finger to clear food from the cheek, and repeat instructions for swallowing. ________ T. BERENSON, RN

Implementation (Documentation)

2/2 0745 Weighed 109 lbs using standing scale. Up in chair for breakfast. Places food on R side of mouth with spoon. Given instructions for swallowing as identified in care plan. ________ V. HILL, RN

Evaluation (Documentation)

0830 Mouth suctioned twice. Food still under tongue after several swallowing attempts. States, "I can't feel where the food's at." Used a mirror to visualize retained food. Able to swallow food after finger sweep. Ate half of breakfast. States, "I'm so discouraged. I don't think I'll ever be able to eat in public again." ________ V. HILL, RN

KEY CONCEPTS

- Nutrition is the process by which the body uses food. Malnutrition results from inadequate consumption of nutrients.
- The components of basic nutrition include adequate amounts of calories, proteins, carbohydrates, fats, vitamins, and minerals.
- Some factors that affect nutritional needs include age, height and weight, growth, activity, and health status.
- The food pyramid is a guide for promoting a healthy intake of food. It recommends the number of servings and the portion sizes for meat or its substitute, dairy products, fruits, vegetables, and grain products to acquire 2000 calories per day.

FOCUS ON OLDER ADULTS

- The nutritional status of older adults is affected by medical conditions, adverse medication effects, functional impairments, and psychosocial conditions, such as dementia, depression, and social isolation.
- Diminished senses of smell and taste interfere with an older adult's appetite and nutritional intake.
- Older adults often consume diets that are high in carbohydrates and other low-cost food items.
- Because older adults require fewer calories, they need to consume nutrient-dense foods such as meat, fruits, vegetables, and dairy products.
- Oral and dental problems are common in older adults and interfere with adequate nutrition.
- Older adults are encouraged to get dental care every 6 months and to practice good dental hygiene daily.
- Dry mouth (xerostomia), a common problem in older adults, is often due to medications or the effects of disease. A dry mouth interferes with chewing, swallowing, and the enjoyment of eating. People with dry mouth are encouraged to drink adequate amounts of noncaffeinated and nonalcoholic beverages.
- Older adults are likely to have chronic conditions, such as arthritis, and visual and hearing impairments, affecting their ability to perform activities of daily living for meeting their nutritional needs.
- Taking multiple medications increases the incidence of food–drug interactions among older adults. Some medications also cause constipation, diarrhea, loss of appetite, and other problems that interfere with the intake, digestion, and absorption of food.
- Oral infections, poorly fitting dentures, or vitamin deficiencies can cause a painful or burning tongue and other difficulties that interfere with eating.
- Dysphagia among older adults is often caused by neurologic conditions including a stroke, esophageal disorders such as dilated or constricted esophagus, or increased pressure from abdominal disorders.
- Some older adults have difficulty obtaining and preparing nutritious meals because of socioeconomic barriers such as low income and an inability to get to the grocery store.
- Environmental barriers such as high counters and cupboards prevent some older adults from storing and preparing a variety of foods.
- Psychosocial impairments such as dementia or depression interfere with food preparation, consumption, and enjoyment.
- Homebound older adults may benefit from receiving home-delivered meals. The nutrition of older adults who are isolated, depressed, or cognitively impaired may improve with participation in a group meal program. Home-delivered meals and group meal programs are widely available and are funded through the Older Americans Act. The National Eldercare Locator (800-667-1116) provides information about these programs.
- Low-income older adults are referred to their local Office or Commission on Aging for assistance in obtaining food stamps.
- For older adults with dementia, depression, or impaired vision, a home health nurse or a responsible person should check the refrigerator and freezer for spoiled and outdated food items at least weekly.

- Nutrition labels must indicate the serving size in household measurements and the daily value for specific nutrients per serving. They must meet specified criteria if they make health-related claims for the product.
- Protein complementation is the practice of combining two or more plant protein sources to obtain all the essential amino acids required for healthy nutrition.
- A diet history is the information obtained by asking a person to describe his or her eating habits and factors that may affect nutrition.
- Data that provide objective information about a person's nutritional status include anthropometric measurements, physical examination data, and results from laboratory tests.
- Problems commonly identified after performing a nutritional assessment include weight problems, anorexia, nausea, vomiting, and stomach gas.
- Common hospital diets are regular, light, soft, mechanical soft, full liquid, and clear liquid, and various therapeutic modifications to these diets.
- Nurses are generally responsible for ordering and canceling diets for patients, serving and collecting meal trays, helping patients eat, and recording the percentage of food eaten.
- Nurses must know the type of diet prescribed for each patient, the purpose for the diet, and its characteristics.
- The nutritional status of older adults is affected by age-related physical changes, underlying medical conditions, adverse effects of medication therapy, functional impairments, psychosocial conditions, and socioeconomic and environmental barriers.

CRITICAL THINKING EXERCISES

- Design a dinner menu for a young, middle-aged, and older adult that meets the daily requirements in the food pyramid but also reflects the patient's unique age-related differences.
- Take your own anthropometric measurements or those of another person, and analyze the information according to the norms provided in this chapter. Based on your analysis, what recommendations are appropriate?
- A patient tells the nurse that she eats the following every day: cereal, milk, and banana for breakfast; a sandwich made with processed meat, mayonnaise, and a soft drink for lunch; a candy bar in the late afternoon; and meat, potatoes, a vegetable, and a glass of milk for supper. In the late evening, she snacks on potato chips. Using the food pyramid, what recommendations would you make to improve this patient's nutrition?

SUGGESTED READINGS

Evans-Stoner N. Guidelines for care of the patient on home nutrition support. Nursing Clinics of North America 1997;32(4):769–775.

Evans-Stoner N. Nutritional assessment: a practical approach. Nursing Clinics of North America 1997;32(4):637–650.

Food and Drug Administration. Better life for special diets. FDA Consumer Publication #98-221. Washington DC, 1998. *www.fda/gov/fdac/foodlabel/special.html*

Galica LA. Parenteral nutrition. Nursing Clinics of North America 1997; 32(4):705–717.

Gamsa H. In it together: anorexia nervosa. Nursing Times 1997;93(31):30.

Gauwitz DF. How to protect the dysphagic stroke patient. American Journal of Nursing 1995;95(8):34–38.

Gerrior JL, Bell SJ, Wanke CA. Oral nutrition for the patient with HIV infection. Nursing Clinics of North America 1997;32(4):813–830.

Grace C. Nutrition and weight reduction. Nursing Times 1998;94(24):1–6.

Green C. Unhappy eater. Nursing Times 1997;93(31):24–25.

Herbert S. A team approach to the treatment of dysphagia. Nursing Times 1996;92(50):26–29.

Hudson P, Evans M. Vegetarian nutrition for pregnant women. Nursing Times 1997;93(33):50–51.

Kapp MB, Cox MJ. Views on providing nutrition and hydration. Journal of Gerontological Nursing 1998;24(7):7–8.

Kayser-Jones J. Mealtime in nursing homes: the importance of individualized care. Journal of Gerontological Nursing 1996;22(3):26–53.

Kayser-Jones J, Schell E. The effect of staffing on the quality of care at mealtime. Nursing Outlook 1997;45(2):64–72.

Keller VE. Management of nausea and vomiting in children. Journal of Pediatric Nursing: Nursing Care of Children and Families 1995;10(5):280–286.

King S. A brittle future—osteoporosis: a recognized complication of chronic anorexia nervosa in women. Nursing Times 1998;94(1):23–24.

Lord LM. Enteral access devices. Nursing Clinics of North America 1997; 32(4):685–704.

McConnel EA. Clinical do's and don'ts: administering parenteral nutrition. Nursing 1998;28(7):18.

Miller A. Know how: vitamins and minerals. Nursing Times 1997;93(34): 72–73.

North American Nursing Diagnosis Association. NANDA nursing diagnoses: definitions and classifications, 1999–2000. Philadelphia, NANDA, 1999.

Office of Disease Prevention and Health Promotion. Healthy people 2010. Washington DC, 1999.

Palmer D, MacFie J. Nutrition. Alternative intake: peripheral parenteral nutrition. Nursing Times 1997;93(49):62–66.

Petty C, Ferguson D, Landford MC. Management decisions: taking charge. What's to eat? Cancer patients help decide. RN 1998;61(10):23–24.

Purdy KS, Dwyer JT, Holland M, Goldberg DL, Dinardo J. You are what you eat. Pediatric Nursing 1996;22(5):391–401.

Rexrode KM, Carey VJ, Hennekens CH, et al. Abdominal adiposity and coronary heart disease in women. Journal of the American Medical Association 1998;280(21):1843–1848.

Salladay SA. Ethical problems. Withdrawing treatment: all or nothing. Nursing 1998;28(10):28.

Selanders LC. The power of environmental adaptation. Florence Nightingale's original theory for nursing practice. Journal of Holistic Nursing 1998;16 (2):227–243.

U.S. Department of Agriculture and U.S. Department of Health and Human Services. Nutrition and your health: dietary guidelines for Americans, 4th ed. Washington DC, 1995.

Whitmer MM. Hospice news. Dietary considerations for clients. Caring 1996;15(2):60–62.

Widell JA, Stevenson SS. Planning good nutrition on a low budget. Home Health 1998;28(10):64hh1–64hh2.

World Health Organization. Preventing and managing the global epidemic of obesity. Geneva, WHO, 1997. In National Institutes of Health. Clinical guidelines on the identification, evaluation, and treatment of overweight and obesity in adults. Publication #98-4083. Washington DC, NIH, 1998.

SKILL 14-1

SERVING AND REMOVING MEAL TRAYS

Suggested Action	Reason for Action
Assessment	
Check on the usual time for meals.	Facilitates planning nursing care
Determine which patients are undergoing tests, or for some other reason must have food withheld.	Ensures that therapeutic outcomes are not affected by eating
Note the type of diet currently prescribed for each patient.	Follows the patient's therapeutic management plan
Review the Kardex for information concerning patients' food allergies or food intolerances.	Reduces the potential for adverse reactions.
Planning	
Prepare patients so they are ready to eat at the designated time.	Ensures that food is served at its appropriate temperature
Meet patients' needs for comfort, hygiene, and elimination before the meal arrives.	Promotes appetite and eating
Help patients to a sitting position.	Assists ambulatory patients to a comfortable position
Implementation	
Wash hands before serving trays.	Prevents transmission of microorganisms
Deliver trays, one by one, as soon as possible.	Facilitates the enjoyment of eating through prompt delivery of food at its intended temperature
Compare the name on the tray with the name on the patient's identification bracelet, or ask the patient to identify himself or herself by name.	Avoids dietary errors
Place the tray so it is facing the patient.	Provides ease of access to food
Uncover the food and check its appearance.	Ensures that the tray is complete, orderly, and tidy
Assist the patient as necessary with opening cartons and preparing food.	Demonstrates consideration and facilitates independence
Replace food that is objectionable, or request special additional items from the dietary department.	Demonstrates respect for unique needs
Check if the patient has any further requests, like adjustment of the pillows or donning eyeglasses, before leaving the room.	Reduces inconveniences during meal time
Make sure the signal cord is handy in case a need arises later.	Provides a means for summoning assistance
Check on the patient's progress from time to time.	Indicates a willingness to provide assistance
Remove the food tray when the patient is finished eating.	Restores order and cleanliness to the environment
Record the amount of fluid consumed from the dietary tray on the bedside flow sheet, if the patient's fluid intake is being monitored.	Ensures accurate fluid assessment
Note the percentage of food that the patient has eaten.	Ensures that dietary intake is documented according to JCAHO using precise current standards rather than vague terms such as *good*, *fair*, and *poor*

continued

SKILL 14-1

SERVING AND REMOVING MEAL TRAYS *Continued*

Suggested Action	Reason for Action
Assist the patient to brush and floss his or her teeth, if desired.	Removes food residue that may support microbial growth
Place the patient in a position of comfort.	Demonstrates care and concern

Evaluation

- Patient states that hunger is satisfied.
- Majority of food is consumed.

Document

- Type of diet and percentage of food consumed

SAMPLE DOCUMENTATION*

Date and Time Ate 100% of mechanical soft diet with need for assistance. ____________ SIGNATURE/TITLE

CRITICAL THINKING

- Discuss ways that a tray of food can be made visually attractive to entice a patient to eat.
- Describe nursing actions that might be appropriate if a patient ate none or only some of the food that was served.

* *In many agencies the percentage of consumed food is recorded on a flow sheet or checklist. Other pertinent data are recorded within the medical record.*

SKILL 14-2

FEEDING A PATIENT

Suggested Action	Reason for Action
Assessment	
Compare the dietary information on the Kardex with the medical record.	Ensures accuracy in therapeutic management
Verify that food or fluids are not being temporarily withheld.	Prevents delaying or having to cancel diagnostic tests
Determine whether the patient's fluid intake is being measured.	Ensures accurate documentation of data
Assess the patient to determine what or how much assistance is necessary.	Aids in identifying specific problems and selecting nursing interventions
Review the medical record to see how well and how much the patient has eaten during previous meals, and weight trends.	Helps in establishing realistic goals and evaluating progress
Review the characteristics of the diet order.	Helps in determining whether the correct food is being served
Analyze the purpose for the prescribed diet.	Assists in evaluating therapeutic responses

continued

SKILL 14-2

FEEDING A PATIENT *Continued*

Suggested Action	Reason for Action
Assess the patient's needs for elimination or relief from pain, nausea, fatigue.	Identifies unmet physiologic needs
Check the medication record for drugs that must be administered before or with meals.	Facilitates optimal drug absorption and reduces drug side effects
Planning	
Set realistic goals for how much food the patient will eat and how much the patient will participate with self-feeding.	Establishes criteria for evaluating patient responses
Select appropriate nursing measures for promoting patient comfort, such as administering an analgesic.	Helps resolve problems that, if ignored, may interfere with eating
Complete priority responsibilities for assigned patients.	Allows a period during which feeding is uninterrupted
Provide oral hygiene and handwashing before the tray is served.	Controls the transmission of microorganisms; promotes appetite and aesthetics
Prepare medications that must be given before or with meals, or delegate that responsibility.	Coordinates drug and nutritional therapy
Clear clutter and soiled articles from the eating area.	Promotes orderliness and a sanitary environment
Implementation	
Wash hands before preparing food.	Prevents transmission of microorganisms
Obtain or clean special utensils or containers that have been adapted for use by a patient with a physical disability, such as a fork to which a hand grip has been attached.	Promotes independence and self-reliance
Raise the head of the bed to a sitting position, or assist patient to a chair.	Promotes safety by facilitating swallowing
Check that the correct diet and tray are served to the correct patient.	Indicates responsibility and accountability for therapeutic management
Cover the patient's upper chest and lap with a napkin or towel.	Protects bedclothes and linen
Sit beside or across from patient.	Promotes socialization and communication
Uncover the food, open cartons, season food.	Increases gastric secretions and motility
Encourage the patient to assist, to the limit of his or her abilities.	Maintains or supports independence and self-care
Avoid rushing.	Communicates a relaxed atmosphere while eating
Collaborate with the patient on which foods are desired before loading a fork or spoon.	Accommodates individual preferences
Provide manageable amounts of food with each bite.	Prevents choking or airway obstruction
For a stroke patient, direct the food toward the unparalyzed side of the mouth.	Places food in an area where there is feeling and muscle control for chewing and swallowing
Give the patient time to chew thoroughly and swallow.	Chewing aids digestion by grinding the food and mixing it with saliva and enzymes.
Let the patient indicate when ready for more food or a sip of beverage.	Promotes an independent locus of control

continued

SKILL 14-2

FEEDING A PATIENT *Continued*

Suggested Action	Reason for Action
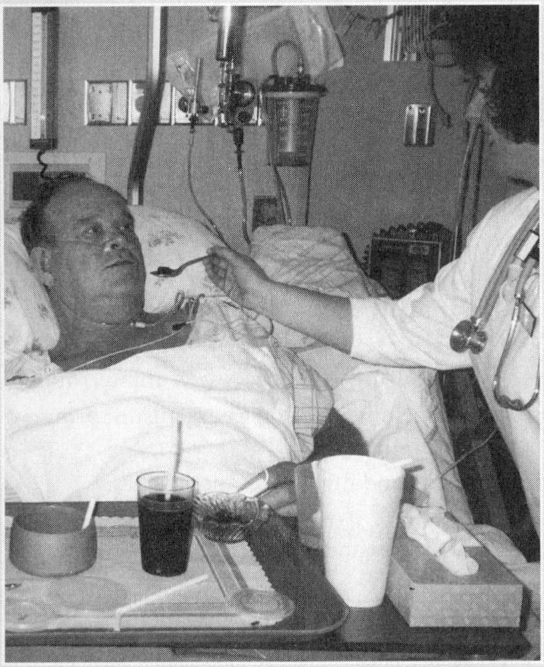 **Feeding a patient. (Courtesy of Ken Timby.)**	
Talk with the patient about pleasant subjects.	Combines eating with socialization
Record fluid intake if the patient's intake is being measured.	Documents essential assessment data
Remove the tray and make the patient comfortable. It is best for patients to remain in a sitting or semisitting position for at least 30 minutes after eating unless there is a medical reason for doing otherwise.	A sitting position prevents the reflux of stomach contents into the esophagus and reduces the potential for aspiration.
Offer the patient an opportunity for oral hygiene.	Removes sugar and starches that support microbial growth and tooth decay
Estimate the amount of food that has been eaten.	Provides data for determining current and future nutritional needs

Evaluation

- Patient eats approximately 75% of meal.
- Patient maintains body weight.
- Patient participates at maximum capacity.

Document

- Type of diet
- Percentage of food consumed*
- Tolerance of food
- Patient's ability to participate
- Problems encountered with chewing or swallowing
- Approaches taken to resolve problems

continued

SKILL 14-2

FEEDING A PATIENT *Continued*

SAMPLE DOCUMENTATION

Date and Time Stated "I'm full" after consuming 75% of full liquid diet. Unable to hold spoon or glass, but could direct straw into mouth. ________________________ SIGNATURE, TITLE

CRITICAL THINKING

- What techniques could a nurse recommend if a family member assumed responsibility for feeding a person being cared for in the home?
- What food modifications are appropriate if the person being fed has no teeth or dentures?
- What actions are useful for ensuring that food is maintained at the desired temperature, both hot and cool?

** In many agencies the percentage of consumed food is recorded on a flow sheet or checklist. Other pertinent data are recorded within the medical record.*

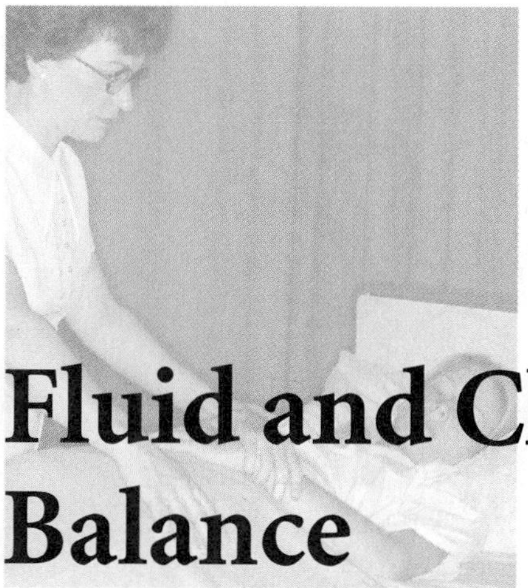

CHAPTER 15

Fluid and Chemical Balance

CHAPTER OUTLINE

NURSING GUIDELINES

INCREASING ORAL INTAKE
RESTRICTING ORAL FLUIDS
SELECTING A VENIPUNCTURE SITE
REMOVING AIR BUBBLES FROM IV TUBING
DISCONTINUING AN IV INFUSION
ADMINISTERING TPN

SKILLS

SKILL 15-1: RECORDING INTAKE AND OUTPUT
SKILL 15-2: PREPARING INTRAVENOUS SOLUTIONS
SKILL 15-3: STARTING AN INTRAVENOUS INFUSION
SKILL 15-4: CHANGING IV SOLUTION CONTAINERS
SKILL 15-5: CHANGING IV TUBING
SKILL 15-6: INSERTING A MEDICATION LOCK
SKILL 15-7: ADMINISTERING A BLOOD TRANSFUSION

NURSING CARE PLAN

FLUID VOLUME DEFICIT

KEY TERMS

active transport
air embolism
anions
cations
circulatory overload
colloid solutions
colloidal osmotic pressure
colloids
crystalloid solutions
dehydration
drop factor
electrochemical neutrality
electrolytes
emulsion
extracellular fluid
facilitated diffusion
filtration
fluid imbalance
hydrostatic pressure
hypertonic solution
hypervolemia
hypoalbuminemia
hypotonic solution
hypovolemia
infiltration
infusion pump
intake and output
intermittent venous access device
interstitial fluid
intracellular fluid
intravascular fluid
intravenous fluids
ions
isotonic solution
needleless systems
nonelectrolytes
osmosis
parenteral nutrition
passive diffusion
peripheral parenteral nutrition
phlebitis
ports
pulmonary embolus
third-spacing
thrombus formation
total parenteral nutrition
venipuncture
volumetric controller

LEARNING OBJECTIVES

An understanding of the content within this chapter will be evidenced by the student's ability to:

- Name four components of body fluid.
- List five physiologic transport mechanisms for distributing fluid and its constituents.
- Name 10 assessments that provide data about a patient's fluid status.
- Describe three methods for maintaining or restoring fluid volume.
- Describe four methods for reducing fluid volume.
- List six reasons for administering intravenous fluids.
- Differentiate between crystalloid and colloid solutions, and give examples of each.
- Explain the terms isotonic, hypotonic, and hypertonic when used in reference to intravenous solutions.
- List four factors that affect the choice of tubing used to administer intravenous solutions.

- Name three techniques for infusing intravenous solutions.
- Discuss at least five criteria for selecting a vein when administering intravenous fluid.
- List seven complications associated with intravenous fluid administration.
- Discuss two purposes for inserting an intermittent venous access device.
- Identify three differences between administering blood and crystalloid solutions.
- Name at least five types of transfusion reactions.
- Explain the concept of parenteral nutrition.

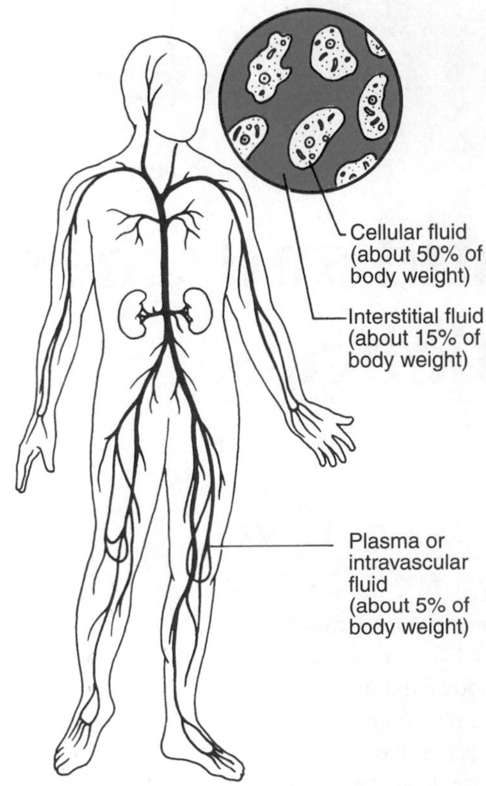

FIGURE 15–1. Average distribution of body fluid.

Body fluid is a mixture of water, chemicals called electrolytes and nonelectrolytes, and blood cells. Water, the vehicle for transporting these substances, is the very essence of life. Because water is not stored in any great reserve, daily replacement is the key to maintaining survival. In this chapter, the mechanisms for maintaining fluid balance and restoring fluid volume and the components in body fluid are discussed.

Body Fluid

WATER

The human body is composed of approximately 45% to 75% water. Body water is normally supplied and replenished from three sources: drinking liquids, consuming food, and metabolizing nutrients. Once the water is absorbed, it is distributed among various locations, called compartments, within the body.

Fluid Compartments

Body fluid is located in two general compartments. **Intracellular fluid** (fluid inside cells) represents the greatest proportion of water in the body. The remaining body fluid, **extracellular fluid** (fluid outside cells), is further subdivided into **interstitial fluid** (fluid in the tissue space between and around cells) and **intravascular fluid** (watery plasma, or serum, portion of blood) (Fig. 15-1). The percentage of water in these compartments varies with age and gender (Table 15-1).

ELECTROLYTES

Electrolytes (chemical compounds, such as sodium and chloride, that are dissolved, absorbed, and distributed in body fluid and possess an electrical charge) are obtained from dietary sources of food and beverages. They are essential for maintaining cellular, tissue, and organ functions. For example, electrolytes affect fluid balance and complex chemical activities such as muscle contraction and the formation of enzymes, acids, and bases (refer to the discussion of minerals in Chap. 14).

Collectively, electrolytes are called **ions** (substances that carry either a positive or negative electrical charge). **Cations** (electrolytes with a positive charge) and **anions** (electrolytes with a negative charge) are present in equal amounts overall, but their concentrations vary in each of the body's fluid compartments (Table 15-2). For example, there are more potassium ions inside cells than outside.

Electrolytes are measured in the serum of blood specimens, and the amount is reported in *milliequivalents* (mEq). When one or more cations or anions become excessive or deficient, an electrolyte imbalance occurs and can lead to dangerous physiologic problems. In many situations, changes in fluid volumes are accompanied by electrolyte imbalances.

TABLE 15–1. **Percentages of Body Fluid According to Age and Gender**

Fluid Compartment	Infants	Adult Men	Adult Women	Elderly
Intravascular	4%	4%	5%	5%
Interstitial	25%	11%	10%	15%
Intracellular	48%	45%	35%	25%
Total	77%	60%	50%	45%

TABLE 15–2. **Major Serum Electrolytes**

Electrolyte	Chemical Symbol	Cation/Anion	Normal Serum Level	Predominant Compartment
Sodium	Na	Cation	135–148 mEq/L	ECF
Potassium	K	Cation	3.5–5.0 mEq/L	ICF
Chloride	Cl	Anion	90–110 mEq/L	ECF
Phosphate	PO_4	Anion	1.7–2.6 mEq/L	ICF
Calcium	Ca	Cation	2.1–2.6 mEq/L	ICF
Magnesium	Mg	Cation	1.3–2.1 mEq/L	ICF
Bicarbonate	HCO_3	Anion	22–26 mEq/L	ICF

ECF, extracellular compartment; ICF, intracellular compartment

NONELECTROLYTES

Nonelectrolytes (chemical compounds that remain bound together when dissolved in a solution) do not conduct electricity. The chemical end-products of carbohydrate, protein, and fat metabolism—namely glucose, amino acids, and fatty acids—provide a continuous supply of nonelectrolytes.

In the absence of metabolic disease, as long as a person consumes adequate amounts of nutrients, a stable amount of nonelectrolytes circulating in body fluid is maintained. Deficiency states occur when body fluid is lost or when the ability to eat is compromised.

BLOOD

Blood consists of 3 liters of plasma, or fluid, and 2 liters of blood cells, for a total circulating volume of 5 liters. Blood cells include erythrocytes, or red blood cells; leukocytes, or white blood cells; and platelets, also known as thrombocytes. For every 500 red blood cells, there are approximately 30 platelets and 1 white blood cell (Fischbach, 1996).

Any disorder that alters the volume of body fluid, whether it is fluid retention or loss, also affects the plasma volume of blood. Blood cell volume is affected by chronic bleeding or hemorrhage, infection, chemicals or conditions that destroy the blood cells once they have been produced, and disorders that affect the bone marrow's production of blood cells. Deficits in either fluid or cell volume are treated by administering fluid, whole blood or packed cells, or individual blood components.

FLUID AND ELECTROLYTE DISTRIBUTION MECHANISMS

Although fluid compartments are identified separately, water and the substances dissolved therein continuously circulate throughout all areas of the body. The movement and relocation of water and substances within body fluid are governed by physiologic transport mechanisms such as osmosis, filtration, passive diffusion, facilitated diffusion, and active transport (Fig. 15-2).

Osmosis

Osmosis (process that regulates the distribution of water) controls the movement of fluid from one location to another. Under the influence of osmosis, water moves through a semipermeable membrane like those surrounding body cells, capillary walls, and body organs and cavities, from an area where the fluid is more dilute to another area where the fluid is more

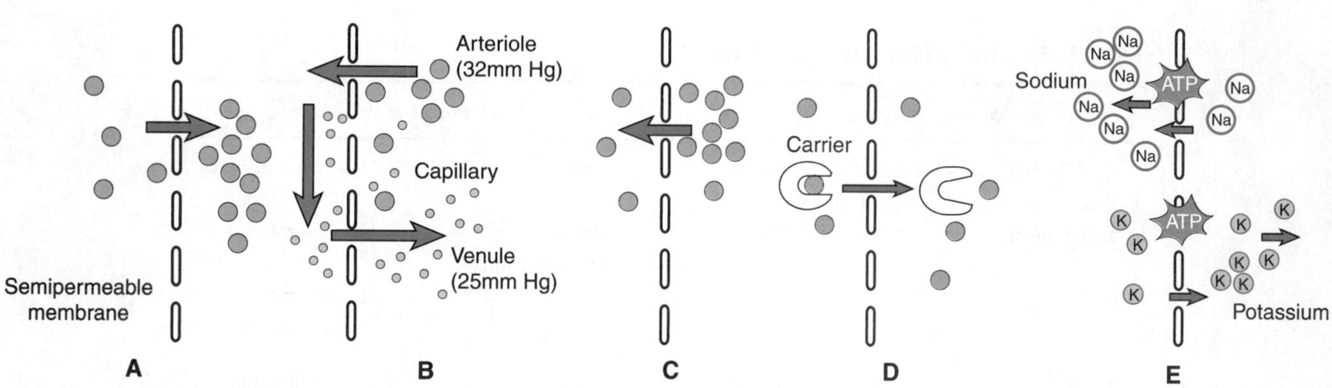

FIGURE 15–2. (*A*) Osmosis. (*B*) Filtration. (*C*) Passive diffusion. (*D*) Facilitated diffusion. (*E*) Active transport.

concentrated. Once the fluid is of equal concentration on both sides of the membrane, the transfer of fluid between compartments does not change appreciably, except volume for volume.

Osmosis is influenced by the presence and quantity of colloids on either side of the semipermeable membrane. **Colloids** (undissolved protein substances) such as albumin and blood cells within body fluids do not readily pass through membranes. Their very presence produces **colloidal osmotic pressure** (force for attracting water) that influences fluid volume in any given fluid location.

Filtration

Filtration (process that regulates the movement of water and substances from a compartment where the pressure is higher to one where the pressure is lower) is another mechanism that influences fluid distribution. The force of filtration is referred to as **hydrostatic pressure** (pressure exerted against a membrane). For example, at the arterial end of a capillary, the fluid is under higher pressure, due to the contraction of the left ventricle, than at the venous end. Consequently, fluid and dissolved substances are forced into the interstitial compartment at the capillary's arterial end. Water is then reabsorbed from the interstitial fluid in comparable amounts at the venous end of the capillary due to colloidal osmotic pressure. Filtration also governs the manner in which the kidney excretes fluid and wastes and then selectively reabsorbs water and substances that need to be conserved.

Passive Diffusion

Passive diffusion (physiologic process in which dissolved substances, such as electrolytes and gases, move from an area of higher concentration to an area of lower concentration through a semipermeable membrane) occurs without the expenditure of energy—hence the word *passive.* Passive diffusion facilitates **electrochemical neutrality** (identical balance of cations with anions) in any given fluid compartment. Like osmosis, passive diffusion remains fairly static once equilibrium is achieved.

Facilitated Diffusion

Facilitated diffusion (process in which certain dissolved substances require the assistance of a carrier molecule to pass from one side of a semipermeable membrane to the other) also regulates chemical balance. Facilitated diffusion distributes substances from an area of higher concentration to one that is lower. Glucose is an example of a substance distributed by facilitated diffusion.

Active Transport

Active transport (process of chemical distribution that requires an energy source) involves a substance called *adenosine triphosphate* (ATP). ATP provides energy to drive dissolved chemicals against the concentration gradient. In other words, it allows chemical distribution from an area of low concentration to one that is higher—just the opposite of passive diffusion.

An example of active transport is the *sodium-potassium pump system* on cellular membranes that regulates the movement of potassium from lower concentrations in the extracellular fluid into cells where it is more highly concentrated. It also moves sodium, which has a lower concentration within the cells, to extracellular fluid, where it is more abundant.

Metabolic disorders that diminish the supply of ATP seriously affect normal cellular functions by impairing the distribution of chemicals within intracellular and extracellular fluid.

FLUID REGULATION

In healthy adults, fluid intake generally averages approximately 2500 mL per day, but it can range from 1800 to 3000 mL per day with a similar volume of fluid loss (Table 15-3). Normal mechanisms for fluid loss are urination, bowel elimination, perspiration, and breathing. Losses from the skin in areas other than where sweat glands are located and from the vapor in exhaled air are referred to as *insensible losses* because they are, for practical purposes, unnoticeable and unmeasurable.

TABLE 15–3. **Daily Fluid Intake and Losses**

Sources of Fluid		Mechanisms of Fluid Loss	
Oral liquids	1,200–1,500 mL/day	Urine	1,200–1,700 mL/day
Food	700–1,000 mL/day	Feces	100–250 mL/day
Metabolism	200–400 mL/day	Perspiration	100–150 mL/day
		Insensible losses	
		Skin	350–400 mL/day
		Lungs	350–400 mL/day
Total	2,100–2,900 mL/day	**Total**	2,100–2,900 mL/day
Average intake	2,500 mL/day	**Average loss**	2,500 mL/day

Under normal conditions, several mechanisms maintain a match between fluid intake and output. For example, as body fluid becomes concentrated, the brain triggers the sensation of thirst, which then stimulates the person to drink. As fluid volume expands, the kidneys excrete a proportionate volume of water to maintain or restore proper balance.

However, there are circumstances in which oral intake or fluid losses are altered. Therefore, nurses assess patients for signs of fluid deficit or excess, particularly in those prone to fluid imbalances (Display 15-1).

Fluid Volume Assessment

Fluid status is assessed using a combination of physical assessment (Table 15-4) and measurement of intake and output volumes.

INTAKE AND OUTPUT

Intake and output (I&O; record of a patient's fluid intake and fluid loss over a 24-hour period) is one tool to assess fluid status. Agencies often specify which types of patients are automatically placed on I&O. Generally they include patients who:

- Have undergone surgery, until they are eating, drinking, and voiding in sufficient quantities
- Are receiving intravenous fluids
- Are receiving tube feedings
- Have some type of wound drainage or suction equipment
- Have urinary catheters, until it can be determined that they have an adequate output or are voiding well after the catheter has been removed

In addition, many agencies allow nurses to order I&O assessment for patients with an actual or potential fluid imbalance problem independently. The nurse discontinues the nursing order when the assessment is no longer indicated but consults with the physician if it has been medically ordered.

Each agency has a specific I&O form that is kept at the bedside so that the type of fluid and amounts can be conveniently recorded throughout the day (Fig. 15-3). The amounts are subtotaled at the end of each shift, or more frequently in critical care areas. The grand total is documented in a designated area in the medical record—for example, on the graphics sheet with other vital sign information.

Fluid Intake

Fluid intake is the sum of all fluid consumed by a patient or instilled into the body. It includes:

- All the liquids a patient drinks
- The liquid equivalent of melted ice chips, which is half of the frozen volume

TABLE 15–4. **Signs of Fluid Imbalance**

Assessment	Fluid Deficit	Fluid Excess
Weight	Weight loss ≥ 2 lbs/24 hr	Weight gain ≥ 2 lbs/24 hr
Blood pressure	Low	High
Temperature	Elevated	Normal
Pulse	Rapid, weak, thready	Full, bounding
Respirations	Rapid, shallow	Moist, labored
Urine	Scant, dark yellow	Light yellow
Stool	Dry, small volume	Bulky
Skin	Warm, flushed, dry Poor skin turgor	Cool, pale, moist Pitting edema
Mucous membranes	Dry, sticky	Moist
Eyes	Sunken	Swollen
Lungs	Clear	Crackles, gurgles
Breathing	Effortless	Dyspnea, orthopnea
Energy	Weak	Fatigues easily
Jugular neck veins	Flat	Distended
Cognition	Reduced	Reduced
Consciousness	Sleepy	Anxious

DISPLAY 15–1

Conditions that Predispose to Fluid Imbalances

Fluid Deficit

- Starvation
- Impaired swallowing
- Vomiting
- Gastric suction
- Diarrhea
- Laxative abuse
- Potent diuretics
- Hemorrhage
- Major burns
- Draining wounds
- Fever and sweating
- Exercise and sweating
- Environmental heat and humidity

Fluid Excess

- Kidney failure
- Heart failure
- Rapid administration of intravenous fluid or blood
- Administration of albumin
- Corticosteroid drug therapy
- Excessive intake of sodium
- Pregnancy
- Premenstrual fluid retention

24 HOUR INTAKE/OUTPUT RECORD

DATE	WEIGHT	TIME	TYPE OF WEIGHT
2-17	137#	0700	☒ STANDING ☐ CHAIR ☐ BED
CVP READING: TIME / READING	TIME / READING	TIME / READING	

INTAKE 7-3 SHIFT

Time	Oral	IV	Piggyback	Blood	Tube/Feed
0730	100	600			
0900		↓	50		
1130	240	↓			
1300		↓	50		
8 HR TOTAL	340	600	100		
		8° GRAND TOTAL			1040

OUTPUT 7-3 SHIFT

Time	Irrig.	Urine	NG	Emesis	Other	Tube	Tube	BM
0700		250						
0800				100				
1200		300						
1400		400						
		950		100				
							8° GRAND TOTAL	1050

INTAKE 3-11 SHIFT

Time	Oral	IV	Piggyback	Blood	Tube/Feed
1600	30				
1700		600	50		
1730	30	↓			
2000	100	↓			
8 HR TOTAL	160	600	50		
		8° GRAND TOTAL			810

OUTPUT 3-11 SHIFT

Time	Irrig.	Urine	NG	Emesis	Other	Tube	Tube	BM
1530				50				
1800		200						
2200		300						
		500		50				
							8° GRAND TOTAL	550

INTAKE 11-7 SHIFT

Time	Oral	IV	Piggyback	Blood	Tube/Feed
0030	30	600			
		↓			
8 HR TOTAL	30	600			
		8° GRAND TOTAL			630
		24° GRAND TOTAL			2480

OUTPUT 11-7 SHIFT

Time	Irrig.	Urine	NG	Emesis	Other	Tube	Tube	BM
0100		300						
0400		200						
0600		100						
		600						
							8° GRAND TOTAL	600
							24° GRAND TOTAL	2200

FORM 96 (9/92) CIRRUS 3025

24 HOUR INTAKE / OUTPUT RECORD

FIGURE 15–3. Intake and output volumes are recorded throughout a 24-hour period and subtotaled at the end of each 8-hour shift.

- Foods that are liquid by the time they are swallowed, such as gelatin, ice cream, and thin cooked cereal
- Fluid infusions, such as intravenous solutions
- Fluid instillations (for example, those administered through feeding tubes or tube irrigations)

Fluid volumes are recorded in mL. The approximate equivalent for 1 ounce is 30 mL, a teaspoon is 5 mL, and a tablespoon is 15 mL. Packaged beverage containers such as milk cartons usually indicate the specific fluid volume on the label. Commonly, hospitals and nursing homes identify the volume equivalents contained in the cups, glasses, and bowls used to serve food and beverages from the dietary department (Display 15-2). If an equivalency chart is not available, the nurse should use a calibrated container (Fig. 15-4) to measure specific amounts; estimated volumes are usually inaccurate.

Fluid Output

Fluid output is the sum of liquid eliminated from the body, including:

- Urine
- Emesis (vomitus)
- Blood loss
- Diarrhea
- Wound or tube drainage
- Aspirated irrigations

In some cases where accurate assessment is critical to a patient's treatment, the nurse weighs wet linens, pads, diapers, or dressings and subtracts the weight of a similar dry item. An estimate of fluid loss is based on the equivalent: 1 pound (0.47 kg) = 1 pint (475 mL).

Patient cooperation is needed for accurate I&O records. Therefore, patients whose I&O volumes are being recorded are informed about the purpose and goals for fluid replacement or restrictions and the ways they can assist in the procedure.

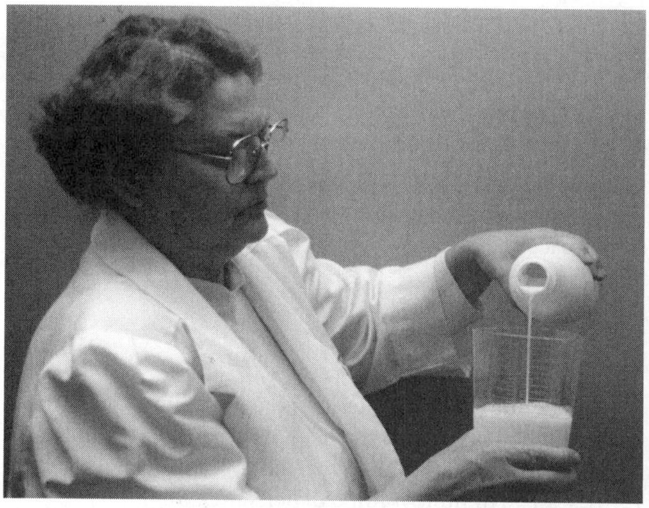

FIGURE 15–4. Calibrated containers used to measure liquid volumes. (Courtesy of Ken Timby.)

Patient Teaching

Recording Intake and Output

Teach the patient or the family to do the following:

- Write down the amount or notify the nurse whenever oral fluid is consumed.
- Use a common household measurement, such as 1 glass or cup, to describe the volume consumed, or refer to an equivalency chart.
- Do not let a staff person remove a dietary tray until the fluid amounts have been recorded.
- Do not empty a urinal or urinate directly into the toilet bowl.
- Make sure that a measuring device is in the toilet bowl if the bathroom is used for voiding (Fig. 15-5).
- If a urinal needs to be emptied, call the nurse or empty its contents into a calibrated container.
- Use a container such as a bedpan or bedside commode if diarrhea occurs. Notify the nurse to measure the contents before it is emptied.
- If vomiting occurs, use an emesis basin rather than the toilet.

Suggested actions for maintaining an I&O record are provided in Skill 15-1.

DISPLAY 15–2

Volume Equivalents for Common Containers

Container	Volume (mL)
Teaspoon	5
Tablespoon	15
Juice glass	120
Drinking glass	240
Coffee cup	210
Milk carton	240
Water pitcher	900
Paper cup	180
Soup bowl	200
Cereal bowl	120
Ice cream cup	120
Gelatin dish	90

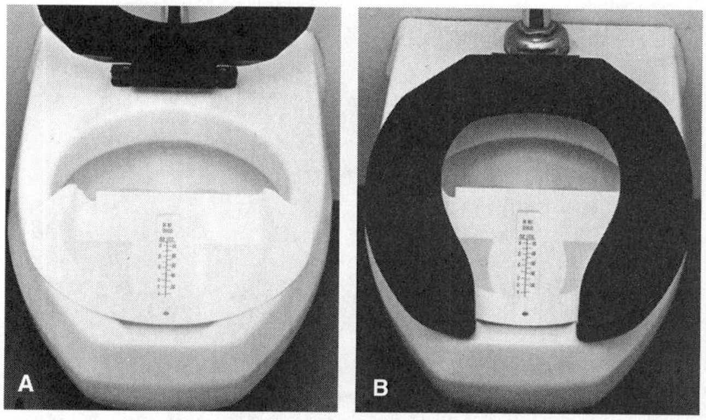

FIGURE 15–5. (*A*) The toilet seat is raised to insert a calibrated container. (*B*) The urine is collected in the container. (Courtesy of Ken Timby.)

Common Fluid Imbalances

Fluid imbalance (general term describing any of several conditions in which the body's water is not in the proper volume or location within the body) can be life-threatening. Common fluid imbalances include hypovolemia, hypervolemia, and third-spacing.

HYPOVOLEMIA

Hypovolemia (low volume in the extracellular fluid compartments), if untreated, results in **dehydration** (fluid deficit in both extracellular and intracellular compartments) (Fig. 15-6). Causes of fluid volume deficits include:

- Inadequate fluid intake
- Fluid loss in excess of fluid intake
- Translocation of large volumes of intravascular fluid to the interstitial compartment or to areas with only potential spaces, such as the peritoneal cavity, pericardium, and pleural space

Fluid balance is restored by treating the cause of hypovolemia, increasing oral intake, administering intravenous fluid replacements, controlling fluid losses, or a combination of these measures.

Nursing Guidelines For

Increasing Oral Intake

☑ Explain to the patient the reasons for increasing consumption of oral fluids.
RATIONALE: This facilitates patient cooperation.

☑ Obtain a list of beverages the patient enjoys drinking.
RATIONALE: This promotes patient compliance.

☑ Develop a schedule for providing small portions of the total fluid volume over a 24-hour period.
RATIONALE: Scheduling ensures that the final goal is reached by meeting short-term goals.

☑ Plan to provide the bulk of the projected fluid intake at times when the patient is awake.
RATIONALE: This avoids disturbing sleep.

☑ Offer verbal recognition and frequent feedback, or design a method for demonstrating the patient's progress—for example, a bar graph or pie chart.
RATIONALE: Positive reinforcement encourages compliance and maintains goal-directed efforts.

☑ Keep fluids handy at the bedside and place them in containers the patient can handle.
RATIONALE: Availability and convenience promote compliance.

☑ Vary the types of fluid, serving glass, or container frequently.
RATIONALE: This reduces boredom and maintains interest in working toward the goal.

☑ Serve fluids in small containers and in small amounts.
RATIONALE: This avoids overwhelming the patient.

☑ Ensure that fluids are at an appropriate temperature.
RATIONALE: This promotes pleasure and enjoyment.

☑ Include gelatin, popsicles, ice cream, and sherbet as alternatives to liquid beverages (if allowed).
RATIONALE: These items provide texture and serve as an alternative to items that are sipped or consumed from a glass.

HYPERVOLEMIA

Hypervolemia (higher-than-normal volume of water in the intravascular fluid compartment) is another example of a fluid imbalance. As the excess volume of fluid is distributed to the interstitial space, edema may be noted. When fluid accumulates in dependent areas of the body (those influenced by gravity), the tissue pits (forms indentations) when compressed (see Chap. 12). Edema (Fig. 15-7) does not usually occur unless there is a 3-liter excess in body fluid. Hypervolemia can lead to **circulatory overload** (severely compromised heart function) if it remains unresolved.

Fluid balance is restored by treating the disorder contributing to the increased fluid volume, by restricting or lim-

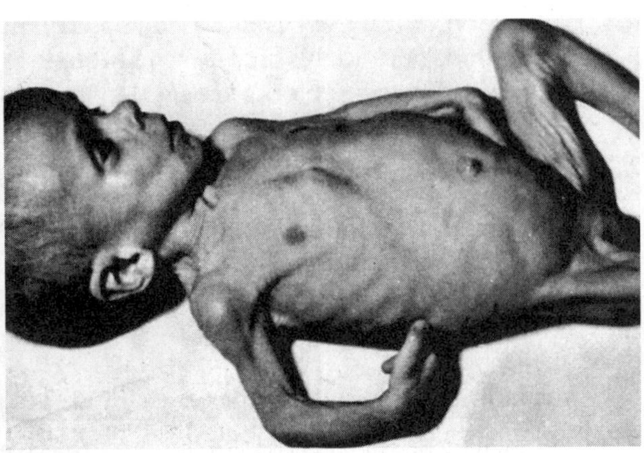

FIGURE 15–6. A severe case of dehydration.

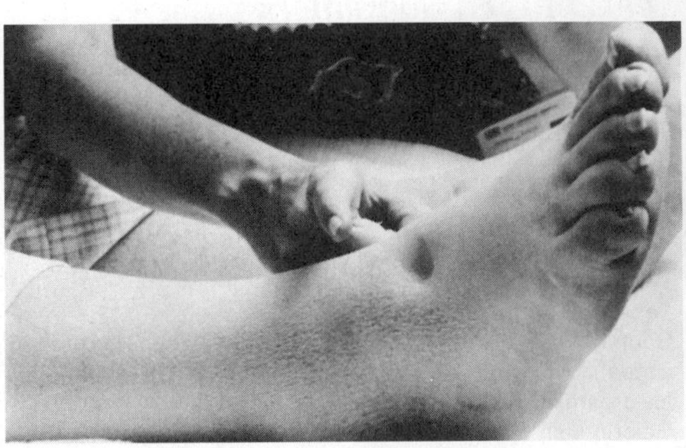

FIGURE 15–7. Evidence of pitting edema.

iting oral fluids, reducing salt consumption (Display 15-3), discontinuing intravenous fluid infusions or reducing the infusing volume, administering drugs that promote urine elimination, or a combination of these interventions.

Nursing Guidelines For

Restricting Oral Fluids

- Explain the purpose for the restrictions.
  RATIONALE: This promotes patient cooperation.
- Identify the total amount of fluid the patient may consume, using measurements with which the patient is familiar.
  RATIONALE: An explanation helps the patient understand the extent of the restrictions.
- Work out a plan for distributing the permitted volume over a 24-hour period with the patient.
  RATIONALE: Including the patient in planning promotes cooperation.
- Ration the fluid so that the patient will be able to consume beverages between meals as well as at mealtimes.
  RATIONALE: This schedule ensures that the patient's thirst will be relieved.
- Avoid sweet drinks and foods that are dry or salty.
  RATIONALE: This reduces thirst and the desire for fluid.
- Serve liquids at their proper temperature.
  RATIONALE: This demonstrates concern for the patient's pleasure and enjoyment.
- Offer ice chips as an occasional substitute for liquids.
  RATIONALE: Ice chips appear to contain more liquid than they actually do, and eating them prolongs the time over which the fluid is consumed.
- Provide water or other fluid in a plastic squeeze bottle or spray atomizer.
  RATIONALE: These devices provide only a small volume of fluid.
- Help the patient with frequent oral hygiene.
  RATIONALE: Oral hygiene relieves thirst, moistens oral mucous membranes, and prevents drying and chapping of lips.
- Allow the patient to rinse the mouth with water but not swallow it.
  RATIONALE: Rinsing reduces thirst and keeps the mouth moist.

DISPLAY 15-3

Foods High in Salt (Sodium)

- Processed meats such as frankfurters and cold cuts
- Smoked fish
- Frozen egg substitutes
- Peanut butter
- Dairy products, especially hard cheese
- Powdered cocoa or hot chocolate mixes
- Canned vegetables, especially sauerkraut
- Pickles
- Tomato and tomato–vegetable juice
- Canned soup and bouillon
- Boxed casserole mixes
- Baking mixes
- Salted snack foods
- Seasonings such as catsup, gravy mixes, soy sauce, monosodium glutamate (MSG), pickle relish, tartar sauce

THIRD-SPACING

Third-spacing (movement of intravascular fluid to nonvascular fluid compartments, where it becomes trapped and useless) is generally manifested by tissue swelling or fluid that accumulates in a body cavity such as the peritoneum (Fig. 15-8). Third-spacing is commonly associated with disorders in which albumin levels are low. Causes of **hypoalbuminemia** (deficit of albumin in the blood) include liver failure, chronic kidney disease, and disorders in which the capillary and cellular permeability is altered, such as burns and severe allergic reactions.

Depletion of fluid in the intravascular space may lead to hypotension and shock; thus, fluid therapy becomes challenging. The priority is to restore the circulatory volume by providing intravenous fluids, sometimes in large volumes at rapid rates. Blood transfusions or the administration of albumin by intravenous infusion is also used to restore colloidal osmotic pressure and pull the trapped fluid back into the intravascular space. When this occurs, patients who were previously hypovolemic can suddenly become hypervolemic. Patients who receive albumin replacement are monitored closely for signs of circulatory overload.

Intravenous Fluid Administration

Policies and practices vary concerning how much responsibility practical/vocational nurses assume with intravenous

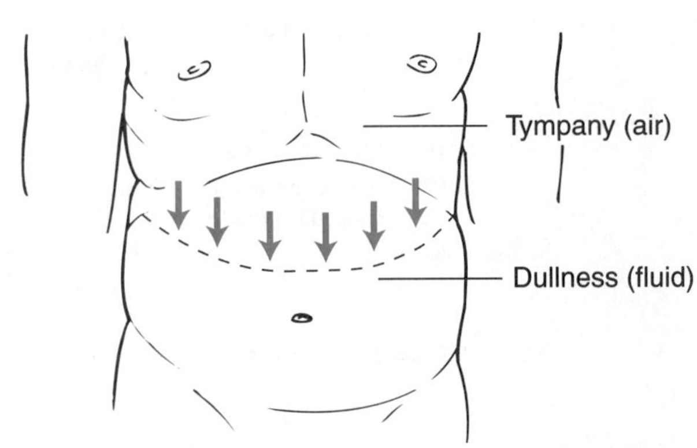

FIGURE 15-8. Fluid accumulation within the peritoneal cavity. Dullness on percussion indicates fluid, whereas tympany indicates air.

fluid therapy. The discussion that follows is provided to meet the needs of nurses who are expected to administer intravenous fluids.

Intravenous (IV) **fluids** (solutions infused into a patient's vein) are used to:

- Maintain or restore fluid balance when oral replacement is inadequate or impossible
- Maintain or replace electrolytes
- Administer water-soluble vitamins
- Provide a source of calories
- Administer drugs (see Chap. 35)
- Replace blood and blood products

TYPES OF SOLUTIONS

There are two types of IV solutions: crystalloid and colloid. **Crystalloid solutions** (water and other uniformly dissolved crystals, such as salt and sugar) and **colloid solutions** (water and molecules of suspended substances, such as blood cells, and blood products such as albumin) are commonly administered intravenously.

Crystalloid Solutions

Crystalloid solutions are classified as isotonic, hypotonic, and hypertonic (Table 15-5), depending on the concentration of dissolved substances in relation to plasma. The concentration of the solution influences the osmotic distribution of body fluid (Fig. 15-9).

Isotonic Solutions

An **isotonic solution** (one that contains the same concentration of dissolved substances as normally found in plasma) is generally administered to maintain fluid balance in patients who may not be able to eat or drink for a short period of time. Because of its equal concentration, an isotonic solution does not cause any appreciable redistribution of body fluid.

Hypotonic Solutions

A **hypotonic solution** (one that contains fewer dissolved substances than normally found in plasma) is administered to patients with fluid losses in excess of fluid intake, such as those who have diarrhea or vomiting. Because hypotonic

TABLE 15–5. **Types of Crystalloid Intravenous Solutions**

Solution	Components	Special Comments
Isotonic Solutions		
0.9% saline, also called normal saline	0.9 g of sodium chloride/100 mL of water	Amounts of sodium and chloride are physiologically equal to those found in plasma
5% dextrose and water, also called D_5W	5 g of dextrose (glucose/sugar)/100 mL of water	Isotonic when infused but the glucose metabolizes quickly, leaving a solution of dilute water
Ringer's solution or lactated Ringer's	Water and a mixture of sodium, chloride, calcium, potassium, bicarbonate, and in some cases lactate	Electrolyte replacement in amounts similar to those found in plasma. The lactate, when present, helps maintain acid–base balance.
Hypotonic Solutions		
0.45% sodium chloride, or also called half-strength saline	0.45 g of sodium chloride/100 mL of water	Smaller ratio of sodium and chloride than found in plasma, causing it to be less concentrated in comparison
5% dextrose in 0.45% saline	5 g of dextrose and 0.45 sodium chloride/100 mL of water	A quick source of energy from sugar, leaving a hypotonic salt solution
Hypertonic Solutions		
10% dextrose in water, also called $D_{10}W$	10 g of dextrose/100 mL of water	Twice the concentration of glucose than in plasma
3% saline	3 g of sodium chloride/100 mL of water	Dehydration of cells and tissues from the high concentration of salt in the plasma
20% dextrose in water	20 g of dextrose/100 mL water	Rapid increase in the concentration of sugar in the blood, causing a fluid shift to the intravascular compartment

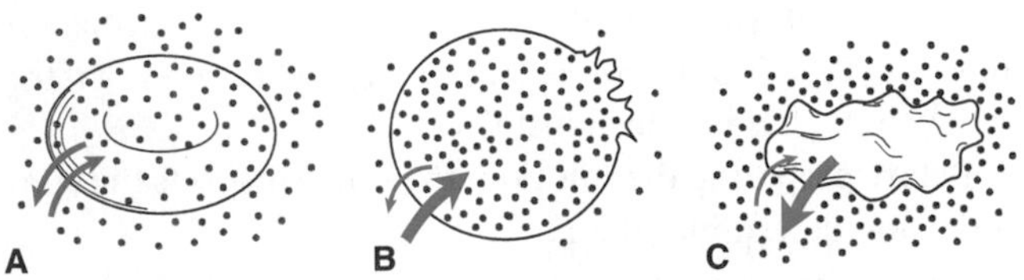

FIGURE 15–9. (*A*) Isotonic solutions. (*B*) Hypotonic solutions. (*C*) Hypertonic solutions. (Timby BK, Scherer JS, Smith, NJ.: Introductory Medical–Surgical Nursing, 7th ed, p 245. Philadelphia, Lippincott Williams & Wilkins, 1999)

solutions are dilute, the water in the solution passes through the semipermeable membrane of blood cells, causing them to swell. This temporarily increases blood pressure as it expands the circulating volume. The water also passes through capillary walls and becomes distributed within other body cells and the interstitial spaces. Hypotonic solutions, therefore, are an effective way to rehydrate patients with fluid deficits.

Hypertonic Solutions

A **hypertonic solution** (one that is more concentrated than body fluid) draws cellular and interstitial water into the intravascular compartment. This causes cells and tissue spaces to shrink. Hypertonic solutions are not used very frequently, except in extreme cases where it is necessary to reduce cerebral edema or expand the circulatory volume rapidly.

Colloid Solutions

Colloid solutions are used to replace circulating blood volume, because the suspended molecules pull fluid from other compartments. Examples of colloid solutions are blood, blood products, and solutions known as plasma expanders.

Blood

Whole blood and packed cells are probably the most common types of colloid solutions. One unit of whole blood contains approximately 475 mL of blood cells and plasma and 60 to 70 mL of preservative and anticoagulant (Smeltzer & Bare, 1996). Packed cells have most of the plasma removed and are preferred for patients who need cellular replacement but do not need, or may be harmed by, the administration of additional fluid.

Most of the blood given to patients comes from public donors. In some cases—for example, when a person anticipates the potential need for blood in the near future or when procedures are used to reclaim blood from wound drainage—the patient's own blood may be reinfused (see Chap. 27).

Blood Products

Several types of blood products are available for patients who need specific substances but do not need all the fluid or cellular components in whole blood (Table 15-6).

Blood Substitutes Because some people, such as Jehovah's Witnesses, object to receiving blood on religious grounds, and because of the risks for bloodborne diseases, such as hepatitis and AIDS, scientists have been working on perfecting blood substitutes. A chemical group called perfluorocarbons appears promising. Perfluorocarbons have been tested and used on a limited basis as an artificial substitute for human blood. The first of its kind, Fluosol DA, produced undesirable side effects: in clinical trials, recipients had a diminished resistance to infection and an increased risk for bleeding. Second-generation blood substitutes, such as Oxygent and Oxyfluor, are undergoing clinical trials. The data show that in smaller volumes, these new blood substitutes have avoided the need to replace 1 to 2 units of blood.

Other applications for perfluorocarbons are being explored because they have a smaller molecular size than red blood cells. This unique characteristic permits oxygen-carrying molecules

TABLE 15–6. **Types of Blood Products**

Blood Product	Description	Purpose for Administration
Platelets	Disk-shaped cellular fragments that promote coagulation of blood	Restores or improves the ability to control bleeding
Granulocytes	Types of white blood cells	Improves the ability to overcome infection
Plasma	Serum minus blood cells	Replaces clotting factors or increases intravascular fluid volume by increasing colloidal osmotic pressure
Albumin	Plasma protein	Pulls third-spaced fluid by increasing colloidal osmotic pressure
Cryoprecipitate	Mixture of clotting factors	Treats blood clotting disorders such as hemophilia

to pass through blood vessels that have been narrowed due to blood clots. Therefore, perfluorocarbons may be able to restore oxygen to tissues with impaired circulation, such as the brain after a stroke or the heart after a heart attack. Scientists theorize that the same effect could be used in the treatment of patients with sickle-cell crisis: pain could be relieved by oxygenating tissues whose blood supply is obstructed by sickled red blood cells. This same chemical could prolong the preservation of organs for transplantation and could improve the oxygenation of cancer cells, making them more vulnerable to standard treatments.

Besides perfluorocarbons, other substances are being tested in the search for a safe, effective substitute for whole blood. For example, solutions containing just hemoglobin have been used successfully in animals. Attempts are being made to recycle outdated red blood cells in donated blood by sealing them within a lipid capsule; this product is referred to as microencapsulated hemoglobin. With continued research, these substances, such as PolyHeme and Hemosol, may improve the treatment of disorders that previously required blood transfusions. Perfecting a blood substitute may reduce the need for human blood donors while decreasing the risk of bloodborne viral diseases.

Plasma Expanders

Various types of nonblood solutions are used to pull fluid into the vascular space. Two examples are dextran 40 (Rheomacrodex) and hetastarch (Hespan). These two substances are polysaccharides—large, insoluble complex carbohydrate molecules. When mixed with water, they form colloidal solutions. Because the suspended particles cannot move through semipermeable membranes when given intravenously, they attract water from other fluid compartments. The desired outcome is to increase the blood volume and raise the blood pressure. Consequently, plasma expanders are used as an economical and virus-free substitute for blood and blood products when treating hypovolemic shock.

PREPARATION FOR ADMINISTRATION

Regardless of the prescribed solution, the nurse prepares the solution for administration, performs a venipuncture, regulates the rate of administration, monitors the infusion, and discontinues the administration when fluid balance is restored.

Solution Selection

IV solutions are commonly stored in plastic bags containing 1000, 500, 250, 100, and 50 mL of solution. A few solutions are stocked in glass containers. The physician specifies the type of solution, additional additives, and the volume (in mL/hr) for infusing the solution. To reduce the potential for infection, IV solutions are replaced every 24 hours, even if the total volume has not been instilled.

Before preparing the solution, the nurse inspects the container and determines that:

- The solution is the one prescribed by the physician.
- The solution is clear and transparent.
- The expiration date has not elapsed.
- No leaks are apparent.
- A separate label is attached, identifying the type and amount of other drugs added to the commercial solution.

Tubing Selection

All IV tubing consists of a spike for accessing the solution, a drip chamber for holding a small amount of fluid, a length of plastic tubing with one or more ports for adding IV medications (see Chap. 35), and a roller or slide clamp to regulate the rate of infusion (Fig. 15-10).

The nurse then selects from several options:

- Primary (long) or secondary (short) tubing
- Vented or unvented tubing
- Microdrip (small drops) or macrodrip (large drop) chamber
- Unfiltered or filtered tubing
- Needle or needleless access ports

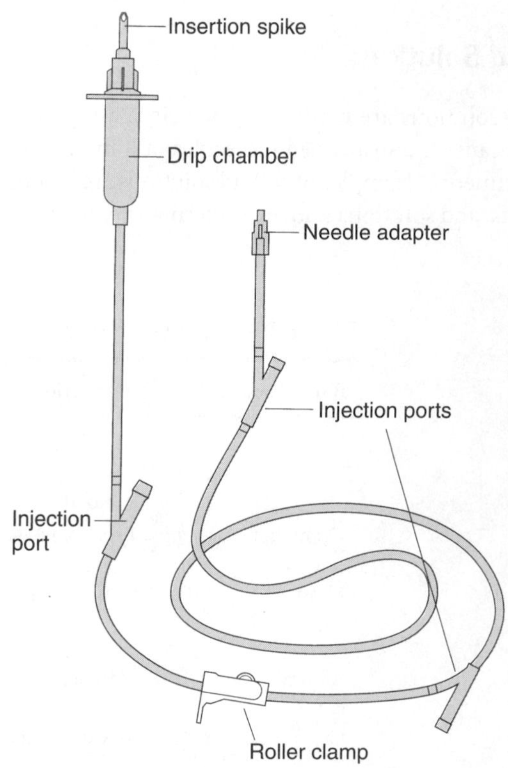

FIGURE 15–10. Basic intravenous tubing.

Primary Versus Secondary Tubing

Primary tubing is approximately 110″ (2.8 m) long; secondary tubing is 37″ (94 cm) long. These measurements vary among manufacturers. Primary tubing is used when the tubing must span the distance from a solution that hangs several feet above the infusion site. Secondary tubing, which is shorter, is used for administering smaller volumes of solution into a port within the primary tubing.

Vented Versus Unvented Tubing

Vented tubing draws air into the container; unvented tubing does not (Fig. 15-11). The choice depends on the type of container in which the solution is packaged. Vented tubing is necessary for administering solutions packaged in rigid glass containers; if unvented tubing is inserted into a glass bottle, the solution will not leave the container. Plastic bags of IV solutions do not need vented tubing, because the container collapses as the fluid infuses.

Drop Size

Drop size refers to the size of the opening through which the fluid is delivered into the tubing. The nurse determines whether it is more appropriate to use macrodrip tubing, which produces large drops, or microdrip tubing, which produces very small drops. When a solution infuses at a fast rate, such as 125 mL/hr, it is generally easier to count fewer, larger drops than smaller ones. When the solution must infuse very precisely or at a slow rate, smaller drops are preferred.

Microdrip tubing, regardless of manufacturer, delivers a standard volume of 60 drops/mL. Macrodrip tubing manufacturers, however, have not been consistent in designing the size of the opening. Therefore, the nurse must read the package label to determine the **drop factor** (number of drops/mL). Some common drop factors are 10, 15, and 20. The drop factor is important in calculating the infusion rate and is discussed later in this chapter.

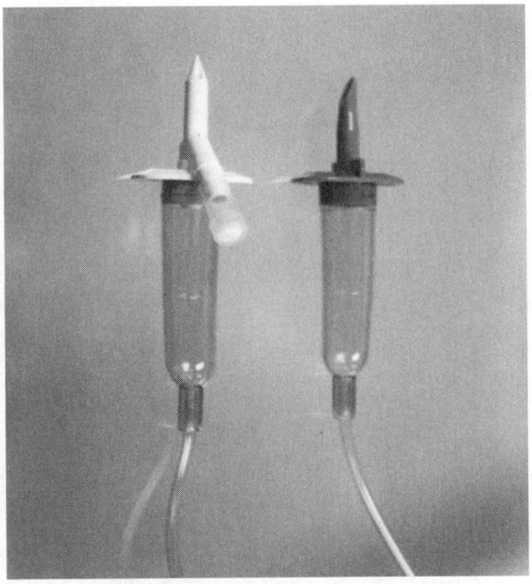

FIGURE 15–11. Vented (*left*) and unvented (*right*) tubing. (Courtesy of Ken Timby.)

Filters

An in-line filter (Fig. 15-12) removes air bubbles as well as undissolved drugs, bacteria, and large substances. Filtered tubing is generally used when:

- Administering parenteral nutrition
- The patient is at high risk for infection
- Infusing IV solutions to pediatric patients
- Administering blood and packed cells

Needle or Needleless Access Ports

Traditionally, the **ports** (sealed openings) in IV tubing were designed for access with a needle. However, this method contributes to the estimated 800,000 to 1 million needle-stick injuries among health care workers each year (Josephson, 1998). To reduce the incidence of work-related injuries and the potential for infection with bloodborne pathogens, **needleless systems** (IV tubing that eliminates the need for access needles) are preferred.

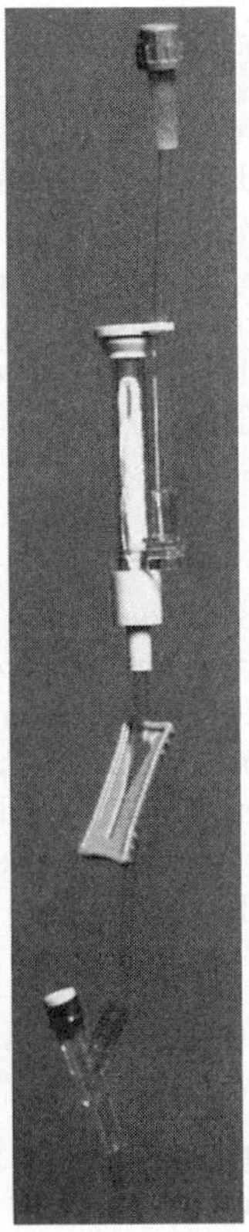

FIGURE 15–12. An in-line filter removes air bubbles as well as undissolved debris that is 0.22 microns in diameter or larger. (Courtesy of Ken Timby.)

With a needleless system, the nurse uses a blunt cannula to pierce the resealable port each time entry into the tubing is needed (see Chap. 35). A needleless access port can be pierced with a needle a limited number of times without altering its integrity, but a port that requires a needle for access cannot be punctured with a blunt cannula.

INFUSION TECHNIQUES

IV infusions are administered either by gravity alone or with an infusion device, an electric or battery-operated machine that regulates and monitors the administration of IV solutions. The use of an infusion device may affect the type of tubing used.

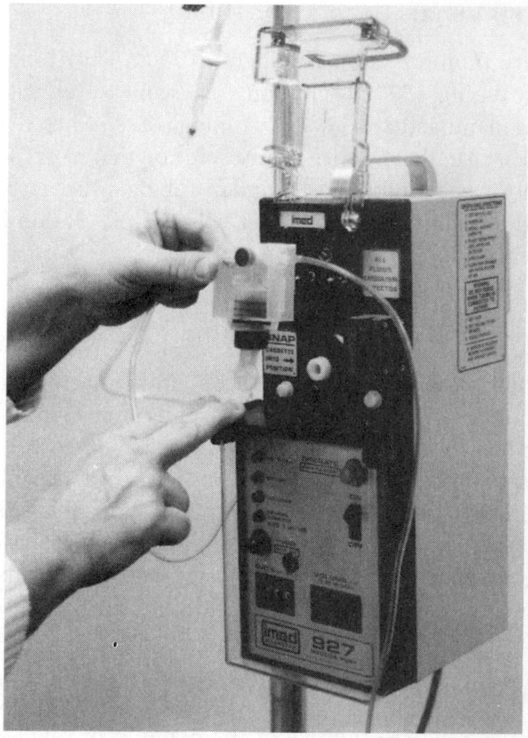

FIGURE 15–13. Special tubing with a cassette is inserted into this electronic infusion pump. (Courtesy of Ken Timby.)

Gravity Infusion

Generally, most basic types of tubing can be used for infusing a solution by gravity. The height of the IV solution rather than the tubing is the most important factor affecting gravity infusions.

To overcome the pressure in the patient's vein, which is higher than atmospheric pressure, the solution is elevated at least 18″ to 24″ (45 to 60 cm) above the site of the infusion. The height of the solution affects the rate of flow: the higher the solution, the faster the solution infuses, and vice versa.

Electronic Infusion Devices

There are two general types of infusion devices: infusion pumps and volumetric controllers. Both are programmed to deliver a preset volume per hour. They trigger audible and visual alarms if the infusion is not progressing at the rate intended. They also sound an alarm when the infusion container is nearly empty, when air is detected within the tubing, or when an obstruction or resistance occurs in delivering the fluid.

Infusion Pumps

An **infusion pump** (infusion device that uses pressure to infuse solutions) requires special tubing that contains a device such as a cassette to create sufficient pressure to push fluid into the vein (Fig. 15-13). The machine adjusts the pressure according to the resistance it meets. This can be a disadvantage because if the catheter or needle within the vein becomes displaced, the pump continues to infuse fluid into the tissue for a period of time.

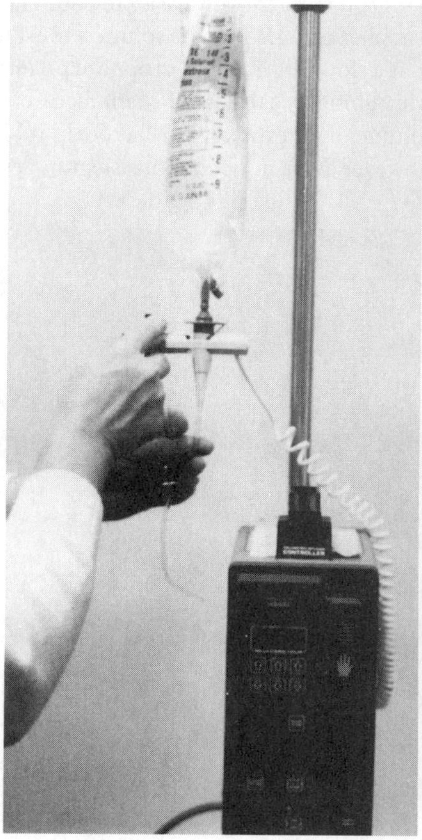

FIGURE 15–14. A volumetric controller monitors and regulates the infusion of intravenous solutions. (Courtesy of Ken Timby.)

Volumetric Controllers

A **volumetric controller** (electronic infusion device that instills IV solutions by gravity; Fig. 15-14) mechanically compresses the tubing at a certain frequency to infuse the solution at a precise, preset rate. Volumetric controllers may or may not require special tubing.

Some models allow the nurse to program the infusion of more than one simultaneous infusion of solutions. In some cases, when one container of fluid finishes infusing, the controller automatically resumes infusing another solution.

The solution and tubing are prepared before accessing the vein with a needle or catheter. Skill 15-2 describes how to prepare an IV solution for administration.

VENIPUNCTURE

Venipuncture (accessing the venous system by piercing a vein with a needle) is a nursing responsibility when a peripheral vein (one distant from the heart) is used. When performing a venipuncture, the nurse assembles needed equipment, inspects and selects an appropriate vein, and inserts the venipuncture device.

Venipuncture Devices

Several devices are used to access a vein: a butterfly needle, an over-the-needle catheter (most common), or a through-the-needle catheter (Fig. 15-15).

Venipuncture devices are available in various diameters or gauges; the larger the gauge number, the smaller the diameter. The diameter of the venipuncture device should always be smaller than the vein into which it will be inserted to reduce the potential for occluding blood flow. An 18-, 20-, or 22-gauge is the size most often used for adults.

Besides a device for puncturing the vein, the following items are needed: clean gloves; tourniquet; antiseptic swabs to cleanse the skin; transparent dressing to cover the puncture site; and adhesive tape to secure the venipuncture device and tubing. The use of antibiotic or antimicrobial ointment at the site varies; agency policy is followed. An armboard may be needed to prevent the patient from dislodging the venipuncture device.

Vein Selection

The veins in the hand and forearm are most commonly used for inserting a venipuncture device (Fig. 15-16); scalp veins are used for infants and small children.

Nursing Guidelines For

Selecting a Venipuncture Site

- ☑ Use veins on the nondominant side.
  RATIONALE: This reduces the potential for dislodging the device due to movement and use.
- ☑ Do not use foot and leg veins.
  RATIONALE: Using foot and leg veins restricts mobility and increases the potential for blood clots.
- ☑ If possible, do not use a vein on the side of previous breast surgery or one in which vascular surgery has been performed for kidney dialysis.
  RATIONALE: Using such veins further compromises circulation and increases the potential for infection and poor healing.
- ☑ Choose a vein in a location that will be unaffected by joint movement.
  RATIONALE: A venipuncture device in such a location could become displaced more easily.
- ☑ Look for a large vein, if a large-gauge needle or catheter is necessary.
  RATIONALE: Matching the needle and vein size prevents compromising circulation.
- ☑ Avoid using veins on the inner surface of the wrist.
  RATIONALE: This prevents pain and discomfort.
- ☑ Look for a vein proximal to the current site or in the opposite hand or arm.
  RATIONALE: This promotes healing and decreases the risk of fluid leaking from the vein into the tissue.
- ☑ Feel and look for a vein that is fairly straight.
  RATIONALE: It is easier to thread the device into a straight vein.
- ☑ Do not use a vein that appears inflamed, or if the skin over the area looks impaired in any way.
  RATIONALE: Use of such a site creates additional trauma.

Once the general site is selected, the nurse applies a tourniquet to select a specific vein (Fig. 15-17). Display 15-4 identifies several techniques for promoting vein distention.

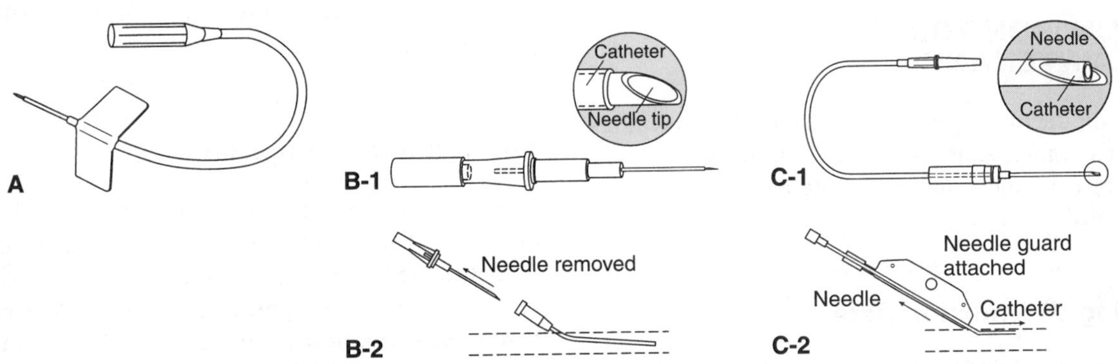

FIGURE 15–15. Venipuncture devices. (*A*) Butterfly needle. (*B-1*) Over-the-needle catheter. (*B-2*) Needle removed. (*C-1*) Through-the-needle catheter. (*C-2*) A needle guard covers the tip of the needle, which remains outside the skin.

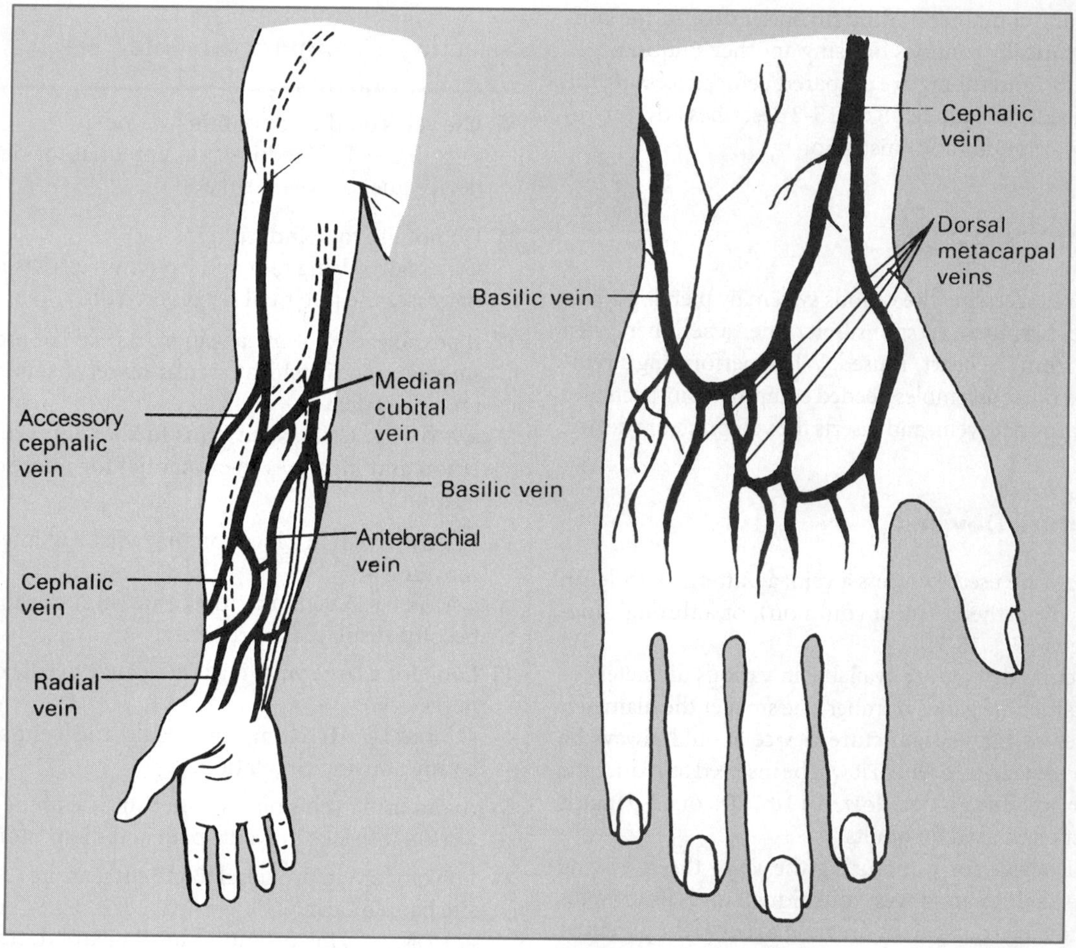

FIGURE 15–16. Potential venipuncture sites.

A blood pressure cuff can be substituted for a rubber tourniquet. Whichever technique is used, the radial pulse should be palpated to indicate that arterial blood flow is being maintained.

Venipuncture Device Insertion

Skill 15-3 describes the technique for inserting an over-the-needle catheter within a vein.

INFUSION MONITORING AND MAINTENANCE

Once the venipuncture is performed and the solution is infusing, the nurse regulates the rate of infusion, assesses for complications, cares for the venipuncture site, and replaces equipment as needed.

Regulating the Infusion Rate

The nurse is responsible for calculating, regulating, and maintaining the rate of infusion according to the physician's order. If an infusion device is being used, the electronic equipment is programmed in mL/hr. If the solution is being infused without an electronic infusion device, the rate is calculated in drops (gtt) per minute. Formulas for calculating infusion rates are provided in Display 15-5.

For gravity infusions, the nurse counts the number of drops falling into the drip chamber per minute. By adjusting the roller clamp, the number of drops is increased or decreased until the infusion rate matches the calculated rate. Thereafter, the nurse monitors the time strip on the side of the container at hourly intervals to ensure that the infusion is instilling at the prescribed rate.

Assessing for Complications

Complications associated with the infusion of IV solutions (Table 15-7) are circulatory overload, in which the intravascular volume becomes excessive, **infiltration** (escape of IV fluid into the tissue), **phlebitis** (inflammation of a vein), **thrombus formation** (stationary blood clot), **pulmonary embolus** (blood clot that travels to the lung), infection (growth of microorganisms at the site or within the blood

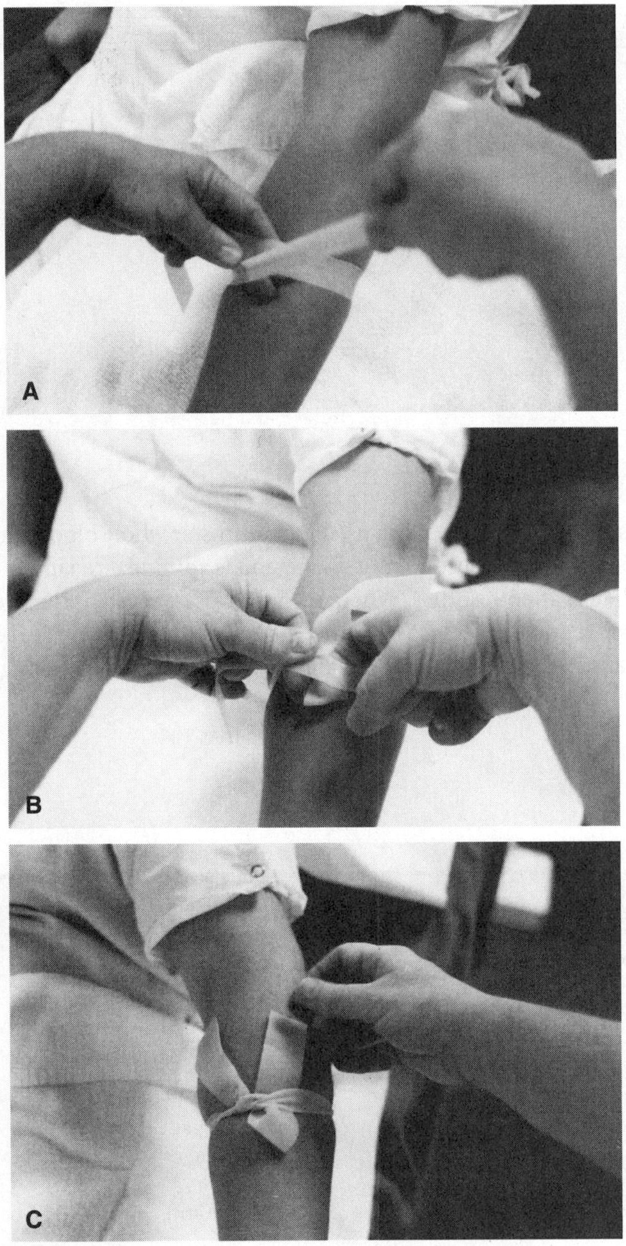

FIGURE 15–17. (*A*) To apply a tourniquet, the ends are pulled tightly in opposite directions. (*B*) Then one end is tucked beneath the other. (*C*) This allows it to be released easily by pulling one of the free ends. (Courtesy of Ken Timby.)

stream), and **air embolism** (bubble of air traveling within the vascular system).

The minimum quantity of air that may be fatal to humans is not known. Animal research indicates that fatal volumes of air are much larger than the quantity present in the entire length of infusion tubing. The average infusion tubing holds about 5 mL of air, an amount not ordinarily considered dangerous. Patients, however, are often frightened when they see air in the tubing, and every effort is made to remove air bubbles.

DISPLAY 15–4

Techniques for Promoting Vein Distention

- Apply a tourniquet or blood pressure cuff tightly about the arm.
- Have the patient make a fist and pump the fist intermittently.
- Tap the skin over the vein several times.
- Lower the patient's arm to promote distal pooling of blood.
- Stroke the skin in the direction of the fingers.
- Apply warm compresses for 10 minutes to dilate veins, and then reapply the tourniquet.

Nursing Guidelines For

Removing Air Bubbles from IV Tubing

- ☑ Flush the line with IV solution before inserting the adaptor into the venipuncture device.
  RATIONALE: This action purges air from the tubing.
- ☑ Tighten the roller clamp if small bubbles are observed.
  RATIONALE: This action prevents continued forward movement of the air.
- ☑ Tap the tubing below the air bubbles (Fig. 15-18).
  RATIONALE: This promotes upward movement of the air above the fluid in the drip chamber.
- ☑ Milk the air in the direction of the drip chamber or filter, if one is incorporated within the tubing.
  RATIONALE: This pushes the air physically to an area where it can be trapped or released.
- ☑ Wrap the tubing around a circular object, like a pencil, starting below the trapped air.
  RATIONALE: This moves the air toward the drip chamber, where it can escape from the liquid into the empty air space.
- ☑ Insert the needle and barrel of a syringe within a port below the air, and open the roller clamp.
  RATIONALE: This siphons fluid and air from the tubing as it passes by the bevel of the needle.

Caring for the Site

Because the venipuncture is a type of wound, it is important to inspect the site at routine intervals. Its appearance is documented daily in the patient's record. A common practice is to change the dressing over the venipuncture site every 24 to 72 hours, according to the agency's infection control policy (see Chap. 28).

DISPLAY 15–5

Formulas for Calculating Infusion Rates

When using an infusion device:

$$\frac{\text{Total volume in mL}}{\text{Total hours}} = \text{mL/hr}$$

Example:

$$\frac{1{,}000\ \text{mL}}{8\ \text{hr}} = 125\ \text{mL/hr}$$

When infusing by gravity:

$$\frac{\text{Total volume in mL}}{\text{Total time in minutes}} \times \text{drop factor*} = \text{gtt/min}$$

$$\frac{1{,}000\ \text{mL}}{480\ \text{min}} \times 20 = 42\ \text{gtt/min}$$

**The macrodrip drop factor varies among manufacturers.*

Replacing Equipment

Solutions are replaced when they finish infusing or every 24 hours, whichever occurs first (Skill 15-4). IV tubing is changed every 72 hours, depending on agency policy, with some exceptions. Tubing used to instill parenteral nutrition is replaced daily. Tubing used to administer whole blood can be reused for a second unit, if one unit is administered immediately after the other. Whenever tubing is changed, it is more convenient to replace both the solution and the tubing at the same time. Skill 15-5 describes how to replace just the tubing, which is generally more difficult.

TABLE 15–7. **Complications of Intravenous (IV) Therapy**

Complication	Signs and Symptoms	Cause(s)	Action
Infection	Swelling Discomfort Redness at site Drainage from site	Growth of microorganisms	Change site. Apply antiseptic and dressing to previous site. Report findings.
Circulatory overload	Elevated blood pressure Shortness of breath Bounding pulse Anxiety	Rapid infusion Reduced kidney function Impaired heart contraction	Slow the IV rate. Contact the physician. Elevate the patient's head. Give oxygen.
Infiltration	Swelling at the site Discomfort Decrease in infusion rate Cool skin temperature at the site	Displacement of the venipuncture device	Restart the IV. Elevate the arm.
Phlebitis	Redness, warmth, and discomfort along the vein	Administration of irritating fluid Prolonged use of the same vein	Restart the IV. Report findings. Apply warm compresses.
Thrombus formation	Swelling Discomfort Slowed infusion	Stasis of blood at the catheter, needle tip, or vein	Restart the IV. Report findings. Apply warm compresses.
Pulmonary embolus	Sudden chest pain Shortness of breath Anxiety Rapid heart rate Drop in blood pressure	Movement of previously stationary blood clot to the lungs	Stay with the patient. Call for help. Administer oxygen.
Air embolism	Same as pulmonary embolus	Failure to purge air from the tubing	Same as for pulmonary embolus, but also place the patient's head lower than the feet. Position the patient on left side.

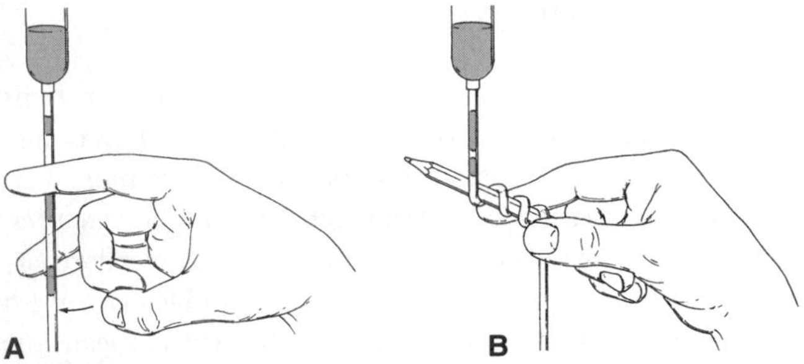

FIGURE 15–18. Removing air bubbles. (*A*) Tapping the tubing may help air bubbles rise into the drip chamber. (*B*) Twisting the tubing around a pencil or other object may displace air bubbles toward the drip chamber.

DISCONTINUATION OF AN INTRAVENOUS INFUSION

IV infusions are discontinued when the solution has infused and no more is scheduled to follow. Alternatively, the venipuncture device is temporarily capped but kept patent with the use of an intermittent venous access device, also known as a medication lock.

Nursing Guidelines For

Discontinuing an IV Infusion

☑ Wash hands.
RATIONALE: Handwashing reduces the spread of microorganisms.

☑ Clamp the tubing and remove the tape that held the dressing and venipuncture device in place.
RATIONALE: This facilitates removal without leaking fluid.

☑ Don gloves.
RATIONALE: Wearing gloves prevents contact with blood.

☑ Gently press a gauze square over the site of entry.
RATIONALE: The gauze will absorb blood.

☑ Remove the catheter or needle by pulling it out without hesitation, following the course of the vein.
RATIONALE: This prevents discomfort and injury to the vein.

☑ Apply pressure to the injection site for 30 to 45 seconds while elevating the forearm (Fig. 15-19).
RATIONALE: Pressure and elevation control bleeding.

☑ Cover the site with a dressing.
RATIONALE: A dressing reduces the potential for infection.

☑ Remove gloves when the bleeding has been controlled, and wash your hands again.
RATIONALE: Handwashing removes microorganisms.

☑ Flex and extend the arm or hand several times.
RATIONALE: This helps the patient regain sensation and mobility.

☑ Record the amount of fluid infused during the current shift on the I&O sheet.
RATIONALE: The nurse is responsible for documenting fluid intake volumes.

☑ Document and sign a notation on the patient's record indicating the time the infusion was discontinued and the condition of the venipuncture site.
RATIONALE: This action demonstrates responsibility and accountability for patient care.

INSERTION OF AN INTERMITTENT VENOUS ACCESS DEVICE

An **intermittent venous access device** (sealed chamber that provides a means for administering IV medications or solutions on a periodic basis; Fig. 15-20) is inserted into a venipuncture device. An intermittent venous access device is also called a saline lock or a heparin lock because the chamber is filled with either of these solutions and periodically flushed with one or the other to prevent blood from clotting at the tip of the catheter or needle.

Intermittent venous access devices are used when the patient:

- No longer needs continuous infusions of fluid
- Needs intermittent administration of IV medication
- May need emergency IV fluid or medications if his or her condition deteriorates

These devices are replaced when the venipuncture site is changed. Skill 15-6 describes how to insert an intermittent venous access device and ensure its patency. The use of a medication lock when administering IV drugs is discussed in Chapter 35.

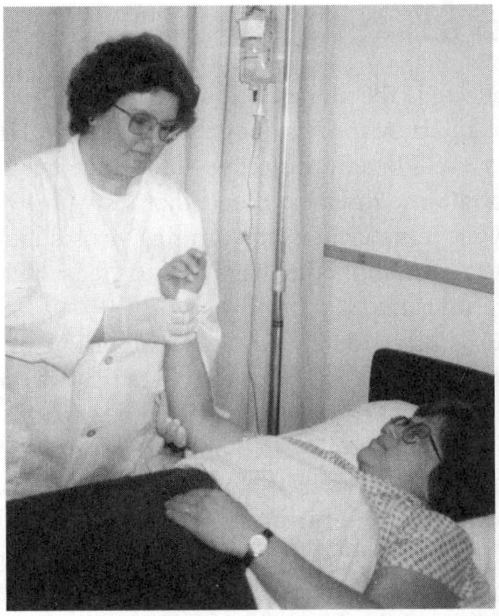

FIGURE 15–19. Applying pressure to the venipuncture site. (Courtesy of Ken Timby.)

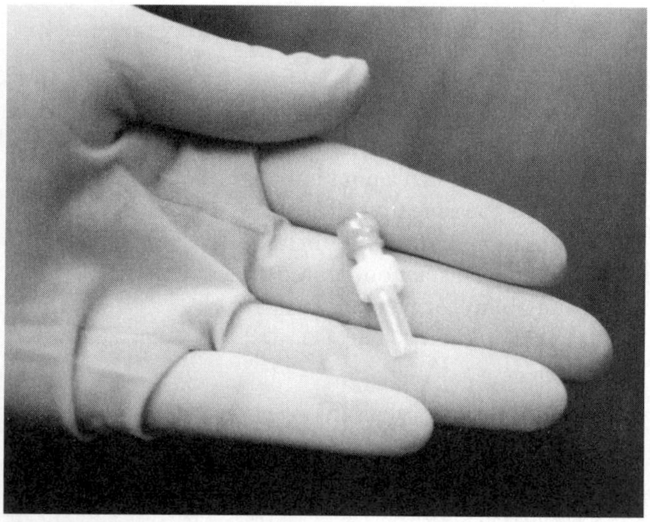

FIGURE 15–20. Intermittent venous access device. (Courtesy of Ken Timby.)

Blood Administration

Blood is collected, stored, and checked for safety and compatibility before it is administered as a transfusion.

BLOOD COLLECTION AND STORAGE

Blood donors are screened to ensure they are healthy and will not be endangered by the temporary loss in blood volume. Refrigerated blood can be stored for 21 to 35 days, after which it is discarded.

BLOOD SAFETY

Once collected, the donated blood is tested for syphilis, hepatitis, and human immunodeficiency virus (HIV) antibodies to exclude administering blood that may transmit these bloodborne diseases. Blood that tests positive is discarded. Unfortunately, disease-carrying viruses may remain undetected if the antibodies have not reached a high enough level to be measured.

The U.S. Blood Safety Council, a division of the Department of Health and Human Services that was created in 1999, has made policies regarding potential hepatitis C infection by blood transfusions. All blood collection agencies must notify persons who received blood before 1987 if the donation came from a donor who has tested positive for hepatitis C since 1990. This policy is being implemented to promote early diagnosis and treatment of infected but nonsymptomatic transfusion recipients.

BLOOD COMPATIBILITY

There are several hundred differences among the proteins present in the blood of a donor and recipient. They can cause minor or major transfusion reactions. One of the most dangerous differences involves the antigens, or protein structures, on membranes of red blood cells. Antigens determine the characteristic blood group—A, B, AB, and O—and Rh factor. Rh positive means the protein is present; Rh negative means the protein is absent.

Before donated blood is administered, the blood of the potential recipient is typed and mixed, or cross-matched, with a sample of the stored blood to determine whether the two are compatible. To avoid an incompatibility reaction, it is best to administer the same blood group and Rh factor. Exceptions are listed in Table 15-8.

Type O blood is considered the universal donor because it lacks both A and B blood group markers on its cell membrane. Therefore, type O blood can be given to anyone because it will not trigger an incompatibility reaction when given to recipients with other blood types. Persons with type AB blood are referred to as universal recipients because their red blood cells have proteins compatible with types A, B, and O.

Rh-positive persons may receive Rh-positive or Rh-negative blood, because the latter does not contain the sensitizing protein. However, Rh-negative persons should never receive Rh-positive blood.

BLOOD TRANSFUSION

Before blood is administered, vital signs are obtained and documented to provide a baseline for comparison should the patient have a transfusion reaction. Each patient who receives blood has a color-coded bracelet with identifying numbers that must correlate with those on the unit of blood. IV medications are never infused through tubing that is being used to administer blood.

TABLE 15–8. **Blood Groups and Compatible Types**

Blood Groups	Percentage of Population	Compatible Blood Types
A	41%	A and O
B	9%	B and O
O	47%	O
AB	3%	AB, A, B, and O
Rh+	85% whites 95% African Americans	Rh+ and Rh–
Rh–	15% whites 5% African Americans	Rh– only

Blood transfusions require special equipment and monitoring for potential complications.

Blood Transfusion Equipment

There are certain standards for the gauge of the catheter or needle and the type of tubing used to transfuse blood.

Catheter or Needle Gauge

Because blood contains cells in addition to water, it is generally infused through a 16 to 20-gauge—preferably an 18-gauge—catheter or needle. Using a smaller gauge increases the potential for prolonging the infusion beyond 4 hours, and 4 hours is the maximum safe period for administering one unit of blood.

Blood Transfusion Tubing

Blood is administered through tubing referred to as a Y-set (Fig. 15-21). There are two branches at the top of the tubing; one is used for administering normal saline solution, the other for administering blood. Normal saline (0.9% sodium chloride) is the only solution used when administering blood because other types of solutions destroy red blood cells. The two branches of the Y-set join above a filter that removes clotted blood and dead cell debris. The normal saline is always administered before the blood is hung and follows after the blood has been infused. It is also used during the infusion if the patient has a transfusion reaction.

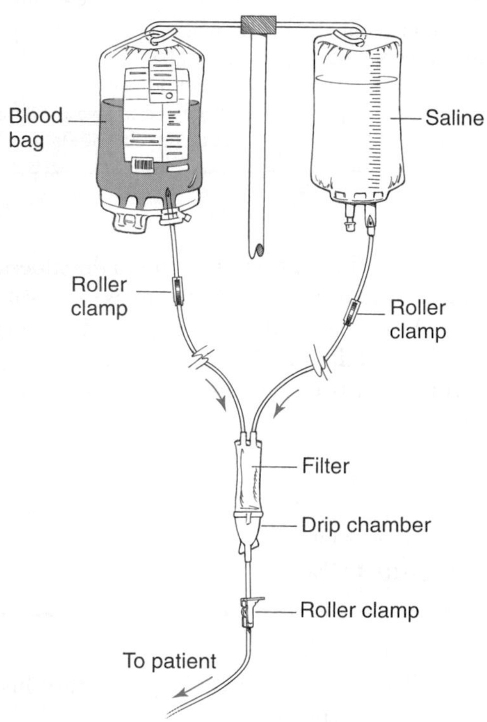

FIGURE 15–21. Blood transfusion tubing.

Skill 15-7 describes how to administer a blood transfusion.

TRANSFUSION REACTIONS

Serious transfusion reactions generally occur within the first 5 to 15 minutes of the infusion, so the nurse usually remains with the patient during this critical time. However, because a transfusion reaction can occur at any time, patients are monitored frequently during a transfusion and are instructed to call for assistance if they feel any unusual sensations (Table 15-9).

Parenteral Nutrition

The term *parenteral* means "a route other than enteral or intestinal." Therefore, **parenteral nutrition** (nutrients, such as protein, carbohydrate, fat, vitamins, minerals, and trace elements, that are administered intravenously) is provided by other than the oral route. Depending on the concentration of these substances, parenteral nutrition is administered through an IV catheter in a peripheral vein or through a catheter that terminates in a central vein near the heart.

PERIPHERAL PARENTERAL NUTRITION

Peripheral parenteral nutrition (isotonic or hypotonic IV nutrient solution instilled in a vein distant from the heart) is not extremely concentrated and hence can be infused through peripheral veins. It provides temporary nutritional support of approximately 2000 to 2500 calories daily. It can meet a person's metabolic needs when oral intake is interrupted for 7 to 10 days, or it can be used as a supplement during a transitional period as the patient begins to resume eating.

TOTAL PARENTERAL NUTRITION

Total parenteral nutrition (TPN; hypertonic solution of nutrients designed to meet almost all the caloric and nutritional needs of patients) is preferred for patients who are severely malnourished or who may not be able to consume food or liquids for a long period of time. Display 15-6 lists patients who may benefit from TPN.

Because TPN solutions are extremely concentrated, they must be delivered to an area where they are diluted in a fairly large volume of blood. This excludes peripheral veins. TPN solutions are infused through a catheter inserted into the sub-

TABLE 15–9. **Transfusion Reactions**

Type of Reaction	Signs and Symptoms	Cause(s)	Action
Incompatibility	Hypotension, rapid pulse rate, difficulty breathing, back pain, flushing	Mismatch between donor and recipient blood groups	Stop the infusion of blood. Infuse the saline at a rapid rate. Call for assistance. Administer oxygen. Raise the feet higher than the head. Be prepared to administer emergency drugs. Send first urine specimen to laboratory. Save the blood and tubing.
Febrile	Fever, shaking chills, headache, rapid pulse, muscle aches	Allergy to foreign proteins in the donated blood	Stop the blood infusion. Start the saline. Check vital signs. Report findings.
Septic	Fever, chills, hypotension	Infusion of blood that contains microorganisms	Stop the infusion of blood. Start the saline. Report findings. Save the blood and tubing.
Allergic	Rash, itching, flushing, stable vital signs	Minor sensitivity to substances in the donor blood	Slow the rate of infusion. Assess the patient. Report findings. Be prepared to give an antihistamine.
Moderate chilling	No fever or other symptoms	Infusion of cold blood	Continue the infusion. Cover and make the patient comfortable.
Overload	Hypertension, difficulty breathing, moist breath sounds, bounding pulse	Large volume or rapid rate of infusion; inadequate cardiac or kidney function	Reduce the rate. Elevate the head. Give oxygen. Report findings. Be prepared to give a diuretic.
Hypocalcemia (low calcium)	Tingling of fingers, hypotension, muscle cramps, convulsions	Multiple blood transfusions containing anticalcium agents	Stop the blood infusion. Start saline. Report findings. Be prepared to give antidote, (calcium chloride).

DISPLAY 15–6

Candidates for Total Parenteral Nutrition

- Patients who have not eaten for 5 days and are not likely to eat during the next week
- Patients who have had a 10% or more loss of body weight
- Patients exhibiting self-imposed starvation (anorexia nervosa)
- Patients with cancer of the esophagus or stomach
- Patients with postoperative gastrointestinal complications
- Patients with inflammatory bowel disease in an acute stage
- Patients with major trauma or burns
- Patients with liver and renal failure

clavian or jugular vein; the tip terminates in the superior vena cava. This type of a catheter is referred to as a central venous catheter (Fig. 15-22). Sometimes a peripherally inserted central catheter is used; this long catheter is inserted in a peripheral arm vein, but its tip terminates in the superior vena cava as well (Fig. 15-23).

Nursing Guidelines For

Administering TPN

☑ Weigh the patient daily.
RATIONALE: The patient's weight helps monitor his or her response to treatment.

☑ Use tubing that contains a filter.

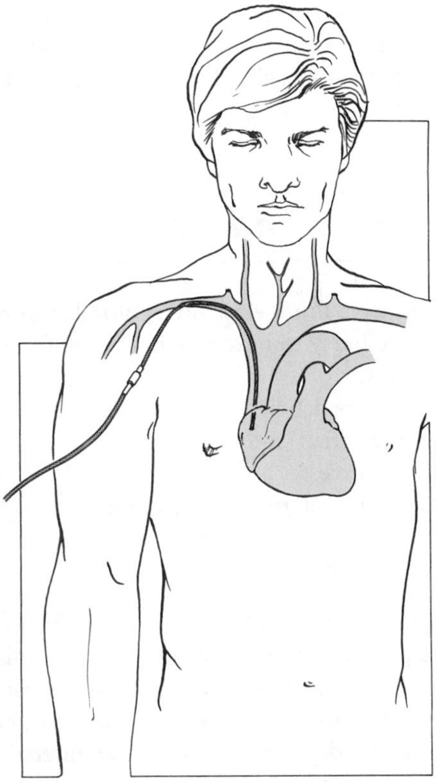

FIGURE 15–22. Central venous catheter inserted into the subclavian vein and threaded into the superior vena cava.

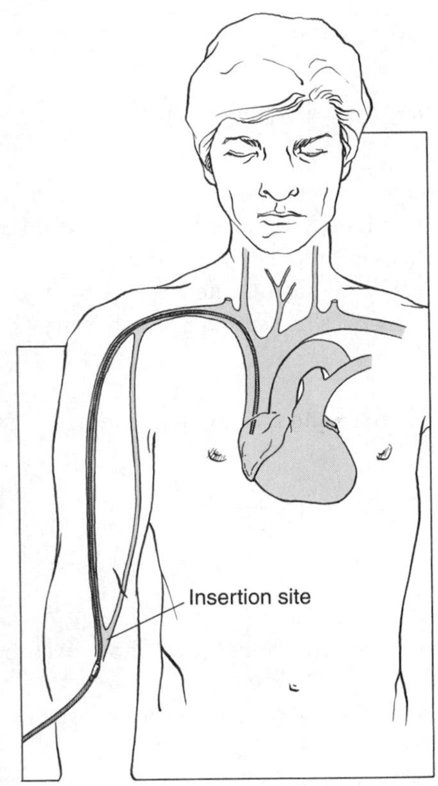

FIGURE 15–23. Peripherally inserted central catheter with distal tip in the superior vena cava.

RATIONALE: Filters absorb air and bacteria, two potential complications associated with the use of central venous catheters.

- ☑ Change TPN tubing daily.
  RATIONALE: Changing tubing reduces the potential for infection.
- ☑ Tape all connections in the tubing and central catheter.
  RATIONALE: Taping prevents accidental separation and reduces the potential for an air embolism.
- ☑ Clamp the central catheter and have the patient bear down whenever separating the tubing from its catheter connection.
  RATIONALE: This action prevents an air embolism.
- ☑ Use an infusion pump to administer TPN solution.
  RATIONALE: An infusion pump monitors and regulates precise fluid volumes.
- ☑ Infuse initial TPN solutions gradually (25 to 50 mL/hr).
  RATIONALE: Gradual administration allows time for physiologic adaptation.
- ☑ Never increase the rate of infusion to make up for an uninfused volume, unless the physician has been consulted.
  RATIONALE: Speeding up the infusion tends to increase blood sugar levels.
- ☑ Monitor intake and especially urine output.
  RATIONALE: High blood glucose levels can trigger diuresis (increased urine excretion), resulting in outputs greater than intake.
- ☑ Monitor capillary blood glucose levels (see Chap. 13).
  RATIONALE: Blood glucose may not be adequately metabolized without the additional administration of insulin.
- ☑ Wean the patient from TPN gradually.
  RATIONALE: Weaning prevents a sudden drop in blood sugar levels.

LIPID EMULSIONS

An **emulsion** (mixture of two liquids, one of which is insoluble in the other) can be administered parenterally. The combination allows a vehicle for administering lipids, or fat, which is often missing from parenteral nutritional solutions. A parenteral lipid emulsion is a mixture of water and fats in the form of soybean or safflower oil, egg yolk phospholipids, and glycerin.

Lipid solutions, which look milky white (Fig. 15-24), are given intermittently with TPN solutions. They provide additional calories and promote adequate blood levels of fatty acids. Lipid solutions are administered peripherally or in a port in the central catheter below the filter and close to the vein. If the lipid solution is squeezed or mixed with TPN solutions in larger volumes than those moving through the

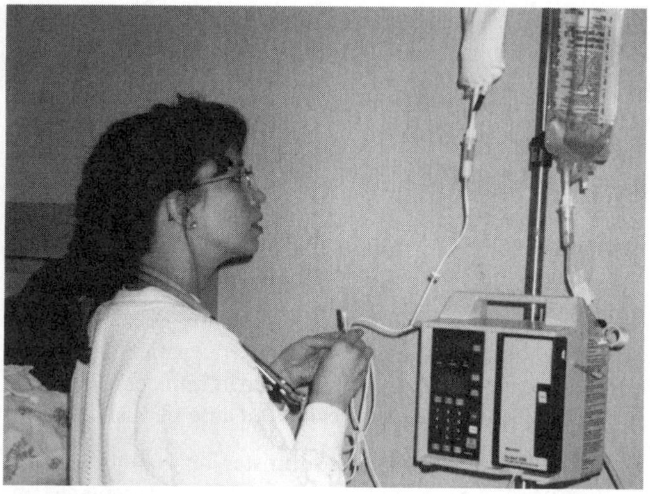

FIGURE 15–24. Administration of lipid emulsion. (Courtesy of Ken Timby.)

catheter, the lipid molecules tend to "break" and separate in the solution.

The patient receiving an administration of lipids may have an adverse reaction within 2 to 5 hours of the infusion (Dudek, 1997). Common manifestations include fever, flushing, sweating, dizziness, nausea, vomiting, headache, chest and back pain, dyspnea, and cyanosis. Delayed reactions (up to 10 days later) are characterized by enlargement of the liver and spleen accompanied by jaundice, reduced white blood cell and platelet counts, elevated blood lipid levels, seizures, and shock.

Nursing Implications

Patients who have fluid, electrolyte, blood, and nutritional imbalances are likely to have one or more of the following nursing diagnoses:

- Feeding self-care deficit
- Fluid volume deficit
- Fluid volume excess
- Risk for altered oral mucous membrane
- Risk for impaired skin integrity
- Knowledge deficit

The nursing care plan illustrates the nursing process as it applies to a patient with Fluid volume deficit. This diagnostic category is defined by the North American Nursing Diagnosis Association (1999) as "the state in which an individual experiences decreased intravascular, interstitial and/or intracellular fluid."

Nursing Care Plan

Fluid Volume Deficit

Assessment

Subjective Data

States, "I've been living on the streets. I don't have a job. I haven't eaten in several days."

Objective Data

56-year-old homeless man brought to the Emergency Department after being found by police wandering and confused near Main St. Outdoor daytime temperatures have been in the 90° ranges. Height 5′10″, weight 137 lbs. States usual weight is around 160 lbs. T—100° orally, P—100 and weak, R—28. Oral mucous membranes are dry. Able to void 50 mL of dark, amber urine. BP 100/68 in R. arm while sitting up. Skin is dry and tents for >5 seconds when compressed.

Diagnosis

Fluid Volume Deficit related to inadequate oral intake and increased fluid loss.

Plan

Goal

The patient's oral fluid intake will be 1,500–3,000 mL in the next 24 hours (8/15).

Orders: 8/14

1. Compile a list of food and fluid likes and dislikes.
2. Provide a minimum of 100 to 200 mL/hour of preferred liquids every hour over the next 16 hours. Avoid disturbing hours of sleep.
3. Request dietary department to send foods that are good sources of sodium, such as milk, cheese, bouillon, ham.
4. Refer to Salvation Army shelter for the homeless before discharge

R. Armstrong, RN

continued

Nursing Care Plan ***Fluid Volume Deficit*** *Continued*

Implementation (Documentation)	8/14	1000	States "I like just about anything. I'm so thirsty. A big, cool glass of lemonade sounds wonderful right now." Also lists ginger ale and orange juice as favorite beverages. Dietary department notified to send sodium-rich foods for next 24 hours. Discharge planner notified for referral to Salvation Army. ______ L. O'CONNELL, LPN
		1030	200 mL of orange juice provided and consumed. Weakness and tremors of the hand noted. Able to use a straw with glass. ______ L. O'CONNELL, LPN
Evaluation (Documentation)		1230	Ate macaroni and cheese, sausage, stewed tomatoes, and whole milk for lunch. ______ L. O'CONNELL, LPN
		1430	Total oral fluid intake since 1000 has been 1,000 mL. Urine is lighter in color. Voided a total of 600 mL since admission. Vital signs improving; see graphic sheet for specifics. Discharge planner will visit in A.M. 8/15. ______ L. O'CONNELL, LPN

FOCUS ON OLDER ADULTS

- Because older adults are likely to have chronic conditions affecting the heart and kidneys, they are at risk for fluid and electrolyte imbalances.
- Diuretic medications, often prescribed for older adults with cardiovascular disorders, increase the risk for fluid and electrolyte imbalances.
- Mobility limitations, cognitive impairments, and impaired ability to perform activities of daily living can lead to fluid deficits in older adults who do not maintain adequate food and fluid intake independently.
- Because age-related changes diminish the sensation of thirst, older adults are encouraged to drink fluids even when they do not feel thirsty.
- More fluid may be consumed if it is offered by the nurse, rather than asking if the older adult would like a drink.
- Because caffeine acts as a diuretic, older adults are encouraged to drink noncaffeinated beverages.
- To maintain adequate consumption of nutrients, it is best to offer fluids to older adults at times other than meals. Distending the stomach with liquids creates a sensation of satiety (fullness) and thereby reduces the consumption of food.
- Older adults may restrict their fluid intake under the mistaken notion that this will reduce incontinence. This practice contributes to incontinence by increasing bladder irritability and increases the risks for urinary tract infection, postural hypotension, falls, and injuries.
- Assessment for fluid and electrolyte imbalances is important for any older adult who has a change in mental status.
- When older adults must fast before certain procedures, increased oral fluid intake in the hours before beginning fluid restrictions is emphasized to prevent dehydration.
- Because the skin of older adults is less elastic, assessment of skin turgor is more accurate over the sternum. Additional indicators of dehydration in older adults include mental status changes, concentrated urine, dry mucous membranes, low urine output, and elevated hematocrit, hemoglobin, serum sodium, and blood urea nitrogen (BUN).
- Nurses need to monitor closely the response of older adults to intravenous infusions because many older adults cannot tolerate volumes that are safely administered to younger adults.
- Dehydration in older adults may be a consequence or indicator of abuse or neglect.

KEY CONCEPTS

- Body fluid is a mixture of water, chemicals called electrolytes and nonelectrolytes, and blood cells.
- Body fluid is distributed inside cells, called the intracellular compartment, and outside cells, called the extracellular compartment; the latter is further subdivided into the fluid between cells (interstitial fluid) and within blood (intravascular fluid).
- Fluid and the components within it are distributed within each of the fluid compartments by means of osmosis, filtration, passive diffusion, facilitated diffusion, and active transport.
- Fluid volume status is assessed by measuring a patient's intake and output, obtaining daily weights, obtaining vital signs, monitoring bowel elimination patterns and stool characteristics, observing the color of urine, and

assessing skin turgor, the condition of the oral mucous membranes, lung sounds, and level of consciousness.

- Fluid volume is restored by treating the underlying disorder, increasing oral intake, administering IV fluid replacements, controlling fluid losses, or a combination of all of these measures.
- Fluid volume excess is reduced or eliminated by treating the underlying disorder, restricting or limiting oral fluids, reducing salt consumption, discontinuing IV fluid infusions or reducing the infusing volume, administering drugs that promote urine elimination, or a combination of these interventions.
- IV fluids are administered to maintain or restore fluid balance, maintain or replace electrolytes, administer water-soluble vitamins, provide calories, administer drugs, and replace blood and blood products.
- Crystalloid solutions are mixtures of water and substances such as salt and sugar that totally dissolve. Colloid solutions are mixtures of water and suspended, undissolved substances such as blood cells.
- An isotonic solution has the same concentration of dissolved substances as plasma; a hypotonic solution has fewer dissolved substances; and a hypertonic solution is more concentrated than plasma.
- When selecting tubing for administering IV solutions, the nurse must consider whether to use primary or secondary tubing and vented or unvented tubing, which drop size is most appropriate, and whether a filter is needed.
- IV fluids may be infused by gravity or with the assistance of an infusion device, such as a pump or volumetric controller.
- When selecting a vein for venipuncture, the nurse gives priority to one in the nondominant hand or arm that is fairly straight, is larger than the needle or catheter gauge, is likely to be undisturbed by joint movement, and appears unimpaired by previous trauma or use.
- Complications of IV fluid therapy include infiltration, phlebitis, infection, circulatory overload, thrombus formation, pulmonary embolus, and air embolism.
- An intermittent venous access device is used in patients who require intermittent IV fluid or medication administration or for emergency access to the vascular system.
- When administering blood, the nurse assesses vital signs before and during the transfusion; uses no smaller than a 20-gauge needle or catheter, normal saline solution, and Y-set tubing; and infuses the blood within 4 hours or less.
- During a blood transfusion, the nurse monitors the patient closely for incompatibility; febrile, septic, and allergic reactions; chilling; circulatory overload; and signs of hypocalcemia.
- Parenteral nutrition is a technique for providing nutrients, such as protein, carbohydrate, fat, vitamins, minerals, and trace elements, intravenously rather than orally.

CRITICAL THINKING EXERCISES

- When calculating a patient's I&O, you find that the patient has had a total intake of 1000 mL and output of 750 mL. What other assessment findings are you likely to observe?
- What nursing interventions would you plan to restore the patient's fluid imbalance in the previous situation? What criteria would indicate that the patient's fluid imbalance has been corrected?
- Several people involved in a serious motor vehicle accident are brought to the emergency department. All of the victims have lost a great deal of blood. Identify methods for restoring their fluid volume and the substances, including possible blood products and blood groups, that may be used for patients who have type A, B, O, and AB blood, with Rh-positive antigens.

SUGGESTED READINGS

Angeles T. IV rounds. How to prevent phlebitis. Nursing 1997;27(1):26.

Belcaster A. Action stat. Venous air embolism. Nursing 1997;27(4):33.

Bove LA. Restoring electrolyte balance: sodium & chloride. RN 1996;59(1):25.

Chang TMS. Modified hemoglobin blood substitutes: present status and future perspectives. Biotechnology Annual Review 1998;4:75–112.

Clinical update. Local anesthesia: taking the sting out of venipuncture. Nursing 1998;28(10):48–51.

Dudek S. Nutrition handbook for nursing practice, 3d ed. Philadelphia, Lippincott-Raven, 1997.

Fischbach FT. Manual of laboratory and diagnostic tests, 5th ed. Philadelphia, Lippincott-Raven, 1996.

Fitzpatrick L, Fitzpatrick T. Blood transfusion: keeping your patient safe. Nursing 1997;27(8):34–41.

Jacobson AF. Research for practice. Prolonging the life of IV sites. American Journal of Nursing 1997;97(4):22.

Josephson DL. Intravenous infusion therapy for nurses. Albany, Delmar Publishers, 1998.

Macklin D. How to manage PICCs. American Journal of Nursing 1997; 97(9):26–33.

Masoorli S. Guide to medical devices. What to look for in an infusion pump. Nursing 1996;26(8):24p, 24r.

NANDA nursing diagnoses: definitions and classification, 1999–2000. Philadelphia, NANDA, 1999.

O'Donnell ME. Assessing fluid and electrolyte balance in elders. American Journal of Nursing 1995;95(11):40–46.

Pettit DN, Kraus V. The use of gauze versus transparent dressings for peripheral intravenous catheter sites. Nursing Clinics of North America 1995; 30(3):495–506.

Roth D. IV rounds. Venipuncture tips for geriatric patients. Nursing 1997; 27(10):69.

Sandrock J. Critical care. Treating traumatic hypovolemia: which fluid to choose? Nursing 1998;28(1):32cc1–32cc4.

Skokal W. Infusion pump update: no time to keep up with the ever-changing field of infusion devices? Here's an overview of what's new on the market. RN 1997;60(10):35–39.

Smeltzer SC, Bare BG. Brunner and Suddarth's textbook of medical-surgical nursing, 8th ed. Philadelphia, Lippincott-Raven, 1996.

SKILL 15-1

RECORDING INTAKE AND OUTPUT

Suggested Action	Reason for Action
Assessment	
Check the Kardex or listen in report to determine whether an assigned patient is on I&O.	Ensures compliance with the plan for care
Verify during report how much IV fluid has been accounted for from any currently infusing solution.	Indicates the credited volume for calculating fluid intake at the end of the shift
Review the nursing care plan for any previously identified fluid problem and nursing orders for specific interventions.	Promotes continuity of care
Review the patient's medical record and analyze the trends in I&O, vital sign measurements, laboratory findings, and weight records.	Aids in analyzing trends in fluid status
Perform a physical assessment to obtain data that reflects the patient's fluid status (see Table 15-4).	Provides current data
Inspect all tubings and drains to ensure they are patent (open).	Ensures that methods for instilling or removing fluids are functional
Notice whether all suction containers or drainage containers were emptied at the end of the previous shift.	Ensures accurate record keeping
Determine how much the patient understands about I&O measurements, fluid intake goals, or fluid restrictions.	Verifies whether additional teaching is needed
Look for a calibrated container and bedside I&O record.	Facilitates keeping accurate data
Obtain a collection device for inside the toilet if the patient has none and uses the toilet for urinary elimination.	Facilitates measuring voided urine
Measure the amount of water in the patient's bedside carafe at the beginning of the shift.	Provides a baseline for measuring fluid consumed in addition to that served at regular meal times
Planning	
Place the patient on I&O or plan to measure I&O if the patient is at high risk for fluid imbalance or the assessment data suggests a problem.	Demonstrates safe and appropriate nursing care
Identify the goal for fluid intake or restriction. A minimum of 1,000 mL in 8 hours is not unrealistic for a patient in fluid deficit. An amount prescribed by the physician or an intake equal to the patient's previous hourly output may be used as a guideline for fluid restrictions.	Provides a target for patient care
Implementation	
Explain or reinforce the purpose and procedures that will be followed for measuring I&O.	Facilitates patient cooperation
Record the volume for all fluids consumed from the dietary tray and other sources of oral liquids.	Contributes to accurate assessment records
Make sure that all IV fluids or tube feedings are being administered at the prescribed rate.	Ensures compliance with medical therapy

continued

SKILL 15–1

RECORDING INTAKE AND OUTPUT *Continued*

Suggested Action	Reason for Action
Ensure that the nurse who adds additional IV fluid containers also records the volume when the infusion is complete or replaced.	Ensures accurate record keeping
Keep track of the fluid volumes used to irrigate drainage tubes or flush feeding tubes.	Ensures accurate record keeping
Measure and record the volume of voided urine. Although urine is not considered a vehicle for the transmission of bloodborne microorganisms, gloves are worn as standard precautions.	Ensures accurate record keeping and reduces the transmission of microorganisms
Measure and record the volume of urine collected in a catheter drainage bag near the end of the shift.	Ensures accurate record keeping

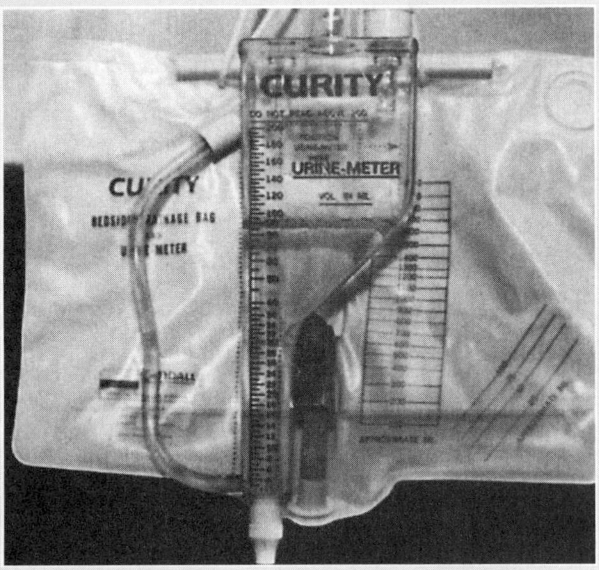

Urine drainage bag. (Courtesy of Ken Timby.)

Suggested Action	Reason for Action
Wear gloves to measure liquid stool or other body fluids and record their measured amounts.	Prevents the transmission of microorganisms and provides assessment data
Wash your hands thoroughly after removing and disposing of the gloves.	Reduces the presence and potential transmission of microorganisms
Check the volume remaining in currently infusing IV fluids; subtract the remaining volume from the credit provided at the beginning of the shift.	Ensures accurate assessment data
Total all fluid intake volumes and all fluid output volumes for the current 8-hour shift, and record the amounts.	Ensures accurate record keeping
Compare the data to determine whether the intake and output are approximately the same and whether the goals for fluid intake or restrictions have been met.	Demonstrates concern for safe and appropriate care
Report major differences in I&O to the nurse in charge or the patient's physician.	Demonstrates concern for safe and appropriate care

continued

SKILL 15-1

RECORDING INTAKE AND OUTPUT *Continued*

Suggested Action	Reason for Action
Review the plan of care and make revisions if the goals have not been met or if additional nursing interventions seem appropriate.	Demonstrates responsibility and accountability
Report the I&O volumes, IV fluid credit amount, and any other pertinent data to the nurse who will be assuming responsibility for the patient's care.	Demonstrates responsibility and accountability

Evaluation

- Intake approximates output.
- Goals for fluid intake or restriction have been met.
- Significant data have been reported.
- The patient's fluid status justifies continuing the care as planned, or the care plan has been revised.

Document

- Date and time
- Intake and output volumes for the previous 8 hours

SAMPLE DOCUMENTATION*

Date and Time Fluid intake for the previous 8 hours is 1,200 mL and output is 1,000 mL.

______________________________ SIGNATURE/TITLE

CRITICAL THINKING

- Calculate the fluid intake in milliliters for the following 8-hour period based on the volumes contained in your agency's dietary utensils, or use the equivalents in Display 15-2:

  The patient consumes: 1 juice glass of orange juice, 1 carton of milk, 1 cup of coffee, 1 bowl of soup, 1 dish of jello, 1 glass of water; the patient receives 100 mL IV infusion of solution containing an antibiotic.
- Evaluate the above total and indicate whether this is a sufficient intake to maintain fluid balance, assuming the patient will continue to receive a similar amount during the remaining 16 hours.
- What assessment findings suggest that a patient is at risk for fluid volume deficit?

* These data are generally recorded on a graphic flow sheet rather than in the narrative nursing notes; however, for teaching purposes, this example has been provided.

SKILL 15-2

PREPARING INTRAVENOUS SOLUTIONS

Suggested Action	Reason for Action
Assessment	
Check the medical order for the type, volume, and projected length of fluid therapy.	Ensures accuracy and guides the selection of equipment
Determine whether the solution is in a bag or bottle and whether the infusion will be administered by gravity or infusion device.	Affects the selection of tubing
Review the patient's medical record for information on the risk for infection.	Determines need for filtered tubing
Read the label on the solution at least three times.	Helps prevent errors
Planning	
Mark a time strip and attach it to the side of the container (see Fig. A).	Facilitates monitoring

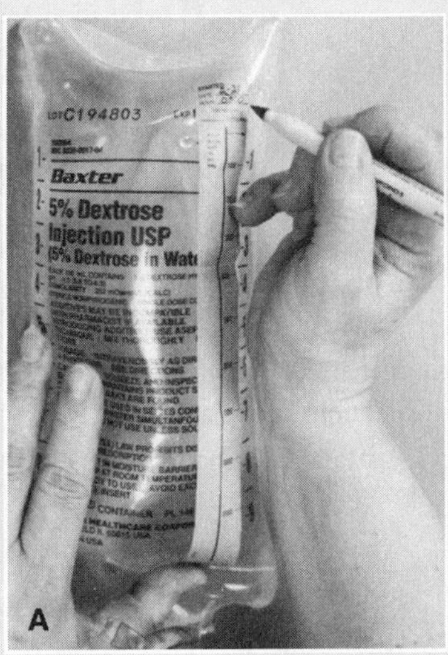

Marking a time strip. (Courtesy of Ken Timby.)

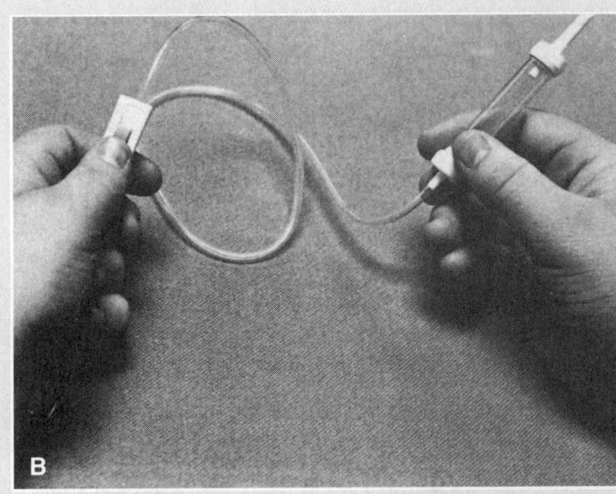

Tightening the roller clamp. (Courtesy of Ken Timby.)

Suggested Action	Reason for Action
Implementation	
Wash your hands.	Reduces the transmission of microorganisms
Select the appropriate tubing and stretch it once it has been removed from the package.	Straightens the tubing by removing bends and kinks
Tighten the roller clamp (see Fig. B).	Aids in filling the drip chamber

continued

SKILL 15-2

PREPARING INTRAVENOUS SOLUTIONS *Continued*

Suggested Action	Reason for Action
Remove the cover from the access port.	Provides access for inserting the spike
Insert the spike by puncturing the seal on the container (see Fig. C).	Provides an exit route for fluid
Hang the solution container from an IV pole or suspended hook.	Inverts the container
Squeeze the drip chamber, filling it no more than half full (see Fig. D).	Leaves space to count the drops when regulating the rate of infusion

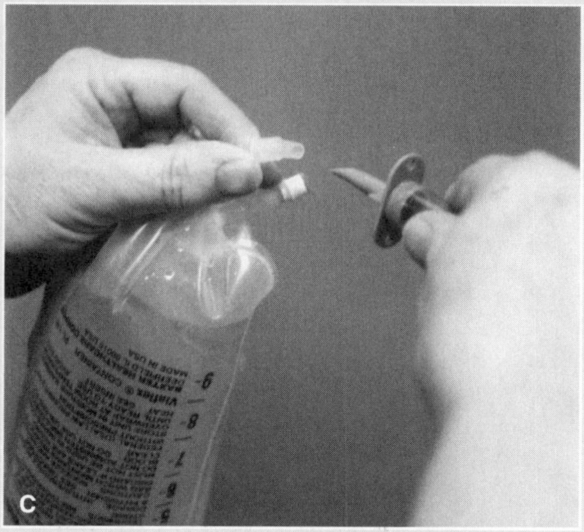

Inserting the spike. (Courtesy of Ken Timby.)

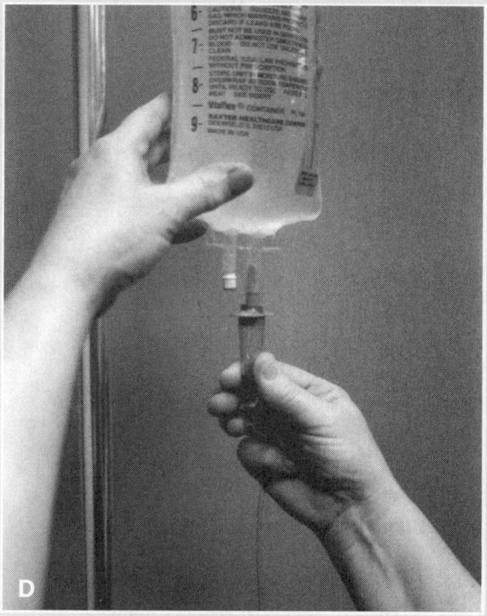

Squeezing the drip chamber. (Courtesy of Ken Timby.)

Release the roller clamp.	Flushes air from the tubing
Invert ports within the tubing as the solution approaches (see Fig. E).	Displaces air that may be trapped in the junction
Tighten the roller clamp when all the air has been removed.	Prevents loss of fluid
Attach a piece of tape or a label on the tubing giving the date, time, and your initials.	Provides a quick reference for determining when the tubing needs to be changed
Take the solution and tubing to the patient's room.	Facilitates administration

continued

SKILL 15–2

PREPARING INTRAVENOUS SOLUTIONS *Continued*

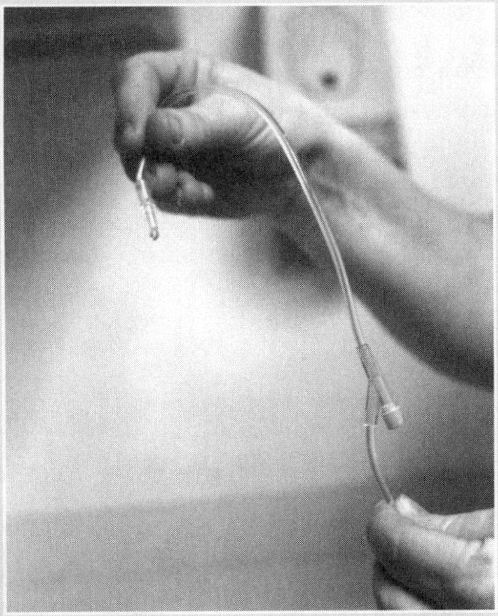

E

Inverting all the ports. (Courtesy of Ken Timby.)

Evaluation

- Solution and tubing are properly labeled.
- Tubing has been purged of air.

Document

- Date and time
- Type and volume of solution
- Rate of infusion once venipuncture has been performed
- Location of venipuncture site

SAMPLE DOCUMENTATION

Date and Time 1,000 mL of 5% D/W infusing at 125 mL/hr through IV in L. forearm.

_______________________________________ SIGNATURE/TITLE

CRITICAL THINKING

- A nurse asks you to prepare a time strip that will be attached to a 1-L bag of IV solution. If the solution will infuse over 8 hours, at what volumes will you mark the hourly increments?
- If a nurse asks you to obtain a 1-L container of 5% dextrose in water, what assessments will you perform when inspecting the container?
- Discuss the type of tubing you would select when preparing to administer a continuous infusion of IV crystalloid solution that is available in a plastic container. The rate of the infusion is 100 mL/hour and the patient has a healthy immune system.

SKILL 15-3

STARTING AN INTRAVENOUS INFUSION

Suggested Action	Reason for Action
Assessment	
Check the identity of the patient.	Prevents errors
Review the patient's medical record to determine whether there are any allergies to iodine or tape.	Influences supplies that will be used and modifications in the procedure
Inspect and palpate several potential venipuncture sites (see Fig. A).	Provides an alternative if the first attempt is unsuccessful
Planning	
Bring all the necessary equipment to the bedside (see Fig. B).	Promotes organization and efficient time management

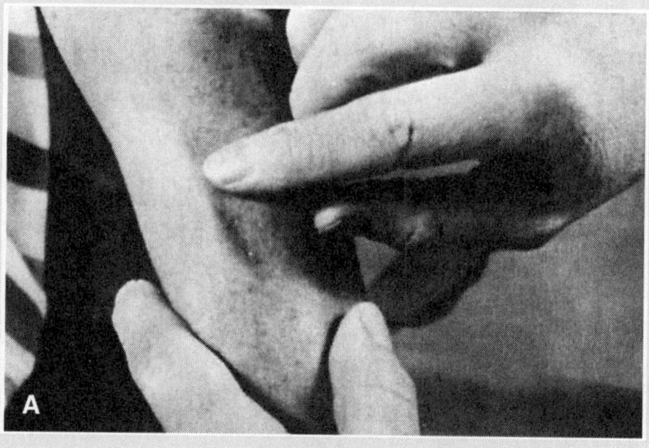

Palpating veins.

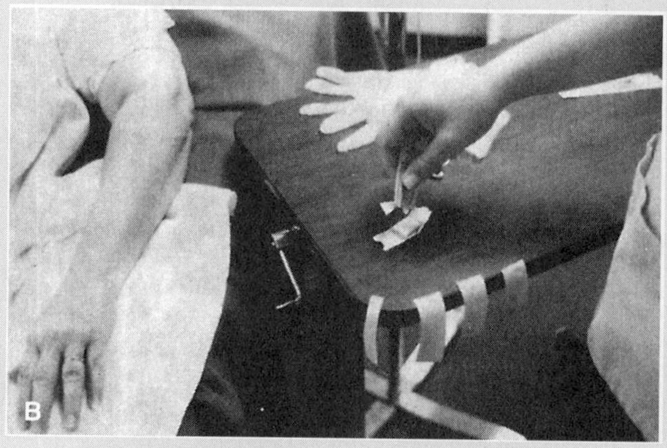

Preparing supplies. (Courtesy of Ken Timby.)

Suggested Action	Reason for Action
Position the patient on his or her back or in a sitting position.	Promotes comfort and facilitates inspection of the arm
Place an absorbent pad beneath the hand or arm.	Prevents having to change bed linen if the site bleeds
Select a site most likely to facilitate the purpose for the infusion and comply with the criteria for vein selection.	Facilitates continuous fluid administration and minimizes potential complications
Clip body hair at the site if it is excessive.	Facilitates visualization and reduces discomfort when adhesive tape is removed
Apply topical anesthetic such as Numby Stuff or EMLA cream.	Provides local anesthesia to insertion site to minimize pain associated with a needle stick
Tear strips of tape, open the package with the venipuncture device, and place antiseptic ointment on an opened Band-Aid or gauze square, based on the agency's policy.	Saves time and ensures that the venipuncture device is not displaced once it is inserted. The application of antimicrobial ointment is controversial and is dependent on agency policy
Implementation	
Wash your hands.	Reduces the number of microorganisms
Apply a tourniquet or a blood pressure cuff 2″ to 4″ (5 to 10 cm) above the vein that will be used.	Distends the vein

continued

SKILL 15-3

STARTING AN INTRAVENOUS INFUSION *Continued*

Suggested Action	Reason for Action
Use an antimicrobial solution such as Betadine and/or alcohol to cleanse the skin, starting at the center of the site outward 2″ to 4″ (see Fig. C).	Reduces the potential for infection
Allow the antiseptic to dry.	Potentiates the effectiveness of antiseptic and prevents burning when the needle is inserted
Don clean gloves.	Provides a barrier for bloodborne viruses
Use the thumb to stretch and stabilize the vein and soft tissues about 2″ (5 cm) below the intended site of entry (see Fig. D).	Helps straighten the vein and prevents it from moving about underneath the skin

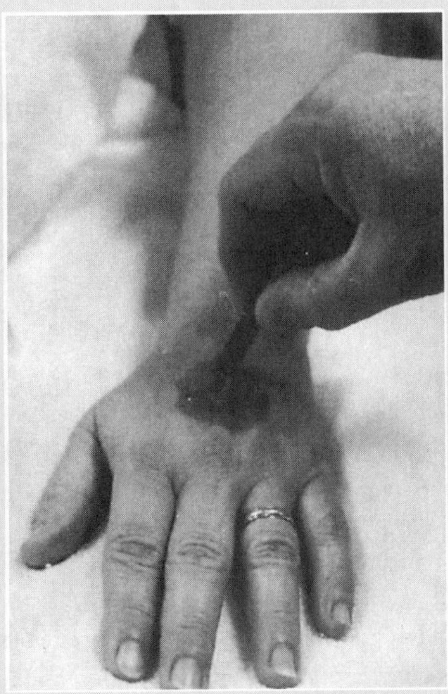

C

Cleaning the site. (Courtesy of Ken Timby.)

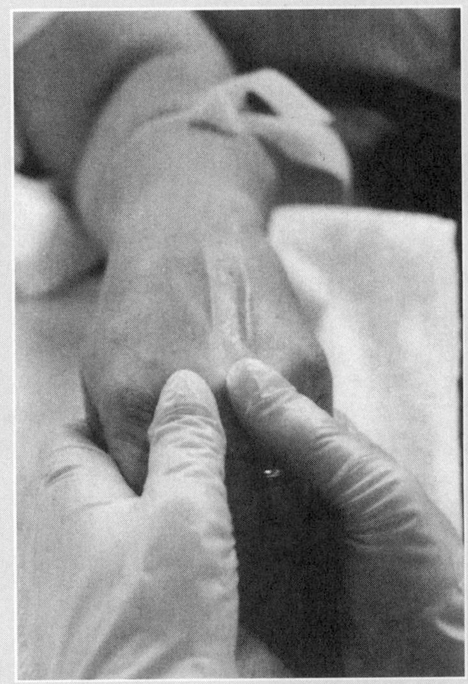

D

Stabilizing the vein. (Courtesy of Ken Timby.)

Suggested Action	Reason for Action
Position the venipuncture device with the bevel up and at approximately a 45° angle above or to the side of the vein (see Fig. E).	Facilitates piercing the vein

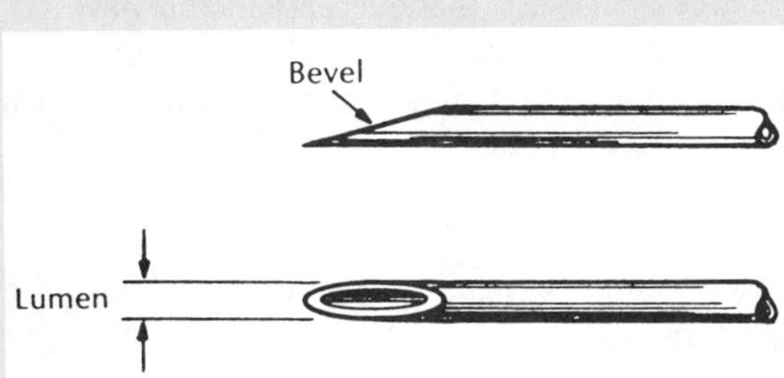

E

Placing the bevel up.

continued

SKILL 15-3

STARTING AN INTRAVENOUS INFUSION *Continued*

Suggested Action	Reason for Action
Warn the patient just before inserting the needle.	Prepares the patient for discomfort
Feel for a change in resistance and look for blood to appear behind the needle.	Indicates the vein has been pierced
Once blood is observed, advance the needle about ⅛″ to ¼″ (see Fig. F).	Positions the catheter tip within the inner wall of the vein

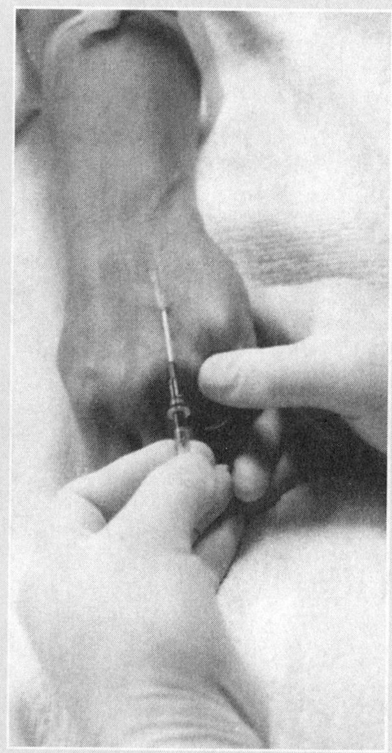

F

Advancing the needle tip. (Courtesy of Ken Timby.)

Suggested Action	Reason for Action
Withdraw the needle slightly so that the tip is within the catheter.	Prevents puncturing the outside of the vein wall
Slide the catheter into the vein until only the end of the infusion device can be seen.	Ensures full insertion of the catheter
Release the tourniquet.	Reduces venous pressure and restores circulation
Apply pressure over the internal tip of the catheter.	Limits blood loss
Remove the protective cap covering the end of the IV tubing and insert it into the end of the venipuncture device.	Facilitates infusing the solution
Release the roller clamp and begin infusing solution slowly.	Clears blood from the venipuncture device before it can clot
Remove gloves when there is no longer a potential for direct contact with blood.	Facilitates handling tape

continued

SKILL 15-3

STARTING AN INTRAVENOUS INFUSION *Continued*

Suggested Action	Reason for Action
Place a small amount of antiseptic ointment onto the site or dressing.	Reduces the potential for infection. However, the application of antimicrobial ointment is controversial. Agency policy must be followed.
Secure the catheter by criss-crossing a piece of tape from beneath the tubing (see Fig. G).	Prevents catheter displacement
Cover the entire site with additional strips of tape, taking care to loop and secure the tubing (see Fig. H).	Prevents tension on the tubing that may cause displacement

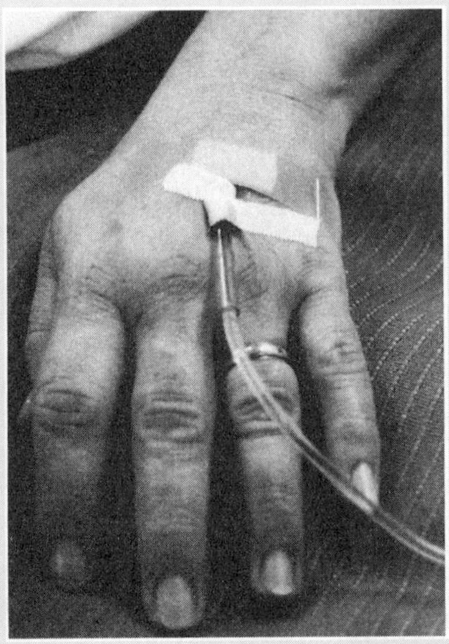

G

Stabilizing catheter. (Courtesy of Ken Timby.)

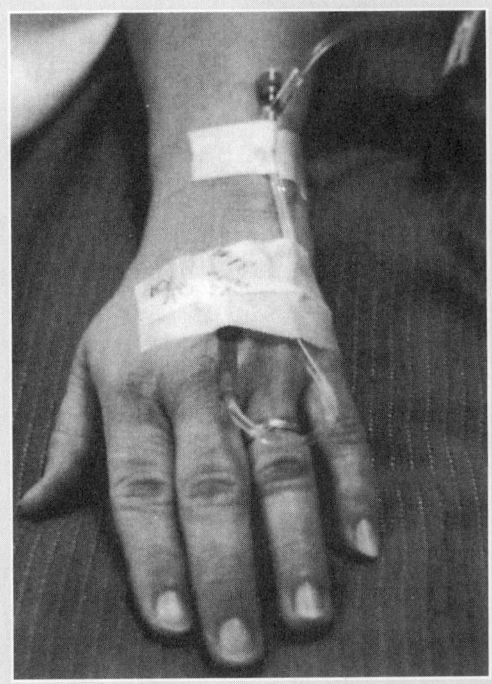

H

Securing the tubing.

Suggested Action	Reason for Action
Write the date, time, gauge of the catheter, and your initials on the outer piece of tape.	Provides a quick reference for determining when the site must be changed
Tighten or release the roller clamp to regulate the rate of fluid infusion.	Facilitates compliance with the medical order

Evaluation

- A flashback of blood was observed before advancing the catheter.
- Minimal discomfort and blood loss occurred.
- Fluid is infusing at the prescribed rate.

Document

- Date and time
- Gauge and type of venipuncture device
- Site of venipuncture
- Type and volume of solution
- Rate of infusion

continued

SKILL 15-3

STARTING AN INTRAVENOUS INFUSION *Continued*

SAMPLE DOCUMENTATION

Date and Time #20 gauge over-the-needle catheter inserted into vein in L. forearm. 1,000 mL 0.9% saline infusing at 42 gtt/min. ______________________ SIGNATURE/TITLE

CRITICAL THINKING

- You have been informed that an assigned patient needs an IV infusion. Discuss factors that will influence the anatomic location for performing the venipuncture.
- What suggestions can you offer if it is difficult to distend a patient's veins before performing a venipuncture?
- After a venipuncture has been performed and the solution is infusing, the nurse records the date, the size of the venipuncture device, and initials. What information is missing? Explain why the missing information is essential.

SKILL 15-4

CHANGING IV SOLUTION CONTAINERS

Suggested Action	Reason for Action
Assessment	
Assess the volume that remains in the infusing container and the rate at which it is infusing.	Helps establish when the solution will need to be replaced
Check the medication record or physician's orders to determine what solution is to follow the current infusion.	Ensures compliance with the medical order
Planning	
Obtain the replacement solution well in advance of needing it.	Ensures that the infusion will be uninterrupted
Attach a time strip to the new container indicating the date, your initials, and the hourly infusion volumes.	Avoids having to complete this responsibility later
Organize patient care to change the container when the current infusion becomes low.	Demonstrates efficient time management
Implementation	
Check the identity of the patient.	Prevents errors
Wash your hands.	Reduces the transmission of microorganisms
Tighten the roller clamp slightly or slow the rate of infusion on an infusion device.	Slows the rate of infusion so that the drip chamber remains filled with solution
Remove the almost-empty solution container from the suspension hook with the tubing still attached.	Facilitates separating the tubing from the container
Invert the empty solution container and pull the spike free.	Prevents minor loss of remaining solution

continued

SKILL 15–4

CHANGING IV SOLUTION CONTAINERS *Continued*

Suggested Action	Reason for Action
Deposit the empty bag in a lined waste receptacle.	Keeps the environment clean and orderly
Remove the seal from the replacement solution container.	Provides access to the port
Insert the spike into the port of the new container.	Provides a route for infusing fluid
Hang the new container from the suspension hook on the IV standard or infusion device.	Restores height to overcome venous pressure
Inspect for the presence of air within the tubing; remove it, if present.	Reduces the potential for air embolism or an alarm from an infusion device detecting air
Readjust the roller clamp or reprogram the infusion device to restore the prescribed rate of infusion.	Demonstrates compliance with the medical order

Evaluation

- Solution container is replaced.
- Infusion continues.

Document

- Volume infused from previous container on I&O record
- Time, volume, type of solution, and signature on the medication record or wherever the agency specifies documenting the administration of IV solutions
- Condition of the patient

SAMPLE DOCUMENTATION

Date and Time 1,000 mL lactated Ringer's instilling at 42 gtt/min. Dressing over venipuncture is dry and intact. No swelling or discomfort in the area of the infusing fluid.

______________________________ SIGNATURE/TITLE

CRITICAL THINKING

- Explain the nursing actions you would use if air bubbles are evident in the tubing when the container of solution is changed.
- Discuss what actions a nurse should take if the wrong type of IV solution is hung at the time of replacement. Assume that the solution has been infusing for several hours before the discrepancy is noted.

SKILL 15-5

CHANGING IV TUBING

Suggested Action	Reason for Action
Assessment	
Determine the agency's policy for changing IV tubing.	Demonstrates responsibility for complying with infection control policies
Check the date and time on the label attached to the tubing.	Determines the approximate time when the tubing must be changed
Determine whether the solution container will need to be replaced before the time expires on the tubing.	Facilitates changing both the container and tubing at the same time
Planning	
Obtain appropriate replacement tubing and supplies for changing the dressing.	Ensures that equipment will be available and ready when needed
Attach a new label to the tubing indicating the date and time the tubing is changed and your initials.	Provides a quick reference for determining when the tubing must be changed again
Implementation	
Wash your hands.	Reduces the transmission of microorganisms
Tear strips of adhesive tape and dressing materials and place them in a convenient location.	Facilitates dexterity later in the procedure
Open the new package containing the tubing, stretch the tubing, and tighten the roller clamp.	Prepares the tubing for insertion into the solution container
Remove the solution container from the suspension hook with the tubing still attached.	Facilitates separating the tubing from the container
Invert the solution container and pull the spike free.	Prevents minor loss of remaining solution
Secure the spike to the IV pole with a strip of previously torn tape.	Facilitates continued infusion
Insert the spike from the new tubing into the container of solution.	Provides a route for the fluid
Squeeze the drip chamber to fill it half full, open the roller clamp, and purge the air from the tubing.	Prepares the tubing for use
Remove the tape and dressing from the venipuncture site.	Provides access to the venipuncture device
Don gloves.	Provides a barrier from contact with blood
Tighten the roller clamp on the expired tubing.	Temporarily interrupts the infusion
Stabilize the hub of the venipuncture device and separate the tubing from it.	Prevents accidental removal of the catheter or needle from the vein
Remove the cap from the end of the new tubing and attach it to the end of the venipuncture device.	Connects the venipuncture device to the tubing without contaminating the tip of the tubing
Continue to hold the venipuncture device with one hand while releasing the roller clamp on the new tubing.	Re-establishes the infusion
Replace the dressing on the venipuncture site, and secure the tubing.	Covers the site and keeps the tubing and venipuncture device from being pulled out
Readjust the rate of infusion.	Complies with the medical order

continued

SKILL 15-5

CHANGING IV TUBING *Continued*

Suggested Action	Reason for Action
Write the date, time, and your initials on the new dressing, and include the gauge of the venipuncture device and original date of insertion.	Provides a quick reference for determining future nursing responsibilities for infection control
Dispose of the expired tubing in a lined receptacle.	Maintains a clean and orderly environment

Evaluation

- Tubing is replaced.
- Solution continues to infuse at the prescribed rate.

Document

- Date and time
- Assessment findings of venipuncture site
- Dressing change

SAMPLE DOCUMENTATION

Date and Time No redness, swelling, or tenderness at venipuncture site in L. forearm. Dressing changed following replacement of IV tubing. ______________________________ SIGNATURE/TITLE

CRITICAL THINKING

- Discuss why it is advantageous to change the IV tubing and container of solution at the same time, rather than doing each at separate times.
- Discuss the potential hazards to the patient and nurse that can occur when changing the tubing during IV infusions.

SKILL 15-6

INSERTING A MEDICATION LOCK

Suggested Action	Reason for Action
Assessment	
Confirm that the physician has written an order to discontinue the continuous infusion of IV fluid and insert a medication lock.	Demonstrates responsibility and accountability for carrying out medical orders
Check the patient's identity.	Prevents errors
Inspect the site for signs of redness, swelling, or drainage.	Provides data indicating whether the site can be maintained or whether a new venipuncture should be performed
Observe whether the infusion is instilling at the predetermined rate.	Indicates whether the vein and catheter are patent (open)
Determine whether the patient understands the purpose and technique for inserting a medication lock.	Indicates the need for patient teaching

continued

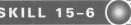

SKILL 15-6

INSERTING A MEDICATION LOCK *Continued*

Suggested Action	Reason for Action
Planning	
Assemble necessary equipment, which includes the medication lock, syringe containing 2 mL of sterile normal saline (0.9% sodium chloride) or heparinized saline (10 U per mL or 100 U per mL, depending on the agency's policy), alcohol swabs, gloves, and supplies for changing or reinforcing the dressing over the site.	Promotes organization and efficient time management
Implementation	
Wash your hands.	Reduces the spread of microorganisms
Fill the chamber of the medication lock with saline or heparin solution.	Displaces air from the empty chamber
Loosen the tape over the dressing to expose the connection between the hub of the catheter or needle and the tubing adapter; also remove the tape that is stabilizing the tubing to the patient's arm.	Facilitates removing the tubing from the patient
Loosen the protective cap from the end of the medication lock.	Maintains sterility while preparing for the insertion of the lock
Don clean gloves.	Provides a barrier from contact with blood
Tighten the roller clamp on the tubing and stop the infusion pump or controller if one is being used.	Prevents leakage of fluid when the tubing is removed
Apply pressure over the tip of the catheter or needle (see Fig. A).	Controls or prevents blood loss
Remove the tip of the tubing from the venipuncture device and insert the medication lock (see Fig. B).	Seals the opening in the catheter or needle
Screw the lock onto the end of the catheter or needle.	Stabilizes the connection
Swab the rubber port on the medication lock with alcohol.	Cleanses the port

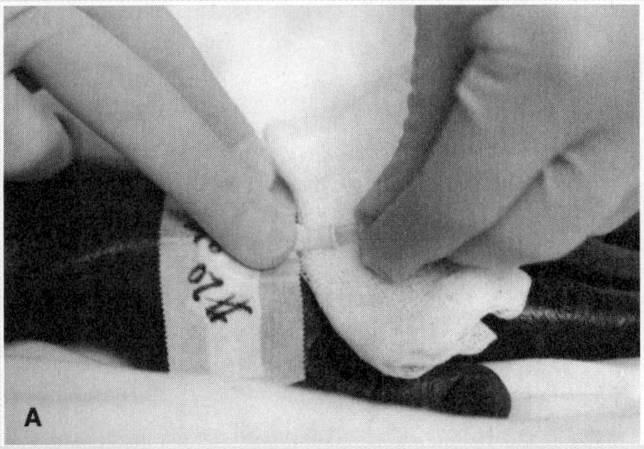

A

Applying pressure over the catheter tip. (Courtesy of Ken Timby.)

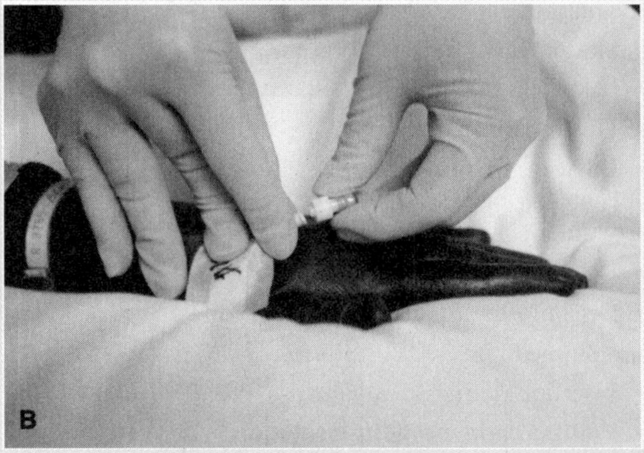

B

Inserting the device. (Courtesy of Ken Timby.)

continued

SKILL 15-6

INSERTING A MEDICATION LOCK *Continued*

Suggested Action	Reason for Action
Pierce the port with the needle on the syringe or blunt needleless adapter and gradually instill 2 mL of saline or heparin until the syringe is almost empty (see Fig. C).	Clears blood from the venipuncture device and lock before it can clot

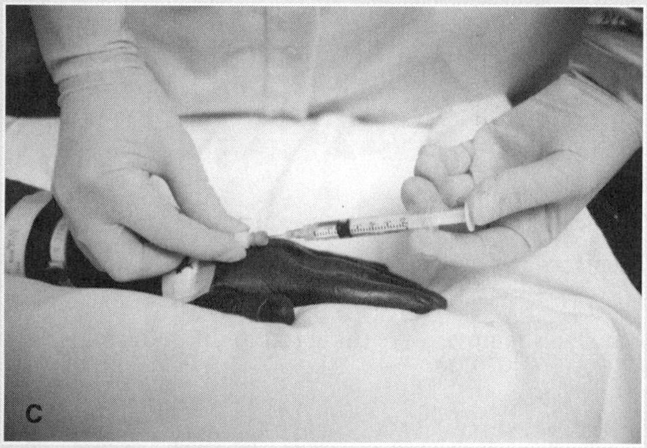

Instilling saline or heparin solution. (Courtesy of Ken Timby.)

Suggested Action	Reason for Action
Begin to remove the needle from the port as the last volume of solution is instilled; clamp or pinch the tubing, or press over the venipuncture device before removing a needleless adapter.	Continues the application of positive pressure (pushing effect) rather than negative pressure (pulling effect) during the time the syringe is removed. Negative pressure pulls blood into the catheter or needle tip, which may cause an obstruction.
Retape or secure the dressing.	Reduces the possibility that the lock and catheter may be accidentally dislodged
Plan to flush the lock at least every 8 hours with 1 or 2 mL of flush solution (either saline or heparin solution) when it is not used, or after each use.	Ensures continued patency

Evaluation

- Site appears free of inflammation.
- Patency is maintained.
- Flush solution instills easily.
- Device is stabilized.

Document

- Date and time
- Discontinuation of infusing solution
- Volume of infused IV solution
- Insertion of medication lock
- Volume and type of flush solution
- Assessment findings

continued

SKILL 15-6

INSERTING A MEDICATION LOCK *Continued*

SAMPLE DOCUMENTATION

Date and Time Infusion of 5%D/W discontinued. 700 mL of IV solution infused. Medication lock inserted into IV catheter in R. hand and flushed with 2 mL of normal saline. No redness, swelling, or discomfort at site. ________________________________ SIGNATURE, TITLE

CRITICAL THINKING

- Discuss advantages for using a medication lock as they relate to both the patient and the nurse.
- Discuss possible reasons why the flush solution will not instill into a medication lock, techniques for preventing the contributing causes, and subsequent nursing action(s) if the device cannot be flushed.

SKILL 15-7

ADMINISTERING A BLOOD TRANSFUSION

Suggested Action	Reason for Action
Assessment	
Check the patient's identity.	Prevents errors
Determine whether a special signed consent is required.	Complies with legal responsibilities
Check the size of the current venipuncture device if an IV is infusing.	Indicates whether another venipuncture must be performed
Review the medical record for results of type and cross-match.	Indicates whether blood is available in the blood bank
Take temperature, pulse, respirations, and blood pressure within 30 minutes of obtaining blood.	Provides a baseline for comparison during the transfusion
Planning	
Complete major nursing activities before starting the infusion of saline unless the blood must be given immediately.	Avoids disturbing the patient once the blood is being administered
Plan to perform a venipuncture or start the infusion of saline just before obtaining the blood.	Prevents administering fluid unnecessarily
Obtain necessary equipment, including a 250-mL container of normal saline (0.9% NaCl) and a Y-set.	Complies with the standards of care for administering blood
Tighten the roller clamp on one branch of the Y-tubing and the roller clamp below the filter.	Prepares the tubing for purging with saline
Insert the unclamped branch of the Y-set into the container of saline and squeeze the drip chamber until it and the filter are half full.	Moistens the filter and fills the upper portion of the tubing with saline
Release the lower clamp and flush air from the remaining section of tubing.	Reduces the potential for infusing a bolus of air
Implementation	
Perform the venipuncture or connect the Y-set to the present venipuncture device, if it is a 16–20 gauge.	Provides access to the venous circulation and ensures that blood will move freely through the catheter or needle

continued

SKILL 15-7

ADMINISTERING A BLOOD TRANSFUSION *Continued*

Suggested Action	Reason for Action
Begin the infusion of saline.	Ensures that the site is patent and that there will be no delay once the unit of blood is obtained
Go to the blood bank to pick up the unit of blood, making sure to take a form identifying the patient.	Prevents mistaken identity when releasing the matched blood
Double-check the information on the blood bag with the cross-matched information on the lab slip with the blood bank personnel.	Prevents releasing the wrong unit of blood or blood that is not a compatible blood group and Rh factor
Check that the blood has not passed the expiration date.	Ensures maximum benefit from the transfusion
Inspect the container of blood and reject the blood if it appears dark black or has obvious gas bubbles inside.	Indicates deteriorated or tainted blood
Plan to give the blood as soon as it is brought to the unit.	Demonstrates an understanding that blood must be infused within 4 hours after being released from the blood bank
Rotate the blood, but do not shake or squeeze the container, if the serum has separated from the cells.	Avoids damaging intact cells
At the bedside, check the label on the blood bag with the numbers on the patient's wristband with a second nurse; sign in the designated areas on the transfusion record.	Reduces the potential for administering incompatible blood
Spike the container of blood.	Provides a route for administering the blood
Tighten the roller clamp on the saline branch of the tubing and release the roller clamp on the blood branch.	Fills the tubing and filter with blood
Regulate the rate of infusion at no more than 50 mL/hr for the first 15 minutes (check the drop factor to determine the rate in gtt/min).	Establishes a slow rate of infusion so the nurse can monitor for and respond to signs of a transfusion reaction
Increase the rate after the first 15 minutes so as to complete the infusion in 2–4 hours if a second assessment of vital signs is basically unchanged and if no signs of a reaction have occurred.	Increases the rate of administration to infuse the unit within a safe period of time
Assess the patient at 15- to 30-minute intervals during the transfusion.	Ensures patient safety
Clamp the tubing from the blood and release the clamp on the saline when the blood has infused.	Flushes blood cells from the tubing
Take vital signs one more time.	Documents the condition of the patient at the completion of the blood administration
Tighten the roller clamp below the filter when the tubing looks reasonably clear of blood.	Prevents leaking when the IV is discontinued
Don gloves.	Provides a barrier from contact with blood
Loosen the tape covering the venipuncture site and remove the catheter, or remove the blood tubing and reconnect the previously infusing solution.	Discontinues the infusion or restores previous fluid therapy
Apply a dressing or Band-Aid over the venipuncture site if the IV is discontinued.	Prevents infection
Dispose of the blood container and tubing according to agency policy.	Blood is a biohazard and requires special bagging to ensure that others will not accidentally come in direct contact with the blood.

continued

SKILL 15-7

ADMINISTERING A BLOOD TRANSFUSION *Continued*

Evaluation

- Entire unit of blood is administered within 4 hours.
- Patient demonstrates no evidence of transfusion reaction, or
- Reactions have been minimized by appropriate interventions.
- Infusion is discontinued or previous orders are resumed.

Document

- Venipuncture procedure, if initiated for the administration of blood
- Preinfusion vital signs
- Names of nurses who checked armband and blood bag container
- Time blood administration began
- Rate of infusion during first 15 minutes and remaining period of time
- Signs of reaction, if any, and nursing actions
- Periodic vital sign assessments
- Time blood infusion completed
- Volume of blood and saline infused

SAMPLE DOCUMENTATION

Date and Time #18 gauge over-the-needle catheter inserted into L. forearm and connected to 250 mL of 0.9% saline infusing at 21 mL/hr. T—98^2 (tympanic), P—90, R—22, BP 116/64 in R. arm while lying flat. One unit of type O+ whole blood #684381 obtained from the blood bank and checked by E. Rogers, RN, and D. Baker, RN. Blood bag and wrist band information found to be compatible. Blood infusing at 50 mL/hr for 15 minutes. Rate increased to 125 mL/hr during remainder of infusion. Blood transfusion completed at 1600. No evidence of transfusion reaction. T—98^2 (tympanic), P—86, R—20, BP 122/70 in R. arm at end of transfusion. Total of 100 mL of saline and 500 mL of blood infused before IV discontinued.

______________________________ SIGNATURE/TITLE

CRITICAL THINKING

- A patient you are caring for is scheduled to receive a blood transfusion shortly. What are your plans for assessing the patient before, during, and after the transfusion? What is the basis for your assessment concerns?
- If a patient receiving a blood transfusion suddenly develops hypotension and tachycardia, and you observe flushing and dyspnea, what nursing actions are appropriate? Rank the nursing actions in order of priority.

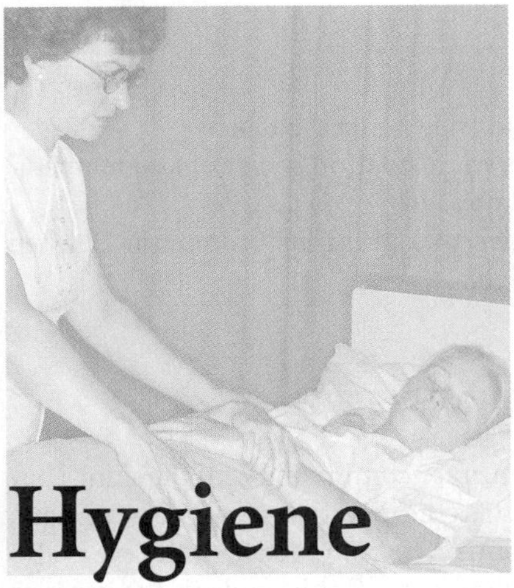

CHAPTER 16

Hygiene

CHAPTER OUTLINE

NURSING GUIDELINES

BATHING PATIENTS
SHAVING PATIENTS

SKILLS

SKILL 16-1: PROVIDING A TUB BATH OR SHOWER
SKILL 16-2: ADMINISTERING PERINEAL CARE
SKILL 16-3: GIVING A BED BATH
SKILL 16-4: GIVING ORAL CARE TO UNCONSCIOUS PATIENTS
SKILL 16-5: SHAMPOOING HAIR

NURSING CARE PLAN

SELF-CARE DEFICIT, BATHING/HYGIENE

KEY TERMS

bag bath
bed bath
bridge
caries
cuticles
dentures
gingivitis
hygiene
integument
ophthalmologist
optometrist
oral hygiene
partial bath
perineal care
periodontal disease
plaque
podiatrist
sordes
tartar
towel bath

LEARNING OBJECTIVES

An understanding of the content within this chapter will be evidenced by the student's ability to:

- Define the term hygiene.
- Name five hygiene practices that most people perform regularly.
- Give two reasons why a partial bath is more appropriate for older adults than daily bathing.
- List at least three advantages to towel or bag baths.
- Name two situations in which shaving with a safety razor is contraindicated.
- Name three items that are recommended for oral hygiene.
- Identify two methods for preventing the chief hazard in providing oral hygiene for an unconscious patient.
- Describe two techniques for preventing damage to dentures during cleaning.
- Describe two methods for removing hair tangles.
- Name two types of patients for whom nail care is provided with extreme caution.
- Name four visual and hearing devices.
- List two alternatives for patients who cannot insert or care for their own contact lenses.
- Discuss four reasons for sound disturbances experienced by people who wear hearing aids.
- Describe an infrared listening device.

Hygiene (practices that promote health through personal cleanliness) is fostered through activities such as bathing, oral care, cleaning and maintaining fingernails and toenails, and shampooing and grooming hair. It also applies to the care and maintenance of devices such as eyeglasses and hearing aids to ensure continued and proper function.

Hygiene practices and needs differ according to age, inherited characteristics of the skin and hair, cultural values, and health problems. This chapter provides suggestions for carrying out hygiene practices when providing patient care. Principles that refer to the patient environment, including bed-making skills, are discussed in Chapter 17.

The Integumentary System

Most hygiene practices are based on maintaining or restoring a healthy integumentary system. The word **integument** (covering) is the origin for the collective structures that cover the surface of the body and its openings. The integumentary system includes the skin, mucous membranes, hair, and nails. Because the mouth, or oral cavity (which is lined with mucous membrane), also contains teeth, a discussion of this accessory structure is also included.

SKIN

The skin consists of the epidermis, dermis, and subcutaneous layers (Fig. 16-1). The *epidermis,* or outermost layer, contains dead skin cells that form a tough protein called *keratin.* Keratin serves to protect the underlying layers and structures within the skin. The cells in the epidermis are continuously shed and replaced from the *dermis,* or true skin, which contains most of the secretory glands (Table 16-1). The *subcutaneous layer* separates the skin from skeletal muscles. It contains fat cells, blood vessels, nerves, and the roots of hair follicles and glands.

The structures that make up the skin carry out functions such as:

- Protecting inner structures of the body from injury and infection
- Regulating body temperature
- Maintaining fluid and chemical balance
- Providing sensory information such as pain, temperature, touch, and pressure
- Assisting in converting preforms of vitamin D when exposed to sunlight

MUCOUS MEMBRANES

The mucous membranes are continuous with the skin. They line body passages such as the digestive, respiratory, urinary, and reproductive systems. The conjunctiva of the eye is also lined with mucous membrane. Goblet cells in the mucous membranes secrete *mucus,* a slimy substance that keeps the membranes soft and moist.

HAIR

Each hair is a thread of keratin. Hair is formed from cells at the base of a single follicle. Although hair covers the entire body, its amount, distribution, color, and texture vary considerably among males and females, infants and adults, and ethnic groups.

Besides contributing to an individual's unique appearance, hair basically helps to prevent heat loss. As heat escapes from the skin, it becomes trapped in the air between the hairs. Body heat is further maintained by the contraction of small muscles around the hair follicles, commonly described as goose bumps.

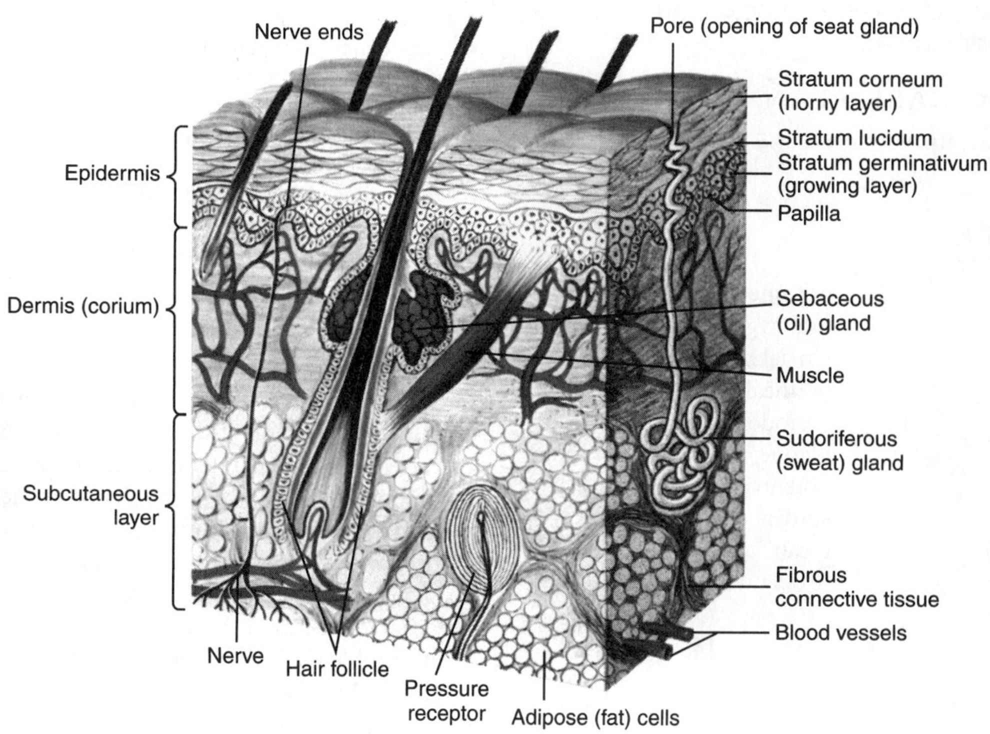

FIGURE 16–1. Cross-section of the skin.

TABLE 16–1. **Types of Skin Glands**

Gland	Location	Secretion	Purpose
Sudoriferous	Throughout the dermis and subcutaneous layers, especially in the axilla and groin	Sweat	Regulate body temperature Excrete body waste
Ceruminous	Ear canals	Cerumen	Perform protective functions; cerumen has antimicrobial properties
Sebaceous	Throughout the dermis	Sebum	Lubricate skin and hair
Ciliary	Eyelids	Sweat and sebum	Protect lid margin and lubricate eyelash follicles

Sebaceous glands in the hair follicle release sebum, an oily secretion that adds weight to the shafts of hair, causing them to flatten against the skull. Oily hair further attracts dust and debris.

The texture, elasticity, and porosity of hair are inherited characteristics influenced by the amount of keratin and sebum produced. To alter the basic structure that has been genetically inherited, some people use chemicals to curl, relax, or lubricate their hair.

NAILS

Fingernails (Fig. 16-2) and toenails are also made of keratin, which, in concentrated amounts, gives them their tough texture. Fingernails and toenails provide some protection to the digits. Normal nails are thin, pink, and smooth. The free margin ordinarily extends from the end of each finger or toe, and the skin around the nails is intact. Changes in the shape, color, texture, thickness, and integrity of the nails provide evidence of local injury or infection and even systemic diseases (see Chap. 12).

TEETH

Teeth, the enamel of which is a keratin structure, are present beneath the gums at birth. The exposed portion of each tooth is referred to as the *crown;* the portion within the gum is the *root* (Fig. 16-3).

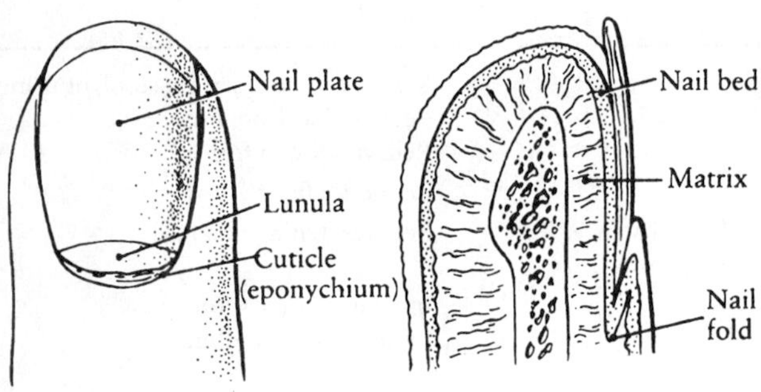

FIGURE 16–2. External and cross-sectional views of a nail.

The teeth begin to erupt at about 6 months of age and continue to do so for 2 or 2.5 more years. As the jaw grows, the *deciduous teeth* (baby teeth) are replaced by *permanent teeth.* Adults have 28 to 32 permanent teeth, depending on whether the third molars (wisdom teeth) are present.

Healthy teeth are firmly fixed within the gums. Their alignment, which is related to jaw structure, is generally a result of heredity. Although the teeth are white originally, they become discolored from chronic consumption of coffee or tea, tobacco use, or the use of certain drugs, such as tetracycline antibiotics taken during childhood.

The integrity of the teeth largely depends on the person's oral hygiene practices, diet, and general health. Saliva, which moistens food and begins its digestive processes, tends to keep the teeth clean and inhibits bacterial growth. However, the accumulation of food debris, especially sugar, and **plaque** (substance composed of mucin and other gritty substances in saliva) supports the growth of mouth bacteria. The combination of sugar, plaque, and bacteria eventually erodes the tooth enamel, causing **caries** (cavities).

Tartar (hardened plaque) is more difficult to remove and may lead to **gingivitis** (inflammation of the gums). The pockets of gum inflammation promote **periodontal disease** (condition that results in destruction of the tooth-supporting structures and jawbone).

Hygiene Practices

The teeth are prone to decay if uncared for, and the integument contains many types of secretory glands that produce odors and attract debris. Therefore, hygiene measures are beneficial for maintaining personal cleanliness and healthy structures of the integument. Although there are wide variations, most Americans include bathing, shaving, brushing the teeth, shampooing, and nail care among their hygiene practices.

BATHING

Bathing is a hygiene practice in which a cleansing agent, such as soap, and water are used to remove sweat, oil, dirt, and

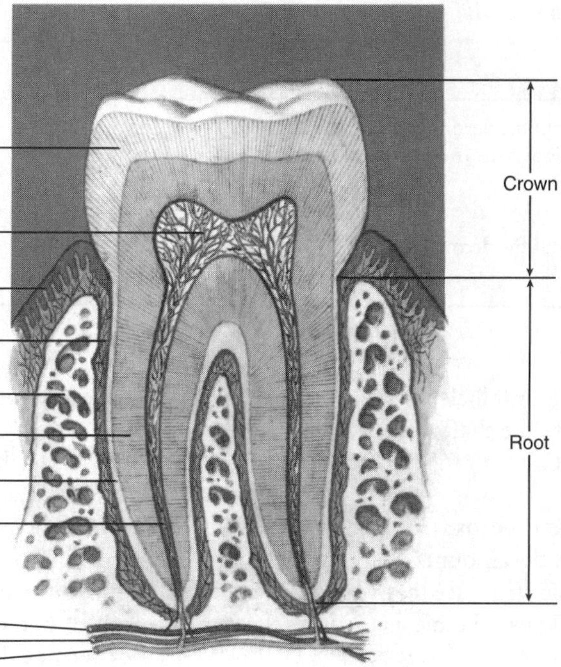

FIGURE 16–3. Cross-section of a tooth. (Cohen B: Medical terminology: An illustrated guide, p 165. Philadelphia, JB Lippincott, 1997)

microorganisms from the skin. Although restoring cleanliness is the primary objective for bathing, there are several other benefits:

- Eliminating body odor
- Reducing the potential for infection
- Stimulating circulation
- Providing a refreshed and relaxed feeling
- Improving self-image

In addition to bathing for hygiene purposes, other types of baths are administered (Table 16-2). In general, however, most bathing is done in a tub or shower, at a sink, or at the bedside.

Tub Bath or Shower

If the safety risks are negligible and there are no contraindications, the nurse encourages patients to bathe independently in a tub or shower (Skill 16-1). In most hospitals and nursing homes, bathing facilities are equipped with a variety of rails and handles to promote patient safety.

Partial Bath

A daily bath or shower is not always necessary—in fact, for older adults, who do not perspire as much as younger adults

TABLE 16–2. **Therapeutic Baths**

Type	Description	Purpose
Sitz bath	Immersion of the buttocks and perineum in a small basin of continuously circulating water	Removes blood, serum, stool, or urine Reduces local swelling Relieves discomfort
Sponge bath	Applications of tepid water to the skin	Reduces a fever
Medicated bath	Soaking or immersing in a mixture of water and another substance, such as baking soda (sodium bicarbonate), oatmeal, or cornstarch	Relieves itching or a rash
Whirlpool bath	Warm water that is continuously agitated within a tub or tank	Improves circulation Increases joint mobility Relieves discomfort Removes dead tissue

and who are prone to having dry skin, frequent washing with soap further depletes the oil from the skin. Therefore, sometimes partial bathing is appropriate. A **partial bath** (washing only the areas of the body that are subject to the greatest soiling or sources of body odor) is generally confined to the face, hands, and axillae. Partial bathing is done at a sink or with a basin at the bedside.

Sometimes the *perineum,* the area around the genitals and rectum, requires special or frequent cleansing in addition to bathing. **Perineal care** (peri-care; techniques used for cleansing the perineum) is especially important after a vaginal delivery or gynecologic or rectal surgery so that the impaired skin is kept as clean as possible. It is also appropriate whenever male or female patients have bloody drainage, urine, or stool that collects in this area.

When providing perineal care, nurses must:

- Prevent direct contact between themselves and the secretions or excretions that are present
- Cleanse so that secretions and excretions are removed from less-soiled to more-soiled areas

These principles help prevent the transfer of infectious microorganisms to the nurse and to uncontaminated areas on or within the patient (Skill 16-2).

Bed Bath

Patients who cannot take a tub bath or shower independently are given a bed bath. During a **bed bath** (washing with a basin of water at the bedside), the patient may actively assist with some aspects of bathing.

Nursing Guidelines For Bathing Patients

☑ Ask the patient whether he or she uses special soap, lotion, or other hygiene products.
RATIONALE: Determining the patient's preferences individualizes care.

☑ Wear gloves if there is any potential for direct contact with blood, drainage, or other body fluid.
RATIONALE: Gloves reduce the potential for acquiring an infection.

☑ Keep the patient covered during the bath.
RATIONALE: Covering the patient demonstrates respect for modesty.

☑ Wash cleaner areas of the body first and dirtier areas last.
RATIONALE: This reduces the spread of microorganisms.

☑ Encourage the patient to participate at whatever level is appropriate.
RATIONALE: Participation promotes independence and self-esteem.

☑ Monitor the patient's tolerance of activity.
RATIONALE: If the activity becomes too strenuous, it should be stopped and continued later.

☑ Inspect the body for skin disorders as it is being washed (Table 16-3).
RATIONALE: Bathing provides an excellent opportunity for physical assessment.

☑ Communicate with the patient, and use the opportunity to do informal health teaching.
RATIONALE: Talking demonstrates respect for the patient as a person, rather than an object being washed; teaching promotes health.

☑ Wash one part of the body at a time.
RATIONALE: Exposing only one part prevents chilling.

☑ Place a towel under the part of the body being washed.
RATIONALE: A towel will absorb moisture.

☑ Use firm but gentle strokes.
RATIONALE: Gentle strokes avoid friction that may damage the skin.

☑ Wash and dry well between folds of skin.
RATIONALE: Effective washing removes debris and microorganisms from areas where they are apt to breed.

☑ Keep the washcloth wet, but not so wet that it drips.
RATIONALE: This demonstrates concern for the patient's comfort.

☑ Wash areas that are more soiled, such as the anus, last.
RATIONALE: Washing soiled areas last prevents transferring microorganisms to cleaner areas of the body.

☑ Remove all soap residue.
RATIONALE: Removing soap prevents drying the skin and possible itching.

☑ Dry the skin after it has been rinsed.
RATIONALE: Drying the skin prevents chilling.

☑ Replace the water as it cools.
RATIONALE: Using warm water shows concern for the patient's comfort.

☑ Apply an emollient lotion to the skin after bathing.
RATIONALE: A lotion restores lubrication to the skin.

Skill 16-3 explains how to give a bed bath.

In some agencies, two variations of the traditional bed bath—the towel bath and the bag bath—are being used because they save time and money. Display 16-1 lists their advantages.

Towel Bath

A **towel bath** (technique for bathing in which a single large towel is used to cover and wash a patient) requires a towel

TABLE 16–3. **Examples of Integumentary Disorders**

Condition	Description	Patient Teaching
Acne	Inflammation of sebaceous glands and hair follicles on the face, upper chest, and back	Keep the face clean. Refrain from touching or squeezing lesions. Avoid the use of oily cosmetics.
Contact dermatitis	Allergic sensitivity evidenced by red skin rash and itching	Avoid scratching or wearing clothing made of irritating fibers, such as wool. Use tepid water and hypoallergenic or glycerin soap when bathing. Pat the skin dry; do not rub.
Furuncle (boil)	Raised pustule, usually in the neck, axillary, or groin area, that feels hard and painful	Keep hands away from the infected lesion. Use separate face cloth and towels than others in family; launder personal bath items in hot water and bleach. Wash hands thoroughly before and after applying medication to the skin.
Psoriasis	Noninfectious chronic skin disorder that appears as elevated silvery scales over elbows, knees, trunk, and scalp that shed. Acute episodes occur between periods of relief.	Follow medical regimen, which may be life-long. Be wary of advertised remedies that promise a cure or quick relief, because they rarely do.
Pediculosis (lice infestation)	Brown crawling insects that move over the scalp and skin and deposit yellowish-white eggs on hair shafts including pubic area. Skin bite causes itching.	Inspect the skin carefully; adult lice move quickly from light. Look for eggs (nits) on hairs $1/4''$ to $1/20''$ from the scalp or skin surface. Do not share clothing, combs, brushes; lice are spread by direct contact. Use a pediculocide (chemical that kills lice), in addition to a lice comb and manual removal. Do not use hair conditioner: it coats the hair and protects the nits.
Scabies	Infestation with an itch mite that burrows within the webs and sides of fingers, around arms, axilla, waist, breast, lower buttocks, and genitalia	Bathe thoroughly in the morning and at night. Apply prescribed medication after bathing. Don clean clothes after bathing. Avoid skin-to-skin contact with uninfected people.
Tinea capitis, pedis, corporis, and cruris	Fungal infection in the scalp, feet, body, or groin that appears as a ring or cluster of papules or vesicles that itch, become scaly, cracked, and sore	Use separate bathing and grooming articles. Keep body areas dry, especially in folds of skin. Wear clothing that promotes evaporation of perspiration.
Skin cancer	Newly pigmented growth or change in existing skin lesion, especially where skin is chronically exposed to sun	See a physician for examination and possible biopsy. Avoid direct sun exposure between 10 AM and 4 PM. Recommend using a sun screen of SPF $\geq$15. Wear a wide-brimmed hat. Do not use artificial tanning facilities.
Fungal nail infection	Thick, yellowed, rough-appearing toenails or fingernails; can spread from one nail to others	Consult a physician about prescription drugs, which are approximately 50% effective. Wear leather shoes, and alternate pairs to reduce damp shoe conditions. Be aware that the fungus can be spread by unsanitary utensils used in the application of artificial fingernails. Seek professional nail care from a podiatrist.
Candidiasis	Yeast infection of the mouth or vagina. Oral candidiasis appears as white patches or red spots on the tongue, gums, or throat. Vaginal candidiasis appears as a thick, cottage cheese–like discharge that causes itching and burning.	Follow directions for oral or topical anti-fungal medications. Swish antifungal mouth rinses, retain the solution in the mouth as long as possible, and then swallow the rinse. Avoid simple sugars and alcohol, because they promote growth of yeast. Eat yogurt that contains live *Lactobacillus acidophilus* to restore a balance of helpful to harmful microbes.

DISPLAY 16-1

Advantages of Towel or Bag Baths

- Reduces the potential for skin impairment because the nonrinsable cleanser lubricates rather than dries the skin
- Prevents the transmission of microorganisms that may be growing in wash basins
- Reduces the spread of microorganisms from one part of the body to another because separate cloths or regions of the towel are used
- Preserves the integrity of the skin because friction is not used while drying the skin
- Promotes self-care among patients who may lack the strength or dexterity to wet, wring, and lather a washcloth
- Saves time compared to conventional bathing
- Promotes comfort because the moist towel or cloths are used so quickly they are warmer when applied

measuring 3 feet × 7.5 feet, or a bath sheet. No basin or soap is used. The towel is prefolded and moistened with approximately a half-gallon (2 L) of water heated to 115° to 120°F (46.1° to 48.8°C) and 1 ounce (30 mL) of no-rinse liquid cleanser. The nurse unfolds the towel so that it covers the patient (Fig. 16-4), and a separate section is used to wipe each part of the body, beginning at the feet and moving upward. The soiled areas of the towel are folded to the inside as each area is bathed, and the skin is allowed to air-dry for 2 to 3 seconds. Once the front of the body is washed, the nurse positions the patient on the side and repeats the procedure. The towel is unfolded in such a manner that the clean surface covers the patient. The back is bathed, then the buttocks. When the towel bath is complete, the bed linen is changed.

Bag Bath

A **bag bath** (technique for bathing that involves the use of 8 to 10 premoistened, warmed, disposable cloths contained in a plastic bag) is another alternative to bed baths. The cloths in the bag contain a no-rinse *surfactant* (a substance that reduces surface tension between the skin and surface contaminants) and an *emollient/humectant* (a substance that attracts and traps moisture in the skin), but no soap. The bag and its contents are warmed in a microwave or warming unit or are

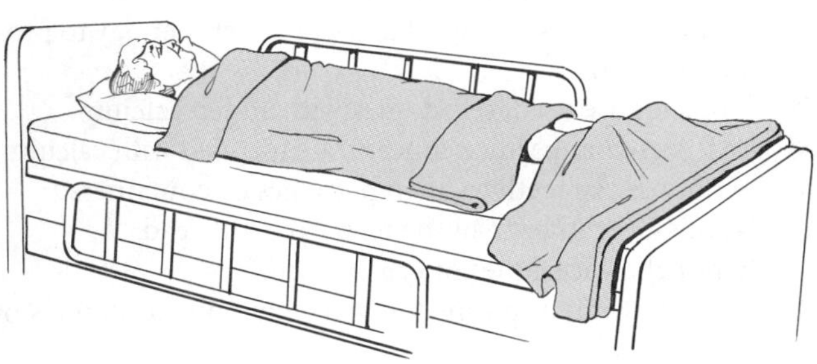

FIGURE 16–4. Giving a towel bath.

set in a container of warm water before being used. At the bedside, a separate cloth is used to wash each part of the body. Air-drying circumvents the need for a towel.

SHAVING

Shaving removes unwanted body hair. In the United States, most men shave their face daily and most women shave their axillae and legs regularly, but personal or cultural differences must be respected. The nurse asks each patient about his or her preferences before assuming otherwise.

Shaving is accomplished with an electric or a safety razor. In some circumstances, use of a safety razor is contraindicated (Display 16-2) and an electric or battery-operated razor is used. When the patient cannot shave, the nurse assumes responsibility for this hygiene practice.

Nursing Guidelines For

Shaving Patients

- ☑ Prepare a basin of warm water, soap, face cloth, and towel.
  RATIONALE: These supplies are needed for wetting, rinsing, and lathering the face.
- ☑ Wash the skin with warm, soapy water.
  RATIONALE: Washing removes oil, helping to raise the shafts of hair.
- ☑ Lather the skin with soap or shaving cream.
  RATIONALE: Use of soap or shaving cream reduces the surface tension as the razor is pulled across the skin.
- ☑ Start at the upper areas of the face (or other area of the body that requires shaving) and work down (Fig. 16-5).
  RATIONALE: This progression provides more control of the razor.

DISPLAY 16-2

Contraindications to Using a Safety Razor

Use of a safety razor is contraindicated for patients:

- Receiving anticoagulants (drugs that interfere with clotting)
- Receiving thrombolytic agents (drugs that dissolve blood clots)
- Taking high doses of aspirin
- With blood disorders such as hemophilia
- With liver disease who have impaired clotting
- With rashes or elevated or inflamed skin lesions about the face
- Who are suicidal

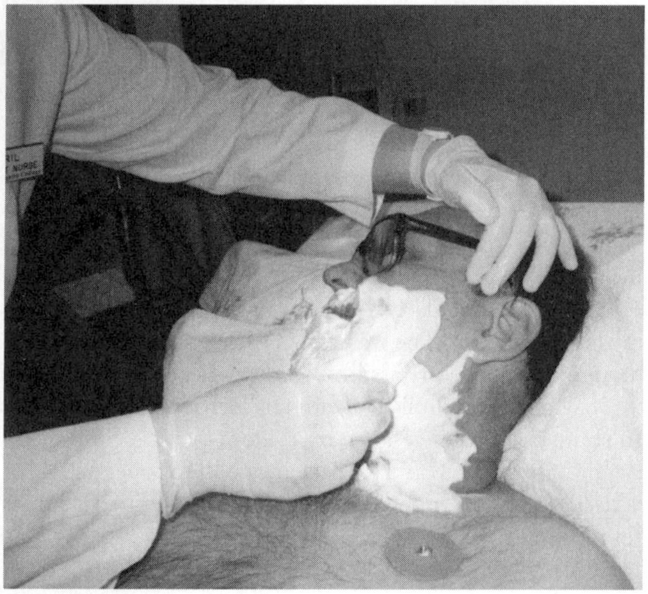

FIGURE 16–5. Shaving a patient's face. (Courtesy of Ken Timby.)

- Pull the skin taut below the area to be shaved.
  RATIONALE: This evens the level of the skin.
- Pull the razor in the direction of hair growth.
  RATIONALE: Shaving with hair reduces the potential for irritating the skin.
- Use short strokes.
  RATIONALE: Short strokes provide more control of the razor.
- Rinse the razor after each stroke, or as hair accumulates.
  RATIONALE: Rinsing keeps the cutting edge of the razor clean.
- Rinse the remaining soap or shaving cream from the skin.
  RATIONALE: Rinsing reduces the potential for drying the skin.
- Apply direct pressure to areas that seem to bleed, or apply alum sulfate (styptic pencil) at the site of bleeding.
  RATIONALE: Pressure or alum helps promote clotting.
- Apply aftershave lotion, cologne, or cream to the shaved area, if the patient desires it.
  RATIONALE: The alcohol in lotion and cologne reduces and retards microbial growth in the tiny abrasions caused by the razor; cream restores oil to the skin.

ORAL HYGIENE

Oral hygiene (practices used to clean the mouth, especially the teeth) includes brushing and flossing the teeth. Dentures and bridges also require special cleaning and care.

Tooth Brushing and Flossing

Patients who are alert and physically capable generally attend to their own oral hygiene. For patients confined to bed, the nurse assembles the necessary items—a toothbrush, toothpaste, a glass of water, an emesis basin, and floss.

Most dentists recommend using a soft-bristled toothbrush and toothpaste. Flossing removes plaque and food debris from the surfaces of teeth that the brush does not reach. The choice of unwaxed or waxed floss is a personal one. Waxed floss is thicker and more difficult to insert between teeth; unwaxed floss frays more quickly.

Although conscientious oral hygiene does not prevent dental problems completely, it reduces the chance that they will occur. Therefore, patients need to learn how to maintain the structure and integrity of their natural teeth.

Patient Teaching For

Reducing Dental Disease and Injuries

Teach the patient or family to do the following:

- Brush and floss the teeth as soon as possible after each meal, using the following techniques:
- Moisten the toothbrush and apply toothpaste.
- Hold the toothbrush at a 45° angle to the teeth.
- Brush the front and back of all the teeth from the gum line toward the crown of the teeth, using circular motions (Fig. 16-6).
- Brush back and forth over the chewing surfaces of the molars.
- Rinse the mouth periodically to flush loosened debris.
- Wrap an 18″ length of floss around the middle fingers of each hand.
- Slide the floss between two teeth until it is next to the gum.
- Move the floss back and forth.
- Repeat flossing with new sections of the floss until all the teeth have been flossed, including the outer surface of the last molar.
- Use a tartar-control toothpaste or rinse containing fluoride.
- If brushing is impossible, rinse the mouth with water after eating.
- Use a battery-operated oral irrigating device, which uses pulsating jets of water to flush debris from teeth, bridges, or braces.
- Eat fewer sweets, such as soft drinks containing sugar, candy, gum that contains fructose or another form of sugar, pastries, and sweet desserts.
- Eat more raw fruits and vegetables, which naturally remove plaque and other food as they are chewed.
- Eat two or three servings of dairy products per day to provide calcium.
- If antacids are used, select ones with added calcium.
- Use frozen orange juice concentrate fortified with calcium.
- Do not use the teeth to open packages or containers.
- Use scissors rather than the teeth to cut thread.
- Do not chew ice cubes or crushed ice.
- Avoid chewing unpopped or partially popped kernels of popcorn.
- Have dental check-ups at least every 6 months.

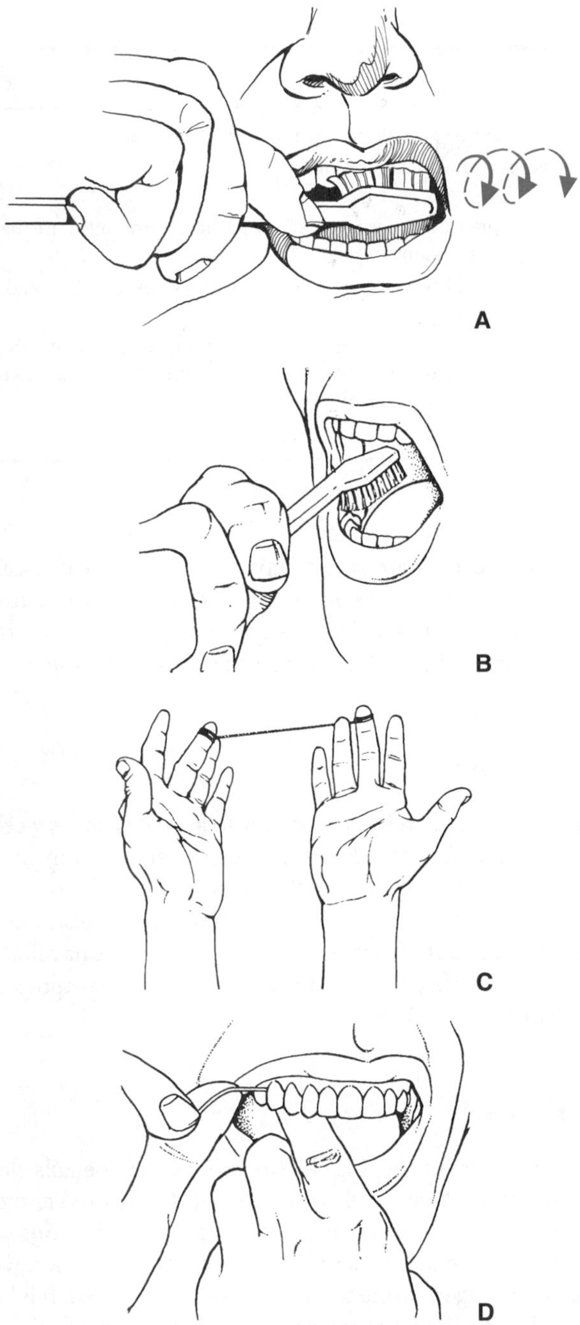

FIGURE 16-6. (*A*) Brushing toward crown of teeth. (*B*) Brushing chewing surfaces. (*C*) Preparing floss for use. (*D*) Using floss; about ½ inch of approximately 18 inches of wrapped floss is used at any one time.

Oral Care for Unconscious Patients

Oral hygiene is not neglected because a patient is unconscious. In fact, because unconscious patients are not salivating in response to seeing, smelling, and eating food, they need oral care even more frequently than conscious patients. **Sordes** (dried crusts containing mucus, microorganisms, and epithelial cells shed from the mucous membrane) are common on the lips and teeth of unconscious patients.

Toothbrushing is the preferred technique for providing oral hygiene for unconscious patients (Skill 16-4). However, patients who are not alert are at risk for aspirating (inhaling) saliva and liquid oral hygiene products into their lungs. Aspirated liquids predispose patients to pneumonia. Therefore, the nurse uses special precautions to avoid getting fluid in the patient's airway.

In addition to toothbrushing, the mouth is moistened and refreshed with oral swabs. Various substances are used for oral hygiene, depending on the circumstances and assessment findings for each patient (Table 16-4).

Denture Care

Dentures (artificial teeth) substitute for a person's lower or upper set of teeth, or both. A **bridge** (dental appliance that replaces one or several teeth) is fixed permanently to other natural teeth so that it cannot be removed, or it is fastened with a clasp that allows it to be detached from the mouth.

For patients who cannot remove their own dentures, the nurse dons gloves and uses a dry gauze square or clean face cloth to grasp and free the denture from the mouth (Fig. 16-7). Dentures and removable bridges are cleaned with a toothbrush, toothpaste, and cold or tepid water. Care is taken to hold dentures over a plastic basin or towel so they will not break if dropped.

Dentists recommend that dentures and bridges remain in place except while they are being cleaned. Keeping dentures and bridges out for long periods permits the gum lines to change, affecting the fit. If the dentures or bridge are removed during the night, they are stored in a covered cup. Plain water is most often used to cover dentures when they are not in the mouth, but some add mouthwash or denture cleanser to the water.

HAIR CARE

Sometimes patients need assistance with grooming or shampooing their hair.

Hair Grooming

The following are recommendations for grooming patients' hair:

- Try to use the hairstyle a patient prefers.
- Brush the hair slowly and carefully to avoid damaging it.
- Brush the hair to increase circulation and distribution of sebum.
- Use a wide-toothed comb, starting at the ends of the hair rather than from the crown downward if the hair is matted or tangled.
- Apply a conditioner or alcohol to loosen tangles.

TABLE 16–4. **Optional Substances for Oral Care**

Substance	Use
Antiseptic mouthwash diluted with water	Reduces bacterial growth in the mouth; freshens breath
Equal parts of baking soda and table salt in warm water, or baking soda mixed with normal saline	Removes accumulated secretions
One part hydrogen peroxide to 10 parts of water	Releases oxygen and loosens dry sticky particles; prolonged use may damage tooth enamel
Milk of magnesia	Reduces oral acidity; dissolves plaque, increases flow of saliva, and soothes oral lesions
Lemon and glycerin swabs	Increases salivation and refreshes the mouth; glycerin may absorb water from the lips and cause them to become dry and cracked if used for more than several days
Petroleum jelly	Lubricates lips

- Use oil on the hair if it is dry. Many preparations are available, but pure castor oil, olive oil, and mineral oil are satisfactory.
- Braiding the hair helps prevent tangles.
- If hair loss occurs from cancer therapy or some other disease or medical treatment, provide the patient with a turban or baseball cap.

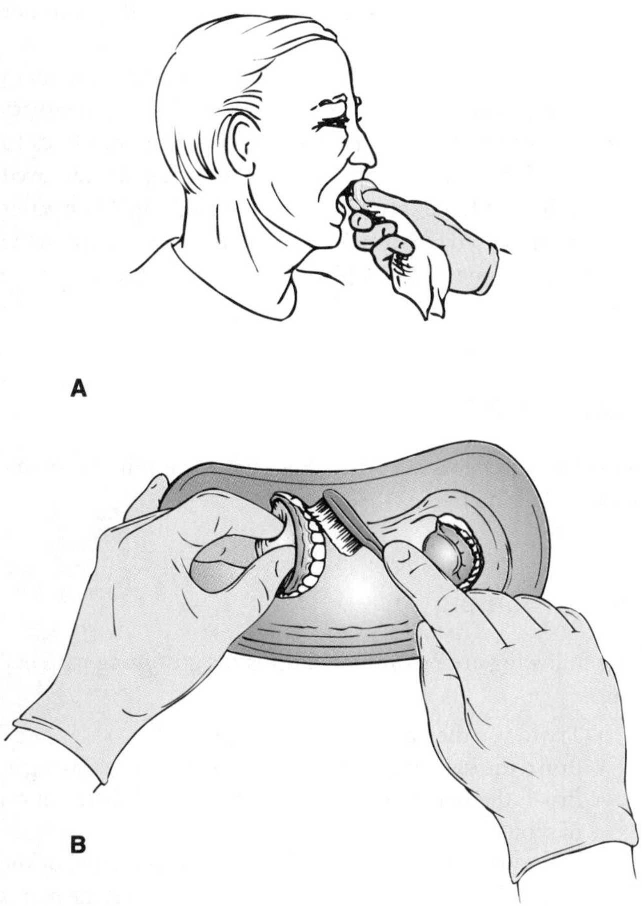

FIGURE 16–7. (*A*) Removing an upper denture. (*B*) Cleaning dentures.

- Avoid using hairpins or clips that may injure the scalp.
- Obtain the patient's or family's permission before cutting the hair if it is hopelessly tangled and cutting seems to be the only solution for providing adequate grooming.

Shampooing

Hair is washed as often as necessary to keep it clean. A weekly shampoo is sufficient for most people, but shampooing more or less often will not damage the hair.

Long-term health care facilities often employ beauticians and barbers, but if professional services are unavailable, the nurse or delegated nursing staff member shampoos the patient's hair (Skill 16-5).

NAIL CARE

Nail care involves keeping the fingernails and toenails clean and trimmed. Patients who have diabetes, impaired circulation, or thick nails are at risk for vascular complications secondary to trauma. The services of a **podiatrist** (person with special training in caring for feet) are often indicated. It is best to check with the patient's physician before cutting fingernails or toenails.

If there are no contraindications, nails are cared for in the following manner:

- Soak the hands or feet in warm water to soften the keratin and loosen trapped debris.
- Clean under the nails with a wooden orange stick or other sturdy but blunt instrument.
- Push **cuticles** (thin edge of skin at the base of the nail) downward with a soft towel.
- Use a file, emery board, metal clippers, or manicure scissors to trim long fingernails.
- Trim toenails straight across to avoid sharp or jagged points, which may injure the adjacent skin (Fig. 16-8).

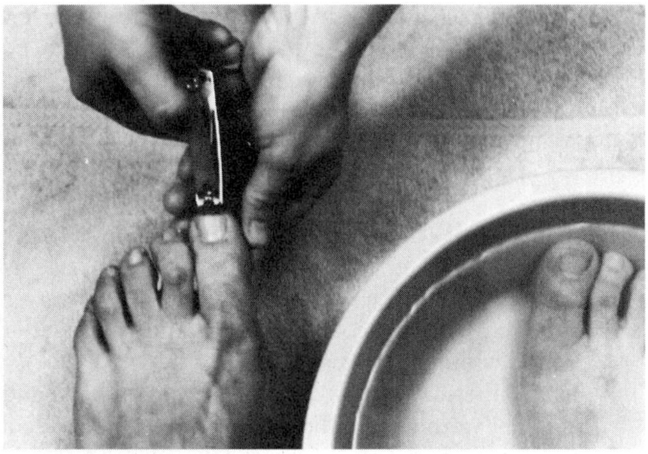

FIGURE 16–8. Foot care. (Courtesy of Ken Timby.)

To keep the skin and nails soft and supple, lotion or an emollient cream is applied after bathing and nail care. If foot perspiration is a problem, a prescribed antifungal, deodorant powder is used. Because impaired skin, especially about the feet, is often slow to heal and susceptible to infection, any abnormal assessment findings are reported immediately. To avoid injuring the feet, patients should wear sturdy slippers or clean socks and supportive shoes.

Visual and Hearing Devices

Visual and hearing devices such as eyeglasses and hearing aids improve communication and socialization. Both represent a considerable financial investment. If they become damaged or broken, the temporary loss deprives patients of full sensory perception. Therefore, they should be well maintained and safely stored when not in use.

Although eyeglasses and hearing aids are not body structures, they are worn in close contact with the body for long periods. Consequently, they tend to collect secretions, dirt, and debris, which may interfere with their function and use. Therefore, the nurse cares for these devices at the same time that other hygiene measures are provided.

EYEGLASSES

Prescription lenses are made of glass or plastic. Plastic lenses weigh much less but are more easily scratched. Glass lenses are more apt to break if dropped. When not in use, eyeglasses should be stored in a soft case or should be rested on the frame.

Glass and plastic lenses are cleaned as follows:

- Hold the eyeglasses by the nose or ear braces.
- Run tepid water over both sides of the lenses (hot water damages plastic lenses).
- Wash the lenses with soap or detergent.
- Rinse with running tap water.
- Dry with a clean, soft cloth, such as a handkerchief. Do not use paper tissues, because some contain wood fibers and pulp can scratch the lenses.

Some prefer to use commercial glass cleaner, but this is not necessary.

CONTACT LENSES

A contact lens is a small plastic disk placed directly on the cornea. Contact lenses are usually worn in both eyes, but some patients who have had cataract surgery on one eye wear a single contact lens or a single contact lens and eyeglasses. The nurse should not assume that someone who wears eyeglasses does not use a contact lens, and vice versa.

Several types of contact lenses are available: hard, soft, or gas permeable (Fig. 16-9). All contact lenses (except disposable types, which are worn for approximately 1 week and then discarded) need to be removed for cleaning, eye rest, and disinfection. People who are not conscientious about following a routine for contact lens care risk infection, eye abrasion, and permanent damage to the cornea.

When caring for a patient who wears contact lenses, the nurse should have the patient remove and insert the lenses and care for them according to his or her established routine. For patients who cannot do so, the nurse may assist with the removal of the lenses or should consult the patient's **ophthalmologist** (medical doctor who treats eye disorders) or **optometrist** (person who prescribes corrective lenses) about

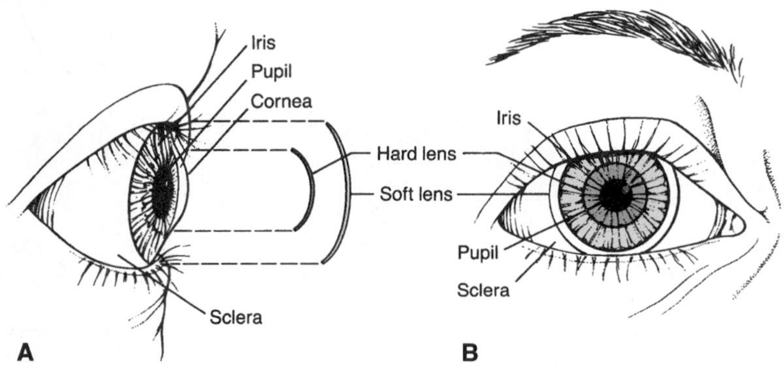

FIGURE 16–9. Location and size of hard and soft contact lenses. (*A*) Side view. (*B*) Front view.

alternatives for promoting adequate vision and safety. Some people, when ill, may resume wearing eyeglasses temporarily, use a magnifying glass, or do without any visual aid.

Contact Lens Removal

Before removing contact lenses, the nurse obtains an appropriate storage container. Commercial containers are available. Because the lens prescriptions may be different for each eye, the container is labeled "left" and "right." The patient's head is elevated and a towel is placed over the chest to prevent loss or damage to the contact lenses. The techniques for removing soft contact lenses are different than for hard contact lenses.

To remove a soft contact lens, the lens is moved from the cornea to the sclera by sliding it into position with a clean, gloved finger. When the lens is repositioned, the lid margins are compressed together toward the lens. Compression bends the pliable lens, allowing air to enter beneath it. The air releases the lens from the surface of the eye. The loosened lens is then gently grasped between the thumb and forefinger for removal. Soft lenses dry and crystallize if exposed to air, so they are immediately placed in a soaking solution in the storage container.

To remove a hard contact lens, the blink method is the most common technique. The patient is positioned and prepared similarly as for removing soft contact lenses. The lens is left in place on the cornea. The thumb and a finger are placed on the center of the upper and lower lids. Slight pressure is applied to the lids as the patient is instructed to blink. Blinking separates the hard lens from the cornea. If the blink method is unsuccessful, an ophthalmic suction cup is placed on the lens, and gentle suction lifts the lens from the eye. After removal, the lenses are soaked in the storage container.

ARTIFICIAL EYES

An artificial eye is a plastic shell that acts as a cosmetic replacement for the natural eye (Fig. 16-10). There is no way to restore vision once the natural eye is removed. The artificial eye and the socket into which it is placed need to be cleaned occasionally. If the patient cannot care for the artificial eye, the nurse removes it by depressing the lower eyelid until the lid margin is wide enough to allow the artificial eye to slide free. The eye socket is irrigated with water or saline before reinserting the artificial eye.

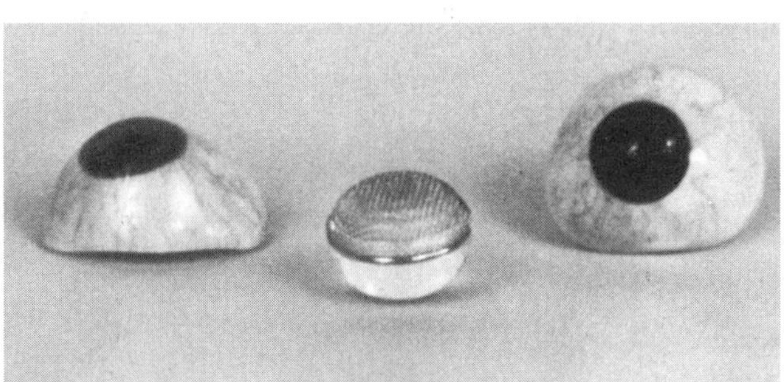

FIGURE 16–10. Front and side views of an artificial eye. The round implant (*center*) is positioned permanently within the bony orbit from which the natural eye has been removed. Only the cosmetic shell (*left* and *right*) is removed for cleaning. (Courtesy of Ken Timby.)

HEARING AIDS

There are three types of hearing aids:

- In-the-ear devices are small, self-contained aids that fit entirely within the patient's ear.
- Behind-the-ear devices consist of a microphone and amplifier worn behind the ear that delivers sound to a receiver within the ear.
- Body aid devices use electrical components, enclosed in a case carried somewhere on the body, to deliver the sound via a wire connected to an ear mold receiver (Fig. 16-11).

In-the-ear and behind-the-ear models are most common. Behind-the-ear models can be attached to an eyeglass frame. Body aids are used primarily by those with a severe hearing loss or those unable to care for a small device. Hearing aids are powered by small mercury or zinc batteries that need to be replaced after 100 to 200 hours of use.

Most patients insert and remove their own hearing aids, but the nurse may need to assess and troubleshoot problems that develop (Table 16-5). Patients and their families need to know how to maintain the hearing aid.

Patient Teaching For

Maintaining a Hearing Aid

Teach the patient and family to do the following:

- ▷ Keep a supply of extra batteries on hand.
- ▷ Avoid exposing the electrical components to extreme heat, water, cleaning chemicals, or hair spray.

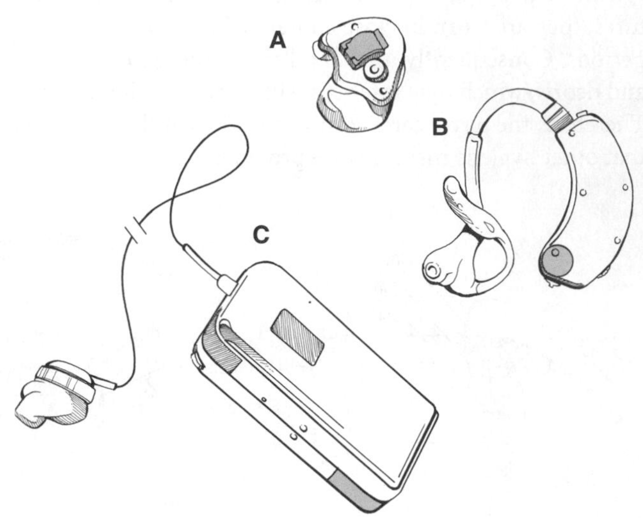

FIGURE 16–11. Types of hearing aids: (*A*) in-the-ear, (*B*) behind-the-ear, and (*C*) body aid.

TABLE 16–5. **Troubleshooting Hearing Aid Problems**

Problem	Possible Causes	Action
Reduced or absent sound	Weak or dead battery	Test and replace battery.
	Incorrect battery position	Match the positive pole of the battery to the positive symbol in the case.
	Cracked tubing leading to the receiver	Repair tubing.
	Broken wire between body aid and receiver	Repair wire.
	Accumulation of cerumen in the ear	Clean the ear.
	Cerumen plugging the receiver	Remove cerumen with an instrument called a wax loop, tip of a pin, or needle on a syringe.
	Ear congestion due to an upper respiratory infection	Consult the physician about administering a decongestant.
	Damaged electrical components	Have the device inspected by a person who services hearing aids.
Shrill noise, called *feedback*, caused by conditions that return sound to the microphone	Malposition or failure to insert the receiver fully in the ear	Remove and reinsert.
	Kinked receiver tubing	Remove and untwist.
	Excessive volume	Reduce volume control.
	Hearing aid left on while removed from the ear	Turn hearing aid off or replace it in the ear.
Garbled sound	Poor battery contact	Check battery for correct size; make sure the battery compartment is closed; clean metal contact points with an emery board.
	Dirty components	Clean with a soft cloth.
	Debris in the on/off switch	Move the switch back and forth several times.
	Corroded battery	Remove and replace.
	Cracked case	Repair or replace.

- Wipe the outer surface of a body aid or behind-the-ear case occasionally.
- Turn the hearing aid off when it is not being worn to prolong the life of the battery.
- Store the hearing aid in a safe place where it will not fall or become lost.

Infrared Listening Devices

Infrared listening devices (IRLDs) resemble earphones attached to a hand-held receiver. They are an alternative to conventional hearing aids. An IRLD converts sound into infrared light and sends it via a wall- or ceiling-mounted receiver to the person wearing the listening device. The light is converted back into an auditory stimulus. IRLDs are being used by people who need help hearing lectures, television, or live performances. Some geriatric centers are installing IRLDs in rooms used for social and recreational activities.

One advantage of an IRLD over a conventional hearing aid is that an IRLD reduces background noise. Background noise is a common reason people give for not wearing their hearing aids. However, IRLDs cannot be used outdoors, in rooms that contain many windows, or in rooms that are brightly lit, because infrared light jams the signal, causing audio interference.

Nursing Implications

Patients who require assistance with personal hygiene may have a variety of nursing diagnoses:

- Self-care deficit, bathing/hygiene
- Self-care deficit, dressing/grooming
- Activity intolerance
- Risk for impaired skin integrity

The nursing care plan is a care plan for a patient with a nursing diagnosis of Self-care deficit, bathing/hygiene, defined in the NANDA taxonomy (1999) as "impaired ability to perform or complete bathing/hygiene activities for oneself."

Nursing Care Plan: *Self-Care Deficit: Bathing/Hygiene*

Assessment

Subjective Data
States, "I can't bathe myself and I need help brushing my teeth."

Objective Data
52-year-old woman admitted for the repair of fractures sustained as a result of falling down the basement stairs of home. Arm cast on right. Right hand is dominant. Uses exposed right thumb and fingers for grasping objects. Right elbow not enclosed within cast and has full range of motion. Left arm in traction and suspension.

Diagnosis

Self-care deficit: bathing/hygiene related to musculoskeletal impairment as manifested by the inability to use hands effectively for performing hygiene independently

Plan

Goal
The patient will report feeling clean and refreshed after assistance with daily bathing and mouth care.

Orders: 6/2
1. Provide daily bed bath at a convenient time for patient.
2. Use patient's own castile soap.
3. Place small towel in rt. hand for assisting with drying face and chest.
4. Provide a gown with sleeves that fasten with snaps.
5. Apply deodorant and powder to underarms daily.
6. Turn toward the arm in traction for washing back and buttocks.
7. Provide mouth care after each meal as follows:
   - Wrap and tape washcloth around handle of toothbrush so patient can grasp it with fingers and thumb of right hand.
   - Apply toothpaste to toothbrush.
   - Set emesis basin and glass of water with straw on overbed table.

_____ V. MILLER, RN

Implementation (Documentation)

6/3 0845 Brushed own teeth after breakfast. _____ L. COOK, LPN

0900 Complete bed bath administered using castile soap. Able to assist with drying upper body. Hair under arms shaved. Deodorant and powder applied in axillae. Skin is pink, warm, and intact. No redness around edges of cast. Able to turn without difficulty to left side for back care. _____ L. COOK, LPN

Evaluation (Documentation)

0930 States, "I feel so much better about seeing my doctor and visitors after I've gotten cleaned up in the morning." _____ L. COOK, LPN

FOCUS ON OLDER ADULTS

- Poor hygiene and grooming in older adults is often a sign of dementia, depression, abuse, or neglect.
- Older adults do not need to bathe as frequently as younger adults because they have diminished perspiration and sebum production.
- Older adults with limited range of motion in their joints from arthritis require assistance with hygiene. Long-handled bath sponges or hand-held shower attachments help to maintain independence.
- If older adults are not rushed, chilled, or exposed, they are more receptive to assistance with their personal hygiene.
- Nonskid strips on the floor of bathtubs and showers, along with strategically placed handles and grab bars, help reduce the risk of falls for older adults when bathing.
- A tub/shower seat is an important safety measure for older adults who have mobility limitations or difficulty maintaining their balance.
- Soap, which is extremely drying to the skin is used sparingly. A mild, superfatted, nonperfumed soap such as castile, Dove, Tone, or Basis is preferred.
- Bath oils can be added to a water basin when administering a bed bath to an older adult. However, oils are not used in showers or bathtubs because the oil increases the risk for falls.
- Skin care products containing alcohol or perfumes are avoided because they tend to aggravate dry skin conditions that are common in older adults. These agents also can cause allergic reactions.
- The fingernails of older adults are kept trimmed and smooth because older adults are more susceptible to skin tears and scratches.
- When drying the skin of older adults, gentle patting motions rather than harsh, rubbing motions are preferred.
- Because older adults are likely to have diminished temperature sensation, the temperature of bath water is checked with the wrist before older adults immerse in it.
- Older adults who are cognitively impaired may be fearful of bathing, especially in a tub or shower.
- Increasing oral fluid intake or adding humidity to the air reduces the discomfort of dry skin experienced by older adults.
- Modifying clothing with Velcro closures, front zippers, elastic waists, and oversized buttons and buttonholes facilitates an older adult's ability to dress and undress independently.
- Lower extremity skin and nail problems are prevented by encouraging older adults to purchase sturdy shoes and replace or repair them as they become worn.
- Thorough inspection of the feet of older adult patients is essential because they may have ulcerations or other lesions of which they are unaware.
- Benign skin lesions such as seborrheic keratoses (tan to black raised areas on the trunk) and senile lentigines (brown, flat patches on the face, hands, and forearms) are common in older adults.
- Tooth loss is common in older adults due to periodontal disease.
- Older adults are more susceptible to impacted cerumen (ear wax), a common cause of hearing loss. Over-the-counter ear drops such as Debrox are used to prevent and treat this condition. Irrigation of the ear with body-temperature tap water followed by instillation of a drying agent such as 70% alcohol may be necessary for removal of impacted cerumen.

KEY CONCEPTS

- Hygiene refers to practices that promote health through personal cleanliness.
- Hygiene practices that most people perform regularly include bathing, shaving, oral hygiene, hair care, and nail care.
- A partial bath is more appropriate for older adults rather than a daily tub bath or shower, because they do not perspire as much as young adults and soap tends to dry their skin.
- Towel and bag baths add lubrication to the skin; avoid friction, which preserves skin integrity; reduce the transmission of microorganisms from one part of the body to another; save time; provide more opportunity for self-care; and promote comfort because of the warmth of the liquid.
- Use of a safety razor is contraindicated for patients who have clotting disorders, those receiving anticoagulants and thrombolytics, and those who are depressed and suicidal.
- Most dentists recommend using a soft-bristled toothbrush, tartar-control toothpaste with fluoride, and dental floss.
- The chief hazard in providing oral hygiene for unconscious patients is aspiration of liquid into the lungs. To prevent aspiration, unconscious patients are positioned on the side with the head lower than the body. Oral suction equipment is used to remove liquid from the mouth.
- To prevent damage during cleaning, dentures are held over a plastic or towel-lined container, and cold or tepid water is used.
- Hair can be detangled by applying conditioner, using a wide-toothed comb, and combing from the end of the hair toward the scalp.
- The physician is consulted about nail care for patients with diabetes or poor circulation.
- Daily hygiene also includes cleaning and caring for visual or hearing devices such as eyeglasses, contact lenses, artificial eyes, or hearing aids.
- Patients who cannot insert and care for contact lenses may consider wearing eyeglasses, using a magnifying lens, or doing without while they are ill.
- The sound produced by a hearing aid may be altered due to dead or weak batteries, batteries that are not making full contact, corroded batteries, malposition within the ear, excessive volume, impacted cerumen, and dirty or damaged components.
- Infrared listening devices are an alternative to hearing aids. They convert sound into infrared light and then reconvert the light to sound through a receiver worn in a headset with earphones.

CRITICAL THINKING EXERCISES

- You have been assigned to two patients: a 75-year-old woman who is unconscious after a stroke and a 38-year-old male mechanic being treated for an ulcer. How do their hygiene needs differ?
- You are responsible for inspecting long-term care facilities, such as nursing homes. What criteria should health care agencies meet in relation to bath facilities and hygiene policies to receive a positive evaluation?

SUGGESTED READINGS

Dose AM. The symptom experience of mucositis, stomatitis, and xerostomia. Seminars in Oncology Nursing 1995;11:248–255.

Freeman EM. International perspectives on bathing. Journal of Gerontological Nursing 1997;23(5):40–59.

Hearing aids: advances in design improve sound quality. Mayo Clinic Health Letter 1998;16(6):4.

Hearing aid management. School Nurse News 1998;15(1):10.

Hector LM, Touhy TA. The history of the bath: from art to task? Reflections for the future. Journal of Gerontological Nursing 1997;23(5):7–15.

Held-Warmkessel J. Chemotherapy complications. Nursing 1998;28(4):41–46.

Hoeffer B, Rader J, McKenzie D, Lavelle M, Steward B. Reducing aggressive behavior during bathing cognitively impaired nursing home residents. Journal of Gerontological Nursing 1997;23(5):16–23.

Jupitur T, Spivey V. Perception of hearing loss and hearing handicap on hearing aid use by nursing home residents. Geriatric Nursing 1997;18(5): 201–208.

Kraker K, Vajdik C. Designing the environment to make bathing pleasant in nursing homes. Journal of Gerontological Nursing 1997;23(5):50–51.

Lake A. Prevention of complications related to contact lens wear. Nursing Times 1996;92(20):36–38.

Making bathing pleasant for your patients. Journal of Gerontological Nursing 1997;23(5):5.

Maurizio SJ, Rogers JL. Prevention update. Oral hygiene for the home care patient. Caring 1997;16(3):54–55.

Miller R. Helping impaired elderly patients get through a bath. RN 1995;58(12):65.

Moore J. Assessment of nurse-administered oral hygiene. Nursing Times 1995;91(1):40–41.

NANDA nursing diagnoses: definitions and classification, 1999–2000. Philadelphia, NANDA, 1999.

Potts HW, Richie MF, Kaas MJ. Resistance to care. Journal of Gerontological Nursing 1996;22(11):11–16.

Rader J, Lavelle M, Hoeffer B, McKenzie D. Individualizing the bathing process. Journal of Gerontological Nursing 1996;22(3):32–38.

Ryan S. Dry mouth misery. Practice Nurse 1996;11(3):183–185.

Shuster J. Adverse drug reaction. Anticholinergics and cavities. Nursing 1997;27(1):71.

Skewes SM. Bathing: it's a tough job. Journal of Gerontological Nursing 23(5):1997;45–59.

Winslow EH, Jacobson AF. Reducing disruptive behavior during bathing. American Journal of Nursing 1997;97(2):20–21.

SKILL 16-1

PROVIDING A TUB BATH OR SHOWER

Suggested Action	Reason for Action
Assessment	
Check the Kardex or nursing care plan for hygiene directives.	Ensures continuity of care
Assess the patient's level of consciousness, orientation, strength, and mobility.	Provides data for evaluating the patient's ability to carry out hygiene practices independently
Check for gauze dressings, plaster cast, or electrical or battery-operated equipment; determine whether they can be protected with waterproof material or whether they are safe if they become wet.	Maintains safety of the patient and ensures integrity of treatment devices
Determine if and when any laboratory or diagnostic procedures are scheduled.	Aids in time management
Check the occupancy, cleanliness, and safety of the tub or shower.	Helps in organizing the plan for care

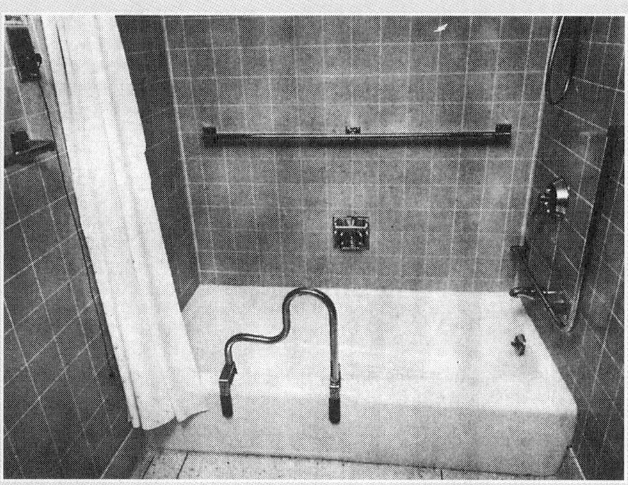

Tub and shower equipped for patient safety.

Suggested Action	Reason for Action
Planning	
Clean the tub or shower if necessary.	Reduces the potential for spreading microorganisms
Consult with the patient about a convenient time for tending to hygiene needs.	Promotes cooperation between the patient and nurse and patient participation in decision making
Assemble supplies: floor mat, towels, face cloth, soap, clean pajamas or gown.	Demonstrates organization and efficient time management
Implementation	
Escort the patient to the shower or bathing room.	Shows concern for the patient's safety
Demonstrate how to operate the faucet and drain.	Ensures the patient's safety and comfort
If the patient cannot operate the faucet, fill the tub approximately half full with water 105° to 110°F (40° to 43°C), or adjust the shower to a similar temperature.	Demonstrates concern for the patient's safety and comfort
Place a "do not disturb" or "in use" sign on the outer door.	Ensures privacy

continued

SKILL 16–1

PROVIDING A TUB BATH OR SHOWER *Continued*

Suggested Action	Reason for Action
Help the patient into the tub or shower if assistance is needed by: • Placing a chair next to the tub • Having the patient swing his or her feet over the edge of the tub • Lean forward, grab a support bar, and raise the buttocks and body until it can be lowered within the tub	Reduces the risk of falling
Have the patient sit on a stool or seat in the tub or shower, if the patient will have difficulty exiting from the tub or may become weak while bathing.	Ensures safety

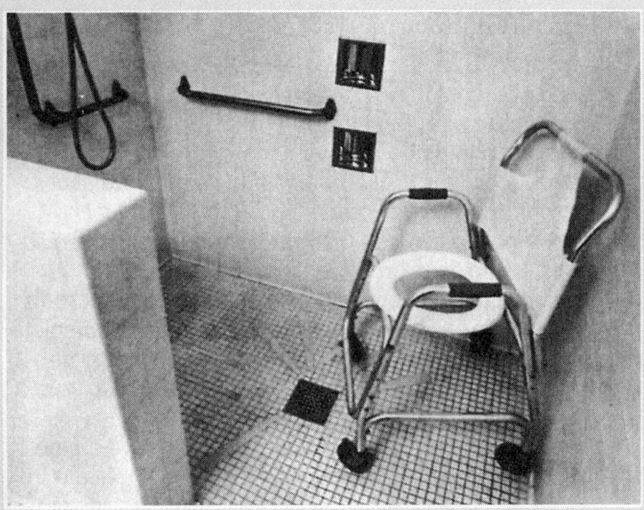

Shower chair.

Suggested Action	Reason for Action
Show the patient how to summon help.	Promotes safety
Stay close at hand.	Ensures proximity in case patient needs assistance.
Check on the patient at frequent intervals by knocking on the door and waiting for a response.	Shows respect for privacy yet concern for safety
Escort the patient back to his or her room after the bath or shower.	Demonstrates concern for safety and welfare
Clean the tub or shower with an antibacterial agent and dispose of soiled linen in its designated location.	Reduces the spread of microorganisms and demonstrates concern for the next person to use the tub or shower
Remove the "in use" sign from the door.	Indicates that the bathing room is unoccupied

Evaluation

- Patient is clean.
- Patient remains uninjured.

Document

- Date and time
- Tub bath or shower

continued

SKILL 16-1

PROVIDING A TUB BATH OR SHOWER *Continued*

SAMPLE DOCUMENTATION*

Date and Time Tub bath taken independently. ______________________ SIGNATURE/TITLE

CRITICAL THINKING

- What suggestions might you offer to convalescing patients who will be responsible for bathing and safety in their own home? What home safety devices might they purchase? How might they reduce the risk of falling?
- How would you respond to a patient who believes that daily bathing is unnecessary or even unhealthy?

* Generally, routine hygiene measures are documented on a checklist, but for teaching purposes an example of narrative charting has been provided.

SKILL 16-2

ADMINISTERING PERINEAL CARE

Suggested Action	Reason for Action
Assessment	
Inspect the genital and rectal areas of the patient.	Provides data for determining whether perineal care is necessary
Planning	
Wash your hands.	Reduces the spread of microorganisms
Gather gloves, soap, water, and clean cloths or antiseptic wipes or a container of cleansing solution in a squeeze bottle, and several towels or absorptive pads.	Provides a means of removing debris and microorganisms
Explain the procedure to the patient.	Reduces anxiety and promotes cooperation
Pull the privacy curtain.	Demonstrates respect for modesty
Place the patient in a dorsal recumbent position and cover with a bath blanket (see Fig. A).	Provides access to the perineum
While the patient holds the top of the blanket, pull and fan-fold the top linen to the foot of the bed.	Maintains patient modesty and keeps upper linen clean and dry
For a female patient, place a disposable pad beneath the buttocks or place the patient on a bedpan; for a male patient, place a disposable pad under the penis and beneath the buttocks.	Aids absorption of liquid that may drip during cleansing
Implementation	
Bend the female patient's knees and spread the legs.	Exposes area for cleansing
Put on gloves.	Prevents contact with blood, secretions, or excretions
Separate the folds of the labia and wash from the pubic area toward the anus (see Fig. B). Never go back over an area that has already been cleaned.	Cleanses in a direction from less soiled to more soiled areas of the body; prevents reintroducing microorganisms into previously cleaned areas
Use a clean area of the cloth or a separate antiseptic wipe for each stroke.	Avoids resoiling areas that have already been cleaned

continued

SKILL 16-2

ADMINISTERING PERINEAL CARE *Continued*

Suggested Action	Reason for Action
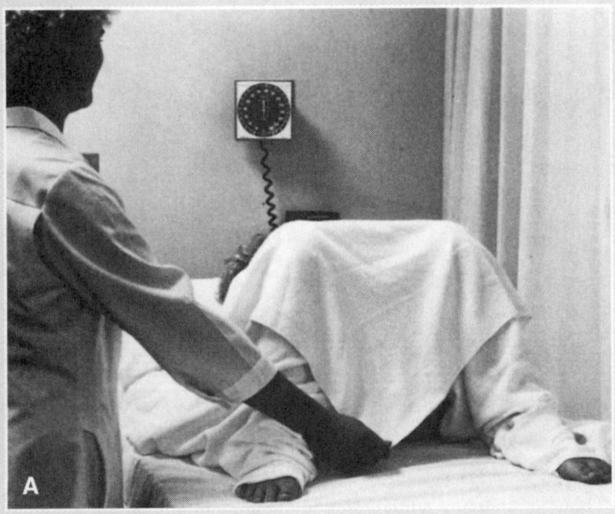 **Positioning and draping the patient. (Courtesy of Ken Timby.)**	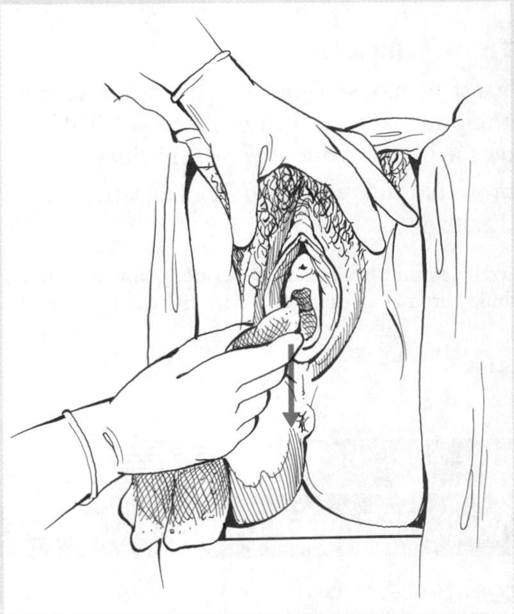 **Cleansing the labia.**
Wash debris from the outside of a urinary catheter, if one exists, especially where it is in contact with mucous membrane and genital tissue.	Reduces the numbers and growth of microorganisms that may ascend to the bladder
Squeeze the antiseptic solution container, if one is used, starting at the upper areas of the labia downward toward the anus (see Fig. C).	Ensures that solution will drain toward more soiled areas of the body; prevents reintroducing microorganisms into previously cleaned areas

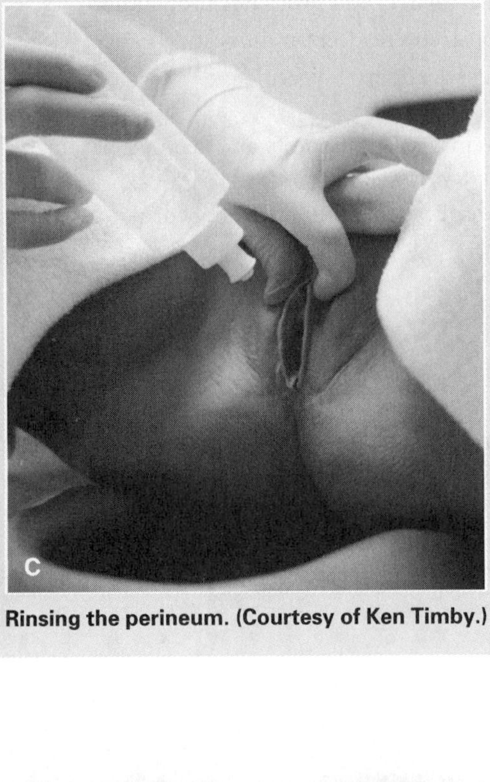

Rinsing the perineum. (Courtesy of Ken Timby.)

continued

SKILL 16-2

ADMINISTERING PERINEAL CARE *Continued*

Suggested Action	Reason for Action
For males, grasp the penis and retract the foreskin if the patient is uncircumcised.	Facilitates removing debris and secretions that may be trapped beneath the fold of skin
Clean the tip of the penis using circular motions (see Fig. D). Never go back over an area that has already been cleaned.	Keeps the urethral opening clean
Replace the foreskin.	Prevents trauma
Wipe the shaft of the penis toward the scrotum (see Fig. E).	Keeps microorganisms and debris from the urethral opening
Spread the legs and wash the scrotum.	Removes debris where it may be trapped and harbor microorganisms

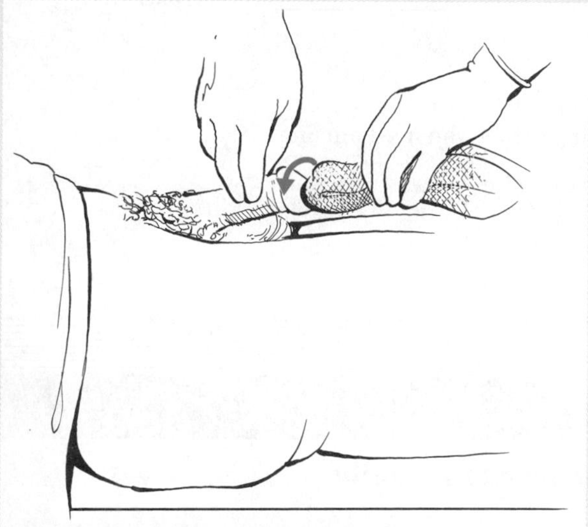

D

Cleansing the glans penis.

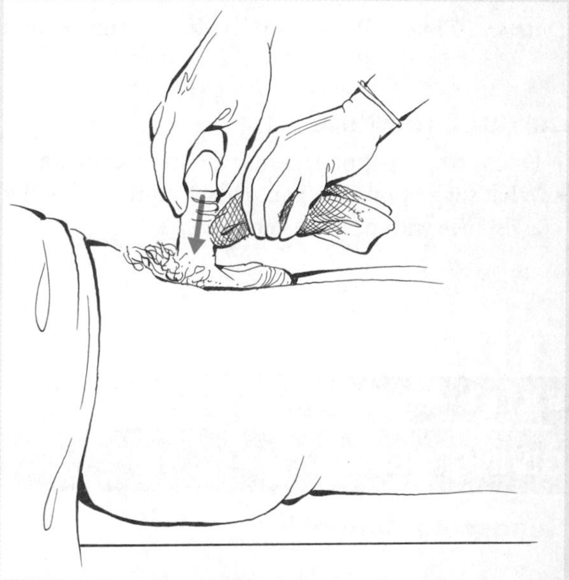

E

Cleansing the shaft of the penis.

Suggested Action	Reason for Action
Pat the skin dry with a towel.	Removes excess moisture
Turn the patient to the side and wash from the perineum toward the anus.	Cleans in a direction toward more soiled areas of the body
Rinse and pat the skin dry.	Prevents skin irritation from soap residue and retained moisture; a warm, dark, moist environment contributes to fungal skin infections
Apply a clean absorbent perineal pad to patients who are menstruating or have other types of vaginal or rectal drainage.	Promotes cleanliness and reduces contact between the skin and moist drainage
Remove damp towels, place an absorbent disposable pad beneath the patient if drainage is excessive, and cover the patient with bed linen.	Restores comfort; protects linen from becoming soiled
Deposit wet cloths, soiled wipes, and towels in an appropriate container.	Controls the spread of microorganisms
Empty and rinse the bedpan.	Controls the spread of microorganisms
Remove gloves and wash your hands again.	Reduces the spread of microorganisms
Attend to the comfort and safety of the patient.	Demonstrates concern for the patient's welfare

continued

SKILL 16-2

ADMINISTERING PERINEAL CARE *Continued*

Evaluation

- Genital, perineal, and rectal areas are clean and dry.
- Cleansing has been from lesser to more soiled areas of the body.
- There has been no direct contact with drainage, secretions, or excretions.
- Soiled articles have been properly disposed.

Document

- Date and time
- Care provided
- Description of drainage and tissue

SAMPLE DOCUMENTATION

Date and Time Peri-care provided to remove moderate amount of bloody drainage coming from vagina. Perineal tissue is intact. ________________________ SIGNATURE/TITLE

CRITICAL THINKING

- Discuss the types of patients who may require assistance with perineal care.
- What suggestions can you make for promoting the dignity of patients who need nursing assistance with perineal care?

SKILL 16-3

GIVING A BED BATH

Suggested Action	Reason for Action
Assessment	
Check the Kardex or nursing care plan for hygiene directives.	Ensures continuity of care
Inspect the skin for signs of dryness and presence of drainage or secretions.	Provides data for determining whether a complete or partial bath is appropriate
Planning	
Consult with the patient to determine a convenient time for tending to hygiene needs.	Promotes cooperation between the patient and nurse; allows patient participation in decision making
Assemble supplies: bath blanket, towels, face cloths, soap, wash basin, clean pajamas or gown, clean bed linen, other hygiene articles such as deodorant or antiperspirant, and a razor for males.	Demonstrates organization and efficient time management
Implementation	
Wash your hands.	Reduces the spread of microorganisms
Pull the privacy curtain.	Demonstrates respect for modesty
Raise the bed to an appropriate height.	Reduces muscle strain on the back when providing care

continued

SKILL 16-3

GIVING A BED BATH *Continued*

Suggested Action	Reason for Action
Remove extra pillows or positioning devices and place the patient on his or her back.	Prepares the patient for washing the anterior body surface.
Cover the patient with a bath blanket.	Shows respect for the patient's modesty and provides warmth
Remove the patient's gown.	Facilitates washing the patient
While the patient holds the top of the bath blanket, pull and fan-fold the top linen to the bottom of the bed, or remove the linen, fold it, and lay it on a chair.	Keeps linen, which may be reused, clean
If linen is too soiled to be reused, place it in a laundry hamper.	Reduces the spread of microorganisms
Hold dirty linen away from contact with your uniform.	Reduces the spread of microorganisms
Fill a basin with 105° to 110°F (40° to 43°C) water and place the basin on the overbed table.	Provides comfortably warm water for bathing within easy access
Wet the washcloth and fold it to fashion a mitt (see Fig. A).	Keeps water from dripping from the margins of the cloth
Wipe each eye with a separate corner of the mitt from the nose toward the ear (see Fig. B).	Prevents getting soap in the eyes

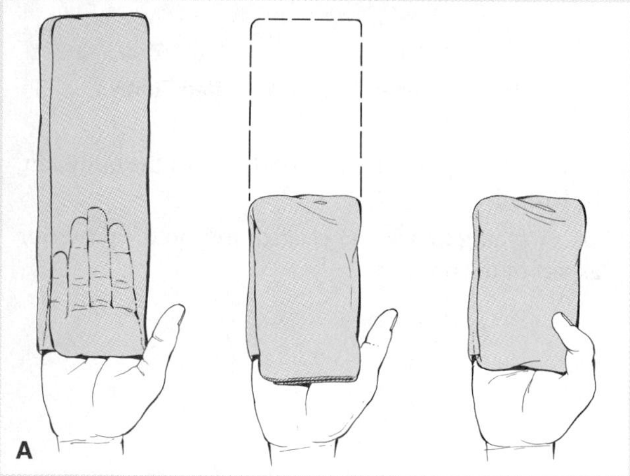

Making a mitt.

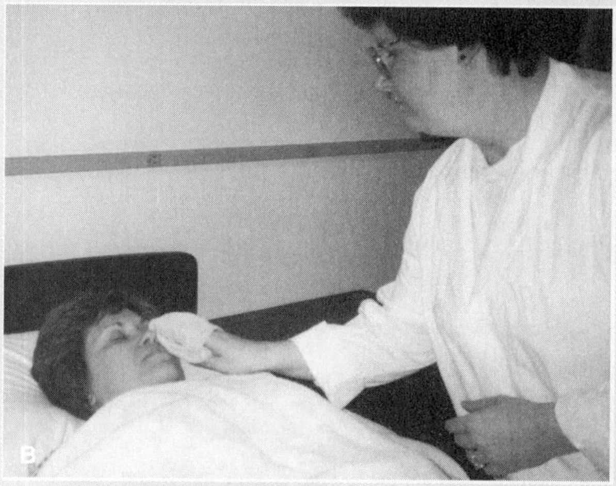

Wiping the eyes. (Courtesy of Ken Timby.)

Suggested Action	Reason for Action
Lather the wet washcloth with soap and finish washing the face.	Removes oil, sweat, and microorganisms
Rinse the washcloth and remove soapy residue from the face, then dry well.	Prevents drying the skin
Bathe each of the patient's arms separately; the axillae may be included now or when the chest is washed (see Fig. C).	Cleanses soiled material and keeps the patient from becoming too chilled
Offer to apply deodorant or antiperspirant after the axillae have been washed.	Demonstrates respect for the patient's usual hygiene practices; reduces perspiration and body odor
Place each hand in the basin of water as it is washed (see Fig. D).	Facilitates more thorough washing than just using the washcloth

continued

SKILL 16-3

GIVING A BED BATH *Continued*

Suggested Action	Reason for Action
Discard and replace the water in the wash basin; rinse the washcloth well or replace it with a clean one.	Eliminates debris, microorganisms, and soap residue, and increases the warmth of the water in preparation for washing cleaner areas of the body
Wash the chest, abdomen, each leg, and then the feet, following the steps described for the upper body (see Fig. E).	Follows the principle of washing from cleaner to more soiled areas

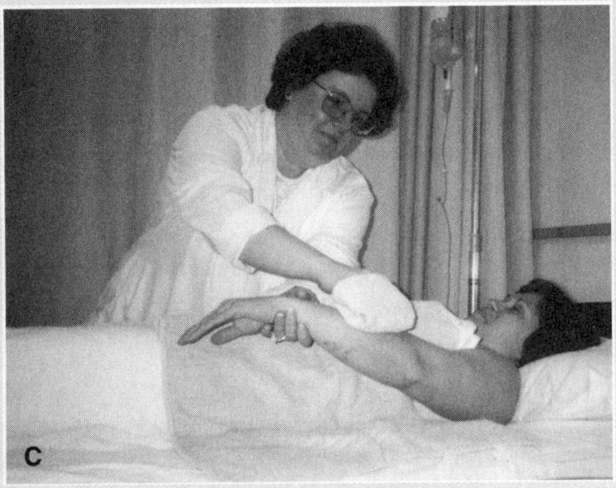

Washing the arm. (Courtesy of Ken Timby.)

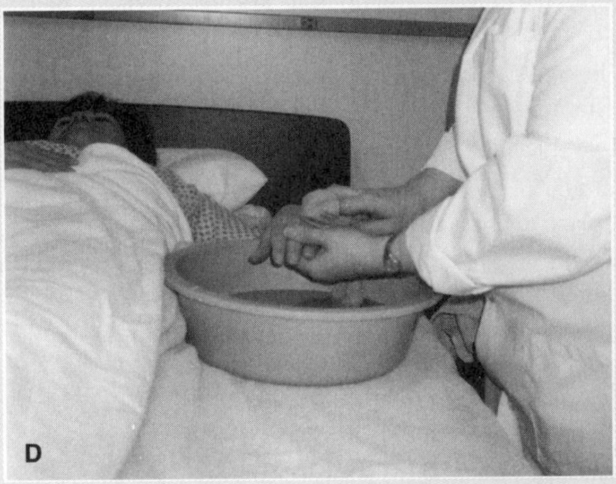

Washing a hand. (Courtesy of Ken Timby.)

Suggested Action	Reason for Action
Help the patient onto his or her side.	Repositions the patient so the posterior of the body can be bathed
Change the water and bathe the patient's back.	Allows washing to begin at cleaner area on the posterior aspect of the body

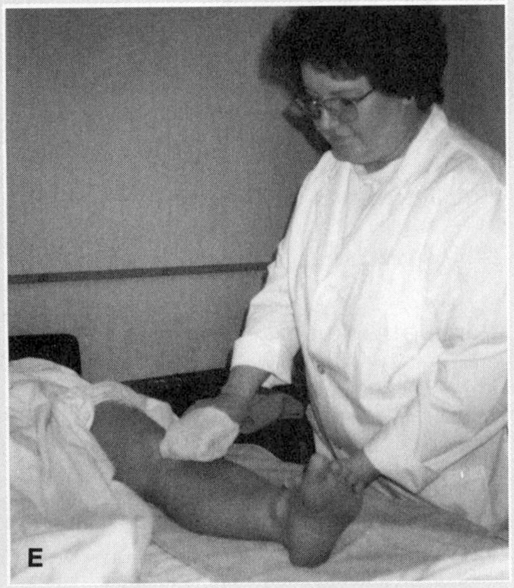

Washing a leg. (Courtesy of Ken Timby.)

continued

SKILL 16-3

GIVING A BED BATH *Continued*

Suggested Action	Reason for Action
Offer to apply lotion and provide a back rub.	Improves circulation and relaxes the patient
Don gloves and wash the buttocks, genitals, and anus last. Dry thoroughly.	Reduces the potential for contact with lesions or drainage that may contain infectious microorganisms. Prevents moisture accumulation.
Discard the water and wipe the basin dry.	Controls the growth and spread of microorganisms
Remove gloves and help the patient don a fresh gown.	Restores comfort and modesty

Evaluation

- Patient is completely bathed.
- Patient experiences no discomfort or intolerance of activity.

Document

- Date and time
- Type and extent of hygiene
- Response of the patient
- Assessment findings observed during bath

SAMPLE DOCUMENTATION*

Date and Time Complete bed bath given. Able to wash face and genitals independently. Skin is intact. No dyspnea noted during bath. ________________ SIGNATURE/TITLE

CRITICAL THINKING

- Which method of bathing (shower, tub bath, bed bath) is appropriate for the following patients: (1) a 75-year-old woman with arthritis of the hips; (2) a 60-year-old man with frequent seizures; (3) a 65-year-old man who becomes short of breath with exertion; (4) a 72-year-old woman recovering from pneumonia. Explain the reasons for your answers.

* Generally, routine hygiene measures are documented on a checklist, but for teaching purposes an example of narrative charting has been used.

SKILL 16-4

GIVING ORAL CARE TO UNCONSCIOUS PATIENTS

Suggested Action	Reason for Action
Assessment	
Check the nursing care plan about the frequency of oral hygiene.	Maintains continuity of care
Inspect the patient's mouth.	Helps determine equipment and supplies needed
Look for oral hygiene supplies that may already be at the patient's bedside.	Controls costs

continued

SKILL 16-4

GIVING ORAL CARE TO UNCONSCIOUS PATIENTS *Continued*

Suggested Action	Reason for Action
Planning	
Arrange to brush the patient's teeth once per shift and provide additional oral care at least every 2 hours.	Promotes a schedule for removing plaque and microorganisms and moistening and refreshing the mouth
Assemble the following equipment: toothbrush, toothpaste, suction catheter, water, bulb syringe, padded tongue blade, emesis basin, towel or absorbent pad, and gloves. Some agencies may stock a toothbrushing device connected directly to a suction catheter (see Fig. A).	Promotes organization and efficient time management

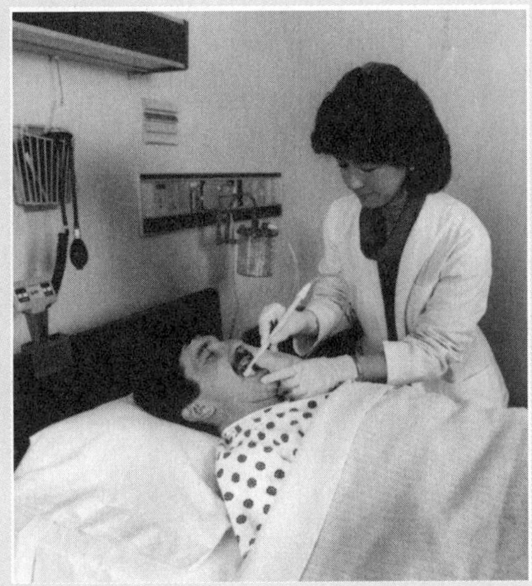

A

Special toothbrush with suction attachment. (Courtesy of Trademark Medical, Fenton, MO.)

Suggested Action	Reason for Action
Implementation	
Explain to the patient what you are about to do.	Reduces anxiety if the patient has the cognitive capacity to understand
Position the patient on his or her side with the head slightly lowered.	Prevents liquids from draining into the airway
Place a towel beneath the head.	Absorbs liquids
Connect a Yankeur suction tip or suction catheter to a portable or wall-mounted suction source.	Promotes safety
Spread toothpaste over a moistened toothbrush.	Prepares the toothbrush for use
Don gloves.	Prevents direct contact with blood or microorganisms in the mouth
Use a tongue blade or lower the patient's chin to open the mouth and separate the teeth (see Fig. B).	Serves as a safe substitute for the nurse's fingers
Brush all the surfaces of the teeth with the toothbrush.	Removes plaque and microorganisms
Instill water and suction the mouth with a bulb syringe or Yankeur suction device (see Fig. C).	Removes debris and reduces the potential for aspiration

continued

SKILL 16-4

GIVING ORAL CARE TO UNCONSCIOUS PATIENTS *Continued*

Suggested Action	Reason for Action

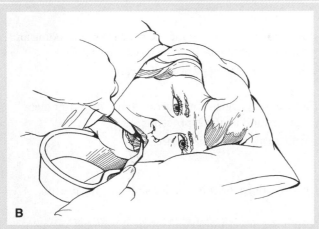

Brushing with tongue blade separating teeth.

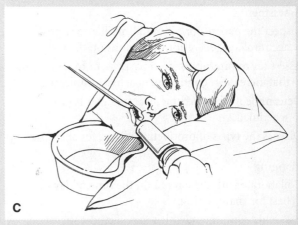

Rinsing and suctioning.

Suggested Action	Reason for Action
Clean and store oral hygiene supplies.	Restores cleanliness and order to the patient environment
Remove wet towel and gloves; restore patient to a position of comfort and safety.	Demonstrates concern for the patient's dignity and welfare

Evaluation
- The teeth are clean.
- The oral mucosa is smooth, pink, moist, and intact.
- Safety is maintained.

Document
- Date and time
- Assessment findings if significant
- Type of oral care
- Unusual events, such as choking, that occurred, and nursing action that was taken
- Outcome of any nursing action

SAMPLE DOCUMENTATION*

Date and Time Teeth brushed and mouth rinsed. Liquid suctioned from the mouth using a Yankeur suction catheter. No choking during oral care. Lung sounds are clear bilaterally.

________________________________ SIGNATURE/TITLE

CRITICAL THINKING
- Compare independent oral hygiene performed by a patient and that administered by a nurse for a dependent patient. How are they similar; how are they different?

* Generally, routine hygiene measures are documented on a checklist, but for teaching purposes an example of narrative charting has been used.

SKILL 16-5

SHAMPOOING HAIR

Suggested Action	Reason for Action
Assessment	
Inspect the patient for oily and limp hair or signs of accumulating secretions or lesions on the scalp.	Provides data to determine the need for shampooing and what supplies may be appropriate to use
Assess for respiratory symptoms, pain, or other conditions that increase or contribute to activity intolerance.	Aids in establishing priorities for care
Determine if and when medical treatments or tests are scheduled.	Ensures that hygiene measures will not interrupt therapeutic or diagnostic procedures
Discuss the types of products available for shampooing.	Facilitates individualized care
Planning	
Collaborate with the patient on the time of day that is best for shampooing.	Involves the patient in the decision-making process
Assemble equipment, which may include: shampoo, conditioner, hair oil treatment, towels, water pitcher, shampoo basin or trough.	Promotes organization and efficient time management

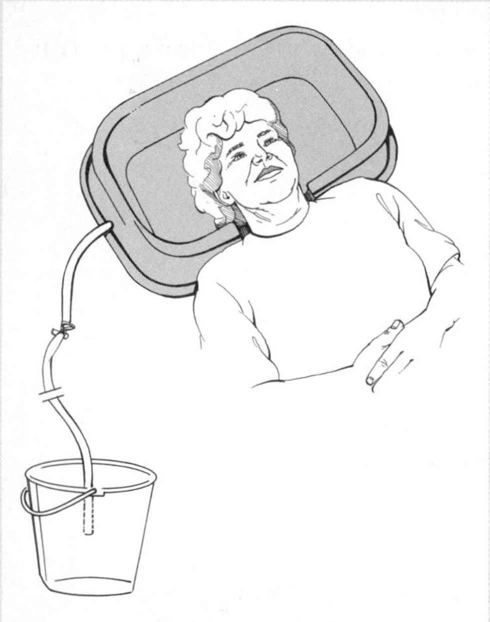

Shampooing the hair.

Suggested Action	Reason for Action
Implementation	
Close the door to the room and pull the privacy curtain.	Reduces the potential for chilling and promotes respect for privacy
Remove the pillow and protect the upper area of the bed with towels; cover the patient's chest and shoulders with a towel.	Absorbs moisture
Don gloves if there are any open lesions about the head.	Prevents direct contact with blood or secretions
Wet the hair thoroughly and apply shampoo.	Dilutes and distributes the shampoo

continued

SKILL 16-5

SHAMPOOING HAIR *Continued*

Suggested Action	Reason for Action
Work the shampoo into a lather.	Facilitates cleansing throughout the hair
Rinse the hair with water.	Removes oil and shampoo from the hair
Apply conditioner if requested and available.	Relaxes the hair and reduces tangles
Wrap the head with a dry towel and fluff the hair.	Absorbs water and shortens the drying time
Remove and discard gloves when there is no threat for direct contact with blood or secretions.	Facilitates hair care
Comb, braid, or style the hair according to the patient's preference.	Promotes self-esteem
Clean and store shampooing supplies.	Restores cleanliness and order to the patient environment

Evaluation

- The hair is clean and dry.

Document

- Date and time
- Assessment findings
- Type of care
- Response of the patient

SAMPLE DOCUMENTATION

Date and Time Scalp and hair appear oily. Skin is intact. Bed shampoo provided. Hair dried, combed, and styled in braids. Scalp is clean and intact. No evidence of chilling, fatigue, or discomfort during shampoo. States, "I feel so much better." ____________________ SIGNATURE/TITLE

CRITICAL THINKING

- Discuss how hair loss or neglect of hair care affects the psyche (emotional health and self-esteem).
- Discuss how hair care is modified if the patient has pediculosis (lice).
- Describe differences in hair care for African-American patients.

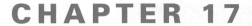

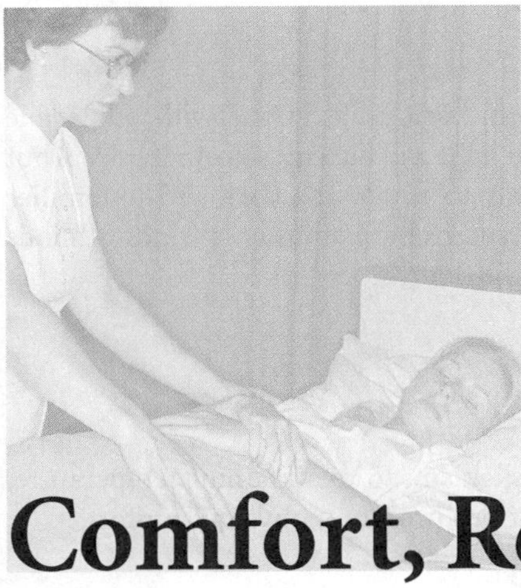

CHAPTER 17

Comfort, Rest, and Sleep

CHAPTER OUTLINE

The Patient Environment
Sleep and Rest
Sleep Assessment
Sleep Disorders
Nursing Implications

NURSING GUIDELINES

FACILITATING PROGRESSIVE RELAXATION

SKILLS

SKILL 17-1: MAKING AN UNOCCUPIED BED
SKILL 17-2: MAKING AN OCCUPIED BED
SKILL 17-3: GIVING A BACK MASSAGE

NURSING CARE PLAN

SLEEP PATTERN DISTURBANCE

KEY TERMS

apnea
bruxism
cataplexy
circadian rhythm
climate control
comfort
drug tolerance
environmental psychologist
humidity
hypersomnia
hypersomnolence
hypnogogic hallucinations
hypnotic
hypopnea
hypoxia
insomnia
jet lag
massage
mattress overlay
melatonin
microsleep
multiple sleep latency test
narcolepsy
nocturnal enuresis
nocturnal polysomnography
occupied bed
parasomnia
photoperiod
phototherapy
progressive relaxation
relative humidity
rest
restless legs syndrome
sedative
sleep
sleep apnea/hypopnea syndrome
sleep diary
sleep paralysis
sleep rituals
sleep–wake cycle disturbance
somnabulism
stimulants
sundown syndrome
sunrise syndrome
thermoregulation
tranquilizer
unoccupied bed
ventilation

LEARNING OBJECTIVES

An understanding of the content within this chapter will be evidenced by the student's ability to:

- Differentiate between comfort, rest, and sleep.
- Describe four ways to modify the patient environment to promote comfort, rest, and sleep.
- List four standard furnishings in each patient room.
- State at least five functions of sleep.
- Name the two phases of sleep and describe their differences.
- Describe the general trend in sleep requirements as a person ages.
- Name 10 factors that affect sleep.
- List four categories of drugs that affect sleep.
- Name four techniques for assessing sleep patterns.
- Describe four categories of sleep disorders.
- Discuss at least five techniques for promoting sleep.
- Name two nursing measures that promote relaxation.
- Discuss unique characteristics of sleep among older adults.

C**omfort** (state in which a person is relieved of distress) facilitates **rest** (waking state characterized by reduced activity and mental stimulation) and **sleep** (state of arousable unconsciousness). One of the factors that contributes to comfort is a safe, clean, and attractive environment. This chapter addresses measures for ensuring that the setting for patient care is one that promotes a sense of well-being. It includes measures for maintaining the order and cleanliness of the patient's bed and room, and describes nursing interventions that facilitate rest and sleep.

The Patient Environment

The term *environment,* as it is used here, refers to the room where the patient receives nursing care and the furnishings within it. But in a broader sense, the health care facility's location and design involve many other subtle elements that influence the consumer's overall impression of the institution.

Most patients are unaware of the thought and consideration that go into their surroundings. Accessible parking, lighting inside and outside the physical plant, landscaping, barriers that reduce traffic noise, and signs that help patients find their way around the building create a positive appeal among those in need of health care.

PATIENT ROOMS

Patient rooms resemble bedrooms but are no longer the bare, white, sterile environments of a few decades ago. Thanks to **environmental psychologists** (specialists who study how the environment affects behavior), patient rooms are now brighter, more colorful, and tastefully decorated. The wall and floor treatments, lighting, and mechanisms for maintaining climate control are practical and conducive to comfort.

Walls

Blue and colors with blue tints, such as mauve and light green, promote relaxation, so these color schemes are preferred within health care settings and patient rooms. If they are not used exclusively, they are integrated into wallpaper trim and decorative accessories such as framed pictures. The art often depicts country scenes and peaceful images.

Floors

Because noise interferes with comfort, the hallways and work stations are carpeted in most agencies. The floors in patient rooms have tile or linoleum surfaces to facilitate cleaning spills.

Lighting

Adequate lighting, both natural and artificial, is important to the comfort of patients and nursing personnel. Newer buildings have large window areas, atriums, skylights, and enclosed courtyards to facilitate exposure to sunlight as a technique for reducing stress.

Bright artificial light facilitates nursing care but is not conducive to patient comfort. Therefore, most patient rooms have multiple lights in various locations with adjustable intensity. Because dim light and darkness promote sleep, but injuries are more likely to occur in a dark and unfamiliar environment, patient rooms have adjustable window blinds and night lights near the floor.

Climate Control

Climate control (mechanisms for maintaining temperature, humidity, and ventilation) promotes physical comfort.

Temperature and Humidity

Most patients are comfortable when the room temperature is 68° to 74°F (20° to 23°C). Newer buildings provide thermostats in each room so that the temperature can be adjusted to suit the patient.

Humidity (amount of moisture in the air) and **relative humidity** (ratio between the amount of moisture in the air and the greatest amount of water vapor the air can hold at a given temperature) affect comfort. At a relative humidity of 60%, the air contains 60% of its potential water capacity. A relative humidity of 30% to 60% is comfortable for most patients.

If the environmental temperature becomes greater than the skin temperature, evaporation is the only mechanism for regulating body temperature. Evaporation is reduced when humidity levels rise because air that is almost or fully saturated with water cannot absorb additional moisture. Therefore, instead of evaporating, sweat accumulates and drips from the skin.

Many agencies are air-conditioned. Electric fans and dehumidifiers are not always an adequate substitute but may be used if air conditioners are not available. In buildings where the air is dry, moisture can be added to the environment with a humidifier or a cool mist machine. Patients who have ineffective **thermoregulation** (ability to maintain stable body temperature) may feel hot or cold even when the temperature and humidity are optimal.

Ventilation

At home, **ventilation** (movement of air) is accomplished by opening windows or using ceiling fans. In hospitals and nursing homes, however, open windows are a fire and safety hazard and ceiling fans spread infectious microorganisms. Consequently, ventilation is usually accomplished through a system of air ducts that circulate air in and out of each patient room.

Poorly ventilated rooms and buildings tend to smell bad. Removing soiled articles, emptying bedpans and urinals, and opening privacy curtains and room doors help reduce odors. An alternative is to use an air freshener or deodorant; in general, though, scented sprays substitute one odor for another, and ill patients generally find any strong smell disagreeable. Nurses should be conscientious about their own hygiene, should not wear overpowering perfume, and should not smell of cigarette smoke.

ROOM FURNISHINGS

Manufacturers of hospital furnishings attempt to design equipment that is both attractive and practical (Fig. 17-1). The bed and its components, the mattress and pillow, chairs, the overbed table, and the bedside stand must be safe, durable, and comfortable.

The Bed

Hospital beds are adjustable—that is, the height and position of the head and knees can be changed either electronically or manually. Adjusting the bed promotes comfort, enables self-care, or facilitates a therapeutic position (see Chap. 23). Hospital beds are usually kept in their lowest position except when patients are receiving nursing care or when bed linens are being changed. Skill 17-1 describes how to make an **unoccupied bed** (changing linen when the bed is empty).

Full or half siderails are attached to the bed frame. There is controversy as to whether raised siderails are a risk or benefit, because some patients climb over them rather than seek nursing assistance. Siderails are considered a form of physical restraint in long-term care facilities, and their use must be justified (Omnibus Budget Reconciliation Act of 1987; see Chap. 18).

Some beds have removable headboards (Fig. 17-2). This facilitates resuscitation efforts if the patient goes into respiratory or cardiac arrest. Removing the headboard gives the code team responders better access for airway intubation. Placing the headboard under the patient's upper body allows more effective cardiac compression than possible on a mattress (see Chap. 37).

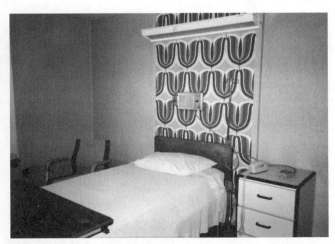

FIGURE 17–1. Typical hospital room furnishings. (Courtesy of Ken Timby.)

Mattress

Many people equate the comfort of a bed with the quality of the mattress. A good mattress adjusts to the shape of the body while supporting it. A mattress that is too soft alters the alignment of the spine, causing some people to awaken feeling sore from muscle and joint strain.

Hospital mattresses are generally made of tough materials that will withstand long-term use. Because mattresses are not sterilized between uses, they are covered with a waterproof coating that withstands cleaning with strong antimicrobial solutions.

Occasionally **mattress overlays** (layers of foam or other devices placed on top of the mattress; Fig. 17-3) are used to promote comfort or to keep the skin intact (see Chap. 23). Display 17-1 lists the patients for whom a mattress overlay or therapeutic mattress of foam, gel, air, or water is appropriate.

Pillows

Pillows are primarily used for comfort, but they also are used to elevate a part of the body, relieve swelling, promote breathing, or help maintain a therapeutic position (see Chap. 23). Pillows are stuffed with foam, *kapok* (a mass of silky fibers), or feathers.

Bed Linen

The linen used for most hospital beds includes:

- Mattress pad
- Bottom sheet, which is sometimes fitted
- Optional drawsheet, which is placed beneath the patient's hips
- Top sheet
- Blanket, depending on the preference of the patient
- Spread
- Pillow case

Some hospitals use printed sheets to provide a more homelike atmosphere.

To control expenses, bed linen may not be changed every day, but any linen that is wet or soiled is changed as frequently as necessary. Sometimes folded sheets or disposable, absorbent pads are placed between the patient and the bottom sheet to avoid the need to change the entire bed when linen becomes soiled. Skill 17-2 explains how to make an **occupied bed** (changing linen while the patient remains in bed).

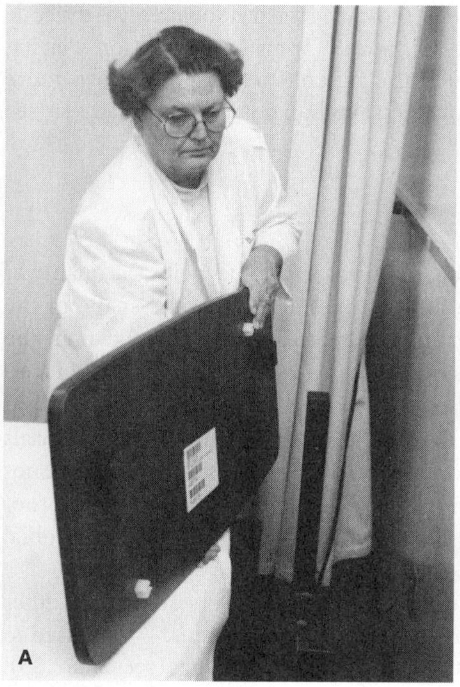
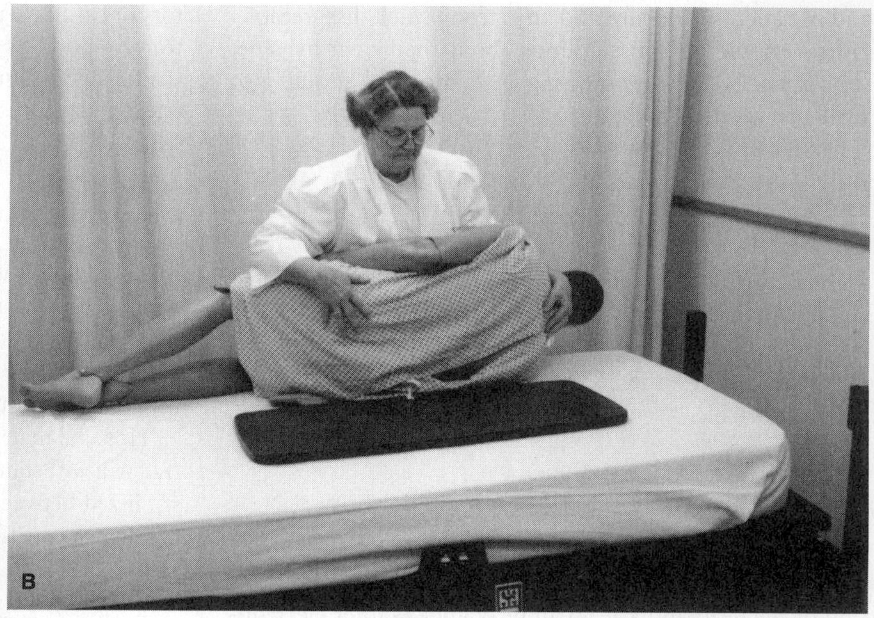

FIGURE 17–2. (*A*) The nurse removes the headboard from a standard hospital bed. (*B*) The headboard is placed beneath a patient before resuscitation.

Privacy Curtain

A privacy curtain is a long fabric partition, mounted from the ceiling. It can be drawn completely around each patient's bed. The privacy curtain is used to preserve the patient's dignity and modesty whenever it is necessary to examine or expose the patient for care. It also is used to shield a patient from being observed while using a urinal or bedpan.

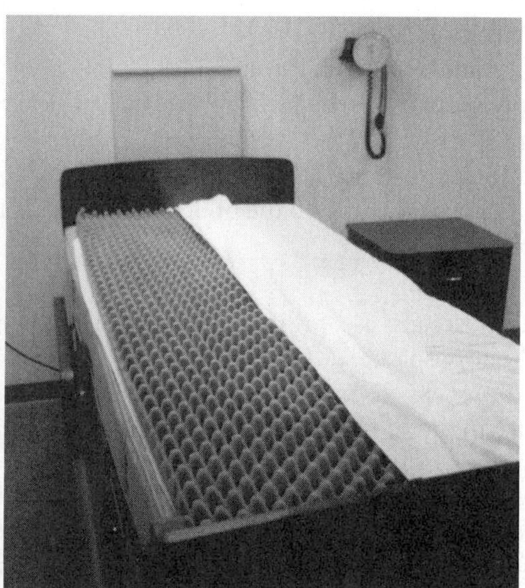

FIGURE 17–3. Egg crate mattress overlay. (Courtesy of Ken Timby.)

Overbed Table

An overbed table is a portable, flat platform positioned over the lap of a patient. The height of the table is adjustable depending on whether the bed is in a high or low position. The overbed table makes it convenient for the patient to eat while in bed and to perform personal hygiene or other activities requiring a flat surface. Nurses also use the overbed table to hold equipment when providing patient care. There is often a concealed compartment in the overbed table that may contain a mounted mirror and a place for personal items (hairbrush, comb, cosmetic bag, razor, or book).

Bedside Stand

A bedside stand is actually a small cupboard. It usually contains a drawer for personal items and two shelves. The upper

DISPLAY 17–1

Patient Criteria for Mattress Overlay or Therapeutic Mattress

- Complete immobility
- Limited mobility
- Impaired skin integrity
- Inadequate nutritional status
- Incontinence of stool and/or urine
- Altered tactile perception
- Compromised circulatory status

shelf is used to store the patient's bath basin, soap dish, soap, and a kidney-shaped basin called an emesis basin. The lower shelf is used to store a bedpan, urinal, and toilet paper. The elimination utensils are kept separate from the hygiene supplies to reduce the transmission of microorganisms. A carafe of water and a drinking container are placed atop the bedside stand.

Chairs

There is generally at least one chair per patient in each room. Hospital chairs usually are straight-backed to facilitate good postural support. The best sitting position is when the hips, knees, and ankles are all at 90° angles. There may be one upholstered chair in each patient room. Although upholstered chairs are more comfortable, some patients find that rising from them is difficult.

Sleep and Rest

No matter how comfortable the physical environment or how attractive and homelike the furnishings, recuperation may be sabotaged or prolonged by failure to promote rest and sleep. Although sleep requirements vary, alterations in sleep patterns can have serious physical and emotional consequences.

FUNCTIONS OF SLEEP

Besides promoting emotional well-being, sleep enhances various physiologic processes. Although the exact mechanisms are not totally understood, the restorative functions of sleep can be inferred from the effects of sleep deprivation (Display 17-2). Sleep is believed to play a role in:

- Reducing fatigue
- Stabilizing mood
- Improving blood flow to the brain
- Increasing protein synthesis
- Maintaining the disease-fighting mechanisms of the immune system
- Promoting cellular growth and repair
- Improving the capacity for learning and memory storage

DISPLAY 17–2

Effects of Chronic Sleep Deprivation

- Reduced physical stamina
- Altered comfort, such as headache and nausea
- Impaired coordination, especially of fine motor skills
- Loss of muscle mass and weight
- Increased susceptibility to infection
- Slower wound healing
- Decreased pain tolerance
- Poor concentration
- Impaired judgment
- Unstable moods
- Suspiciousness

SLEEP PHASES

Sleeping is divided into two phases: *nonrapid eye movement* (NREM) *sleep* and *rapid eye movement* (REM) *sleep.* These names come from the fact that there are periods during sleep when eye movements are either subdued or energetic.

Nonrapid eye movement sleep is also called *slow wave sleep,* because during this phase electroencephalographic (EEG) waves appear as progressively slower oscillations. The REM phase of sleep is referred to as *paradoxical sleep* because the EEG waves appear similar to those produced during periods of wakefulness, but it is the deepest stage of sleep. Thus, NREM sleep is characterized as quiet sleep and REM sleep as active sleep.

Sleep Cycles

During sleep, people pass back and forth through four distinct stages of NREM sleep and the REM phase of sleep. The characteristics and lengths of each phase are identified in Table 17-1. NREM sleep normally precedes REM sleep, the phase during which most dreaming occurs. Although the length of time spent in any one phase or stage varies according to age and other variables, most people cycle back and forth from stages 2, 3, and 4 of NREM to REM phases four to six times during the night.

SLEEP REQUIREMENTS

Sleep requirements vary among different age groups. The need for sleep decreases with age, although there are individual differences (Table 17-2). According to the National Sleep Foundation (1994), older adults tend to sleep fewer hours at night but take one or two daytime naps. On the average, they also awaken for a few seconds as many as 150 times a night and fully awaken at least once for urination. Younger adults awaken briefly five times a night without the need for urination.

FACTORS AFFECTING SLEEP

The amount and quality of sleep can be affected by changes in the amount and intensity of light, activity, the environ-

TABLE 17–1. **Characteristics of Sleep Phases**

Sleep Phase	Length	Features
NREM	50–90 minutes	Deep, restful, dreamless sleep
Stage 1	A few minutes	Light sleep, easily aroused Gradual reduction in vital signs
Stage 2	10–20 minutes	Deeper relaxation Can be awakened with effort
Stage 3	15–30 minutes	Early phase of deep sleep Snoring Relaxed muscle tone Little or no physical movement Difficult to arouse
Stage 4	15–30 minutes; shortens toward morning	Deep sleep Sleep-walking, sleep-talking, and bedwetting may occur
REM	20-minute average; lengthens toward morning	Darting eye movements Very difficult to awaken Vivid, colorful, emotional dreams Loss of muscle tone; jaw relaxes; tongue may fall to the back of the throat Vital signs fluctuate Irregular respirations Pauses in breathing for 15–20 seconds Absence of snoring Muscle twitching Gastric secretions increase Men may have erections

ment, motivation, emotions and moods, food and beverages, illness, and drugs (Table 17-3).

Light

The sleep–wake cycle is influenced by daylight and darkness. **Circadian rhythm** (phenomena that cycle on a 24-hour basis) is a term derived from two Latin words: *circa* (about) and *dies* (day). Thus, drowsiness and sleep correlate with the circadian rhythm of the setting sun and night. Wakefulness corresponds with sunrise and daylight.

Researchers (Rosenthal et al., 1984) have suggested that the cycles of wakefulness followed by sleep are linked to a photosensitive system involving the eyes and the pineal gland in the brain (Fig. 17-4). In the absence of bright light, the pineal gland secretes **melatonin** (hormone that induces drowsiness and sleep); light triggers the suppression of melatonin secretion.

TABLE 17–2. **Sleep Requirements**

Age	Total Sleep Time	Percentage in REM
Newborn	16–20 hours/day	50%
3 months – 1 year	14–15 hours/day	35%
Toddler	12 hours/night plus 1 or 2 naps	No data
Preschool	9–12 hours/night	No data
5 – 6 years	11 hours/night	20%
11 years	9 hours/night	No data
Adolescent	7–9 hours/night	25%
Adult	7–9 hours/night	20%–25%
Elderly	7–9 hours/night	13%–15%

Activity

Activity, especially exercise, increases fatigue and the need for sleep. Activity appears to increase both REM and NREM sleep, especially the deep sleep of the fourth stage of NREM. However, if physical activity occurs just before bedtime, it has a stimulating rather than relaxing effect.

Environment

Most people sleep best in their usual environment: they develop a preference for a particular pillow, mattress, and blankets. They also tend to adapt to the unique sounds of where they live, such as traffic, trains, and the hum of appliance motors or furnaces.

TABLE 17–3. **Factors Affecting Sleep**

Sleep-Promoting Factors	Sleep-Suppressing Factors
Darkness, dim light	Sunlight, bright light
Consistent sleep schedule	Inconsistent sleep schedule
Secretion of melatonin	Suppression of melatonin
Familiar sleep environment	Strange sleep environment
Optimal warmth and ventilation	Cold, hot, stuffy room
Performance of sleep rituals	Disturbance of sleep rituals
Sedative, hypnotic drugs	Stimulant drugs
Depression	Depression, anxiety, worry
Relaxation	Activity
Satiation	Hunger, thirst
Proteins containing L-tryptophan	Protein-deficient diets
Excessive alcohol consumption	Metabolism of alcohol
Comfort	Pain, nausea, full bladder
Quiet	Noise
Effortless breathing	Difficulty breathing

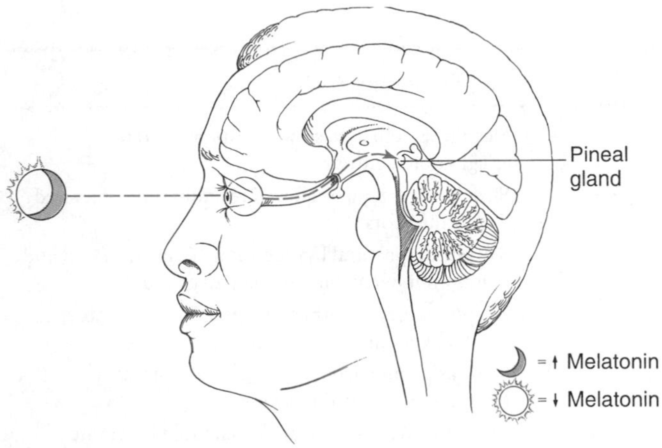

FIGURE 17–4. The sleep–wake cycle is influenced by a photosensitive light system.

In addition, sleep is induced by repeating **sleep rituals** (habitual activities performed before retiring). Sleep rituals include eating a light snack, watching television, reading, and performing hygiene. Therefore, when the environment is altered or the activities performed before bedtime are disturbed—as they are on vacation or in the hospital—the ability to fall asleep and remain asleep is affected.

Motivation

When there is no particular reason to stay awake, sleep generally occurs easily. But if the desire to remain awake is strong, such as when a person wishes to participate in something interesting or important, the desire to sleep can be overcome.

Emotions and Moods

Depressive disorders are classically associated with an inability to sleep or the tendency to sleep more than usual. Also, emotions such as anger, fear, anxiety, and dread interfere with sleep. All are more than likely the result of changes in the types and amounts of neurotransmitters that affect the sleep–wake center in the brain.

Sometimes sleeplessness is conditioned—that is, anticipating sleeplessness, a characteristic pattern of some chronic insomniacs, actually reinforces it (a self-fulfilling prophesy). The expectation that the onset of sleep will be difficult increases the person's anxiety. The anxiety then floods the brain with stimulating chemicals that interfere with relaxation, a prerequisite for natural sleep.

Food and Beverages

Hunger or thirst interferes with sleep. The consumption of particular foods and beverages may also promote or inhibit the ability to sleep.

Sleep is facilitated by a chemical known as L-tryptophan that is found in protein foods such as milk and dairy products. The recommendation to drink warm milk to induce sleep may have originally been an anecdotal observation of its **hypnotic** (sleep-producing) effect. L-Tryptophan is also present in poultry, fish, eggs, and to some extent in plant sources of protein such as legumes.

Alcohol is a depressive drug that promotes sleep, but it tends to reduce normal REM and deep sleep stages of NREM sleep. As alcohol is metabolized, stimulating chemicals that were blocked by the sedative effects of the alcohol surge forth from neurons, causing early awakening.

Beverages containing caffeine, a central nervous system stimulant, cause wakefulness. Caffeine is present in coffee, tea, chocolate, and most cola drinks.

Illness

Almost any illness is accompanied by stress, anxiety, and discomfort, any one of which can alter normal sleep patterns. In the hospital, other factors that contribute to sleep loss or fragmentation of sleep include being aroused by the noise from equipment, being awakened for nursing activities, and being disturbed by unfamiliar sounds such as loud talking, elevators, dietary carts, and housekeeping equipment.

Several medical disorders involve symptoms that are aggravated at night or can disturb sleep. For example, ulcers tend to be more painful during the night because hydrochloric acid is increased during REM sleep. In fact, pain of any kind is more distressing when there are few distractions. Conditions that are worsened by lying flat in bed, such as some cardiac, respiratory, and musculoskeletal disorders, contribute to sleeplessness.

Drugs

Caffeine and alcohol, which have already been discussed, are nonprescription drugs that affect sleep. Some prescribed drugs can also promote or interfere with sleep. **Sedatives** and **tranquilizers** (drugs that produce a relaxing and calming effect) promote rest, a precursor to sleep. Hypnotics are drugs that induce sleep. **Stimulants** (drugs that excite structures in the brain) cause wakefulness (Table 17-4).

Some sedatives and hypnotics have a paradoxical effect when administered to older adults: they tend to produce wakefulness instead of sleep. Also, people who take sedative and hypnotic drugs for a period of time tend to develop **drug tolerance** (diminished effect from the drug at its usual dosage range). Without realizing the danger, these people may increase the dose of the drug or the frequency of its administration to achieve the same effect first experienced at a lower dose. Increasing the dose or frequency has potentially life-threatening consequences.

TABLE 17–4. **Drugs That Affect Sleep**

Drug Category	Drug Family	Example	Adverse Reactions
Sedatives	Barbiturates	Phenobarbital (Luminal)	Sleepiness, lethargy, slowed respiratory rate, agitation, confusion
	Antihistamines	Diphenhydramine (Benadryl)	Sleepiness, dizziness, slowed reaction time, impaired coordination
	Antipsychotics	Haloperidol (Haldol)	Sleepiness, postural hypotension, abnormal facial and mouth movements, stiff gait, dry mouth
Tranquilizers	Benzodiazepines	Alprazolam (Xanax)	Sleepiness, dry mouth, constipation, slowed heart rate, hypotension, liver damage
Hypnotics	Barbiturates	Pentobarbital (Nembutal)	Same as phenobarbital, daytime drowsiness
	Nonbarbiturates	Temazepam (Restoril)	Dizziness, lethargy during the day
Stimulants	Amphetamines	Dextroamphetamine (Dexedrine)	Insomnia, restlessness, anorexia, rapid heart rate
	Amphetamine-like	Methylphenidate (Ritalin)	Nervousness, insomnia, rash, anorexia, nausea

When sedatives, tranquilizers, and hypnotics are abruptly discontinued, they cause a period of intense stimulation that interferes with sleep.

Some drugs, such as diuretics, which increase the formation of urine, may awaken patients with a need to empty the bladder. For this reason, diuretics are generally administered early in the morning so that the peak effect has diminished by bedtime.

Sleep Assessment

Many people blame inadequate sleep for daytime fatigue, or they underestimate the actual amount of time they sleep. A more accurate sleep pattern assessment can be obtained through sleep questionnaires, sleep diaries, polysomnographic evaluation, and a multiple latency sleep test.

QUESTIONNAIRES

Several questionnaires have been developed to help identify sleep patterns. Questionnaires are either designed to obtain specific information or are unstructured to give the person more freedom to respond. The data can be gathered during interviews, or the questions can be answered independently in the form of a self-report.

Examples of questions for the patient include:

- When you think about your sleep, what kinds of impressions come to mind?
- Is there anything about your sleep that bothers you?
- Do you fall asleep at inappropriate times?
- Do you wake feeling rested?
- How long does it take you to fall asleep?
- Do you feel stiff and sore in the morning?
- Have you been told that you stop breathing while asleep?
- Do you fall sleep during physical activities?
- What do you do to help yourself sleep well?

Members of the patient's household are asked:

- Does the patient snore or gasp for air when sleeping?
- Does the patient kick or thrash around while sleeping?
- Does the patient sleep-walk?

SLEEP DIARY

A **sleep diary** (daily account of sleeping and waking activities) is compiled by the patient or by personnel in a sleep disorder clinic. The patient notes the times he or she is asleep, describes daily activities during each 15-minute waking period, completes a 24-hour log of consumed food and beverages, and notes when any medications are taken. These self-kept diaries generally cover a 2-week period.

Although sleep diaries are inexpensive and simple to compile, Rogers et al. (1993) found that they varied in accuracy and reliability. Therefore, sleep assessments include other objective diagnostic techniques for gathering data to ensure that sleep disorders and their etiologies are accurately identified.

NOCTURNAL POLYSOMNOGRAPHY

Nocturnal polysomnography (technique used to obtain physiologic data during nighttime sleep) is performed during an entire night's sleep. It generally takes place in a sleep disorder clinic, but it is now possible to conduct the study at the patient's home; a technician monitors a computerized recording system up to 60 feet away.

Dime-sized sensors attached to the head and body (Fig. 17-5) record:

- Brain waves
- Eye movements

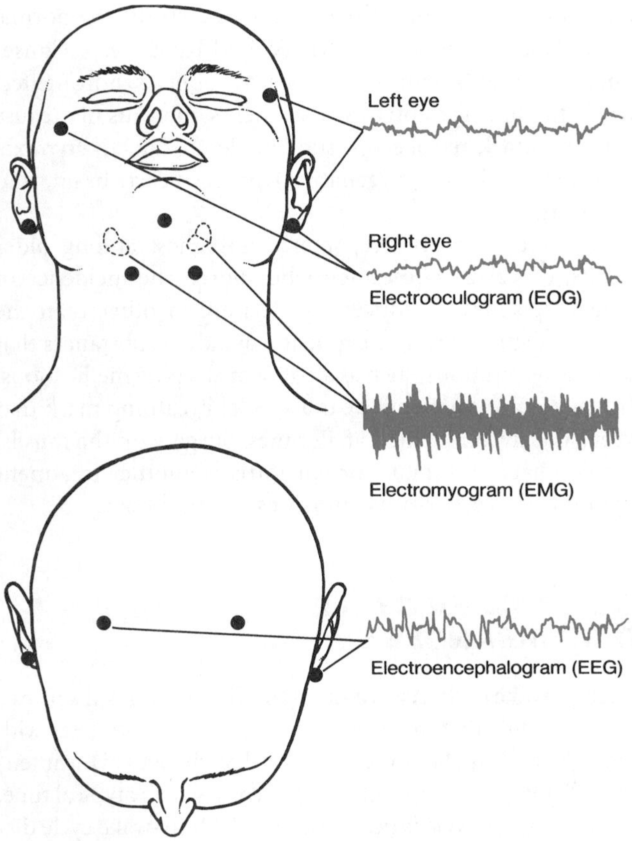

FIGURE 17–5. Normal sleep patterns and sleep disorders are evaluated by collecting physiologic data.

- Muscle tone
- Limb movement
- Body position
- Nasal and oral airflow
- Chest and abdominal respiratory effort
- Snoring sounds
- Oxygen level in the blood

The diagnostic data are compared with the patterns and characteristics of normal sleep cycles to help diagnose sleep disorders.

MULTIPLE SLEEP LATENCY TEST

A **multiple sleep latency test** (assessment of daytime sleepiness) is another helpful study. The person undergoing this test is asked to take a daytime nap at 2-hour intervals while attached to sensors similar to those used in polysomnography. The patient is allowed to nap for about 20 minutes. The nap periods are repeated four or five times throughout the day.

Patients who have certain sleep disorders causing daytime sleepiness have a short latency period—that is, they fall asleep in less than 5 minutes. Most well-rested persons take an average of 15 minutes before they experience the onset of daytime sleep.

Experiencing early REM sleep is also a pathologic finding that can be detected during a multiple sleep latency test. A REM period normally does not occur for at least an hour and after cycling through the first four stages of NREM. Therefore, REM should not occur during a 20-minute test nap.

Sleep Disorders

About 25 million Americans have a sleep disorder of one type or another (Oldham, 1995), but many of them do not seek treatment. Most problems are short-lived, but some sleep disorders are both chronic and serious. There are four categories of sleep disorders: insomnia, hypersomnias, sleep–wake cycle disturbances, and parasomnias.

INSOMNIA

Insomnia (difficulty falling asleep or staying asleep, or awakening early) results in feeling unrested the next day. Almost everyone has had insomnia. Most cases of insomnia resolve themselves in less than 3 weeks. According to the American Psychiatric Association (1994), insomnia is considered a sleep disturbance if it occurs at least three times a week for at least a month. Although chronic insomnia can be treated with hypnotic drugs, it is helpful to start treatment with nonpharmacologic interventions.

Patient Teaching For

Promoting Sleep

Teach the patient or the family to do the following:

- Resist napping during the day.
- Use the bed and bedroom just for sleeping.
- Perform sleep rituals.
- Go to bed and get up at approximately the same time, even on weekends or days off.
- If you cannot get to sleep for more than 20 to 30 minutes, get out of bed and do something else, such as reading.
- Try a bedtime relaxation tape that plays soothing music, sounds of nature, or a constant background sound (white noise).
- Exercise regularly during the day, but not late in the evening.
- Avoid alcohol, nicotine, and caffeine.
- Eat dairy products and other proteins daily.
- Modify the temperature and ventilation in the bedroom according to personal preferences.
- Use earplugs or eyeshades to reduce environmental noise or light.
- Avoid using nonprescription or prescription sleeping pills unless they have been recommended by a physician. Hypnotics should be used on a short-term basis only.

- Try drinking chamomile tea, which some claim improves sleep.
- Follow label directions on any medications.
- If a diuretic drug is prescribed, take it early in the morning.

HYPERSOMNIAS

Hypersomnia (sleep disorder characterized by feeling sleepy despite getting a normal amount of sleep) includes two conditions: narcolepsy and sleep apnea/hypopnea syndrome.

Narcolepsy

Narcolepsy (sleep disorder characterized by the sudden onset of daytime sleep, short NREM period before the first REM phase, and pathologic manifestations of REM sleep) is a disabling condition. It should not to be confused with **hypersomnolence** (excessive sleeping for long periods of time as in Washington Irving's 1819 American folk story, *Rip Van Winkle*).

Although the diagnosis of narcolepsy generally requires a multiple sleep latency test and polysomnography, its symptoms help to distinguish it from other conditions that cause sleepiness. For example, the sleepiness of narcolepsy is accompanied by abnormalities of REM sleep that include:

- **Sleep paralysis** (the person cannot move for a few minutes just before falling asleep or awakening)
- **Cataplexy** (sudden loss of muscle tone, triggered by an emotional change such as laughing or anger)
- **Hypnogogic hallucinations** (dreamlike auditory or visual experiences while dozing or falling asleep)

Narcoleptic symptoms diminish with age in about a third of those affected. If untreated, the patient may become involved in motor vehicle or occupational accidents. Prescribed stimulant drugs, such as methylphenidate (Ritalin) or dextroamphetamine (Dexedrine), help improve alertness. Antidepressants reduce the symptoms associated with atypical REM sleep.

Sleep Apnea/Hypopnea Syndrome

Apnea (cessation of breathing) and **hypopnea** (hypoventilation) are manifestations of a second form of hypersomnia, **sleep apnea/hypopnea syndrome** (sleep disorder in which the sleeper stops breathing or the breathing slows for 10 seconds or longer, five or more times per hour; Dantzker and Steinberg, 1994). This is discussed further in Chapter 20.

During the apneic or hypopneic periods, ventilation is reduced and blood oxygenation drops. The accumulation of carbon dioxide and the fall in oxygen cause brief periods of awakening throughout the night. This disturbs the normal transitions and periods of NREM and REM sleep. Consequently, patients with sleep apnea/hypopnea syndrome feel tired after having slept; or worse, their symptoms may cause a heart attack, stroke, or sudden death due to **hypoxia** (decreased cellular oxygenation) of the heart, brain, and other organs.

The incidence of sleep apnea is highest among older adults, especially obese men who snore. The incidence of apneic episodes is reduced by sleeping in other than the supine position, losing weight, and avoiding substances that depress respirations, such as alcohol or sleeping medications. In severe cases, patients wear a special breathing mask that keeps the alveoli inflated at all times. Surgery on the tonsils, uvula, pharynx, tongue, or epiglottis is another treatment option when conservative measures are ineffective.

SLEEP–WAKE CYCLE DISTURBANCES

A **sleep–wake cycle disturbance** (condition that results from a sleep schedule that involves daytime sleeping) interferes with biologic rhythms. Sleeping is triggered by changes in the intensity of light. When exposure to light comes at an atypical time, the sleep–wake cycle is desynchronized. Sleep–wake cycle disorders occur among shift workers, jet travelers, and those diagnosed with *seasonal affective disorder,* a cyclical mood disorder believed to be linked to diminished exposure to sunlight.

Shift Work

Those who work evenings or nights or who switch from one shift to another are especially prone to unsynchronized sleep–wake cycles. The indoor lighting to which most shift workers are exposed is not bright enough to suppress melatonin; consequently, many shift workers fight to stay awake. Some experience **microsleep** (unintentional sleep lasting 20 to 30 seconds). Statistics show that shift workers are more prone to errors and accidents due to sleepiness (Centers for Disease Control & Prevention, 1997; DeHart, 1993). Most people who work night shifts never completely adapt to the reversal of day and night activities, no matter how long the pattern is established.

Jet Travel

Jet travel causes a sudden change in the currently established **photoperiod** (number of daylight hours) to which a person is accustomed. Consequently, travelers often describe having **jet lag** (emotional and physical changes experienced when arriving in a different time zone). Many travelers have difficulty falling or staying asleep, but jet lag is more transient than shift work. Some travelers re-establish normal sleep–wake cycles, but it takes at least 1 day for each time zone that is crossed when traveling east, slightly less when traveling west.

Seasonal Affective Disorder

Seasonal affective disorder is characterized by hypersomnolence, lack of energy when awake, increased appetite accompanied by cravings for sweets, and weight gain. The symptoms begin during the darker winter months and disappear as the number of daylight hours increases in the spring. In some ways, the disorder resembles the hibernation patterns in bears and other animals.

Some suggest that seasonal affective disorder is due to excessive melatonin. To counteract the symptoms, **phototherapy** (technique for suppressing melatonin by stimulating light receptors in the eye) is prescribed. The artificial light used in phototherapy is at least 2,000 to 2,500 lux, the equivalent of the bright light measured on a sunny spring day. The lights are used for 2 to 6 hours each day to simulate the number of daylight hours during sunnier months (Display 17-3). Phototherapy usually relieves symptoms within 3 to 5 days, but symptoms tend to recur in the same amount of time if phototherapy is abruptly discontinued.

PARASOMNIAS

Parasomnias (conditions associated with activities that cause arousal or partial arousal, usually during transitions in NREM periods of sleep) are not life-threatening, but they disturb others in the household—most significantly, the bed partner. Some examples of parasomnias are:

- **Somnambulism** (sleep-walking)
- **Nocturnal enuresis** (bedwetting)
- Sleep-talking
- Nightmares and night terrors
- **Bruxism** (grinding of the teeth)
- **Restless legs syndrome** (movement typically in the legs [but occasionally in the arms or other body parts] to relieve disturbing skin sensations)

Restless legs syndrome, also known as nocturnal myoclonus, may be the most disabling parasomnia. The symptoms keep the person awake or prevent continuous sleep. Eventually, sleep deprivation affects the person's life, damaging work productivity and personal relationships. Medical etiologies, such as iron deficiency, kidney failure, and peripheral nerve pathology, can mimic the manifestations of restless legs syndrome. Once these conditions are diagnostically eliminated, the condition is confirmed with polysomnography.

Conservative treatment of the parasomnias include implementing safety measures for sleep-walkers (stair gates, security locks on doors and windows), mouth devices for bruxism, lifestyle changes, nutritional support, and good sleep hygiene. In severe cases, drug therapy is used.

DISPLAY 17-3

Components of Phototherapy

To relieve the symptoms of seasonal affective disorder, the patient:

- Initiates a schedule of full-spectrum* light exposure beginning in October–November
- Removes eyeglasses or contact lenses that have ultraviolet filters
- Sits within 3 feet of the artificial light for approximately 2 hours soon after awakening from sleep
- Glances at the light periodically but may engage in other activities such as reading or handiwork
- Repeats the exposure to light after sundown (to simulate extending the daylight hours) up to a cumulative time of 3 to 6 hours a day
- Continues the pattern of light exposure until spring

** Full-spectrum light simulates the energy of bright natural sunlight.*

Nursing Implications

After assessing patient comfort and sleep patterns and the accompanying symptoms, nurses identify one or more nursing diagnoses that require interventions:

- Fatigue
- Impaired bed mobility
- Sleep pattern disturbance
- Sleep deprivation
- Relocation stress syndrome
- Risk for injury
- Impaired gas exchange

The nursing care plan is an example of how the nursing process has been used to develop a plan of care for a patient with Sleep pattern disturbance, defined in the NANDA taxonomy (1999) as a "time-limited disruption of sleep (natural, periodic suspension of consciousness) amount and quality."

Several sleep-promoting nursing measures, such as maintaining sleep rituals, reducing the intake of stimulating chemicals, promoting daytime exercise, and adhering to a regular schedule for retiring and awakening, have already been discussed. Two additional methods that are beneficial are assisting the patient with progressive relaxation exercises and providing a back massage.

PROGRESSIVE RELAXATION

Progressive relaxation is a therapeutic exercise in which a person actively contracts and then relaxes muscle groups. The technique is used to break the worry–tension cycle that interferes with relaxation.

Nursing Guidelines For
Facilitating Progressive Relaxation

- ☑ Select a room that is quiet, private, and dimly lit.
  RATIONALE: Such a setting reduces stimulation of the arousal center in the brain, which responds to noise, bright lights, and activity.
- ☑ Encourage the patient to assume a comfortable position; this usually involves lying down or sitting.
  RATIONALE: Sitting or lying down provides external support for the body, which facilitates muscle relaxation.
- ☑ Advise the patient to avoid talking and instead listen to the suggestions that will follow.
  RATIONALE: Advising the patient to take a passive role reduces performance anxiety (worry about appearing incompetent or foolish).
- ☑ Instruct the patient to close the eyes and consciously focus on breathing.
  RATIONALE: Closing the eyes blocks visual stimuli; focusing on breathing helps turn the patient's attention away from distracting thoughts and feelings.
- ☑ Tell the patient to inhale deeply through the nose and exhale slowly out the mouth. Repeat the activity several times.
  RATIONALE: This breathing oxygenates the blood and brain and reduces the heart rate.
- ☑ Tell the patient to tighten the muscles in an area of the body, such as the foot, and hold the position for at least 5 seconds.
  RATIONALE: Tightening a muscle depletes the level of stimulating neurotransmitters.
- ☑ Direct the patient to relax the tensed muscles and focus on the pleasant feeling.
  RATIONALE: Focusing on the pleasant feeling directs the cortex's attention to the desired outcome and raises the patient's awareness.
- ☑ Proceed with sequence after sequence of muscle contraction followed by relaxation until all muscle groups in the body have been exercised.
  RATIONALE: Continued tensing and relaxation leads to higher planes of relaxation.
- ☑ Continue suggesting throughout that the patient focus on how relaxed or weightless he or she feels.
  RATIONALE: These verbal cues reinforce relaxation.
- ☑ Tell the patient that as you reach zero after counting backward from 10, he or she can begin to move.
  RATIONALE: This provides a gradual end to the relaxation period.

Patients can learn to perform progressive relaxation exercises independently using self-suggestion. Some patients eventually omit the muscle contraction phase and go directly to progressive relaxation of muscle groups.

BACK MASSAGE

Massage (stroking the skin) promotes two desired outcomes: it relaxes tense muscles and improves circulation (Skill 17-3). Massage is performed using a variety of stroking techniques (Table 17-5). Stimulating strokes are omitted if the purpose is to relax the patient.

KEY CONCEPTS

- Comfort is a state in which a person is relieved of distress. Rest is a waking state characterized by reduced activity and mental stimulation. Sleep is a state of arousable unconsciousness.
- Some environmental factors that promote comfort, rest, and sleep are colorful walls and room decor, reduced noise, increased amount of natural sunlight, and a comfortable climate.
- Standard furnishings in all patient rooms are the bed, the overbed table, the bedside stand, and at least one chair.
- Sleep is a basic human need. Among other things, it reduces fatigue, stabilizes mood, increases protein syn-

TABLE 17–5. **Massage Techniques**

Technique	Description	Method
Effleurage	To skim the surface	The hands are used to make a circular pattern using long strokes over the massaged area.
Pétrissage	To knead	The skin is lifted and compressed or pulled in opposing directions.
Frôlement	To brush	The skin is lightly touched with the fingertips.
Tapotement	To tap	The skin is lightly struck with the sides of the hands.
Vibration	To set in motion	The skin is moved rhythmically with open or cupped palms, causing the tissue to quiver.
Friction	To rub	The skin is pulled from opposite directions using the thumbs and fingers.

Nursing Care Plan: *Sleep Pattern Disturbance*

Assessment

Subjective Data

States, "I feel so tired. It seems that it takes forever to fall asleep. It's been 2 weeks since I've gotten more than 4 hours of sleep. I'm so worried I'll never go home again."

Objective Data

63-year-old woman admitted to nursing home for intermediate care after repair of a fractured hip. Yawns frequently, naps rather than participating in activities. Asks for and receives barbiturate hypnotic each night, which is often repeated several hours later.

Diagnosis

Sleep pattern disturbance related to excessive stimulating neurochemicals secondary to anxiety over rehabilitation

Plan

Goal

The patient will begin sleeping within 30 minutes of going to bed and remain asleep for a minimum of 6 hours within 10 days (by 3/15).

Orders: 3/5

1. Awaken patient at 0730, her usual time for rising.
2. Substitute decaffeinated coffee or tea at meals and offer an alternative for food items containing chocolate.
3. Discourage daytime napping for the next 5 days.
4. Supervise ambulation with a walker for at least 20 minutes three times a day, the last being no later than 1930.
5. Provide yogurt, vanilla pudding, custard, or some other dairy product at approximately 2200.
6. Let patient stay up until 2330, her usual bedtime.
7. Hold sleeping medication and give a back massage instead.

J. HALEY, RN

Implementation (Documentation)

3/5 1800–2300 Served decaffeinated coffee with supper. Peanut butter cookies substituted for chocolate brownie. At 1900, walked the length of the hall three times, which took 25 minutes. Ate a dish of vanilla ice cream at 2200. Assisted with hygiene and changing into gown and bathrobe. Watching television in room. — P. ROGERS, LPN

Evaluation (Documentation)

3/5 2330 Assisted to bed. — C. VARGAS, LPN

3/6 0000 Observed to be sleeping. — C. VARGAS, LPN

thesis, promotes cellular growth and repair, and improves the capacity for learning and memory storage.

- There are two phases of sleep: nonrapid and rapid eye movement sleep. During nonrapid eye movement (NREM) sleep and its four subdivisions, the body is active, but the brain is not. During rapid eye movement (REM) sleep, the body is physically inactive, but the brain is highly active.
- As humans age, they sleep fewer hours and spend less time in REM sleep. Newborns spend 16 to 20 hours of each day sleeping, approximately half in the REM phase. Older adults require 7 to 9 hours of sleep and spend only 13% to 15% in the REM phase.
- The amount and quality of sleep can be affected by circadian rhythms, activity, the environment, motivation, emotions and moods, food and beverages, illness, and drugs.
- There are four major categories of drugs that either promote or interfere with sleep. Sedatives and tranquilizers produce a relaxing and calming effect, hypnotics induce sleep, and stimulants excite structures in the brain, causing wakefulness.
- Sleep questionnaires, sleep diaries, polysomnographic evaluations, and the multiple sleep latency test are techniques used to assess sleep patterns.
- Sleep disorders fall into four major categories: insomnia (difficulty falling asleep or staying asleep, or early-

FOCUS ON OLDER ADULTS

- Older adults who move to an institutional setting, such as a nursing home or assisted living facility, are usually more comfortable with their own bed furnishings and personal mementos and belongings.
- Older adults tend to prefer warmer temperatures.
- Older adults with cognitive impairments may feel that environmental temperatures are uncomfortably warm or cool, even when the temperature is comfortable for others.
- Insomnia and hypersomnia are often manifestations of depression among older adults.
- Because of age-related changes, older adults have more difficulty falling asleep, awaken more readily, and spend less time in the deeper stages (including the dream stage) of sleep. As a consequence, older adults often feel tired, complain of sleep problems, and spend more time in bed without actually sleeping.
- Using night lights rather than bright room lights is preferred if an older adult arises during the night. Bright lights stimulate the brain and interfere with efforts to resume sleep.
- The National Institutes of Health (1990) recommends that sleep disorders in older adults be managed without hypnotic medications.
- Some older adults who are cognitively impaired develop **sundown syndrome** (onset of disorientation as the sun sets) (Display 17-4). Others develop **sunrise syndrome** (early-morning confusion), which is associated with inadequate sleep or the effects of sedative and hypnotic medications.
- Family members, especially spouses, may experience sleep disturbances if an older adult snores, gets up during the night, or wanders.
- It is important to identify potential sources of sleep disturbances among older adults such as discomfort, emotional or medical conditions, uncomfortable environment, and the effects of caffeine, alcohol, or medications (see Table 17-4).
- Chronic conditions may interfere with sleep by causing pain, difficulty breathing, or frequent urination. Interventions to control these condition help to improve sleep.
- Hypnotic agents tend to have paradoxical effects in older adults—that is, they have a stimulating effect or cause mental changes.
- Because hypnotic medications reduce the amount of REM sleep, older adults are likely to have nightmares and other sleep cycle disturbances for several weeks after hypnotics are discontinued.
- Although hypnotic medications are effective initially, tolerance usually develops, sometimes within a few days.
- Many hypnotic medications, particularly those that have a very long half-life such as flurazepam (Dalmane), tend to cause daytime drowsiness. Examples of hypnotics with shorter half-lives that are better tolerated by older adults include triazolam (Halcion), temazepam (Restoril), and zolpidem (Ambien).
- Older adults with limited mobility may sleep better if they participate in chair or water exercises during the day.
- Older adults are encouraged to use any of the following relaxation techniques before bedtime: imagery, meditation, deep breathing, progressive relaxation, soothing music, body or foot massage, chair rocking, reading nonstimulating materials, or watching nonstimulating television.
- Short daytime naps and rest periods, usually less than 2 hours in duration, can restore energy for an older adult without interfering with nighttime sleep.

morning awakening), hypersomnias (conditions resulting in daytime sleepiness despite adequate nighttime sleep), sleep–wake cycle disturbances (resulting from desynchronized periods of sleeping and wakefulness), and parasomnias (associated with activities that cause arousal or partial arousal, usually during transitions in NREM periods of sleep).

- Sleep is promoted by exercising regularly during the day; avoiding alcohol, nicotine, and caffeine; performing sleep rituals; going to bed and getting up at about the same time every day; and getting out of bed if sleep does not come easily and returning after some nonstimulating activity.
- To promote relaxation, which facilitates the onset of sleep, nurses assist patients with progressive relaxation exercises or provide a back massage.
- Older adults tend to have. more difficulty falling asleep, they awaken more readily, and they spend less time in the deeper stages of sleep. This explains why some older adults feel tired even though they have slept an appropriate length of time.

DISPLAY 17–4

Characteristics of Sundown Syndrome

- Alert and oriented during the day
- Onset of disorientation as the sun sets
- Disorganized thinking
- Restlessness
- Agitation
- Perseveration (ruminating over the same repetitive thought)
- Wandering about

CRITICAL THINKING EXERCISES

- List features in the exterior and interior environment of an agency where you have clinical experience that attract or detract from its image as a place for comfort and rest.
- If you were a patient, what items in the health care environment would you find important in supporting your comfort, rest, and sleep?
- Discuss possible effects of suffering from a sleep disorder or living with a person who has a sleep disorder.
- Develop a sleep assessment tool that incorporates questions to identify all four categories of sleep disorders.

SUGGESTED READINGS

American Psychiatric Association. Statistical manual of mental disorders, 4th ed. Washington DC, APA, 1994.

Ball MC, Hanger HC, Thwaites JH. Bed rails: a barrier to independence? Clinical Rehabilitation 1997;11(4):347–349.

Bangura K. Dying for a snooze: sleep deprivation. Nursing Times 1998; 94(21):28–30.

Capezuti E, Talerico KA, Strumpf N, et al. Individualized assessment and intervention in bilateral siderail use. Geriatric Nursing: American Journal of Care for the Aging 1998;19(6):322–330.

Clark PE, Clark MJ. Therapeutic touch: is there a scientific basis for practice? American Journal of Nursing 1995;95(7):17.

Cender D, Gelhot A, Phillips B, et al. Daytime drowsiness: is a drug to blame? Journal of Respiratory Diseases 1998;19(8):617–629.

Centers for Disease Control & Prevention, National Institute for Occupational Safety and Health. Plain language about shift work. USDHHS, 1997.

Czeisler CA, Johnson MP, Duffy JF, Brown EN, Ronda JM, Kronauer RE. Exposure to bright light and darkness to treat physiologic maladaptation to night work. New England Journal of Medicine May 3, 1990:1253–1307.

Dantzker DR, Steinberg H. Pulmonary and critical care medicine. Journal of the American Medical Association 1994(271):1709–1710.

DeHart RL. Limits and fatigue. Journal of the American Medical Association November 10, 1993:2230.

Erwin J. Staying alert: how shift work affects nurses' health. NurseWeek (California statewide edition) 1998;11(23):13

Frasca-Beaulieu K. Interior design for ambulatory care facilities: how to reduce stress and anxiety in patients and families. Journal of Ambulatory Care Management 1999;2(1):67–73.

Geyer N. The need for comfort, rest and sleep. Nursing News 1998;22(4): 56–58.

Geyer N. Facilitating comfort, rest and sleep. Nursing News 1998;22(7):10–11.

Hallock D. Interpreting symptoms: obstructing sleep apnea. American Journal of Nursing 1998;98(7):22.

Hawley K, Cates M. Paws for comfort. Nursing 1998;28(2):57.

Hope KW. The effects of multisensory environments on older people with dementia. Journal of Psychiatric and Mental Health Nursing 1998;5(5): 377–385.

James M, Tremea MO, Jones JS, et al. Can melatonin improve adaptation to night shift? American Journal of Emergency Medicine 1998;16(4): 367–370.

Kelly M. Omnibus Budget Reconciliation Act of 1987; a policy analysis. Nursing Clinics of North America 1989;24(3):791–794.

Legal questions. Sundown syndrome: showing no restraint. Nursing 1998; 25(9):66.

Lempkin P. Sleep disorders: home sleep studies provide new options. Caring 1996;15(9):68–72.

MacLeod V, Shneerson J. Narcolepsy: nursing the sleeping sickness. Nursing Times 1998;94(22):48–50.

Mantle F. Sleepless and unsettled: alternative therapies. Nursing Times 1996; 92(23):46–47.

Meehan TC. Therapeutic touch as a nursing intervention. Journal of Advanced Nursing 1998;28(1):117–125.

NANDA nursing diagnoses: definitions and classification, 1999–2000. Philadelphia, NANDA, 1999.

National Institutes of Health Consensus Development Conference: Treatment of sleep disorders in older people. NIH consensus statement, 1990.

National Sleep Foundation. The nature of sleep and its disorders. Los Angeles, 1994.

Nelson EA. Mattresses: the patient's view. Professional Nurse 1997; 13(1):5.

Oldham JM. The Columbia University College of Physicians & Surgeons complete home medical guide, 3rd ed. Victoria, British Columbia, Crown Publishers, 1995.

Omnibus Budget Reconciliation Act of 1987: Conference report to accompany HR 3545. Washington DC, U.S. Government Printing Office, 1987.

Pagel JF, Zafralotfi S, Zammit G. How to prescribe a good night's sleep. Patient Care 1997;31(4):87–102.

Patient care: the right bed can help your patient. RN 1998;61(1):16C–16D.

Pope DS. Music, noise, and the human voice in the nurse–patient environment. Image: The Journal of Nursing Scholarship 1995;27(4): 291–295.

Rogers A, Caruso C, Aldrich M. Reliability of sleep diaries for assessment of sleep/wake patterns. Nursing Research 1993;42(6):368–371.

Rosenthal NE, Sack DA, Gillin C, et al. Seasonal affective disorder. Archives of General Psychiatry 1984(41):72–80.

Routasalo P. Non-necessary touch in the nursing care of elderly people. Journal of Advanced Nursing 1996;23:904–911.

Sleep and aging. http://www. sleep foundation.org/publications/sleepage.html.

Smith DA. Sleep disorders in the elderly. Annals of Long-Term Care 1998;6(6):36–42.

Tetlow S. Bed and mattress choice. Community Nurse 1997;3(8):31–32.

SKILL 17–1

MAKING AN UNOCCUPIED BED

Suggested Action	Reason for Action
Assessment	
Check the Kardex or nursing care plan to determine the patient's activity level.	Determines whether the patient can be out of bed during bedmaking
Inspect the linen for moisture or evidence of soiling.	Indicates what and how much of the linen must be changed
Planning	
Plan to change the linen after the patient's hygiene needs have been met.	Reduces the potential for getting the clean linen wet or soiled
Wash your hands; use gloves if there is a potential for direct contact with blood, stool, or other body fluids.	Reduces the transmission of microorganisms
Bring necessary bed linen to the room.	Demonstrates organization and efficient time management
Place the clean linen on a clean, dry surface such as the back of a chair (see Fig. A).	Reduces transmission of microorganisms to clean supplies
Assist the patient from the bed.	Facilitates bedmaking
Implementation	
Raise the bed to a high position and lower siderails.	Prevents postural and muscular strain
Remove equipment attached to the bed linens, such as the signal cord and drainage tubes, and check for personal items.	Avoids breakage, spills, or loss of personal items
Loosen the bed linen from where it has been tucked under the mattress.	Facilitates removal or retightening
Fold any linen that may be reused and place it on a clean surface.	Promotes efficiency and orderliness
Roll linen that will be replaced so that the soiled surface is enclosed (see Fig. B).	Reduces contact with sources of microorganisms

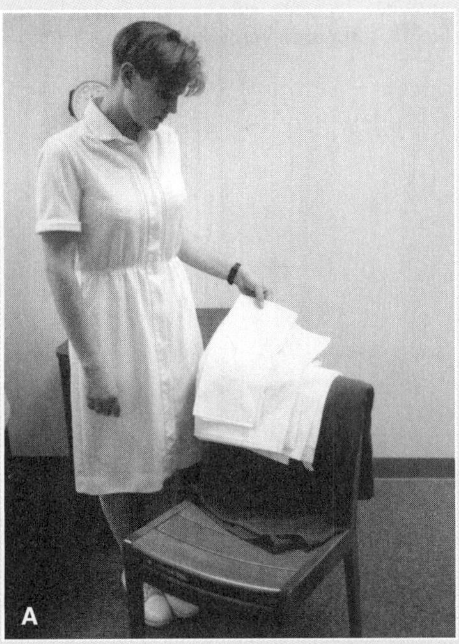

Arranging clean bed linen. (Courtesy of Ken Timby.)

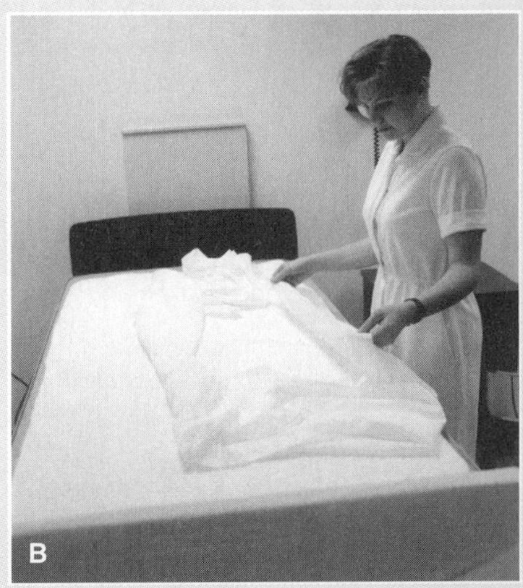

Enclosing soiled side of linen. (Courtesy of Ken Timby.)

continued

MAKING AN UNOCCUPIED BED *Continued*

Suggested Action	Reason for Action
Remove the soiled linen while holding it away from your uniform (see Fig. C).	Prevents transferring microorganisms to your uniform and then to other patients
Place the soiled linen directly into a pillow case, laundry hamper, or self-made pouch from one of the removed sheets (see Fig. D). *Do not place the soiled linen on the floor.*	Keeps the soiled linen from being further contaminated
Remove gloves and wash your hands once contact with body secretions is no longer likely.	Facilitates use of the hands

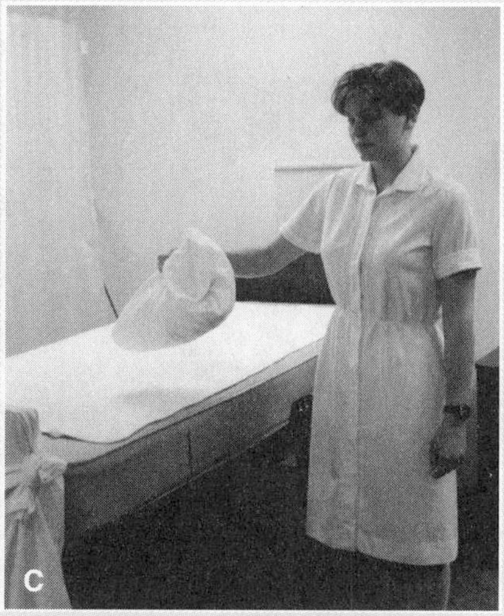

Avoiding contact with uniform. (Courtesy of Ken Timby.)

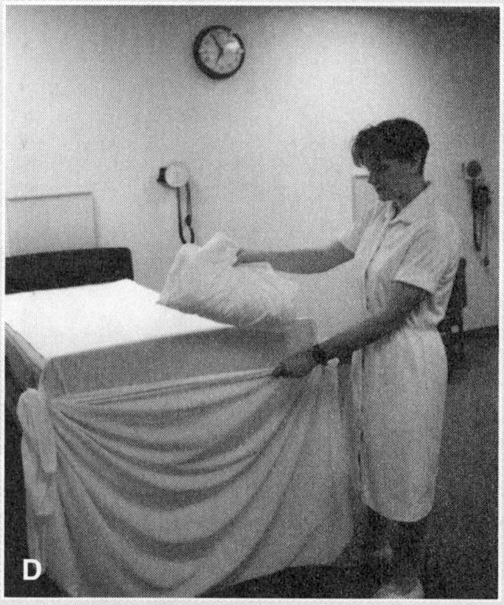

Placing soiled linen in temporary hamper. (Courtesy of Ken Timby.)

Suggested Action	Reason for Action
Reposition the mattress so it is flush with the headboard.	Provides maximum foot room
Tighten any linen that will be reused.	Removes wrinkles, which promotes patient comfort
If the bottom sheet needs changing, center the longitudinal fold and open the layers of folded linen to one side of the bed (see Fig. E).	Reduces postural strain
If using a flat sheet, make sure the flat edge of the hem is flush with the edge of the mattress at the foot end (see Fig. F).	Prevents skin pressure and irritation

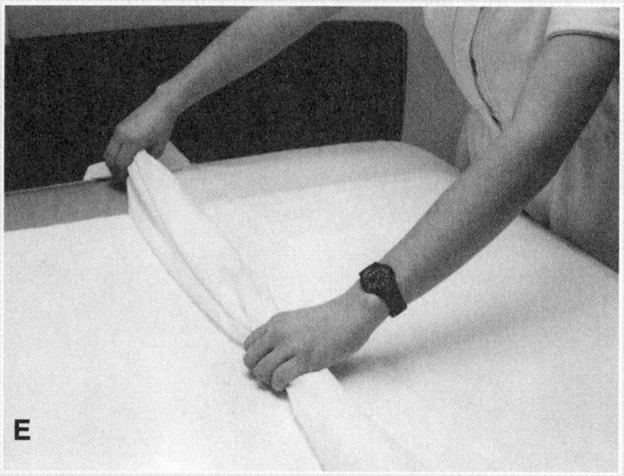

Centering the linen. (Courtesy of Ken Timby).

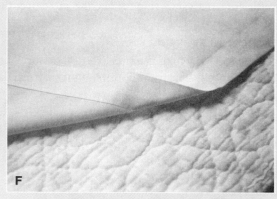

Positioning the hem. (Courtesy of Ken Timby).

continued

SKILL 17–1

MAKING AN UNOCCUPIED BED *Continued*

Suggested Action	Reason for Action
Tuck the upper portion of the sheet under the mattress, or if a fitted sheet is used, position the upper and lower corners of the mattress within the contoured corners of the sheet.	Anchors the bottom sheet
Make a mitered or square corner at the top of the bed if a flat sheet is used (see Fig. G).	Secures the bottom sheet

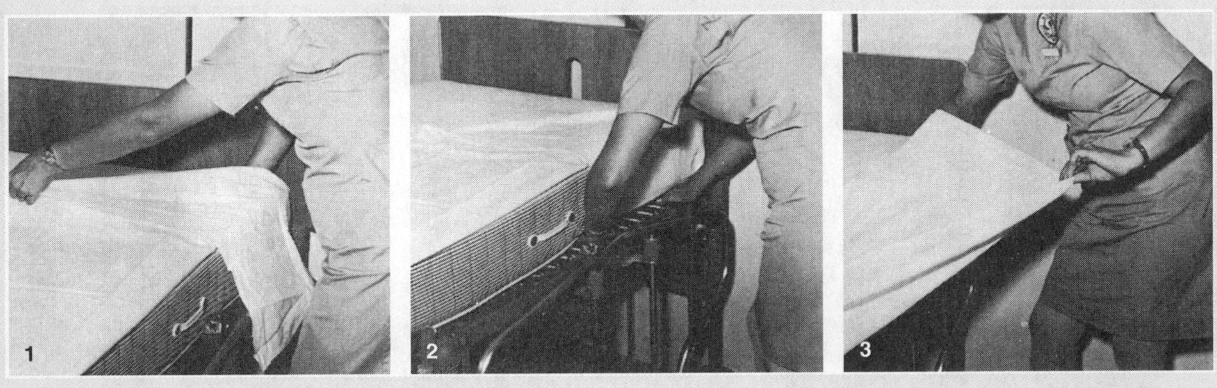

G 1 2 3

(*1*) Fold the edge of the sheet back on itself, forming a triangle; (*2*) tuck the edge hanging from the bed under the mattress; and (*3*) follow by tucking the remaining sheet under the mattress, preserving the mitered triangle at the corner.

Suggested Action	Reason for Action
If the patient is apt to soil the linen with urine or stool, fold a flat sheet horizontally with the smooth edge of the hem toward the foot of the bed, and tuck it in place approximately where the buttocks will be located. Do the same if a draw sheet is available.	Reduces the need to change all of the bottom linen
Position the top linen on one half of the bed at this time, or wait until all of the bottom linen has been secured.	Saves time by reducing the number of moves about the bed
Move to the other side of the bed, pull the linen taut, and tuck the free edges beneath the mattress (see Fig. H).	Secures the bottom linen
Center the top sheet and unfold it to one side, leaving sufficient length at the top for making a fold over the spread.	Provides a smooth edge next to the patient's neck
Add blankets if the patient wishes.	Demonstrates concern for the patient's comfort
Make a toe pleat by folding a small vertical or horizontal envelope of sheet near the bottom of the mattress (see Fig. I).	Keeps pressure off toes

continued

SKILL 17–1

MAKING AN UNOCCUPIED BED *Continued*

Suggested Action	Reason for Action
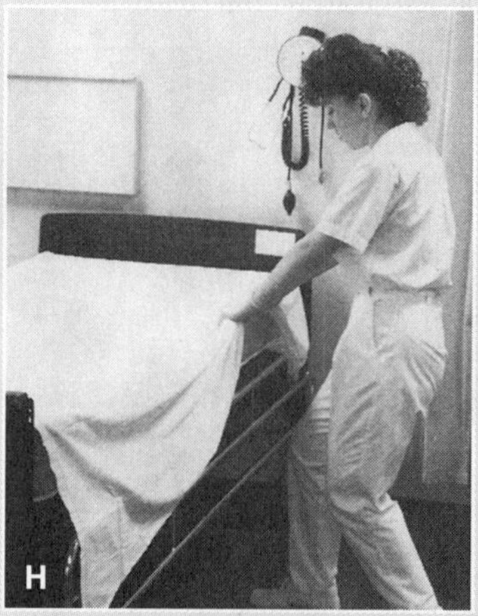 **Pulling the bottom sheet taut. (Courtesy of Ken Timby.)**	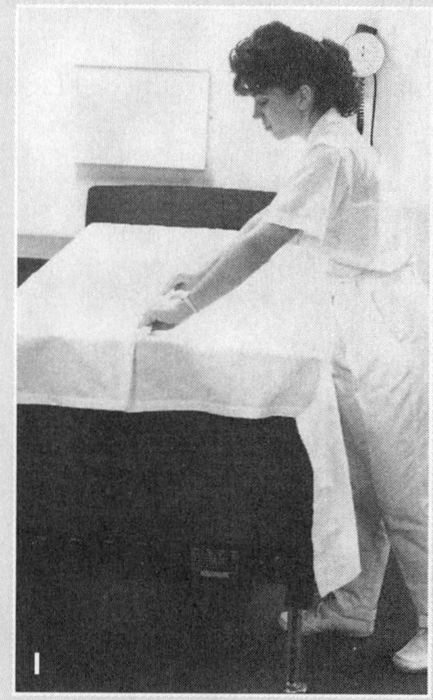 **Making a toe pleat. (Courtesy of Ken Timby.)**
Cover the top sheet with the spread, tuck the excess linen under the bottom of the mattress, and finish with a mitered or square corner.	Secures the top linen
Gather the pillow case as you would hosiery, and slip the case over the pillow (see Fig. J).	Prevents contact between the pillow and your uniform
Place the pillow at the head of the bed with the open end away from the door and the seam of the pillowcase toward the headboard.	Presents a tidy view of the room from the hallway; prevents pressure on the skin around the head and neck

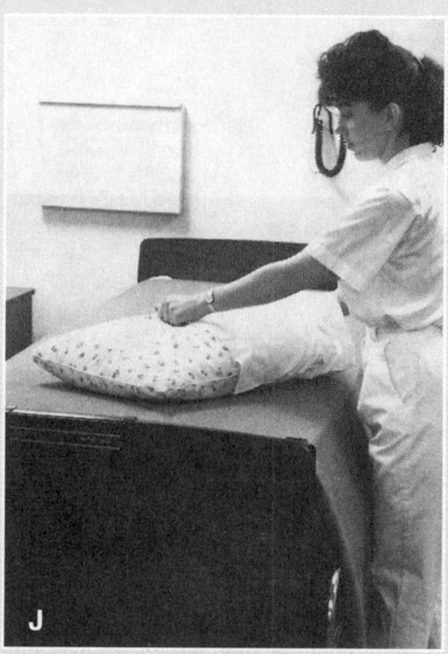

Covering the pillow. (Courtesy of Ken Timby.)

continued

SKILL 17–1

MAKING AN UNOCCUPIED BED *Continued*

Suggested Action	Reason for Action
Fan-fold or pie-fold the top linen toward the foot of the bed (see Fig. K).	Facilitates returning to bed
Secure the signal device on or to the bed (see Fig. L).	Ensures that the patient can receive nursing assistance
Adjust the bed to a low position.	Enables the patient to return to bed
Wash your hands.	Reduces the transmission of microorganisms

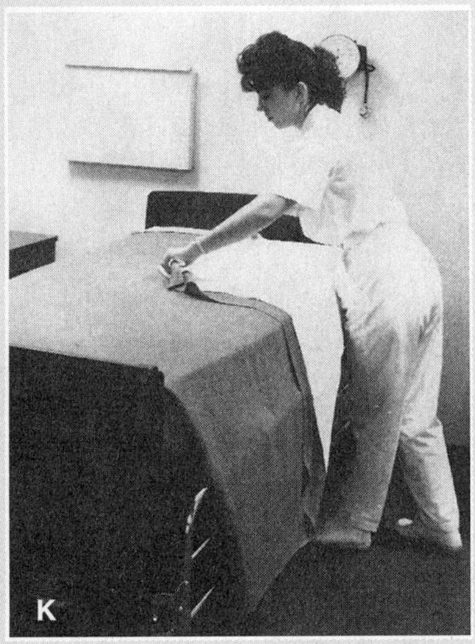

Pie-folding the linen. (Courtesy of Ken Timby.)

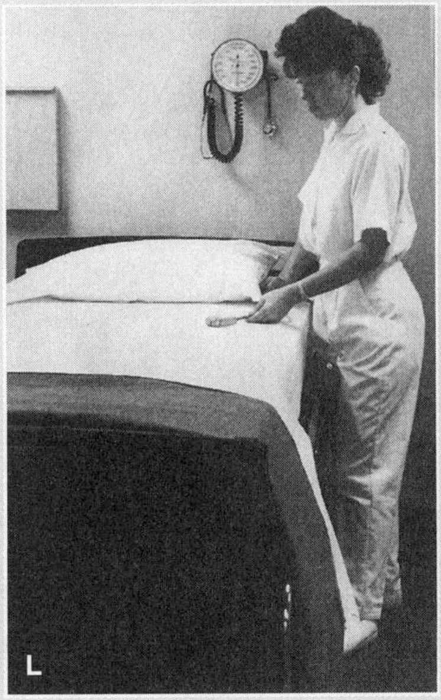

Attaching the signal cord. (Courtesy of Ken Timby.)

Evaluation

- The bed is clean and dry.
- The linen is free of wrinkles.
- The environment is orderly.
- The patient feels comfortable.

Document

- Date and time
- Characteristics of drainage if present
- Any unique measures taken to ensure patient comfort

SAMPLE DOCUMENTATION

Date and Time Menses established. Bed linen changed while shower taken. Given a supply of sanitary napkins. Absorbent pad placed over bottom sheet.

_______________________________ SIGNATURE/TITLE

CRITICAL THINKING

- List situations when it would be appropriate to change some of the linen when providing patient care and those when it is more appropriate to change all the bed linen.
- Discuss expected outcomes that result from having clean, fresh linen on the bed.

SKILL 17-2

MAKING AN OCCUPIED BED

Suggested Action	Reason for Action
Assessment	
Check the Kardex or nursing care plan to confirm that the patient must remain in bed.	Demonstrates compliance with the care plan
Assess the patient's level of consciousness, physical strength, breathing pattern, heart rate, and blood pressure.	Indicates a need for bedrest if abnormal findings are noted, whether it has been prescribed or not
Inspect the linen for moisture or evidence of soiling.	Indicates what and how much of the linen must be changed
Determine who might be available to assist if the patient is too weak or unable to cooperate.	Avoids postural or muscular injury and ensures the comfort and safety of the patient
Planning	
Plan to change the linen after the patient's hygiene needs have been met.	Reduces the potential for getting the clean linen wet or soiled
Wash your hands; use gloves if there is a potential for direct contact with blood, stool, or other body fluids.	Reduces the transmission of microorganisms
Bring necessary bed linen to the room.	Demonstrates organization and efficient time management
Place the clean linen on a clean, dry surface such as the back of a chair.	Reduces transmission of microorganisms to clean supplies
Implementation	
Explain what you plan to do.	Informs the patient and promotes cooperation
Raise the bed to a high position.	Prevents postural and muscular strain
Cover the patient with a bath blanket or leave the top sheet loosened but in place.	Maintains warmth and demonstrates respect for modesty
Fold the top sheet or spread if it will be reused and place it on a clean surface.	Promotes efficiency and orderliness
Unfasten equipment attached to the bottom linen and check for personal items.	Avoids breakage, spills, or loss of personal items
Loosen the bed linen from where it has been tucked under the mattress.	Facilitates removal or retightening
Lower the rail on the side of the bed where you are standing and roll the patient toward the opposite side rail.	Provides room for making the bed while ensuring the safety of the patient
Roll the soiled bottom sheets as close to the patient as possible.	Facilitates removal
Proceed to unfold and tuck the bottom sheet and drawsheet on the vacant side of the bed, as described in Skill 17-1.	Remakes half of the bed with clean linen
Fold the free edges of the sheet under the folded portion of the soiled sheets.	Keeps the clean sheet from becoming soiled; facilitates pulling the sheets from under the patient
Raise the siderail and move to the opposite side of the bed.	Prevents postural and muscular strain
Lower the siderail in your new position and help the patient roll over the mound of sheets.	Helps reposition the patient on the clean side of the bed

continued

SKILL 17-2

MAKING AN OCCUPIED BED *Continued*

Suggested Action	Reason for Action
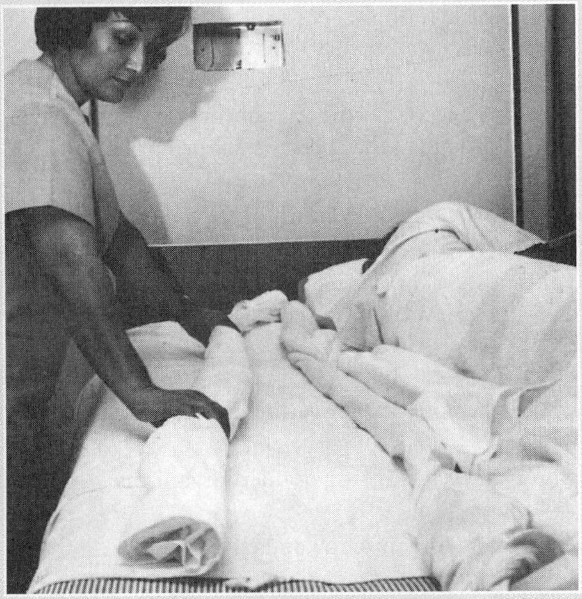 Changing linen on half of the bed.	
Pull the soiled laundry close to the edge of the bed and the clean linen close beside it.	Reduces the mound of linen in the center of the bed
Remove the soiled linen and place it into a pillow case or pouch that is off the floor.	Keeps the soiled linen from becoming further contaminated
Pull the clean bottom sheet until it is unfolded from beneath the patient.	Promotes patient comfort
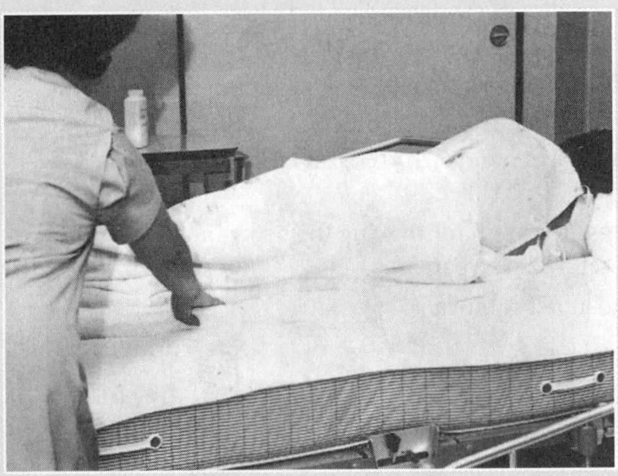 Pulling clean linen through.	
Miter or square the upper corner of the sheet; pull and tuck the free edges under the mattress.	Secures the clean sheets
Assist the patient to the middle of the bed.	Ensures comfort and safety

continued

SKILL 17–2

MAKING AN OCCUPIED BED *Continued*

Suggested Action	Reason for Action
Straighten or replace the top sheet, blankets, and spread; remove and replace the pillowcase if necessary.	Restores comfort and orderliness to the environment
Reposition the patient according to the therapeutic regimen or comfort.	Demonstrates compliance with the care plan; shows concern for patient comfort
Lower the height of the bed and raise the remaining siderail if appropriate.	Reduces the potential for injury
Dispose of the soiled linen in a laundry hamper outside the room.	Restores order to the room and ensures that the linen will be collected for laundering
Wash your hands.	Reduces the transmission of microorganisms

Evaluation

- The bed is clean and dry.
- The linen is free of wrinkles.
- The environment is orderly.
- The patient feels comfortable.

Document

- Date and time
- Characteristics of drainage if present
- Measures taken to ensure patient comfort.

SAMPLE DOCUMENTATION

Date and Time Unresponsive even to painful stimuli. Complete bed bath given followed by linen change. Repositioned on L side with head at a 45° elevation. Full siderails raised. Bed in low position. ________________ SIGNATURE/TITLE

CRITICAL THINKING

- What observations would you make to determine the bedmaking competency performed by unlicensed assistive personnel?
- Discuss the actions you would take if while making an occupied bed, the patient became short of breath, nauseated, or uncomfortable.
- Explain how you might alter the application or type of bed linen if your patient tended to chill easily, perspired profusely, or had difficulty changing positions.

SKILL 17-3

GIVING A BACK MASSAGE

Suggested Action	Reason for Action
Assessment	
Observe whether the patient is still awake 30 minutes after retiring for sleep.	Indicates a delay in the usual onset of sleep
Determine whether the patient is experiencing pain, has a need for bladder or bowel elimination, is hungry, is too warm or cold, or has any other physical or environmental problem that may be easily overcome.	Eliminates all but psychophysiologic etiologies as the cause for sleeplessness
Check the patient's medical record to determine whether there are any conditions for which a backrub would be contraindicated, such as fractured ribs or a back injury.	Demonstrates concern for the safety and comfort of the patient
Ask the patient if he or she would like a back massage.	Allows the patient an opportunity to participate in decision making
Planning	
Obtain lotion or an alternative substance such as alcohol or powder if the patient's skin is oily.	Demonstrates organization and efficient time management
Use gloves if there are any open, draining lesions on the skin.	Provides a barrier against bloodborne microorganisms
Reduce environmental stimuli, such as bright lights and loud noise.	Decreases stimulation of the wake center in the brain
Implementation	
Pull the privacy curtain around the patient's bed.	Demonstrates respect for modesty
Raise the bed to an appropriate height to avoid bending at the waist.	Reduces back strain
Wash your hands; don gloves if appropriate.	Reduces the spread of microorganisms
Help the patient lie on his or her abdomen or side, and untie the hospital gown or remove it completely.	Provides access to the back
Instruct the patient to breathe slowly and deeply in and out through an open mouth.	Promotes ventilation and relaxation
Squirt a generous amount of lotion into your hands and rub them together.	Warms the lotion
Place the entire surface of the hands on either side of the lower spine and move them upward over the shoulders and back again using long, continuous strokes. Repeat the stroke pattern several times.	Uses *effleurage* to promote relaxation
Apply firmer pressure with the upstroke and lighter pressure during the downstroke.	Enhances relaxation by alternating pressure and rhythm
Make smaller circular strokes up and down the length of the back with the thumbs.	Uses *friction* to improve blood flow and remove chemicals that accumulate in contracted muscles

continued

SKILL 17–3

GIVING A BACK MASSAGE *Continued*

Suggested Action	Reason for Action
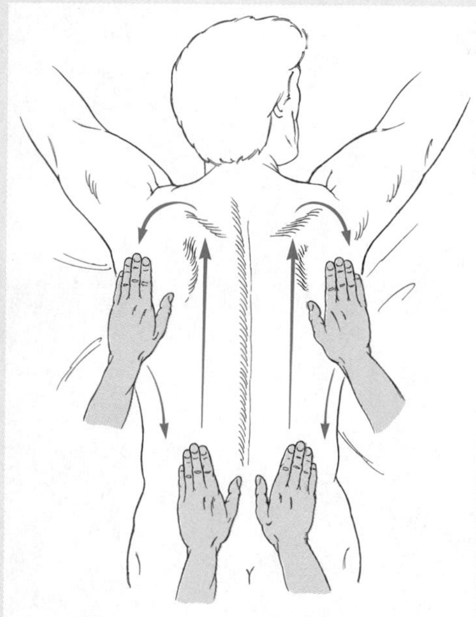 Effleurage.	
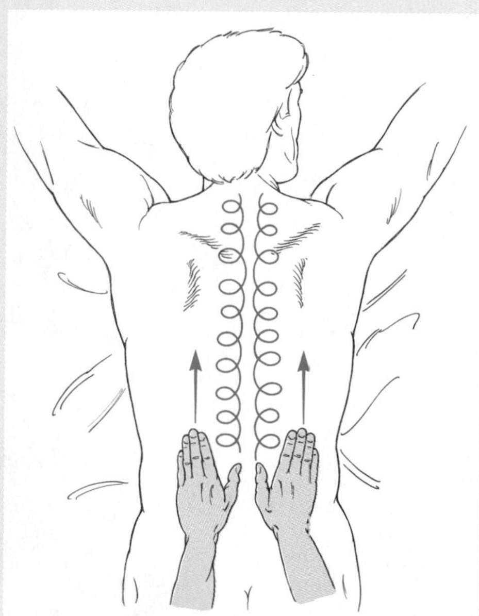 Friction.	
Lift and gently compress tissue with the fingers, starting at the base of the spine and ending at the neck and shoulder areas.	Utilizes *pétrissage* to increase blood circulation
Pull the skin in opposite directions in a kneading fashion to lift and stretch the skin from the base of the spine to the shoulder areas.	Uses another pétrissage technique to reduce the tension in muscles and improve circulation

continued

SKILL 17-3

GIVING A BACK MASSAGE *Continued*

Suggested Action	Reason for Action

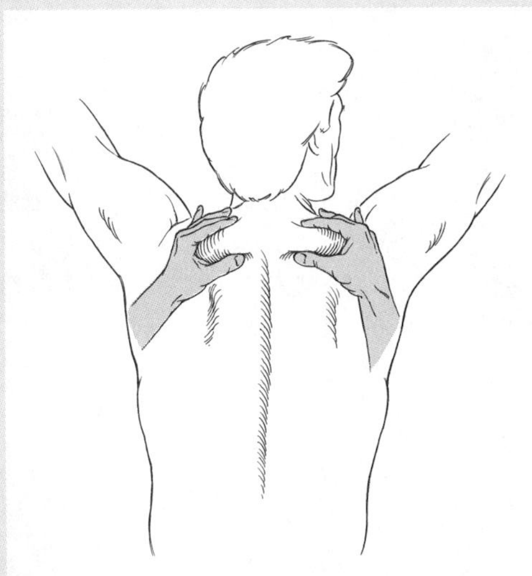

Pétrissage.

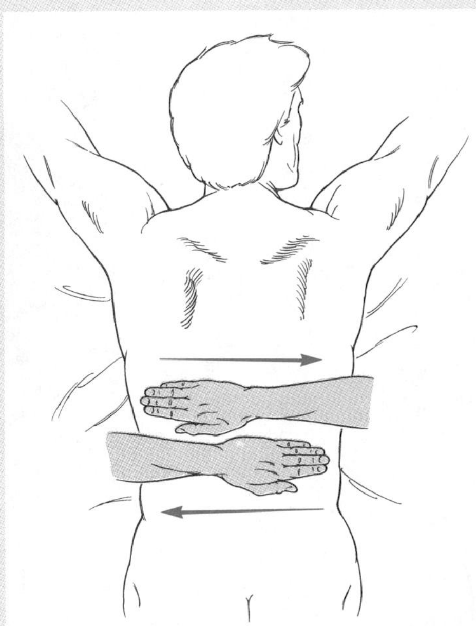

Kneading.

End the backrub by lightly stroking the length of the back, gradually lightening the pressure as the fingers are move downward.	Uses *frôlement* to prolong the sensation of relaxation
Lightly cover the patient and lower the bed.	Extends the period of relaxation by reducing activity and may induce NREM sleep

continued

SKILL 17-3

GIVING A BACK MASSAGE *Continued*

Suggested Action	Reason for Action

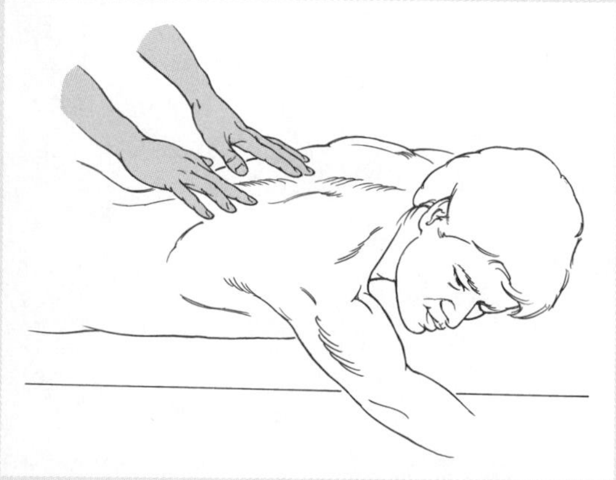

Frôlement.

Evaluation

- Patient feels relaxed.
- Sleep is promoted.

Document

- Date and time of back massage
- Response of patient

SAMPLE DOCUMENTATION

Date and Time Unable to sleep. Assisted to bathroom to void. Light snack of graham crackers and milk provided. Back massaged for 10 minutes. Observed to be sleeping 20 minutes later. ______________ SIGNATURE/TITLE

CRITICAL THINKING

- Describe techniques for maximizing the positive effects of a back massage.
- Discuss as many techniques as possible that could be used to evaluate whether a back massage achieved its purpose.
- List situations in which a back massage could be a therapeutic nursing intervention and the rationale for implementing it.

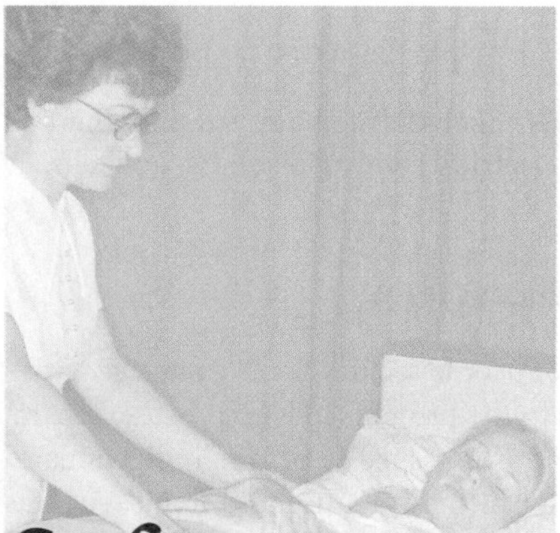

Safety

CHAPTER 18

CHAPTER OUTLINE

Age-Related Safety Factors
Environmental Hazards
Restraints
Nursing Implications

NURSING GUIDELINES

USING A FIRE EXTINGUISHER

SKILLS

SKILL 18-1: USING PHYSICAL RESTRAINTS

NURSING CARE PLAN

RISK FOR INJURY

KEY TERMS

asphyxiation	macroshock
drowning	microshock
electrical shock	poisoning
environmental hazards	restraint alternatives
fire plan	restraints
latex sensitivity	safety
latex-safe environment	thermal burn

LEARNING OBJECTIVES

An understanding of the content within this chapter will be evidenced by the student's ability to:

- Give an example of one common injury that predominates at each stage of development, from infancy through older adulthood.
- Name six injuries that are due to environmental hazards.
- Identify at least two methods for reducing latex sensitization.
- List four areas of responsibility that are incorporated into most fire plans.
- Describe the indications for using each class of fire extinguishers.
- Discuss five measures for preventing burns.
- Name three common causes of asphyxiation.
- Discuss two methods for preventing drowning.
- Explain why humans are susceptible to electrical shock.
- Discuss three methods for preventing electrical shock.
- Name at least six common substances associated with poisonings.
- Discuss four methods for preventing poisonings.
- Discuss the benefits and risks of using physical restraints.
- Explain the basis for enacting restraint legislation and JCAHO accreditation standards.
- Differentiate between a restraint and a restraint alternative.
- Give at least four criteria for applying a physical restraint.
- Describe two areas of concern when an accident happens.
- Explain why older adults are prone to falling.

S**afety** (measures that prevent accidents or unintentional injuries) is a major nursing responsibility. This chapter deals with factors that place people at risk for injury, environmental hazards in the home and health care agency, and nursing measures that keep patients safe.

Age-Related Safety Factors

No age group is immune to accidental injury, but there are distinct differences among age groups because of their varying levels of cognitive function and judgment, activity and mobility, degree of supervision, and the design and safety devices in physical surroundings.

INFANTS AND TODDLERS

Infants rely on the safety consciousness of their adult caretakers. They are especially vulnerable to injuries resulting from falling off changing tables or being unrestrained in automobiles. Toddlers are naturally inquisitive, more mobile than infants, and fail to understand the danger of climbing. Consequently, they are often the victims of accidental poisoning, falls from high chairs or down stairs, burns, electrocution from exploring outlets or manipulating electric cords, and drowning in swimming pools.

SCHOOL-AGED CHILDREN AND ADOLESCENTS

School-aged children are physically active, which makes them prone to play-related injuries. Many adolescents suffer sports-related injuries because they participate in physically challenging activities—sometimes without adequate protective equipment—before their musculoskeletal systems can withstand the stress. Adolescents also tend to be impulsive and take risks as a result of peer pressure.

ADULTS

Adults are at risk for injuries from ignoring safety issues, fatigue, sensory changes, and the effects of disease. The types of injuries suffered by young, middle-aged, and older adults depend on their social, developmental, and physical differences (Table 18-1).

Environmental Hazards

Examples of **environmental hazards** (potentially dangerous conditions in the physical surroundings) in the home and health care environment include latex sensitization, thermal burns, asphyxiation, electrical shock, poisoning, and falls.

LATEX SENSITIZATION

Increasing numbers of people are developing **latex sensitivity** (allergic response to the proteins in latex). Latex, natural rubber sap whose origin is a species of tree indigenous to Brazil, is a component of many household items, such as balloons, envelope glue, erasers, and carpet backing, as well as health care products. The widespread use of precautions to prevent bloodborne infections, such as AIDS and hepatitis B and C, has contributed to a rise in the number of latex-sensitive people. This is due, in part, to repeated exposure to latex in medical gloves and other equipment (Display 18-1). Patients who are predisposed include those with a history of asthma and allergies to other substances, multiple surgeries, and recurring medical procedures.

Types of Latex Reactions

Sensitization follows latex exposure via the skin, mucous membranes, inhalation, ingestion, injection, or wound management. The two forms of allergic reactions to latex or the chemicals used in its manufacture are:

- Contact dermatitis, a delayed localized skin reaction that occurs within 6 to 48 hours and lasts several days

TABLE 18–1. **Age-Related Factors Affecting Adult Safety**

Adult Group	Contributing Factors	Common Types of Injuries
Young adults	Alcohol and drug abuse Emancipation from parental supervision Naiveté about workplace hazards	Motor-vehicle accidents Boating accidents Head and spinal cord injury Eye injuries, chemical burns, traumatic amputations, soft tissue and back injuries
Middle-aged adults	Failure to use safety devices Overexertion and fatigue Disregard for use of seat belts and car safety harnesses Lack of expertise in performing home maintenance or repairs	Physical trauma (see above) Burns and asphyxiation related to nonfunctioning smoke, heat, and carbon monoxide detectors
Older adults	Visual impairment Urinary urgency Postural hypotension Reduced coordination Impaired mobility Inadequate home maintenance Mental confusion Impaired temperature regulation	Falls Poisoning /medication errors Hypothermia and hyperthermia Scalds and burns

DISPLAY 18–1

Common Items Containing Latex

Medical gloves	Intravenous injection ports
Band-Aids	Nondisposable sheet protectors
Bulb syringes	Stethoscope tubing
Medication vial stoppers	Tourniquets
Urinary catheters	Elastic (Jobst) stockings
Condoms	Mattress covers
Wound drains	Dental bands
Endoscopes	Blood pressure cuff and tubing

- Immediate hypersensitivity, an instantaneous or fairly prompt systemic reaction manifested by swelling, itching, respiratory distress, hypotension, and death in severe cases

Sensitized people can also develop a cross-reaction to fruits and vegetables such as avocados, bananas, almonds, peaches, kiwi, tomatoes, and others because the molecular structure in latex and other plant substances is similar.

Safeguarding Patients and Personnel

One of the best techniques for preventing latex sensitization and allergic reactions is to minimize or eliminate latex exposure. Health care agencies are providing personnel with more than one type of gloves (Table 18-2). If latex gloves are used, nurses should avoid using oil-based hand creams or lotions and should wash their hands thoroughly after glove removal to reduce the transfer of latex proteins to others and objects in the environment.

Other measures to protect patients and personnel include:

- Obtaining an allergy history, and a sensitivity to latex in particular
- Flagging the chart and room door and attaching an allergy-alert identification bracelet on latex-sensitive patients
- Locating patients with a latex allergy in a private room or **latex-safe environment** (room stocked with latex-free equipment and wiped clean of glove powder)
- Stocking a latex-safe cart containing synthetic gloves and latex-free patient care and resuscitation equipment in the room of a patient sensitive to latex

TABLE 18–2. **Types of Medical Gloves**

Type	Advantages	Disadvantages
Latex		
Powdered latex	Inexpensive Elastic Adequate barrier against bloodborne pathogens	Release latex protein allergen into the air via powder
Low-powder latex	Less potential for airborne distribution of latex and chemical proteins	Unproven ability to prevent sensitization
Powder-free latex	Reduced sensitization of nonallergic individuals from lack of airborne distribution of latex allergen	Deposit latex protein on surface environment; causing symptoms in sensitized individuals Slightly more expensive than powdered latex gloves
Low-protein latex	Less latex protein	No significant evidence that use eliminates sensitization
Nonlatex		
Vinyl; powder and powder-free	Similar strength of latex gloves Cost approximately the same as powdered latex gloves	Less durable and more likely to leak than latex Recommend changing after 30 minutes to maintain barrier protection
Nitrile	Better resistance to tears, punctures, and chemical disintegration than latex or vinyl gloves	Possible contact dermatitis from chemicals contained in nitrile More expensive than latex or vinyl
Neoprene	Fit, strength, and barrier protection similar to latex	Contain potentially allergic chemicals More expensive than nitrile gloves
Thermoplastic elastomer	Strength and protection similar or superior to latex	Free of latex or chemical allergens Most expensive of all gloves

- Communicating with personnel in other departments so that they use nonlatex equipment and supplies during diagnostic or treatment procedures
- Promptly reporting allergic events and their possible cause to the agency's administration; administrators are required to report injuries, serious illnesses, or deaths due to unsafe equipment to the Food and Drug Administration
- Referring patients to latex allergy support groups
- Recommending that latex-sensitive patients wear a Medic-Alert bracelet at all times
- Advising latex-sensitive patients to notify their employer's health officer about the allergy in case of a future claim for worker's compensation or a legal case concerning discrimination in the workplace

BURNS

A **thermal burn** (skin injury caused by flames, hot liquids, or steam) is the most common form of burn. Burns also result from contact with caustic chemicals (such as lye), electric wires, or lightning.

Burn Prevention

Because many adults become complacent about safety hazards, the nurse should review burn-prevention measures with patients who are being treated for thermal-related accidents.

Patient Teaching For

Burn Prevention

Teach the patient or the family to do the following:

- Change the batteries in smoke, heat, and carbon monoxide detectors at least every year.
- Equip the home with at least one fire extinguisher.
- Develop an evacuation plan (and an alternate escape route) and a place for family members to meet after exiting a burning home or apartment.
- Practice the evacuation plan periodically.
- Keep all windows and doors barrier-free.
- Identify the location of exits when staying in a hotel.
- Dispose of rags that have been saturated with solvents.
- Keep items away from the pilot lights on the furnace, water heater, or clothes dryer.
- Avoid storing gasoline, kerosene, turpentine, or other solvents.
- Go to public fireworks displays rather than letting children light their own.
- Never smoke when sleepy or around oxygen equipment.
- Use safety matches rather than a lighter; children are less capable of using matches.
- Buy clothing, especially sleepwear, that is made from natural or flame-resistant fabrics.
- Never run if clothing is on fire; instead: stop, drop, and roll.
- Do not overload electrical outlets or circuits.
- Set thermostats on hot water heaters for less than 120°F (48.8°C).
- Keep cords to coffee pots, electric frying pans, or other small cooking appliances above the reach of young children.
- Follow label directions about the use of gloves when using chemicals.
- Flush chemicals with copious amounts of water if they come in contact with skin.
- Go inside if the weather is threatening or you see lightning.
- If you are inside a burning building:
  - Feel if the surface of a door is hot before opening it.
  - Close doors behind you.
  - Crawl on the floor if the room is smoke-filled.
  - Use stairs rather than the elevator.
  - Never go back inside, regardless of whom or what has been left there.
  - Go to a neighbor's home to call the fire department or 911 operator.

Most fire codes require that public buildings, including hospitals and nursing homes, have a functioning sprinkler system. Sprinkler systems help control the fire and limit structural damage.

Fire Plans

To prevent or limit burn injuries in a health care setting, all employees must know and follow the agency's **fire plan** (procedure followed if there is a fire). Compliance with the fire plan is a major component of the Joint Commission on Accreditation of Healthcare Organizations' (JCAHO) inspection. Every accredited health care agency must demonstrate and document that staff members have been trained in the following five areas:

- Specific roles and responsibilities at and away from the fire's point of origin
- Use of the fire alarm system
- Roles in preparing for building evacuation
- Location and proper use of equipment for evacuation or transporting patients to areas of refuge
- Building compartmentalization procedures for containing smoke and fire (Krozek & Scoggins, 1999)

To obtain JCAHO accreditation, staff on each shift must also participate in quarterly fire drills.

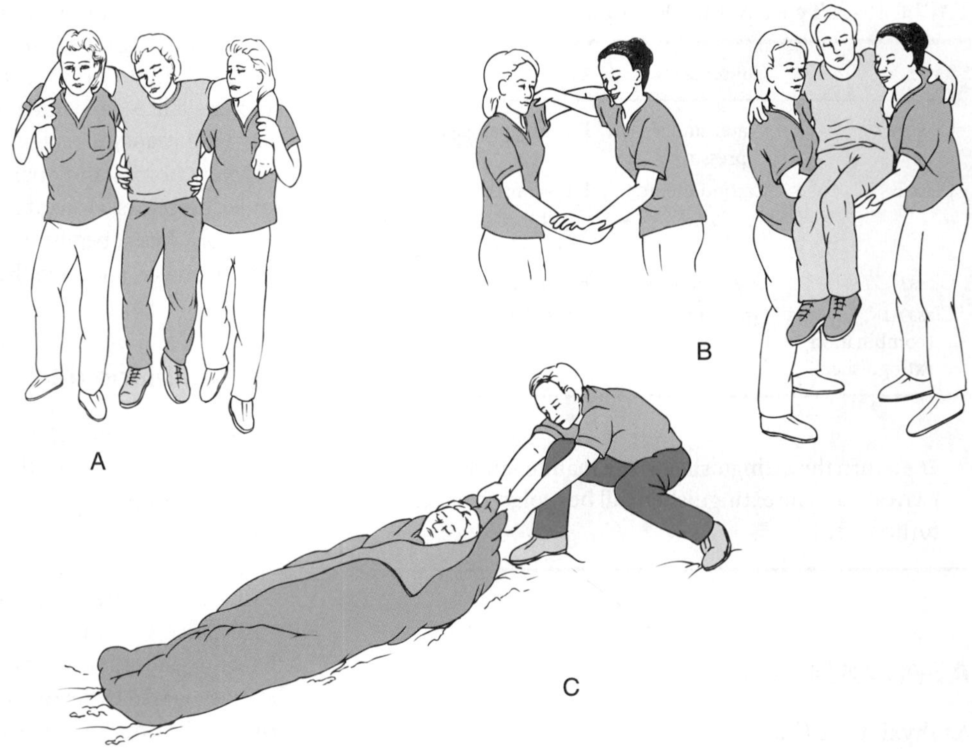

FIGURE 18–1. Evacuation of patients. (*A*) Human crutches; rescuers secure a weak but ambulatory patient's arm and waist. (*B*) Seat carry; rescuers interlock arms and carry a non-ambulatory patient. (*C*) Body drag; rescuer drags an unconscious victim or one who is unable to assist on a blanket or sheet.

Fire Management

The National Fire Protection Association, whose Life Safety Code is the basis for the JCAHO's management standards, recommends using the acronym RACE to identify the basic steps to be taken when managing a fire:

R—Rescue
A—Alarm
C—Confine (the fire)
E—Extinguish

Most health care agencies incorporate these concepts by including the following actions in their fire plan:

- Evacuate patients from the room where the fire is located.
- Inform the switchboard operator of the fire location. He or she will alert personnel over the public address system and notify the fire department.
- Return to the nursing unit when an alarm sounds; do not use the elevator.
- Clear the halls of visitors and equipment.
- Close the doors to patient rooms and stairwells, as well as fire doors between adjacent units. Wait for further directions.
- Place moist towels or bath blankets at the threshold of doors if smoke is leaking.
- Use an appropriate fire extinguisher if necessary.

Rescue and Evacuation

The first priority is to rescue patients in the immediate vicinity of the fire. Those who can walk are led to a safe area, and the room and fire doors are closed after exiting. Those who cannot walk are evacuated by nursing personnel, using a variety of techniques (Fig. 18-1).

Fire Extinguishers

There are four types of fire extinguishers (Table 18-3). Each type is labeled. Nurses must know which type of extinguisher is appropriate for the burning substance, and how to use it.

Nursing Guidelines For

Using a Fire Extinguisher

- ☑ Know the location of each type of fire extinguisher.
  RATIONALE: Knowing where the extinguishers are minimizes response time.
- ☑ Free the extinguisher from its enclosure.
  RATIONALE: The extinguisher must be removed for use.
- ☑ Remove the pin that locks the handle.
  RATIONALE: The pin must be removed for use.
- ☑ Aim the nozzle near the edge, not the center, of the fire.
  RATIONALE: The chemical will contain the fire.
- ☑ Move the nozzle from side to side.
  RATIONALE: Doing so increases the effectiveness of fire control.
- ☑ Avoid skin contact with the contents of the fire extinguisher.
  RATIONALE: The chemicals in the extinguisher can cause injury.

TABLE 18–3. **Types of Fire Extinguishers**

Type	Contents	Use
Class A	Water under pressure	Burning paper, wood, cloth
Class B	Carbon dioxide	Fires caused by gasoline, oil, paint, grease, and other flammable liquids
Class C	Dry chemicals	Electrical fires
Class ABC (combination extinguisher)	Graphite	Fires of any kind

□ Return the extinguisher to the maintenance department.
RATIONALE: The extinguisher will be replaced or refilled for future use.

ASPHYXIATION

Asphyxiation (inability to breathe) can be due to airway obstruction (see Chap. 37), inhalation of noxious gases such as smoke or carbon monoxide, or drowning.

Smoke Inhalation

Smoke can be more deadly than fire. Cigarette smoking has been banned in almost all health care facilities, and consequently smoke inhalation now accounts for less than 10% of fires at these facilities (Fig. 18-2). Although the percentage has been reduced, there is still a risk for fires from smoking; some attribute this to the fact that secretive smokers tend to discard smoldering cigarette butts quickly rather than risk being discovered. Home fires, on the other hand, often occur when smokers fall asleep with a burning cigarette or when children play with matches or lighters.

Many homes and apartment buildings are equipped with smoke detectors. However, some people dismantle their smoke detector when it begins to emit an audible alarm signaling low battery power, and then they fail to replace the batteries.

Carbon Monoxide

Carbon monoxide (CO), an odorless gas, is released during the incomplete combustion of carbon products such as fossil fuels (kerosene, natural gas, wood, and coal—substances commonly used to heat homes). CO, when inhaled, binds with hemoglobin and interferes with the oxygenation of cells. Without adequate ventilation, the consequences can be lethal.

Because CO can be present even without smoke, CO detectors should be installed in all homes, and alarms should be investigated by fire department personnel. Without detectors, victims may be unaware of the presence of CO and may attribute their symptoms to the flu. As their condition deteriorates, they become confused and lapse into a coma, followed by death.

Drowning

Drowning (situation in which fluid occupies the airway and interferes with ventilation) can occur in swimmers and nonswimmers alike. Accidental drownings occur during water activities such as fishing, boating, swimming, and water-skiing.

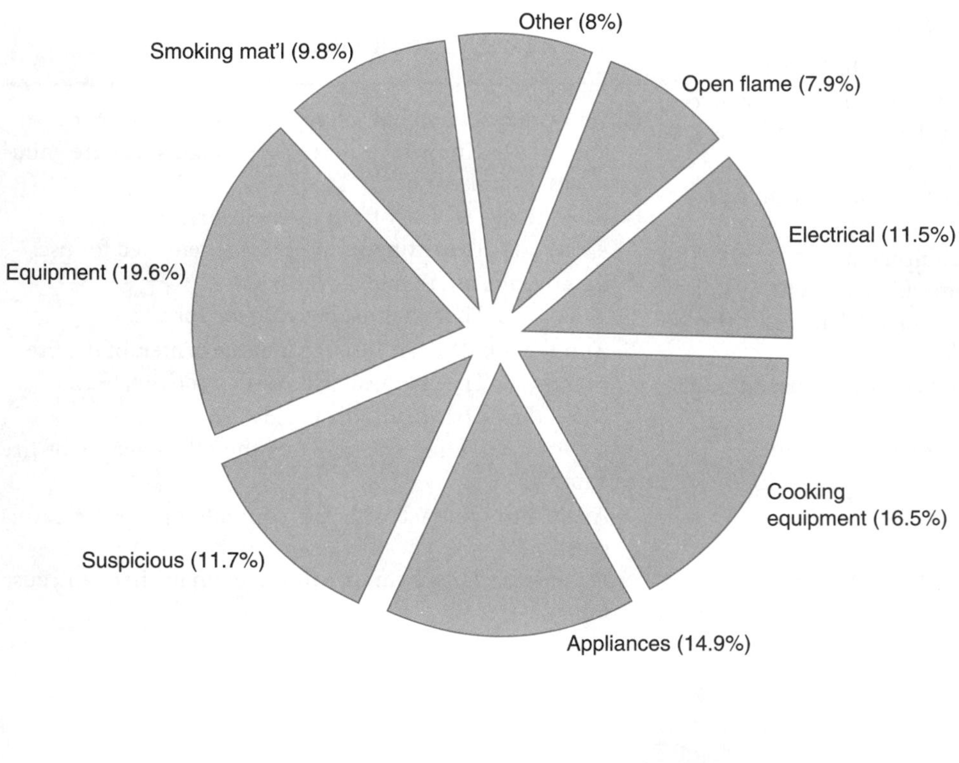

FIGURE 18–2. Smoking statistics as collected by the National Fire Protection Association. (Source: The U.S. Fire Problem Overview Report. Leading Causes and other Patterns and Trends Facilities that Care for the Sick. [1999] Quincy, MA: NFPA.)

Some incidents are linked to alcohol abuse, which tends to interfere with good judgment and promotes risk taking. Other victims overestimate their stamina.

Drownings can also occur at home or in the health care environment. Young children can drown if left momentarily in a bathtub or if they have access to a swimming pool. Swimming pools should be fenced and locked, and children should never be left unattended in a bathtub or pool.

Although the potential for drowning in a health care institution is statistically remote, it can happen. Therefore, any helpless or cognitively impaired patient, young or old, is never left alone in a tub of water, regardless of its depth.
Victims of cold-water drownings are more likely to be resuscitated because the cold lowers their metabolism, conserving oxygen (see Chap. 11). Prevention, however, is far better:

- Learn to swim.
- Never swim alone.
- Wear an approved flotation device.
- Do not drink alcohol when participating in water-related sports.
- Notify a law enforcement officer if boaters appear unsafe.

Resuscitation

Cardiopulmonary resuscitation (CPR), if begun immediately, may be lifesaving for a victim of drowning or asphyxiation (see Chap. 37). Current CPR certification is generally an employment requirement for nurses. Many hospitals teach new parents how to administer CPR (Fig. 18-3).

ELECTRICAL SHOCK

Electrical shock (discharge of electricity through the body) is a potential hazard wherever there are machines and equipment. The body is susceptible to electrical shock because it is composed of water and electrolytes, both of which are good conductors of electricity. A *conductor* is a substance that facilitates the flow of electrical current; an *insulator* is a substance that contains electrical currents so they do not scatter. Electric cords are covered with rubber or some other insulating substance.

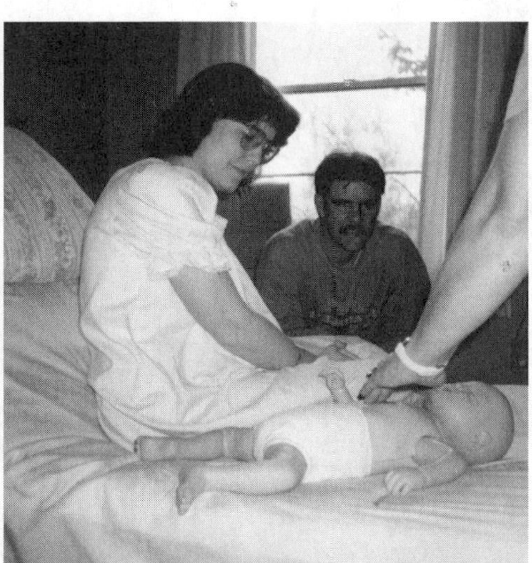

FIGURE 18–3. Parents being taught cardiopulmonary resuscitation as part of discharge planning. (Courtesy of Ken Timby.)

Macroshock (harmless distribution of low-amperage electricity over a large area of the body) feels like a slight tingling. **Microshock** (low-voltage but high-amperage electricity) is not usually felt by a person with intact skin. Intact skin helps to prevent shock and injury because it offers resistance or acts as a barrier between the electrical current and the water and electrolytes within. However, if the skin is wet or its integrity is impaired, the electrical current can be fatal, especially if delivered directly to the heart.

The potential for electrical shock is reduced by using grounded equipment. A *ground* diverts leaking electrical energy to the earth. Grounded equipment is identified by the presence of a three-pronged plug.

In addition to using grounded equipment, other safety measures used to prevent electrical shock include the following:

- Never use an adaptor to bypass a grounded outlet.
- Make sure all outlets and switches have cover plates.
- Plug all machines used for patient care into outlets within 12 feet of each other or within the same cluster of wall outlets (Berger & Williams, 1998).
- Unplug machines if they are no longer necessary.
- Discourage patients from resting electric hair dryers, curling irons, or razors on or near a sink that contains water.
- Do not use a machine that has a frayed or cracked cord or a plug with exposed wires.
- Grasp the plug, not the cord, to unplug it.
- Do not use extension cords.
- Report macroshocks to the engineering department.
- Clean liquid spills as soon as possible.
- Stand clear of the patient and bed during cardiac defibrillation.

POISONING

Poisoning (injury caused by the ingestion, inhalation, or absorption of a toxic substance) is more common in homes than in health care institutions. Accidental poisonings usually occur among toddlers and commonly involve substances located in the bathroom or kitchen (Display 18-2). Many children treated for accidental poisoning have a repeat episode.

There are fewer poisonings in health care facilities because medications are kept locked. By law, chemicals such as liquid antiseptics, intended for external use, are kept separate from other drugs. However, medication errors (see Chap. 32), in which the wrong medication or dose is administered, could be considered a form of poisoning.

DISPLAY 18-2

Common Substances Associated with Childhood Poisonings

Drugs: aspirin, acetaminophen, vitamins with iron, antidepressants, sedatives, tranquilizers, antacid tablets, diet pills, laxatives
Cleaning Agents: bleach, toilet bowl or tank disks, detergents, drain cleaners
Paint Solvents: turpentine, kerosene, gasoline
Heavy Metals: lead paint chips
Chemical Products: glue, shoe polish, antifreeze, insecticides
Cosmetics: hair dye, shampoo, nail polish remover
Plants: mistletoe berries, rhubarb leaves, foxglove, castor beans

Prevention

Curious children should be educated about poisons. Poison control centers offer stickers (Fig. 18-4) that can be used for education and prevention. Parents should place these stickers on toxic substances and should explain that any container displaying a sticker should not be touched. Parents should also be taught to reduce the risk of poisoning in the home.

Patient Education For

Preventing Childhood Poisoning

Teach the parents or caretakers to do the following:
- Install child-resistant latches on cupboard doors.
- Request child-proof caps on all prescription medications.
- Buy chemicals and nonprescription drugs with tamper-proof lids.
- Flush old medications down the toilet.
- Never transfer a toxic substance to a container usually used for food.
- Do not refer to medications as "candy" and do not tell children they taste "yummy."
- Do not keep drugs in your purse.
- Remind grandparents or babysitters to "child-proof" their homes.
- Remove toxic houseplants from the home.
- Keep the home well ventilated when using an aerosol or another substance that leaves lingering fumes in the air.

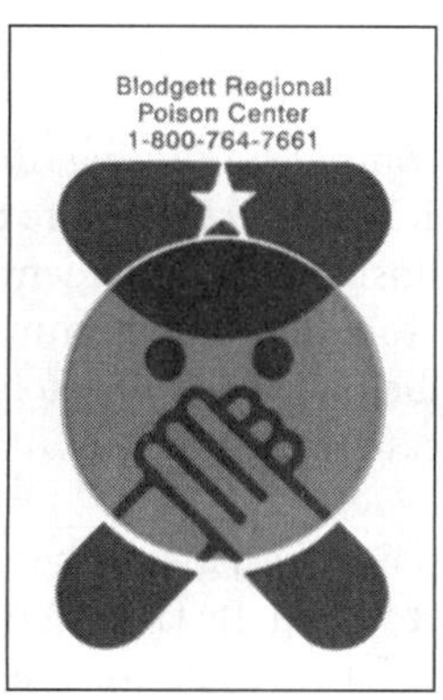

FIGURE 18–4. This sticker provided by poison control centers is used to warn young children about toxic substances in the home.

Adults who cannot administer their own medications safely can use containers that are prefilled by a responsible person (Fig. 18-5).

Treatment

Initial treatment for a suspected poisoning victim involves maintaining breathing and cardiac function. After that, an attempt is made to identify what was ingested, how much was taken, and when it was taken. Definitive treatment depends on the substance, the condition of the patient, and whether the substance is still in the stomach. For ingestions of commercial products that contain multiple ingredients, the poison control center is consulted. Otherwise, treatment follow the decision tree in Figure 18-6.

FALLS

Falls, more than any other injury discussed thus far, are the most common accident experienced by older adults, and they have the most serious consequences for this age group. Approximately 40% of injuries among older adults involve

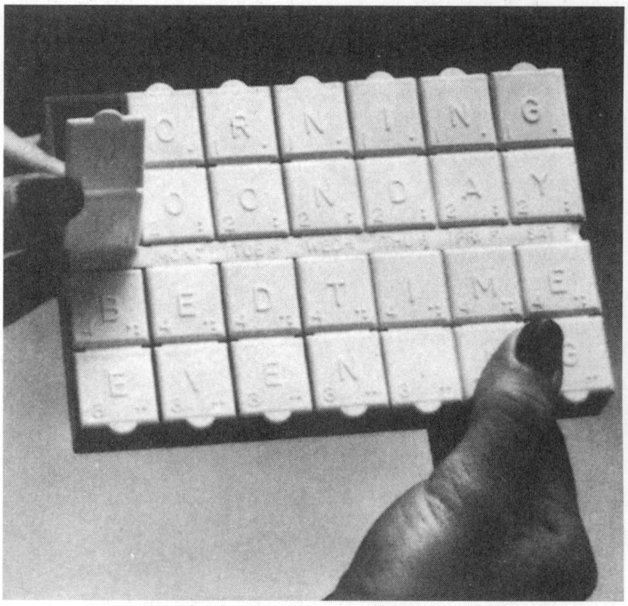

FIGURE 18–5. A pill organizer may help reduce the incidence of medication overdoses. (Courtesy of Apex Medical Corp, Bloomington, MN.)

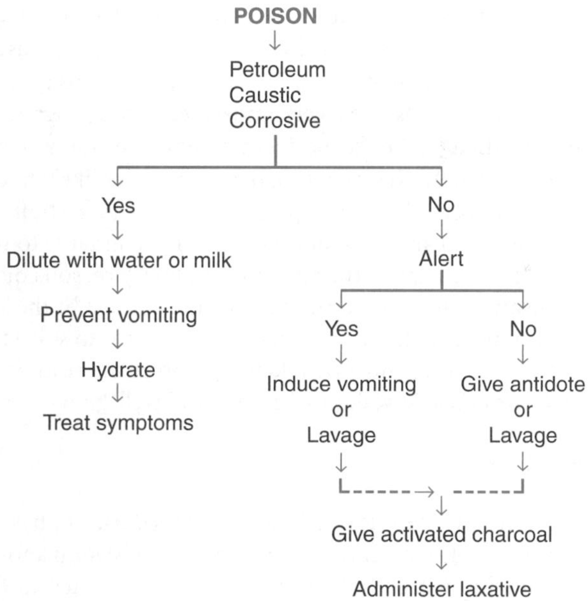

FIGURE 18–6. Decision tree for treating ingested poisons.

falls, and nearly 33% result in hospitalization (Ash et al, 1998). Many adults over 65 die from complications associated with a fall or suffer years of disability, impaired mobility, and pain.

Contributing Factors

Older adults are more prone to falling for several reasons. Many have age-related changes such as visual impairments and disorders affecting gait, balance, and coordination. Some take medications that lower blood pressure, causing them to feel dizzy on rising. Others have urinary urgency and rush to reach the toilet. Other social and environmental factors also contribute to their high incidence of falls. For example, older adults often wear slippers to accommodate swollen feet. Although slippers are more comfortable, less expensive, and less tiring to put on than shoes, they do not offer much support or traction. Clutter may accumulate around the house if the older adult lacks the energy to clean or does not want to discard old items.

For hospitalized older adults, the risk for falls rises. They are in an unfamiliar environment. They must rely on nursing assistance for mobility, and such assistance is not always prompt. Medications and altered health status may cause temporary confusion and poor judgment.

Assessment

Some falls can be prevented by determining which patients are at higher risk. Many long-term care agencies use assessment tools for this purpose (Fig. 18-7). Most of these tools use risk factors to determine which patients need fall-prevention protocols.

Prevention

Different fall-prevention approaches are used in the home and in health care facilities. Measures for preventing falls are modified based on the patient's circumstances.

Risk Factors	Risk Points	Score
Confusion/disorientation	+4	
Depression	+2	
Altered elimination (incontinence, nocturia, frequency)	+1	
Dizziness/vertigo	+1	
Sex = male	+1	
Antiepileptics (any prescribed)	+2	
Benzodiazepines (any prescribed)	+1	
Get-up-and-go (rising from chair) test:		
Able to rise in a single movement	0	
Pushes up, successful in one attempt	+1	
Multiple attempts, but successful	+3	
Unable to rise without assistance	+4	
	FINAL RISK SCORE=	*

* KEY: > 5 High risk for falling

FIGURE 18–7. Hendrich Fall Risk Tool. (Original research in Hendrich A, Nyhuis A, Kippenbrock T, Soja ME. Hospital falls: Development of a predictive model for clinical practice. Applied Nursing Research 1995; 8[3]; 129–139; updated research to be published in 2000. Used with permission of Ann Hendrich, MSN, RN, Methodist Hospital, Indianapolis, IN.)

Patient Teaching For
Preventing Falls

Teach the patient or the family to do the following:
- Keep the environment well lit.
- Install and use handrails on stairs inside and outside the home.
- Place a strip of light-colored adhesive tape on the edge of each stair for visibility.
- Remove scatter rugs.
- Keep extension cords next to the wall.
- Do not wax floors.
- Wear slippers with nonskid soles.
- Keep pathways clutter-free.
- Wear short robes without cloth belts, which may loosen and trip the patient.
- Use a cane or walker if prescribed.
- Replace the tip on a cane as it wears down.
- Stay indoors when the weather is icy or snowy.
- Sit down when using public transportation, even if it means asking someone for his or her seat.
- Install and use grab bars in the shower and near the toilet.
- Place a nonskid mat or decals on the floor of the tub or shower.
- Use soap-on-a-rope or a suspended container of liquid soap to prevent slipping on a loose soap bar.
- Use a flashlight or nightlight when it is dark.
- Make sure that pets are not underfoot.
- Mop up spills immediately.
- Use long-handled tongs to reach high objects rather than climbing on a chair.

Older adults should keep a list of emergency numbers posted by the phone. The elderly person who lives alone may want to become part of a daily phone tree. If he or she does not call in or does not answer a call, someone investigates. Personal response services are also available in which the subscriber wears a wireless, waterproof pendant with a button that can be used to summon help in an emergency. Activating the button places a call to the manufacturer's emergency response center, and once connected the user can carry on a two-way hands-free conversation. Calls for assistance are directed to predetermined people such as family, neighbors, the physician, or emergency personnel. If the user cannot communicate, the center dispatches emergency personnel to the user's location.

Restraints

In health care agencies, fall-prevention measures too often include the use of physical and chemical **restraints** (method of restricting a person's freedom of movement, physical activity, or normal access to his or her body; JCAHO, 1999). The use of restraints is closely regulated. Although the use of restraints is intended to prevent falls and other injuries, their risks, in many cases, outweigh their benefits. Research indicates that restrained patients become increasingly confused; suffer chronic constipation, incontinence, infections such as pneumonia, and pressure ulcers; and experience a progressive decline in their ability to perform activities of daily living (Stone et al, 1999). Restrained patients are more likely to die during their hospital stay than patients who are not restrained.

It is unethical and a violation of JCAHO standards to use physical or chemical restraints for disciplinary reasons or to compensate for limited personnel. Restraints must be the last intervention used after trying all other measures to solve the problem. Measures must be taken to protect the restrained patient's health, safety, dignity, rights, and well-being.

LEGISLATION

After research studies revealed the widespread use of physical restraints in long-term care facilities, federal legislation known as the Nursing Home Reform Law was incorporated in the Omnibus Budget Reconciliation Act (OBRA) in 1987 (Display 18-3). Compliance with the law became mandatory in 1990.

ACCREDITATION STANDARDS

The JCAHO followed the lead of OBRA legislation by developing restraint and seclusion standards in 1991. The standards, which differ for nonpsychiatric and psychiatric institutions, continue to be revised; the most recent revision occurred in 1999. The standards address three areas: agency restraint protocol, medical orders, and patient monitoring and documentation of nursing care.

Restraint Protocol

A *protocol* is a plan or set of steps to be followed when implementing an intervention. During a JCAHO inspection, the accrediting team looks for an agency's protocol for restraint use that has been approved by the medical staff. The protocol

DISPLAY 18–3

OBRA Legislation Addressing Restraints

The Omnibus Reconciliation Act (OBRA) of 1987 specifies that:

> The resident (patient) has the right to be free from any physical restraints imposed or psychoactive drug administered for purposes of discipline or convenience, and not required to treat the resident's (patient's) medical symptoms. . . . Restraints may only be imposed to ensure the physical safety of the resident or other residents and only upon the written order of a physician that specifies the duration and the circumstances under which the restraints are to be used (except in emergency situations which must be addressed in the facility's restraint policy).

must identify the criteria that justify the application and discontinuation of restraints. Restraints are considered appropriate when the patient's behavior jeopardizes treatment. For example, it is acceptable to restrain a patient who attempts to remove an endotracheal tube that facilitates mechanical ventilation. However, less restrictive measures, such as having someone sit with the patient, should be attempted first.

Medical Orders

Nurses can independently apply a restraint in accordance with the established protocol. However, the medical record must show that a licensed independent practitioner (usually a physician) has been notified about its application within 12 hours. A signed written order must be obtained for the use of restraints within 24 hours. The order should specify the type of restraint, the reason for applying the restraint, the criteria for removal, and the duration of use. The medical order must be renewed every 24 hours after examining the patient to determine the need for continued use.

Monitoring and Documentation

The patient's chart must contain documented evidence of frequent and regular nursing assessments of the restrained patient's vital signs, circulation, skin condition, and behavior. In addition, nursing care concerning toileting, nutrition, hydration, and range of motion while the patient is restrained must be recorded. The documented care must reflect the agency's established protocol. Communication with the patient's family regarding the need for restraints should be included in the nursing documentation. When the assessment findings indicate that the patient has improved, the restraint is removed, even if the order has not expired.

RESTRAINT ALTERNATIVES

The intent of both the OBRA legislation and JCAHO standards is to promote **restraint alternatives** (protective or adaptive devices that promote patient safety and postural support, but which the patient can release independently) and eventually restraint-free patient care. Agencies are being challenged to implement interventions that protect patients from injury while ensuring their freedom, mobility, and dignity.

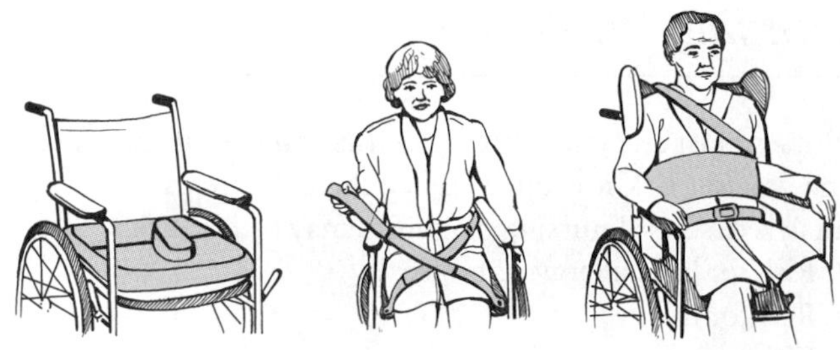

FIGURE 18–8. Examples of restraint alternatives.

Restraint alternatives are generally appropriate for patients who tend to need repositioning to maintain their body alignment or improve their independence and functional status. Some examples include seat inserts or gripping materials that prevent sliding, support pillows, seat belts or harnesses with front-releasing Velcro or buckle closures, and commercial or homemade tilt wedges (Fig. 18-8). If the patient is unaware of or cannot release the restraint alternative, it is considered a restraint.

Other supplementary measures may also reduce the need for restraints. Personnel are encouraged to improve gait training, provide physical exercise, reorient patients, encourage assistive ambulatory devices such as walkers and hall rails, and use electronic seat and bed monitors that sound an alarm when patients get up without assistance. Before considering the use of physical restraints, the patient's response to other alternatives is observed and documented. When patients are in a wheelchair, they must be positioned correctly (Table 18-4).

USE OF RESTRAINTS

Sometimes the use of restraints is justified. To avoid liability, nurses and the personnel that they supervise must demonstrate competency in their safe application. Skill 18-1 explains how to apply restraints and use them appropriately.

TABLE 18–4. **Basic Wheelchair Positioning Principles**

Structure	Front View	Side View
Head	Head/neck centered over trunk midline	Head/ear centered over hip
Shoulders	Level in horizontal line	Top of shoulder over hip
Trunk	Sternum perpendicular to center of pelvis	Spine perpendicular to hip
Pelvis	Tops of hips level in horizontal line	Lumbar curve preserved
Thighs	Knees level in horizontal line	Hip and knee level in horizontal line
Knees	Knees not touching; legs perpendicular to floor	Knees bent 90°; edge of seat 3 inches from knee crease
Feet	Great toes and fifth toes level in horizontal line	Heel and forefoot positioned on footplate; ankle in neutral position

Pang J. Proper patient positioning in wheelchairs. Nursing Update Winter 1994;5(1):2. With permission from J. T. Posey Co., Arcadia, CA.

Nursing Implications

Nurses must recognize safety hazards and identify patients at the greatest risk for injury. Once the data are gathered and analyzed, several nursing diagnoses may be identified.

- Risk for latex allergy response
- Risk for injury
- Risk for trauma
- Impaired walking
- Sensory/perceptual alteration: visual
- Acute confusion
- Chronic confusion
- Impaired environmental interpretation syndrome
- Impaired home maintenance management

The nursing care plan gives sample interventions for a patient with a nursing diagnosis of Risk for injury, defined in the NANDA taxonomy (1999) as "a state in which an individual is at risk of injury as a result of environmental conditions interacting with the individual's adaptive and defensive resources."

Despite appropriate assessments and plans for preventing injuries, accidents still occur. When they do, the nurse's first concerns are the safety of the patient and the potential for allegations of malpractice. Therefore, if an accident occurs, the nurse should do the following:

- Check the patient's condition immediately.
- Call for help if the patient is in danger.
- Begin resuscitation measures if necessary.
- Comfort and reassure the patient.
- Avoiding moving the patient until it is safe to do so.
- Report the accident and assessment findings to the physician.
- Complete an incident report as soon as the patient is stabilized (see Chap. 3).

Nursing Care Plan

Risk for Injury

Assessment

Subjective Data

States, "I'm afraid of falling. I've had some near-misses at home since my last surgery. I get dizzy when I hurry and my feet get all tangled up."

Objective Data

62-year-old man admitted for treatment of pneumonia. Postural hypotension evidenced by a difference of 20 mm Hg in systolic pressure when lying and standing (135/85 lying; 115/80 standing). Fractured hip repaired after a fall during prior hospitalization for eye surgery. Wears eyeglasses at all times while awake. Has a walker but does not consistently use it. Takes a daily diuretic.

Diagnosis

Risk for Injury related to dizziness and impaired mobility

Plan

Goal

The patient will ask for assistance when getting in and out of bed and will use his walker consistently while ambulating throughout hospital stay.

Orders: 7/5

1. Assess BP lying and standing daily @ 0800.
2. Keep the bed in low position.
3. Reinforce the need to use the call signal.
4. Assist to a sitting position until dizziness passes before standing.
5. Keep walker within reach at all times.
6. Help to put on nonskid slippers and glasses for ambulation. ____________ B. JOYNER, RN

Implementation (Documentation)

7/6 0800 Bed in low position. BP 138/82 on R. arm while lying and 125/78 while sitting. Sat for 3 minutes on edge of bed. States, "I don't feel dizzy this morning. It usually hits me in the afternoon after my water pill kicks in." Helped with nonskid sneakers. ____________ J. BUTLER, SN

Evaluation (Documentation)

0830 Tried to walk from bed to bathroom without using walker. Instructed to use the walker at all times. Location of call light in the bathroom identified. Said, "I hate having to depend on you." ____________ J. BUTLER, SN

FOCUS ON OLDER ADULTS

- Older adults have an increased risk for falls, accidents, and fractures because of physiologic age-related changes and disease conditions affecting mobility, balance, and sensory function.
- The National Center for Injury Prevention & Control (1996) reports that falls are the second leading cause of injury-related deaths in adults 65 to 84 and the leading cause of injury-related deaths in adults over 85. Falls are the most common cause of injury and hospital admissions for trauma among the elderly.
- Hospitalizations are nearly twice as long for those who fall compared with those who do not. About half of the patients hospitalized for falling are transferred to a nursing facility (Tideiksaar, 1997).
- *Osteoporosis* (loss of bone mass) increases the risk for fractures, especially in older women. Osteoporotic fractures may occur with little or no trauma and even without a fall.
- Some older adults develop "fallophobia" (exaggerated fear of falling), which inhibits them from engaging in activities that enhance the quality of their life.
- Older adults who have had a previous fall often exhibit a characteristic gait, attributed more to being overly cautious than a result of a prior injury.
- Restraining older adults can be as detrimental to the person as the consequences of a fall. Physical restraints are always considered a last resort, only after all other interventions have been tried.
- Older adults who are confused or otherwise cognitively impaired may need precautions to prevent wandering. Helpful devices include placing a specially designed net with a stop sign across the exit doorway with Velcro, or disguising an exit door by covering it with a curtain or wallpaper that blends in with the surrounding environment.
- Older adults with cognitive impairments need to be protected from accidental ingestion of toxic substances, such as medications and cleaning agents, in households and institutional settings.
- Many types of monitors, identification bracelets (that include a phone number), and alerting/alarm devices are available for use with older adults who are at risk for wandering. Early identification is necessary so that proper precautions can be initiated. Daily documentation of what a person is wearing is helpful should the patient wander and need to be identified.
- The Alzheimer's Association (800-438-4380) sponsors a program called "Safe Return," which facilitates the reporting and return of persons with cognitive impairments who become lost.
- Photographing all residents in a nursing facility may be helpful should they wander off.
- Reflective tape and other distinct markings placed on the floor are helpful in identifying a path to the bathroom for older adults who are confused or disoriented.
- To distract patients from attempting to pull out tubes or interfere with other treatments, it is helpful to keep their hands occupied with stringing large wooden beads or buttons and sorting items.
- Caregivers of older adults benefit from being relieved for periods of time by other family members, community volunteers, or paid caregivers.

KEY CONCEPTS

- Accidental injuries vary according to the victim's stage of development. Because infants must rely on their caretakers, they are susceptible to falls. Poisonings are common among toddlers. School-aged children suffer play-related injuries, and adolescents are often the victims of sport-related injuries. Young adults are commonly involved in motor-vehicle accidents. Middle-aged adults suffer a variety of physical trauma, such as back injuries. Falls are common among older adults.
- Environmental hazards often contribute to injuries and deaths due to latex sensitization, burns, asphyxiation, electrical shock, poisoning, and falls.
- Latex sensitization can be reduced by using nonlatex gloves and medical equipment, washing one's hands after removing latex gloves, and avoiding the use of petroleum-based hand creams or lotions, which retain latex protein on the skin.
- Most fire plans incorporate four steps: rescue those in danger, sound an alarm, confine the fire, and extinguish the blaze.
- There are four classes of fire extinguishers. Class A extinguishers are used for paper, wood, and cloth fires. Class B extinguishers are used on fuels and flammable liquids. Class C extinguishers are used for electrical fires. Class ABC extinguishers can be used on any type of fire.
- Methods of preventing burns include installing and maintaining smoke detectors, developing and practicing a fire evacuation plan, and never going back into a burning building.
- Asphyxiation is commonly caused by smoke inhalation, carbon monoxide poisoning, and drowning.
- Drownings can be prevented by wearing approved flotation devices, avoiding alcohol consumption when around the water, and never swimming alone.
- Humans are susceptible to injury from electrical shock because the human body is predominately composed of water and electrolytes, which are good conductors of electrical current.
- Electrical shock may be prevented by using three-pronged grounded equipment, making sure all cover plates are intact, and replacing equipment that has frayed electrical cords.
- Substances commonly implicated in poisonings include chemicals such as drugs, cleaning agents, paint solvents, heavy metals, cosmetics, and plants.
- Poisonings may be prevented by using child-proof caps on medication bottles, installing latches on storage cupboards, and never transferring a toxic substance to a container generally associated with food.
- Older adults in general are prone to falling because they have gait and balance problems due to age-related changes, visual impairment, postural hypotension, and urinary urgency.
- Although physical restraints prevent falls, they create concomitant risks for constipation, incontinence, infections

such as pneumonia, pressure ulcers, and a progressive decline in the ability to perform activities of daily living.

- The overuse of physical restraints in health care facilities has led to the passage of legislation and accreditation standards regulating their use.
- Restraints are devices that restrict movement; restraint alternatives are protective and adaptive devices that can be independently removed by patients.
- Restraint use may be justified when patients have a history of previous falls or may experience life-threatening consequences, when there has been an unsatisfactory response to restraint alternatives, when patients are seriously impaired mentally or physically, or if their movement must be restricted during a life-threatening event.
- If an accident occurs, the nurse's first concerns are the safety of the patient and the potential for allegations of malpractice.

CRITICAL THINKING EXERCISES

- When discharging an older adult to the care of a family member, what safety measures are appropriate to include in the discharge instructions?
- Without resorting to the use of restraints, how can you prevent falls in a patient with an unsteady gait?
- List some alternatives to restraints when caring for a patient who tends to wander, one who does not ask for but needs assistance with ambulation, and one who has a history of pulling out his or her intravenous catheter.

SUGGESTED READINGS

Andrews P. Using restraints with restraint. Nursing 1998;28(10):6–9.

Ash KL, Macleod P, Clark L. A case control study of falls in the hospital setting. Journal of Gerontological Nursing 1998;24(12):7–15.

Berger KJ, Williams MB. Fundamentals of nursing: collaborating for optimal health, 2nd ed. Norwalk, Appleton & Lange, 1998.

Burt S. What you need to know about latex allergy. Nursing 1998;29 (10):33–39.

DiBartolo V. Nine steps to effective restraint use. RN 1998;61(12):23–24.

Firestone T. Physical restraints: meeting the standards, improving the outcomes. MedSurg Nursing 1998;7(2):121–123.

Janelli LM, Kanski GW, Neary MA. Physical restraints: has OBRA made a difference? Journal of Gerontological Nursing 1994;20(6):17–21.

JCAHO. Comprehensive accreditation manual for hospitals: the official handbook. Oakbrook Terrace, Ill., JCAHO, 1999.

Kobs A. Answering your questions about patient restraints. Nursing 1997;27(12):32hn12.

Kobs A. What's new for 1999? Part II. Nursing Management 1998;29(10):12.

Kobs A. Restraints revisited. Nursing Management 1998;29(1):17–18.

Kohn P. The legal implications of latex allergy. RN 1999;62(1):63–65.

Krozek C, Scoggins A. Meeting environment of care standards on the patient care unit: Part II, amended to comply with 1999 JCAHO standards publication. Glendale, Cinahl Information Systems, 1999.

NANDA nursing diagnoses: definitions and classification, 1999–2000. Philadelphia, NANDA, 1999.

National Center for Injury Prevention & Control. National summary of injury mortality data, 1988–1994. Atlanta, CDC, 1996. http://www.cdc.gov/ncipc/duip/falls.htm

National Fire Prevention Association. Life safety code. Quincy, Mass., NFPA, 1997. http://catalog.nfpa.org

National Fire Prevention Association. The U.S. fire problem overview report. Quincy, Mass., NFPA, 1999.

Omnibus Budget Reconciliation Act of 1987: Conference report to accompany HR 3545. Washington DC, U.S. Government Printing Office, 1987.

Pang J. Proper positioning in wheelchairs. Nursing Update Winter 1994; 5(1):2.

Reith KA, Bennett CC. Restraint-free care. Nursing Management 1998;29 (5):36–40.

Richman D. To restrain or not to restrain? RN 1998;61(7):55–56.

Salladay SA. Restraints: severing the ties that bind. Nursing 1998;28(5):30.

Stone JT, Wyman JF, Salisbury SA. Clinical gerontological nursing: a guide to advanced practice, 2nd ed. Philadelphia, WB Saunders, 1999.

Sullivan-Marx EM. Restraint-free care: how does a nurse decide? Journal of Gerontological Nursing 1996;22(9):7–14.

Terpstra TL, Van Doren E. Reducing restraints: where to start. Journal of Continuing Education in Nursing 1998;29(1):10–16.

Tideiksaar R. Falling in old age: prevention and management, 2d ed. New York, Springer, 1997.

SKILL 18-1

USING PHYSICAL RESTRAINTS

Suggested Action	Reason for Action
Assessment	
Assess the patient's physical and mental status for signs suggesting danger to self or others.	Provides data for determining the need for physical restraints
Consult with staff and family on options other than restraints.	Supports the principle of using less restrictive approaches initially
Observe the patient's response to alternative measures.	Determines the need to revise the current plan for care
Check the chart for a physician's order for the use of restraints.	Complies with JCAHO requirements
Review the agency's restraint policy or procedure if there is no current medical order.	Follows standards for care
Assess the patient's skin and circulation.	Provides a baseline of information for future comparisons
Inspect the restraint that will be used and avoid any that are in poor condition.	Ensures safety
Planning	
Obtain a current order for the use of physical restraints if they are necessary.	Complies with JCAHO guidelines
Choose a restraint compatible with the size of the patient.	Prevents injury
Approach the patient slowly and calmly. Speak in a soft, controlled voice.	Reduces agitation
Use the patient's name and make eye contact.	Helps secure the patient's attention
Explain why restraint is necessary.	Promotes understanding and cooperation
Reassure the patient that the restraints will be discontinued when the possibility for harm no longer exists.	Indicates criteria for releasing restraints
Plan to remove or loosen the restraints at time periods established by agency policy to assess circulation, provide joint mobility, give skin care, assist with elimination, offer food and fluids, and evaluate whether restraints are still needed.	Demonstrates attention to basic physiologic and safety needs; supports the principle that restraints are not applied longer than necessary
Implementation	
Place the patient in a position of comfort with proper body alignment.	Maintains functional position and reduces discomfort
Protect any bony prominences or fragile skin that may be injured by a restraint.	Reduces or prevents injury
Upper Extremity Restraints	
Apply mitts rather than wrist restraints, if possible.	Maintains freedom to move elbows and shoulders
Use soft cloth restraints instead of stiff leather.	Promotes skin integrity
Provide as much length as possible without allowing the patient to pull at tubes or other treatment devices.	Facilitates movement

continued

SKILL 18–1

USING PHYSICAL RESTRAINTS *Continued*

Suggested Action	Reason for Action

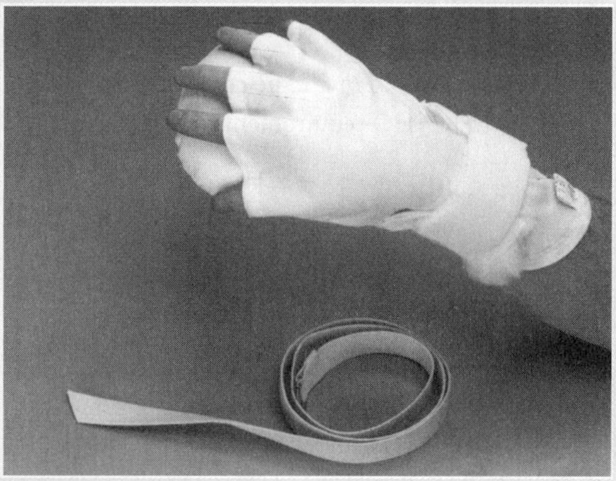

Hand mitts can be applied with or without ties. (Courtesy of the J. T. Posey Co., Arcadia, CA.)

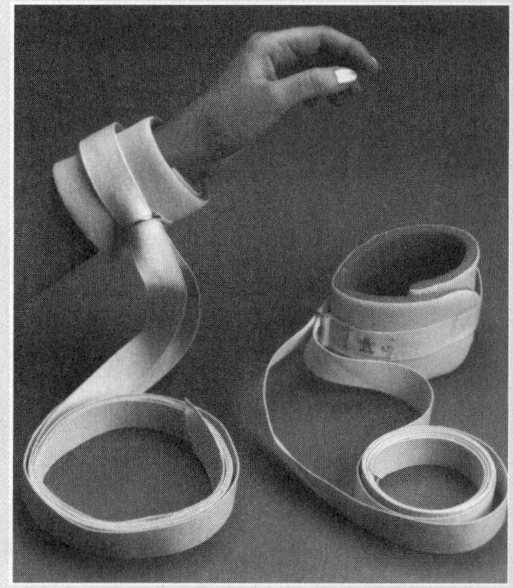

Soft wrist restraints. (Courtesy of the J. T. Posey Co., Arcadia, CA.)

Wheelchair Restraints

Suggested Action	Reason for Action
Avoid back cushions if possible.	Creates the potential for slack if they become dislodged
Make sure the patient's hips are flush with the back of the chair.	Promotes good posture and skeletal alignment
Apply belts snugly over the thighs with at least a 45° angle between the belt and knees.	Minimizes sliding up toward the ribs and compromising breathing

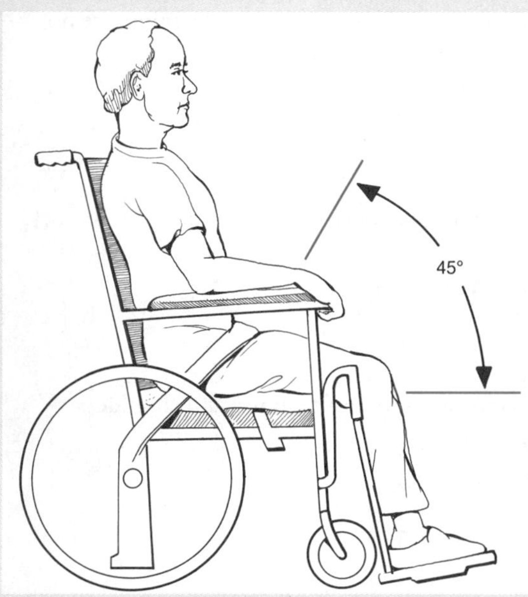

With the lap strap at a 45° angle to the knees, the hips are held toward the back of the chair.

continued

SKILL 18–1

USING PHYSICAL RESTRAINTS *Continued*

Suggested Action	Reason for Action
Apply vests with Velcro or zipper closures at the back; use criss-crossing vests with front closures only on docile patients.	Keeps fasteners out of reach; prevents strangulation
Support the feet on footrests.	Reduces pressure behind the knees and promotes circulation of blood
Tie restraints under the chair, not behind the back.	Prevents suffocation if the patient should slide downward

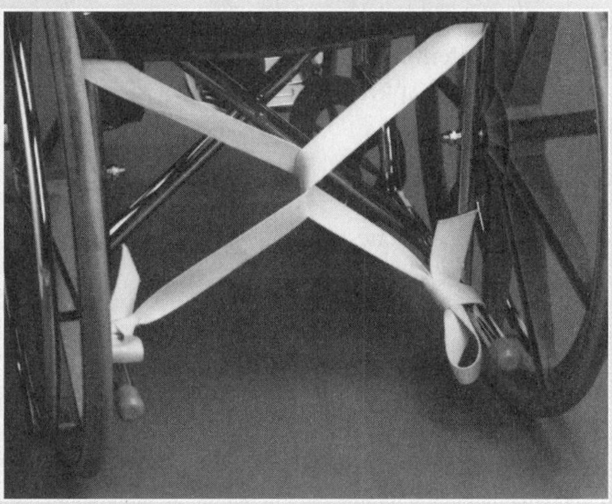

Restraint ties are secured beneath the chair. (Courtesy of the J.T. Posey Co., Arcadia, CA.)

Suggested Action	Reason for Action
Use a quick-release knot when tying any type of restraint.	Facilitates removal should the patient's safety become compromised

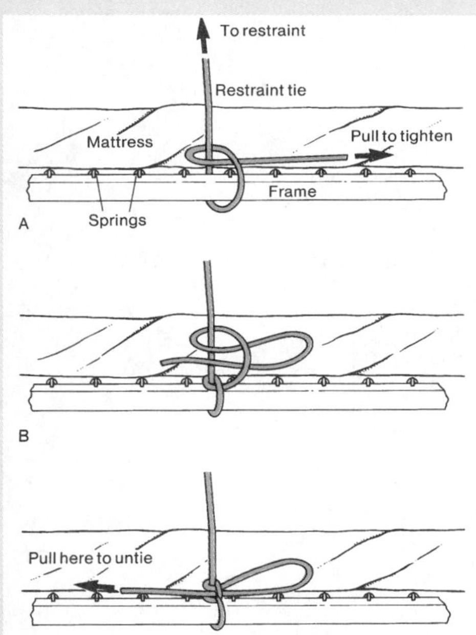

Follow the sequence in steps A, B, and C to tie a quick-release knot.

continued

SKILL 18-1

USING PHYSICAL RESTRAINTS *Continued*

Suggested Action	Reason for Action
Keep the patient in sight whenever restraints are used.	Aids in monitoring the patient's safety
Never restrain a patient to a toilet.	Prevents drowning or falls
Bed Restraints	
Position the patient in the center of the mattress.	Allows maximum movement and proper body alignment
Use full siderails and maintain them in an "up" position while the patient is restrained.	Prevents injury from slipping between or below half rails
Apply siderail covers or pad the rails with soft bath blankets if the patient is extremely restless.	Reduces the potential for becoming caught or injured within the open spaces of the rails
Apply belt restraints snugly at the waist but with enough room to slide an open hand between the device and the patient.	Ensures ventilation
Secure the straps to the moveable part of the bed frame, not the siderails or stationary frame.	Prevents sliding and chest compression

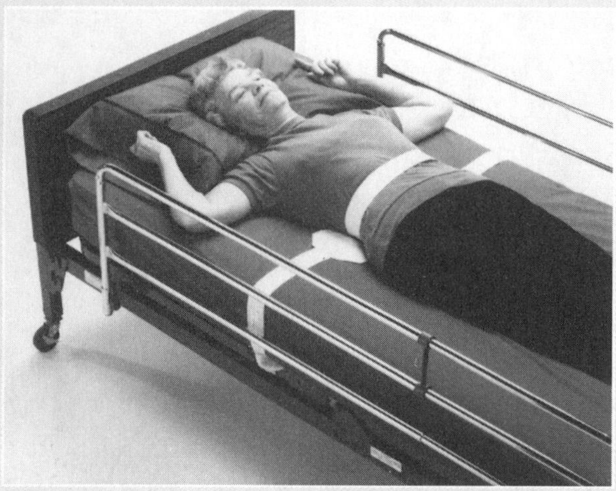

The restraint ties are secured to the moveable portion of the bed frame. (Courtesy of the J.T. Posey Co., Arcadia, CA.)

Suggested Action	Reason for Action
Monitor aggressive, agitated, or restless patients frequently.	Promotes patient safety

Evaluation

- Restraint(s) are applied correctly.
- Patient remains free of injury.
- Restraints are released according to policy.
- Basic needs are met.
- Restraints are discontinued when no longer needed.

Document

- Assessment findings that indicate a need for restraint
- Types of restraint alternatives and the patient's response

continued

SKILL 18-1

USING PHYSICAL RESTRAINTS *Continued*

- Condition of skin, circulation, sensation, and joint mobility before restraint application
- Type of restraint applied
- Communication with physician and responsible family member
- Frequency of release and assessment findings
- Nursing measures used to promote skin integrity and joint flexibility, and to meet nutritional and elimination needs
- Assessments indicating an ongoing need for restraints

SAMPLE DOCUMENTATION

Date and Time Pulling on urinary catheter. Reminded to leave catheter alone. Placed close to nursing station to allow quick intervention. Given a skein of yarn to wrap as a ball to distract patient from catheter. Continues to tug at catheter. Catheter is patent, but urine now appears bloody. Order obtained for soft cloth wrist restraints. Skin over wrists is intact, no edema, full mobility, fingers are warm and pink, can differentiate sharp from dull sensation. Restraints secured to arms of wheelchair. Daughter notified of need to use restraints at this time and concurs with treatment plan. ____________________ SIGNATURE/TITLE

CRITICAL THINKING

- Discuss how you would feel if you or a family member were placed in restraints.
- For what reasons might you sue a nurse who applied restraints?
- List some methods for avoiding a lawsuit when restraints are necessary.

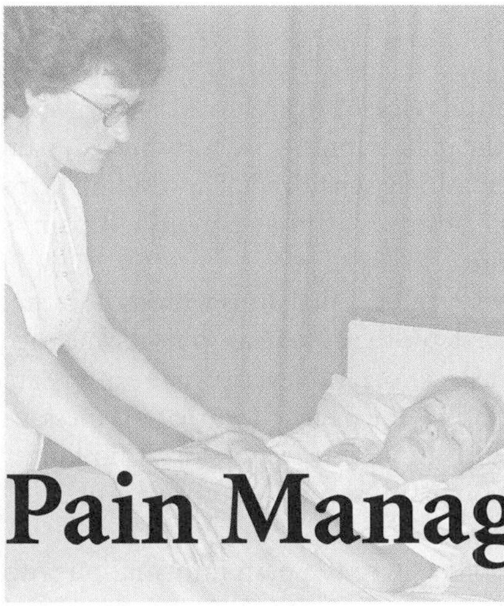

Pain Management

CHAPTER 19

CHAPTER OUTLINE

NURSING GUIDELINES

MANAGING PAIN

SKILLS

SKILL 19-1: PREPARING A PCA INFUSER
SKILL 19-2: OPERATING A TENS UNIT

NURSING CARE PLAN

PAIN

KEY TERMS

acupressure
acupuncture
acute pain
adjuvants
alternative medical therapy
analgesic
biofeedback
bolus
chronic pain
controlled substances
cordotomy
cutaneous pain
distraction
endogenous opioids
equianalgesic dose
gate-control theory
hypnosis
imagery
intractable pain
intraspinal analgesia
loading dose
malingerer
meditation
neuropathic pain
nociceptors
nonopioids
opioids
pain
pain management
pain perception
pain threshold
pain tolerance
patient-controlled analgesia (PCA)
percutaneous electrical nerve stimulation (PENS)
placebo
referred pain
relaxation
rhizotomy
somatic pain
suffering
transcutaneous electrical nerve stimulation (TENS)
visceral pain

LEARNING OBJECTIVES

An understanding of the content within this chapter will be evidenced by the student's ability to:

- Give a general definition of pain.
- Explain the course of pain transmission.
- Explain the difference between pain perception, pain threshold, and pain tolerance.
- Describe the gate-control theory of pain transmission.
- Discuss how endogenous opioids reduce pain transmission.
- Name at least five types of pain.
- Give at least three characteristics that differentiate acute pain from chronic pain.
- List five components of a basic pain assessment.
- Name four common pain-intensity assessment tools used by nurses.
- Identify at least three occasions when it is essential to perform a pain assessment and document assessment findings.
- Name four physiologic mechanisms for managing pain.
- Give three categories of drugs used alone or in combination to manage pain.
- Identify two surgical procedures used when other methods of pain management are ineffective.
- List at least five nondrug, nonsurgical methods for managing pain.
- Discuss the most common reason why patients request frequent administrations of pain-relieving drugs.
- Define addiction.
- Discuss how addiction affects pain management.
- Define placebo and explain the basis for its positive effect.

Pain is probably the major cause of physical distress among patients. This chapter provides information about pain and techniques for pain relief.

Pain

Pain (unpleasant sensation usually associated with disease or injury) causes physical discomfort and is also accompanied by **suffering** (emotional component of pain). Because there is no effective method for validating or invalidating pain, Margo McCaffery (1998), a nursing expert on pain, defines pain as being "whatever the person says it is, and existing whenever the person says it does." Understanding how pain is produced and perceived is essential to finding mechanisms for pain relief.

PAIN TRANSMISSION

The transmission of pain begins with some type of injury that stimulates **nociceptors** (nerve receptors), millions of which are present in the skin, bones, joints, muscles, and internal organs. Nociceptors transmit the pain impulse and other sensory information, such as pressure and temperature changes, using various neurochemicals over spinal pathways to the brain (Fig. 19-1).

Substance P, one type of pain neurotransmitter, stimulates nerve endings at the site of the injury and the spinal cord. Prostaglandin, a chemical released from injured cells, speeds the transmission. As the pain impulses are transmitted, pain receptors become increasingly sensitized. This finding helps to explain the clinical observation that established pain is more difficult to suppress.

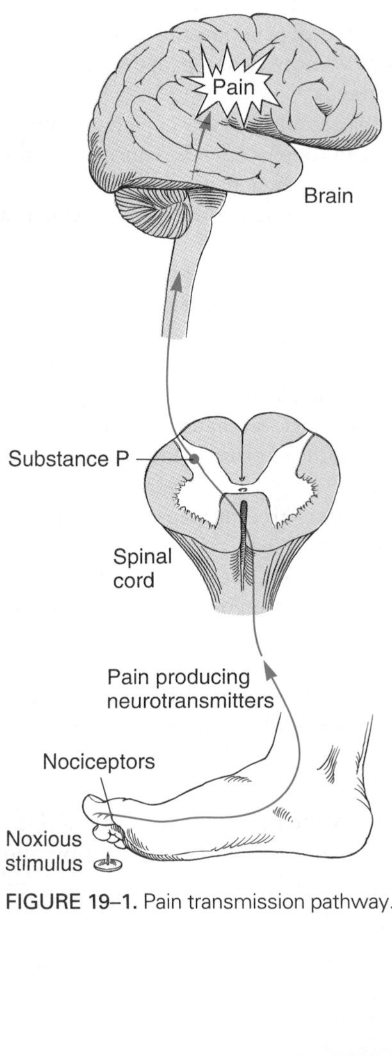

FIGURE 19–1. Pain transmission pathway.

When pain impulses reach the thalamus within the brain, two responses occur. First, the thalamus transmits the message to the cortex, where the location and severity of the injury are identified. Second, it notifies the nociceptors that the message has been received and continued transmission is no longer necessary. A malfunction in this secondary process is one reason why chronic pain lingers.

The cortex proceeds to share the pain information with the limbic system, the structure responsible for emotions. Together, the cortex and the limbic system transform the physiologic data into something that is biopsychosocially unique based on the person's cultural beliefs, current anxiety level, past pain experiences, and overall outlook (Mayo Clinic, 1996).

PAIN PERCEPTION

Pain perception (conscious experience of discomfort) occurs when the **pain threshold** (point at which sufficient pain-transmitting neurochemicals reach the brain) is reached. Surpassing the pain threshold results in awareness of discomfort. Pain thresholds tend to be the same among healthy people, but individuals tolerate or bear the sensation of pain differently. **Pain tolerance** (amount of pain a person endures once the threshold has been passed) is influenced by learned behaviors specific to gender, age, and culture (see Chap. 6).

PAIN THEORIES

Several theories attempt to explain how pain is transmitted (and thus the basis for pain-relieving mechanisms). No one theory is all-encompassing, but one that has attracted a great deal of interest is the gate-control theory (Melzack & Wall, 1965).

Gate-Control Theory

The **gate-control theory** (belief about how pain is transmitted and blocked) proposes that spinal pathways conduct several types of cutaneous (skin) sensations to the brain, but they can conduct only one at a time. While one pathway is occupied with transmitting a sensory neural message through an open "gate," the other gates are closed (Fig. 19-2). The brain, therefore, does not perceive pain while it is preoccupied with other sensory input. This helps to explain how massage, vibration, pressure, heat, cold, and other nondrug mechanisms reduce pain perception.

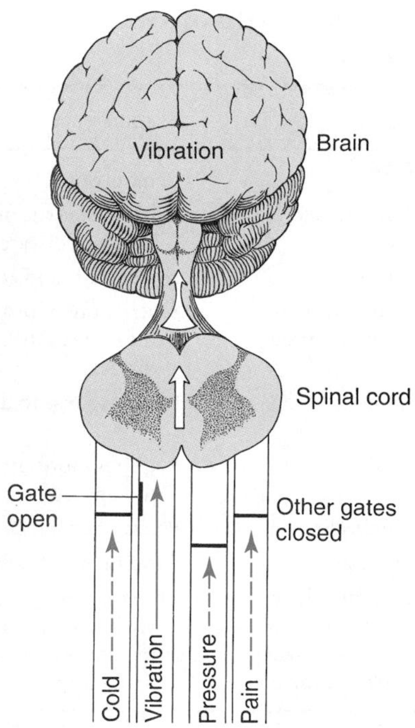

FIGURE 19–2. Depiction of the gate-control theory.

Endogenous Opioids

Another mechanism for diminishing the perception of pain involves **endogenous opioids** (naturally produced morphine-like chemicals). The endogenous opioids *endorphins, dynorphins,* and *enkephalins* reduce pain. Their release is stimulated by two neurotransmitters, serotonin and norepinephrine (see Chap. 5). When endogenous opioids are released, they are thought to bind to sites on the nerve cell's membrane that block the transmission of pain-conducting neurotransmitters such as substance P and prostaglandins (Fig. 19-3).

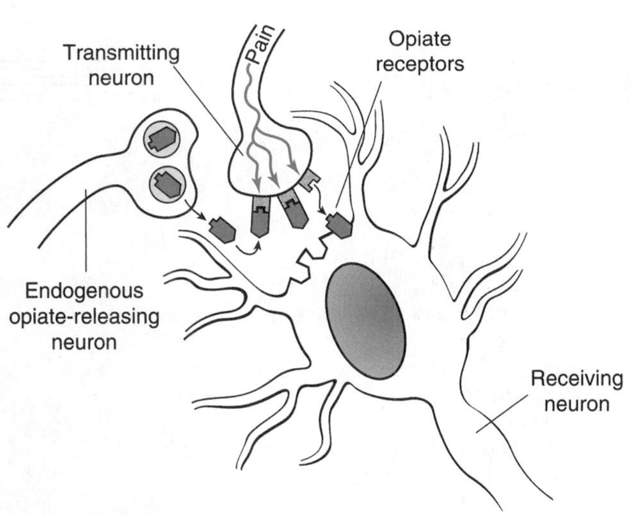

FIGURE 19–3. Mechanism of pain transmission and interference.

TYPES OF PAIN

Not all pain is exactly the same. Five types of pain have been described according to source (cutaneous, visceral, or neuropathic) or duration (acute or chronic).

Cutaneous Pain

Cutaneous pain (discomfort that originates at the skin level) is a commonly experienced sensation resulting from some form of trauma. The depth of the trauma determines the type of sensation felt. According to Bullock and Henze (2000), damage confined to the epidermis produces a burning sensation. At the dermis level, the pain is localized and superficial. Subcutaneous tissue injuries produce an aching, throbbing pain. **Somatic pain** (discomfort generated from deeper connective tissue) develops from injury to structures such as muscles, tendons, and joints.

Visceral Pain

Visceral pain (discomfort arising from internal organs) is associated with disease or injury. It is sometimes referred or poorly localized. **Referred pain** (discomfort perceived in a general area of the body, usually away from the site of stimulation) is not experienced in the exact site where an organ is located (Fig. 19-4). Visceral pain is accompanied by other autonomic nervous system symptoms such as nausea, vomiting, pallor, hypotension, and sweating.

Neuropathic Pain

Neuropathic pain (pain with atypical characteristics) is also called functional pain. This type of pain is often experienced days, weeks, or even months after the source of the pain has been treated and resolved (Copstead, 1995). This has led some to speculate that a dysfunctional chemical message is being transmitted to the brain.

One example of neuropathic pain is *phantom limb pain* or *phantom limb sensation,* in which a person with an amputated limb perceives that the limb still exists and feels burning, itching, and deep pain in tissues that have been surgically removed.

Acute Pain

Acute pain (discomfort that has a short duration) lasts for a few seconds to less than 6 months. It is associated with tissue trauma, including surgery, or some other recent identifiable etiology. Although severe initially, acute pain eases with healing and eventually goes away. The gradual reduction in pain promotes coping with the discomfort because there is a rein-

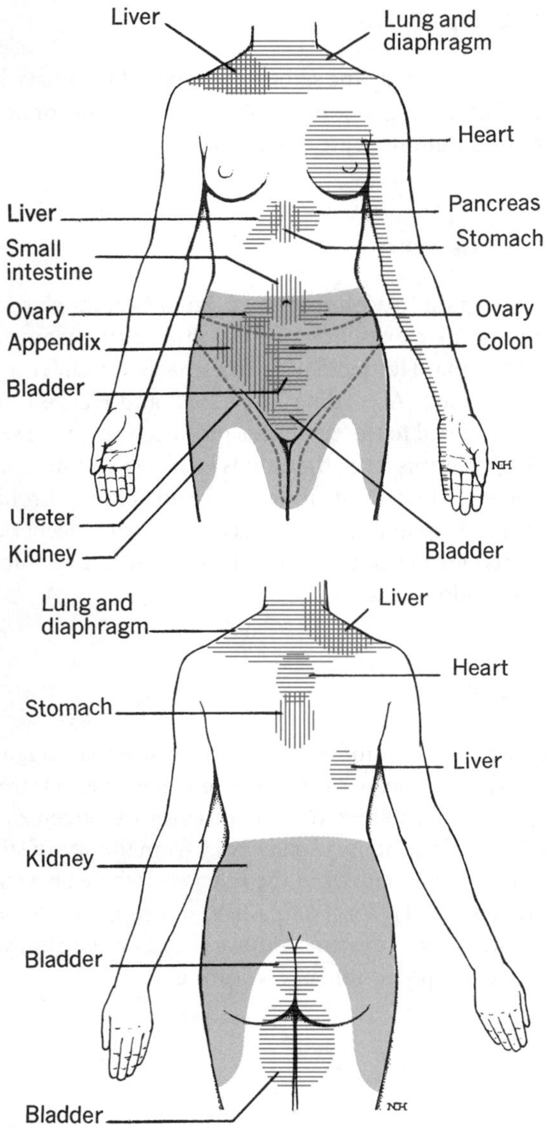

FIGURE 19–4. Areas of referred pain.

forcing belief that the pain will disappear in time. Acute and chronic pain both result in physical and emotional distress and can be intermittent (incorporating periods of relief), but that is where the similarities end.

Chronic Pain

The characteristics of **chronic pain** (discomfort that lasts longer than 6 months) are almost totally opposite from acute pain (Table 19-1). The longer pain exists, the more far-reaching its effects on the sufferer (Display 19-1). Others begin to show negative reactions to the chronic pain sufferer, such as:

- Saying they are tired of hearing about the pain
- Ignoring the sufferer's concerns and complaints
- Getting angry
- Suggesting that the pain has a psychological basis
- Telling the patient he or she is using the pain to manipulate others for selfish purposes
- Criticizing the patient for using drugs "as a crutch"
- Suggesting that the patient is addicted to pain medication (American Pain Society, 1999a)

TABLE 19–1. **Characteristics of Acute and Chronic Pain**

Acute Pain	Chronic Pain
Recent onset	Remote onset
Symptomatic of primary injury or disease	Uncharacteristic of primary injury or disease
Specific and localized	Nonspecific and generalized
Severity associated with the acuity of the injury or disease process	Severity out of proportion to the stage of the injury or disease
Favorable response to drug therapy	Poor response to drug therapy
Requires less and less drug therapy	Requires more and more drug therapy
Diminishes with healing	Persists beyond healing stage
Suffering is decreased	Suffering is intensified
Associated with sympathetic nervous system responses such as hypertension, tachycardia, restlessness, anxiety	Absence of autonomic nervous system responses; manifests depression and irritability

Pain Assessment

Because of the wide variety of types of pain and effects on lifestyle and personal relationships, standardized methods for assessing pain and treating it aggressively are needed. According to the American Pain Society (1999b), "the most

DISPLAY 19–1

Quality-of-Life Activities Affected by Chronic Pain

Exercising
Working around the house
Sleeping
Enjoying hobbies and leisure time
Socializing
Walking
Concentrating
Having sex
Maintaining relationships with family and friends
Working a full day at employment
Caring for children

common reason for unrelieved pain in U.S. hospitals is the failure of staff to routinely assess pain and pain relief." Because no machines or laboratory tests can measure pain, nurses are limited to the subjective information that only patients can supply.

A basic pain assessment includes the patient's description of the *onset, quality, intensity, location,* and *duration* of the pain (Table 19-2). Nurses also ask what other symptoms accompany the pain and what if anything makes it better or worse. During an admission assessment, the nurse also asks questions such as:

- What activities are you unable to do because of pain?
- Do you ever take pain medication? If so, when?
- What are the names and dosages of pain medicine you take?
- What nondrug methods, such as rest, do you use to relieve your pain?
- How does your pain change with self-treatment?
- What are your preferences for managing your pain?
- What pain level is an acceptable goal for you if total pain relief is not possible?

When caring for a patient listed in Display 19-2, the nurse must assess for the presence of behavioral signs that commonly accompany pain, such as:

- Moaning
- Crying
- Grimacing
- Guarded position
- Increased vital signs
- Reduced social interactions
- Irritability
- Difficulty concentrating
- Changes in eating and sleeping

Autonomic nervous system responses such as tachycardia, hypertension, dilated pupils, perspiration, pallor, rapid and shallow breathing, urinary retention, reduced bowel motility, and elevated blood glucose levels may be apparent. Patients with chronic pain are not as likely to manifest autonomic nervous system responses.

DISPLAY 19–2

Underassessed and Undertreated Pain Populations

- Infants
- Children younger than 7 years of age
- Culturally diverse patients
- Patients who are mentally challenged (retarded)
- Patients with dementia (diminished brain function)
- Patients who are hearing- or speech-impaired
- Patients who are psychologically disturbed

ASSESSMENT TOOLS

Pain disorder clinics ask patients to complete a questionnaire to help assess their pain. In the McGill-Melzack Pain Questionnaire, patients are instructed to check the words that best describe their pain (Fig. 19-5). The words are categorized according to the quality of the pain; they also have a numeric value. The total score quantifies the severity of the patient's pain. By comparing changes in the number and types of word choices, pain therapists can evaluate whether the patient is improving.

Nurses can use any of four simpler assessment tools to quantify a patient's pain intensity: a numeric scale, a word scale, a linear scale, and a picture scale (Fig. 19-6). Patients identify how their pain compares with the choices on the scale. One scale is not better than another. A numeric scale is commonly used when assessing adults. The picture scale is best for children and patients who are culturally diverse or mentally challenged. Regardless of the assessment tool used, many patients underrate or minimize their pain intensity.

ASSESSMENT STANDARDS

The American Pain Society has proposed that pain assessment should be considered the fifth vital sign—the patient's

TABLE 19–2. **Components of Pain Assessment**

Characteristic	Description	Examples
Onset	Time or circumstances under which the pain became apparent	After eating, while shoveling snow, during the night
Quality	Sensory experiences and degree of suffering	Throbbing, crushing, agonizing, annoying
Intensity	Magnitude of pain	None, slight, mild, moderate, severe; or numeric scale from 0 to 10
Location	Anatomic site	Chest, abdomen, jaw
Duration	Time span of pain	Continuous, intermittent, hours, weeks, months

McGill - Melzack Pain Questionnaire

Patient's Name ________ Date ________ Time ________ am/pm
Analgesic(s) ________ Dosage ________ Time Given ________ am/pm
________ Dosage ________ Time Given ________ am/pm

Analgesic Time Difference (hours): +4 +1 +2 +3

PRI: S ____ (1-10) A ____ (11-15) E ____ (16) M(S) ____ (17-19) M(AE) ____ (20) M(T) ____ (17-20) PRT(T) ____ (1-20)

1 FLICKERING, QUIVERING, PULSING, THROBBING, BEATING, POUNDING
2 JUMPING, FLASHING, SHOOTING
3 PRICKING, BORING, DRILLING, STABBING, LANCINATING
4 SHARP, CUTTING, LACERATING
5 PINCHING, PRESSING, GNAWING, CRAMPING, CRUSHING
6 TUGGING, PULLING, WRENCHING
7 HOT, BURNING, SCALDING, SEARING
8 TINGLING, ITCHY, SMARTING, STINGING
9 DULL, SORE, HURTING, ACHING, HEAVY
10 TENDER, TAUT, RASPING, SPLITTING
11 TIRING, EXHAUSTING
12 SICKENING, SUFFOCATING
13 FEARFUL, FRIGHTFUL, TERRIFYING
14 PUNISHING, GRUELLING, CRUEL, VICIOUS, KILLING
15 WRETCHED, BLINDING
16 ANNOYING, TROUBLESOME, MISERABLE, INTENSE, UNBEARABLE
17 SPREADING, RADIATING, PENETRATING, PIERCING
18 TIGHT, NUMB, DRAWING, SQUEEZING, TEARING
19 COOL, COLD, FREEZING
20 NAGGING, NAUSEATING, AGONIZING, DREADFUL, TORTURING

PPI
0 No pain
1 MILD
2 DISCOMFORTING
3 DISTRESSING
4 HORRIBLE
5 EXCRUCIATING

PPI ____ COMMENTS:

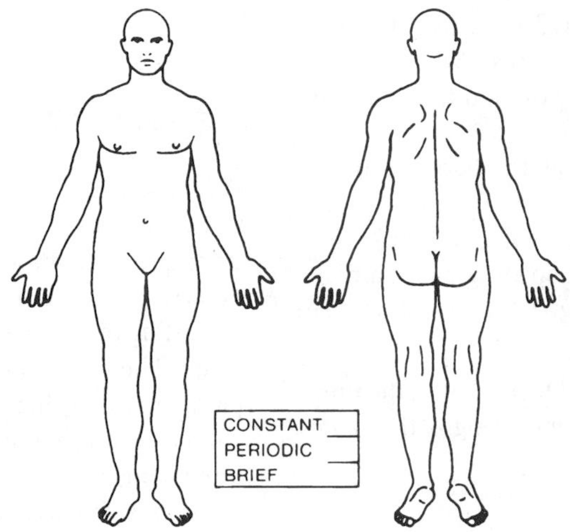

CONSTANT
PERIODIC
BRIEF

ACCOMPANYING SYMPTOMS: NAUSEA, HEADACHE, DIZZINESS, DROWSINESS, CONSTIPATION, DIARRHEA
COMMENTS:

SLEEP: GOOD, FITFUL, CAN'T SLEEP
COMMENTS:

FOOD INTAKE: GOOD, SOME, LITTLE, NONE
COMMENTS:

ACTIVITY: GOOD, SOME, LITTLE, NONE
COMMENTS:

FIGURE 19–5. Individuals with chronic pain use this pain-assessment questionnaire or one like it. Key: PRI(T)—pain rating index total; (S)—sensory terms; (A)—affective terms; (E)—evaluative terms; (M)—miscellaneous descriptors. The abbreviation PPI refers to present pain index, identified according to the words in the last box in the second column.

pain level should be checked and documented every time the nurse assesses temperature, pulse, respiration, and blood pressure. Pain is assessed whenever the nurse considers it appropriate, and routinely in the following circumstances:

- When the patient is admitted
- At least once per shift when pain is an actual or potential problem
- When the patient is at rest, and when involved in a nursing activity
- After each potentially painful procedure or treatment.
- Before implementing a pain-management intervention, such as administering an **analgesic** (pain-relieving drug), and again 30 minutes later

Pain Management

Pain management (techniques for preventing, reducing, or relieving pain) is a major focus for quality improvement programs in health care agencies. To demonstrate the importance of managing pain, the Joint Commission on Accreditation of Healthcare Organizations (JCAHO, 1999) requires evidence that the pain of terminally ill patients is being adequately treated. The American Pain Society, working with the Agency for Health Care Policy and Research (a division of the Department of Health and Human Services), has developed *Standards for the Relief of Acute Pain and Cancer Pain* (Display 19-3). The objective of this collaborative effort is to improve

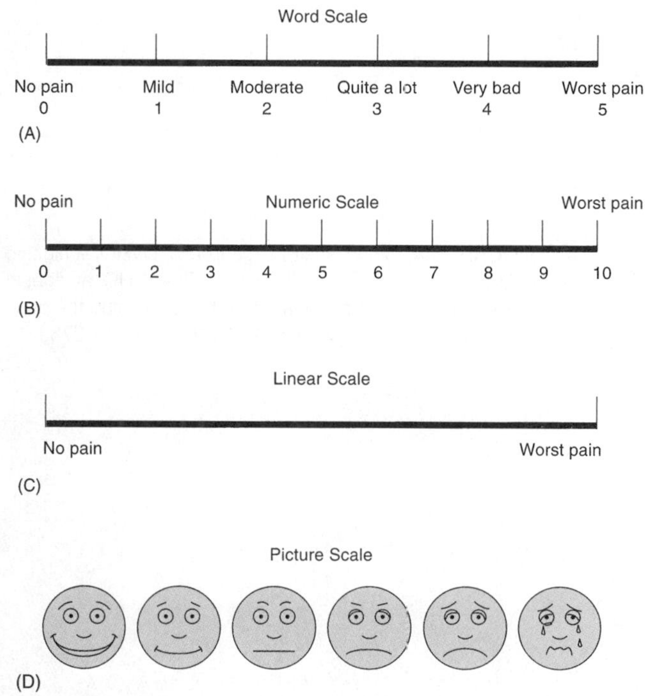

FIGURE 19–6. Pain assessment tools: (*A*) word scale, (*B*) numeric scale, (*C*) linear scale, (*D*) picture scale.

DISPLAY 19-3

Standards for the Relief of Acute Pain and Cancer Pain

Standard I

Acute pain and cancer pain are recognized and effectively treated.

Standard II

Information about analgesics is readily available.

Standard III

Patients are informed on admission, both orally and in writing, that effective pain relief is an important part of their treatment, that their communication of unrelieved pain is essential, and that health professionals will respond quickly to their reports of pain.

Standard IV

Explicit policies for use of advanced analgesic technologies are defined.

Standard V

Adherence to standards is monitored by an interdisciplinary committee.

Reprinted with permission from American Pain Society, Principles of analgesic use in the treatment of acute pain and chronic cancer pain, 4th ed., Skokie, Illinois, 1999.

the way pain is assessed and controlled. The original effort has been expanded to include the assessment and treatment of pain in all patient populations (Dahl et al., 1998).

Most techniques for managing pain fall into one of four general physiologic categories (Table 19-3).

DRUG THERAPY

Drug therapy, either alone or in combination with other therapeutic measures, is the cornerstone of pain management. The World Health Organization (Jadad & Browman, 1995) recommends following a three-tiered drug approach based on the pain intensity and the patient's response to therapy (Fig. 19-7). Physicians prescribe one or more of the following classes of drugs: **nonopioids** (nonnarcotic drugs), **opioids** (narcotic drugs), and **adjuvants** (drugs that assist in accomplishing the desired effect of a primary drug). The choice of drug, its dose, and the timing of medication administration are critical in achieving optimal pain relief.

TABLE 19–3. **Approaches to Pain Management**

Approach	Intervention	Examples
Interrupting pain-transmitting chemicals at the site of injury	Local anesthetics, anti-inflammatory drugs	Procaine, lidocaine, aspirin, ibuprofen, acetaminophen, naproxen, indomethacin
Altering transmission at the spinal cord	Intraspinal anesthesia and analgesia, neurosurgery	Epidural, caudal, rhizotomy, cordotomy, sympathectomy
Using gate-closing mechanisms	Cutaneous stimuli	Massage, acupuncture, acupressure, heat, cold, therapeutic touch, electrical stimulation
Blocking brain perception	Narcotics, nondrug techniques	Morphine, codeine, hypnosis, imagery, distraction

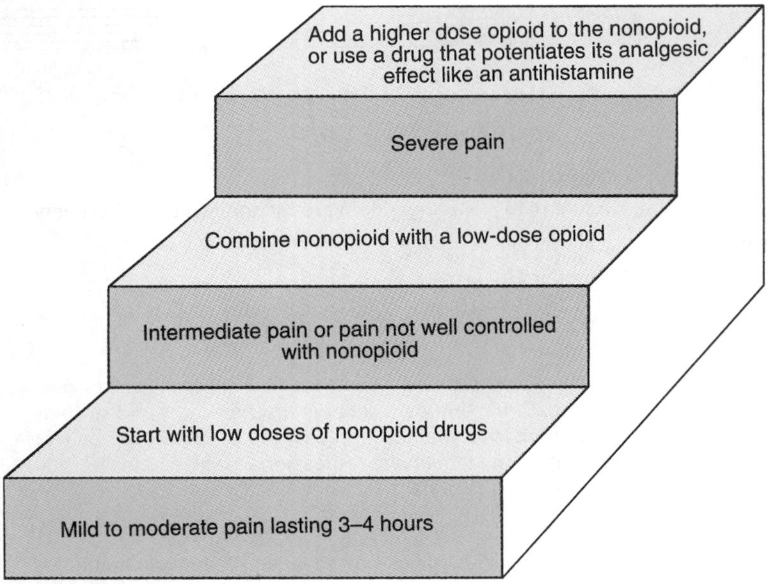
Add a higher dose opioid to the nonopioid, or use a drug that potentiates its analgesic effect like an antihistamine
Severe pain
Combine nonopioid with a low-dose opioid
Intermediate pain or pain not well controlled with nonopioid
Start with low doses of nonopioid drugs
Mild to moderate pain lasting 3–4 hours

FIGURE 19–7. World Health Organization (WHO) analgesic ladder. (Jadad AR, Browman GP: The WHO analgesic ladder for cancer pain management: Stepping up the quality of its evaluation. JAMA 1995; 274[23]; 1870–1873.)

Nonopioid Drugs

Nonopioid drugs include aspirin, acetaminophen (Tylenol), and nonsteroidal anti-inflammatory drugs (NSAIDs), such as ibuprofen (Motrin, Advil, Nuprin), ketoprofen (Orudis KT), and naproxen sodium (Naprosyn, Aleve). These drugs relieve pain by altering neurotransmission peripherally at the site of injury.

One of the newest categories of nonopioid drugs is the cyclooxygenase (COX)-2 inhibitors, such as celecoxib (Celebrex) and rofecoxib (Vioxx). COX is an enzyme: COX-1 protects the gastrointestinal tract and urinary system and COX-2 promotes the production of pain-transmitting and inflammatory chemicals such as prostaglandins. The inhibition of COX-2 results in pain relief. COX-2 inhibiters are superior to older NSAIDs that equally suppress COX-1 and COX-2 enzymes. By inhibiting COX-2 to a greater degree than COX-1, they cause fewer undesirable side effects.

Most nonopioids are very effective at relieving pain caused by inflammation. The exception is acetaminophen, which has limited anti-inflammatory activity; however, it is still an effective analgesic. The efficacy of COX-2 inhibitors for relieving other types of pain, such as headaches and body aches from influenza, is not established.

Except for the new COX-2 inhibitors, almost all the NSAIDs cause gastrointestinal irritation and bleeding, so they should be given with food.

Opioid Drugs

When pain is no longer controlled with a nonopioid, the nonopioid is combined with an opioid—for example, aspirin with codeine or acetaminophen with codeine. **Opioids** (synthetic narcotics) and opiate analgesics, narcotics containing opium or its derivatives, are **controlled substances** (drugs whose prescription and dispensing are regulated by federal law because they have the potential for being abused). Examples are:

- Morphine sulfate
- Codeine sulfate
- Meperidine (Demerol)
- Fentanyl (Duragesic, Sublimaze)

Narcotics interfere with central pain perception (at the brain) and are generally reserved for treating moderate and severe pain. They are administered by the oral, rectal, transdermal, or parenteral (injected) route.

Opioids and opiates cause sedation, nausea, constipation, and respiratory depression. Because of an exaggerated fear of causing addiction (see below), narcotics tend to be underprescribed, even if patients can benefit from their use. When they are used, the same bias leads some nurses to administer the lowest dosage of a prescribed range or to delay administration until the maximum time between dosages has elapsed. Consequently, many patients experience inadequate pain management, which contributes to long-term suffering and disability. In addition, unrelieved pain can lead to pneumonia due to shallow breathing, suppressed coughing, and reduced movement. Psychological effects of unrelieved pain include anxiety, depression, and despair, even to the point of suicide.

Patient-Controlled Analgesia

Patient-controlled analgesia (PCA; intervention that allows patients to self-administer narcotic pain medication) involves the use of an infusion device. PCA is used primarily to relieve acute pain after surgery, but this technology is finding its way into the home health arena, where it is being used by patients with cancer.

PCA has several advantages to both patients and nurses:

- Pain relief is rapid because the drug is delivered intravenously.
- Pain is kept within a constant tolerable level (Fig. 19-8).
- Less drug is actually used, because the pain is continuously controlled with small doses.
- Patients are spared the discomfort of repeated injections.
- Anxiety is reduced, because the patient does not need to wait for the nurse to prepare and administer an injection.
- Side effects are reduced with smaller individual dosages and lower total dosages.
- Patients tend to ambulate and move about more, reducing the potential for complications from immobility.
- Patients can take an active role in their pain management.
- The nurse is free to carry out other nursing responsibilities.

The infusion device is programmed by the nurse so that the patient can receive a **bolus** or **loading dose** (larger dose of drug, administered initially or when pain is exceptionally intense) and additional lower doses at frequent intervals depending on the patient's level of discomfort (Skill 19-1). Once a dose is delivered, the patient cannot administer another dose for a specified amount of time; this period, known as a *lockout,* prevents overdoses.

Intraspinal Analgesia

Intraspinal analgesia (method of relieving pain by instilling a narcotic or local anesthetic via a catheter into the subarachnoid or epidural space of the spinal cord) is another technique for managing pain. The intraspinal analgesic is administered several times per day or as a continuous low-dose infusion. Intraspinal analgesia relieves pain while producing minimal systemic drug effects. In patients who need long-term analgesia, the risk for injuring the subcutaneous tissue with repeated injections (which may eventually lessen drug absorption) is diminished with the use of intraspinal analgesia.

Adjuvant Drugs

Analgesic drugs are combined with a wide range of adjuvant drugs to improve pain control. The categories of adjuvant drugs and examples of each are:

- Antidepressants: tricyclic antidepressants such as amitryptyline (Elavil); selective serotonin reuptake inhibitors such as fluoxetine (Prozac) and paroxetine (Paxil)
- Anticonvulsants: carbamazepine (Tegretol), gabapentin (Neurontin)
- N-methyl-D-aspartate (NMDA) receptor antagonists: dextromethorphan, ketamine (Ketalar)
- Nutritional supplements such as glucosamine

Each category acts by different mechanisms. The antidepressants may produce their analgesic-enhancing effect by increasing norepinephrine and serotonin levels, augmenting the release of endorphins. Anticonvulsants are believed to inhibit the transmission of pain by regulating and potentiating the inhibitory neurotransmitter gamma-aminobutyric acid (GABA) (see Chap. 5). NMDA drugs interfere with the function of nociceptive nerve fibers, perhaps blocking the release of substance P, its nerve-sensitizing properties, and other inflammatory chemicals. Those who favor **alternative medical therapy** (treatment outside the mainstream of traditional medicine) contend that glucosamine slows the breakdown of joint cartilage and promotes its regeneration, relieving pain associated with joint diseases.

Adjuvant drugs are never used as a first-line treatment for pain. However, when they are used as combination drug

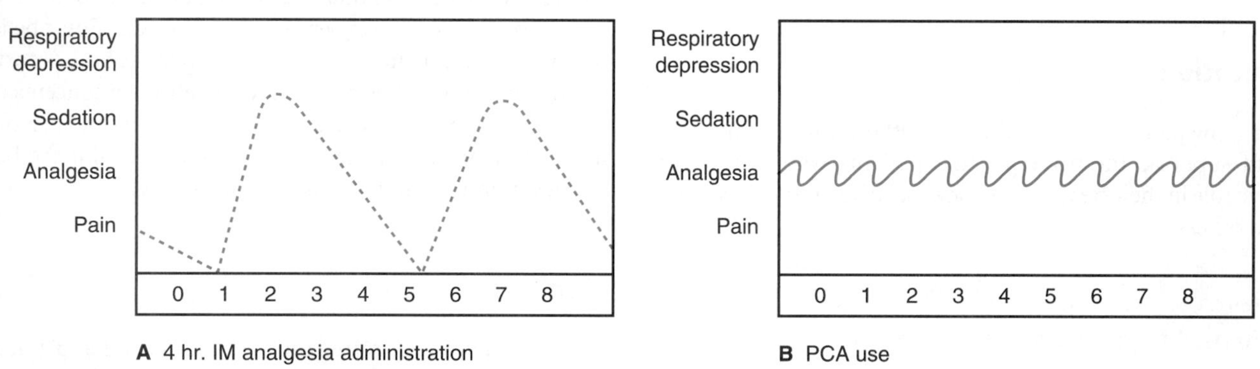

FIGURE 19–8. Pain is less effectively controlled and produces more side effects with (*A*) IM analgesia than with (*B*) patient-controlled analgesia (PCA). (Adapted from Hormer M, Rosen M, Vickers MD, Eds. Patient-Controlled Analgesia. St. Louis, CV Mosby, 1985.)

therapy, the dose of the primary drug can often be decreased. With a lowered opioid dosage, for instance, the patient will have less sedation and fewer undesirable side effects.

SURGICAL APPROACHES

Intractable pain (pain unresponsive to other methods of pain management) can be relieved with surgery. Rhizotomy and cordotomy are neurosurgical procedures that provide pain relief.

A **rhizotomy** (surgical sectioning of a nerve root close to the spinal cord) prevents sensory impulses from entering the spinal cord and traveling to the brain. Generally more than one nerve needs to be sectioned to achieve the desired result. Chemical rhizotomy, using alcohol or phenol, and percutaneous rhizotomy, which uses radiofrequency waves, are nonsurgical alternatives for destroying nerve fibers. A **cordotomy** (surgical interruption of pain pathways in the spinal cord) is accomplished by cutting bundles of nerves. Although the sensation of pain is interrupted with both procedures, the perception of pressure and temperature is also inhibited in the area supplied by the nerves. Consequently, there is a greater risk for unnoticed injury.

NONDRUG/NONSURGICAL INTERVENTIONS

Several additional interventions can be used to help manage pain. Some—education, imagery, distraction, relaxation techniques, and applications of heat or cold—are independent nursing measures. Others—transcutaneous electrical nerve stimulation, acupuncture and acupressure, percutaneous electrical nerve stimulation, biofeedback, and hypnosis—require collaboration with individuals who have specialized training and expertise. The latter interventions are more likely to be used for patients with chronic pain or those in whom acute pain-management techniques have been unsuccessful or are contraindicated.

Education

Educating patients about pain and methods for pain management supports the principle that patients who assume an active role in their treatment achieve positive outcomes sooner than others.

Patient Teaching For

Pain and Its Management

Teach the patient or the family to do the following:

- Ask the doctor what to expect from the disorder or its treatment.
- Discuss pain-control methods that have worked well or not so well before.
- Talk with the doctor and nurses about any concerns you have about pain medicine.
- Identify any drug allergies you have.
- Inform the doctor and nurses about other medicines you take, in case they may interact with pain medications.
- Help the doctor and nurses measure your pain on a pain scale by stating the number or word that best describes the pain.
- Ask for or take pain-relieving drugs when pain begins or before an activity that causes pain.
- Set a pain-control goal, such as having no pain worse than 4 on a scale of 1 to 10.
- Inform the doctor and nurses if the pain medication is not working.
- Perform simple techniques such as abdominal breathing and jaw relaxation to increase comfort.
- Consult with the doctor or nurses about using cold or hot packs or other nondrug techniques to enhance pain control.

Patients should not expect to be totally pain-free, but they should not have to endure severe pain.

Imagery

Imagery (using the mind to visualize an experience) is sometimes referred to as intentional daydreaming. The images a person selects are chosen from pleasant memories. In *guided imagery,* the nurse or another person suggests the image to be used, such as a walk in the woods, and describes the sensory experiences in great detail. Tape recordings for guided imagery and relaxation (discussed later) are also available, but the subject matter and descriptions can become boring when played over and over again. Some prefer to use taped sounds of nature, making it easy to conjure up different images each time.

Physiologically, the process of imagery produces an alteration in consciousness that allows the patient to forget about uncomfortable sensory experiences, such as pain. Some believe that imagery stimulates the visual portion of the brain's cortex, located in the right hemisphere, where abstract concepts and creative activities take place (Fig. 19-9). While the person is imaging, neurotransmitters are released that calm the body physically and promote emotional well-being.

Meditation

Meditation (concentrating on a word or idea that promotes tranquility) is similar to imagery, except the subject matter tends to be more spiritual. Sometimes meditation involves silent repetition of a word, such as "love" or "peace," a prayer, or a statement that reflects a strong personal or reli-

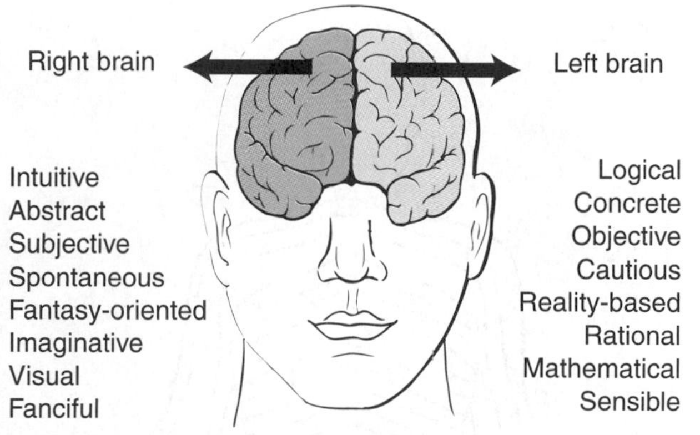

FIGURE 19–9. Right hemispheric functions are utilized during imagery and meditation.

gious belief. Those who use this technique successfully tend to experience a relaxed state with lowered blood pressure and pulse rates.

Distraction

Distraction (intentional diversion of attention) switches the person's focus from an unpleasant sensory experience to one that is neutral or more pleasant. The distraction occurs in the "here and now"; it is not imagined. Examples are talking with someone, watching television, participating in a hobby, and listening to music. The mind can attend to only one stimulus at a time: while the person is occupied with the diversional activity, the brain is blocked from perceiving painful stimuli.

Relaxation

Relaxation (technique for releasing muscle tension and quieting the mind) helps to reduce pain, relieve anxiety, and promote a sense of well-being. Consciously relaxing breaks the circuit among neurons that are overloading the brain with distressing thoughts and painful stimuli. Patients can be taught the following procedure for relaxation.

Patient Teaching For
Relaxation

Teach the patient to do the following:

- Assume a comfortable position, either sitting or lying down.
- Close your eyes and clear your mind.
- Let the chair or bed effortlessly support your body.
- Become aware of how your body feels.
- Take deep abdominal breaths.
- Focus on the rhythm of your breathing.
- Relax with each breath in and out.
- Tighten and then release muscles in sequential parts of your body, such as the toes, feet, lower legs, thighs, and buttocks. Progress toward the face and scalp.
- Visualize healing energy flowing from your feet through your head. Release your worries and discomfort as it passes through.
- Let yourself sleep, if possible.
- At the end of the session, wake up or begin to move gradually.

Heat and Cold

Applications of heat or cold (thermal therapy) are well-established techniques for relieving pain. In some locations of practice, nurses must obtain permission from the physician before using heat or cold.

Pain caused by an injury is best treated initially with cold applications (ice bag or chemical pack). The cold reduces localized swelling and decreases vasodilation, which carries pain-producing chemicals into the circulation. Many believe that cold applications relieve pain faster and sustain pain relief longer. Heat applications (hot water bottle, rice bag [cloth bag containing uncooked rice that is heated in the microwave], or moist packs) are placed over a painful area 24 to 48 hours after the injury.

Thermal applications, whether hot or cold, are never used longer than 20 minutes at any one time (see Chap. 28). The skin is always protected with an insulating layer, such as a cloth or towel. The patient should never go to sleep while a hot or cold pack is in place, and hot and cold applications are contraindicated in areas of the body where circulation or sensation is impaired.

Menthol (Icy Hot, Heet, Ben Gay) and capsaicin (Zostrix; a compound found in red peppers) are chemicals sometimes applied topically. Both increase blood flow in the area of application, creating a warm/cool feeling that lasts for several hours.

Transcutaneous Electrical Nerve Stimulation

Transcutaneous electrical nerve stimulation (TENS; medically prescribed pain-management technique that delivers bursts of electricity to the skin and underlying nerves) is an intervention implemented by nurses (Skill 19-2). The electrical stimulus, generated by a battery-powered stimulator, is perceived by the patient as a pleasant tapping, tingling, vibrating, or buzzing sensation. TENS is used intermittently for 15 to 30 minutes or longer whenever the patient feels a need for it.

For some time, TENS has been used by patients with chronic pain, but today it is being used by surgical patients. Reports of its effectiveness range from "useless" to "fantastic."

No one is sure exactly how TENS works. Some think the gate-control theory explains its effectiveness. Supposedly the transmission of electrical stimuli over larger myelinated nerves takes precedence over the transmission of pain-producing stimuli to the brain. Others believe TENS stimulates the body to release endogenous opioids, and still others suggest that its effectiveness is based on the power of suggestion.

TENS is a nonnarcotic, noninvasive method and has no toxic side effects. It is contraindicated in pregnant women because its effect on the unborn fetus has not been determined. Patients with cardiac pacemakers (especially the demand type), patients prone to an irregular heart beat, and patients with previous heart attacks are not candidates for TENS.

Acupuncture and Acupressure

Acupuncture (pain-management technique in which long, thin needles are inserted into the skin) and **acupressure** (technique that involves tissue compression rather than needles to reduce pain) are based on ancient traditions of Chinese medicine. Both techniques have been demonstrated to prevent or relieve pain, but their exact analgesic mechanisms are not completely understood. Some speculate that these techniques stimulate the body's production of endogenous opioids or that the twisting and vibration of the needles and the pressure applied are forms of cutaneous stimuli that close the gates to pain-transmitting neurochemicals. Acupuncture and acupressure are becoming more accepted as legitimate forms of pain therapy in the United States (National Institutes of Health, 1997).

Percutaneous Electrical Nerve Stimulation

One of the newest innovations in acute and chronic pain management is **percutaneous electrical nerve stimulation** (PENS; pain-management technique involving a combination of acupuncture needles and TENS). Acupuncture-like needles are inserted within soft tissue and an electrical stimulus is conducted through the needles (Fig. 19-10). PENS is considered superior to TENS in providing pain relief because the needles are located closer to nerve endings. PENS therapy is administered three times a week for 30 minutes for a total of 3 weeks (White et al., 1999). The technique has been successful in research trials on patients with low back pain, pain caused by the spread of cancer to bones, shingles (acute herpes zoster viral infection), and migraine headaches.

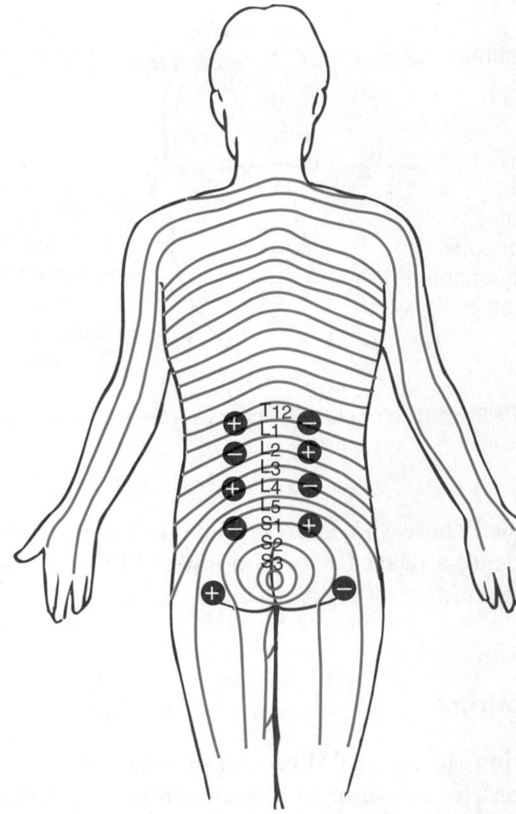

FIGURE 19–10. With PENS therapy, five pairs of electrical stimulating leads (alternating positive and negative current) are connected to needles inserted in the lumbar and sacral regions of the spine.

Biofeedback

Biofeedback (technique in which the patient learns to control or alter a physiologic phenomenon [such as pain, blood pressure, headache, heart rate and rhythm, or seizures]) is used as an adjunct to traditional pain management. Initially, the patient is connected to a physiologic sensing instrument such as a pulse oximeter or an electromyography machine. The instrument produces a visual or audible signal that correlates with the person's heart rate, skin temperature, or muscle tension. The patient is encouraged to reduce or extinguish the signal using whatever mechanism he or she can—generally, by physically relaxing. The feedback from the machine demonstrates to the patient how well he or she is accomplishing the goal. Eventually, patients can learn to control their symptoms without the assistance of the equipment, using self-suggestion alone.

Hypnosis

Hypnosis (therapeutic technique in which a person enters a trancelike state) results in an alteration in perception and memory. During hypnosis, the suggestion is made that the person's pain will be eliminated or the sensation will be experienced in a more pleasant way.

Although self-hypnosis is possible, more often hypnosis is induced with the help of a hypnotherapist. Hypnotherapists receive special clinical training; their professional organizations include the American Society of Clinical Hypnosis and the International Society for Medical and Psychological Hypnosis.

Nursing Implications

Nurses should increase their knowledge about pain, take every patient's pain seriously, and implement measures for treating pain effectively. Whenever a patient's pain is not controlled to his or her satisfaction, the nurse pursues better goal achievement by collaborating with pain experts.

Nursing Guidelines For

Managing Pain

☑ Never doubt the patient's description of pain or need for relief.
RATIONALE: Bias on the nurse's part may lead to withholding prescribed medication or undertreating the symptoms.

☑ Follow the written medical orders for administering pain medications.
RATIONALE: This practice demonstrates compliance with nurse practice acts.

☑ Administer pain-relieving drugs as soon as the need becomes evident.
RATIONALE: Administering drugs promptly reduces the patient's suffering.

☑ Consult the physician if the current drug therapy is not controlling the patient's pain.
RATIONALE: Consulting with the physician demonstrates patient advocacy.

☑ Collaborate with the physician to develop several pain-management options involving combinations of drugs, alternative routes of administration, and different dosing schedules.
RATIONALE: Developing options individualizes pain management.

☑ Support the formation of an interdisciplinary pain-management team (physicians, surgeons, nurses, pharmacists, anesthesiologists, physical therapists, massage therapists, and so forth) who can be consulted on hard-to-manage pain problems.
RATIONALE: Such a group makes available the expertise of a variety of practitioners.

☑ Administer pain medication before an activity that produces or intensifies pain.
RATIONALE: This timing prevents pain, which is much easier than treating it.

TABLE 19–4. **Adult Equianalgesic Doses**

Drug	Intramuscular Dose	Oral Dose	Duration (hours)
Morphine sulfate	10 mg	30–60 mg	3–7
Meperidine (Demerol)	75 mg	300 mg	2–4
Hydromorphone (Dilaudid)	1.5 mg	7.5 mg	4–5
Codeine	120 mg	200 mg	4–6

Karch AM. Lippincott's nursing drug guide. Philadelphia, Lippincott Williams & Wilkins, 1999.

☑ When the patient's pain is continuous, administer analgesic drugs on a scheduled basis rather than irregularly.
RATIONALE: Giving the drugs regularly controls pain when it is at a lower intensity.

☑ Monitor for drug side effects, such as respiratory depression, decreased levels of consciousness, nausea, vomiting, and constipation.
RATIONALE: Careful monitoring demonstrates concern for the patient's safety and comfort.

☑ Consult the professional literature or experts on the **equianalgesic dose** (oral dose that provides the same level of pain relief as a parenteral dose; Table 19-4).
RATIONALE: This prevents undertreatment of pain due to changes in drug absorption or drug metabolism.

☑ Change the patient's position, elevate a swollen limb to reduce swelling, loosen a tight dressing, and assist the patient with bowel or bladder elimination.
RATIONALE: These measures reduce factors that intensify the pain experience.

☑ Implement independent and prescribed nondrug interventions, such as patient teaching, imagery, meditation, distraction, and TENS, as additional techniques for pain management.
RATIONALE: These techniques reduce mild to moderate pain when used alone or potentiate pain management when combined with drug therapy.

☑ Allow rest periods between activities.
RATIONALE: Exhaustion reduces the patient's ability to cope with pain.

Patients with pain are likely to have a variety of nursing diagnoses, including the following:

- Pain
- Chronic pain
- Anxiety
- Fear
- Ineffective individual coping
- Knowledge deficit: pain management

The nursing care plan is an example of how the steps in the nursing process are followed when planning the care of a patient with Pain, a nursing diagnosis defined in the NANDA taxonomy (1999) as "an unpleasant sensory and emotional experience arising from actual or potential tissue damage or described in terms of such damage (International Association for the Study of Pain); sudden or slow onset of any intensity from mild to severe with an anticipated or predictable end and a duration of less than 6 months."

ADDICTION

One of the leading factors interfering with adequate pain management is the fear of addiction. The American Pain Society (1999) defines addiction as "a pattern of compulsive drug use characterized by a continued craving for an opioid and the need to use the opioid for effects other than pain relief." Statistics indicate that the fear of addiction is greater than the reality.

Nurses often assume that requests for frequent doses of narcotics are motivated by a patient's desire to experience the drug's pleasant effects. What may be happening is that the prescribed dose or frequency of administration is not controlling the pain, a phenomenon that occurs as patients develop drug tolerance. Nurses may undertreat the pain or may convince the physician to prescribe a placebo.

PLACEBOS

A **placebo** (inactive substance) is sometimes prescribed as a substitute for an analgesic drug. Placebos can relieve pain, especially when patients have confidence in their health care providers. The trust a patient has in the nurse or physician probably has more to do with the efficacy of placebos than any other factor. Consequently, it is wrong to assume that a patient whose pain is relieved with placebos is addicted or is a **malingerer** (someone who pretends to be sick or in pain). Using deception is considered unethical (American Pain Society, 1999).

Nursing Care Plan: *Pain*

Assessment

Subjective Data

States, "It feels like a semi-truck is parked on my chest. I know I must be having a heart attack." Indicates that pain measures 10 on a scale of 1 to 10.

Objective Data

55-year-old man brought to Emergency Department from work. Holds hands over L. precordial area. Rubs L. arm. Perspires profusely. Startles when staff enter room. Pulse is 108 beats/min and irregular. Blood pressure is 148/92. Respirations are 30/min. Elevated ST segment on cardiac rhythm strip.

Diagnosis

Pain related to possible reduction in oxygen to myocardium

Plan

Goal

That patient will report that his pain is reduced to ≤7 using a 0–10 scale by 9/20.

Orders: 9/19

1. Maintain bed rest.
2. Administer 50% oxygen continuously by mask.
3. Explain all procedures and routines before being performed.
4. Allow wife to remain at bedside as desired.
5. Administer prescribed analgesic as needed. ______________ R. VERCLER, RN

continued

Nursing Care Plan ***Pain*** *Continued*

Implementation (Documentation)	9/19	1400	Face mask applied and oxygen administered at 6 liters per minute. Respirations 28 and labored. Placed in high Fowler's position. ________ N. DUNN, RN
		1415	States, "I feel tightness and aching from my chest into my neck and L. arm. It's still a 10; please do something." ________ N. DUNN, RN
		1420	Nitroglycerin tab given sublingually. Instructed to let tablet remain under tongue for absorption. Explained there may be tingling in the area of the tablet, a headache, and a warm, flushed feeling associated with absorption, but the medication will help more blood get to the heart muscle. Advised to remain in bed for the time being. Wife at bedside holding hands. ________ N. DUNN, RN
		1435	1,000 mL D_5W started IV in L. hand with a #18 angiocath. Running at a keep open rate. No pain relief from nitroglycerin. ________ N. DUNN, RN
		1445	Morphine sulfate 4 mg given IV push for chest pain. ________ N. DUNN, RN
Evaluation (Documentation)		1500	States, "My pain is starting to ease up. It's about an 8½ right now." ________ N. DUNN, RN

FOCUS ON OLDER ADULTS

- Older adults who are depressed or cognitively impaired often focus their complaints on physical symptoms such as pain, discomfort, and fatigue.
- Pain often goes underreported among older adults because they believe that pain is a normal part of aging or that nothing can be done about it.
- Because older adults have more chronic illnesses and disease conditions, they are at higher risk for pain.
- Although it is a common belief that older adults are less sensitive to pain stimuli, recent studies suggest that the intensity and frequency of chronic pain increase with advanced age and that older adults are more likely to have atypical presentations of pain.
- Older adults who are cognitively impaired may not be able to complain of pain or discomfort. Changes in mental status or behavior are primary manifestations of pain in people with dementia.
- When assessing pain in older adults, attention focuses on how the pain or discomfort interferes with their daily function and quality of life.
- Older adults who are depressed, or have chronic conditions or high levels of stress usually have diminished pain tolerance because they have less energy to cope with pain.
- Older adults may endure pain because they do not want to be perceived as a nuisance or a complainer.
- The oral or dermal (topical) route is the preferred route for analgesic drug administration for older adults.
- Topical treatments, such as hot or cold packs, are effective and safe methods of managing musculoskeletal pain.
- Because older adults are more sensitive than younger adults to narcotics, they may respond to lower and less frequent doses.
- Older adults are more likely to develop mental changes from narcotic analgesics, even in low doses.
- Adverse effects of analgesics, even over-the-counter products, are often more dramatic in older adults. Common adverse effects are confusion, disorientation, gastritis, constipation, urinary retention, blurred vision, and gastrointestinal bleeding.
- Although the administration of low doses of antidepressants, anticonvulsants, or stimulants may enhance the effectiveness of analgesics for older adults, these agents also increase the risk of adverse effects and drug interactions.
- Unrelenting pain, such as that associated with cancer, can lead to sleep deprivation, poor nutrition, diminished social interaction, feelings of helplessness, and suicide.
- Vascular pain, a problem experienced by many older adults with diabetes, is often described as "burning."

KEY CONCEPTS

- Pain is an unpleasant sensation usually associated with disease or injury.
- The sensation of pain is transmitted over nerves to peripheral receptors called nociceptors. Once the nerve impulse is transmitted up the spinal cord, it is delivered to the thalamus, cortex, and limbic system areas of the brain.
- The pain threshold is the point at which pain-transmitting neurochemicals reach the brain and cause conscious awareness, known as pain perception. Pain tolerance is

the amount of pain a person endures once the threshold has been reached.

- The gate-control theory of pain proposes that although there are several pathways for transmitting cutaneous information to the brain, the gates to all but one pathway close, permitting only a single stimulus to be transmitted at a time.
- Endogenous opioids are naturally produced chemicals with morphine-like characteristics. It is believed that these chemicals bind to sites on the nerve cell's membrane, blocking the transmission of pain-producing neurotransmitters.
- The five general types of pain are cutaneous pain, visceral pain, neuropathic pain, acute pain, and chronic pain.
- Acute pain differs from chronic pain in its duration, etiology, and response to therapeutic measures.
- When performing a basic pain assessment, the nurse asks the patient to describe the pain's onset, quality, intensity, location, and duration.
- Four commonly used pain-intensity assessment tools are a numeric scale, a word scale, a linear scale, and a picture scale.
- A pain assessment is performed, at a minimum, on admission, once per shift when pain is an actual or potential problem, and before and after implementing a pain-management intervention.
- The physiologic basis for pain management involves interrupting pain-transmitting chemicals at the site of injury, altering pain transmission at the spinal cord, using gate-closing mechanisms, and blocking pain perception in the brain.
- Three categories of drugs used to manage pain are nonopioids, opioids, and adjuvant drugs.
- Rhizotomy and cordotomy are surgical pain-management techniques used when other methods are ineffective.
- Examples of nondrug/nonsurgical methods of pain management are educating patients about pain and its control and using imagery, meditation, distraction, relaxation, and interventions such as applications of heat and cold, transcutaneous electrical nerve stimulation, acupuncture and acupressure, percutaneous electrical nerve stimulation, biofeedback, and hypnosis.
- Patients often request frequent doses of pain-relieving medications because the dosage or schedule for administration is not controlling the pain.
- The fear of addiction leads to inadequate pain management.
- A placebo is an inactive substance given as a substitute for an actual drug. The positive effect some patients have from placebos is probably due to the trust they have in the physician or nurse.

CRITICAL THINKING EXERCISES

- Recall a personal experience involving pain. Describe the factors that intensified the pain and the measures, other than medication, that relieved it. Discuss how this information can be applied to restoring comfort among patients who are in pain.

SUGGESTED READINGS

Allcock N. Factors affecting the assessment of pain: a literature review. Journal of Advanced Nursing 1996;24(6):1144–1151.

American Pain Society. New survey of people with chronic pain reveals out-of-control symptoms, impaired daily lives. Glenview, Ill., Feb. 17, 1999a.

American Pain Society. Principles of analgesic use in the treatment of acute pain and cancer pain, 4th ed. Skokie, Ill., 1999b.

American Pain Society Quality of Care Committee. Quality improvement guidelines for the treatment of acute pain and cancer pain. Journal of the American Medical Association 1995;274(23):1874–1880.

Berkowitz CM. Epidural pain control—your job, too. RN 1997;60(8):22–27.

Bullock BL, Henze R. Focus on pathophysiology, 5th ed. Philadelphia, Lippincott Williams & Wilkins, 2000.

Cancer pain relief and palliative care: report of a WHO expert committee. Geneva, Switzerland, World Health Organization, 1990.

Carr DB, Jacox AK, Chapman CR, et al. Acute pain management: operative or medical procedures and trauma: clinical practice guidelines. Rockville, Md., US Public Health Service, Agency for Health Care Policy and Research, publication 92-0032, 1992.

Caudill MA, Holman GW, Turk D. Effective ways to manage chronic pain. Patient Care 1996;30(11):154–167.

Cerrato P. Acupuncture: where East meets West. RN 1996;59(10):55–57.

Copstead LC. Perspectives on pathophysiology. Philadelphia, WB Saunders, 1995.

Dahl JL, Berry P, Stevenson K, Gordon DB, Ward S. Institutionalizing pain management: making pain assessment and treatment an integral part of the nation's healthcare system. American Pain Society Bulletin 1998;8(4):1–3.

Faries J. Easing your patient's postoperative pain. Nursing 1998;28(6):58–60.

Fuller BF. The process of infant pain assessment. Applied Nursing Research 1998;11(2):62–68.

Harkins SW, Scott R. Pain and presbyalgos. In Birren JE, ed. Encyclopedia of gerontology, vol. 2. San Diego, Academic Press, 1996:247–260.

Jacox A, Carr DB, Payne R, et al. Management of cancer pain: clinical practice guideline No. 9. Rockville, Md., US Public Health Service, Agency for Health Care Policy and Research, publication 94-0592, 1994.

Jadad AR, Browman GP. The WHO analgesic ladder for cancer pain management: stepping up the quality of its evaluation. Journal of the American Medical Association 1995;274(23):1870–1873.

JCAHO. Comprehensive accreditation manual for hospitals: the official handbook. Oakbrook Terrace, Ill., JCAHO, 1999.

Jimenez SL. Pain and comfort—assessment: the key to effective pain management. Journal of Perinatal Education 1998;7(1):35–38.

Kelleher DJ, Rennell B, Kidd BL. The effect of social context on pain measurement. Journal of Musculoskeletal Pain 1998;6(2):77–86.

Magrum LC, Bentzen C, Landmark S. Pain management in home care. Seminars in Oncology Nursing 1996;12(3):202–218.

Mayo Clinic. Managing pain: attitude, medication and therapy are keys to control. Medical Essay, a supplement to Mayo Clinic Health Letter. Rochester, Minn., Mayo Clinic, 1996. http://www.mayohealth.org

McCaffery M. Pain management handbook. Nursing 1997;27(4):42–45.

McCaffery M, Beebe A. Pain: clinical manual for nursing practice, 2d ed. St. Louis, CV Mosby, 1998.
Melzack R, Wall PD. Pain mechanisms: a new theory. Science 1965;150: 971–974.
NANDA nursing diagnoses: definitions and classification, 1999–2000. Philadelphia, NANDA, 1999.
National Institutes of Health. Acupuncture. NIH Consensus Statement 1997; 15(5):1–34.
Pasero CL. Pain ratings: the fifth vital sign. American Journal of Nursing 1997;97(2):15–16.
Pasero CL, McCaffery M. Managing postoperative pain in the elderly. American Journal of Nursing 1996;96(10):39–46.
Pujalte JM, Llavore EP, Ylescupidez FR. Double-blind clinical evaluation of oral glucosamine sulphate in the basic treatment of osteoarthritis. Current Medical Research and Opinion 1980;7:110–114.
Sloman R. Relaxation and the relief of cancer pain. Nursing Clinics of North America 1995;30(4):697–709.
VanCouwenberghe C, Pasero CL. Teaching patients how to use PCA. American Journal of Nursing 1998;98(9):14–15.
White PF, Phillips J, Proctor TJ, Craig WF. Percutaneous electrical nerve stimulation (PENS): a promising alternative medicine approach to pain management. American Pain Society Bulletin 1999;9(2):1–8.
World Health Organization. Cancer pain relief with a guide to opioid availability, 2d ed. Geneva, WHO, 1996.

SKILL 19-1

PREPARING A PATIENT-CONTROLLED ANALGESIA (PCA) INFUSER

Suggested Action	Reason for Action
Assessment	
Check the written medical order for the use of a PCA infusion device, the prescribed drug, the initial loading dose, the dose per self-administration, and the lockout interval.	Provides data for programming the infusion device
Check the patient's wristband.	Prevents medication errors
Assess what the patient understands about PCA.	Indicates the type and amount of teaching that must be provided
Check that the currently infusing intravenous (IV) solution is compatible with the prescribed analgesic.	Avoids incompatibility reactions
Planning	
Obtain the following equipment: infuser, PCA tubing, prefilled medication container.	Promotes organization and efficient time management
Plug the power cord into the electrical wall outlet.	Prolongs the life of the battery
Explain the equipment and how it functions.	Reduces anxiety and promotes independence
Implementation	
Wash your hands.	Reduces the transmission of microorganisms
Attach the PCA tubing to the assembled syringe.	Provides a pathway for delivering the medication

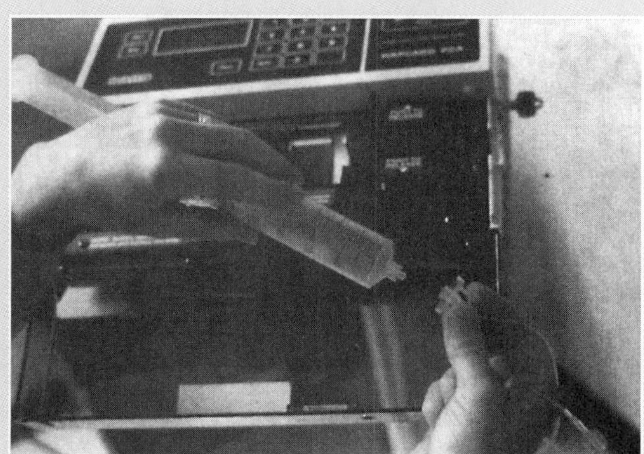

Connecting tubing. (Courtesy of Ken Timby.)

continued

SKILL 19-1

PREPARING A PATIENT-CONTROLLED ANALGESIA (PCA) INFUSER *Continued*

Suggested Action	Reason for Action
Open the cover or door of the infuser and load the syringe into its cradle.	Stabilizes the syringe within the infuser

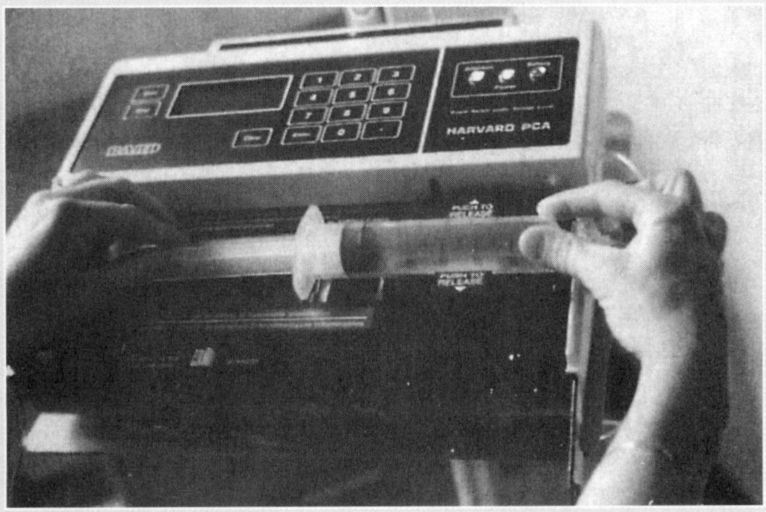

Loading the syringe within the PCA machine. (Courtesy of Ken Timby.)

Suggested Action	Reason for Action
Fill the PCA tubing with fluid.	Displaces air from the tubing

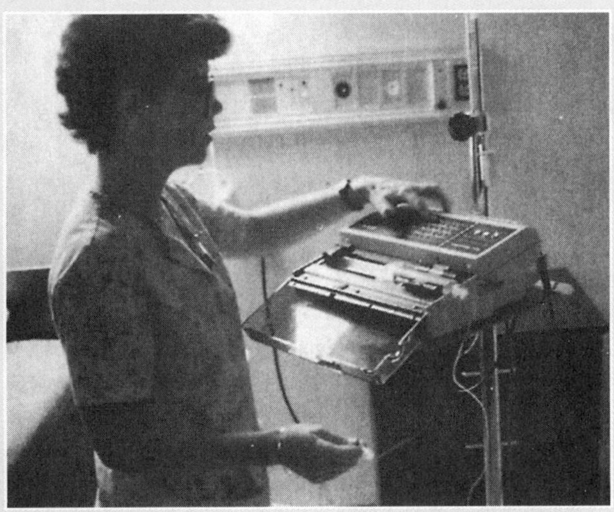

Purging air from intravenous tubing. (Courtesy of Ken Timby.)

Suggested Action	Reason for Action
Connect the PCA tubing to the IV tubing.	Facilitates intermittent administration of medication
Assess the patient's pain.	Provides data from which to evaluate the drug's effectiveness
Set the volume for the prescribed loading dose and administer it to the patient.	Administers a slightly larger dose of the drug to establish a reduced level of pain rather quickly
Program the infuser according to the individual dose and lockout period.	Prevents overdosing

continued

SKILL 19-1

PREPARING A PATIENT-CONTROLLED ANALGESIA (PCA) INFUSER *Continued*

Suggested Action	Reason for Action
Close the security door and lock it with a key.	Prevents tampering

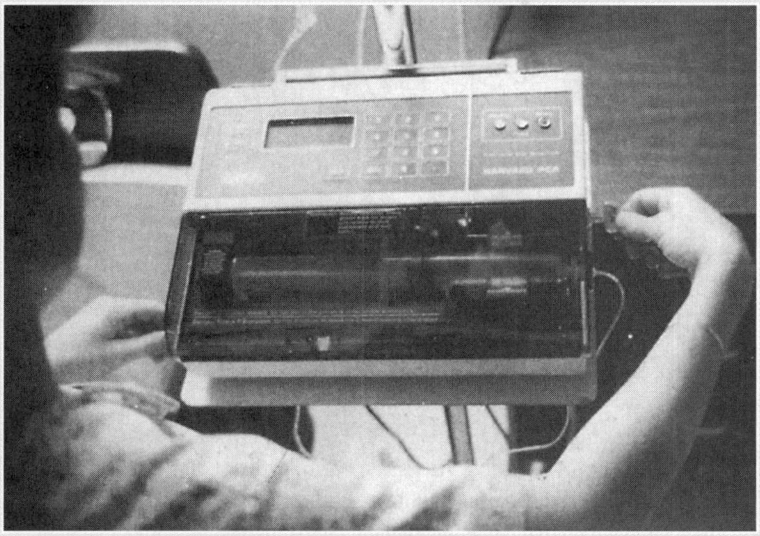

Locking the infuser within the PCA machine. (Courtesy of Ken Timby.)

Suggested Action	Reason for Action
Instruct the patient to press and release the control button each time pain relief is needed.	Educates the patient on how to operate the equipment

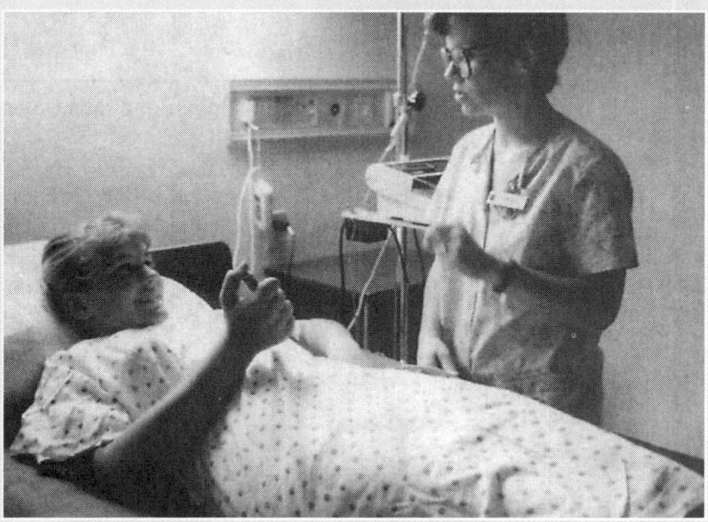

Explaining the use of the PCA infuser. (Courtesy of Ken Timby.)

Suggested Action	Reason for Action
Explain that a bell will sound when the infuser delivers medication.	Provides sensory reinforcement that the machine is working
Assess the patient's pain at least every 2 hours.	Complies with standards of care
Replace the medication syringe when it becomes empty.	Maintains continuous pain management
Change the primary IV solution container every 24 hours.	Complies with infection control policies

continued

SKILL 19-1

PREPARING A PATIENT-CONTROLLED ANALGESIA (PCA) INFUSER *Continued*

Evaluation

- The patient self-administers pain medication.
- The patient's pain is controlled.

Document

- Date and time
- Volume and type of analgesic solution
- Name of analgesic drug
- Initial pain assessment
- Loading dose
- Individual dose and time schedule
- Reassessments of pain
- Total volume self-administered per shift

SAMPLE DOCUMENTATION

Date and Time 30 mL syringe of saline c̄ 30 mg of morphine sulfate inserted within PCA pump. Describes pain around abdominal incision as continuous and stabbing. Rates the pain at a level of 7 on a scale of 0 to 10. Loading dose of 2 mg administered. Infuser programmed to deliver 0.1 mL—the equivalent of 0.1 mg—at no more than 10-minute intervals. Rates pain at a level of 5 within 10 minutes after loading dose. Instructed and observed to self-administer a subsequent dose. ________________________________ SIGNATURE, TITLE

CRITICAL THINKING

- Discuss some explanations for why a patient may be self-administering very few doses of an opioid drug via a PCA infuser.
- Describe some nursing actions that are appropriate if a patient uses the maximum doses of drug with a PCA infuser.

SKILL 19-2

OPERATING A TRANSCUTANEOUS ELECTRICAL NERVE STIMULATION (TENS) UNIT

Suggested Action	Reason for Action
Assessment	
Check the written medical order for providing the patient with a TENS unit.	Demonstrates collaboration with the medical management of patient care
Ask the physician or physical therapist about the best location for electrode placement. Some possible variations are: • On or near the painful site • On either side of an incision • Over cutaneous nerves • Over a joint	Optimizes pain management by individualizing electrode placement
Read the patient's history to determine whether there are any conditions for which the use of a TENS unit is contraindicated.	Demonstrates concern for patient safety
Check the patient's wristband.	Prevents errors and ensures proper patient identification
Assess what the patient understands about TENS.	Indicates the type and amount of teaching that must be provided
Planning	
Obtain the TENS unit and two to four self-adhesive electrodes.	Promotes organization and efficient time management
Explain the equipment and how it functions.	Reduces anxiety and promotes independence
Establish a goal with the patient for the level of pain management desired.	Aids in evaluating the effectiveness of the intervention
Implementation	
Wash your hands.	Reduces the transmission of microorganisms
Peel the backing from the adhesive side of the electrodes.	Facilitates skin contact
Position each electrode flat against the skin.	Enhances contact with the skin for maximum effectiveness

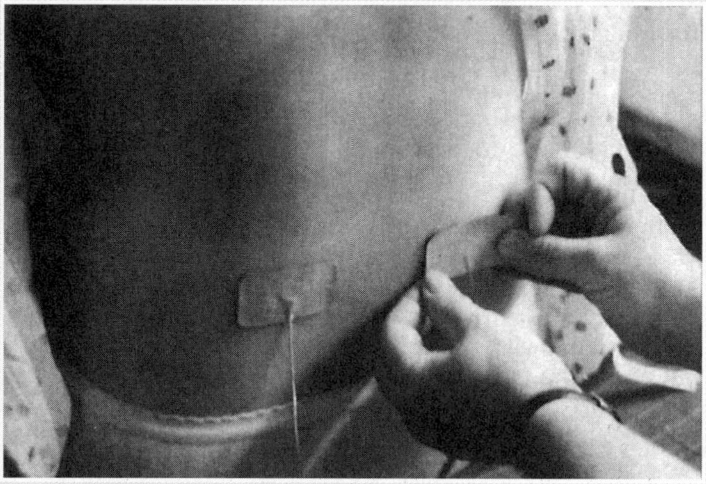

Attaching electrodes. (Courtesy of Ken Timby.)

continued

SKILL 19–2

OPERATING A TRANSCUTANEOUS ELECTRICAL NERVE STIMULATION (TENS) UNIT *Continued*

Suggested Action	Reason for Action
Space the electrodes at least the width of one from the other.	Prevents the potential for burning caused by close proximity of the electrodes
Make sure the settings on the TENS unit are off.	Prevents premature stimulation to the skin
Attach the cord(s) from the electrodes to the outlet jack(s) on the TENS unit, much like a headset connects with a radio.	Completes the circuitry from the electrodes to the battery-operated power unit
Turn the amplitude (intensity) knob on to the lowest setting and assess if the patient can feel a tingling, buzzing, or vibrating sensation.	Helps acquaint the patient with the sensation produced by the TENS unit
Gradually increase the intensity to the point at which the patient experiences a mild or moderately pleasant sensation.	Adjusts intensity according to the patient's response—a high intensity does not always provide the most pain relief; in fact, it may cause discomfort, muscle contractions, or itching

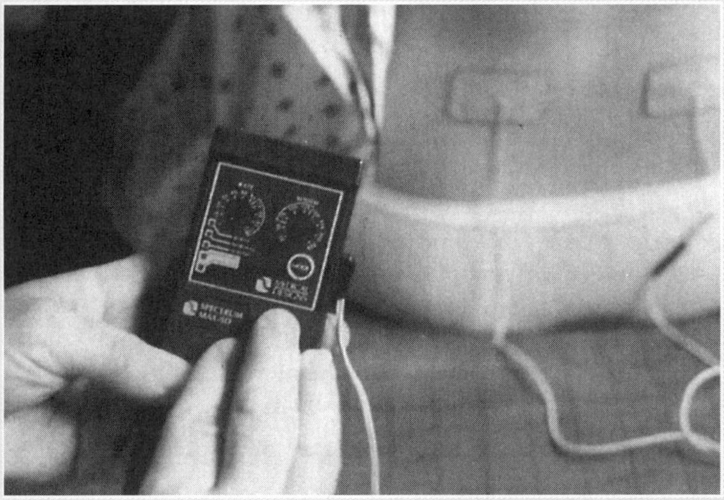

Adjusting the TENS settings. (Courtesy of Ken Timby.)

Suggested Action	Reason for Action
Set the rate (pulses per second) at a low rate and increase upward; a rate of 80 to 125 pulses per second is a conventional setting.	Adjusts the frequency of stimuli according to the patient's comfort and tolerance
Set the pulse width (the duration of each pulsation); a pulse width of 60 to 100 microseconds is usually used for acute pain; but 220 to 250 microseconds at higher amplitudes may be necessary for chronic or intense pain.	Provides wider and deeper stimulation as the pulse width increases
Turn the unit off when a sufficient level of pain relief occurs, and turn it back on when pain reappears.	Tests whether the TENS unit may be sufficient for intermittent rather than continuous use
Turn the unit off and remove the cord from the outlet jacks before bathing the patient.	Reduces hazards from potential contact of electrical equipment with water
Remove the electrode patches periodically to inspect the skin; reapply electrodes if they become loose.	Aids in skin assessment

continued

SKILL 19-2

OPERATING A TRANSCUTANEOUS ELECTRICAL NERVE STIMULATION (TENS) UNIT *Continued*

Suggested Action	Reason for Action
Slightly change the position of the electrodes if skin irritation develops.	Promotes skin integrity
Replace or recharge the batteries as needed.	Maintains function of the unit

Evaluation

- Pain is managed at the goal set by the patient.
- Activity is increased.
- Less pain medication is required.
- Emotional outlook is improved.

Document

- Date and time
- Initial pain assessments
- Location of electrodes
- Power settings
- Length of time TENS unit is in use
- Reassessments of pain 30 minutes after application of unit and at least once per shift
- Time when TENS is stopped or discontinued

SAMPLE DOCUMENTATION

Date and Time Selects the word "severe" from a pain scale of none to severe. Pain is described as "piercing" and continuous. Points to lower spine when asked to identify location of pain. Electrodes placed to the immediate R. and L. of the lumbosacral vertebrae. TENS unit initially set at a rate of 80 pulses per second and a pulse width of 60 microseconds. Used for 30 minutes, at which time rated pain at "moderate." Rate increased to 100 pulses per second with a pulse width of 150. ______________________________ SIGNATURE, TITLE

CRITICAL THINKING

- Give some reasons why a person may object to using TENS as a pain-management technique.
- What types of patients or painful conditions, in your opinion, would benefit from experimenting with a TENS unit for relief?

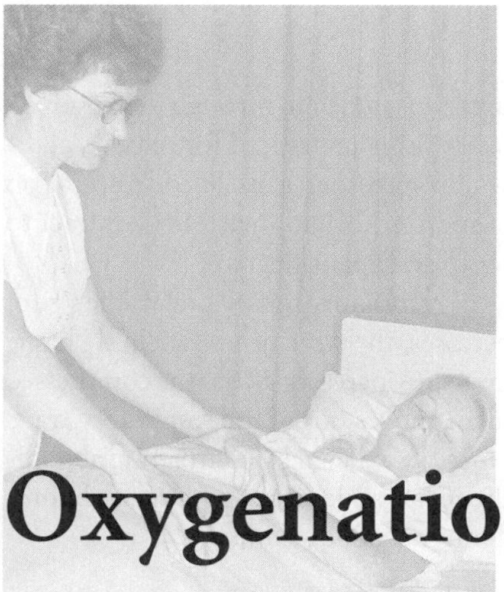

Oxygenation

CHAPTER 20

CHAPTER OUTLINE

Anatomy and Physiology of Breathing
Assessing Oxygenation
Promoting Oxygenation
Oxygen Therapy
Related Oxygenation Techniques
Nursing Implications

NURSING GUIDELINES

ASSISTING WITH AN ABG
ADMINISTERING OXYGEN SAFELY

SKILLS

SKILL 20-1: USING A PULSE OXIMETER
SKILL 20-2: ADMINISTERING OXYGEN
SKILL 20-3: MAINTAINING A WATER-SEAL CHEST TUBE DRAINAGE SYSTEM

NURSING CARE PLAN

INEFFECTIVE BREATHING PATTERN

KEY TERMS

apnea
arterial blood gas
CPAP mask
diaphragmatic breathing
expiration
face tent
flowmeter
Fowler's position
fraction of inspired oxygen
humidifier
hyperbaric oxygen therapy
hypercarbia
hypoxemia
hypoxia
incentive spirometry
inspiration
liquid oxygen units
nasal cannula
nasal catheter
non-rebreather mask
orthopneic position
oxygen analyzer
oxygen concentrator
oxygen tent
oxygen therapy
oxygen toxicity
partial rebreather mask
pulse oximetry
pursed-lip breathing
respiration
simple mask
stent
surfactant
tension pneumothorax
tidaling
transtracheal catheter
T-piece
tracheostomy collar
ventilation
Venturi mask
water-seal chest tube drainage

LEARNING OBJECTIVES

An understanding of the content within this chapter will be evidenced by the student's ability to:

- Explain the difference between ventilation and respiration.
- Differentiate between external and internal respiration.
- Name two methods for assessing the oxygenation status of patients at the bedside.
- List at least five signs of inadequate oxygenation.
- Name two nursing interventions that can be used to improve ventilation and oxygenation.
- Identify four items that may be needed when providing oxygen therapy.
- Name four sources for supplemental oxygen.
- List five common oxygen delivery devices.
- Discuss two hazards related to the administration of oxygen.
- Describe two additional therapeutic techniques that relate to oxygenation.
- Discuss at least two facts concerning oxygenation that affect the care of older adults.

Oxygen, which measures approximately 21% in the Earth's atmosphere, is essential for sustaining life. It is used by each cell of the human body to metabolize nutrients and produce energy. Without oxygen, cell death occurs rapidly.

This chapter describes the anatomic and physiologic aspects of breathing, techniques for assessing and monitoring oxygenation, types of equipment used in oxygen therapy, and skills needed to maintain respiratory function. Techniques for airway management, such as suctioning and other methods for maintaining a patent airway, are in Chapter 36.

Anatomy and Physiology of Breathing

The elasticity of lung tissue allows the lungs to stretch and fill with air during **inspiration** (breathing in) and return to a resting position after **expiration** (breathing out). **Ventilation** (movement of air in and out of the lungs) facilitates **respiration** (exchange of oxygen and carbon dioxide). External respiration takes place at the most distal point in the airway between the alveolar-capillary membranes (Fig. 20-1). Internal respiration occurs at the cellular level by means of hemoglobin and body cells.

The stimulus to breathe, for disease-free people, is triggered chemically and neurologically by increased blood levels of carbon dioxide and hydrogen ions.

MECHANICS OF VENTILATION

Ventilation occurs as a result of pressure changes within the thoracic cavity produced by the contraction and relaxation of respiratory muscles (Fig. 20-2). During inspiration, the dome-shaped diaphragm contracts and moves downward in the thorax. The intercostal muscles move the chest outward by elevating the ribs and sternum. This combination expands the thoracic cavity. Expansion creates more chest space, causing the pressure within the lungs to fall below that in the atmosphere. Because air flows from an area of higher pressure to one of lower pressure, air is pulled in through the nose, filling the lungs. When there is an acute need for oxygen, additional muscles, known as accessory muscles of respiration (the pectoralis minor and sternocleidomastoid) contract to assist with even greater chest expansion.

During expiration, the respiratory muscles relax, the size of the thoracic cavity decreases, the stretched elastic lung tissue recoils, intrathoracic pressure increases due to the compressed pulmonary space, and air moves out of the respiratory tract. Additional air can be forcibly exhaled by contracting abdominal muscles such as the rectus abdominis, transverse abdominis, and external and internal oblique muscles.

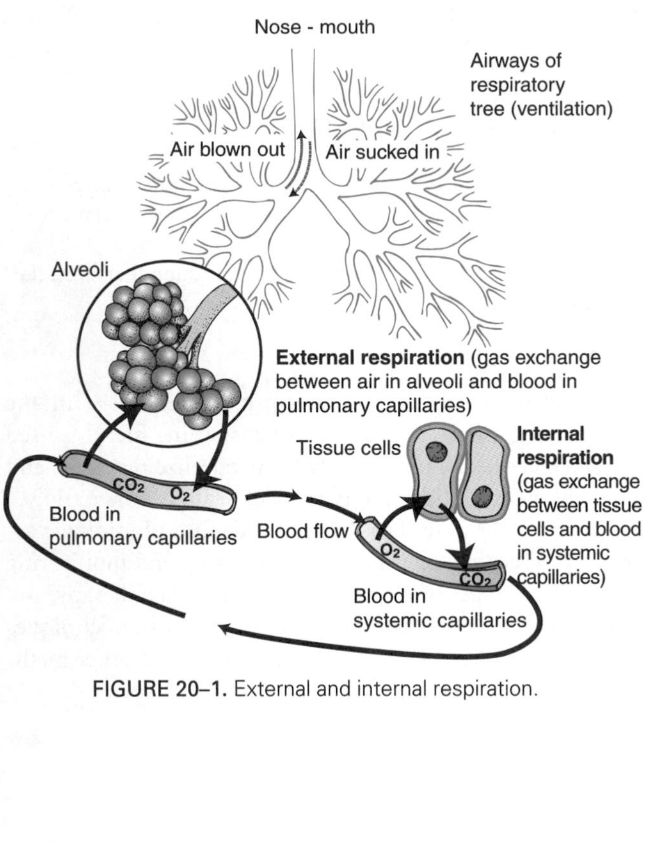

FIGURE 20–1. External and internal respiration.

Assessing Oxygenation

The quality of oxygenation is determined by collecting physical assessment data, monitoring arterial blood gases, and using pulse oximetry. A combination of these helps to identify signs of **hypoxemia** (insufficient oxygen within arterial blood) and **hypoxia** (inadequate oxygen at the cellular level).

PHYSICAL ASSESSMENT

Oxygenation is physically assessed by monitoring the patient's respiratory rate, observing the breathing pattern and effort, checking chest symmetry, and auscultating lung sounds (see Chap. 12). Additional assessments include recording the heart rate and blood pressure, determining the patient's level of consciousness, and observing the color of the skin, mucous membranes, lips, and nailbeds (Display 20-1).

ARTERIAL BLOOD GASES

An **arterial blood gas** assessment (ABG; a laboratory test using arterial blood to assess oxygenation, ventilation, and acid–base balance) measures the partial pressure of oxygen dissolved in plasma (PaO_2), the percentage of hemoglobin that is saturated with oxygen (SaO_2), the partial pressure of carbon dioxide in plasma ($PaCO_2$), the pH of blood, and the level of bicarbonate (HCO_3) ions (Table 20-1). Arterial blood is preferred because arteries have a greater oxygen content than veins and are responsible for carrying oxygen to all the cells. Initial and subsequent ABGs are ordered to assess the patient in acute respiratory distress or to evaluate the progress of a patient receiving medical treatment.

In most situations, the collection of arterial blood is done collaboratively by a laboratory technician and the nurse. The nurse notifies the laboratory of the need for the blood test, records pertinent assessments on the laboratory request

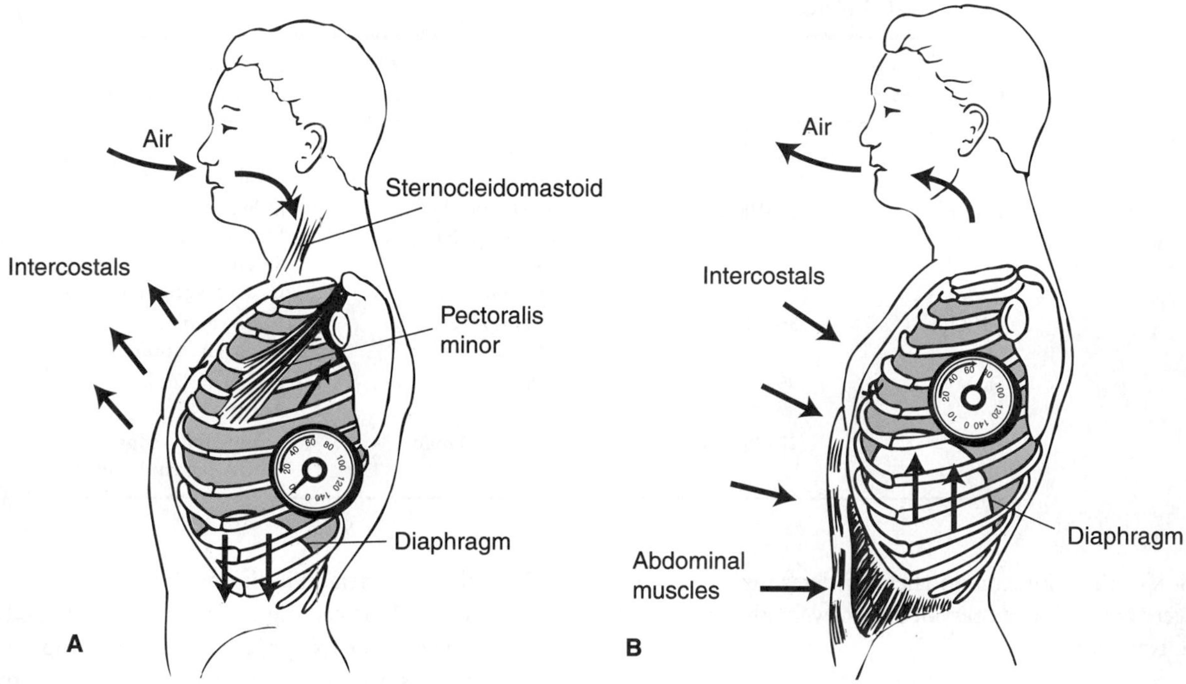

FIGURE 20–2. Ventilation and thoracic pressure changes. (*A*) Inspiration. (*B*) Expiration.

form and in the patient's chart, prepares the patient, assists the laboratory technician who obtains the specimen, and implements measures for preventing complications after the arterial puncture. In emergencies, a nurse who is trained in performing arterial punctures may obtain the specimen.

Nursing Guidelines For

Assisting with an ABG

- ☑ Perform the Allen test before the arterial puncture by doing the following:
  - ☐ Flex the patient's elbow and elevate the forearm where the arterial puncture will be made.
  - ☐ Compress the radial and ulnar arteries simultaneously. (Fig. 20-3*A*).
  - ☐ Instruct the patient to open and close the fist until the palm of the hand appears blanched.
  - ☐ Release pressure from the ulnar artery while maintaining pressure on the radial artery (see Fig. 20-3*B*).
  - ☐ Observe whether the skin flushes or remains blanched.
  - ☐ Release pressure on the radial artery.

  RATIONALE: The Allen test determines whether the hand has an adequate ulnar arterial blood supply should the radial artery become damaged or occluded. The radial artery should *not* be punctured if the Allen test shows absent or poor collateral arterial blood flow, as evidenced by continued blanching after pressure on the ulnar artery has been released. Alternative sites include the brachial, femoral, or dorsalis pedis arteries.

- ☑ Keep the patient at rest for at least 30 minutes before obtaining the specimen, unless the procedure is an emergency.

  RATIONALE: Because an ABG reflects the patient's status at the moment of blood sampling, activity can transiently lower levels of oxygen in the blood and lead to an incorrect interpretation of the test results.

- ☑ Record the patient's current temperature, respiratory rate, and level of activity if other than resting.

  RATIONALE: Increased metabolism and activity affect cellular oxygen demands. Therefore, the data help in interpreting the results of laboratory findings.

- ☑ Record the amount of oxygen the patient is receiving at the time of the test (either room air or prescribed amount) and ventilator settings.

DISPLAY 20–1

Common Signs of Inadequate Oxygenation

- Decreased energy
- Restlessness
- Rapid, shallow breathing
- Rapid heart rate
- Sitting up to breathe
- Nasal flaring
- Use of accessory muscles
- Hypertension
- Sleepiness, confusion, stupor, coma
- Cyanosis of the skin (mucous membranes in dark-skinned patients), lips, and nailbeds

TABLE 20–1. **Values for Arterial Blood Gases**

Component	Normal Range	Abnormal Findings	Indication of Abnormal Findings
pH	7.35–7.45	<7.35 >7.45	Acidosis Alkalosis
PaO_2	80–100 mm Hg	60–80 mm Hg 40–60 mm Hg <40 mm Hg >100 mm Hg	Mild hypoxemia Moderate hypoxemia Severe hypoxemia Hyperoxygenation
$PaCO_2$	35–45 mm Hg	<35 mm Hg >45 mm Hg	Hyperventilation Hypoventilation
SaO_2	95–100%	<95%	Hypoventilation Anemia
HCO_3	22–26 mEq	<22 or >26 mEq	Compensation for acid–base imbalance

RATIONALE: This information helps in determining whether oxygen therapy is necessary or aids in evaluating its current effectiveness.

☑ Hyperextend the wrist over a rolled towel.
RATIONALE: Hyperextension brings the radial artery nearer the skin surface to facilitate penetration.

☑ Comfort the patient during the puncture.
RATIONALE: An arterial puncture tends to be painful unless a local anesthetic is used.

☑ After the specimen is obtained, expel any air bubbles from it.
RATIONALE: This ensures that the only gas present in the specimen is that contained in the blood.

☑ Rotate the collected specimen.
RATIONALE: Rotation mixes the blood with the anticoagulant in the specimen tube, ensuring that the blood sample will not clot before it can be examined.

☑ Place the specimen on ice immediately.
RATIONALE: Blood cells deteriorate outside the body, causing changes in the oxygen content of the sample. Cooling the sample slows cellular metabolism and ensures more accurate test results.

☑ Apply direct manual pressure to the arterial puncture site for 5 to 10 minutes.
RATIONALE: Arterial blood flows under higher pressure than venous blood. Therefore, prolonged manual pressure is necessary to control bleeding.

☑ Cover the puncture site with a pressure dressing composed of several 4″ × 4″ gauze squares and tape.
RATIONALE: Tight mechanical compression provides continued pressure to reduce the potential for arterial bleeding.

☑ Assess the puncture site periodically for bleeding or formation of a hematoma (collection of trapped blood) beneath the skin.

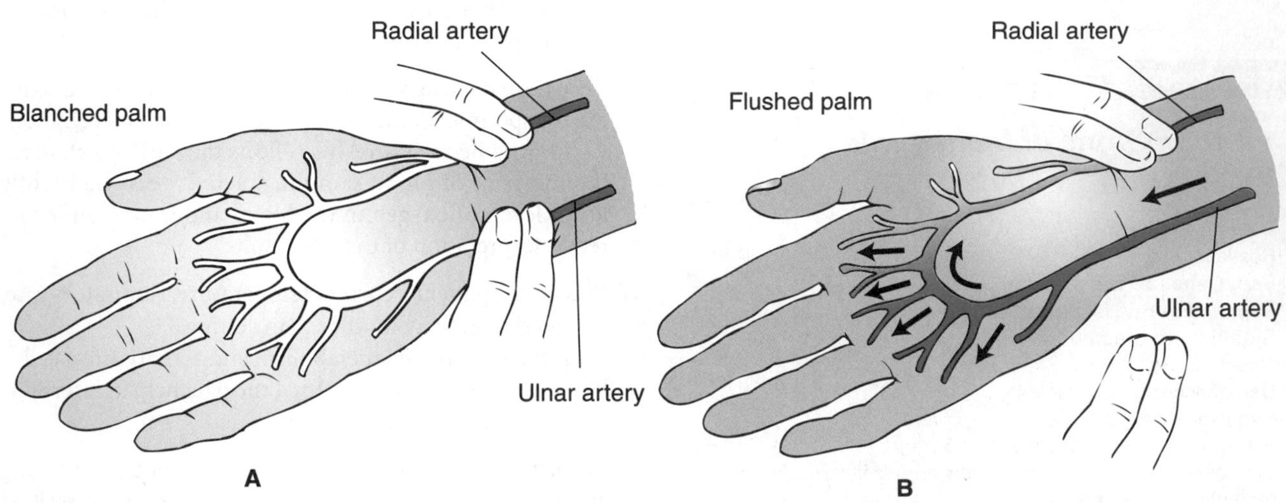

FIGURE 20–3. (*A*) Simultaneous compression of radial and ulnar arteries. (*B*) Pressure on the radial artery released.

RATIONALE: Periodic inspection aids in early identification of arterial bleeding, which can lead to substantial blood loss and discomfort.

☑ Report the laboratory findings to the prescribing physician as soon as they are available.
RATIONALE: Collaboration with the physician assists in making changes in the treatment plan to improve the patient's condition.

PULSE OXIMETRY

Pulse oximetry (a noninvasive, transcutaneous technique for periodically or continuously monitoring the oxygen saturation of blood) is described in Skill 20-1. A pulse oximeter is composed of a sensor and a microprocessor. Red and infrared light are emitted from one side of a spring-tension or adhesive sensor that is attached to a finger, toe, earlobe, or bridge of the nose. The opposite side of the sensor detects the amount of light that is absorbed by hemoglobin. The microprocessor then computes the information and displays it on a machine at the bedside. The measurement of oxygen saturation when obtained by pulse oximetry is abbreviated and recorded as SpO_2 to distinguish it from the SaO_2 measurement obtained from arterial blood.

Based on the oxygen-hemoglobin dissociation curve (Fig. 20-4), it is possible to infer the PaO_2 from the pulse oximetry measurement. The normal SpO_2 is 95% to 100%. A sustained level of less than 90% is cause for concern. If the SpO_2 remains low, oxygen therapy is needed. However, various factors affect the accuracy of the displayed information (Table 20-2). Troubleshooting the equipment, performing current physical assessments, and obtaining an ABG help to confirm the significance of the displayed findings.

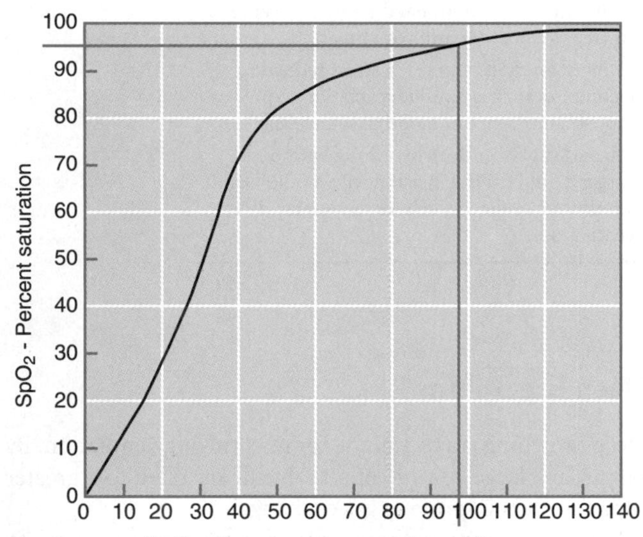

FIGURE 20–4. Draw a line from the SpO_2 in the left column across the graph to the point at which it intersects the curve. Use the numerical scale at the bottom to calculate the PaO_2. In this example, with an SpO_2 of 95%, the PaO_2 is approximately 98 mm Hg.

TABLE 20–2. **Factors That Interfere with Accurate Pulse Oximetry**

Factor	Cause	Remedy
Movement of the sensor	Tremor Restlessness Loss of adhesion	Relocate sensor to another site. Replace sensor or tape in place.
Poor circulation at the sensor site	Peripheral vascular disease Edema Tourniquet effect from taped sensor Vasoconstrictive drug effects	Change the sensor location or type of sensor. Loosen or change sensor location. Discontinue use temporarily.
Barrier to light	Nail polish Thick toenails Acrylic nails	Remove polish. Relocate sensor. Remove nail.
Extraneous light	Direct sunlight Treatment lights	Cover sensor with a towel.
Hemoglobin saturation with other substances	Carbon monoxide poisoning	Discontinue use temporarily

Promoting Oxygenation

Many factors affect ventilation and subsequently respiration (Table 20-3). Two nursing interventions frequently used for promoting oxygenation are positioning and teaching breathing techniques. Adhesive nasal strips can be used to improve oxygenation by reducing airway resistance and improving ventilation.

POSITIONING

Unless contraindicated by their condition, hypoxic patients are placed in high **Fowler's position** (an upright seated position; see Chap. 23). This position eases breathing by allowing the abdominal organs to descend away from the diaphragm. As a result, the lungs have the potential to fill with a greater volume of air.

As an alternative, patients who find breathing difficult may benefit from a variation of Fowler's position called the **orthopneic position** (seated position with the arms supported on pillows or the arm rests of a chair, often leaning forward over the bedside table or a chair back; Fig. 20-5). The

TABLE 20–3. **Factors Affecting Oxygenation**

Fact	Nursing Implication
Adequate respiration depends on a minimum of 21% oxygen in the environment and normal function of the cardiopulmonary system.	Know that patients with cardiopulmonary disorders require more than 21% oxygen to maintain adequate oxygenation of blood and cells.
Breathing can be voluntarily controlled.	Assist patients who are hyperventilating to slow the rate of breathing; teach patients to perform pursed-lip breathing to exhale more completely.
Patients with chronic lung diseases are stimulated to breathe by low blood levels of oxygen, called the hypoxic drive to breathe.	Remember that giving high percentages of oxygen can depress breathing in patients with chronic lung disease. No more than 2–3 L oxygen is safe unless the patient is mechanically ventilated.
Smoking causes increased amounts of inhaled carbon monoxide that compete and bond more easily than oxygen to the hemoglobin.	Keep in mind that patients who smoke have a greater potential for compromised gas exchange and acquiring chronic pulmonary and cardiac diseases.
Nicotine increases the heart rate and constricts arteries.	Teach people who do not smoke never to start. Identify products that are available, such as nicotine skin patches and gum, that can help smokers stop.
Pregnant women who smoke have a risk for low-birth-weight infants because low blood oxygenation affects fetal metabolism and growth.	Promote smoking cessation for pregnant women who are addicted to nicotine.
Pulmonary secretions within the airway and fluid within the interstitial space between the alveoli and capillaries interfere with gas exchange.	Encourage coughing, deep breathing, turning, and ambulating to keep alveoli inflated and the airway clear. Antibiotics, diuretics, and drugs that improve heart contraction reduce fluid within the lungs.
Gas exchange is increased by maximum lung expansion and compromised by any condition that compresses the diaphragm, such as obesity, intestinal gas, pregnancy, and an enlarged liver.	Assist patients to sit up to lower abdominal organs away from the diaphragm. Encourage weight loss, expulsion of gas via ambulation and bowel elimination, and assist with removing abdominal fluid by paracentesis (see Chap. 13) to improve breathing.
Activity and emotional stress increase the metabolic need for greater amounts of oxygen.	Provide rest periods and teach stress reduction techniques such as muscle relaxation to promote maintenance of blood oxygen levels.
Pain associated with muscle movement around abdominal and flank surgical incisions decreases the incentive to breathe deeply and cough forcefully.	Teach and supervise deep breathing before surgery. Support the incision with a pillow and administer drugs that relieve pain to facilitate ventilation.

orthopneic position allows room for maximum vertical and lateral chest expansion and provides comfort while resting or sleeping.

BREATHING TECHNIQUES

Breathing techniques such as deep breathing with or without an incentive spirometer, pursed-lip breathing, and diaphragmatic breathing help patients breathe more efficiently.

Deep Breathing

Deep breathing is a technique for maximizing ventilation. By taking in a large volume of air, alveoli are filled to a greater capacity, thus improving gas exchange.

Deep breathing is therapeutic for patients who tend to breathe shallowly, such as those who are inactive or in pain. To encourage deep breathing, the patient is taught to take in as much air as possible, hold the breath briefly, and exhale slowly. In some cases it is helpful to use an incentive spiro-

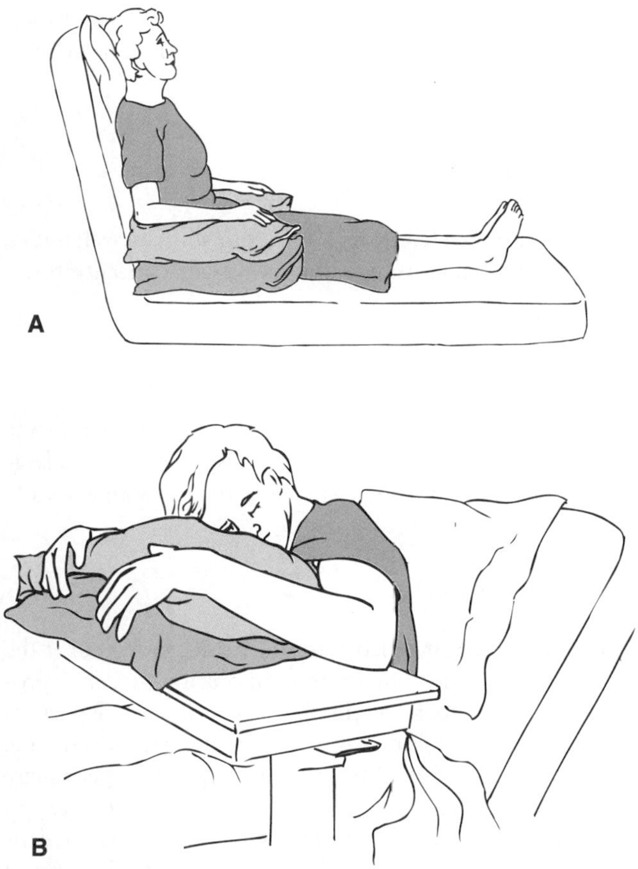

FIGURE 20–5. (*A*) Orthopneic position. (*B*) Alternative orthopneic position.

meter. However, deep breathing alone, if performed effectively, is sufficiently beneficial.

Incentive Spirometry

Incentive spirometry (a technique for deep breathing using a calibrated device) encourages patients to reach a goal-directed volume of inspired air. Although spirometers are constructed in different ways, all are marked in at least 100-milliliter increments and include some visual cue, such as elevation of lightweight balls, to show how much air has been inhaled (Fig. 20-6). The calibrated measurement also helps the nurse evaluate the effectiveness of the patient's breathing efforts.

Patient Teaching For
Using an Incentive Spirometer

Teach the patient to:

- Sit upright unless contraindicated.
- Identify the mark indicating the goal for inhalation.
- Exhale normally.
- Insert the mouthpiece, sealing it between the lips.
- Inhale slowly and deeply until the predetermined volume has been reached.
- Hold the breath for 3 to 6 seconds.
- Remove the mouthpiece and exhale normally.
- Relax and breathe normally before the next breath with the spirometer.
- Repeat the exercise 10 to 20 times per hour while awake or as prescribed by the physician.

Pursed-Lip Breathing

Pursed-lip breathing (a form of controlled ventilation in which the expiration phase of breathing is consciously prolonged) is another technique for improving gas exchange. If done correctly, pursed-lip breathing helps patients eliminate more than the usual amount of carbon dioxide from the lungs. Pursed-lip breathing and diaphragmatic breathing are especially helpful for patients who have chronic lung diseases such as emphysema, which are characterized by chronic hypoxemia and **hypercarbia** (excessive levels of carbon dioxide in the blood).

Pursed-lip breathing is performed as follows:

- Inhale slowly through the nose while counting to three.
- Purse the lips as though to whistle.
- Contract the abdominal muscles.
- Exhale through pursed lips for a count of six or more.

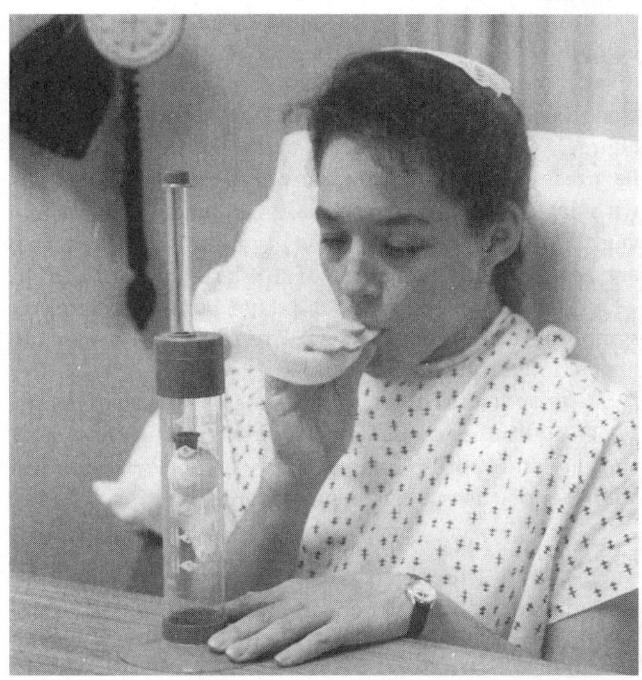

FIGURE 20–6. During deep inhalation, a ball rises in an incentive spirometer.

Expiration should be two to three times longer than inspiration. Not all patients can reach this goal initially, but with practice the length of expiration can increase.

Diaphragmatic Breathing

Diaphragmatic breathing (breathing that promotes the use of the diaphragm rather than the upper chest muscles) is used to increase the volume of air exchanged during inspiration and expiration. With practice, diaphragmatic breathing reduces respiratory effort and relieves rapid, ineffective breathing.

Patient Teaching For

Diaphragmatic Breathing

Teach the patient to:

- Lie down with knees slightly bent.
- Place one hand on the abdomen and the other on the chest.
- Inhale slowly and deeply through the nose while letting the abdomen rise more than the chest.
- Purse the lips.
- Contract the abdominal muscles and begin to exhale.
- Press inward and upward with the hand on the abdomen while continuing to exhale.
- Repeat the exercise for 1 full minute; rest for at least 2 minutes.
- Practice the breathing exercises at least twice a day for a period of 5 to 10 minutes.
- Progress to doing diaphragmatic breathing while upright and active.

Nasal Strips

Adhesive nasal strips, which can be purchased commercially, are used to reduce airflow resistance by widening the breathing passageways of the nose. Increasing the nasal diameter promotes easier breathing. Nasal strips are used by people with ineffective breathing as well as athletes, whose oxygen requirements are increased during sustained exercise. Nasal strips are also used to reduce or eliminate snoring.

Oxygen Therapy

When positioning and breathing techniques are inadequate for keeping the blood adequately saturated with oxygen, oxygen therapy is necessary. **Oxygen therapy** (a therapeutic intervention for administering more oxygen than exists in the atmosphere) is used to prevent or relieve hypoxemia. Oxygen therapy requires an oxygen source, a flowmeter, in some cases an oxygen analyzer or humidifier, and an oxygen delivery device.

OXYGEN SOURCES

Oxygen is supplied from any one of four sources: wall outlet, portable tank, liquid oxygen unit, or oxygen concentrator.

Wall Outlet

Most modern health care facilities supply oxygen through a wall outlet in the patient's room. The outlet is connected to a large central reservoir that is filled with oxygen on a routine basis.

Portable Tanks

When oxygen is not piped into individual rooms, or if the patient needs to leave the room temporarily, oxygen is provided in portable tanks resembling steel cylinders (Fig. 20-7) that hold various volumes under extreme pressure. A large tank of oxygen contains 2,000 pounds of pressure per square inch. Therefore, tanks are delivered with a protective cap to prevent accidental force against the tank outlet. Any accidental force applied to a partially opened outlet could cause the tank to take off like a rocket, with disastrous results. Therefore, oxygen tanks are transported and stored while strapped to a wheeled carrier.

Before oxygen is administered from a portable tank, the tank is "cracked," a technique for clearing the outlet of dust and debris. Cracking is done by turning the tank valve slightly to allow a brief release of pressurized oxygen. The force causes a loud hissing noise, which may be frightening. Therefore, it is best to crack the tank away from the patient's bedside.

Liquid Oxygen Unit

A **liquid oxygen unit** (device that converts cooled liquid oxygen to a gas by passing it through heated coils) is shown in Figure 20-8. These small, lightweight, portable units are used primarily by ambulatory home patients because they allow greater mobility inside and outside the home. Each unit holds approximately 4 to 8 hours' worth of oxygen. However, liquid oxygen is more expensive, the unit may leak during warm weather, and the outlet may become occluded by frozen moisture.

Oxygen Concentrator

An **oxygen concentrator** (machine that collects and concentrates oxygen from room air and stores it for patient use) is illustrated in Figure 20-9. An oxygen concentrator eliminates

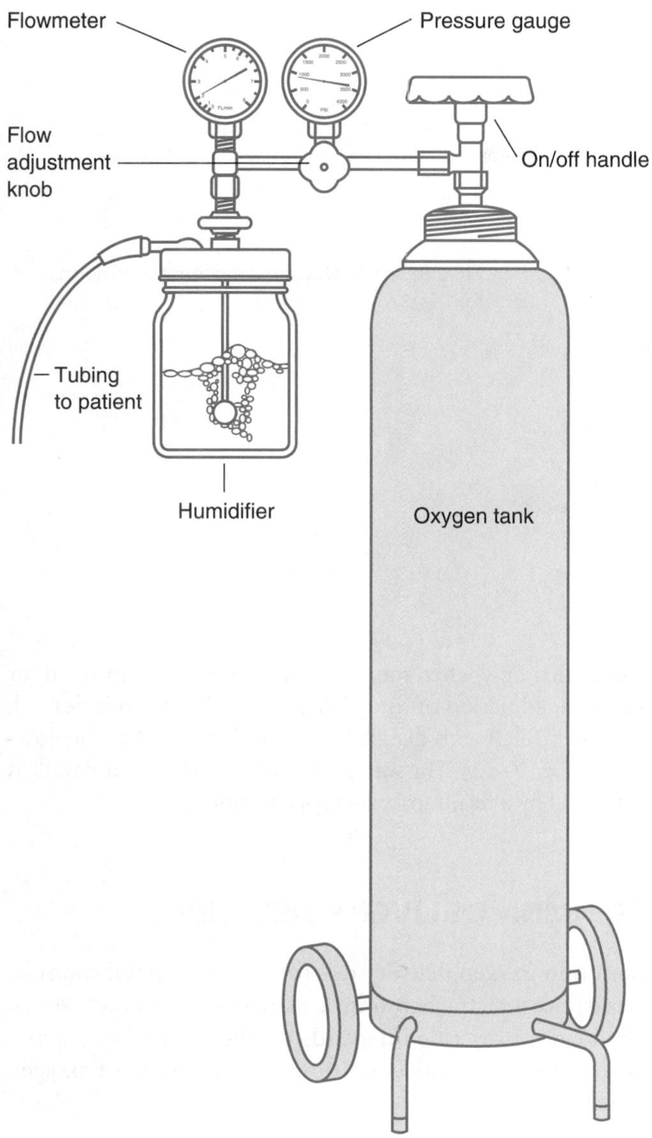

FIGURE 20–7. Portable oxygen tank.

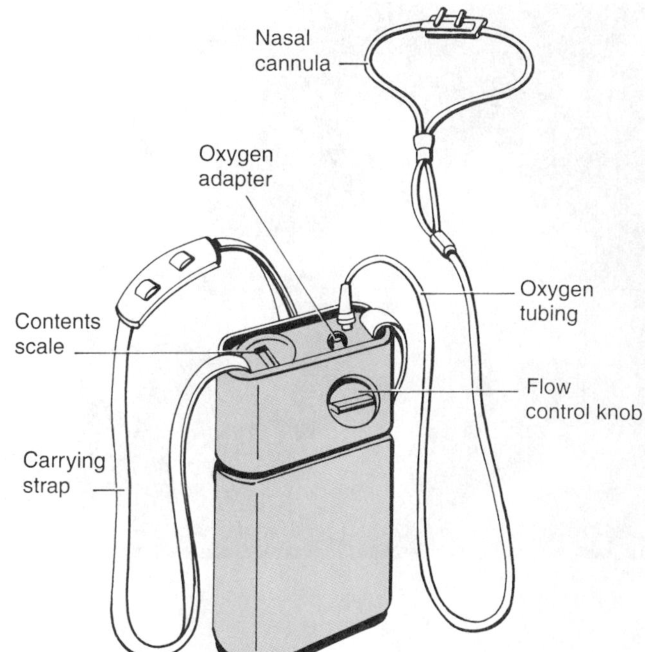

FIGURE 20–8. Liquid oxygen unit.

the need for a central reservoir of piped oxygen or the use of bulky tanks that must be constantly replaced. This type of oxygen source is used in home health care and long-term care facilities primarily because of its convenience and economy.

Although it is more economical than oxygen supplied in portable tanks, the device increases the patient's electric bill. Other disadvantages are that it generates heat from its motor and that it produces an unpleasant odor or taste if the filter is not cleaned regularly. Also, patients must have a secondary source of oxygen available in case of a power failure.

EQUIPMENT USED IN OXYGEN ADMINISTRATION

Besides an oxygen source, other pieces of equipment used during the administration of oxygen are a flowmeter, oxygen analyzer, and humidifier.

Flowmeter

The flow of oxygen is measured in liters per minute (L/min). A **flowmeter** (gauge used to regulate the amount of oxygen delivered to the patient) is attached to the oxygen source (Fig. 20-10). To adjust the rate of flow, the nurse turns the dial until the indicator is directly beside the prescribed amount.

The physician prescribes the concentration of oxygen, also called the **fraction of inspired oxygen** (FIO_2; the portion of oxygen in relation to total inspired gas), as a percentage or as a decimal (for example, 40% or 0.40). The prescription is based on the patient's condition. The Joint Commission on Accreditation of Healthcare Organizations (JCAHO) recommends that oxygen be prescribed as a percentage rather than in L/min because depending on the oxygen delivery device, L/min may provide different percentages of oxygen.

Oxygen Analyzer

An **oxygen analyzer** (device that measures the percentage of delivered oxygen) is used to determine whether the patient is receiving the amount prescribed by the physician (Fig. 20-11). The nurse or respiratory therapist first checks the percentage of oxygen in the room air with the analyzer. If there is a normal mixture of oxygen and other gases in the environment, the analyzer indicates 0.21 (21%). When the analyzer is positioned near or within the device used to deliver oxygen, the reading should register at the prescribed amount (greater than 0.21). If there is a discrepancy, the flowmeter is adjusted to reach the desired amount. Oxygen analyzers are used most

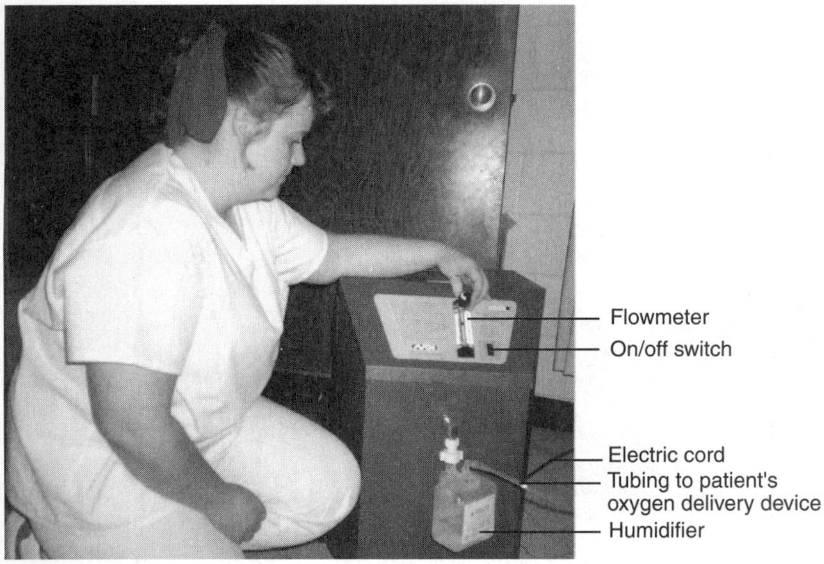

FIGURE 20–9. Oxygen concentrator. (Courtesy of Ken Timby.)

often when caring for newborns in isolettes, children in croup tents, and patients who are mechanically ventilated.

Humidifier

A **humidifier** (device that produces small water droplets) may be used during oxygen administration because oxygen is drying to the mucous membranes. In most cases, oxygen is humidified only when more than 4 L/min is administered for an extended period of time. When humidification is desired, a bottle is filled with distilled water and attached to the flowmeter (Fig. 20-12). The water level is checked daily and refilled as needed by a respiratory therapist or nurse.

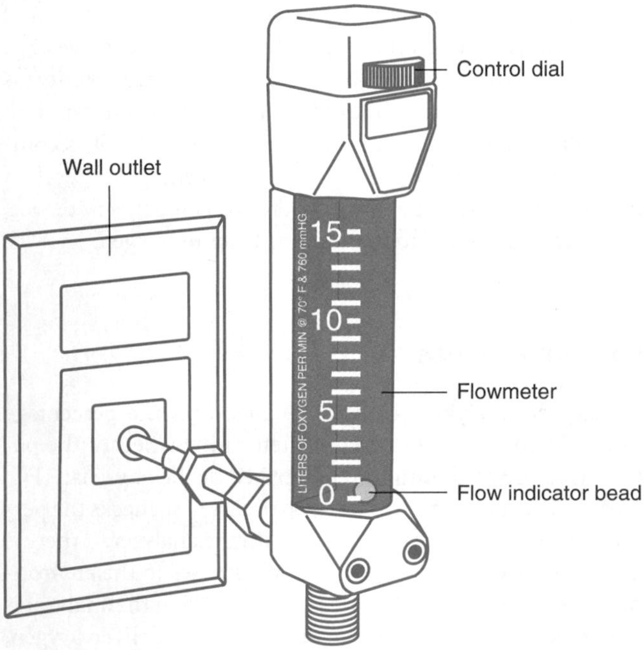

FIGURE 20–10. Flowmeter attached to a wall outlet for oxygen administration.

COMMON DELIVERY DEVICES

Common oxygen delivery devices include a nasal cannula, masks, face tent, tracheostomy collar, or T-piece (Table 20-4). The device prescribed depends on the patient's oxygenation status, physical condition, and amount of oxygen needed.

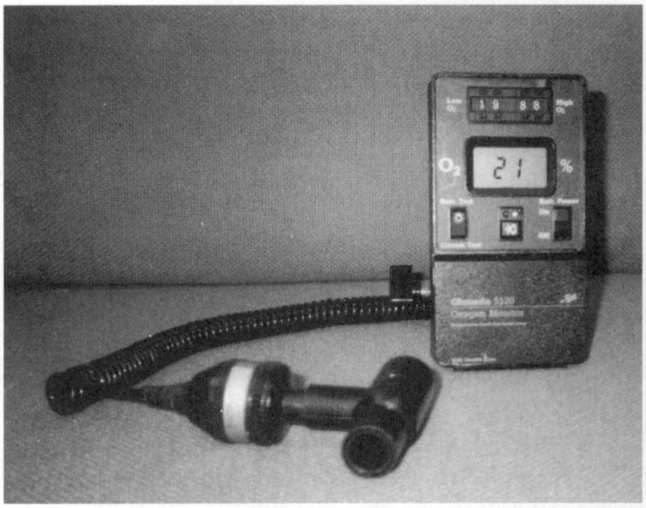

FIGURE 20–11. Oxygen analyzer. (Courtesy of Ken Timby.)

Nasal Cannula

A **nasal cannula** (hollow tube with half-inch prongs placed into the patient's nostrils) is held in place by wrapping the tubing about the ears and adjusting the fit beneath the chin. It provides a means of administering low concentrations of oxygen. Therefore, it is ideal for patients who are not extremely hypoxic or who have chronic lung diseases. High percentages of oxygen are contraindicated for patients with chronic lung disease because they have adapted to excessive levels of retained carbon dioxide, and their drive to breathe is stimulated by low blood oxygen levels. Consequently, if patients with chronic lung disease receive more than 2 to 3 liters of oxygen over a sustained period of time, their respiratory rate slows or even stops.

Masks

Oxygen can be delivered using a simple mask, a partial rebreather mask, a non-rebreather mask, or a Venturi mask.

Simple Mask

A **simple mask** (oxygen delivery device that fits over the nose and mouth) allows atmospheric air to enter and exit through side ports. It is held in place with an elastic strap. The simple mask, like other types of masks, allows the administration of higher levels of oxygen than are possible with a cannula. A simple mask is sometimes substituted for a cannula when a patient has nasal trauma or breathes through the mouth. When a simple mask is used, oxygen is delivered at no less than 5 L/min.

The efficiency of any mask is affected by how well it fits the face. Without a good seal, the oxygen leaks from the mask, thus diminishing its concentration. Other problems are associated with masks as well. All oxygen masks interfere with eating and make verbal communication difficult to understand. Also, some patients become anxious when their nose and mouth are covered because it creates a feeling of being suffocated. Skin care also becomes a priority because masks create pressure and trap moisture.

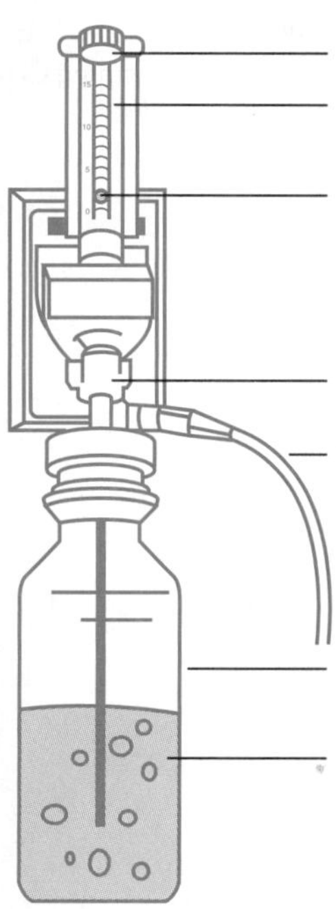

FIGURE 20–12. An oxygen humidifier attached to a flowmeter.

Partial Rebreather Mask

A **partial rebreather mask** (oxygen delivery device through which a patient inhales a mixture of atmospheric air, oxygen from its source, and oxygen contained within a reservoir bag) provides a means for recycling oxygen and venting all the carbon dioxide during expiration from the mask. During expiration, the first third of exhaled air enters the reservoir bag. The portion of exhaled air in the reservoir bag contains a high proportion of oxygen because it comes directly from the upper airways—the gas in this area has not been involved in gas exchange at the alveolar level. Once the reservoir bag is filled, the remainder of exhaled air is forced from the mask through small ports. With a simple mask, some carbon dioxide always remains within the mask and is reinhaled.

Non-rebreather Mask

A **non-rebreather mask** (oxygen delivery device in which *all* the exhaled air leaves the mask rather than partially entering the reservoir bag) is designed to deliver an FIO_2 of 90% to 100%. This type of mask contains one-way valves that allow only oxygen from its source as well as the oxygen in the reservoir bag to be inhaled. No air from the atmosphere is inhaled. All the air that is exhaled is vented from the mask. None enters the reservoir bag. Obviously, patients for whom non-rebreather masks are used are those who require high concentrations of oxygen. They are usually critically ill and may eventually need mechanical ventilation.

Humidification is *not* used when a mask with a reservoir bag is used, despite the high concentrations of oxygen. Also, patients with partial and non-rebreather masks are monitored closely to ensure that the reservoir bag remains partially inflated at all times.

Venturi Mask

A **Venturi mask** (oxygen delivery device that mixes a precise amount of oxygen and atmospheric air), sometimes called a

TABLE 20–4. **Comparison of Oxygen Delivery Devices**

Device	Common Range of Administration	Advantages	Disadvantages
Nasal cannula	2–6 L/min FIO_2 24–40%*	Is easy to apply promotes comfort Does not interfere with eating or talking Is less likely to create feeling of suffocation	Dries nasal mucosa at higher flows May irritate the skin at cheeks and behind ears Is less effective in some patients who tend to mouth breathe Does not facilitate administering high FIO_2 to hypoxic patients

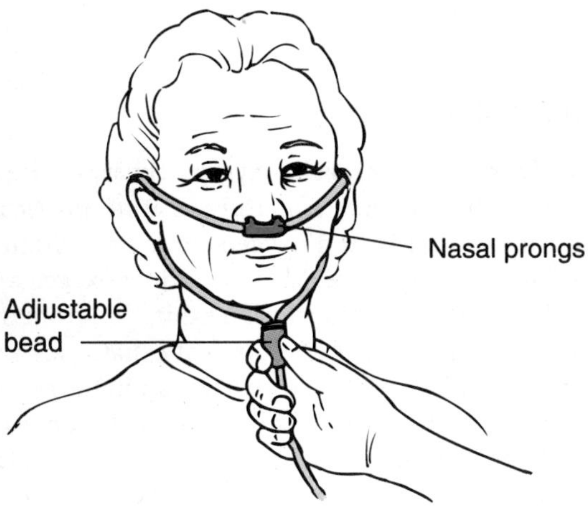

Masks			
Simple	5–8 L/min FIO_2 35–50%*	Provides higher concentrations than possible with a cannula Is effective for mouth breathers or patients with nasal disorders	Requires humidification Interferes with eating and talking Can cause anxiety among those who are claustrophobic Creates a risk for rebreathing CO_2 retained within mask

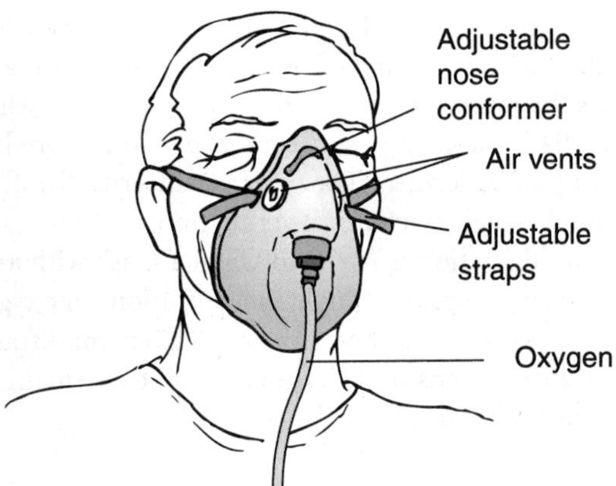

continued

TABLE 20–4. **Comparison of Oxygen Delivery Devices** *Continued*

Device	Common Range of Administration	Advantages	Disadvantages
Partial rebreather	6–10 L/min FIO_2 35–60%*	Increases the amount of oxygen with lower flows	Requires a minimum of 6 L/min Creates a risk for suffocation Requires monitoring to verify that reservoir bag remains inflated at all times
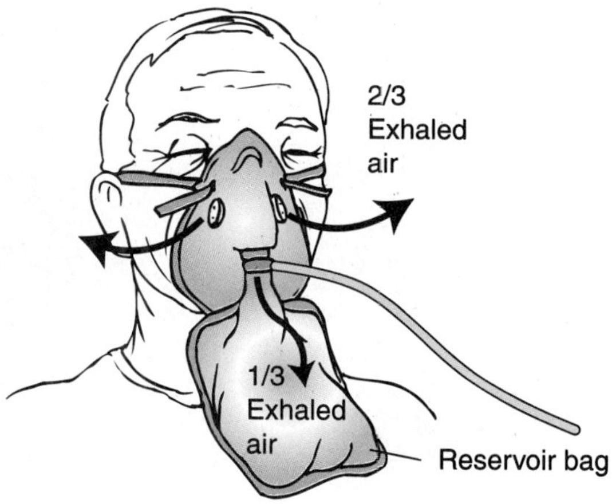			
Non-rebreather	6–10 L/min FIO_2 60–90%*	Delivers highest FIO_2 possible with a mask	See partial rebreather mask Creates a risk of oxygen toxicity
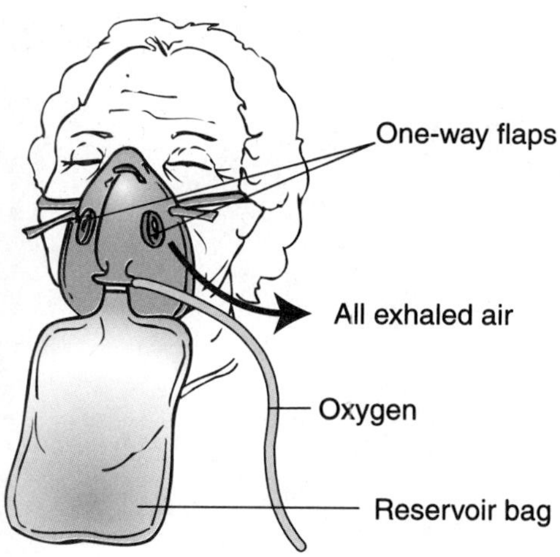			

continued

TABLE 20–4. **Comparison of Oxygen Delivery Devices** *Continued*

Device	Common Range of Administration	Advantages	Disadvantages
Venturi	4–8 L/min FIO_2 24–40%*	Delivers FIO_2 precisely	Permits condensation to form in tubing which diminishes the flow of oxygen

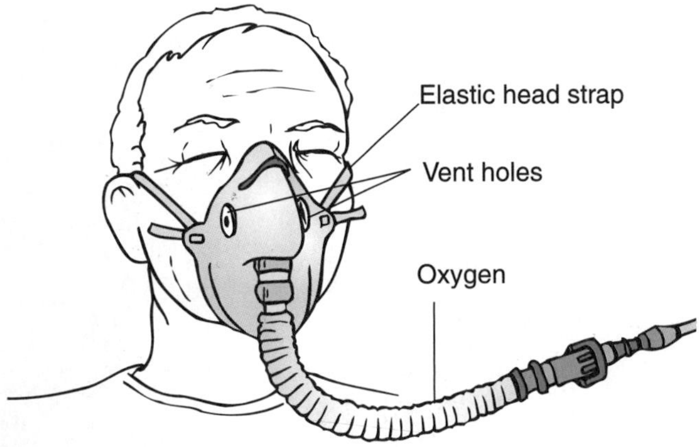

Device	Common Range of Administration	Advantages	Disadvantages
Face tent	8–12 L/min FIO_2 30–55%*	Provides a comfortable fit Is useful for patients with facial trauma and burns Facilitates humidification	Interferes with eating May result in inconsistent FIO_2, depending on environmental loss

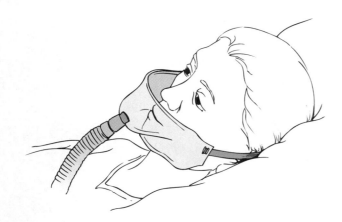

continued

TABLE 20–4. **Comparison of Oxygen Delivery Devices** *Continued*

Device	Common Range of Administration	Advantages	Disadvantages
Tracheostomy collar	4–10 L/min FIO_2 24–100%*	Facilitates humidifying and warming oxygen	Allows water vapor to collect in tubing, which may drain into airway
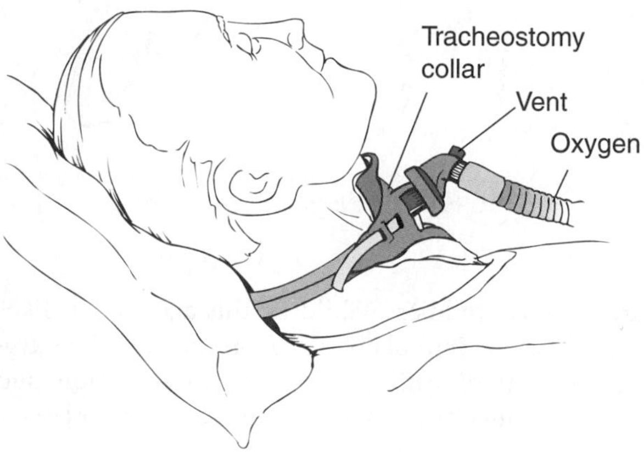			
T-piece	4–10 L/min FIO_2 24–100%*	Delivers any desired FIO_2 with high humidity	May pull on tracheostomy tube Allows humidity to collect and moisten gauze dressing
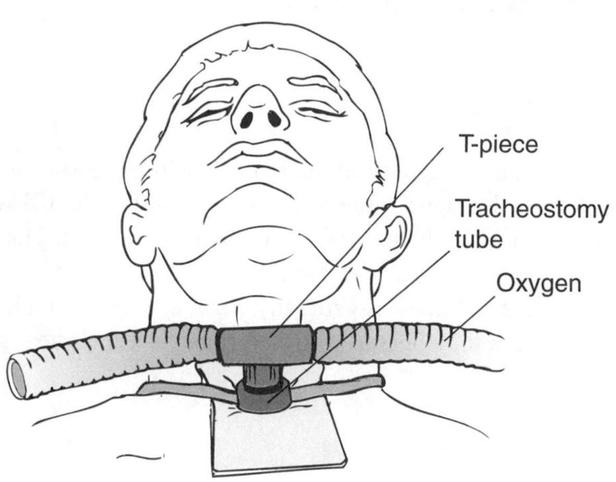			

*Source: American Association for Respiratory Care (AARC).

Venti mask, has a large ringed tube that extends from the mask. Adapters within the tube, which are color-coded or regulated by a dial system, permit only specific amounts of room air to mix with the oxygen. This feature ensures that the Venturi mask delivers the exact amount of prescribed oxygen. Unlike masks with reservoir bags, humidification can be added when a Venturi mask is used.

Face Tent

A **face tent** (device that provides oxygen in an area about the nose and mouth) delivers oxygen without the discomfort of a mask. Because the face tent is open and loose around the face, patients are less likely to feel claustrophobic. An added advantage is that a face mask can be used for patients with facial trauma or burns. A disadvantage is that the amount of oxygen patients actually receive may be inconsistent with what is prescribed due to environmental losses.

Tracheostomy Collar

A **tracheostomy collar** (device that delivers oxygen near an artificial opening in the neck) is applied over a tracheostomy, an opening into the trachea through which a patient breathes (see Chap. 36). Because the warming and moisturizing functions of the nose are bypassed, a tracheostomy collar provides a means for both oxygenation and humidification. The moisture that collects, however, tends to saturate the gauze dressing around the tracheostomy, making it necessary to change it frequently.

T-Piece

A **T-piece** (device that fits securely onto a tracheostomy tube or endotracheal tube) is similar to a tracheostomy collar but is attached directly to the artificial airway. Although the gauze around the tracheostomy usually remains dry, the moisture that collects within the tubing tends to condense and may enter the airway during position changes if it is not drained periodically. Another disadvantage is that the weight of the T-piece, or its manipulation, may pull on the tracheostomy tube, causing the patient to cough or experience discomfort. Skill 20-2 describes how to administer oxygen by common delivery methods.

ADDITIONAL DELIVERY DEVICES

Other methods for delivering oxygen are not as commonly used. Occasionally, oxygen is delivered by means of a nasal catheter, oxygen tent, transtracheal catheter, or continuous positive airway pressure (CPAP) mask.

Nasal Catheter

A **nasal catheter** (tube for delivering oxygen that is inserted through the nose into the posterior nasal pharynx; Fig. 20-13) is used for patients who tend to breathe through the mouth or experience claustrophobia when a mask covers their face. The catheter tends to irritate the nasopharynx, and therefore some patients find it uncomfortable. If a catheter is prescribed, the nurse secures it to the nose to avoid displacement and cleans the nostril with a cotton applicator on a regular basis to remove dried mucus.

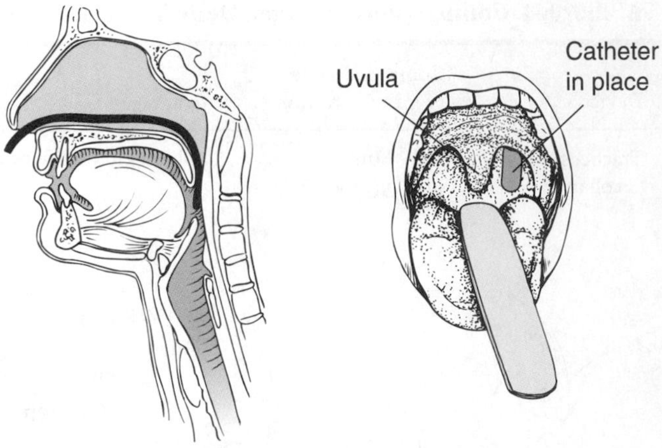

FIGURE 20–13. Nasal catheter placement.

Oxygen Tent

An **oxygen tent** (clear plastic enclosure that provides cooled, humidified oxygen) is more likely to be used in the care of active toddlers. Children this age are less likely to keep a mask or cannula in place but may require oxygenation and humidification for respiratory conditions such as croup or bronchitis. A face hood may be used for less-active infants.

Oxygen concentrations are difficult to control when an oxygen tent is being used. Therefore, when caring for a child in an oxygen tent, the edges of the tent must be tucked securely beneath the mattress to limit opening the zippered access ports so that oxygen does not escape too freely. Oxygen levels must be monitored with an analyzer.

CPAP Mask

A **CPAP mask** (device that maintains positive pressure within the airway throughout the respiratory cycle; Fig. 20-14) keeps the alveoli partially inflated even during expiration. The face mask is attached to a portable ventilator.

This type of mask is generally worn at night to maintain oxygenation for a person who experiences sleep **apnea** (peri-

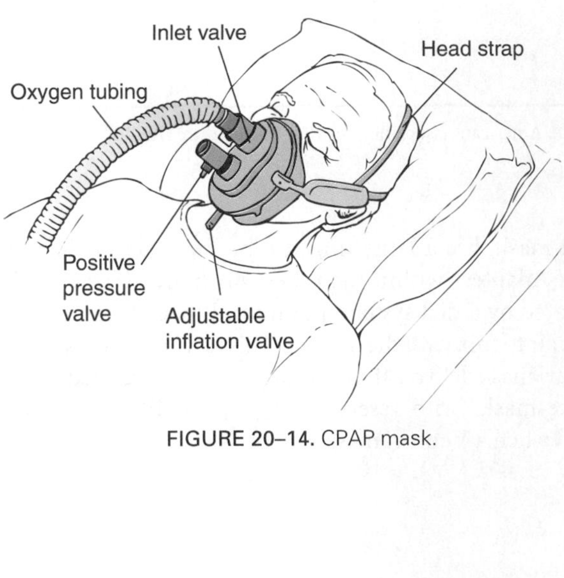

FIGURE 20–14. CPAP mask.

ods during which he or she stops breathing). The residual oxygen within the alveoli continues to diffuse into the blood during apneic episodes that may last 10 or more seconds, as frequently as 10 to 15 times an hour. Sleep apnea is dangerous because falling oxygen saturation levels may precipitate cardiac arrest and death.

Transtracheal Oxygen

Some patients who require long-term oxygen therapy may prefer its administration through a **transtracheal catheter** (hollow tube inserted within the trachea to deliver oxygen; Fig. 20-15). This device is less noticeable than a nasal cannula. The patient is adequately oxygenated with lower flows, decreasing the costs of replenishing the oxygen source.

Before transtracheal oxygen is used, a **stent** (tube that keeps a channel open) is inserted into a surgically created opening and remains there until the wound heals. Thereafter, the stent is removed and the catheter is inserted and held in place with a necklace-type chain. Patients are taught how to clean the tracheal opening and catheter, a procedure performed several times a day. During cleaning, patients administer oxygen with a nasal cannula.

OXYGEN HAZARDS

Regardless of which device is used, oxygen administration involves potential hazards: first and foremost, oxygen's capacity to support fires, and second, the potential for oxygen toxicity.

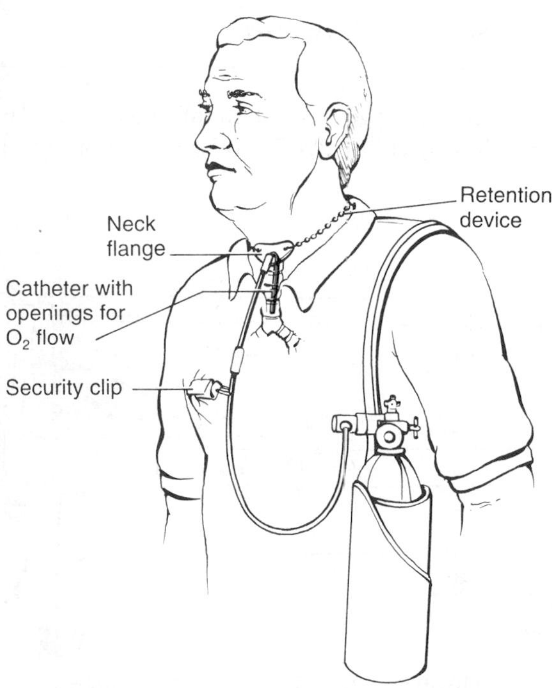

FIGURE 20–15. Transtracheal oxygen administration.

Fire Potential

Oxygen itself does not burn, but it does support combustion—in other words, it contributes to the burning process. Therefore, it is necessary to control all possible sources of open flames or ungrounded electricity.

Nursing Guidelines For

Administering Oxygen Safely

- ☑ Post "Oxygen in Use" signs wherever oxygen is stored or in use.
  RATIONALE: Warns others of potential fire hazard.
- ☑ Prohibit the burning of candles during religious rites.
  RATIONALE: Eliminates a source of open flames.
- ☑ Check that electrical devices have a three-pronged plug (see Chap. 18).
  RATIONALE: Provides a ground for leaking electricity.
- ☑ Inspect electrical equipment for frayed wires or loose connections.
  RATIONALE: Avoids sparks or uncontrolled pathway for electricity.
- ☑ Avoid using petroleum products, aerosol products (such as hair spray), and products containing acetone (such as nail polish remover) where oxygen is used.
  RATIONALE: Prevents ignition of flammable substance.
- ☑ Secure portable oxygen cylinders to rigid stands.
  RATIONALE: Prevents rupturing the tank.

Oxygen Toxicity

Oxygen toxicity (lung damage that develops when oxygen concentrations of more than 50% are administered for longer than 48 to 72 hours) is a potential hazard. The exact mechanism by which hyperoxygenation damages the lungs is not definitely known. One theory is that it reduces **surfactant** (lipoprotein produced by cells in the alveoli that promotes elasticity of the lungs and enhances gas diffusion).

Once oxygen toxicity develops, it is difficult to reverse. Unfortunately, the early symptoms are quite subtle (Display 20-2). The best prevention is to administer the lowest FIO_2 possible for the shortest amount of time.

DISPLAY 20-2

Signs and Symptoms of Oxygen Toxicity

- Non-productive cough
- Substernal chest pain
- Nasal stuffiness
- Nausea and vomiting
- Fatigue
- Headache
- Sore throat
- Hypoventilation

Related Oxygenation Techniques

There are two additional techniques that relate to oxygenation: a water-seal chest tube drainage system and hyperbaric oxygen therapy.

WATER-SEAL CHEST TUBE DRAINAGE

Water-seal chest tube drainage (technique for evacuating air or blood from the pleural cavity) helps to restore negative intrapleural pressure and reinflate the lung. Patients who require water-seal drainage have one or two chest tubes connected to the drainage system.

Several companies provide equipment for water-seal drainage. All these products consist of a three-chamber system (Fig. 20-16):

- One chamber collects blood or acts as an exit route for pleural air.
- A second compartment holds water that prevents atmospheric air from re-entering the pleural space (hence the term "water seal").
- A third chamber, if used, facilitates the use of suction, which may speed the evacuation of blood or air.

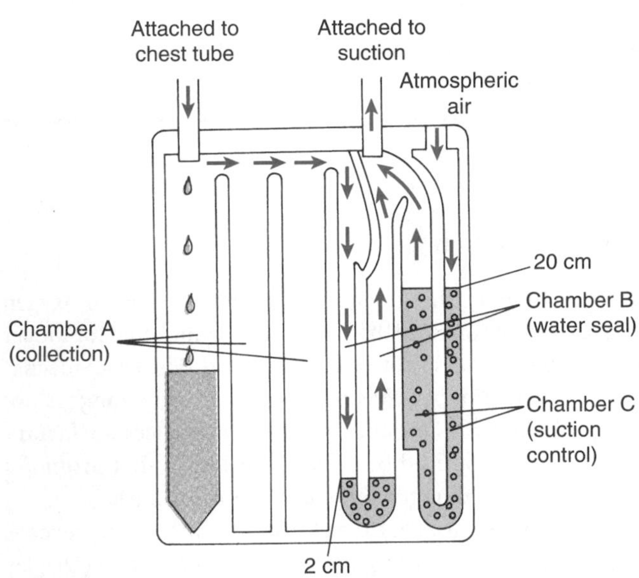

FIGURE 20–16. A three-chambered water-seal drainage system.

One of the most important principles when caring for patients with water-seal drainage is that the chest tube must never be separated from the drainage system unless it is clamped. Even then, the tube is clamped for a brief amount of time. Additional nursing responsibilities are included in Skill 20-3.

HYPERBARIC OXYGEN THERAPY

Hyperbaric oxygen therapy (HBOT) consists of the delivery of 100% oxygen at three times the normal atmospheric pressure within an airtight chamber (Fig. 20-17). Treatments, which last approximately 90 minutes, are repeated over days, weeks, or months of therapy. Providing pressurized oxygen increases the oxygenation of blood plasma from a normal level of 80 to 100 mm Hg to more than 2,000 mm Hg (Collison, 1993). Oxygen toxicity is avoided by providing patients with brief periods of breathing room air.

HBOT helps regenerate new tissue at a faster rate; thus, its most popular use is for promoting wound healing. However, it is also used for treating carbon monoxide poisoning, gangrene associated with diabetes or other conditions of vascular insufficiency, decompression sickness experienced by deep-sea divers, anaerobic infections (especially in burn patients), and a host of other medical conditions.

Nursing Implications

Nurses assess the oxygenation status of patients on a day-by-day and shift-by-shift basis. Therefore, it is not unusual to

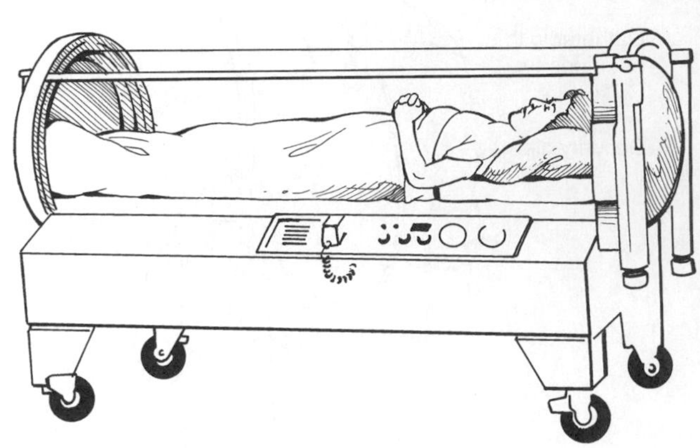
FIGURE 20–17. Hyperbaric oxygen chamber.

identify any one or several of the following nursing diagnoses among patients who are experiencing hypoxemia or hypoxia.

- Ineffective breathing pattern
- Impaired gas exchange
- Anxiety
- Risk for injury (related to oxygen hazards)

Abnormal assessment findings often lead to collaboration with the physician and the prescription for oxygen therapy. The accompanying nursing care plan is one example of how the nursing process applies to a patient with the nursing diagnosis of Ineffective breathing pattern. This diagnostic category is defined in the NANDA taxonomy (1999) as "inspiration and/or expiration that does not provide adequate ventilation." Interventions need to be adapted for older patients, who have unique age-related changes and special teaching needs.

Nursing Care Plan

Ineffective Breathing Pattern

Assessment

Subjective Data

States, "It seems so hard for me to get my breath. I can't work in my flower garden because I get winded when I try to do any gardening. I can't sleep lying down because I can't breathe except sleeping in a chair."

Objective Data

55-year-old woman with a history of smoking 1–2 packs of cigarettes daily for 30 years. Respiratory rate is rapid and shallow at 40 breaths per minute. Using accessory muscles to breathe. Barrel chest noted with diminished lung sounds bilaterally.

Diagnosis

Ineffective breathing pattern related to retention of carbon dioxide secondary to chronic pulmonary damage from long-term cigarette smoking

Plan

The patient will demonstrate an effective breathing pattern by 5/10 as evidenced by a respiratory rate no greater than 32 while performing mild activity such as bathing face, arms, and chest.

Orders: 4/28

1. Provide periods of rest between activities.
2. Elevate the head of the bed up to 90°.
3. Teach how to perform diaphragmatic and pursed-lip breathing and practice same at least b.i.d.
4. Administer oxygen per nasal cannula at 2 L/min. as prescribed by the physician if SpO_2 falls below 90% and is sustained there.
5. Explore nicotine cessation therapy with transdermal skin patches

_______________ R. ANTONIO, RN

Implementation (Documentation)

4/28 1000 Washed upper body and then provided 15 minutes of rest. Respiratory rate at 40 breaths per min. Placed in high Fowler's position. Pulse oximeter shows SpO_2 of 86%. 2 L of oxygen administered per nasal cannula. Discontinued after 30 min. when SpO_2 measured 90%. _______________ S. LUNCEFORD, LPN

Evaluation (Documentation)

1030 Demonstrated diaphragmatic and pursed-lip breathing. Having difficulty performing breathing exercises while lying down. Head raised and technique practiced again. Tolerance and performance improves in seated position.

_______________ S. LUNCEFORD, LPN

FOCUS ON OLDER ADULTS

- Age-related structural changes affecting the respiratory tract in older adults include the following: cartilage in the upper airway structures becomes more rigid due to calcification; the ribs and vertebrae lose calcium; the lungs become smaller and less elastic; the chest wall muscles become weaker and stiffer; alveoli enlarge; and alveolar walls become thinner.
- The following age-related functional changes in the respiratory tract occur: diminished coughing reflex and gag reflex; increased use of accessory muscles for breathing; diminished efficiency of gas exchange in the lungs; and increased mouth breathing and snoring.
- Some changes in lung volumes occur, resulting in a slight decrease in overall efficiency and requiring a greater energy expenditure by older adults. However, because of compensatory changes, such as the increased use of accessory muscles, older adults experience no change in the volume of air in the lungs after maximal inhalation (known as total lung capacity).
- Older adults who smoke or are inactive, debilitated, or chronically ill are at a higher risk for respiratory infections and compromised respiratory function.
- Older adults who smoke need counseling about smoking cessation and information about resources and techniques to assist with smoking cessation.
- Unless contraindicated, older adults need encouragement to maintain a liberal fluid intake (to keep mucous membranes moist) and to engage in regular exercise (to maintain optimal respiratory function).
- Older adults who have lost weight and subcutaneous fat in their cheeks may not receive the prescribed amounts of oxygen by mask because of an inadequate facial seal.
- Older adults who require home oxygen need encouragement to continue socializing with others outside the home to prevent feelings of isolation and depression.
- Older adults are advised to receive annual influenza immunizations and a pneumonia immunization at least once after the age of 65 years. Current guidelines recommend a booster dose for older adults who received their initial immunization 5 or more years ago.

KEY CONCEPTS

- Ventilation is the act of moving air in and out of the lungs. Respiration refers to the mechanisms by which oxygen is delivered to the cells.
- External respiration takes place through alveolar-capillary membranes. Internal respiration occurs at the cellular level via hemoglobin and body cells.
- The oxygenation status of patients can be determined at the bedside by performing focused physical assessments, monitoring ABGs, and using pulse oximetry.
- Five signs of inadequate oxygenation are restlessness, rapid breathing, rapid heart rate, sitting up to breathe, and using accessory muscles.
- Oxygenation can be improved by positioning patients with the head and chest elevated and teaching them to perform breathing exercises.
- When oxygen therapy is prescribed, a source for the oxygen, a flowmeter, an oxygen delivery device, and in some cases an oxygen analyzer or humidifier are all needed.
- Oxygen may be supplied through a wall outlet, in portable tanks, within a liquid oxygen unit, or with an oxygen concentrator.
- Most patients receive oxygen therapy through a nasal cannula, any one of several types of masks, or a face tent. Those who have had an opening created in their trachea may receive oxygen through a tracheostomy collar, T-piece, or transtracheal catheter.
- Whenever oxygen is administered, nurses must be concerned about two hazards: the potential for fire and oxygen toxicity.
- Older adults have unique respiratory risk factors for several reasons. They often have age-related structural and functional changes that may compromise ventilation and respiration.

CRITICAL THINKING EXERCISES

- Discuss some differences between oxygen therapy in a health care setting and that in a home environment.
- Rank the four methods of supplying oxygen, from most advantageous to least. Explain the reasons for the order in which you have ranked them.

SUGGESTED READINGS

Collison L. Hyperbarics, when pressuring patients helps. RN 1993;56(3):42–48.

Gallauresi BA. Device errors. Pulse oximeters. Nursing September 1998;28:31.

Hanson MJS. Caring for a patient with COPD. Nursing December 1997;27:39–46.

Jones S. Oxygen therapy. Community Nurse 1997;3(2):23–24.

Mattice C. Consult stat: The best place to stick a pulse ox sensor. RN 1998;61(5):63–65.

NANDA nursing diagnoses: definitions and classification 1999–2000. Philadelphia: NANDA, 1999.

Nowak TJ, Handford AG. Essentials of pathophysiology, 2d ed. Boston: McGraw-Hill, 1999.

Reynolds JE. Noninvasive ventilation for acute respiratory failure. Journal of Emergency Nursing 1997;23(6):608–610.

Ring L, Danielson E. Patients' experiences of long-term oxygen therapy. Journal of Advanced Nursing 1997;26(2):337–344.

Schakenbach L. Consult stat. Caring for patients with TTO (transtracheal oxygen therapy). RN 1997;60(5):69–70.

SKILL 20-1

USING A PULSE OXIMETER

Suggested Action	Reason for Action
Assessment	
Assess potential sensor sites for quality of circulation, edema, tremor, restlessness, nailpolish, or artificial nails.	Determines where sensor is best applied. The finger is the preferred site, followed by the toe, earlobe, and bridge of the nose. Aids in controlling possible factors that might invalidate monitored findings.
Review the medical history for data indicating vascular or other pathology, such as anemia or carbon monoxide inhalation.	Suggests the potential for unreliable data. There must be adequate circulation, red blood cells, and oxygenated hemoglobin for reliable results.
Check prescribed medications for vasoconstrictive effects.	Impaired blood flow interferes with the accuracy of pulse oximetry.
Determine how much the patient understands about pulse oximetry.	Indicates the need for and type of teaching. The best learning takes place when it is individualized.
Planning	
Explain the procedure to the patient.	Reduces anxiety and promotes cooperation and a sense of security for coping with unfamiliar situations.
Obtain equipment.	Promotes organization and efficient time management, preventing wasted motion and repeating actions.
Implementation	
Wash your hands.	Reduces the transmission of microorganisms. Soap, water, and friction remove surface microorganisms.
Position the sensor so that the light emission is directly opposite the sensor.	Ensures accurate monitoring. Proper light and sensor alignment ensures accurate measurement of red and infrared light absorption by hemoglobin.
Attach the sensor cable to the machine.	Connect the sensor with the microprocessor to ensure proper function
Observe the numeric display, audible sound, and waveform on the machine.	Indicates the equipment is functioning.

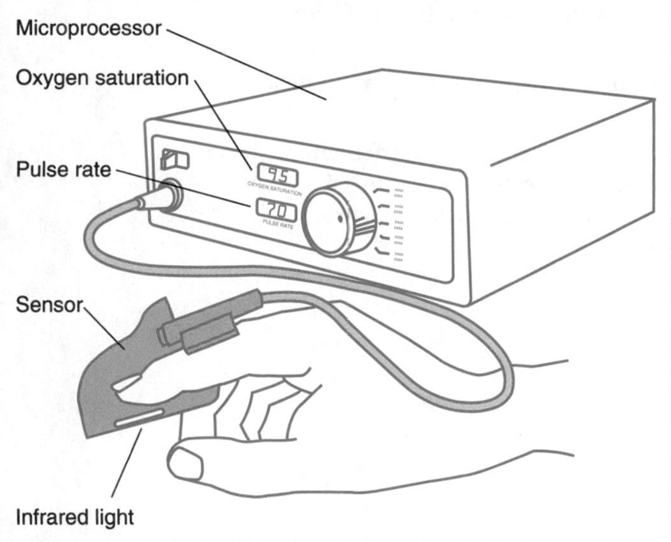

Oximetry equipment and monitor data.

continued

SKILL 20-1

USING A PULSE OXIMETER *Continued*

Suggested Action	Reason for Action
Set the alarms for saturation level and pulse rate according to the manufacturer's directions.	Programs the machine to alert the nurse to check the patient. Spot checks of SpO_2 are appropriate for patients who are stable and receiving oxygen therapy; continuous pulse oximetry is recommended for patients who are unstable and may abruptly experience desaturation.
Move an adhesive finger sensor if the finger becomes pale, swollen, or cold; remove and reapply a spring-tension sensor every 2 hours.	Prevents vascular impairment and skin breakdown because pressure greater than 32 mm Hg leads to tissue hypoxia and cellular necrosis.

Evaluation

- SpO_2 measurements remain within 95–100%.
- Patient exhibits no evidence of hypoxemia or hypoxia.
- SpO_2 measurements correlate with SaO_2 measurements.

Document

- Normal SpO_2 measurements once a shift unless ordered otherwise
- Abnormal SpO_2 measurements when they are sustained
- Nursing measures to improve oxygenation if SpO_2 levels fall below 90% and are prolonged
- Person to whom abnormal measurements have been reported and outcome of communication
- Removal and relocation of sensor
- Condition of skin at sensor site

SAMPLE DOCUMENTATION

Date and Time SpO_2 remains constant at 95–98% with pulse rate that ranges between 80–92 bpm while receiving oxygen by nasal cannula at 4 L/min. Respirations unlabored. Skin under sensor is intact and warm. Nailbed beneath sensor is pink with capillary refill <2 seconds. Spring-tension sensor changed from L. index finger to R. index finger.

________________________________ SIGNATURE/TITLE

CRITICAL THINKING

- Give some examples of factors that affect pulse oximetry measurements and how to facilitate accuracy.
- What level of oxygen saturation and pulse rates are cause for nursing concern and indicate a need for further assessment?
- What actions are appropriate if a patient appears to be hypoxemic, but the pulse oximeter indicates a normal $Sp0_2$? What action(s) would be appropriate if the opposite occurred—i.e., the patient appears normal, but the pulse oximeter reading gives you cause for concern?

SKILL 20-2

ADMINISTERING OXYGEN

Suggested Action	Reason for Action
Assessment	
Perform physical assessment techniques that focus on oxygenation.	Provides a baseline for future comparisons
Monitor the SpO_2 level with a pulse oximeter.	Provides a baseline for future comparisons
Check the medical order for the type of oxygen delivery device, liter flow or prescribed percentage, and whether the oxygen is to be administered continuously or only as needed.	Ensures compliance with the plan for medical treatment, because except in emergencies, oxygen therapy is medically prescribed.
Note whether a wall outlet is available or if another type of oxygen source must be obtained.	Promotes organization and efficient time management
Determine how much the patient understands about oxygen therapy.	Indicates the need for and type of teaching that must be done
Planning	
Obtain equipment, which usually includes a flowmeter, delivery device, and in some cases a humidifier.	Promotes organization and efficient time management
Contact the respiratory therapy department for equipment, if that is agency policy.	Follows interdepartmental guidelines Ensures nursing collaboration with various paraprofessionals to provide patient care
"Crack" the portable oxygen tank if that is the type of oxygen source being used.	Prevents alarming the patient
Explain the procedure to the patient.	Decreases anxiety and promotes cooperation
Eliminate safety hazards that may support a fire or explosion.	Demonstrates concern for safety because open flames, electrical sparks, smoking, and petroleum products are contraindicated when oxygen is in use.
Implementation	
Wash your hands.	Reduces the transmission of microorganisms
Assist the patient to a Fowler's or alternate position.	Promotes optimal ventilation
Attach the flowmeter to the oxygen source.	Provides a means for regulating the prescribed amount of oxygen

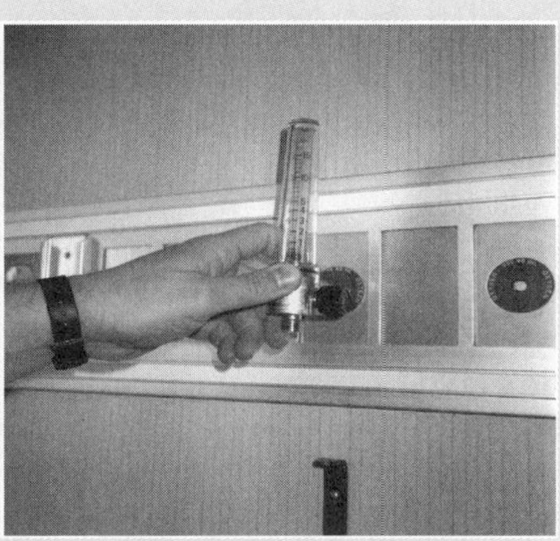

Attaching the flowmeter. (Courtesy of Ken Timby.)

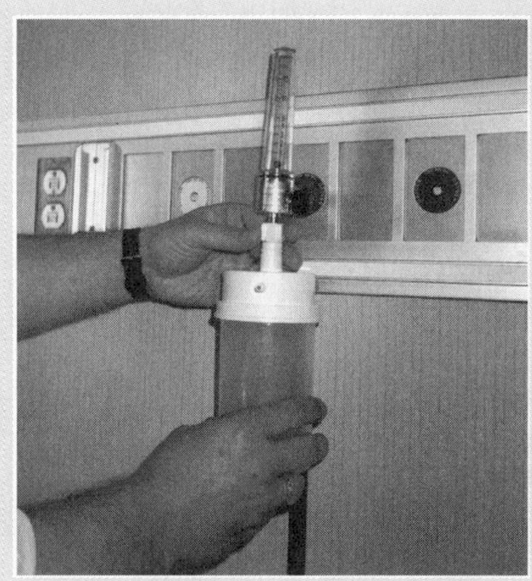

Connecting the humidification bottle. (Courtesy of Ken Timby.)

continued

SKILL 20-2

ADMINISTERING OXYGEN *Continued*

Suggested Action	Reason for Action
Fill a humidifier bottle with distilled water to the appropriate level if administering 4 or more L/min.	Provides moisture because oxygen dries mucous membranes. The potential increases with the percentage being administered.
Connect the humidifier bottle to the flowmeter.	Provides a pathway through which moisture is added to the oxygen
Insert the appropriate color-coded valve or dial the prescribed percentage if a Venturi mask is being used.	Regulates the FIO_2
Attach the distal end of the tubing from the oxygen delivery device to the flowmeter or humidifier bottle.	Provides a pathway for oxygen from its source to the patient

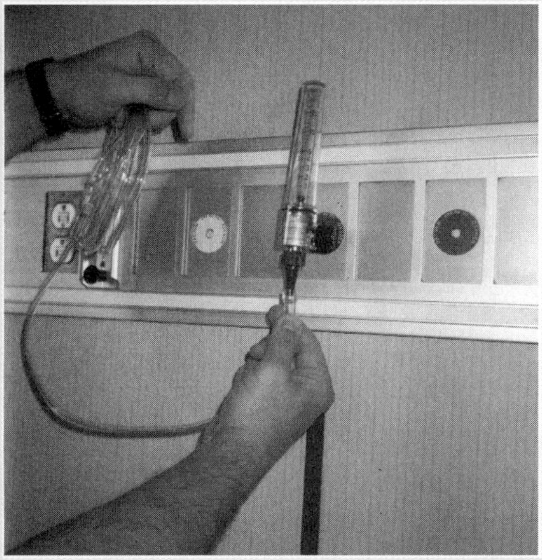

Attaching tubing from the delivery device. (Courtesy of Ken Timby.)

Suggested Action	Reason for Action
Turn on the oxygen by adjusting the flowmeter to the prescribed volume.	Fills the delivery device with oxygen-rich air
Note that bubbles appear in the humidifier bottle, if one is used, or that air is felt at the proximal end of the delivery device.	Indicates that oxygen is being released
Make sure that if a reservoir bag is used, it is partially filled and remains that way throughout oxygen therapy.	Prevents asphyxiation and promotes high oxygenation. A reservoir bag must never become totally deflated during inhalation.
Attach the delivery device to the patient.	Provides oxygen therapy
Drain any tubing that collects condensation.	Maintains a clear pathway for oxygen and prevents accidental aspiration when turning a patient
Remove the oxygen delivery device and provide skin, oral, and nasal hygiene at least every 4–8 hours.	Maintains intact skin and mucous membranes; reduces the growth of microorganisms
Reassess the patient's oxygenation status every 2–4 hours.	Indicates how well the patient is responding to oxygen therapy
Notify the physician if the patient manifests signs of hypoxemia or hypoxia despite oxygen therapy.	Demonstrates concern for safety and well-being of the patient

continued

SKILL 20-2

ADMINISTERING OXYGEN *Continued*

Evaluation

- Respiratory rate is 12–24 breaths per minute at rest.
- Breathing is effortless.
- Heart rate is <100 bpm.
- Patient is alert and oriented.
- Skin and mucous membranes are normal in color.
- SpO_2 is $\geq$ 90%.
- FIO_2 and delivery device correspond to medical order.

Document

- Assessment data
- Percentage or liter flow of oxygen administration
- Type of delivery device
- Length of time in use
- Patient's response to oxygen therapy

SAMPLE DOCUMENTATION

Date and Time Restless, pulse rate 120, resp. rate 32 with nasal flaring. Placed in high Fowler's position. SpO_2 at 85–88%. Simple mask applied with administration of oxygen at 6 L/min. After 15 min. of oxygen therapy is less agitated, pulse rate 100, respiratory rate 28, no nasal flaring noted. SpO_2 at 90%–92%. Oxygen continues to be administered.

________________________________ SIGNATURE/TITLE

CRITICAL THINKING

- List signs and symptoms that suggest a need for oxygen therapy.
- Give examples of oxygen delivery devices and circumstances for their use.
- Explain the difference between a flowmeter and an oxygen analyzer.
- Besides humidifying oxygen, what other nursing measures promote comfort and maintain the integrity of mucous membranes?
- What evidence indicates the patient is well oxygenated?
- What data are important to report to the nurse in charge or the physician about a patient who is receiving oxygen?

SKILL 20-3

MAINTAINING A WATER-SEAL CHEST TUBE DRAINAGE SYSTEM

Suggested Action	Reason for Action
Assessment	
Review the patient's medical record to determine the condition that necessitated inserting a chest tube.	Indicates whether to expect air, bloody drainage, or both; any condition that causes an opening between the atmosphere and the pleural space results in a loss of intrapleural negative pressure and subsequent lung deflation.
Determine whether the physician has inserted one or two chest tubes.	Helps direct assessment; the usual sites for chest tubes are at the 2nd intercostal space in the midclavicular line and in the 5th to 8th intercostal space in the midaxillary line.

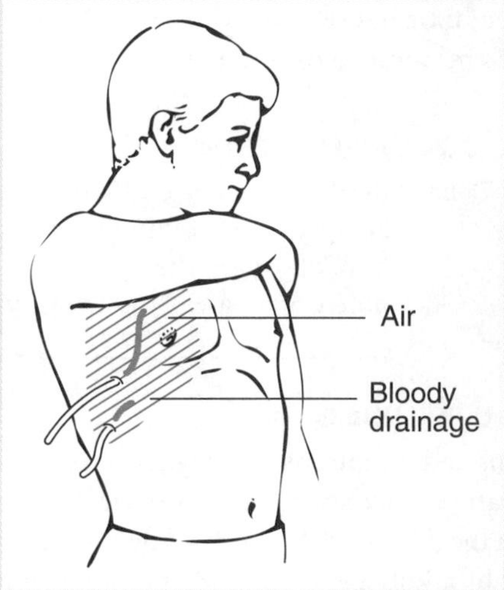

Suggested Action	Reason for Action
Note the date of chest tube(s) insertion.	Provides a point of reference for analyzing assessment data
Check the medical orders to determine whether the drainage is being collected by gravity or with the addition of suction and, if so, how much.	Provides guidelines for carrying out medical treatment; mechanical suction is used when there is a large air leak or when there is a potential for a large accumulation of drainage.
Planning	
Arrange to perform a physical assessment of the patient and equipment as soon as possible after receiving report.	Establishes a baseline and early opportunity for troubleshooting abnormal findings
Locate a roll of tape and container of sterile distilled water.	Facilitates efficient time management for general maintenance of the drainage system
Implementation	
Introduce yourself to the patient and explain the purpose for the interaction.	Reduces anxiety and promotes cooperation
Wash your hands.	Reduces the transmission of microorganisms because conscientious handwashing is one of the most effective methods for preventing infection.

continued

SKILL 20-3

MAINTAINING A WATER-SEAL CHEST TUBE DRAINAGE SYSTEM *Continued*

Suggested Action	Reason for Action
Check to see that a pair of hemostats (instruments for clamping) are at the bedside.	Facilitates checking for air leaks in the tubing or clamping the chest tube in the event the drainage system must be replaced to prevent the re-entry of atmospheric air within the pleural space, thus promoting lung expansion
Turn off the suction regulator, if one is used, before assessing the patient.	Eliminates noise that may interfere with chest auscultation
Assess the patient's lung sounds.	Provides a baseline for future comparison. Because lung sounds cannot be heard in uninflated areas, the presence of lung sounds in previously silent areas indicates re-expansion.
Inspect the dressing for signs that it has become loose or saturated with drainage.	Indicates a need for changing the dressing
Palpate the skin around the chest tube insertion site to feel and listen for air crackling in the tissues.	Indicates subcutaneous air leak and internal displacement of the drainage tube

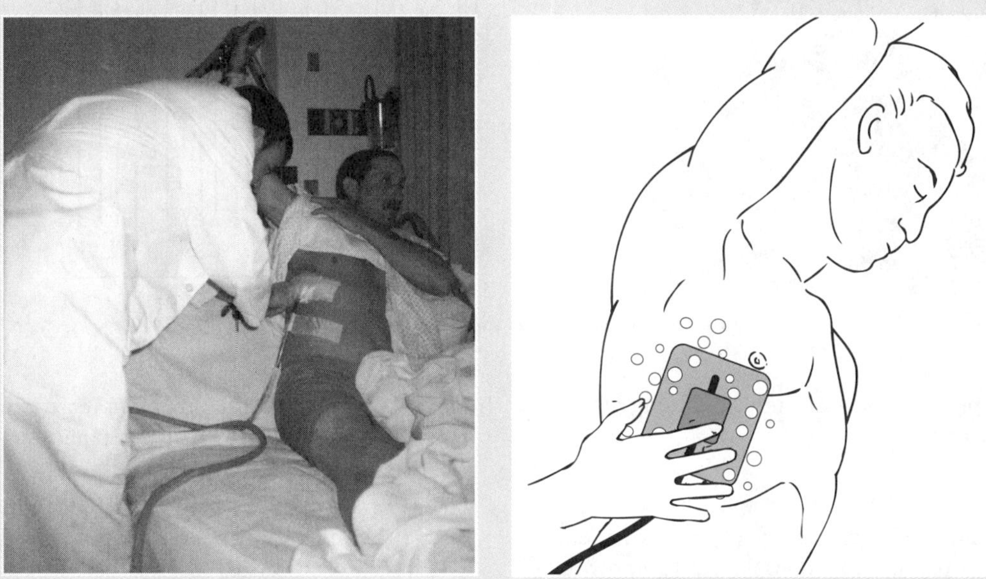

Palpating for air bubbles. (Courtesy of Ken Timby.)

Suggested Action	Reason for Action
Inspect all connections to determine that they are taped and secure.	Indicates appropriate care has been performed and ensures that the drainage system will not become accidentally separated
Reinforce connections where the tape may be loose.	Prevents accidental separation
Check that all of the tubing is unkinked and hangs freely into the drainage system.	Ensures evacuation of air and bloody drainage because fluid cannot drain upward against gravity; neither air nor fluid can pass through a physical obstruction.
Observe the fluid level in the water-seal chamber to see whether it is at the 2-cm level.	Maintains the water seal, preventing the passage of atmospheric air into the pleural space

continued

SKILL 20-3

MAINTAINING A WATER-SEAL CHEST TUBE DRAINAGE SYSTEM *Continued*

Suggested Action	Reason for Action
Add sterile distilled water to the 2-cm mark if the fluid is below standard.	Maintains the water seal
Note whether the water is **tidaling** (the rise and fall of water in the water-seal chamber that coincides with respiration).	Indicates that the tubing is unobstructed and the lung has not completely inflated; results in intrathoracic pressure changes during breathing that cause fluid to rise and fall.

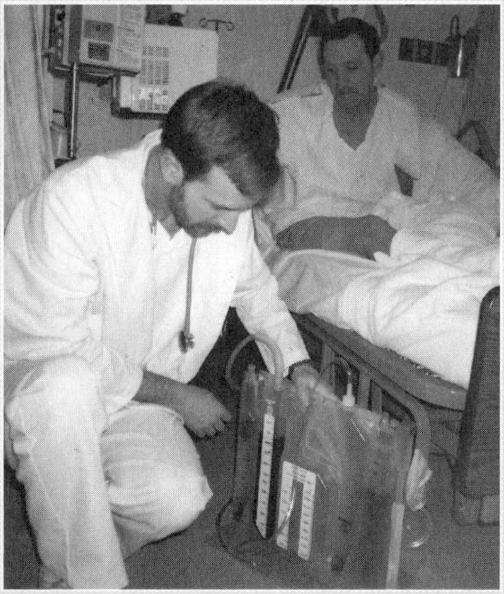

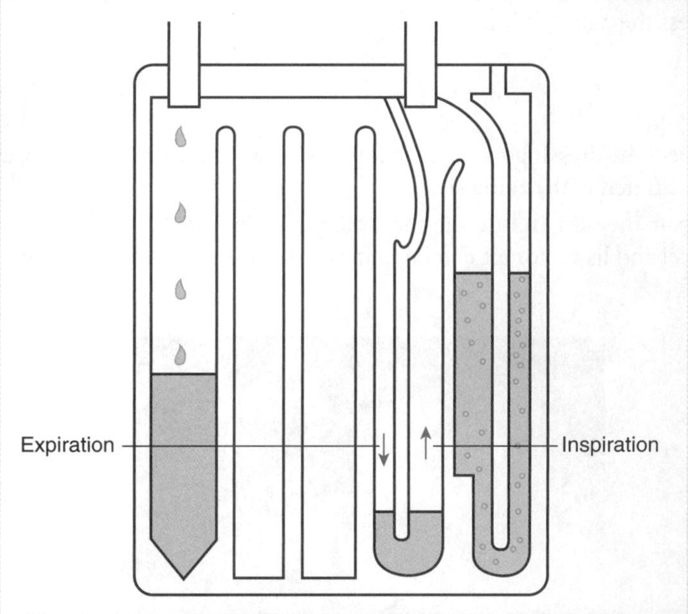

Watching for tidaling. (Courtesy of Ken Timby.)

Suggested Action	Reason for Action
Observe for the presence of continuous bubbling *in the water-seal chamber.*	Indicates an air leak in the tubing or at a connection; constant bubbling is normal and expected *in the suction control chamber* as long as it is used.
If constant bubbling is observed, clamp hemostats at the chest and within a few inches away; observe whether the bubbling stops; continue releasing and reapplying the hemostats toward the drainage system until the bubbling stops.	Provides a means for determining the location of an air leak within the tubing because gas escapes through the path of least resistance.
Apply tape around the tube above where the last clamp was applied when the bubbling stopped.	Seals the origin of the air leak
Note whether the water level in the suction chamber is at 20 cm.	Determines appropriate water level for suction because the depth of water in the suction chamber determines the amount of negative pressure—*not* the pressure setting on the suction source. The usual depth is 20 cm.

continued

SKILL 20-3

MAINTAINING A WATER-SEAL CHEST TUBE DRAINAGE SYSTEM *Continued*

Suggested Action	Reason for Action

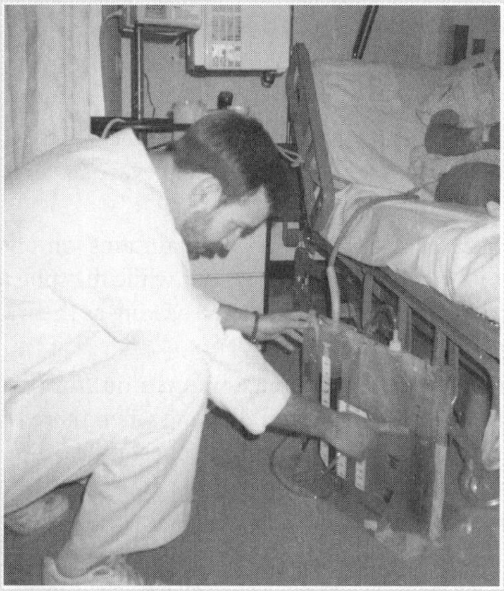
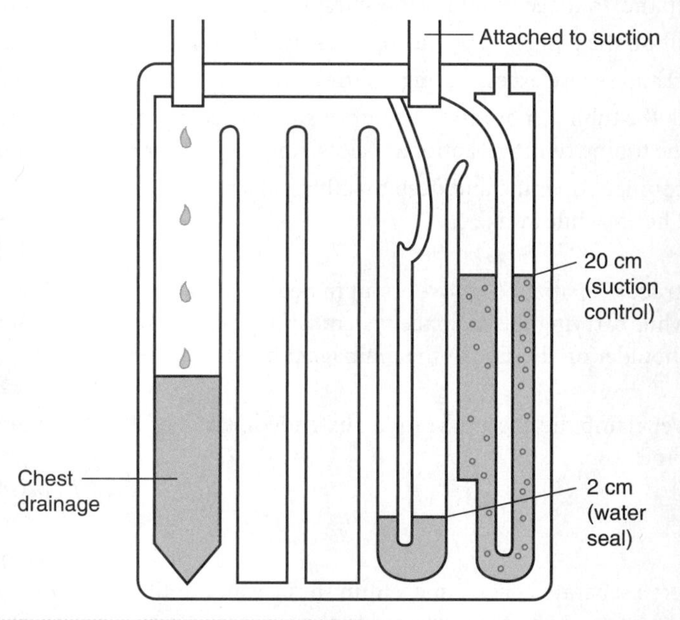

Noting water levels. (Courtesy of Ken Timby.)

Suggested Action	Reason for Action
Add sterile distilled water to the 20-cm mark in the suction control chamber if it has evaporated.	Maintains the standard amount for suction

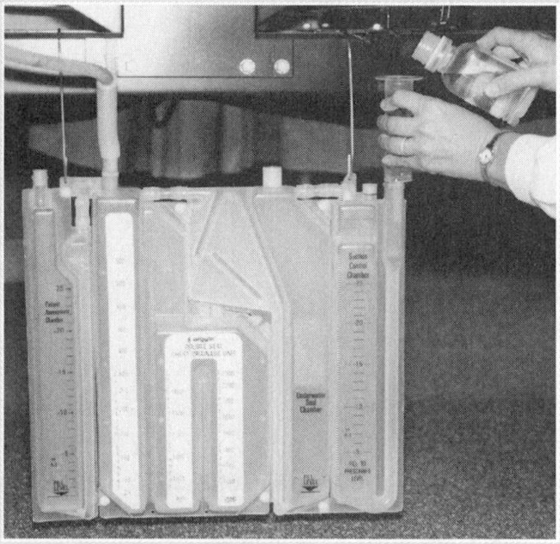

Adding water to the suction control chamber. (Courtesy of Ken Timby.)

Suggested Action	Reason for Action
Regulate the suction so that it produces *gentle* bubbling.	Prevents rapid evaporation and unnecessary noise
Observe the nature and amount of drainage in the collection chamber.	Provides comparative data; more than 100 mL/hr or bright-red drainage is reported immediately.

continued

SKILL 20-3

MAINTAINING A WATER-SEAL CHEST TUBE DRAINAGE SYSTEM *Continued*

Suggested Action	Reason for Action
Keep the drainage system below chest level.	Maintains gravity flow of drainage
Position the patient to avoid compressing the tubing.	Facilitates drainage
Curl and secure excess tubing on the bed.	Avoids dependent loops to facilitate drainage
Milk the tubing, a process of compressing and stripping the tubing to move stationary clots, only if necessary.	Creates extremely high negative intrapleural pressure; milking is never done routinely.
Encourage coughing and deep breathing at least every 2 hours while awake.	Promotes lung reexpansion because the mechanics of breathing and forceful coughing help evacuate air and fluid.
Instruct the patient to move about in bed, ambulate while carrying the drainage system, and exercise the shoulder on the side of the drainage tube(s).	Prevents hazards of immobility and maintains joint flexibility, with no danger to the patient while the tube to the suction source is disconnected as long as the water seal remains intact.
Never clamp the chest tube for an extended period of time.	Predisposes to developing a **tension pneumothorax** (extreme air pressure within the lung when there is no avenue for its escape); Clamping a chest tube *briefly* is safe, for example when changing the entire drainage system.
Insert a separated chest tube within sterile water until it can be reattached and secured to the drainage system.	Provides a temporary water seal to prevent the entrance of atmospheric air, which can recollapse the lung
Prevent air from entering the tube insertion site by covering it with a gloved hand or woven fabric, if the tube is accidentally pulled out.	Reduces the amount of lung collapse
Mark the drainage level on the collection chamber at the end of each shift.	Provides data about fluid loss without the risk of recollapsing the lung.
	Never empty the drainage container.

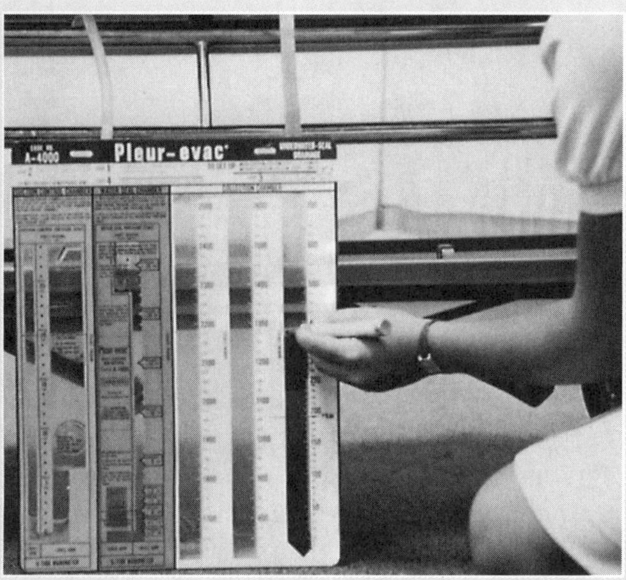

Marking drainage level. (Courtesy of Ken Timby.)

continued

SKILL 20-3

MAINTAINING A WATER-SEAL CHEST TUBE DRAINAGE SYSTEM *Continued*

Suggested Action	Reason for Action

Evaluation

- Patient exhibits no evidence of respiratory distress.
- Dressing is dry and intact.
- Equipment is functioning appropriately.
- Water is at recommended levels.

Document

- Assessment findings
- Care provided
- Amount of drainage during period of care

SAMPLE DOCUMENTATION

Date and Time Upper and lower chest tubes connected to water-seal drainage system. Normal lung sounds heard throughout chest except in apex and base of left lung, where chest tubes are inserted. Tidaling still observed in water-seal chamber. 20 cm of suction maintained. Dark-red chest tube drainage measures a scant 50 mL. Ambulated in hall while disconnected from suction. Performed full range of motion with left shoulder.

_______________________________________ SIGNATURE/TITLE

CRITICAL THINKING

- Identify the chest location and names of normal lung sounds, and describe their characteristics (refer to Chap. 12 for review).
- Discuss how a collapsed lung affects oxygenation.

UNIT SIX

PREVENTING INFECTION

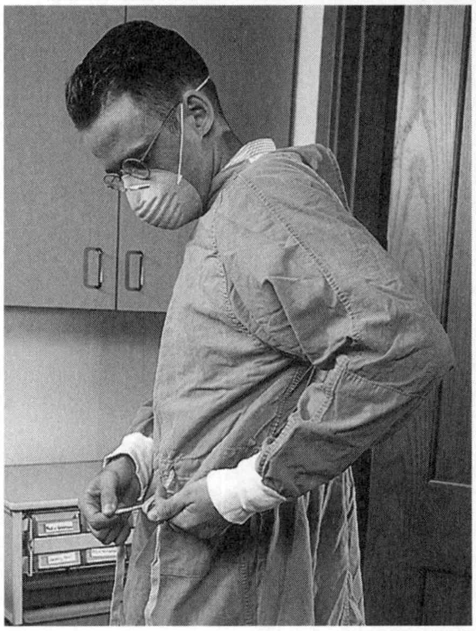

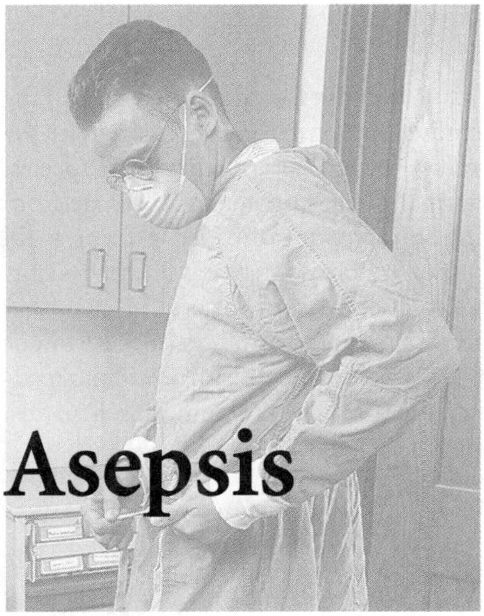

CHAPTER 21

Asepsis

CHAPTER OUTLINE

Microorganisms
Chain of Infection
Asepsis
Nursing Implications

NURSING GUIDELINES

USING A MASK OR FILTER RESPIRATOR
REMOVING GLOVES
CREATING A STERILE FIELD
DONNING A STERILE GOWN

SKILLS

SKILL 21-1: HANDWASHING
SKILL 21-2: DONNING STERILE GLOVES

NURSING CARE PLAN

KNOWLEDGE DEFICIT

KEY TERMS

aerobic bacteria
anerobic bacteria
antimicrobial agents
antiseptics
asepsis
aseptic techniques
biologic defense mechanisms
chain of infection
communicable diseases
community-acquired infections
concurrent disinfection
contagious diseases
disinfectants
exit route
hand antisepsis
handwashing
medical asepsis
microorganisms
mode of transmission
nonpathogens
normal flora
nosocomial infections
opportunistic infections
pathogens
port of entry
reservoir
resident microorganisms
spore
sterile field
sterile technique
sterilization
surgical asepsis
susceptible host
terminal disinfection
transient microorganisms
viral load

LEARNING OBJECTIVES

An understanding of the content within this chapter will be evidenced by the student's ability to:

- Describe microorganisms.
- Name seven specific types of microorganisms.
- Differentiate between nonpathogens and pathogens, resident and transient microorganisms, and aerobic and anaerobic microorganisms.
- Discuss two examples of adaptive changes that some microorganisms have made to ensure their survival.
- Name the six components of the chain of infection.
- Cite examples of biologic defense mechanisms.
- Define nosocomial infection.
- Discuss the concept of asepsis.
- Differentiate between medical and surgical asepsis.
- Identify at least three principles of medical asepsis.
- List five examples of medical aseptic practices.
- Name at least three techniques for sterilizing equipment.
- Identify at least three principles of surgical asepsis.
- List at least three nursing activities that require the application of the principles of surgical asepsis.

Preventing infections is one of the priorities in nursing. This chapter discusses how microorganisms survive and how to use **aseptic techniques** (measures that reduce or eliminate microorganisms).

Microorganisms

Microorganisms (living animals or plants visible only with a microscope) are what most people call germs. What they lack in size, they make up for in numbers. Microorganisms are literally everywhere. They are in the air, soil, and water, as well as on and within virtually everything and everyone.

Once microorganisms invade, one of three events occurs: the body's immune defense mechanisms eliminate them, they reside within the body without causing disease, or they cause an infection or infectious disease. Factors that influence whether an infection develops include the type and number of microorganisms, the characteristics of the microorganism (such as its virulence), and the person's state of health.

TYPES OF MICROORGANISMS

Microorganisms are divided into two main groups: **nonpathogens** (harmless and beneficial microorganisms) and **pathogens** (microorganisms that cause illness). Pathogens and nonpathogens include bacteria, viruses, fungi, rickettsiae, protozoans, mycoplasmas, and helminths.

Pathogens have a high potential for causing infections and **communicable diseases, contagious diseases,** or **community-acquired infections** (infectious diseases that can be transmitted to other people). Examples of communicable diseases are measles, streptococcal sore throat, sexually transmitted diseases, and tuberculosis.

Bacteria

Bacteria are single-celled microorganisms. They appear in a variety of shapes: round (cocci), rod-shaped (bacilli), or spiral (spirochetes) (Fig. 21-1). **Aerobic bacteria** (microorganisms that require oxygen to live) and **anerobic bacteria** (microorganisms that exist without oxygen) demonstrate how varied these life forms have become.

Viruses

Viruses, the smallest microorganisms known to cause infectious diseases, are seen only with an electron microscope. They are filterable, meaning they pass through very small barriers. Viruses are unique because they do not possess all the genetic information necessary to reproduce; they require the metabolic and reproductive materials of other living species. Some can remain dormant in a human and reactivate from time to time, causing an infectious disorder to recur again and again. An example of this phenomenon is the herpes simplex virus that causes cold sores (fever blisters).

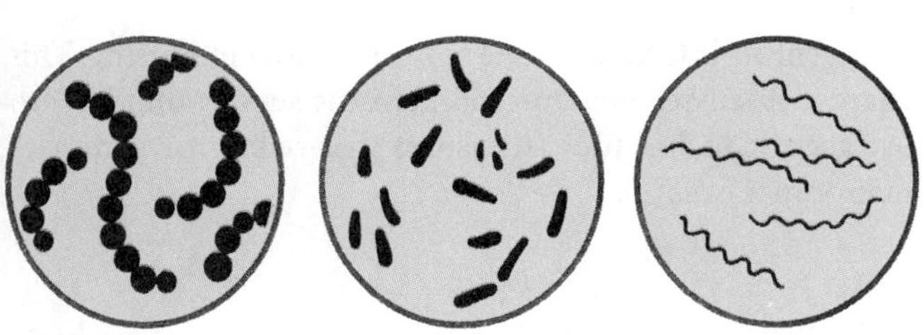

A B C

FIGURE 21–1. Classification of bacteria according to shape: (*A*) cocci, (*B*) bacilli, (*C*) spirochetes. (Timby B, Scherer S, Smith N. Introductory medical-surgical nursing, 7th ed. Philadelphia: Lippincott Williams & Wilkins, 1999.)

Some viral infections, such as the common cold, are minor and self-limiting—that is, they terminate with or without medical treatment. Others, such as rabies, poliomyelitis, hepatitis, and AIDS, are more serious or fatal.

Fungi

Fungi include yeasts and molds. Only a few types of fungi produce infectious diseases in humans. There are three types of fungal (mycotic) infections: superficial, intermediate, and systemic. Superficial fungal infections affect the skin, mucous membranes, hair, and nails. Examples are tinea corporis (ringworm), tinea pedis (athlete's foot), and candidiasis, a vaginal yeast infection. Intermediate fungal infections affect subcutaneous tissues, such as a fungal granuloma, an inflammatory lesion under the skin. Systemic fungi infect deep tissues and organs such as the lungs, causing histoplasmosis, for example.

Rickettsiae

Rickettsiae are microorganisms that resemble bacteria, but like viruses they cannot survive outside another living species. Consequently, infectious rickettsial diseases are transmitted to humans by an intermediate life form such as fleas, ticks, lice, or mites. Lyme disease, transmitted by a tiny deer tick, is a problem in New England, the Mid-Atlantic area, and some north-central states, such as Minnesota, where people live, work, or enjoy activities in wooded areas.

Protozoans

Protozoans are single-celled animals that are classified according to their ability to move. Some protozoans use *ameboid motion;* they extend their cell walls and their intracellular contents flow forward. Other protozoans move by means of *cilia,* hairlike projections, or *flagella,* whiplike appendages. Some cannot move independently at all.

Mycoplasmas

Mycoplasmas are microorganisms that lack a cell wall; they are therefore referred to as *pleomorphic* because they assume a variety of shapes. Mycoplasmas are similar to bacteria but are not related to bacteria. Primarily, these organisms infect the surface linings of the respiratory, genitourinary, and gastrointestinal tracts, causing infectious disorders in these structures.

Helminths

Helminths are infectious worms; some but not all are microscopic. Helminths are classified into three major groups: nematodes (roundworms), cestodes (tapeworms), and trematodes (flukes). Some helminths enter the body in the egg stage, whereas others spend the larval stage in an intermediate life form before finding their way into humans. Helminths mate and reproduce after they invade a species; they are then excreted, and the cycle begins again.

SURVIVAL OF MICROORGANISMS

Each species of microorganisms is unique, but they all share one characteristic: although they are infinitesimally small, they are powerful enough to cause diseases. All they need is a favorable environment in which to thrive. Conditions that promote the survival of most microorganisms include warmth, darkness, oxygen, water, and nourishment. Humans offer all of these and thus are optimal hosts for supporting the growth and reproduction of microorganisms.

Adaptation

Many pathogens have mutated to adapt to hostile environments and unfavorable living conditions. Their adaptability has ensured their survival, and therefore they continue to pose a threat to humans.

One example of biologic adaptation is the ability of some microorganisms to form spores. A **spore** (temporarily inactive microbial life form) resists heat and destructive chemicals and can survive without moisture. Consequently, spores are more difficult to destroy than their more biologically active counterparts. When conditions are favorable, spores can resume growth and reproduction.

Another example of adaptation is the development of antibiotic-resistant bacterial strains of *Staphylococcus aureus, Enterococcus faecalis* and *faecium,* and *Streptococcus pneumoniae.* These strains no longer respond to drugs that once were effective (Display 21-1). Some speculate that resistant species can transmit their resistant genes to totally different microbial species (Reiss, 1996). If that occurs—and some say it already has—the survival of humans is in jeopardy.

DISPLAY 21-1

Causes of Antibiotic Drug Resistance

- Prescribing antibiotics for minor or self-limiting bacterial infections
- Administering antibiotics prophylactically (for prevention) in the absence of an infection
- Failing to take the full course of antibiotic therapy
- Taking someone else's prescribed antibiotic without knowing whether it is effective for one's illness or symptoms
- Prescribing antibiotics for viral infections (antibiotics are ineffective for treating infections caused by viruses)
- Dispersing antibiotic solutions into the environment:
  - — depositing partially empty IV bags containing antibiotic drugs in waste containers
  - — releasing droplets while purging IV tubing attached to secondary bags of antibiotic solution
  - — expelling air from syringes before injecting antibiotics
- Administering antibiotics to livestock, leaving traces of drug residue that humans consume after their slaughter
- Spreading nosocomial pathogens via unwashed or poorly washed hands

Chain of Infection

By interfering with the conditions that perpetuate the transmission of microorganisms, humans can avoid acquiring infectious diseases. The six steps of the **chain of infection** (sequence that enables the spread of disease-producing microorganisms) must occur if pathogens are to be transmitted from one location or person to another. These essential components are:

1. An infectious agent
2. A reservoir for growth and reproduction
3. An exit route from the reservoir
4. A mode of transmission
5. A port of entry
6. A susceptible host (Fig. 21-2)

INFECTIOUS AGENTS

All microorganisms, whether pathogens or nonpathogens, are considered infectious agents, but some are less dangerous than others. Just as other animal species coexist *symbiotically* (for mutual benefit), there are **normal flora** (microorganisms that reside in and on humans) that rarely cause disease. In fact, some are necessary for maintaining healthy body functions. For example, intestinal bacteria play a role in producing vitamin K, which helps control bleeding. Bacteria in the vagina create an acid environment that is hostile to the growth of pathogenic microorganisms.

Unless the supporting host becomes weakened, normal flora remain in check. However, if the host's defenses are weakened, even benign microorganisms take advantage of the situation. Given the chance, normal flora can overwhelm their human host, causing what is termed **opportunistic infections**

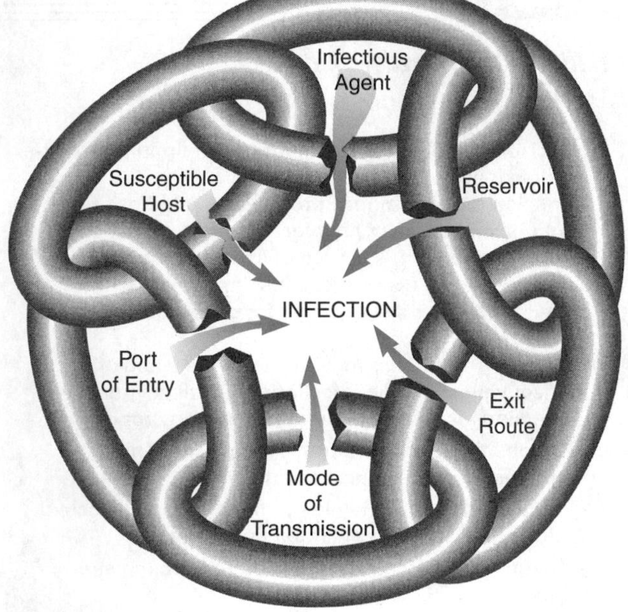

FIGURE 21–2. Chain of infection.

(disorders caused by nonpathogens that occur among people with compromised health). More commonly, however, infections are caused by pathogenic microorganisms that by their very nature produce illness after invading the tissues and organs of the body.

RESERVOIR

A **reservoir** (place where microbes grow and reproduce) provides a haven for sustaining microbial survival. Microorganisms thrive in reservoirs such as living tissue within the superficial crevices of the skin, on shafts of hair, in open wounds, in the blood stream, inside the lower digestive tract, and in nasal passages. Some grow abundantly in stagnant water and uncooked and unrefrigerated food. They are present in intestinal excreta and the organic material in the earth. Goldmann et al. (1996) used the term "silent reservoir" to describe asymptomatic patients who harbor pathogens, especially those resistant to antimicrobial agents—the most dangerous type of all.

EXIT ROUTE

The **exit route** (means by which microorganisms escape from their original reservoir) enables microorganisms to move about. When present in or on humans, they are displaced by handling or touching objects or whenever blood, body fluids, secretions, and excretions are released. In the environment, factors such as flooding and soil erosion also provide a mechanism for escape.

MODE OF TRANSMISSION

A **mode of transmission** (manner in which infectious microorganisms move to another location) is important for survival because most microorganisms lack the means to travel on their own. Microorganisms are transferred by one of five routes: contact, droplet, airborne, vehicle, and vector transmission (Table 21-1).

PORT OF ENTRY

The **port of entry** (site where microorganisms find their way onto or into a new host) facilitates relocation. One of the

TABLE 21–1. **Methods of Transmission**

Route	Description	Example
Contact transmission		
Direct contact	Actual physical transfer from one infected person to another (body surface to body surface contact)	Sexual intercourse with an infected person
Indirect contact	Contact between a susceptible person and a contaminated object	Use of a contaminated surgical instrument
Droplet transmission	Transfer of moist particles from an infected person who is within a radius of 3 feet	Inhalation of droplets released during sneezing, coughing, or talking
Airborne transmission	Movement of microorganisms attached to evaporated water droplets or dust particles that have been suspended and carried over distances greater than 3 feet	Inhalation of spores
Vehicle transmission	Transfer of microorganisms present on or in contaminated items such as food, water, medications, devices, and equipment	Consumption of water contaminated with microorganisms
Vector transmission	Transfer of microorganisms from an infected animal carrier	Diseases spread by mosquitoes, fleas, ticks, or rats

most common ports of entry is openings in the skin or mucous membranes. Microorganisms can also be inhaled, swallowed, introduced into the blood stream, or transferred into body tissues or cavities by means of unclean hands or contaminated instruments.

Biologic Defense Mechanisms

Although microorganisms are present in reservoirs everywhere, they are often prevented from producing infection because of **biologic defense mechanisms** (methods that prevent microorganisms from causing an infectious disorder). These defense mechanisms, present in humans and other animals, reduce susceptibility to infectious diseases. There are two types of biologic defense mechanisms: mechanical and chemical.

Mechanical defense mechanisms are physical barriers that prevent microorganisms from entering the body or that expel microorganisms before they multiply to overwhelming numbers. Examples of mechanical defenses are intact skin and mucous membranes; reflexes such as sneezing, coughing, and vomiting; and infection-fighting blood cells, called phagocytes or macrophages.

Chemical defense mechanisms destroy or incapacitate microorganisms using naturally produced biologic substances. Examples of chemical defenses are enzymes such as lysozyme, which is present in tears, saliva, and other secretions; the acidity of gastric acid; and antibodies. Lysozyme can dissolve the cell wall of some microorganisms. Gastric acid creates an inhospitable microbial environment. Antibodies, complex proteins that are also called immunoglobulins, form when macrophages consume microorganisms and display their distinct cellular markers.

SUSCEPTIBLE HOST

Humans become susceptible to infections when their defense mechanisms are diminished or impaired. A **susceptible host** (one whose biologic defense mechanisms are weakened in some way) is the last link in the chain of infection (Display 21-2). Patients are prime targets for infectious microorganisms because their health is already compromised. Those who are particularly susceptible include patients who:

- Are burn victims
- Have suffered major trauma
- Require invasive procedures such as endoscopy (see Chap. 13)
- Need indwelling equipment such as a urinary catheter
- Receive implantable devices such as intravenous catheters
- Are given antibiotics inappropriately; the inappropriate use of antibiotics promotes microbial resistance
- Are receiving anticancer drugs and anti-inflammatory drugs such as corticosteroids that suppress the immune system
- Are infected with HIV

DISPLAY 21-2

Factors Affecting Susceptibility to Infections

- Inadequate nutrition
- Poor hygiene practices
- Suppressed immune system
- Chronic illness
- Insufficient white blood cells
- Prematurity
- Advanced age
- Compromised skin integrity
- Weakened cough reflex
- Diminished blood circulation

Asepsis

Health care institutions are teeming reservoirs of microorganisms because of the sheer numbers of sick people who are there. Add to this the number of caretakers, equipment, and treatment devices that are in constant flux, and it is easy to understand why infection control is a major concern of health care professionals. It is important to understand and practice methods that will prevent **nosocomial infections** (infections acquired while a person is being cared for in a hospital or other health care agency).

Asepsis (practices that decrease or eliminate infectious agents, their reservoirs, and vehicles for transmission) is the major tactic for controlling infection. Two forms of asepsis, medical asepsis and surgical asepsis, are used to accomplish this goal.

MEDICAL ASEPSIS

Medical asepsis (practices that confine or reduce the numbers of microorganisms), also called *clean technique,* involves the use of measures that interfere with the chain of infection in a variety of ways. The techniques of medical asepsis are based on several principles:

- Microorganisms exist everywhere except on sterilized equipment.
- Frequent handwashing and maintaining intact skin are the best methods for reducing the transmission of microorganisms.
- Blood and body substances are considered major reservoirs of microorganisms.
- Using personal protective equipment such as gloves, gowns, masks, goggles, and hair and shoe covers serves as a barrier to microbial transmission.
- A clean environment reduces the presence of microorganisms.
- Certain areas—the floor, toilets, and the inside of sinks—are considered more contaminated than others. Cleaning should be done from cleaner to dirtier areas.

Examples of medical aseptic practices include using antimicrobial agents, performing handwashing, wearing hospital garments, confining and containing soiled materials appropriately, and keeping the environment as clean as possible. Measures used to control the transmission of infectious microorganisms are discussed in more detail in Chapter 22.

Using Antimicrobial Agents

Antimicrobial agents (chemicals that limit the numbers of infectious microorganisms by destroying them or suppressing their growth) are listed in Table 21-2. Some antimicrobials are used to clean equipment, furniture surfaces, and inanimate objects. Others are applied directly to the skin or administered internally. Examples of antimicrobial agents are antiseptics, disinfectants, and anti-infective drugs.

Antiseptics

Antiseptics (chemicals such as alcohol that inhibit the growth of but do not kill microorganisms) are also known as *bacteriostatic agents.* Antiseptics are generally applied to the skin or mucous membranes. Some are also used as cleansing agents.

Disinfectants

Disinfectants (chemicals that destroy active microorganisms but not spores) also are called *germicides* and *bactericides.* Phenol, household bleach, and formaldehyde are examples of disinfectants. Because they are so strong, they are rarely applied to the skin. Instead, they are used to kill and remove microorganisms from equipment, supplies, floors, and walls.

Anti-infective Drugs

The two groups of drugs used most often to combat infections are antibacterials and antivirals.

Antibacterials, which consist of antibiotics and sulfonamides, are drugs whose chemical actions alter the metabolic processes of bacteria but not viruses. These agents work by damaging or destroying bacterial cell walls or the mechanisms the bacteria need for growth, but they also destroy the bacteria that are part of the body's normal flora. Before the advent of antibacterial therapy, life expectancy was cut short by wound infections, dysentery, and many contagious diseases. Some believe we will return to the days of epidemics, plagues, and pestilence if antibacterial agents can no longer control microorganisms.

Antiviral agents were developed more recently, most likely in response to the rising incidence of bloodborne viral diseases such as AIDS. Antivirals do not destroy the infecting viruses; rather, they control the replication (duplication, copying) of the virus or the release of the virus from the cells. The virus remains alive and is still capable of causing a reactivation of the illness. The goal of antiviral therapy is to limit the **viral load** (numbers of viral copies).

TABLE 21–2. **Antimicrobial Agents**

Type	Mechanism	Example	Use
Soap	Lowers the surface tension of oil on the skin, which holds microorganisms; facilitates removal during rinsing	Dial, Safeguard	Hygiene
Detergent	Acts as soap, except detergents do not form a precipitate when mixed with water	Dreft, Tide	Sanitizing eating utensils, laundry
Alcohol	Injures the protein and lipid structures in the cellular membrane of some microorganisms (70% concentration)	Isopropanol, ethanol	Cleansing skin, instruments
Iodine	Damages the cell membrane of microorganisms and disrupts their enzyme functions; not effective against *Pseudomonas,* a common wound pathogen	Betadine	Cleansing skin
Chlorine	Interferes with microbial enzyme systems	Bleach, Clorox	Disinfecting water, utensils, blood spills
Chlorhexidine	Damages the cell membrane of microorganisms, but is ineffective against spores and most viruses	Hibiclens	Cleansing skin and equipment
Mercury	Alters microbial cellular proteins	Merthiolate, Mercurochrome	Disinfecting skin
Glutaraldehyde	Inactivates cellular proteins of bacteria, viruses, and microbes that form spores	Cidex	Sterilizing equipment

Handwashing

Handwashing (aseptic practice that involves scrubbing the hands with plain soap or detergent, water, and friction) mechanically removes dirt and organic substances. Plain soap or detergents do not have bactericidal activity. Handwashing removes two types of microorganisms: **resident microorganisms** (generally nonpathogens that are constantly present on the skin) and **transient microorganisms** (pathogens picked up during brief contact with contaminated reservoirs).

Although transient microorganisms are more pathogenic, they are more easily removed by handwashing. They tend to cling to grooves and gems in rings, the margins of chipped fingernail polish and broken or separated artificial nails, and long fingernails. Therefore, these items are contraindicated when caring for patients. Without conscientious handwashing, transient microorganisms become residents, thereby increasing the potential for the transmission of infection. Some believe that one explanation for the increase of antimicrobial-resistant pathogens is that the normal flora of patients are being replaced by nosocomial pathogens from health care workers who fail to wash their hands appropriately (Goldmann et al., 1996).

Considering how much the hands are used during patient care, it should come as no surprise that *handwashing is the single most effective way to prevent infections.* Skill 21-1 describes the steps of the handwashing procedure.

There are certain times when handwashing is more important than others (Display 21-3). More time is advised if the hands are visibly soiled, before assisting with a surgical procedure (Table 21-3), or before caring for a newborn or an immunosuppressed patient.

Hand antisepsis (removal and destruction of transient microorganisms) involves the use of products that are stronger than plain soap or detergent, such as antimicrobial soaps or detergents and alcohol-based handrubs. The use of alcohol-based handrubs alone is not a substitute for handwashing, because alcohol does not remove soil or dirt with organic material; however, it does produce antisepsis when the hands are already clean. When handwashing facilities are not available, a towelette containing detergent is used first for cleansing. This is followed by application of an alcohol-based handrub for 10 to 15 seconds, ensuring that all surfaces of the hands are covered.

DISPLAY 21-3

Handwashing Guidelines

Handwashing should be performed:

- When arriving at and leaving work
- Before and after contact with each patient
- Before and after equipment is handled
- Before and after gloving
- Before and after specimens are collected
- Before preparing medications
- Before serving trays or feeding patients
- Before eating
- After toileting, hair combing, or other hygiene
- After cleaning a work area

Personal Protective Equipment

Various garments are used to reduce the transfer of microorganisms between health care personnel and patients: uniforms, scrub suits or gowns, masks, gloves, hair and shoe covers, and protective eyewear. Some of these items are worn

TABLE 21–3. **Differences Between Handwashing and a Surgical Scrub**

Handwashing	Surgical Scrub
Plain wedding band may be worn.	All hand jewelry, including watch, is removed.
Faucets with hand controls are used; elbow, knee, or foot controls are preferred.	Faucets are regulated with elbow, knee, or foot controls.
Liquid, bar, leaflet, or powdered soap or detergent is used.	Liquid antibacterial soap is used; scrubbing devices may be incorporated with antibacterial soap.
Washing lasts a minimum of 10 to 15 seconds.	Scrubbing lasts 2 to 5 minutes, depending on the antibacterial agent and time interval between subsequent scrubs.
Hands are held lower than the elbows during washing, rinsing, and drying.	Hands are held higher than the elbows during washing, rinsing, and drying.
Areas beneath fingernails are washed.	Areas beneath fingernails are cleaned with an orange stick or similar nail cleaner.
Friction is produced by rubbing the hands together.	Friction is produced by scrubbing with a sponge and hand brush.
Hands are dried with paper towels; the paper is used to turn off hand-regulated faucet controls.	Hands are dried with sterile towels.
Clean gloves are donned if the nurse has open skin or if there is a potential for contact with blood or body fluids.	Sterile gloves are donned immediately after the hands are dried.

when caring for any patient regardless of diagnosis or presumed infectious status (see Chap. 22).

Uniforms

Uniforms are worn only while working with patients. Some nurses wear a clean laboratory coat over their uniform to reduce the spread of microorganisms onto or from the surface of clothing worn from home. When caring for patients, a plastic apron or cover gown is worn over the uniform if there is a potential for soiling it with blood or body fluids. When a cover is not worn, care is taken to avoid touching the uniform with any soiled items, such as bed linen. After work, the uniform is changed as soon as possible to avoid exposing the public to the microorganisms present on work clothing.

Scrub Suits and Gowns

Scrub suits and gowns are hospital garments worn in lieu of a white uniform. Their use is mandatory in some areas of a hospital—the nursery, operating room, and delivery room. Use of these garments prevents personnel from bringing microorganisms into the hospital environment on their clothes. Employees in other departments sometimes wear their own scrub suits or gowns because they are comfortable and practical. Personnel who work in mandatory-wear areas don scrub suits and gowns when they arrive for work. Cover gowns are worn over the scrubs when taking coffee or lunch breaks.

Masks

Masks cover the nose and mouth (Fig. 21-3) and are worn to prevent the spread of microorganisms by droplet and airborne transmission. To prevent the transmission of infectious agents that cause tuberculosis, the Centers for Disease Control and Prevention (Garner, 1996) recommends the use of a high-efficiency mask called a high-efficiency particulate air (HEPA) filter respirator (Fig. 21-4) or other types of masks that meet similar standards for filtering particles.

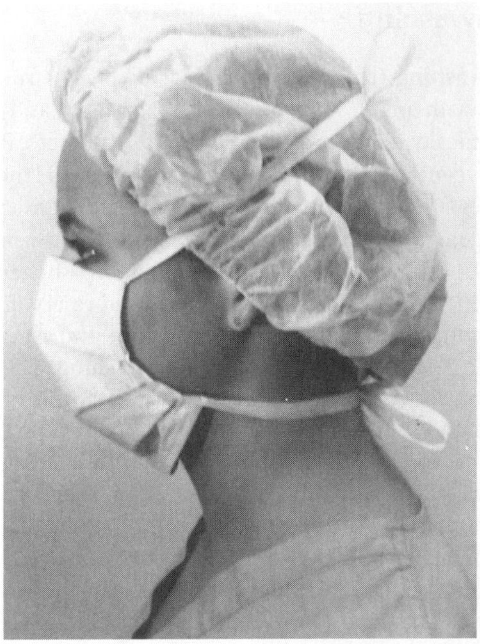

FIGURE 21–3. Face mask and hair cover. (Courtesy of Ken Timby.)

Nursing Guidelines For
Using a Mask or Filter Respirator

- ☑ Wear a mask if there is a risk for coughing or sneezing within a radius of 3 feet.
  RATIONALE: The mask blocks the route of exit.
- ☑ Wear a mask or filter respirator if there is a potential for acquiring diseases caused by droplet or airborne transmission.
  RATIONALE: The mask blocks the port of entry.
- ☑ Position the mask or respirator so it covers the nose and mouth.
  RATIONALE: The mask provides a barrier to nasal and oral ports of entry.
- ☑ Tie the upper strings of a mask snugly at the back of the head and the lower strings at the back of the neck.
  RATIONALE: Proper placement reduces the exit and entry routes for microorganisms.

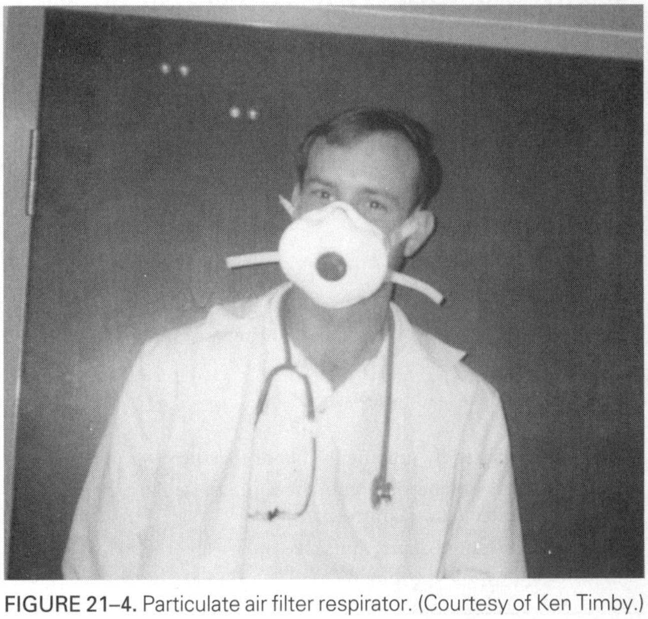

FIGURE 21–4. Particulate air filter respirator. (Courtesy of Ken Timby.)

☑ Avoid touching the mask or respirator once it is in place.
RATIONALE: Touching the mask transfers microorganisms to the hands.

☑ Change the mask or respirator every 20 to 30 minutes or when it becomes damp; filter respirators can be worn multiple times.
RATIONALE: Changing the mask preserves its effectiveness.

☑ Touch only the strings of the mask or the respirator strap during removal.
RATIONALE: Touching the mask transfers microorganisms to the hands.

☑ Discard used masks or respirators into a lined or waterproof waste container.
RATIONALE: Proper disposal reduces the transmission of microorganisms to others.

☑ Perform handwashing after removing a mask or respirator.
RATIONALE: Handwashing removes microorganisms from the hands.

Gloves

Clean gloves, sometimes called examination gloves, are used in the following circumstances:

- As a barrier to prevent direct hand contact with blood, body fluids, secretions, excretions, mucous membranes, and nonintact skin
- As a barrier to protect patients from microorganisms transmitted from nursing personnel when performing procedures or care involving contact with the patient's mucous membranes or nonintact skin
- When there is a potential transfer of microorganisms from one patient or object to another patient during subsequent nursing care

Examination gloves are generally made of latex or vinyl, although other types of gloves are available (see Chap. 18). Latex and vinyl gloves are equally protective with nonvigorous use, but latex gloves have some advantages. They stretch and mold to fit the wearer almost like a second layer of skin, permitting greater flexibility with movement. Perhaps most importantly, they can reseal tiny punctures.

Unfortunately, some nurses and patients are allergic to latex. Reactions vary and range from annoying symptoms such as skin rash, flushing, itching and watery eyes, and nasal stuffiness to life-threatening swelling of the airway and low blood pressure. Nurses who are sensitive to latex can wear alternative types of gloves, or they can wear a double pair of vinyl gloves when there is a high risk for contact with blood or body fluids.

Gloves are changed if they become perforated, after a period of use, and between the care of patients. Vinyl gloves are not as protective after 5 minutes of wear. By using aseptic techniques, gloves are removed without directly touching their more contaminated outer surface.

Nursing Guidelines For
Removing Gloves

☑ Grasp one of the gloves at the upper, outer edge at the wrist (Fig. 21-5).
RATIONALE: This maintains a barrier between contaminated surfaces.

☑ Stretch and pull the upper edge of the glove downward while inverting the glove as it is removed.
RATIONALE: This action encloses the soiled surface, blocking a potential exit route for microorganisms.

☑ Insert the fingers of the ungloved hand within the inside edge of the other glove.
RATIONALE: The inside edge is the cleaner surface of the glove.

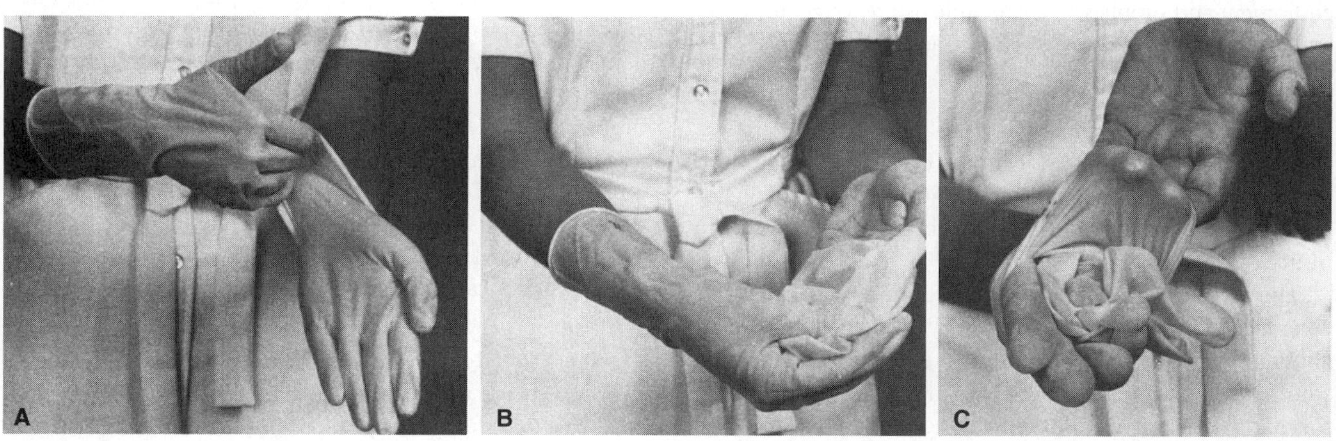

FIGURE 21–5. (*A*) Pulling at cuff. (*B*) Inverting the glove. (*C*) Enclosing contaminated surfaces.

☑ Pull the second glove inside out while enclosing the first glove within the palm.
RATIONALE: This action contains the reservoir of microorganisms.

☑ Place the gloves within a lined waste container.
RATIONALE: Proper disposal confines the reservoir of microorganisms.

☑ Wash hands immediately after gloves are removed.
RATIONALE: Handwashing removes transient and resident microorganisms that have proliferated within the warm, dark, moist environment inside the gloves.

Hair and Shoe Covers

Hair and shoe covers reduce the transmission of pathogens that are present on the hair or shoes. These garments are generally worn during surgery or when a baby is delivered.

Shoe covers are fastened so that they cover the open ends of pant legs. Hair covers should envelop the entire head. Men with beards or long sideburns wear specially designed head covers that resemble a cloth or paper helmet.

Even though hair covers are not required during general nursing care, health care workers should keep their hair short or contained with a clip, rubber band, or some other means.

Protective Eyewear

Protective eyewear is worn when there is a possibility that body fluids will splash into the eyes. Goggles are worn along with a mask, or a multipurpose face shield is used (Fig. 21-6).

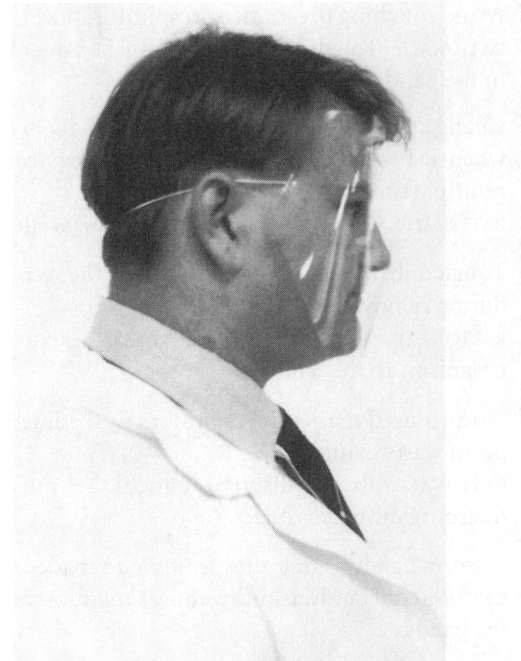

FIGURE 21–6. Face shield. (Courtesy of Ken Timby.)

Confining Soiled Articles

Several medically aseptic practices are used in hospitals to contain reservoirs of microorganisms, especially those on soiled equipment and supplies. They include using designated clean and dirty utility rooms and various waste receptacles.

Utility Rooms

There are at least two utility rooms on each nursing unit: one is designated as a clean room and the other is considered dirty. Soiled articles must not be placed in the clean utility room.

The dirty or soiled utility room contains covered waste receptacles, at least one large laundry hamper, and a flushable hopper. This room also houses equipment for testing stool or urine. A sink is located in the soiled utility room for handwashing and for rinsing grossly contaminated equipment.

Waste Receptacles

Various methods are used to contain soiled articles until they can be disposed of. Most patients have a paper bag at their bedside for tissues or other small, burnable items. Waste baskets are generally lined with plastic. Suction and drainage containers are kept covered and are emptied at least once each shift. Most patient rooms have a wall-mounted puncture-resistant container for needles or other sharp objects (Fig. 21-7).

Keeping the Environment Clean

Health agencies employ laundry staff and housekeeping personnel to assist with cleaning. In general, if soiled linen is bagged appropriately or handled with gloves, the detergents and heat from the water and the dryer produce laundry that is sufficiently clean and free of pathogenic organisms.

Housekeeping personnel are responsible for collecting and disposing of accumulated refuse and for performing concurrent and terminal disinfection. **Concurrent disinfection** (measures that keep the patient environment clean on a daily basis) is carried out by housekeepers who follow the principles of medical asepsis:

- Less soiled areas are cleaned before grossly dirty ones.
- Floors are wet-mopped and furniture is damp-dusted to avoid distributing microorganisms on dust and air currents.

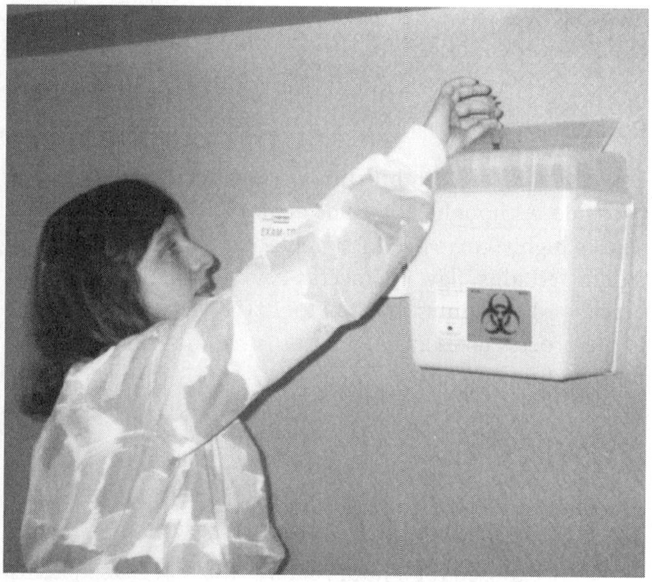

FIGURE 21–7. Sharps container. (Courtesy of Ken Timby.)

- Solutions used for mopping are discarded frequently in a flushable hopper.
- Clean items are never placed on the floor.

Terminal disinfection (measures used to clean the patient environment after discharge) is more thorough than concurrent disinfection. It includes scrubbing the mattress and the insides of drawers and bedside stands.

Nurses who work in the home health setting can teach the patient and family simple aseptic practices for cleaning contaminated articles.

Patient Teaching For

Cleaning Potentially Infectious Equipment

Teach the patient and family to do the following:

- Wear waterproof gloves when handling items that are heavily contaminated or if there are open skin areas on the hands.
- Designate one container for the sole purpose of cleaning contaminated articles.
- Disassemble and rinse reusable equipment as soon as possible after use.
- Rinse grossly contaminated items first under cool, running water; hot water causes protein substances in body fluids to thicken or congeal.
- Soak reusable items in a solution of water and detergent or disinfectant if a thorough cleaning is not immediately possible.
- Use a sponge, scrub brush, or cloth to create friction and loosen dirt, body fluids, and microorganisms from the surface of contaminated articles.
- Force sudsy water through the hollow channels of items to remove debris.
- Rinse washed items well under running water.
- Drain rinsed equipment and air dry.
- Wash hands after cleaning equipment.
- Store clean, dry items in a covered container or in a clean, folded towel.

Surgical Asepsis

Surgical asepsis (measures that render supplies and equipment totally free of microorganisms) and **sterile technique** (practices that avoid contaminating microbe-free items) begin with the process of sterilization.

STERILIZATION

Sterilization (physical and chemical techniques that destroy all microorganisms, including spores) of equipment is done within the health agency or by manufacturers of hospital supplies. Labels on commercially sterilized equipment identify a safe use date.

Physical Sterilization

Microorganisms and spores are destroyed physically by using radiation or heat (boiling water, free-flowing steam, dry heat, and steam under pressure).

Radiation

Ultraviolet radiation can kill bacteria, especially the organism that transmits tuberculosis. However, this process is generally combined with other methods of asepsis because its efficiency depends on circulating organisms by air currents from lower areas of a room to wall- or ceiling-mounted units (Centers for Disease Control and Prevention, 1994). Exposure to sunlight was used in the past to eliminate microorganisms.

Boiling Water

Boiling water is a convenient way to sterilize items used in the home. To be effective, contaminated equipment needs to be boiled for 15 minutes at 212°F (100°C)—longer in places at higher altitudes.

Free-Flowing Steam

Free-flowing steam is a method in which items are exposed to the heated vapor that escapes from boiling water. It requires the same temperature and time requirements as the boiling method. Free-flowing steam is not as reliable as boiling because it is difficult to expose all the surfaces of some contaminated items to the steam.

Dry Heat

Dry heat, or hot air sterilization, is similar to baking items in an oven. To destroy microorganisms with dry heat, temperatures of 330° to 340°F (165° to 170°C) are maintained for at least 3 hours. Dry heat is a good technique for sterilizing sharp instruments and reusable syringes because moist heat damages cutting edges and the ground surfaces of glass. Dry heat prevents rusting of objects that are not made of stainless steel.

Steam Under Pressure

Steam under pressure is the most dependable method for destroying all forms of organisms and spores. The *autoclave* is the type of pressure steam sterilizer that most health care agencies use (Fig. 21-8). Pressure makes it possible to achieve much hotter temperatures than the boiling point of water or free-flowing steam. Heat-sensitive tape that changes color or displays a pattern when exposed to high temperatures is used on sterilized packages as a visual indicator that the wrapped item is sterile.

Chemical Sterilization

Both gas and liquid chemicals are used for sterilizing invasive equipment. Until peracetic acid was perfected as a sterilizing agent, sterilization using liquid chemicals was difficult to accomplish, and some questioned its reliability. The use of peracetic acid, however, is gaining popularity as a reliable method for sterilizing heat-sensitive instruments such as endoscopes.

Gas sterilization using ethylene oxide gas is a traditional method for destroying microorganisms. It is preferred if items are likely to be damaged by heat or moisture or if no better method is available.

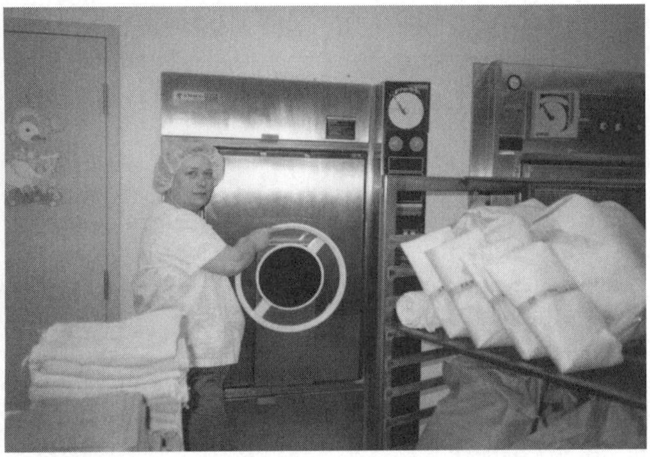

FIGURE 21–8. Autoclave. (Courtesy of Ken Timby.)

Peracetic Acid

Peracetic acid is a combination of acetic acid and hydrogen peroxide. Although early trials demonstrated that peracetic acid is highly corrosive, new methods of buffering it have eliminated this flaw. Peracetic acid sterilizes equipment quickly—12 minutes at 122° to 131°F (50° to 55°C); the entire process takes approximately a half hour from start to finish (Alfa et al., 1998).

Ethylene Oxide Gas

Ethylene oxide gas destroys a broad spectrum of microorganisms, including spores and viruses, when contaminated items are exposed for 3 hours at 86°F (30°C). Gassed items, however, must be aired for 5 days at room temperature or 8 hours at 248°F (120°C) to remove traces of the gas, which can cause chemical burns.

PRINCIPLES OF SURGICAL ASEPSIS

Surgical asepsis is based on the premise that once equipment and areas are free of microorganisms, they can remain in that state if contamination is prevented. Consequently, health care professionals observe the following principles:

- Sterility is preserved by touching one sterile item with another that is sterile.
- Once a sterile item touches something that is not, it is considered contaminated.
- Any partially unwrapped sterile package is considered contaminated.
- If there is a question about the sterility of an item, it is considered unsterile.
- The longer the time since sterilization, the greater the probability that the item is no longer sterile.
- A commercially packaged sterile item is not considered sterile past its recommended expiration date.
- Once a sterile item is opened or uncovered, it is only a matter of time before it becomes contaminated.
- The outer 1″ margin of a sterile area is considered a zone of contamination.
- A sterile wrapper, if it becomes wet, wicks microorganisms from its supporting surface, causing contamination.
- Any opened sterile item or sterile area is considered contaminated if it is left unattended.
- Coughing, sneezing, or excessive talking over a sterile field causes contamination.
- Reaching across an area that contains sterile equipment has a high potential for causing contamination and is therefore avoided.

- Sterile items that are located or lowered below waist level are considered contaminated because they are not within critical view.

The principles of surgical asepsis are observed during surgery, when performing invasive procedures such as inserting urinary catheters, and when caring for open wounds. Practices that involve surgical asepsis include creating a sterile field, adding sterile items to the sterile field, and donning sterile gloves.

Creating a Sterile Field

A **sterile field** (work area free of microorganisms) is formed using the inner surface of a cloth or paper wrapper that holds sterile items, much like a tablecloth. The field enlarges the area where sterile equipment or supplies are placed. When opening the sterile package, the nurse is careful to keep the inside of the wrapper and its contents sterile.

Nursing Guidelines For

Creating a Sterile Field

☑ Remove objects from the area where the field will be created.
RATIONALE: Removing unsterile items provides room for working without accidental contamination.

☑ Wash hands.
RATIONALE: Handwashing reduces the numbers of microorganisms on the hands.

☑ Place the wrapped package on a surface at or above waist level.
RATIONALE: This placement keeps sterile items within sight.

☑ Position the package so that the outermost triangular edge of the wrapper can be moved away from the front of the body (Fig. 21-9).
RATIONALE: This placement prevents reaching over the sterile area.

☑ Unfold each side of the wrapper by touching the area that will be in direct contact with the table or stand, or touch no more than the outer 1″ of the edge of the wrapper.
RATIONALE: This action maintains a sterile zone.

☑ Unfold the final corner of the wrapper by pulling it toward the body.
RATIONALE: This action avoids reaching over an uncovered sterile area.

Adding Items to a Sterile Field

Sometimes it is necessary to add sterile items or sterile solutions to the sterile field.

Sterile Items

Agency-sterilized items or those that have been commercially prepared are added to the sterile field. The former are generally wrapped in a cloth towel. The cloth wrapper is unwrapped as described in the previous nursing guidelines, except the nurse supports the wrapped item in one hand rather than placing it on a solid surface. Each of the four corners is held to prevent the edges of the wrap from hanging loosely (Fig. 21-10). The unwrapped item is placed on the sterile field and the cloth cover is discarded.

Commercially prepared supplies, such as sterile gauze squares, are enclosed in paper wrappers. The paper cover usually has two loose flaps that extend above the sealed edges. By separating the flaps, the sterile contents are dropped onto the sterile field (Fig. 21-11).

Sterile Solutions

Sterile solutions, such as normal saline, come in a variety of volumes. Some containers are sealed with a rubber cap or a screw top. Either is replaced if the inside surface is contami-

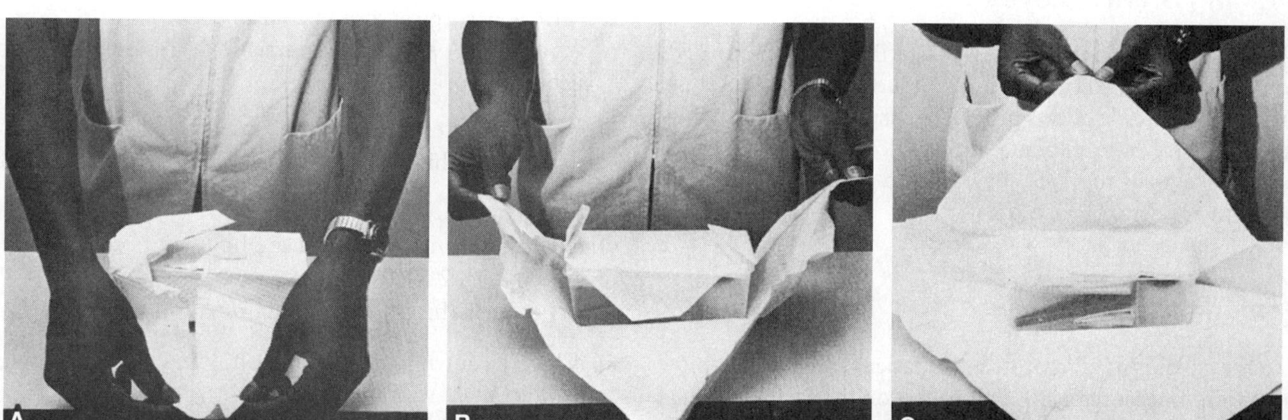

FIGURE 21–9. (*A*) Unfolding away from the body. (*B*) Unfolding the sides. (*C*) Unfolding toward the body.

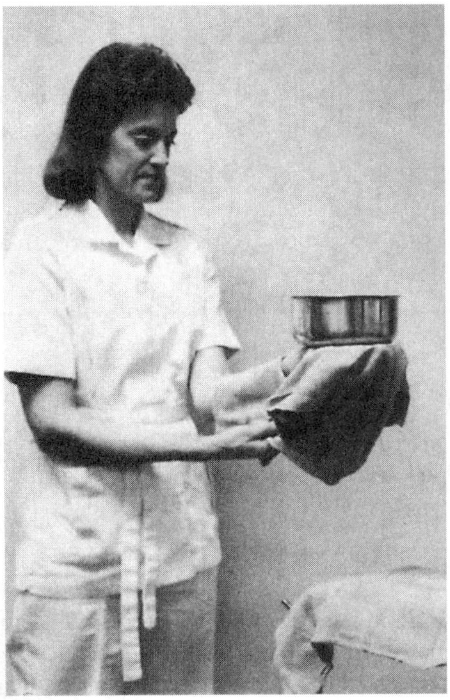

FIGURE 21–10. Adding a sterile basin. (Courtesy of Ken Timby.)

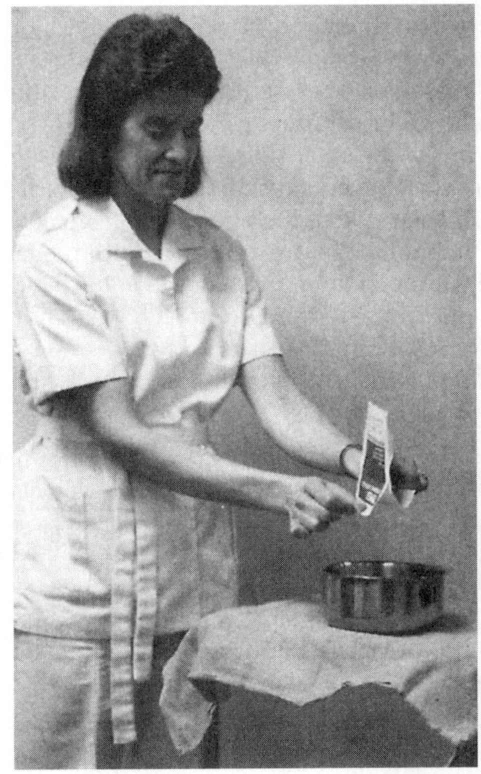

FIGURE 21–11. Adding sterile gauze. (Courtesy of Ken Timby.)

nated. To avoid contamination, the cap is placed upside down on a flat surface or held during pouring.

Before each use of a sterile solution, a small amount of the solution is poured and discarded to wash away airborne contaminants from the mouth of the container. This is called *lipping* the container.

When pouring the sterile solution, the container is held in front of the nurse. The nurse avoids touching any sterile areas within the field. The height of the container is controlled to avoid splashing the sterile field, causing a wet area of contamination (Fig. 21-12). Sterile solutions are replaced on a daily basis even if the entire volume is not used.

Donning Sterile Gloves

When applied correctly (Skill 21-2), sterile gloves can be used to handle sterile equipment and supplies without contaminating them. Sterile gloves provide a barrier to the transmission of microbes to patients. Sterile gloves are included in some packages of supplies; they are also packaged separately in glove wrappers.

Donning a Sterile Gown

A sterile gown is used to protect the patient and sterile equipment from microorganisms that collect on the surface of uniforms, scrub suits, or scrub gowns. Sterile gowns are required during surgery and delivery of infants. They are used during other sterile procedures as well.

Sterile gowns are made of cloth and are laundered and sterilized after each use. Before wrapping a gown for sterilization, it is folded so that its inside surface can be touched while putting it on. To avoid contamination, the following guidelines are observed.

Nursing Guidelines For

Donning a Sterile Gown

- ☑ Apply a mask and hair cover.
  RATIONALE: This sequence prevents contamination of the hands after they are washed.
- ☑ Perform a surgical scrub (see Table 21-3).
  RATIONALE: A surgical scrub removes resident and transient microorganisms.
- ☑ Pick up the sterile gown at the inner neckline.
  RATIONALE: This action preserves the sterility of the outer gown.
- ☑ Hold the gown away from the body and other unsterile objects (Fig. 21-13)
  RATIONALE: This prevents contamination.
- ☑ Allow the gown to unfold while holding it high enough to avoid contact with the floor.
  RATIONALE: This prevents contamination.

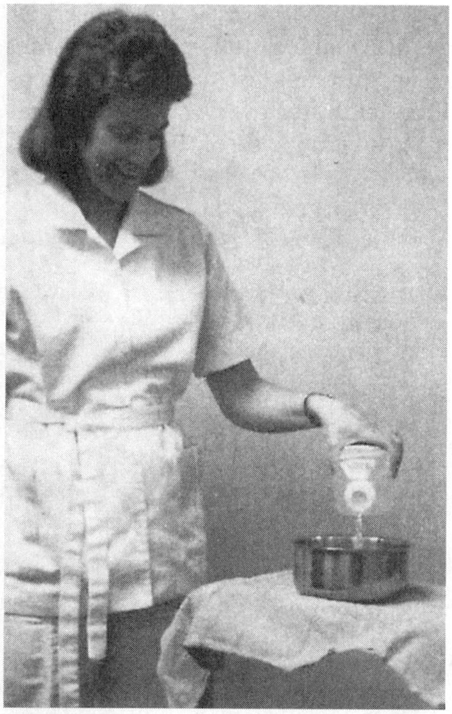

FIGURE 21–12. Adding sterile solution. (Courtesy of Ken Timby.)

☑ Insert an arm within each sleeve without touching the outer surface of the gown.
RATIONALE: This action maintains sterility.

☑ Have an assistant pull at the inside of the gown to adjust the fit, expose the hands, and then tie it closed.
RATIONALE: This action preserves the sterility of the front of the gown.

☑ Don sterile gloves.
RATIONALE: Wearing sterile gloves ensures the sterile condition of the hands and cuff of the gown.

Nursing Implications

Everyone is susceptible to infections, especially if sources of microorganisms among personnel and patients, equipment, and the agency environment are not controlled. Pertinent nursing diagnoses are generally identified when caring for particularly susceptible patients.

- Risk for infection
- Risk for infection transmission
- Altered protection
- Delayed surgical recovery
- Knowledge deficit

The nursing care plan illustrates how aseptic principles are incorporated into a teaching plan for the nursing diagnosis of Knowledge deficit. The NANDA taxonomy (1999) defines knowledge deficit as an absence or deficiency of cognitive information related to a specific topic. Carpenito (1999) used the definition "the state in which an individual or group experiences a deficiency in cognitive knowledge or psychomotor skills concerning the condition or treatment plan." Some have argued that this nursing diagnosis is erroneously used because it is more often an etiology than a nursing diagnosis (Jenny, 1987).

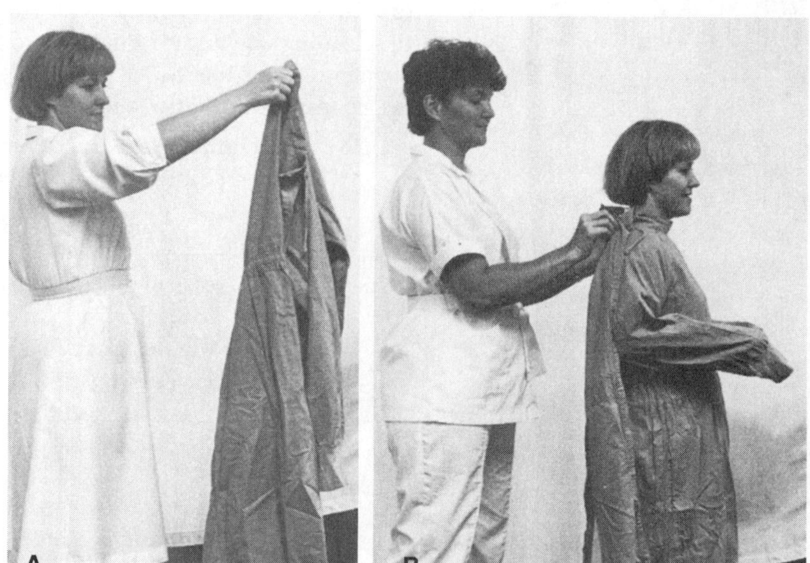

FIGURE 21–13. (*A*) Unfolding a sterile gown. (*B*) Assisting with donning a sterile gown. (Courtesy of Ken Timby.)

Nursing Care Plan

Knowledge Deficit

Assessment

Subjective Data

States, "The school nurse sent this note home saying there's been a case of hepatitis in my daughter's fifth-grade class. Isn't that what drug users get? Should I keep my daughter home from school? What will prevent her from catching it?" Daughter is not experiencing any anorexia or tenderness in right upper quadrant.

Objective Data

11-year-old girl in the fifth grade. Public health department confirms one case of hepatitis A at school. TPR is currently normal. Liver is not palpable. Denies nausea or diarrhea. Sclera of OU are white. Freshly voided urine is light yellow and tests negative for bilirubin with a chemstrip . Will receive gamma globulin injection today.

Diagnosis

Knowledge deficit: cause and prevention of hepatitis A related to unfamiliarity with infectious disease transmission

Plan

Goal

The child will satisfactorily return a demonstration of handwashing and mother will list at least three signs and symptoms of hepatitis A by the end of this office visit.

Orders: 11/17

1. Explain that hepatitis A is spread primarily from stool of an infected person to the mouth of a susceptible person.
2. Provide the following information and ask mother to recall at least three signs and symptoms:
   a. Hepatitis B is usually associated with IV drug use and contaminated blood.
   b. The incubation period of hepatitis A is 25 to 30 days.
   c. Handwashing is an excellent preventive measure when performed before eating and after each use of the toilet; staying home from school is not necessary.
   d. Signs and symptoms include low-grade fever, reduced activity, loss of appetite, nausea, abdominal pain, dark urine, light-colored stool, and yellowing of the skin and white portion of the eyes.
3. Demonstrate handwashing and observe return demonstration, emphasizing the following:
   a. Turn handles of school faucet on using a paper towel and let water run.
   b. Wet hands and lather with liquid soap from a hand-pump dispenser.
   c. Rub lathered hands for at least 10 to 15 seconds.
   d. Rinse, letting water flow from wrists to fingers.
   e. Dry hands with paper towel.
   f. Use a paper towel to turn faucet handle off.____________________ A. JOHNSON, RN

Implementation (Documentation)

11/7 1630 Differentiated between hepatitis A and B. States, "I'm so relieved that this case isn't caused by sharing drug needles." Provided with additional information on hepatitis as identified in care plan. Handwashing demonstration given.____________________ A. JOHNSON, RN

Evaluation (Documentation)

1645 Mother recalled the following signs and symptoms: fever, loss of appetite, nausea, and yellowing of eyes and skin. Child performed handwashing procedure as demonstrated. Given immune serum globulin injection in L. vastus lateralis muscle.____________________ A. JOHNSON, RN

FOCUS ON OLDER ADULTS

- Conscientious handwashing is necessary when caring for all patients, but it is especially important with older adults because they are more susceptible to infections.
- Maintaining intact skin is an excellent first-line defense against acquiring nosocomial infections, but one that is often compromised among older adults.
- People who are debilitated or over 75 are at higher risk for infections, particularly those that are resistant to antibiotics.
- According to surveillance surveys conducted by the Centers for Disease Control and Prevention, many nursing home residents, older hospitalized patients, and health care personnel are colonized with antibiotic-resistant bacteria (Shoevin & Young, 1992).
- Older adults are more likely to have life-threatening consequences of infections than younger adults. For example, mortality rates from pneumonia show an age-related increase from a rate of 24 per 100,000 people aged 60 to 64 years to 1,032 per 100,000 for people aged 85 and older. (Calahan & Wolinsky, 1996).
- Nursing home residents tend to develop infections involving the skin, urinary tract, and respiratory tract.
- Because of the increased susceptibility of older adults to urinary tract infections, the use of indwelling catheters is avoided whenever possible.
- Older adults are more susceptible to pneumonia, influenza, and tuberculosis than their younger counterparts. For example, the incidence of tuberculosis in community-living older adults is twice that of the general population; for older adults in nursing homes, the incidence is four times that in the general population (Miller, 1999).
- Infections are often transmitted to vulnerable older adults through equipment reservoirs such as indwelling urinary catheters, humidifiers, and oxygen equipment or through incisional sites such as those for intravenous tubing, parenteral nutrition, or tube feedings. Use of proper aseptic techniques is essential to prevent the introduction of microorganisms.
- When caring for older patients, attention to perineal hygiene and handwashing is a priority because opportunistic infections from organisms in the stool may develop.
- Older adults and all personnel in health care settings should obtain annual immunizations against influenza; older adults should be immunized against pneumonia.
- Visitors with respiratory infections need to avoid contact with older adults until their symptoms have subsided, or they need to wear a mask.
- Health care workers who are ill should take sick leave rather than expose susceptible patients to infectious organisms.

KEY CONCEPTS

- Microorganisms are living animals or plants that can be seen only with a microscope.
- Some examples of microorganisms are bacteria, viruses, fungi, rickettsiae, protozoans, mycoplasmas, and helminths.
- Nonpathogens are generally harmless microorganisms, whereas pathogens have a high potential for causing infections and contagious diseases. Resident microorganisms are generally nonpathogens that are always present on the skin. Transient microorganisms are generally pathogens that are more easily removed through handwashing. Aerobic microorganisms require oxygen for survival, whereas anaerobic microorganisms do not.
- Some microorganisms have ensured their survival by developing the capacity to form spores and resist antibiotic drug therapy.
- The components of the chain of infection are an infectious agent, a reservoir for growth and reproduction, an exit route from the reservoir, a mode of transmission, a port of entry, and a susceptible host.
- Susceptibility to infectious agents is reduced by several biologic defenses such as intact skin and mucous membranes; reflexes such as sneezing, coughing, and vomiting; infection-fighting blood cells; enzymes such as lysozyme, which is present in tears, saliva, and other secretions; the acidity of gastric acid; and antibodies.
- Nosocomial infections are those acquired by previously uninfected patients while they are being cared for in a health care facility.
- Asepsis refers to practices that decrease the numbers of infectious agents, their reservoirs, and vehicles for transmission.
- Medical asepsis involves practices that confine or reduce the presence of microorganisms.
- Principles of medical asepsis include the following: frequent handwashing and maintaining intact skin are the best methods for reducing the transmission of microorganisms; the use of personal protective equipment (gloves, gown, mask, goggles, and hair and shoe covers) provides barriers that interferes with the transmission of microorganisms; and a clean environment reduces the numbers of microorganisms.
- Examples of medical aseptic practices include using antimicrobial agents, washing hands, wearing hospital garments, confining soiled articles, and keeping the environment clean.
- Surgical asepsis involves measures that render supplies and equipment totally free of microorganisms and practices that avoid contamination during their use.
- Surgical asepsis involves sterilization measures such as ultraviolet radiation, heat, or chemicals.
- Three of the principles of surgical asepsis are as follows: sterility is preserved by touching one sterile item with another one that is sterile; once a sterile item touches something that is not, it is considered contaminated; and any partially unwrapped sterile package is considered contaminated.
- Principles of surgical asepsis are applied when nurses create a sterile field, add supplies or liquids to a sterile field, and don sterile gloves.

CRITICAL THINKING EXERCISES

- Use the chain of infection to trace the transmission of a common cold from one person to another.
- Describe methods of medical asepsis that are helpful in controlling the chain of infection of the common cold.
- If the rate of patient infections increased on a nursing unit, what would you investigate to determine the contributing factors?
- If the cause of nosocomial infections is related to inadequate handwashing among health care personnel, give some suggestions for correcting the problem.

SUGGESTED READINGS

Alfa MJ, DeGagne P, Olson N, Hizon R. Comparison of liquid chemical sterilization with peracetic acid and ethylene oxide sterilization for long narrow lumens. American Journal of Infection Control 1998;26(5):469–477.

Association of Operating Room Nurses. Recommended practices for high-level disinfection. AORN Journal 1999;69(3):591–598.

Calahan CM, Wolinsky FD. Hospitalization for pneumonia among older adults. Journal of Gerontology 1996;51A(6):M276–282.

Carpenito LJ. Nursing diagnoses: application to clinical practice, 8th ed. Philadelphia, Lippincott Williams & Wilkins, 1999.

Centers for Disease Control and Prevention. Guidelines for preventing the transmission of tuberculosis in health-care facilities. Morbidity and Mortality Weekly Report 1994;43(RR13):1–132.

CDC releases final HCW infection guidelines. Hospital Employee Health 1998;17(10):121–122.

Citarella BB, Mueller CJ. Antibiotic-resistant bacteria: safe practices. Caring 1998;17(4):22–24.

Controlling vancomycin-resistant staphylococcal infections: new CDC guidelines. Journal of Critical Illness 1998;13(7):439.

Follow these guidelines for resistant *S. aureus.* Healthcare Benchmarks 1997;4(11):164–165.

Garner JS. Guidelines for isolation precautions in hospitals. Atlanta, Centers for Disease Control and Prevention, 1996.

Garner JS, Favero MS. Guideline for handwashing and hospital environmental control. Atlanta, Centers for Disease Control and Prevention, 1985.

Goldmann DA, Weinstein RA, Wenzel RP, et al. Strategies to prevent and control the emergence and spread of antimicrobial-resistant microorganisms in hospitals: a challenge to hospital leadership. Journal of the American Medical Association 1996;275(3):234–241.

Griffiths-Jones A. Putting up a united front: combatting methicillin-resistant *S. aureus.* Nursing Times 1996;92(19):61–62.

Highlights of CDC's proposed guidelines. OR Manager 1998;14(8):16–17.

Hoffman M. Regulatory update. CDC guidelines for infection precautions. Caring 1997;16(9):58–60.

Jenny J. Knowledge deficit: not a nursing diagnosis. Image 1987;19(4):184–185.

Larson EL. APIC guideline for handwashing and hand antisepsis in health care settings. American Journal of Infection Control 1995;23(4):251–269.

Martone WJ. Spread of vancomycin-resistant enterococci: why did it happen in the United States? Infection Control and Hospital Epidemiology 1998;19(8):539–545.

Mathias JM. APIC guideline recommends shortened surgical scrub. OR Manager 1995;11(11):13.

Miller CA. Nursing care of older adults, 3d ed. Philadelphia, Lippincott Williams & Wilkins, 1999.

NANDA nursing diagnoses: definitions and classification, 1999–2000. Philadelphia, NANDA, 1999.

Norman EM. Critical questions. Fingernails and microflora. American Journal of Nursing 1998;98(10):16HH.

Rees J. Infection control. Washing instructions. Nursing Times 1997;93(37):74.

Reiss PJ. Battling the super bugs. RN 1996;59(3):36–40.

Rice R. Home health care. Infection control in the home: 1998 update. Geriatric Nursing: American Journal of Care for the Aging 1998; 19(5):297–300.

Rutala WA. APIC guidelines for infection control practice. American Journal of Infection Control 1996;24(4):313–342.

Rutala WA. Practical healthcare epidemiology. Disinfection and sterilization of patient-care items. Infection Control and Hospital Epidemiology 1996;17(6):377–384.

Schneider NJ. Infection control. How to safely clean surgical instruments. American Journal of Nursing 1997;97(2):59.

Shales DM, Gerding DN, John JF Jr, et al. SHEA position paper on the prevention of antimicrobial resistance: guidelines for the prevention of antimicrobial resistance in hospitals. Infection Control and Hospital Epidemiology 1997;18(4):275–291.

Shoevin J, Young MS. MRSA: Pandora's box for hospitals: methicillin-resistant *Staphylococcus aureus.* American Journal of Nursing 1992;92:48–52.

Thompson BL, Dwyer DM, Ussery XT, et al. Handwashing and glove use in a long-term care facility. Infection Control and Hospital Epidemiology 1997;18(2):97–103.

SKILL 21-1

HANDWASHING

Suggested Action	Reason for Action
Assessment	
Review the medical record to determine whether it is appropriate to perform handwashing for longer than 10 to 15 seconds	Demonstrates concern for immunosuppressed patients, newborns, or other susceptible hosts
Check that there are soap and paper towels near the sink and that a waste receptacle is nearby.	Promotes effective handwashing and disposal of paper towels; bar soap is supplied in small cakes, which are changed frequently and placed on a drainable holder to avoid colonization with microorganisms; liquid soap is stored in closed containers that are replaced, or cleaned, dried, and refilled on a regular schedule.
Planning	
Trim long fingernails.	Reduces the reservoir where the majority of hand flora reside; prevents tearing gloves
Remove all jewelry; a plain, *smooth* wedding band can be worn; roll up long sleeves.	Facilitates removing transient and resident microorganisms; bacterial counts are higher when rings are worn during patient care.
Explain the purpose for handwashing to the patient.	Reinforces and demonstrates concern for patient safety
Implementation	
Turn on the water using faucet handles, elbow, knee, or foot controls (see Fig. A).	Serves as a wetting agent and facilitates lathering; enhances organization and prevents contamination of hands after they are washed.

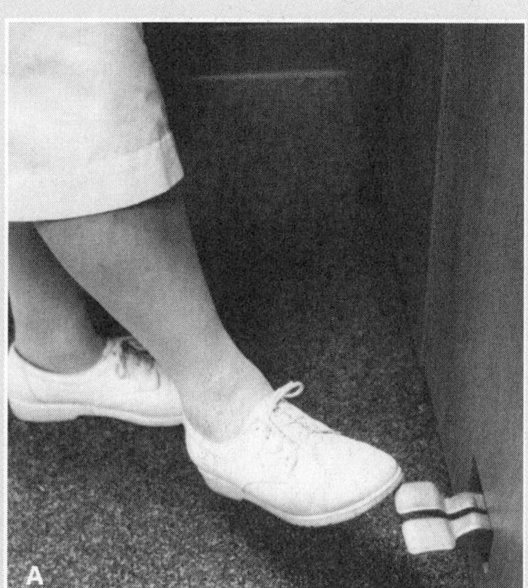

Using foot controls. (Courtesy of Ken Timby.)

Suggested Action	Reason for Action
If a lever-operated paper towel dispenser is available, activate it to dispense the paper towel.	Sinks with electronic sensors decrease hand contamination before and after handwashing, but they are not generally available in most health care agencies.

continued

SKILL 21–1

HANDWASHING *Continued*

Suggested Action	Reason for Action
Wet your hands with comfortably warm water from the wrists toward the fingers (see Fig. B).	Allows water to flow from the least contaminated area to the most contaminated area

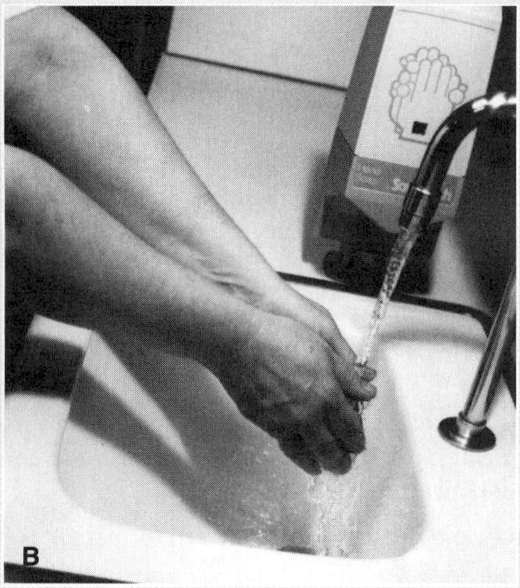

Wetting hands. (Courtesy of Ken Timby.)

Suggested Action	Reason for Action
Avoid splashing water from the sink onto your uniform	Prevents transferring microorganisms to clothing via a wicking action
Dispense about 3 to 5 mL (1 tsp) of liquid soap into your hands, or wet a cake of bar soap.	Provides an agent for emulsifying body oils and releasing microorganism.
Work the soap into a lather and generate friction (see Fig. C).	Expands the volume and distribution of the soap; begins to soften the keratin layer of the skin: loosens debris and directs soap into crevices of skin.

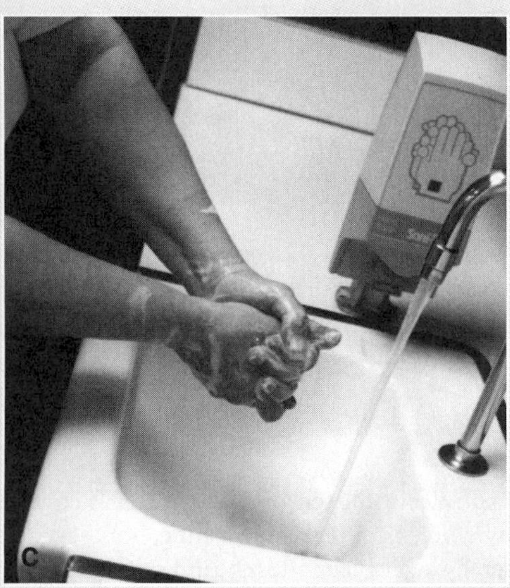

Working up a lather and generating friction. (Courtesy of Ken Timby.)

continued

SKILL 21-1

HANDWASHING *Continued*

Suggested Action	Reason for Action
Rinse the bar soap, if used, and replace it within a drainable soap dish.	Flushes microorganisms from the surface of the soap; drained bar soap is less likely to support growth of microorganisms.
Rub the lather vigorously over all surfaces of the hands, including thumbs and backs of fingers and hands, and under the fingernails.	Frees microorganisms that are lodged in skin creases and crevices
Rinse the soap from your hands by letting the water run from the wrists toward the fingers (see Fig. D).	Avoids transferring microorganisms to cleaner areas
Stop the flow of water if it is controlled by an elbow or knee lever, or a foot pedal (see Fig. E).	Terminates the flow of water without recontaminating the hands

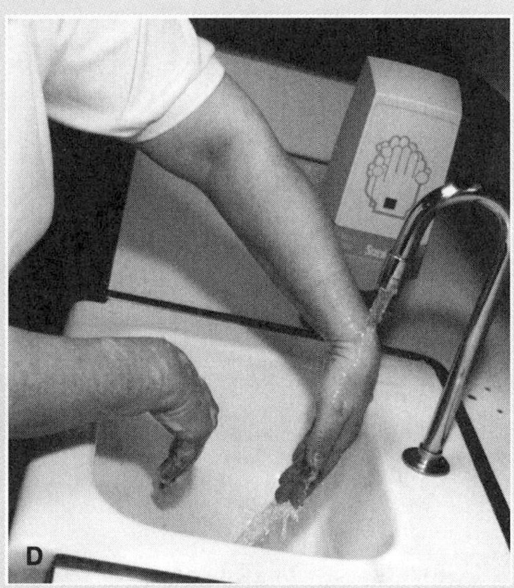

Rinsing hands. (Courtesy of Ken Timby.)

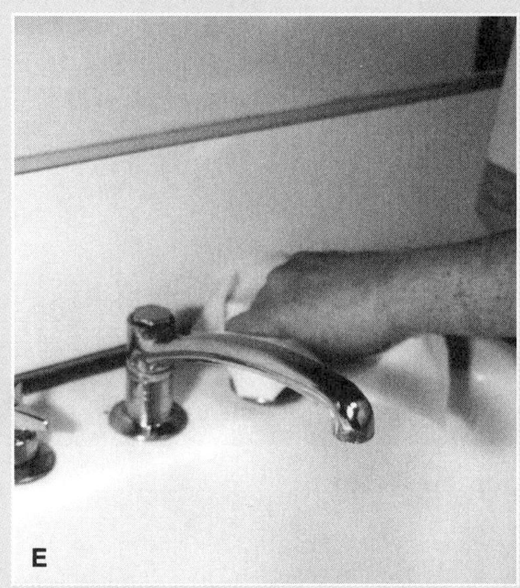

Turning off hand controls. (Courtesy of Ken Timby.)

Suggested Action	Reason for Action
Hold your draining hands lower than your wrists.	Promotes drainage by gravity flow toward the fingers
Dry your hands thoroughly with paper towels or similar item.	Prevents chapping.
	Cloth towels are the least desirable method of drying because they are prone to contamination. A warm air dryer (rarely available in patient environments) is the best. Paper towels dispensed from a holder mounted high enough to avoid splash contamination are acceptable and effective.
Turn the hand controls of the faucet off using a paper towel.	Prevents recontamination of washed hands
Apply hand lotion from time to time.	Maintains the integrity of the skin because skin that becomes irritated and abraded from frequent handwashing increases the risk of acquiring pathogens by direct skin contact.

continued

SKILL 21-1

HANDWASHING *Continued*

Evaluation

- Handwashing has met time requirements.
- Hands are clean.
- Skin is intact.

Document

Because handwashing is performed so frequently, it is not documented, but it is expected as a standard for care among all health care personnel.

CRITICAL THINKING

- Discuss actions for ensuring appropriate handwashing before and after taking care of a patient in his or her home. Use a scenario in which the patient has bar soap that rests on the bathroom sink and terrycloth hand towels that are shared by others in the family.
- You have agreed to volunteer as a nurse in a wilderness camp or as a member of a humanitarian group, like the Peace Corps, in an underdeveloped country. What plans will you make so that you can perform appropriate handwashing?

SKILL 21-2

DONNING STERILE GLOVES

Suggested Action	Reason for Action
Assessment	
Determine whether the procedure requires surgical asepsis.	Complies with infection control measures
Read the contents of prepackaged sterile equipment to determine whether sterile gloves are enclosed.	Indicates whether extra supplies are needed
Discover how much the patient understands about the subsequent procedure.	Provides a basis for teaching
Planning	
Explain what is about to take place to the patient.	Promotes understanding and cooperation
Select a package of sterile gloves of the appropriate size.	Ensures ease when donning and using gloves
Remove unnecessary items from the overbed table or bedside stand.	Ensures an adequate, clean work space
Implementation	
Perform handwashing.	Reduces the potential for transmitting microorganisms
Open the outer wrapper of the gloves.	Provides access to inner wrapper
Place the inner wrapper so that the left glove is on your left side, and the same for the right.	Facilitates donning gloves

continued

SKILL 21–2

DONNING STERILE GLOVES *Continued*

Suggested Action	Reason for Action

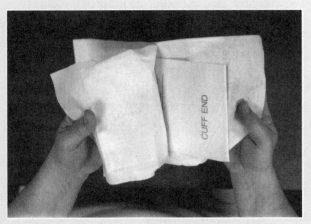

Opening glove wrapper. (Courtesy of Ken Timby.)

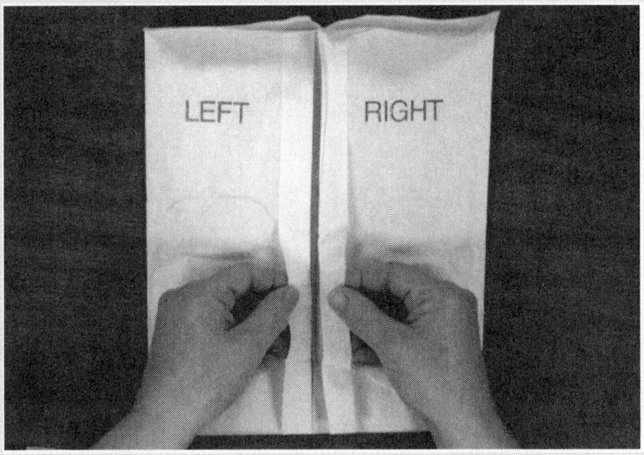

Positioning inner wrapper. (Courtesy of Ken Timby.)

Suggested Action	Reason for Action
Pick up one glove at the folded edge of the cuff using your thumb and fingers.	Avoids contaminating the outer surface of the glove

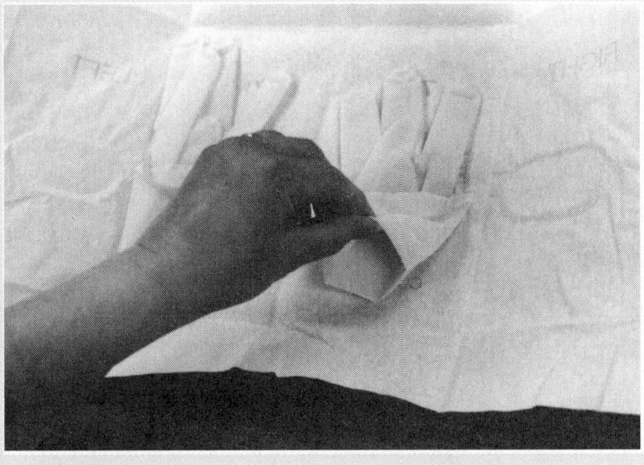

Picking up first glove. (Courtesy of Ken Timby.)

continued

SKILL 21-2

DONNING STERILE GLOVES *Continued*

Suggested Action	Reason for Action
Insert your fingers while pulling and stretching the glove over your hand, taking care not to touch the outside of the glove to anything that is nonsterile.	Avoids contaminating the outer surface of the glove
Unfold the cuff so the glove extends above the wrist, but touch only the surface that will be in direct contact with the skin.	Extends the sterile area
Insert the gloved hand beneath the sterile folded edge of the remaining glove.	Maintains sterility of each glove

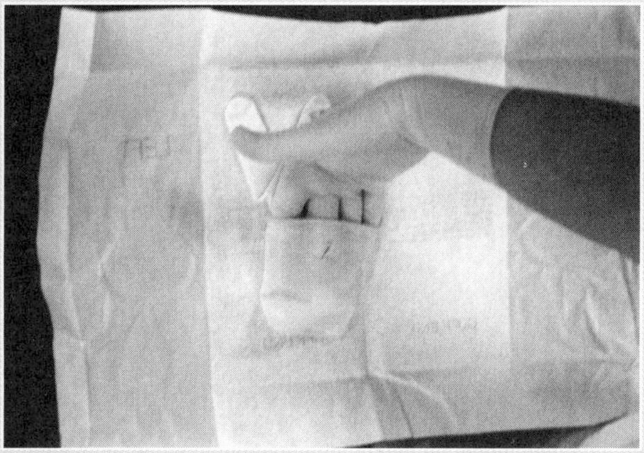

Picking up second glove. (Courtesy of Ken Timby.)

Suggested Action	Reason for Action
Insert the fingers within the second glove while pulling and stretching it over the hand.	Facilitates donning the glove
Take care to avoid touching anything that is not sterile.	Maintains sterility
Maintain your gloved hands at or above waist level.	Prevents the potential for contamination
Repeat the procedure if contamination occurs.	Protects the patient from acquiring an infection

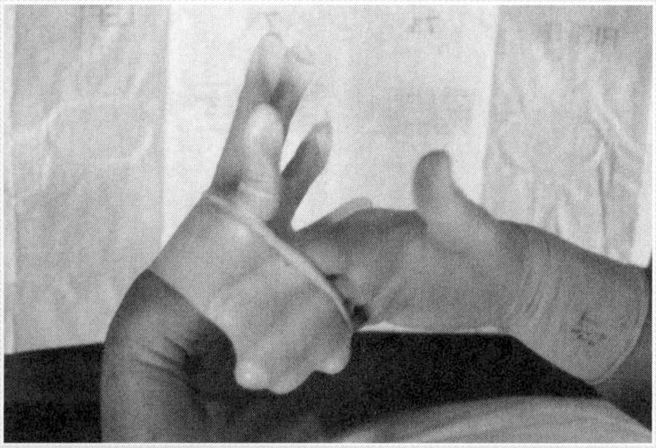

Pulling on second glove. (Courtesy of Ken Timby.)

continued

SKILL 21-2

DONNING STERILE GLOVES *Continued*

Evaluation

- Gloves are donned
- Sterility is maintained

Document

- The procedure that was performed
- Outcome of procedure

SAMPLE DOCUMENTATION

Date and Time Sterile dressing changed over abdominal incision. Wound edges are approximated, with no evidence of redness or drainage. ______________________ SIGNATURE, TITLE

CRITICAL THINKING

- Based on the principles of surgical asepsis and guidelines for creating a sterile field, what is your opinion about observing that a nurse touched an area about 0.5″ in the outside border of the inner glove wrapper before donning sterile gloves?
- What is the best action to take if while donning sterile gloves, a nurse touches the thumb of an already gloved finger to his or her ungloved wrist?

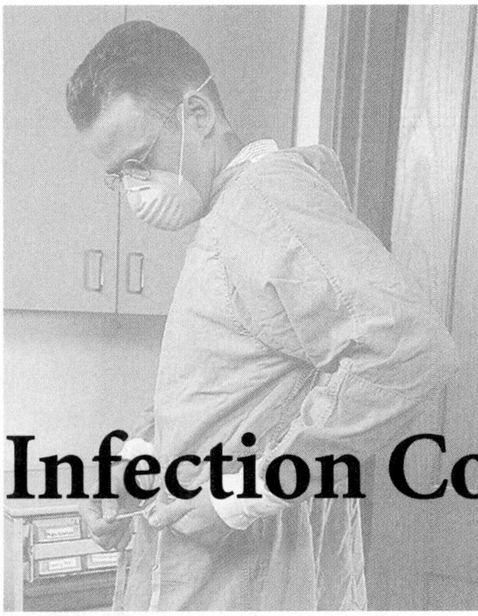

CHAPTER 22

Infection Control

CHAPTER OUTLINE

Infection
Infection Control Precautions
Infection Control Measures
Psychological Implications
Nursing Implications

NURSING GUIDELINES

PROVIDING SENSORY STIMULATION

SKILLS

SKILL 22-1: REMOVING PERSONAL PROTECTIVE EQUIPMENT

NURSING CARE PLAN

RISK FOR INFECTION TRANSMISSION

KEY TERMS

airborne precautions
colonization
contact precautions
double-bagging
droplet precautions
infection
infection control precautions
infectious diseases
personal protective equipment
standard precautions
transmission-based precautions

LEARNING OBJECTIVES

An understanding of the content within this chapter will be evidenced by the student's ability to:

- Explain the meaning of infectious diseases.
- Differentiate between infection and colonization.
- List five stages in the course of an infectious disease.
- Define infection control measures.
- Name two major techniques for infection control.
- Discuss situations in which standard precautions and transmission-based precautions are used.
- Describe the rationale for using airborne, droplet, and contact precautions.
- Explain the purpose of personal protective equipment.
- Discuss the rationale for removing personal protective equipment in a specific sequence after caring for a patient with an infection.
- Explain how double-bagging is performed.
- List two psychological problems common among patients with infectious diseases.
- Provide at least three teaching suggestions for preventing infections.
- Discuss one unique characteristic of older adults in relation to infectious diseases.

Infectious diseases (diseases spread from one person to another) are also called *contagious* or *communicable diseases* and *community-acquired infections.* They were once the leading cause of death, but because of vaccines, aggressive public health measures, and advances in drug therapy, that is no longer true. Nevertheless, infectious diseases have not disappeared. In fact, the microorganisms that cause tuberculosis, gonorrhea, and some forms of wound and respiratory infections have developed drug-resistant strains (see Chap. 21). Add to that the current epidemic of AIDS, an infectious disease spread by HIV in blood and some body fluids (Display 22-1), and it is clear that the war against pathogens has not been won.

This chapter discusses precautions that confine the reservoir of infectious agents and block their transmission from one host to another. To understand the concepts of infection control, it is important to understand the chain of infection (see Chap. 21) and the course of an infection.

Infection

Infection (condition that results when microorganisms cause injury to a host) differs from **colonization** (condition in which microorganisms are present, but the host does not manifest

DISPLAY 22–1

Facts and Myths About the Transmission of HIV

Facts

HIV is transmitted by:

- Having unprotected vaginal, anal, or oral sexual contact with an infected person
- Sharing needles or syringes with an infected person
- Acquiring a needle-stick injury with the blood of an infected person (see Chap. 34)
- Receiving transfusions of infected blood or blood products
- Being born to or breast-fed by an HIV-infected mother
- Having contact with the blood of an infected person through unsterilized equipment for ear-piercing, tattooing, acupuncture, dental procedures, safety razors, or toothbrushes
- Contacting blood of an infected person through an open cut or splashes into the mucous membranes such as the eyes or inside of the nose

Myths

HIV is *not* transmitted by:

- Donating blood
- Being bitten by insects
- Sharing cups and eating utensils
- Inhaling droplets from sneezes or coughs
- Hugging, touching, or closed-mouth kissing an infected person
- Sharing telephones or computer keyboards
- Going to any public place with people infected with HIV
- Using public drinking fountains or toilet seats

Centers for Disease Control and Prevention. Divisions of HIV/AIDS Prevention; The human immunodeficiency virus and its transmission. CDC National AIDS Clearing House, Rockville, MD. http://www.cdc.gov/nchstp/hiv_aids/pubs/facts/transmis.htm, last updated July 1997, accessed 7/99; Ten things to know about HIV/AIDS. http://hivinsite.ucsf.edu/social/misc_documents/2098.346f.html, Nov 13, 1997, accessed 7/99.

any signs or symptoms of infection). Regardless of whether the host is infected or colonized, pathogens and infectious diseases can be transmitted to others.

Infections progress through distinct stages (Table 22-1). The characteristics and length of each stage may differ depending on the infectious agent. For example, the incubation period for the common cold is approximately 2 to 4 days before symptoms appear, but it make take months or years before a person infected with HIV demonstrates symptoms of AIDS.

Infection Control Precautions

Infection control precautions (physical measures designed to curtail the spread of infectious diseases) are essential when caring for patients. Infection control precautions require knowledge of the mechanisms by which an infectious disease is transmitted and the methods that will interfere with the chain of infection. The Centers for Disease Control and Prevention (1996) has established guidelines for two major categories of infection control precautions: standard precautions and transmission-based precautions.

STANDARD PRECAUTIONS

Standard precautions (measures for reducing the risk of microorganism transmission from both recognized and unrecognized sources of infection) are used when caring for all patients, regardless of diagnosis or infection status (Display 22-2).This precautionary system combines methods previously known as *universal precautions* and *body substance isolation.* The use of standard precautions reduces the potential for transmitting bloodborne pathogens and those from moist body substances (feces, urine, sputum, saliva, wound drainage, and other body fluids). Standard precautions are followed whenever there is the potential for contact with:

- Blood
- All body fluids except sweat, regardless of whether they contain visible blood

TABLE 22–1. **The Course of Infectious Diseases**

Stage	Characteristic
Incubation period	Infectious agent reproduces, but there are no recognizable symptoms. The infectious agent may, however, exit the host at this time and infect others.
Prodromal stage	Initial symptoms appear, which may be vague and nonspecific. They may include mild fever, headache, and loss of usual energy.
Acute stage	Symptoms become severe and specific to the tissue or organ that is affected. For example, tuberculosis is manifested by respiratory symptoms.
Convalescent stage	The symptoms subside as the host overcomes the infectious agent.
Resolution	The pathogen is destroyed. Health improves or is restored.

DISPLAY 22–2

Standard Precautions

- Wash hands after touching blood, body fluids, secretions, excretions, and contaminated items, regardless of whether gloves are worn (see Chap. 21).
- Wash hands immediately after gloves are removed.
- Wear clean nonsterile gloves when touching blood, body fluids, secretions and excretions, and contaminated items, and also before touching mucous membranes and nonintact skin.
- Wear a mask and eye protection or a face shield during procedures and patient care activities that are likely to generate splashes or sprays of blood, body fluids, secretions, and excretions.
- Wear a clean nonsterile gown during procedures and patient care activities that are likely to generate splashes or sprays of blood, body fluids, secretions, or excretions or cause soiling of clothing.
- Handle used patient-care equipment soiled with blood, body fluids, secretions, and excretions in a manner that prevents skin and mucous membrane exposures, contamination of clothing, and transfer of microorganisms to other patients and environments.
- Ensure that reusable equipment is not used for the care of another patient until it has been appropriately cleaned and reprocessed, discard single-use items properly (see Chap. 21).
- Follow procedures for adequate routine care, cleaning, and disinfection of environmental surfaces, beds, bed rails, bedside equipment, and other frequently touched surfaces.
- Handle, transport, and process linen soiled with blood, body fluids, and secretions and excretions in a manner that prevents skin and mucous membrane exposures, contamination of clothing, and transfer of microorganisms to other patients and environments.
- Prevent injuries when using needles, scalpels, and other sharp devices after procedures and when cleaning and disposing of instruments.
- Avoid removing, recapping, bending, or breaking used needles; never point the needle toward a body part.
- Use a one-handed "scoop" method for covering a needle, special syringes with a retractable protective guard or shield for enclosing a needle, or blunt-point (needleless) syringes (see Chaps. 34 and 35).
- Place disposable and reusable syringes and needles, scalpel blades, and other sharp items in puncture-resistant containers as close as practical to the area where the items were used.
- Place reusable syringes in a puncture-resistant container for transport to the reprocessing area.
- Use mouthpieces, resuscitation bags, or other ventilation devices as an alternative to mouth-to-mouth resuscitation methods in areas where the need for resuscitation is predictable.
- Locate a patient who contaminates the environment or who does not (or cannot be expected to) assist in maintaining appropriate hygiene or environmental control in a private room, or consult with infection control personnel on other alternatives if a private room is not available.

Adapted from: Garner JS. Guideline for isolation precautions in hospitals, Part II. Recommendations for isolation precautions in hospitals. American Journal of Infection Control 1996; 24(1):32–45; Centers for Disease Control and Prevention. (1996) Guideline for isolation precautions in hospitals. CDC Publication 96138102. Atlanta, GA, National Center for Infectious Diseases.

- Nonintact skin
- Mucous membranes

TRANSMISSION-BASED PRECAUTIONS

Transmission-based precautions (measures for controlling the spread of infectious agents from patients known to be or suspected of being infected with highly transmissable or epidemiologically important pathogens [Centers for Disease Control and Prevention, 1996]) are also called *isolation precautions.* The three types of transmission-based precautions are airborne precautions, droplet precautions, and contact precautions (Table 22-2). These three types replace the earlier categories of strict isolation, contact isolation, respiratory isolation, tuberculosis (AFB) isolation, enteric precautions, and drainage/secretion precautions. The decision to use one or a combination of precautions is based on the mechanism of transmission of the pathogen. One or more categories of transmission-based precautions are used concurrently when diseases have multiple routes of transmission.

Transmission-based precautions are required for various lengths of time, depending on the nature of the infecting microorganisms. Some precautions, with the exception of standard precautions, are discontinued when culture findings are negative, when a wound or lesion stops draining, or after the initiation of effective therapy. Sometimes they are employed throughout treatment.

Airborne Precautions

Airborne precautions (measures that reduce the risk of transmitting airborne infectious agents) block pathogens 5 microns or smaller that are present in the residue of evaporated droplets that remain suspended in the air, as well as those attached to dust particles.

Droplet Precautions

Droplet precautions (measures that block pathogens within moist droplets larger than 5 microns) are used to reduce patho-

TABLE 22–2. **Transmission-Based Precautions**

Type of Precaution	Patient Placement	Protection	Examples of Diseases
Airborne	Private room or in a room with a similarly infected patient Negative air pressure* Six to 12 air changes per hour Discharge of room air to environment or filtered before being circulated	Follow standard precautions. Keep door closed; confine patient to room. Wear a mask for airborne pathogens or OSHA-approved high-efficiency air filter respirator in the case of tuberculosis. Place a mask on the patient if transport is required.	Tuberculosis Measles (rubeola)
Droplet	Private room, or in a room with a similarly infected patient or one in which there is at least 3 feet between other patients and visitors	Follow standard precautions. Leave door open or closed. Wear a mask when entering the room depending on agency policy, but always when within 3 feet of the patient. Place a mask on the patient if transport is required.	Influenza Rubella Streptococcal pneumonia Meningococcal meningitis
Contact	Private room, or in a room with similarly infected patient, or Consult with an infection control professional if the above options are not available.	Follow standard precautions. Don gloves before entering the room. Change gloves during patient care after contact with infective material that contains high concentrations of microorganisms. Remove gloves before leaving the room. Perform handwashing with an antimicrobial agent immediately after removing gloves. Do not touch potentially contaminated surfaces or items in the immediate environment after glove removal and handwashing. Wear a gown when entering the room if there is the possibility that your clothing will touch the patient, environmental surfaces, or items in the room, or if the patient is incontinent or has diarrhea, an ileostomy, a colostomy, or wound drainage not contained by a dressing. Remove the gown before leaving the environment. Avoid transporting the patient, but, if transport is required, use precautions that minimize transmission. Clean bedside equipment and patient care items daily. Use items such as a stethoscope, sphygmomanometer, and other assessment tools exclusively for the infected patient; clean and disinfect them before use for another patient.	Gastrointestinal, respiratory, skin, or wound infections that are drug-resistant Gas gangrene Acute diarrhea Acute viral conjunctivitis Draining abscess

* Negative air pressure pulls air from the hall into the room when the door is opened, as opposed to positive air pressure, which pulls room air into the hall.

Centers for Disease Control and Prevention. Guideline for isolation precautions in hospitals. CDC Publication 96138102. Atlanta, National Center for Infectious Diseases, 1996.

gen transmission from close contact (usually 3 feet or less) between an infected person or a person who is a carrier of a droplet-spread microorganism and others. Microorganisms carried on droplets commonly exit the body during coughing, sneezing, talking, and procedures such as airway suctioning (see Chap. 36) and bronchoscopy. Airborne precautions are used because droplets do not remain suspended in the air.

Contact Precautions

Contact precautions (measures used to block the transmission of pathogens by direct or indirect contact) is the final category of transmission-based precautions. Direct contact involves skin-to-skin contact with an infected or colonized person. Indirect contact occurs by touching a contaminated intermediate object in the patient's environment. Additional precautions are necessary if the microorganism is antibiotic-resistant.

Infection Control Measures

Infection control measures involve the use of **personal protective equipment** (garments that block the transfer of pathogens from one person, place, or object to oneself or others) and techniques that serve as barriers to transmission (Fig. 22-1). Depending on the type of precautions being used, all or some of the following measures are used:

- Locating a patient and equipping a room so that the pathogens are confined to one area
- Using personal protective equipment such as cover gowns, face-protection devices, air filter respirators, and gloves to prevent spreading microorganisms through direct and indirect contact
- Disposing of contaminated linen, equipment, and supplies in such a way that pathogens are not transferred to others
- Using infection control measures to prevent pathogens from spreading when transporting laboratory specimens or patients

PATIENT CARE ENVIRONMENT

The patient care environment includes the room designated for the care of a patient with an infectious disease and the equipment and supplies that are essential to controlling transmission of the pathogens.

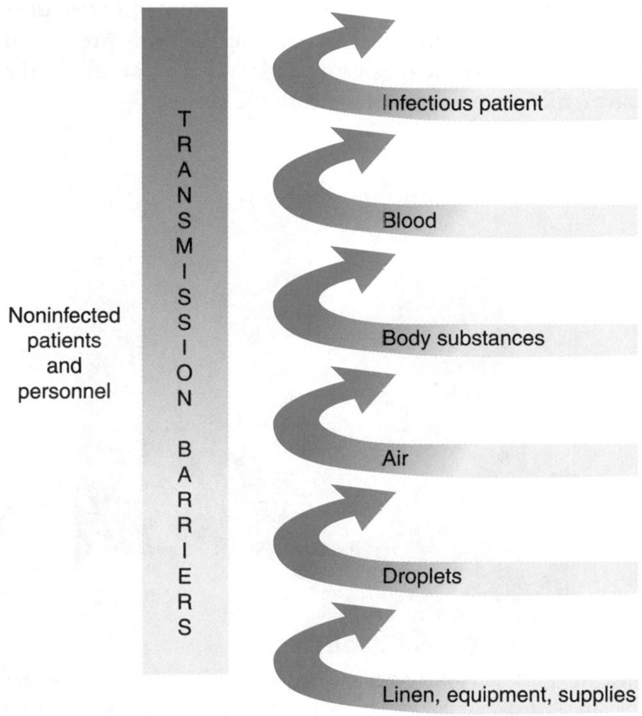

FIGURE 22–1. Blocking sources of infectious disease transmission.

Infection Control Room

Except when standard precautions are used, most infectious or potentially infectious patients are assigned to a private room. Infection control personnel can offer alternatives if a private room is not available (see Table 22-2). The door to the room is kept closed to control air currents and the circulation of dust particles.

The room has a private bathroom so that contaminated liquids and biodegradable solids can be flushed. A sink is also located in the room for handwashing.

An instruction card stating that isolation precautions are required is posted on the door or nearby at eye level (Fig. 22-2). Nurses are responsible for teaching visitors how to comply with the infection control measures.

In accord with the principles of medical asepsis, housekeeping personnel clean the infectious patient's room last to avoid transferring organisms on the wet mop to other patient areas. The mop head, if not disposable, is deposited with the soiled linen. The mop handle is wiped with a disinfectant. Solutions used for cleaning are flushed down the toilet.

Equipment and Supplies

The infection control room contains the same equipment and supplies as any other hospital room, with a few modifications. Equipment that would ordinarily be used for several noninfected patients, such as a stethoscope and sphygmomanometer, is left in the patient's room whenever possible. This prevents the need to clean and disinfect the items each time they are removed.

For the same reason, disposable thermometers are preferred. If a glass thermometer is used, it is cleaned after use and then stored in a container of disinfectant at the patient's bedside; the disinfectant is replaced regularly (see Chap. 11). Electronic or tympanic thermometers are disinfected to make them safe for the next patient.

Items such as a container for soiled laundry (Fig. 22-3), lined waste containers, and liquid soap dispensers are also placed in the room.

PERSONAL PROTECTIVE EQUIPMENT

Infection control measures involve the use of one or more items for personal protection. Personal protective equipment, also called barrier garments (Fig. 22-4), includes gowns, masks, respirators, goggles or face shields, and gloves (see Chap. 21). These items are located just outside the patient's room or in an anteroom (Fig. 22-5).

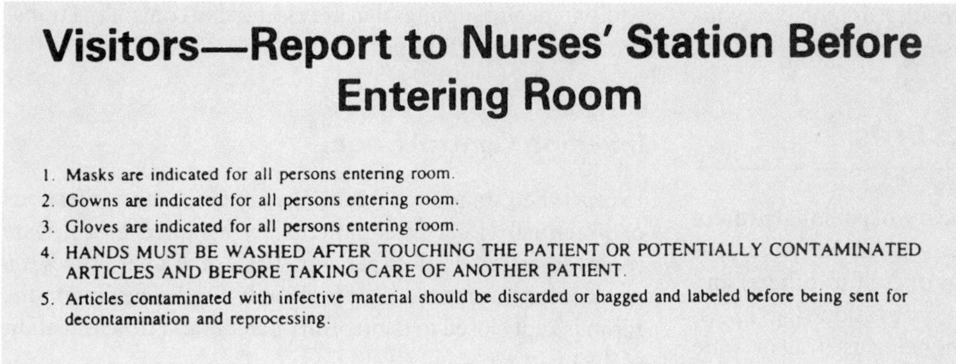

Visitors—Report to Nurses' Station Before Entering Room

1. Masks are indicated for all persons entering room.
2. Gowns are indicated for all persons entering room.
3. Gloves are indicated for all persons entering room.
4. HANDS MUST BE WASHED AFTER TOUCHING THE PATIENT OR POTENTIALLY CONTAMINATED ARTICLES AND BEFORE TAKING CARE OF ANOTHER PATIENT.
5. Articles contaminated with infective material should be discarded or bagged and labeled before being sent for decontamination and reprocessing.

FIGURE 22–2. Door instructional card.

Cover Gowns

Cover gowns are worn for two reasons: they prevent contamination of clothing and protect the skin from contact with blood and body fluids, and when they are removed after direct care of the infectious patient, they reduce the possibility of transmitting pathogens from the patient, the patient's environment, or contaminated objects.

Many types of cover gowns exist, but all have the following common characteristics:

- They open in the back to reduce inadvertent contact with the patient and objects.
- They have close-fitting wrist bands to help avoid contaminating the forearms.
- They fasten at the neck and waist to keep the gown securely closed, thus covering all of the wearer's clothing (Fig. 22-6).

A cover gown is worn only once and then discarded. Discarded cloth gowns are placed in the patient's laundry hamper, removed with the soiled linen, and then washed before being used again. Disposable paper gowns are placed in a waste container and incinerated.

Face-Protection Devices

Depending on the mode of transmission of the pathogen, health care personnel wear a mask or high-efficiency air filter respirator, goggles, or a face shield (see Chap. 21). These items are always applied before entering the patient's room.

Gloves

Gloves are required when an infectious disease is transmitted by direct contact or contact with blood and body substances. They are always donned before or immediately on entering the patient's room. After one use, they are discarded.

Gloves are not a total and complete barrier to microorganisms. They are easily punctured and can leak; the potential for leakage increases with the stress of use.

Wearing gloves does not replace the need for handwashing after they are removed. Hands can be contaminated during glove removal, and microorganisms that were present on the hands before gloving grow and multiply rapidly in the warm, moist environment beneath the gloves.

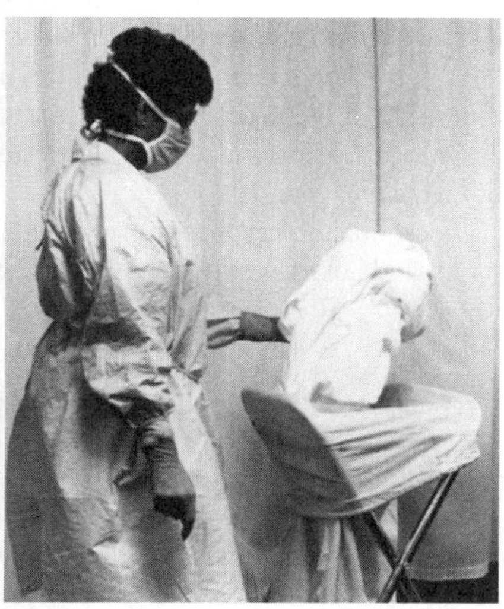

FIGURE 22–3. Containing soiled laundry. (Courtesy of Ken Timby.)

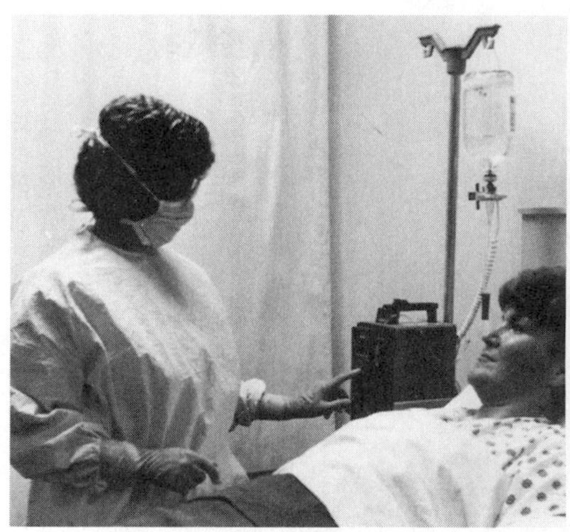

FIGURE 22–4. Personal protective equipment provides a barrier for transmission of infectious microorganisms. (Courtesy of Ken Timby.)

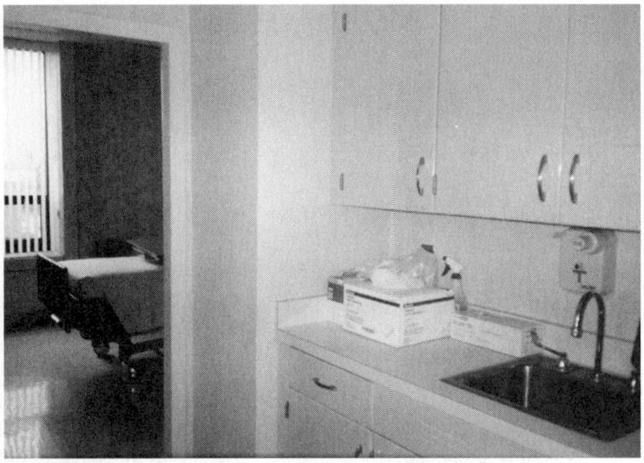

FIGURE 22–5. An anteroom outside the infection control room. (Courtesy of Ken Timby.)

Removing Personal Protective Equipment

Regardless of which garments are worn, an orderly sequence is followed for removing them (Skill 22-1). The goal is to leave the patient's room without contaminating oneself or one's uniform. The procedure involves making contact between two contaminated surfaces or two clean surfaces. Garments that are most contaminated are removed first, preserving the clean uniform underneath.

The technique can be modified to accommodate the removal of any combination of equipment. The most important nursing action is to perform thorough handwashing before leaving the patient's room and before touching any other patient, personnel, environmental surface, or patient care items.

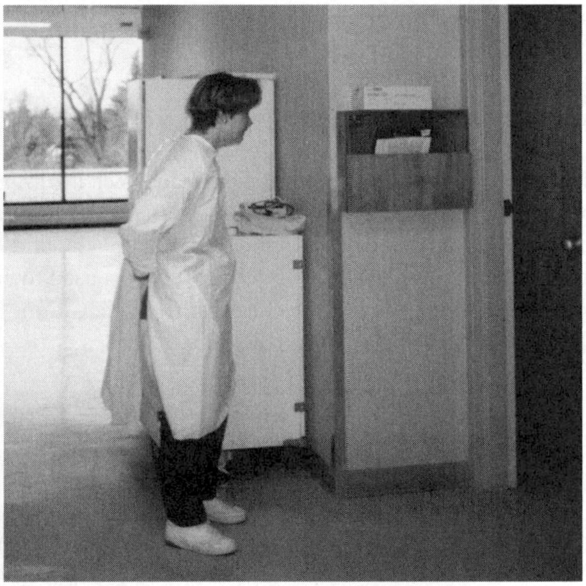

FIGURE 22–6. Donning a cover gown. (Courtesy of Ken Timby.)

DISPOSING OF CONTAMINATED LINEN, EQUIPMENT, AND SUPPLIES

Receptacles in the patient's room are used to collect contaminated items. Soiled waste containers are emptied at the end of each shift or more often if their contents accumulate. To avoid spreading pathogens, some items are double-bagged.

Double-bagging (infection control measure in which one bag of contaminated items, such as trash or laundry, is placed within another) requires two people. One person bags the items and deposits the bag in a second bag held by another person outside the patient's room. The person holding the second bag prevents contamination by manipulating the bag underneath a folded cuff (Fig. 22-7).

The Centers for Disease Control and Prevention (1996) has relaxed its recommendation concerning double-bagging. Its revised position is that one bag is adequate if the bag is sturdy and the articles are placed in the bag without contaminating the outside of the bag. Otherwise double-bagging is used.

DISCARDING BIODEGRADABLE TRASH

Biodegradable trash is refuse that will decompose naturally into less complex compounds. It includes items such as uncon-

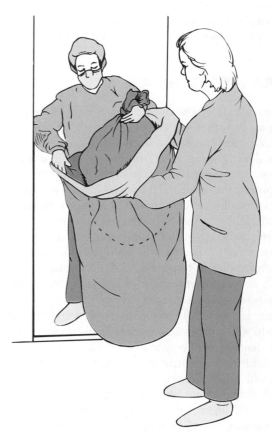

FIGURE 22–7. Double-bagging technique.

sumed beverages, paper tissues, the contents of drainage collectors, urine, and stool. All of these items can be flushed down the toilet in the patient's room. Chemicals and filtration methods in sewage treatment centers are sufficient for destroying pathogens in human wastes.

Bulkier items are placed in a lined trash container and removed from the room by single-or double-bagging. Moist items such as soiled dressings are wrapped so that during their containment, pathogens cannot be transferred by flying or crawling insects. Eventually, the bag and its contents are destroyed by incineration, or they are autoclaved. Autoclaved items can be safely disposed of in landfills.

REMOVING REUSABLE ITEMS

To reduce the need for disinfection of reusable items, disposable equipment and supplies such as plastic bedpans, basins, eating utensils, and paper plates and cups are used as much as possible. If reusable items are necessary for care, they are cleaned with an antimicrobial disinfectant, bagged, and sterilized using heat or chemicals (see Chap. 21).

DELIVERING LABORATORY SPECIMENS

Specimens are delivered to the laboratory in sealed containers in a plastic biohazard bag. When the testing is complete, most specimens are flushed, incinerated, or sterilized.

TRANSPORTING PATIENTS

Patients with infectious diseases may need to be transported to other areas, such as the x-ray department. During transport, methods must be used to prevent the spread of pathogens either directly or indirectly from the patient. For example, to prevent the exit of pathogens from the patient onto transport equipment, the surface of the wheelchair or stretcher is protected from direct patient contact by lining it with a clean sheet or bath blanket. A second one is used to cover as much of the patient's body as possible during transport. A mask or respirator is worn by the patient if the pathogen is transmitted by the airborne or droplet route (Fig. 22-8). Any hospital personnel having direct contact with the patient use personal protective equipment similar to that used in patient care.

Interdepartmental coordination is important. The department to which the patient is transported is made aware that the patient has an infectious disease. This facilitates the expeditious care of the patient and avoids unnecessary waiting in areas with other patients.

When the patient returns, the nurse deposits the soiled linen in the linen hamper in the patient's room, touching only the outside surface of the protective covers. Some agencies also spray or wash the transport vehicle with disinfectant before reuse.

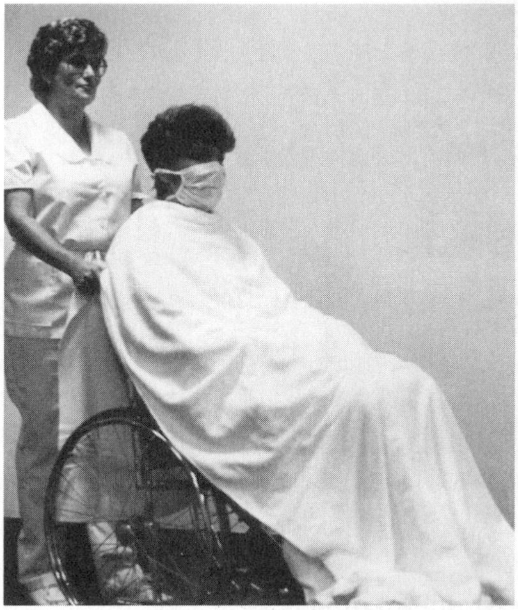

FIGURE 22–8. Transporting an infectious patient. (Courtesy of Ken Timby.)

Psychological Implications

Although infection control measures are necessary, they often leave patients feeling shunned or abandoned. Patients with infectious diseases continue to need human contact and interaction, both of which are often minimal because of the elaborate precautions taken on entering and leaving the room. Fearful family and friends may avoid visiting, and patients are restricted from leaving their room. Measures are needed to relieve the patient's feelings of isolation by providing social interaction and sensory stimulation.

PROMOTING SOCIAL INTERACTION

When transmission-based precautions are in effect, it is important to plan frequent contact with the patient. Visitors are encouraged to come as often as the agency's policies and the patient's condition permit. Every opportunity is used to emphasize that as long as the infection control precautions are followed, visitors are not likely to acquire the disease.

COMBATTING SENSORY DEPRIVATION

Sensory deprivation results when a person experiences insufficient sensory stimulation or is exposed to sensory stimulation that is continuous and monotonous. The goal is to provide a variety of sensory experiences at intervals.

Nursing Guidelines For
Providing Sensory Stimulation

- ☑ Move the bed to various places in the room, or periodically rearrange the furnishings in the room.
  RATIONALE: Such a change provides a new perspective for the patient.
- ☑ Position the patient so he or she can look out the window.
  RATIONALE: Having something different to look at reduces boredom.
- ☑ Encourage the patient to use the telephone.
  RATIONALE: Telephone calls allow social interaction.
- ☑ Communicate using the intercom system if it is inconvenient to enter the room.
  RATIONALE: This shows that the nurse is paying attention to the patient.
- ☑ Converse with the patient about current events in the world.
  RATIONALE: Conversation stimulates the patient's thought processes.
- ☑ Help the patient select television or radio programs.
  RATIONALE: Watching TV or listening to the radio engages the patient's attention.
- ☑ Change the location of equipment that produces monotonous sounds.
  RATIONALE: Changing the location will vary the volume or pitch of the noise.
- ☑ Encourage the patient to be active, within the confines of the room.
  RATIONALE: Activity provides a means of stimulation.
- ☑ Encourage activities that can be done independently, such as reading, working crossword puzzles, playing solitaire, and putting picture puzzles together.
  RATIONALE: Such activities are diverting.
- ☑ Offer a wide choice of foods with different flavors, temperatures, and textures.
  RATIONALE: Eating a variety of foods stimulates oral and olfactory sensations.
- ☑ Use touch appropriately by giving a backrub or changing the patient's position.
  RATIONALE: Touch produces tactile stimulation.

Nursing Implications

Caring for patients with infectious diseases involves meeting both their physical and emotional needs. Some frequently identified nursing diagnoses include the following:

- Risk for infection
- Altered protection
- Risk for infection transmission
- Impaired social interaction
- Social isolation
- Risk for loneliness
- Diversional activity deficit
- Powerlessness
- Fear

The nursing care plan demonstrates how the nursing process is applied when caring for a patient with the nursing diagnosis of Risk for infection transmission. This diagnostic category is not currently approved by the the North American Nursing Diagnosis Association, but Carpenito (1999) defined it as "the state in which an individual is at risk for transferring an opportunistic or pathogenic agent to others."

Nurses also play a pivotal role by teaching measures to prevent infection.

Patient Teaching For
Preventing Infections

Teach the patient and family to do the following:

- ▷ Bathe daily and perform other forms of personal hygiene, such as oral care.
- ▷ Keep the home environment clean and uncluttered.
- ▷ Use diluted household bleach (1:10 or 1:100) as a disinfectant.
- ▷ Obtain appropriate adult immunizations (tetanus vaccine at 10-year intervals, influenza vaccine yearly). A pneumococcal pneumonia immunization lasts a lifetime or revaccination is required every 5 years for extremely high-risk people.
- ▷ Investigate necessary vaccines, water purification techniques, and foods to avoid when traveling outside the United States.
- ▷ Practice a healthy lifestyle, such as eating the recommended number of servings from the Food Pyramid (see Chap. 14).
- ▷ Perform frequent handwashing, especially before eating, after contact with nasal secretions, and after using the toilet.
- ▷ Use disposable tissues rather than a cloth handkerchief for nasal and oral secretions.
- ▷ Avoid sharing personal care items such as washcloths and towels, razors, and cups.
- ▷ Stay home from work or school when ill rather than exposing others to infectious pathogens.
- ▷ Take over the task of cooking if the family member who usually cooks is ill.
- ▷ Keep food refrigerated until use.
- ▷ Cook food thoroughly.
- ▷ Avoid crowds and public places during outbreaks of influenza.
- ▷ Follow infection control instructions when visiting hospitalized family members and friends.
- ▷ Comply with drug therapy when prescribed.

Nursing Care Plan: Risk for Infection Transmission

Assessment

Subjective Data

States, "The health department informed me that my preemployment TB test was positive and my chest x-ray showed some suspicious cavities. The doctor put me in the hospital until my sputum tests are complete."

Objective Data

30-year-old man who is a recent immigrant from India presents with a nonproductive cough and an unexplained weight loss of 7 lbs in 1 month. No current fever.

Diagnosis

Risk for infection transmission related to airborne spread of pathogen causing tuberculosis

Plan

Goal

Will comply with infection control measures and accurately describe postdischarge drug therapy and medical follow-up by time of discharge.

Orders: 5/11

1. Follow airborne transmission precautions until sputum culture is negative; follow standard precautions throughout length of stay.
2. Post infection control measures on room door.
3. Wear a particulate filter respirator during patient care.
4. Teach patient to cover nose and mouth with a paper tissue when coughing, sneezing, or laughing, and dispose of it in a paper bag.
5. Directly observe patient taking prescribed drug therapy.
6. Explain the purpose of combination drug therapy and the need to continue uninterrupted administration to avoid treatment failure and development of drug-resistant strain.
7. Direct patient to provide a sputum specimen at the public health department within 2 to 3 weeks (5/28 to 6/1) if discharged earlier.
8. Recommend TB skin testing for close family members or friends.

________________ L. STRONG, RN

Implementation (Documentation)

5/11 1130 Placed in private infection control room. Instruction card posted. Explained the purpose for wearing a respirator mask. Instructed on how to use tissues when coughing, sneezing, and laughing. Paper bag for tissue disposal taped to siderail of bed. ________________ L. CUPP, LPN

Evaluation (Documentation)

2000 Spent 15 minutes talking with patient during the time of medication administration. Using paper tissues as instructed. Concerned that immigration sponsor has not visited and how illness will affect visa status. Left a message with social worker about contacting sponsor. ________________ L. STONER, LPN

FOCUS ON OLDER ADULTS

- Decreased lymphocyte cells and diminished antibody response increase an older adult's susceptibility to infectious disease.
- Chronic diseases reduce the ability of older adults to resist infections.
- Symptoms of infections tend to be more subtle among older adults, and infections are more likely to have a rapid course once they become established. Common manifestations of infections in older adults include changes in behavior and mental status.
- Because older adults tend to have a lower "normal" or baseline temperature, a temperature that is in the normal range may actually be elevated for an older adult. Assessment and documentation of the older adult's normal temperature is important so accurate comparisons are made when assessing for an elevated temperature.
- Early detection of an infectious process requires prompt treatment to prevent the need for admitting older adults to acute care settings.
- Infections are often the major reason for admitting nursing home residents to hospitals (Jackson & Schafer, 1993).
- Poor nutrition and inadequate fluid intake increase the risk for infections in older adults.
- All long-term care facilities are required to test each resident on admission and each new employee for tuberculosis.
- In many long-term care facilities and other institutional settings, the limited number of private rooms and sinks for handwashing increases the risk for the transmission of pathogens among residents.
- Older adults who are cognitively impaired need more assistance with complying with infection control measures.

KEY CONCEPTS

- Infectious diseases, also called community-acquired, contagious, or communicable diseases, are spread from one person to another.
- An infection is a condition that results when microorganisms cause injury to their host. Colonization refers to a condition in which microorganisms are present, but the host is not damaged and has no signs or symptoms.
- Infectious diseases usually follow five stages: incubation, prodromal, acute, convalescent, and resolution.
- Infection control measures are designed to curtail the spread of infectious diseases.
- The two major categories of infection control measures are standard precautions and transmission-based precautions.
- Standard precautions are measures for reducing the risk of microorganism transmission from both recognized and unrecognized sources of infection.
- Transmission-based precautions are measures to control the spread of infectious agents from patients known to be or suspected of being infected with pathogens.
- The three categories of transmission-based precautions are airborne precautions, droplet precautions, and contact precautions.
- Airborne precautions are used to block very small pathogens that remain suspended in the air or are attached to dust particles. Droplet precautions are used to block larger pathogens contained within moist droplets. Contact precautions are used to block the transmission of pathogens by direct or indirect contact.
- Personal protective equipment is defined as garments that block the transfer of pathogens from a person, place, or object to oneself or others.
- When removing personal protective equipment, an orderly sequence is followed, accompanied by handwashing, to prevent self-contamination and transmission of pathogens to others.
- Double-bagging is an infection control measure for removing contaminated items such as trash or laundry from the patient's environment. It involves placing one bag within another held by someone outside the patient's room.
- Patients with infectious diseases often have decreased social interaction and sensory deprivation because they are confined to their room.
- To prevent infections, people should obtain appropriate immunizations; practice a healthy lifestyle, such as eating the recommended number of servings from the Food Pyramid; and avoid sharing personal items such as washcloths and towels, razors, and cups.
- Symptoms of infectious disorders tend to be more subtle in older adults.

CRITICAL THINKING EXERCISES

- Discuss the similarities between the transmission and control of infections in day care centers for young children and nursing home facilities that house older adults.
- Explain why new cases of AIDS occur despite the fact that its mode of transmission is known.

SUGGESTED READINGS

Bailey EM. Infection control. Exposure to bloodborne pathogens. American Journal of Nursing 1998;98(3):67–68.

Carpenito LJ. Nursing diagnosis: application to clinical practice, 8th ed. Philadelphia, Lippincott Williams & Wilkins, 1999.

Centers for Disease Control and Prevention. Divisions of HIV/AIDS Prevention. The human immunodeficiency virus and its transmission. Rockville, Md., CDC National AIDS Clearing House. http://www:cdc.gov/nchstp/hiv_aids/pubs/facts/transmis.htm, last updated July 1997, accessed 7/99.

Centers for Disease Control and Prevention. Guideline for isolation precautions in hospitals. CDC Publication 96138102. Atlanta, National Center for Infectious Diseases, 1996.

Cole A. Special report: gloves: the pros and cons. Nursing Times 1997;93(6): 44–46.

Danner K. Standard precautions. Computers in Nursing 1998;16(3):131–132.

Freeman CD. Antimicrobial resistance: implications for the clinician. Critical Care Nursing Quarterly 1997;20(3):21–35.

Garner JS. Guidelines for isolation precautions in hospitals. American Journal of Infection Control 1996;24(1):24–52.

Hoffman M. CDC guidelines for infection precautions. Caring 1997;16(9): 58–62.

Jackson MM, Shafer K. Identifying clues to infections in nursing home residents. Journal of Gerontological Nursing 1993;19:33–42.

Kenny P. Managing HIV infection: how to bolster your patient's fragile health. Nursing 1996;26(8):26–37.

Lancaster A. New guidelines protect caregivers from infectious diseases . . . standard precautions. RN 1996;59(3):62.

Marx JF. Teaching your patient about isolation precautions. Nursing 1998;28(5):hn20–21.

Recommended practices for standard and transmission-based precautions in the perioperative practice setting. AORN Journal 1999;62(2):404–411.

Teach nurses the ABCs of bag technique. Homecare Education Management 1996;1(8):98–99.

Ten things to know about HIV/AIDS. http://hivinsite.uscf.edu/social/misc_documents/2098.346f.html, Nov. 13, 1997, accessed 7/99.

West KH, Cohen ML. Standard precautions—a new approach to reducing infection transmission in the hospital setting. Journal of Intravenous Nursing 1997;20(6S):S7–S10.

SKILL 22–1

REMOVING PERSONAL PROTECTIVE EQUIPMENT

Suggested Action	Reason for Action
Assessment	
Determine which type of infection control precautions are being used.	Indicates whether garments must be removed and discarded within the room
Note if there is sufficient soap and paper towels, a laundry hamper, and a lined waste receptacle within the room.	Provides a means for washing and confining soiled garments
Planning	
Make sure that all direct care of the patient has been completed.	Avoids having to don barrier garments a second time
Implementation	
Untie the waist closure if it is fastened at the front of the cover gown before removing gloves.	Provides hand protection while touching a part of the gown that is considered grossly contaminated
Remove gloves and discard them in a lined waste container.	Confines grossly contaminated items
Wash hands (see Chap. 21).	Removes microorganisms
Remove mask (see Chap. 21) and other disposable face-protection items and discard them in the waste container.	Confines contaminated items
Untie or unfasten the neck closure of the cover gown.	Prevents contaminating the back of the uniform and the hands
Remove the gown, but avoid touching the front, by either inserting your fingers at the shoulder or sliding a finger under the cuff and pulling the sleeve down.	Prevents gross contamination of the hands

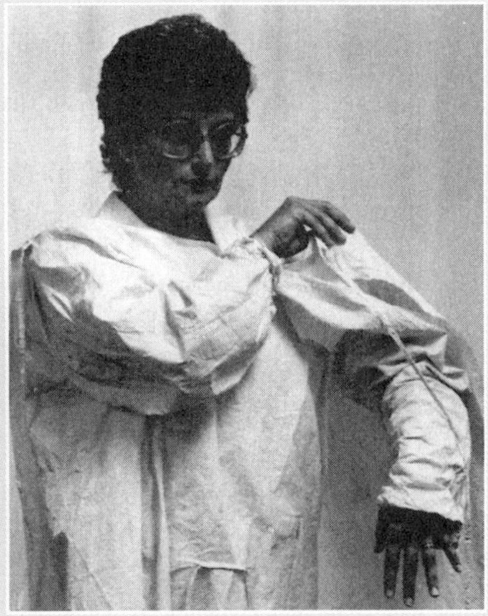

Removing a cover gown. (Courtesy of Ken Timby.)

continued

SKILL 22-1

REMOVING PERSONAL PROTECTIVE EQUIPMENT *Continued*

Suggested Action	Reason for Action
Fold the soiled side of the gown to the inside while holding it away from your uniform.	Prevents contamination of the hands and uniform
Roll up the gown and discard it in the waste container, if it is constructed of paper. If the gown is made of cloth, discard it in the laundry hamper in the room.	Confines contaminated garments
Wash hands.	Removes microorganisms that may have been inadvertently transferred during mask and gown removal
Use a clean paper towel to open the room door.	Protects clean hands from recontamination
Discard the paper towel in the waste container in the patient's room.	Confines contaminated material
Leave the room, taking care not to touch anything.	Prevents recontamination
Go directly to the utility room and wash your hands one final time.	Removes microorganisms; it is always safer to overdo than underdo any practice that controls the spread of pathogens

Evaluation

- Appropriate personal protective equipment was worn.
- Garments were removed with the least contamination possible.
- Handwashing was performed appropriately.

Document

- Type of transmission-based precautions being followed
- Care provided
- Response of patient

SAMPLE DOCUMENTATION

Date and Time Contact precautions followed. Assisted with bath while wearing gloves and gown. States, "I wish the door to my room could be left opened. It gets rather boring in here." Reinforced the purpose for keeping the door closed. _______________ SIGNATURE, TITLE

CRITICAL THINKING

- List the personal protective equipment that is required when assisting patients with hygiene who have (1) measles, (2) meningococcal meningitis, and (3) a draining wound infection.
- In each of the three examples above, describe infection control measures that are appropriate before exiting the patient's room.
- You are caring for a patient with streptococcal pneumonia. Discuss whether you would wear a mask when delivering mail to the patient.

UNIT SEVEN

ASSISTING THE INACTIVE PATIENT

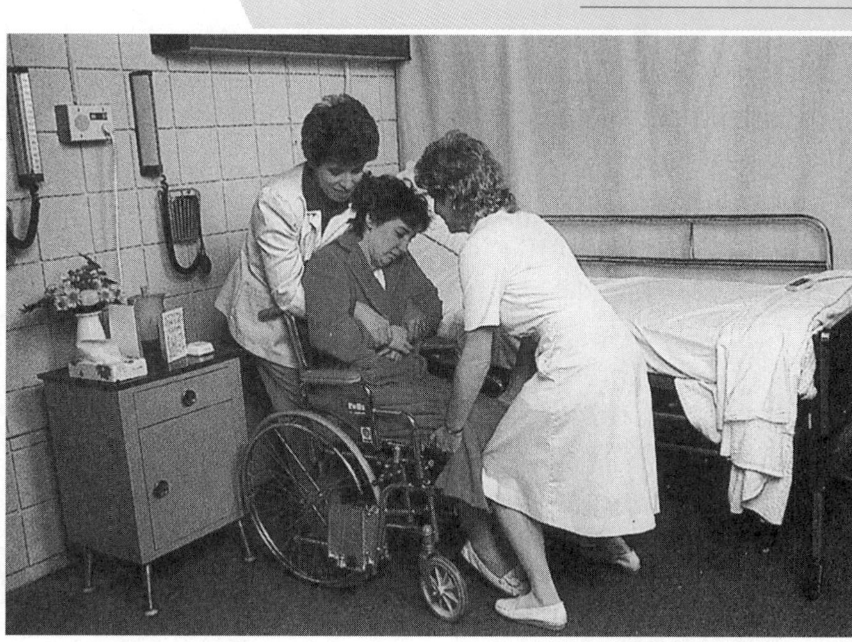

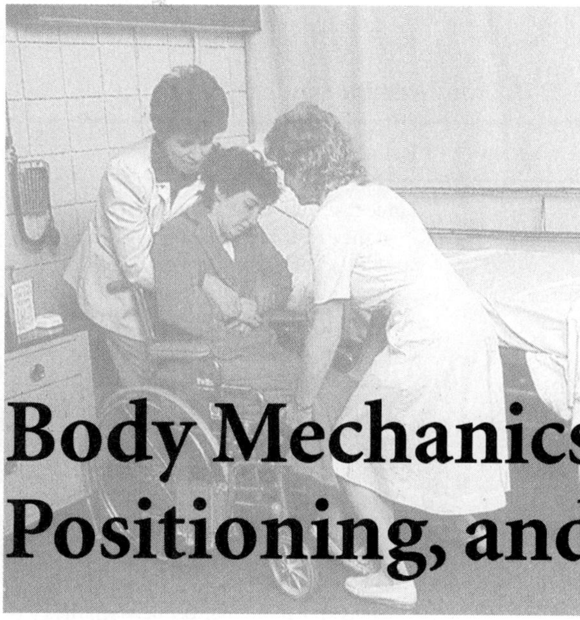

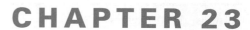

CHAPTER 23

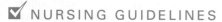

Body Mechanics, Positioning, and Moving

CHAPTER OUTLINE

NURSING GUIDELINES

SKILLS

NURSING CARE PLAN

KEY TERMS

alignment
anatomic position
balance
base of support
bed board
body mechanics
center of gravity
contractures
disuse syndrome
energy
ergonomics
foot drop
Fowler's position
functional mobility
functional position
gravity
lateral oblique position
lateral position
line of gravity
muscle spasms
neutral position
posture
prone position
repetitive strain injuries
shearing
Sims' position
supine position
transfer

LEARNING OBJECTIVES

An understanding of the content within this chapter will be evidenced by the student's ability to:

- Identify characteristics of good posture in a standing, sitting, or lying position.
- Describe three principles of correct body mechanics.
- Explain the purpose of ergonomics.
- Give at least two examples of ergonomic recommendations in the workplace.
- Describe at least 10 signs or symptoms associated with the disuse syndrome.
- Describe six common patient positions.
- Explain the purpose of five different positioning devices used for safety and comfort.
- Name one advantage for each of three different pressure-relieving devices.
- Discuss four types of transfer devices.
- Give at least five general guidelines that apply to transferring patients.

Inactivity leads to a deterioration of health. Multiple complications can occur among people with limited activity and movement (Table 23-1). The consequences of inactivity are collectively referred to as **disuse syndrome** (signs and symptoms that result from inactivity). The potential for disuse syndrome is reduced when nursing care includes activities such as positioning and moving patients. However, nurses can become injured if they fail to use good posture and body mechanics while performing these activities.

TABLE 23–1. **Dangers of Inactivity**

Systems	Effects
Muscular	Weakness Decreased tone/strength Decreased size (atrophy)
Skeletal	Poor posture Contractures Foot drop
Cardiovascular	Impaired circulation Thrombus (clot) formation Dependent edema
Respiratory	Pooling of secretions Shallow respirations Atelectasis (collapsed alveoli)
Urinary	Oliguria (scanty urine) Urinary tract infections Calculi (stone) formation Incontinence (inability to control elimination)
Gastrointestinal	Anorexia (loss of appetite) Constipation Fecal impaction
Integumentary	Pressure sores
Endocrine	Decreased metabolic rate Decreased hormonal secretions
Central nervous	Sleep pattern disturbances Psychosocial changes

TABLE 23–2. **Basic Terminology**

Term Definition	Example
Gravity	Force that pulls objects toward the center of the earth. The pull of gravity causes objects, such as an item dropped from the hand, to fall to the ground. It causes water to drain to its lowest level.
Energy	Capacity to do work. Energy is used to move the body from place to place. Energy is required to overcome the force of gravity.
Balance	Steady position with weight. A person falls when off balance.
Center of gravity	Point at which the mass of an object is centered. The center of gravity for a standing person is the center of the pelvis and about halfway between the umbilicus and the pubic bone.
Line of gravity	Imaginary vertical line that passes through the center of gravity. The line of gravity in a standing person is a straight line from the head to the feet through the center of the body.
Base of support	Area on which an object rests. The feet are the base of support when a person is in a standing position.
Alignment	Parts of an object being in proper relationship to one another. The body is in good alignment in a position of good posture.
Neutral position	The position of a limb that is turned neither toward nor away from the body's midline.
Anatomic position	Frontal and back views with arms at the sides and palms forward.
Functional position	Position in which an activity is performed properly and normally. In the hand, the wrists are slightly dorsiflexed between 20 and 35 degrees and the proximal finger joints are flexed between 45 and 60 degrees, with the thumb in opposition and alignment with the pads of the fingers.

This chapter describes how to position and move patients to prevent complications associated with inactivity and discusses methods for protecting nurses from work-related injuries. Basic terms are defined in Table 23-2.

Maintaining Good Posture

Posture (position of the body, or the way in which it is held) affects a person's appearance, stamina, and ability to use the musculoskeletal system efficiently. Good posture, whether in a standing, sitting, or lying position, distributes gravity through the center of the body over a wide base of support (Fig. 23-1). Good posture is important for both patients and nurses.

When a person performs work while using poor posture, **muscle spasms** (sudden, forceful, involuntary muscle contractions) often result. They occur more often when muscles are strained and forced to work beyond their capacity.

STANDING

To maintain good posture in a standing position (Fig. 23-2):

- Keep the feet parallel, at right angles to the lower legs, and about 4″ to 8″ (10 to 20 cm) apart.
- Distribute weight equally on both feet to provide a broad base of support.
- Bend the knees slightly to avoid straining the joints.
- Maintain the hips at an even level.
- Pull in the buttocks and hold the abdomen up and in to keep the spine properly aligned. This position supports the abdominal organs and reduces strain on both back and abdominal muscles.
- Hold the chest up and slightly forward and extend or stretch the waist to give internal organs more space and maintain good alignment of the spine.
- Keep the shoulders even and centered above the hips.
- Hold the head erect with the face forward and the chin slightly tucked.

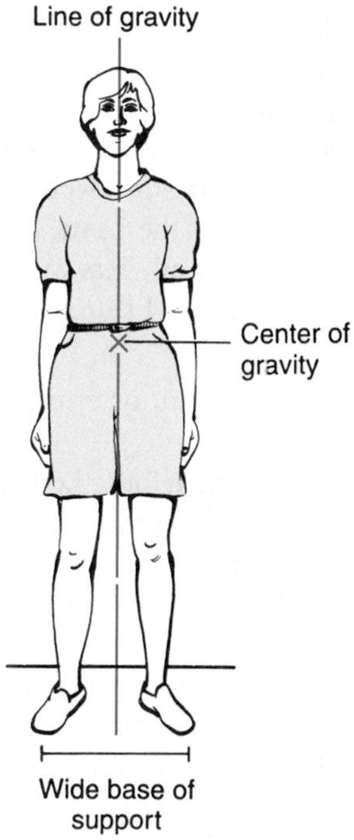

FIGURE 23–1. With good posture, gravity is aligned through the center of the body. A wide stance provides a stable base for support.

SITTING

In a good sitting position (Fig. 23-3), the buttocks and upper thighs become the base of support. Both feet rest on the floor. The knees are bent and the popliteal area is free from the edge of the chair to avoid interfering with distal circulation.

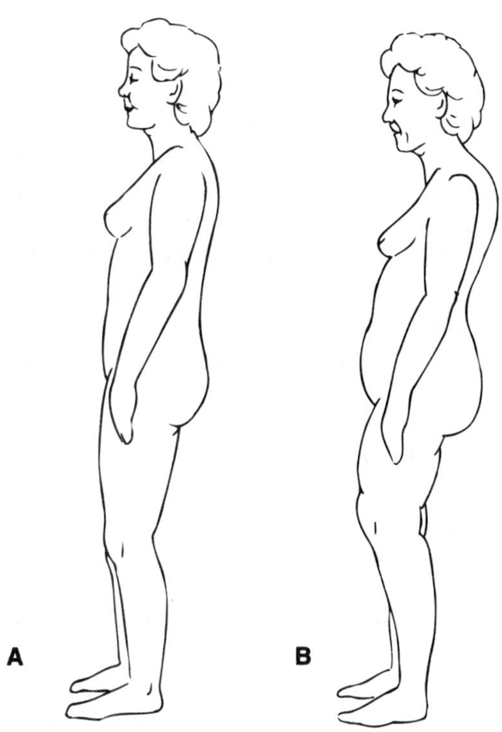

FIGURE 23–2. (*A*) Good standing posture. (*B*) Poor standing posture.

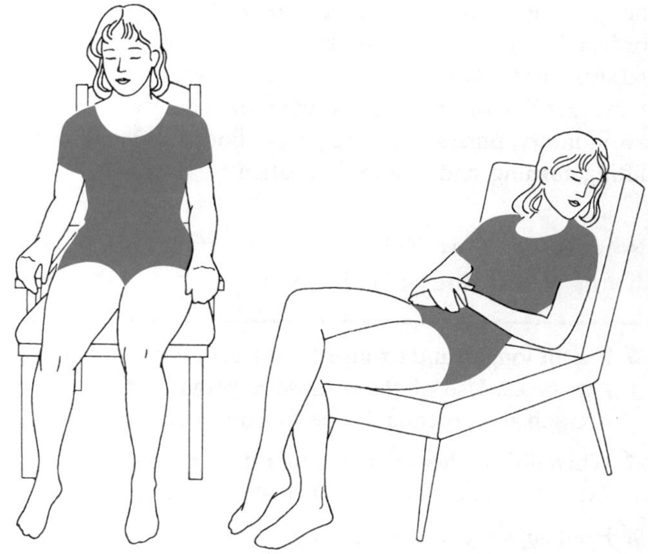

FIGURE 23–3. (*A*) Correct sitting posture. (*B*) Incorrect sitting posture. (Courtesy of Lowren West, New York, NY.)

LYING DOWN

Good posture in a lying position looks the same as a standing position, except the person is horizontal (Fig. 23-4). The head and neck muscles are in a neutral position, centered between the shoulders. The shoulders are level, whereas the arms, hips, and knees are slightly flexed, with no compression of the arms or legs under the body. The trunk is straight and the hips are level. The legs are parallel to each other, with the feet at right angles to the leg.

Body Mechanics

The use of proper **body mechanics** (efficient use of the musculoskeletal system) increases muscle effectiveness, reduces

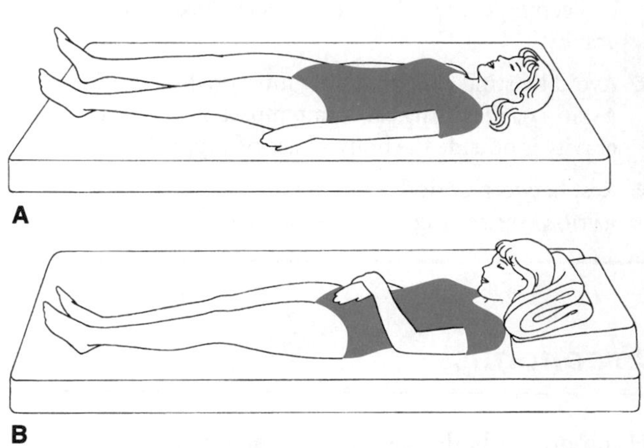

FIGURE 23–4. (*A*) Correct lying posture. (*B*) Incorrect lying posture. (Courtesy of Lowren West, New York, NY.)

fatigue, and helps to avoid **repetitive strain injuries** (disorders that result from cumulative trauma to musculoskeletal structures). Basic principles of body mechanics are important regardless of a person's occupation or daily activities. To avoid injury, nurses must use proper body mechanics when lifting, turning, and positioning patients.

Nursing Guidelines For

Using Good Body Mechanics

- ☑ Use the longest and strongest muscles of the arms and legs.
  RATIONALE: Use of these muscles provides the greatest strength and potential for performing work.
- ☑ When lifting a heavy load, center it over the feet.
  RATIONALE: Such positioning creates a base of support.
- ☑ Hold objects close to the body.
  RATIONALE: Doing so increases balance.
- ☑ Bend the knees.
  RATIONALE: Bending the knees prepares the spine to accept the weight of the load.
- ☑ Contract the abdominal muscles and make a long midriff.
  RATIONALE: This protects the muscles of the abdomen and pelvis and prevents strain and injury to the abdominal wall.
- ☑ Push, pull, or roll objects whenever possible rather than lifting them.
  RATIONALE: Lifting requires more effort.
- ☑ Use body weight as a lever to assist with pushing or pulling an object.
  RATIONALE: This reduces muscle strain.
- ☑ Keep feet apart for a broad base of support.
  RATIONALE: This stance lowers the center of gravity, which promotes stability.
- ☑ Bend the knees and keep the back straight when lifting an object, rather than bending over from the waist with straight knees.
  RATIONALE: This stance makes best use of the longest and the strongest muscles in the body, and improves balance by keeping the weight of the object close to the center of gravity.
- ☑ Avoid twisting and stretching muscles during work.
  RATIONALE: Twisting can strain muscles because the line of gravity is outside the body's base of support.
- ☑ Rest between periods of exertion.
  RATIONALE: Resting promotes work endurance.

Ergonomics

Using proper body mechanics is one component of preserving the integrity of the body. The other component is applying and implementing **ergonomics** (specialty field of engineering science devoted to promoting comfort, performance, and health in the workplace). Ergonomics is used to improve the design of the work environment and equipment. The National Institute for Occupational Safety and Health (NIOSH), a division of the Centers for Disease Control and Prevention, requires employers to comply with many ergonomic recommendations. Examples of ergonomic recommendations are:

- Use assistive devices to lift or transport heavy items or patients.
- Use alternative equipment for tasks that require repetitive motions—for instance, headsets or automatic staplers.
- Position equipment no more than 20° to 30° away—about an arm's length—to avoid reaching or twisting the trunk or neck.
- Use a chair with good back support. It should be high enough so the user's feet can be placed firmly on the floor. There should be room for two fingers between the edge of the seat and the back of the knees. Arm rests should allow a relaxed shoulder position.
- Keep the elbows flexed no more than 100 to 110 degrees, or use wrist rests to keep the wrists in neutral position when working at a computer.
- Work under nonglare lighting.

Many employers require workers to wear a back belt, which theoretically increases intra-abdominal pressure and reduces stress on the lower back. However, according to NIOSH (1997), claims that back belts reduce back injuries remain unproven.

Positioning Patients

Good posture and body mechanics and ergonomically designed features are especially helpful when inactive patients require positioning and moving. An inactive patient's position is changed to relieve pressure on bony areas of the body and to promote **functional mobility** (alignment that maintains the potential for movement and ambulation). General principles for positioning are as follows:

- Change the inactive patient's position at least every 2 hours.
- Enlist help if needed.
- Raise the bed to an appropriate height.
- Remove pillows and positioning devices.
- Unfasten drainage tubes from the bed linen.
- Turn the patient as a complete unit to avoid twisting the spine.
- Place the patient in good alignment, with joints slightly flexed.
- Replace pillows and positioning devices.
- Support limbs in a functional position.

- Use elevation to relieve swelling or promote comfort.
- Provide skin care after repositioning.

COMMON POSITIONS

Six body positions are commonly used when caring for bedridden patients: supine, lateral, lateral oblique, prone, Sims', and Fowler's.

Supine Position

The **supine position** (one in which the person lies on the back) is illustrated in Figure 23-5A. There are two primary concerns associated with the supine position: prolonged pressure, especially at the end of the spine, leads to skin breakdown, and gravity, combined with pressure on the toes from bed linen, creates a potential for **foot drop** (permanent dysfunctional position caused by shortening of the calf muscles and lengthening of the opposing muscles on the anterior leg; Fig. 23-6). Foot drop hinders ambulation because it interferes with a person's ability to place the heel on the floor. The supine position, however, is recommended as a way to reduce the incidence of sudden infant death syndrome among newborns (Carroll & Siska, 1998; Lockeridge, 1997).

Lateral Position

With the **lateral position** (side-lying position; see Fig. 23-5B), foot drop is of less concern because the feet are not pulled down by gravity, as they are when the patient is supine. However, unless the upper shoulder and arm are supported, they may rotate forward and interfere with breathing.

Lateral Oblique Position

In the **lateral oblique position** (a variation of the side-lying position), the patient lies on the side with the top leg placed in 30 degrees of hip flexion and 35 degrees of knee flexion (see Fig. 23-5C). The calf of the top leg is placed behind the midline of the body on a support such as a pillow. The back is supported and the bottom leg is in neutral position. This position produces less pressure on the hip than a strictly lateral position and reduces the potential for skin breakdown.

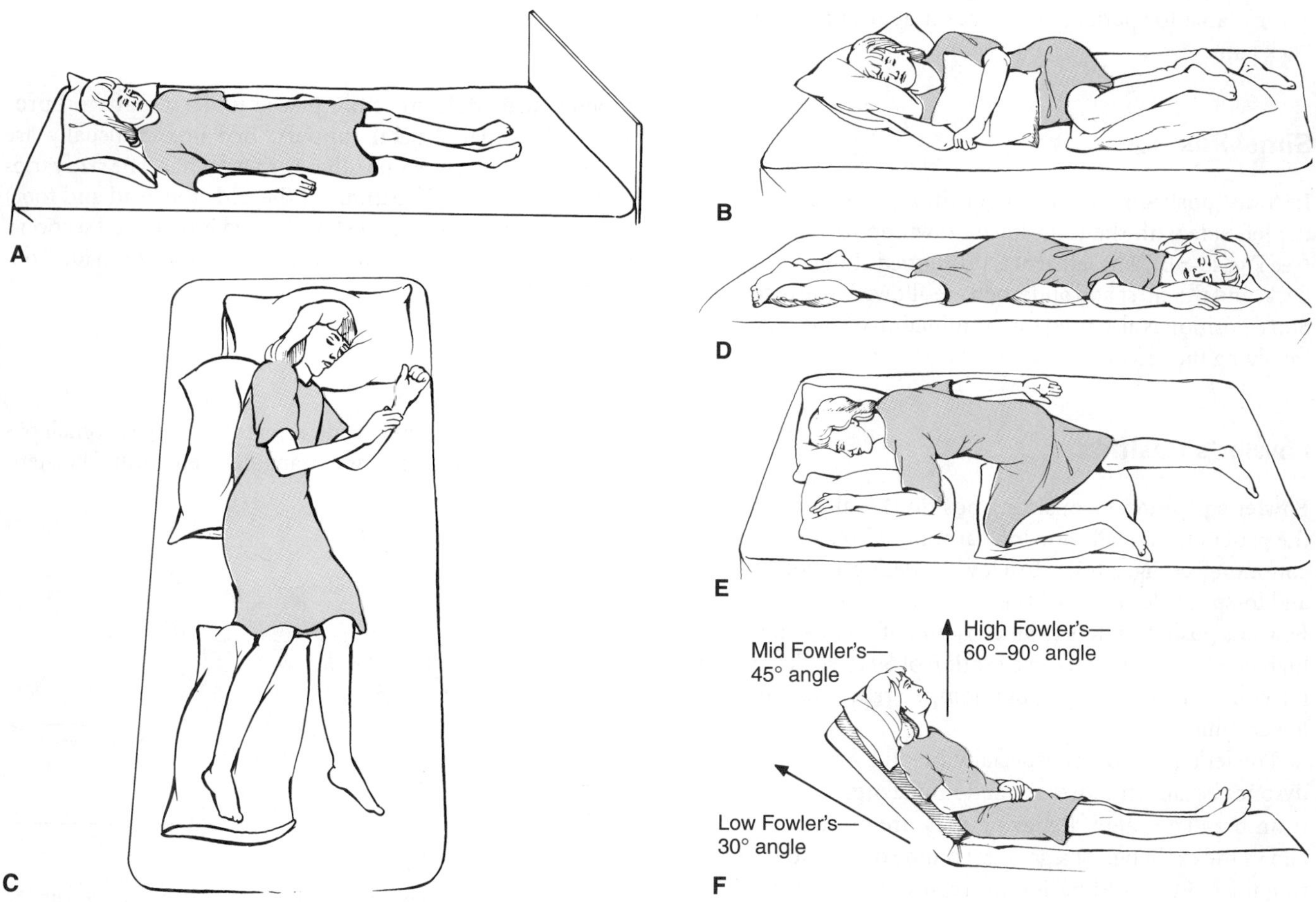

FIGURE 23–5. (*A*) Supine position. (*B*) Lateral position. (*C*) Lateral oblique position. (*D*) Prone position. (*E*) Sims' position. (*F*) Fowler's position.

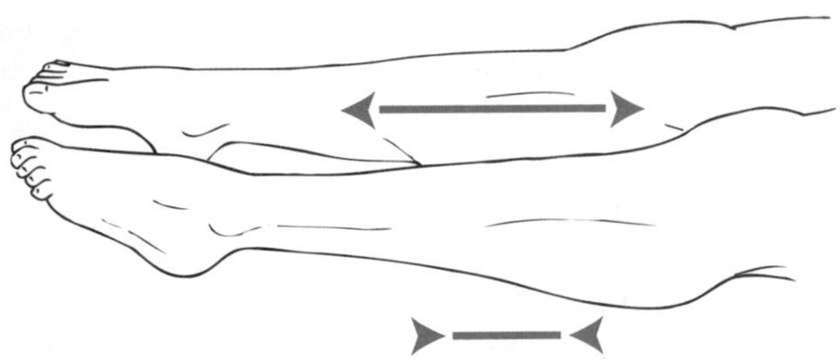

FIGURE 23–6. Foot drop.

Prone Position

The **prone position** (one in which the patient lies on the abdomen; see Fig. 23-5D) is an alternative position for the person with skin breakdown due to pressure ulcers (see Chap. 28). The prone position also provides good drainage from bronchioles, stretches the trunk and extremities, and keeps the hips in an extended position. The prone position improves arterial oxygenation in critically ill patients with adult respiratory distress syndrome and others who are mechanically ventilated (Lasater-Erhard, 1995; Mure et al., 1997; Vollman, 1997). However, the prone position poses a nursing challenge for assessing and communicating with patients, and it is uncomfortable for patients with recent abdominal surgery or back pain.

Sims' Position

In **Sims' position** (semiprone position), the patient lies on the left side with the right knee drawn up toward the chest (see Fig. 23-5E). The left arm is positioned along the patient's back, and the chest and abdomen are allowed to lean forward. Sims' position is also used for examination of and procedures involving the rectum and vagina (see Chap. 13).

Fowler's Position

Fowler's position (semisitting position) makes it easier for the patient to eat, talk, and look around. Three variations are common (see Fig. 23-5F). In a low Fowler's position, the head and torso are elevated to 30 degrees. A mid-Fowler's or semi-Fowler's position refers to an elevation of up to 45 degrees. A high Fowler's position is an elevation of 60 to 90 degrees. The knees may not be elevated, but doing so relieves strain on the lower spine.

Fowler's position is especially helpful for patients with dyspnea because it causes the abdominal organs to drop away from the diaphragm. Relieving pressure on the diaphragm allows the exchange of a greater volume of air. However, sitting for a prolonged period decreases blood flow to tissues in the coccyx area and increases the risk of pressure ulcers in that area.

POSITIONING DEVICES

Many devices are available to help maintain good body alignment in bed and prevent discomfort or pressure. However, any position, no matter how comfortable or anatomically correct, must be changed frequently.

Adjustable Bed

The adjustable bed (see Chap. 17) can be raised or lowered and allows the position of the head and knees to be changed. The high position makes it easier to perform nursing care. Raising the head of the bed helps the patient look around without twisting and bending. It also promotes drainage of the upper lobes of the lungs and prepares the patient for eventually standing and walking. The low position enables an independent patient to get in and out of bed safely (Fig. 23-7).

Mattress

A comfortable, supportive mattress is firm but flexible enough to permit good body alignment. A nonsupportive mattress promotes an unnatural curvature of the spine.

Bed Board

A **bed board** (rigid structure placed under a mattress) provides additional skeletal support. Bed boards usually are made of plywood or some other firm material. The size varies with the situation. If sections of the bed (the head and foot) can be raised, the board must be divided into hinged sections. For home use, full bed boards can be purchased or made from sheets of plywood.

Pillows

Pillows are used to support and elevate a body part. Small pillows, such as contour pillows, triangular wedges, and bolsters,

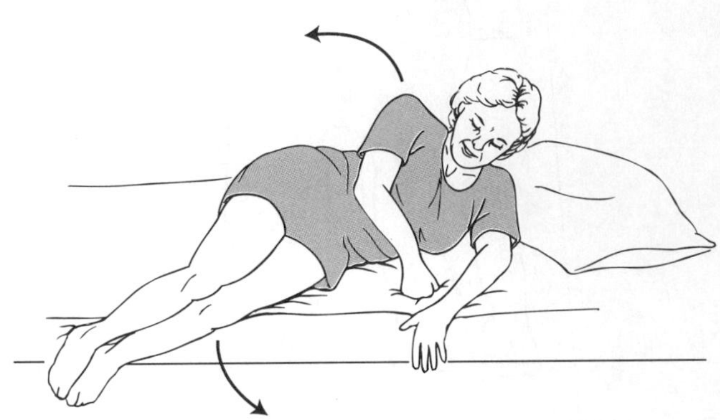

FIGURE 23–7. Grasping the mattress and pushing down with the other hand is an independent technique for sitting on the edge of the bed in preparation for ambulating.

are ideal for supporting and elevating the head, extremities, and shoulders. For home use, oversized pillows are useful for elevating the upper part of the body if an adjustable bed is not available.

Turning Sheet

A turning sheet that extends from the upper back to mid-thighs is a helpful positioning device. It prevents friction when moving, lifting, and turning the patient from side to side. A turning sheet is created by folding a flat sheet in quarters and placing it under the patient. The sheet is rolled close to the sides of the patient's body during repositioning. Working as a team, nurses use the sheet to slide and roll the patient to an alternate position. Care is taken to keep the sheet dry and free of wrinkles to prevent skin breakdown.

Trochanter Rolls

Trochanter rolls (Fig. 23-8) prevent the legs from turning outward. The trochanters are the bony protrusions at the head of the femur near the hip. Placing a positioning device at the trochanters helps prevent the leg from rotating outward.

Nursing Guidelines For

Using a Trochanter Roll

- ☑ Fold a sheet lengthwise in half or in thirds and place it under the patient's hips.
  RATIONALE: The sheet should anchor the body in correct position.
- ☑ Place a rolled-up bath blanket or two bath towels under each end of the sheet that extends on either side of the patient.
  RATIONALE: This provides support to the trochanters.
- ☑ Roll the sheet around the blanket so that the end of the roll is underneath.
  RATIONALE: This action prevents unrolling.
- ☑ Secure the rolls next to each hip and thigh.
  RATIONALE: The rolls prevent external rotation of the hip.
- ☑ Permit the leg to rest against the trochanter roll.
  RATIONALE: This position allows normal alignment of the hips, preventing internal or external rotation.

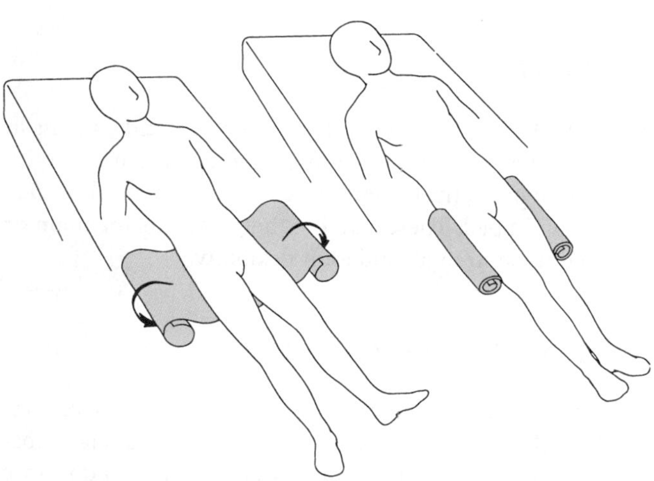

FIGURE 23–8. Placement of trochanter rolls.

Hand Rolls

Hand rolls (Fig. 23-9) are devices that preserve the patient's functional ability to grasp and pick up objects. Hand rolls prevent **contractures** (permanently shortened muscles that resist stretching) of the fingers. They keep the thumb positioned slightly away from the hand and at a moderate angle to the fingers. The fingers are kept in a slightly neutral position rather than a tight fist. A rolled-up washcloth or a ball can be used as an alternative to commercial hand rolls. Hand rolls are removed regularly to facilitate movement and exercise.

Foot Boards and Foot Splints

Foot boards and foot splints are devices that prevent foot drop by keeping the feet in a functional position. Some commercial foot boards have supports that prevent outward rotation of the foot and lower leg (Fig. 23-10A).

If the patient is short and cannot reach a foot board, a foot splint is used (see Fig. 23-10B). A foot splint allows more variety in body positioning while maintaining the foot in a functional position. Some nurses have patients wear ankle-high tennis shoes while in bed to prevent foot drop. The shoes are removed regularly, and proper foot care is given.

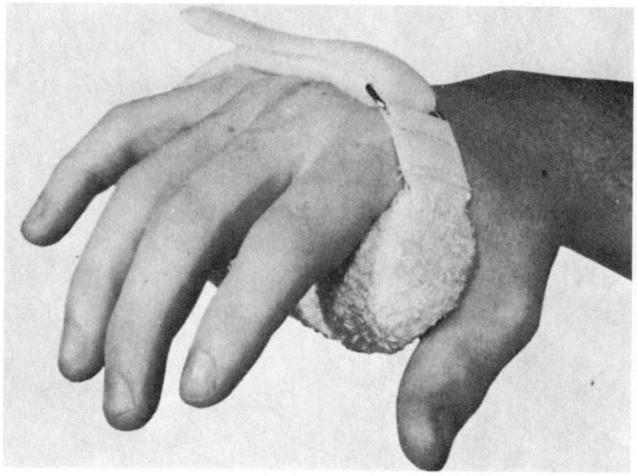

FIGURE 23–9. Hand roll. (Courtesy of the J. T. Posey Company, Arcadia, CA.)

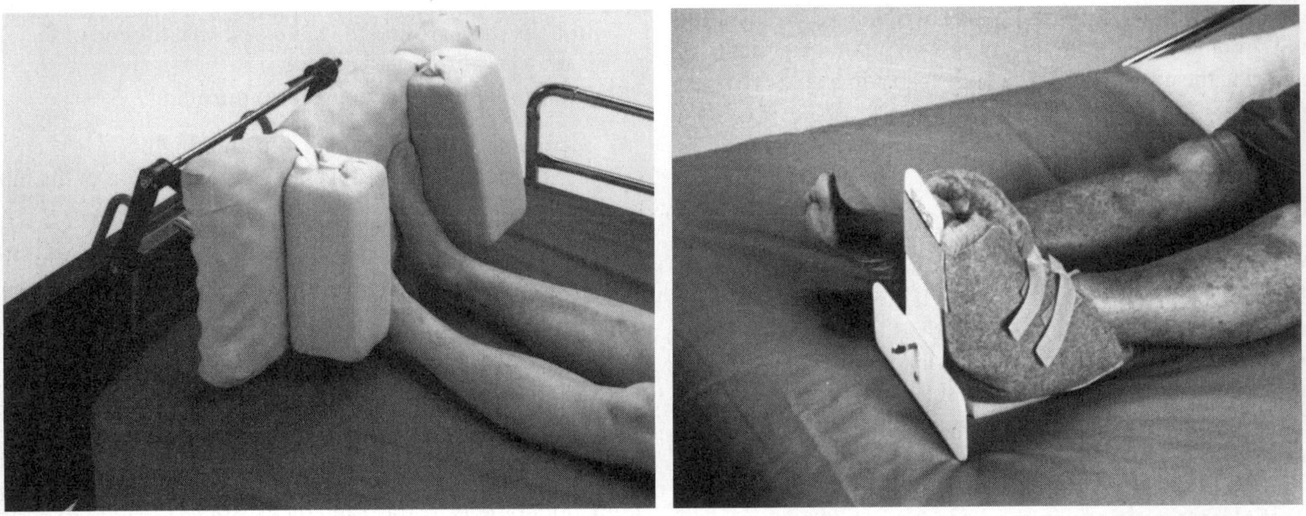

FIGURE 23–10. (*A*) Foot board with lateral supports. (Courtesy of the J. T. Posey Company, Arcadia, CA.) (*B*) Foot splint. (© 1994 Total Care, Gaithersburg, MD.)

If a foot splint or foot board is not available, a pillow and large sheet can be used. The pillow is rolled in the sheet, and the ends of the sheet are twisted before being tucked under the foot of the mattress. A pillow support does not provide the firmness of a board or splint, so it should be replaced as soon as possible with a sturdier device.

Trapeze

A trapeze is a triangular piece of metal hung by a chain over the head of the bed (Fig. 23-11). The patient grasps the trapeze to lift the body and move about in bed. Unless arm movement or lifting is undesirable, a trapeze is an excellent device for helping a bedridden patient increase his or her activity.

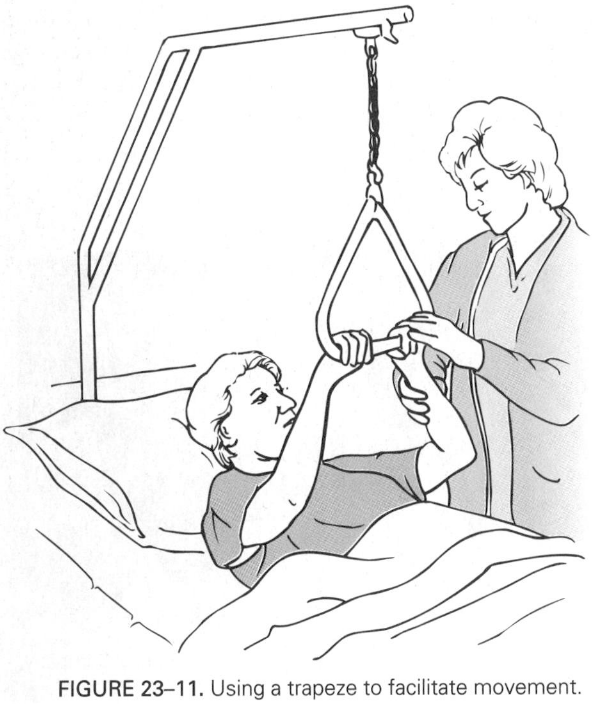

FIGURE 23–11. Using a trapeze to facilitate movement.

TURNING AND MOVING PATIENTS

Patients who cannot change from one position to another independently, and those who need help doing so, need nursing assistance. Good turning and moving skills are important to prevent injury to the nurse and the patient, who may weigh more than the nurse. Skill 23-1 describes the process of repositioning and moving patients.

Protective Devices

Items such as siderails, mattress overlays, cradles, and specialty beds protect the inactive patient from harm or complications.

SIDERAILS

Siderails (Fig. 23-12) are a valuable device to aid patients in changing their position and moving about while in bed. With siderails in place, the patient can safely turn from side to side and sit up in bed. These activities help patients maintain or regain muscle strength and joint flexibility.

MATTRESS OVERLAYS

Mattress overlays are accessory items made of foam, or containing gel, air, or water, that are placed over a standard hospital mattress. They are used to reduce pressure and restore skin integrity (see Chap. 28).

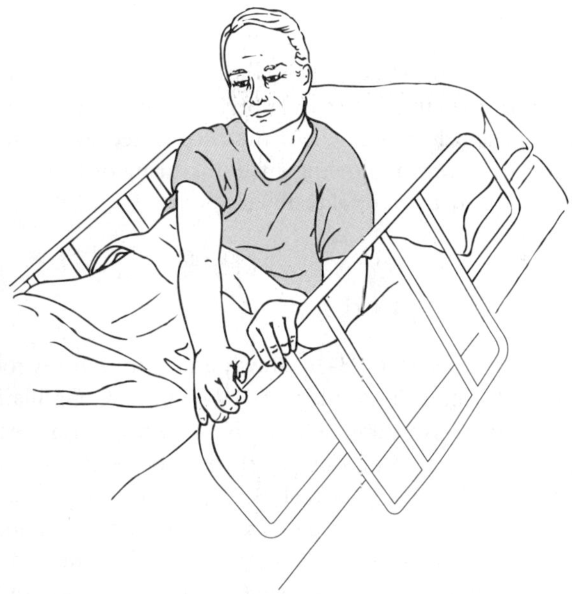

FIGURE 23–12. Using siderails to change position.

Foam and Gel Mattresses

Several types of foam mattresses, made of latex or polyethylene, are available. Foam acts like a layer of subcutaneous tissue because it conforms to the patient's body and acts like a cushion. Consequently, it redistributes pressure over a greater area, thus reducing the compressive effect on skin and tissue. Foam also contains channels and cells filled with air, allowing for evaporation of moisture and escape of heat.

Some foam mattresses are convoluted or made with a series of elevations and depressions, resembling an egg crate (see Chap. 17) or waffle. The density of the foam and the manner in which the foam is formed determine the degree of pressure reduction.

Egg-crate foam mattresses provide minimal pressure reduction and are recommended for comfort only. Thicker, waffle-shaped foam mattresses offer greater pressure reduction and can be used to prevent skin breakdown.

Gel is an alternative substance used to fill cushions and mattresses. It differs from foam in that it suspends and supports the body part. Gel and foam cushions are placed in wheelchairs to prevent the "hammock effect"—the posterior and lateral compression that occurs when sitting in a slinglike seat.

Static Air Mattress

A static air pressure mattress is filled with a fixed volume of air. It is similar in appearance to those used for recreational purposes. It suspends the patient on a buoyant surface, distributing the pressure on the underlying tissue. However, if the mattress becomes underinflated, its effectiveness as a pressure-relieving device is lost. Because plastic is nonabsorbent, air mattresses permit less evaporation of moisture than foam. Also, sharp objects can damage the integrity of the mattress.

Alternating Air Mattress

An alternating air mattress (Fig. 23-13) is similar to a static one, with one exception: every other channel inflates as the next one deflates. The process is then reversed. Through the wavelike redistribution of air, pressure over bony prominences is cyclically relieved. This repetitive process promotes blood flow and keeps the tissue supplied with oxygen. The tubing connecting the mattress to its motor-driven compressor must not become kinked. Some patients also are disturbed by the noise.

Water Mattress

A water mattress supports the body and equalizes the pressure per square inch over its surface. The pressure-relieving effect is maintained regardless of any shift in the patient's position. Many claim that sleeping on a waterbed produces a feeling of tranquility, which may provide beneficial emotional effects. Water mattresses are heavy; therefore, the floor and the bed frame must be able to support the weight. Puncturing leads to damage. Filling and emptying, although done infrequently, are time-consuming.

CRADLE

A cradle is a metal frame that is secured to the mattress or placed on top of the mattress. It forms a shell over the patient's lower legs to keep bed linen off the feet or legs. A cradle is often used for patients with burns, painful joint disease, and fractures of the leg.

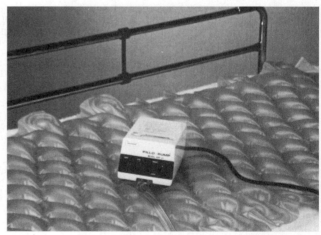

FIGURE 23–13. Alternating air mattress. (© 1994 Total Care, Gaithersburg, MD.)

SPECIALTY BEDS

Specialty beds such as low–air-loss beds, air-fluidized beds, oscillating support beds, and circular beds offer more functions than standard hospital beds. Like mattress overlays, they are used to relieve pressure and to prevent other problems associated with inactivity and immobility (Table 23-3).

Low–Air-Loss Bed

A low–air-loss bed (Fig. 23-14) contains inflated air sacs within the mattress. It maintains capillary pressure well below that which can interfere with blood flow. Regardless of changes in body position, the mattress selectively responds by redistributing the air to maintain low pressure to all skin areas.

Air-Fluidized Bed

An air-fluidized bed (Fig. 23-15) contains a collection of tiny beads within a mattress cover. The beads are blown upward on warm air. When suspended, the dry beads take on the characteristics of fluid, allowing the patient to float on the lifted beads. Excretions and secretions drain away from the body and through the beads, thereby preventing skin irritation and maceration from moisture. The pressure-relieving effects of this type of bed have been shown to speed the healing of severely impaired tissue.

An air-fluidized bed is better used for a patient who is likely to remain in bed for long periods. Fluid balance may become a problem because of the accelerated evaporation caused by the warm, blowing air. Puncturing or tearing the mattress is also a potential problem.

Oscillating Support Bed

An oscillating bed (Fig. 23-16) slowly and continuously rocks the patient from side to side in a 124-degree arc. Oscillation relieves skin pressure and helps to mobilize respiratory secretions. Foam-covered supports applied to the head, arms, and legs prevent sliding and skin **shearing** (force exerted against the surface and layers of the skin as tissues slide in opposite but parallel directions). Compartments within the bed are removed temporarily to facilitate assessment and care of the posterior body.

Circular Bed

A circular bed supports the patient on a 6-or 7-foot anterior or posterior platform suspended across the diameter of the frame (Fig. 23-17). This type of bed allows the patient to

TABLE 23–3. **Pressure-Relieving Devices**

Device	Examples	Indications for Use
Foam mattress or gel cushion	Egg crate Geo-Matt Spencegel pad	Intact skin and minimal risk for breakdown Changes in position occur spontaneously or require minimal assistance.
Static air, alternating air, or water mattress	TENDER Cloud Sof-Care Pulsair Lotus	At some risk for skin breakdown, or A superficial or single deep break in skin but pressure easily relieved Need for prolonged bed rest with immobilization
Oscillating support bed	Roto Rest Tilt and Turn Paragon 9000	At high risk for systemic effects of immobility, such as pneumonia and skin breakdown Combination of the following:
Low–air-loss bed	KinAir FLEXICAIR Mediscus	Impaired skin Continued existence of risk factors for further skin breakdown Alternative positions limited, less than adequate, or impossible Assistance required for frequent transfers from bed
Air-fluidized bed	CLINITRON FluidAir	Combination of the following: Impaired skin Continued existence of risk factors for further skin breakdown Alternative positions limited, less than adequate, or impossible Seldom transferred from bed
Circular bed	CircOlectric	Current or high risk for skin breakdown because of multiple trauma, especially if it involves the head, neck, or spine Burns that require frequent dressing changes or topical applications

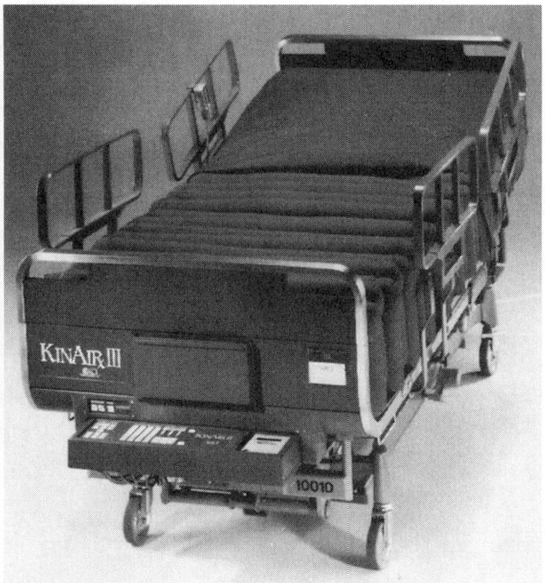

FIGURE 23–14. Low-air-loss bed. (Courtesy of Kinetic Concepts, Inc., San Antonio, TX.)

remain passively immobilized during a position change. The bed has the capacity to rotate the patient, who is sandwiched between the anterior and posterior frames, in a 180-degree arc. Turning permits access to the patient for nursing care. Patients are taught how to operate the bed to make minor adjustments in their position. This promotes a sense of control among otherwise dependent patients.

Transferring Patients

Transfer (moving a patient from place to place) refers to moving a patient from bed to a chair or stretcher and back to bed again. The patient assists in an *active* transfer. A transfer done entirely by others or by mechanical means is a *passive* transfer.

TRANSFER DEVICES

Several devices are available to help transfer patients from one location to another. The use of a transfer handle, transfer belt, transfer board, or mechanical lift helps decrease the potential for injuries to the patient and nurse. Transfer devices are especially helpful when caring for patients who fear falling or lack confidence in the ability of personnel to transfer them safely and comfortably.

Transfer Handle

Some patients with disabilities find that a transfer handle helps them remain active and independent (Fig. 23-18) A transfer handle fits between the mattress and bed frame or box spring and serves as a combination grab bar and handrail to support the patient's weight while exiting and returning to bed. A transfer handle is not considered a restrictive device, like siderails, because the patient is free to move about. It promotes activity and mobility for many who are physically challenged.

Transfer Belt

A transfer belt is a padded device worn around the patient's waist. Its handles provide a means of gripping and supporting the patient. This device is designed for patients who can bear weight and help with the transfer, but are unsteady. It may also be used as a walking belt to provide safety and security while assisting a patient with ambulation (see Chap. 26).

Transfer Board

A transfer board serves as a supportive bridge between two surfaces, such as the bed and a wheelchair or a wheelchair and a car seat. The low-friction board, which is about 30″ long and 8″ wide, is positioned so that the patient's

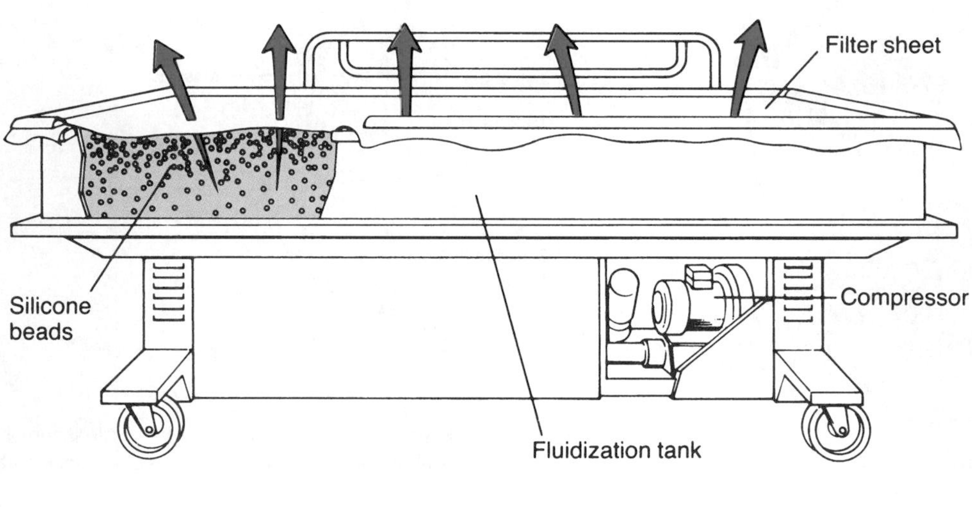

FIGURE 23–15. Air-fluidized bed.

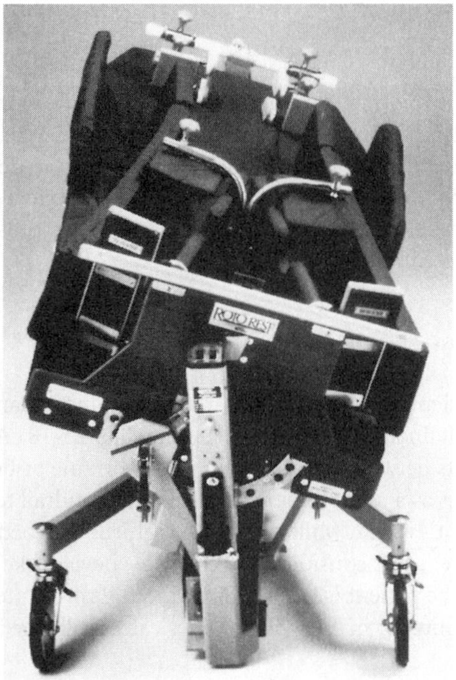

FIGURE 23–16. Oscillating bed. (Courtesy of Kinetic Concepts, Inc., San Antonio, TX.)

buttocks can slide across what would otherwise be an open space or a gap in height between two surfaces. Some patients with strong arm and upper body muscles are able to use a transfer board independently. For patients who need assistance, a transfer belt is used in conjunction with a transfer board. Full-body transfer boards also are available for moving supine patients to a stretcher or x-ray table.

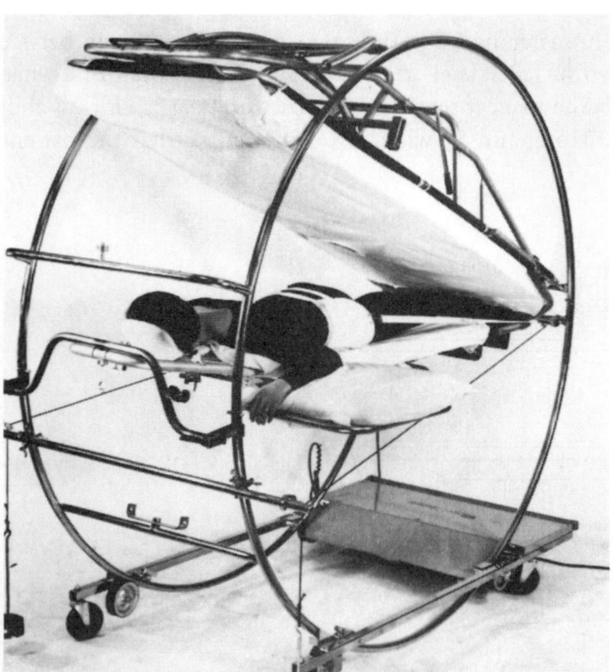

FIGURE 23–17. Circular bed.

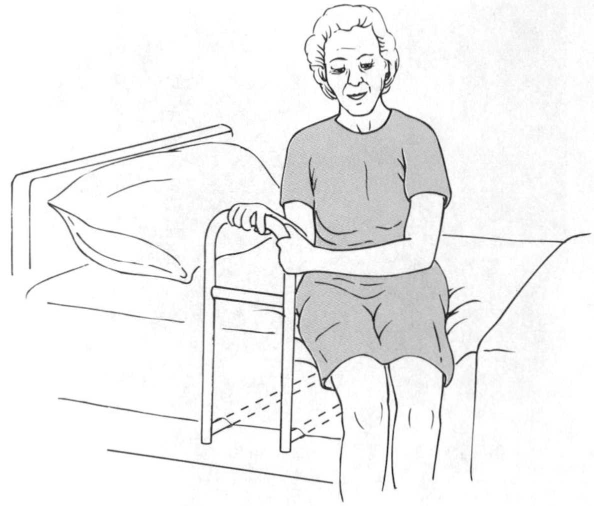

FIGURE 23–18. A transfer handle.

Mechanical Lift

A mechanical lift (Fig. 23-19) helps move large patients or those who have limited ability to assist from the bed to a chair, toilet, or tub, and back again. Both electric and hydraulic models are available, with a lifting capacity of 350 to 600 lbs. Using a mechanical lift enables a caregiver to raise and lower patients secured in a canvas sling, and move them about on a wheeled frame. The wheels are locked when a stationary position is desired, such as when lowering a patient into place.

PATIENT TRANSFER

If the patient cannot assist with a transfer and no transfer device is available, two people can lift the patient from bed into a chair (Fig. 23-20). However, this method is the least

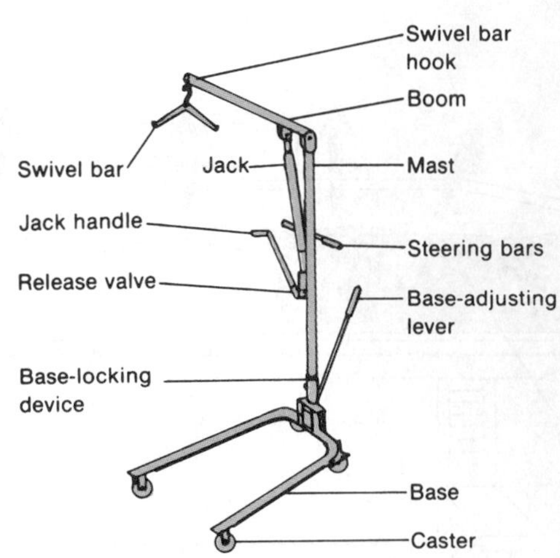

FIGURE 23–19. A mechanical lift. (Smith-Temple J, Johnson J: Nurse's guide to clinical procedures. 3rd ed. Philadelphia: Lippincott Williams & Wilkins, 1998.)

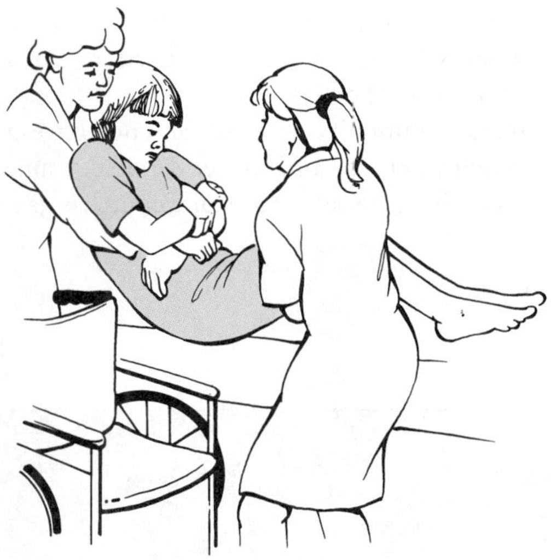

FIGURE 23–20. Passive transfer to a wheelchair.

desirable because of the risk of patient or nurse injury. Nursing personnel should use assistive devices, observe the nursing guidelines that follow, and use the recommendations in Skill 23-2 when transferring patients.

Nursing Guidelines For

Assisting with Patient Transfer

- ☑ Be realistic about how much you can safely lift.
  RATIONALE: Not exceeding one's capabilities demonstrates good judgment.
- ☑ Always practice good body mechanics.
  RATIONALE: Using good body mechanics reduces the potential for injury.
- ☑ Put on braces and other supportive devices before getting a patient out of bed.
  RATIONALE: This maximizes time management.
- ☑ Have the patient wear shoes or nonskid slippers.
  RATIONALE: Appropriate footwear provides support and prevents foot injuries.
- ☑ Plan to transfer patients across the shortest distance.
  RATIONALE: A short transfer reduces the potential for injury.
- ☑ Make sure that the patient's stronger leg, if there is one, is nearest the chair to which the patient is transferring.
  RATIONALE: This action ensures safety.
- ☑ Stand on the side of the bed to which the patient will be moving.
  RATIONALE: This position helps the nurse assist the patient.
- ☑ Explain to the patient what will be done, step by step, and solicit the patient's help as much as possible.
  RATIONALE: These actions inform the patient, encourage self-help, and reduce the workload.

Nursing Implications

During the initial and subsequent patient assessments, the nurse determines the patient's level of dependence on nursing assistance. One scale for quantifying the patient's status is shown in Display 23-1. The nurse selects positioning, transfer, and protective devices according to whether the patient is independent or requires partial or total assistance.

Various nursing diagnoses may apply to inactive patients.

- Impaired physical mobility
- Risk for injury
- Risk for disuse syndrome
- Risk for perioperative positioning injury
- Impaired transfer ability
- Impaired bed mobility
- Risk for impaired skin integrity

The nursing care plan illustrates how the steps in the nursing process are applied when caring for a patient with the nursing diagnosis of Risk for disuse syndrome. The NANDA taxonomy (1999) describes this diagnostic category as "a state in which an individual is at risk for deterioration of body systems as the result of prescribed or unavoidable musculoskeletal inactivity."

While providing nursing care, there may be opportunities to teach patients and their caregivers about techniques that promote activity or reduce the potential for complications from inactivity.

Patient Teaching For

Promoting Activity and Mobility

Teach the patient and family to do the following:

- ▷ Balance periods of activity with periods of rest.
- ▷ Become aware of the dangers of inactivity.
- ▷ Allow adequate time for performing activities.
- ▷ Join a club that involves social activities.
- ▷ Develop hobbies or recreational interests.
- ▷ Become a volunteer at the hospital, your church, or a municipal group.

DISPLAY 23–1

Levels of Functional Status

0 = Completely independent
1 = Requires use of assistive device
2 = Needs minimal help
3 = Needs assistance and/or some supervision
4 = Needs total supervision
5 = Needs total assistance or unable to assist (Carpenito, 1997)

- Join a local group—a coffee club, needlework group, football friends, or bingo or card players.
- Remove objects that might pose a safety hazard, such as throw rugs or electrical cords. Make sure chair legs are not in the way. Promptly mop up any water spilled on the floor.
- Rent or purchase hospital equipment from a medical supply company.
- Investigate the loan of equipment for homebound terminal patients from national organizations such as the American Cancer Society.
- Ask about community services that encourage independent living, such as homemaker services, trained dogs, Meals on Wheels, social services, and church organizations.

Nursing Care Plan

Risk for Disuse Syndrome

Assessment

Subjective Data

States, "Please don't move me; just let me alone."

Objective Data

82-year-old woman recuperating from the surgical repair of a fractured left femur. Weight approximately 95 pounds; occasional incontinence of bladder and bowel; skin translucent and dry; incision line clean and dry with good approximation; skin staples removed yesterday; reddened area on right hip approximately 2.5 × 3 cm; unable to turn self; non-weight bearing; regular mattress; overhead trapeze in place.

Diagnosis

Risk for disuse syndrome

Plan

Goal

The patient will demonstrate

- Intact skin/tissue integrity
- Full range of joint motion
- Negative Homans' sign
- Bowel, bladder, and renal functioning within normal limits by 1/22.

Orders: 1/20

1. Reposition q 2 h around the clock.
2. Provide clean, dry, and wrinkle-free bedding at all times.
3. Use incontinence pads on bed continuously.
4. Assist to bedside commode q 4 h when awake.
5. Use foam mattress on bed.
6. Use trochanter rolls for supine positioning.
7. Use foot board.
8. Encourage active exercise with use of trapeze t.i.d.
9. Vary daily routine when possible.
10. Include the patient in planning the daily routine.
11. Teach family how to turn and position the patient. ________ J. Scales, RN

Implementation (Documentation)

1/21 0745 Right side-lying; incontinent of dark, foul-smelling urine. Reddened area approximately 2.5 × 3 cm over right trochanter. Skin cleansed; lotion applied to right hip. Incision line on left hip dry and pink. Repositioned to back; trochanter rolls in place. Served breakfast: consumed 50% of diet. ________ J. Scales, RN

Evaluation (Documentation)

1/21 1400 Able to move about in bed with assistance of trapeze. Area on right trochanter 2 × 2.5 cm; skin translucent and dry. Incision line on left hip dry and pink. States appetite "getting better." Urine continues concentrated; cranberry juice encouraged. ________ J. Scales, RN

FOCUS ON OLDER ADULTS

- Muscle strength, endurance, and coordination decline by the seventh or eighth decade. Older adults need to maintain as much mobility as possible to prevent disability.
- Older adults require extra time and assistance during positioning, transferring, and ambulating.
- Older adults may be afraid of falling and may limit their mobility because of this fear.
- Bone demineralization increases the risk of fractures for older adults.
- Falls, fractures, and degenerative bone diseases have a serious economic impact on older adults.
- Older adults who are cognitively impaired generally have difficulty following directions regarding positioning and transferring. Keeping instructions simple, giving only one direction at a time, and using demonstrations to supplement verbal instructions are helpful.
- Disuse syndrome is a serious threat to the older adult, and aggressive efforts are made to prevent it. For example, older adults who have been on bed rest for more than 1 day may benefit from physical therapy to help them regain their mobility.

KEY CONCEPTS

- When standing, keep the feet parallel and distribute weight equally on both feet to provide a broad base of support.
- When sitting, the buttocks and upper thighs are the base of support on the chair; both feet rest on the floor.
- Correct posture for lying down is the same as for standing, but in the horizontal plane; body parts are in neutral position.
- Principles of correct body mechanics include the following: distribute gravity through the center of the body over a wide base of support; push, pull, or roll objects rather than lifting them; and hold objects close to the body.
- Ergonomics is a field of engineering science devoted to promoting comfort, performance, and health in the workplace by improving the design of the work environment and equipment that is used. Two examples of ergonomic recommendations are to use assistive devices when lifting or transporting heavy items, and to use alternatives for tasks that require repetitive motions.
- Disuse syndrome is associated with weakness, atony, poor alignment, contractures, foot drop, impaired circulation, atelectasis, urinary tract infections, anorexia, and pressure sores.
- Common patient positions are supine (on the back), lateral (on the side), lateral oblique (on the side with slight hip and knee flexion), prone (on the abdomen), Sims' (semiprone position on the left side with the right knee drawn up toward the chest), and Fowler's (semisitting or sitting position).
- Positioning devices include the following: adjustable bed—allows the position of the head and knees to be changed; pillows—provide support and elevate a body part; trochanter rolls—prevent legs from turning outward; hand rolls—maintain function of the hand and prevent contractures; and foot boards—keep the feet in normal walking position.
- Pressure-relieving devices include the following: siderails—help patients change position; mattress overlays—reduce pressure and restore skin integrity; and cradle—keeps linen off patient's feet or legs.
- Devices used to help transfer patients include a transfer handle, a transfer belt, a transfer board, and a mechanical lift.
- Guidelines to follow when transferring patients include the following: know the patient's diagnosis, capabilities, weaknesses, and activity level; be realistic about how much you can safely lift; transfer patients across the shortest distance possible; solicit the patient's help; and use smooth rather than jerky movements.

CRITICAL THINKING EXERCISES

- You observe one of your coworkers using incorrect body mechanics while giving patient care. How would you approach this coworker? What suggestions would you give?
- List nursing activities that predispose to work-related injuries. How can the risk of injury be reduced during each?

SUGGESTED READINGS

Blue CL. Preventing back injury among nurses. Orthopaedic Nursing 1996;15(6):9–22.

Carpenito LJ. Nursing diagnosis: application to clinical practice, 7th ed. Philadelphia, Lippincott-Raven, 1997.

Carroll JL, Siska ES. SIDS: counseling parents to reduce the risk. American Family Physician 1998;57(7):1566–1572.

DeRoyal Orthopedic Group. The assessment of knowledge and application of proper body mechanics in the workplace. Orthopaedic Nursing 1997; 16(1):66–69.

Fleisher I, Bryant D. Evaluating replacement mattresses. Nursing Management 1997;28(8):38–41.

Gassett RS, Hearne B, Keelan B. Ergonomics and body mechanics in the workplace. Orthopedic Clinics of North America 1996;27(4):861–879.

Hoshowsky VM. Surgical positioning. Orthopaedic Nursing 1998;17(5): 55–65.

Lasater-Erhard M. The effect of patient position on arterial oxygen saturation. Critical Care Nurse 1995;15(5):31–36.

Lockeridge T. Now I lay me down to sleep: SIDS and infant sleep positions. Neonatal Network: Journal of Neonatal Nursing 1997;16(7):25–31.

Morris DG, Matthay MA. ARDS: improving oxygenation with prone ventilation. Journal of Critical Illness 1998;13(12):750–751.

Mure M, Martling CR, Lindahl SG. Dramatic effect on oxygenation in patients with severe acute lung insufficiency treated in the prone position. Critical Care Medicine 1997;25:1539–1544.

NANDA nursing diagnoses: definitions and classification, 1999–2000. Philadelphia, NANDA, 1999.

National Institute for Occupational Safety and Health. Do back belts prevent injury? http://www.cdc.gov/niosh/backbelt.html, updated 6/1997, accessed 7/1999.

Nelson EA. Mattresses: the patient's view. Professional Nurse 1997;13(1):5.
Norman EM. Positioning patients to promote oxygenation. American Journal of Nursing 1997;97(8):16.
Owen BD, Welden N, Kane J. What are we teaching about lifting and transferring patients? Research in Nursing and Health 1999;22(11):3–13.
Patient care: the right bed can help your patient. RN 1998;61(1):16C–16D.
Pring J, Millman P. Evaluating pressure-relieving mattresses. Journal of Wound Care 1998;7(4):177–179.
Rogers JL, Maurizio SJ. Education and training. Body mechanics and transfers for health care providers. Caring 1997;16(12):86–88.
Sander R. Lifting. Elderly Care 1998;10(6):25–30.
Ullin SS, Chaffin DB, Patellos CL, et al. A biomedical analysis of methods used for transferring totally dependent patients. SCI Nursing 1997;14(1): 19–27.
Vollman KM. Critical care nursing technique. Prone positioning for the ARDS patient. Dimensions of Critical Care Nursing 1997;16(4): 184–193.

SKILL 23-1

TURNING AND MOVING A PATIENT

Suggested Action	Reason for Action
Assessment	
Assess for risk factors that may contribute to inactivity.	Indicates a need to reposition more frequently
Determine the time of the last position change.	Ensures following the plan for care
Assess physical ability to assist in turning, positioning, or moving.	Determines if additional help is needed
Inspect for the presence of drainage tubes and equipment.	Ensures that they will not be displaced or cause discomfort to the patient
Planning	
Explain the procedure to the patient.	Increases cooperation and decreases anxiety
Remove all pillows and current positioning devices.	Reduces interference during repositioning
Raise the bed to a comfortable working height.	Prevents back strain by maintaining the center of gravity
Secure extra help if needed.	Ensures safety
Close the door or draw the bedside curtain.	Demonstrates respect for privacy
Implementation	
Turning the Patient From Supine to Lateral or Prone Position	
Wash hands.	Reduces the transmission of microorganisms
Lower the siderail and move the patient to one side of the bed.	Provides room when turning
Raise the siderail.	Ensures safety
Move to the other side of the bed and lower the siderail on that side.	Facilitates assistance and ease in working
Flex the patient's far knee over the near one with the arms across the chest.	Aids in turning and protects the patient's arms
Spread your feet, flex your knees, and place one foot behind the other.	Provides a broad base of support
Place one hand on the patient's shoulder and one on the hip on the far side.	Facilitates turning
Roll the patient toward you.	Reduces effort
Replace pillows behind the back and between the legs and under the upper arm.	Aids in maintaining position and provides comfort
Raise the siderails and lower the height of the bed.	Ensures safety

continued

SKILL 23-1

TURNING AND MOVING A PATIENT *Continued*

Suggested Action	Reason for Action

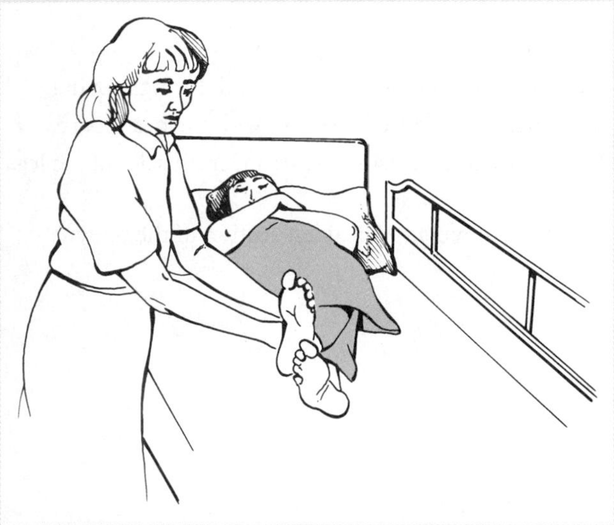

Positioning arms and legs.

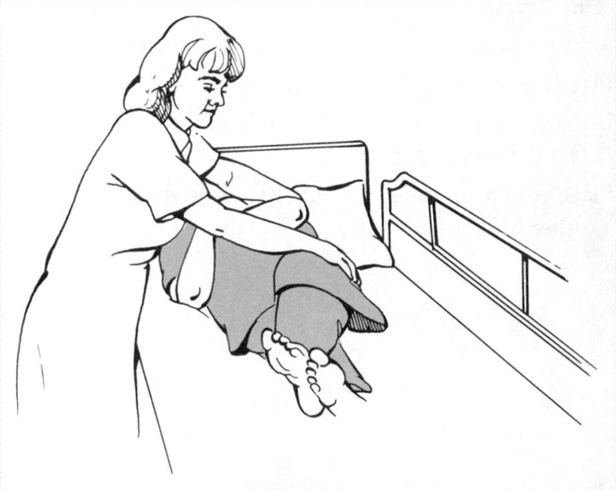

Turning the patient.

For a Prone Position

Begin as described earlier for the lateral position. — Follows same principles

Have the patient turn his or her head opposite to the direction for rolling and leave the arms extended at each side. — Prevents pressure on the face and arms during and after repositioning

Shift your hands from the posterior of the shoulder and hip to the anterior as the patient rolls onto his or her abdomen. — Controls the speed with which the patient is repositioned

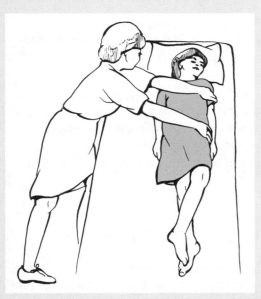

Preparing for prone positioning.

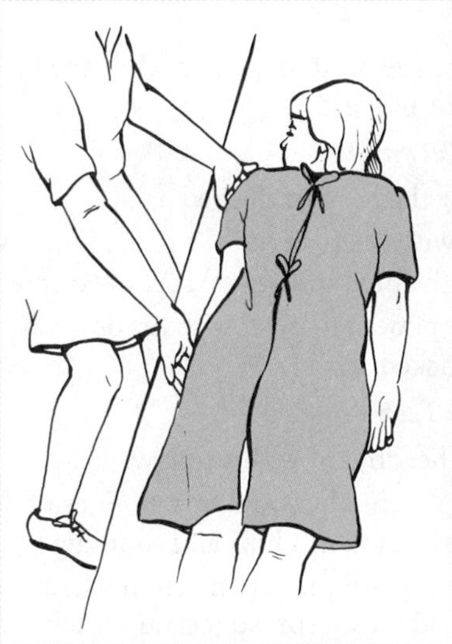

Bracing the patient during turning.

Center the patient in bed. — Prevents pressure on arms

Arrange pillows. — Provides for comfort and support

Raise the siderails and lower the height of the bed. — Ensures safety

continued

SKILL 23-1

TURNING AND MOVING A PATIENT *Continued*

Suggested Action	Reason for Action
Moving the Mobile Patient up in Bed (One-Nurse Technique)	
Remove pillow from under the patient's head.	Prevents strain on the neck and head during moving
Place the pillow against the headboard.	Cushions the head from contact with the headboard
Instruct the patient to bend both knees while keeping the feet flat on the bed.	Aids in assisting by using the stronger muscles of the legs
Place your arm under the patient's shoulders and the other under the hips.	Facilitates moving the heaviest section of the body

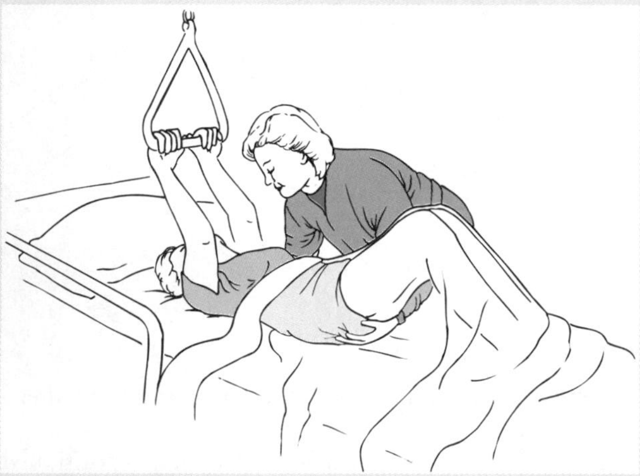

Supporting the upper and mid-sections of the body.

Suggested Action	Reason for Action
Bend your hips and knees, and spread your feet.	Provides a wide base of support and makes use of stronger muscles in the legs rather than the back
Rock toward the head of the bed while the patient pushes with his or her feet.	Creates momentum to facilitate moving
Alternate Technique	
Stand facing the head of the bed.	Facilitates moving upward
Lock arms with the patient.	Uses combined strength of patient and nurse
Bend from the hips and knees; spread your feet.	Follows principles of good body mechanics
Instruct the patient to push with his or her legs while pulling locked arms.	Coordinates momentum and effort to move upward
Two-Nurse Technique	
Protect the headboard with a pillow.	Ensures patient safety
Stand facing each other on opposite sides of the bed between the patient's hips and shoulders.	Distributes weight equally between nurses
Lock hands beneath the patient's buttocks and shoulders.	Doubles the muscular strength
Bend hips and knees; spread feet; and rock toward the head of the bed.	Follows principles of good body mechanics and provides momentum to facilitate moving
Move the patient up on reaching a previously agreed signal, such as the count of three.	Promotes coordination of effort

continued

SKILL 23-1

TURNING AND MOVING A PATIENT *Continued*

Suggested Action	Reason for Action

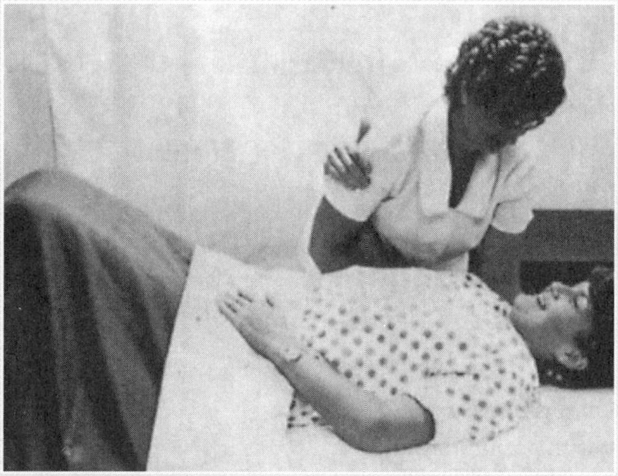

Locking arms. (Courtesy of Ken Timby.)

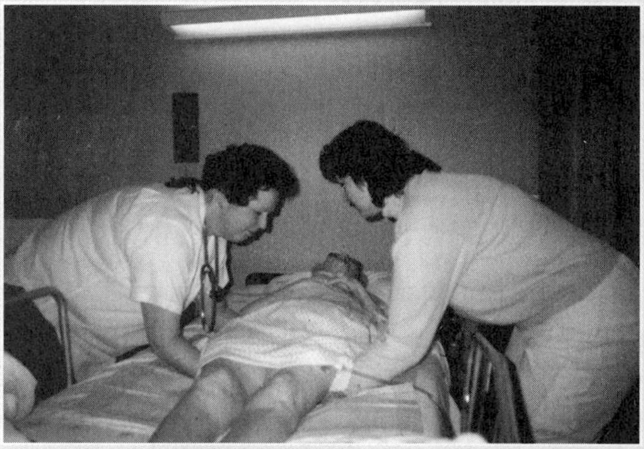

Locking hands. (Note: for purposes of illustration, the cover used to maintain privacy has been removed.) (Courtesy of Ken Timby.)

Using a Turning Sheet

Suggested Action	Reason for Action
Stand opposite one another on each side of the bed.	Facilitates distributing the patient's weight equally between nurses
Roll the turning sheet close to the patient.	Acts as a sling to slide the patient upward

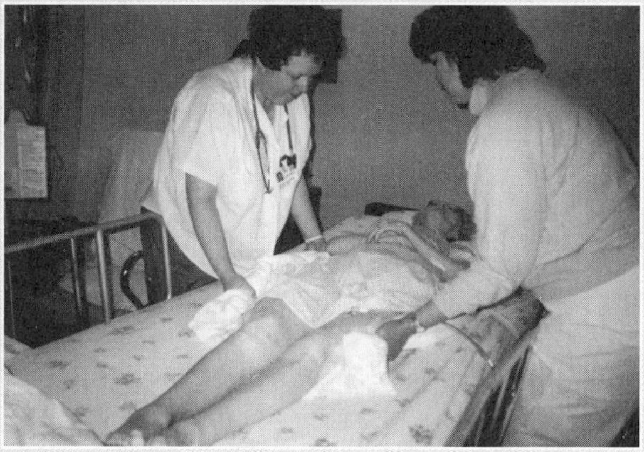

Rolling the turning sheet. (Note: for purposes of illustration, the cover used to maintain privacy has been removed.) (Courtesy of Ken Timby.)

Suggested Action	Reason for Action
Bend hips and knees; spread feet.	Follows principles of good body mechanics
Rock back and forth in unison; move the patient up in bed on reaching an agreed signal.	Coordinates efforts

Evaluation

- Movement is achieved.
- Patient is comfortable.
- Pressure is relieved.
- Joints and limbs are supported.

continued

SKILL 23–1

TURNING AND MOVING A PATIENT *Continued*

Document

- Frequency of turning and moving
- Positions used
- Use of positioning devices
- Assistance required
- Patient's response

SAMPLE DOCUMENTATION

Date and Time Position changed q 2 h from supine to R and L lateral positions with assistance of patient. Pillows used to support limbs and maintain positions. Foot board in place. No shortness of breath noted. No evidence of discomfort during repositioning.

____ SIGNATURE, TITLE

CRITICAL THINKING

- Discuss some advantages and disadvantages for any two patient positions.
- You are assigned to a patient who is weak and unable to assist with positioning and turning. In addition to the usual hospital bed, what else will you obtain to facilitate moving and repositioning your patient?

SKILL 23–2

TRANSFERRING PATIENTS

Suggested Action	Reason for Action
Assessment	
Check the Kardex, nursing care plan, and medical orders for activity level.	Complies with the plan for care
Assess strength and mobility of the patient.	Determines the need for additional personnel or a mechanical lifting device.
Planning	
Consult with the patient on the preferred time for getting out of bed.	Helps patient participate in decision-making
Locate a straight-backed chair, wheelchair, or stretcher to which the patient will be transferred.	Facilitates efficient time management
Arrange the chair or stretcher next to or close to the bed on the patient's stronger side, if there is one.	Ensures safety
Lock the wheels of the bed, wheelchair, or stretcher.	Prevents rolling and ensures safety
Explain how the transfer will be accomplished.	Reduces anxiety and promotes cooperation
Implementation	
From Bed to Chair	
Assist the patient to a sitting position on the side of the bed.	Reduces dizziness; enables the patient to stand

continued

SKILL 23-2

TRANSFERRING PATIENTS *Continued*

Suggested Action	Reason for Action
Help the patient to don a bathrobe and nonskid slippers.	Ensures warmth, modesty, and safety
Place the chair parallel to the bed on the patient's stronger side; raise the foot rests if a wheelchair is used.	Provides easy access
Apply a transfer belt or other assistive device, if needed.	Reduces the risk for falling

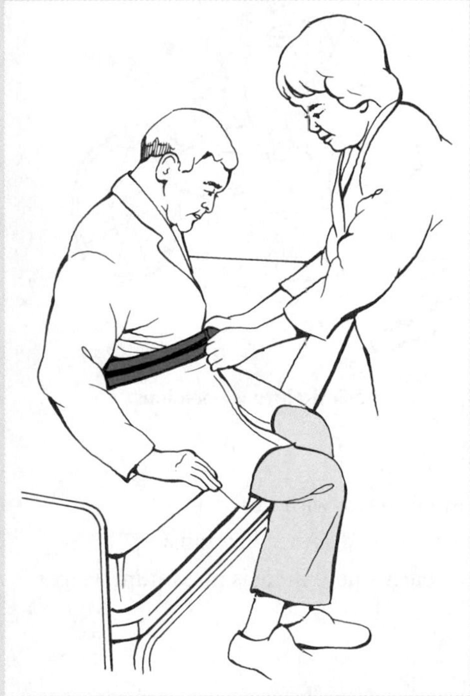

Applying a transfer belt.

Suggested Action	Reason for Action
Grasp the transfer belt or reach under the patient's arms.	Helps support the upper body
Instruct the patient to grasp your shoulders.	Gives the patient leverage for rising
Bend the hips and knees; brace the patient's knees.	Stabilizes the patient and follows principles of good body mechanics
Rock the patient to a standing position at an agreed signal while encouraging the patient to straighten his or her knees and hips.	Provides momentum and reduces the need to lift the patient
Pivot the patient with his or her back toward the chair.	Positions the patient for sitting
Tell the patient to step back until he or she feels the chair at the back of the legs.	Places the patient in close proximity with the chair
Instruct the patient to grasp the arms of the chair while you stabilize his or her knees and lower the patient into the chair.	Promotes safety
Support the feet on the foot rests.	Facilitates good posture

continued

SKILL 23-2

TRANSFERRING PATIENTS *Continued*

Suggested Action	Reason for Action

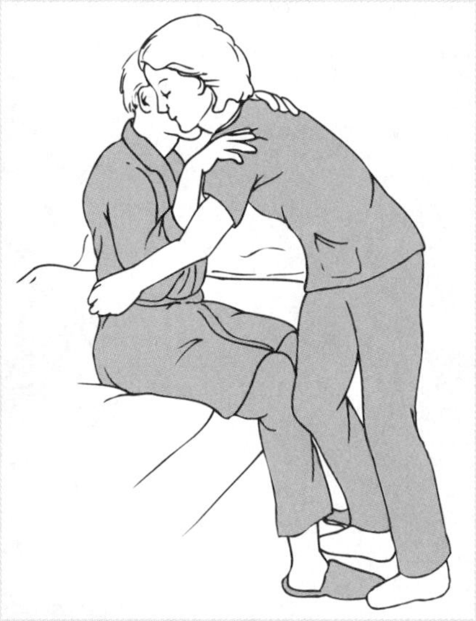

Bracing the patient's knees.

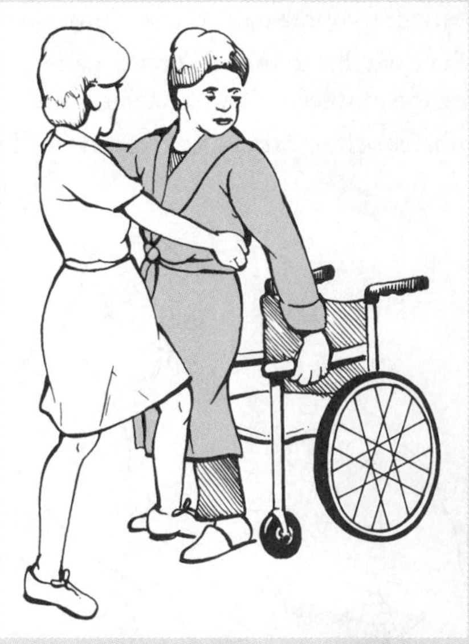

Backing into wheelchair.

Using a Transfer Board

Remove an arm from the wheelchair.	Reduces interference with transfer
Slide the patient to the edge of the bed.	Maintains shortest distance for transfer
Angle the transfer board from the patient's buttocks and hips down toward the seat of the chair.	Places the board where there is maximum weight

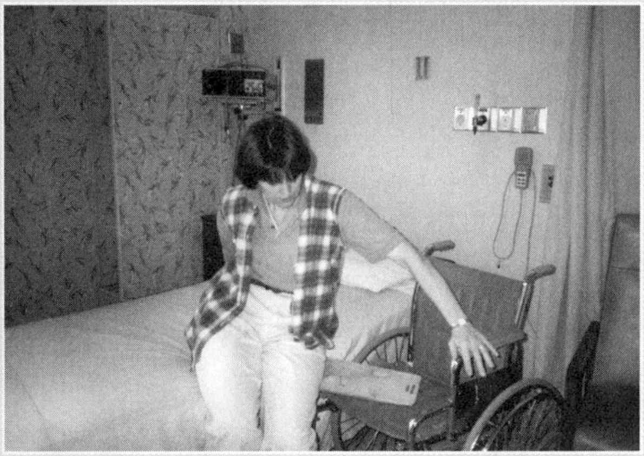

Using a transfer board. (Courtesy of Ken Timby.)

Raise the bed to a sitting position and grasp the patient under the axillae.	Supports upper body
Have an assistant support the lower legs at the knees.	Prevents injury
Slide the patient down the transfer board into the seat of the chair at an agreed-on signal.	Reduces the need to lift patient

continued

SKILL 23-2

TRANSFERRING PATIENTS *Continued*

Suggested Action	Reason for Action
Using a Mechanical Lift	
Raise the bed to a height that places the patient near the nurse's center of gravity.	Reduces the risk for back injury
Lock the brakes on the bed.	Prevents the bed from moving and causing injury
Place the canvas sling under the patient from the shoulders to mid-thigh.	Positions the sling where it will support the greatest mass of the patient
Move the lift device on the same side of the bed as the chair or stretcher to which the patient will be transferred.	Facilitates safety when the patient and equipment are within close proximity
Position the boom on the lift over the patient's torso.	Enables attachment of lifting chains to the canvas sling
Lock the wheels on the lift.	Stabilizes the lift in place
Attach the hooks on the lifting chain or straps to the holes in the canvas sling.	Connects the lift to the patient
Position the patient's arms across his or her chest.	Protects the patient's arms and hands from being injured
Pump the jack handle to elevate the patient to about 6″ above the mattress.	Aids in assessing whether the patient is properly and safely within the sling

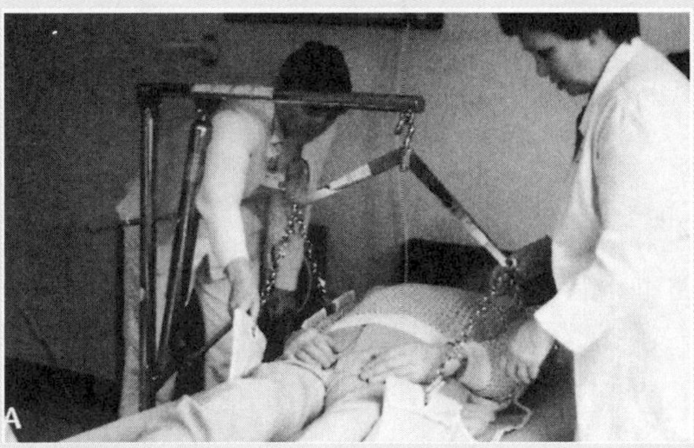

A

Positioning the lift and patient. (Craven R, Hirnle C: Fundamentals of nursing: Human health and function. 3rd ed. Philadelphia: Lippincott Williams & Wilkins, 2000.)

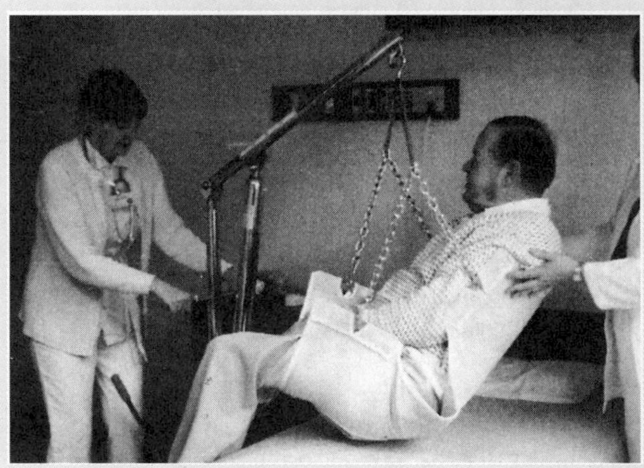

Raising the patient.

Suggested Action	Reason for Action
Unlock the wheels on the lift and move the lifted patient directly over the chair or stretcher.	Relocates the patient to the desired location
Relock the wheels of the lift.	Ensures safety of the patient
Release the jack handle slowly.	Lowers the patient from suspended position
Remove the lifting chains, but leave the canvas sling in place beneath the patient.	Facilitates returning the patient to bed
From Bed to a Stretcher Using a Sheet	
Place the patient in a supine position.	Maintains alignment
Loosen the bottom sheet or place a folded sheet beneath the patient's hips. Roll the sheet close to the patient's body.	Aids in sliding the patient without causing friction
Raise the bed to the same height as the stretcher.	Facilitates movement

continued

SKILL 23-2

TRANSFERRING PATIENTS *Continued*

Suggested Action	Reason for Action
Lower the siderail, position the stretcher parallel with the bed, and lock the wheels.	Maintains the shortest distance for transfer
Place the patient's arms over his or her chest.	Prevents injury
Have an assistant stand by the stretcher and grasp one side of the rolled sheet.	Facilitates pulling the patient
Climb onto the mattress next to the patient's buttocks and hips.	Enables use of stronger muscles in arms and thighs
Have the assistant pull the sheet while lifting together at a prearranged signal.	Facilitates coordination and reduces workload

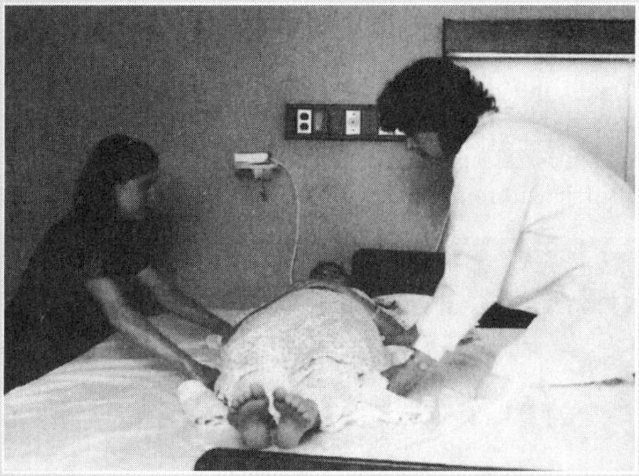

Using a lift sheet. (Craven RF, Hirnle CJ: Fundamentals of nursing: Human health and function. 3rd ed. Philadelphia: Lippincott Williams & Wilkins, 2000)

Evaluation

- Patient is relocated.
- No injury to patient or personnel.

Document

- Method of transfer
- Response of patient

SAMPLE DOCUMENTATION

Date and Time Transferred from bed to wheelchair by standing and pivoting with weight bearing on right leg. Transient pain experienced in left hip during transfer. Refused pain medication. Up in chair approximately 1 hr. ______________________ SIGNATURE, TITLE

CRITICAL THINKING

- List the various methods for transferring patients in a sequence from the one you think is least likely to cause injury to the nurse to the one with the greatest potential.
- In your clinical experience, which method for transferring patients is used most and which is used least? If the method that is used most is different from the method you identified as safest, discuss reasons for the disparity.

CHAPTER 24

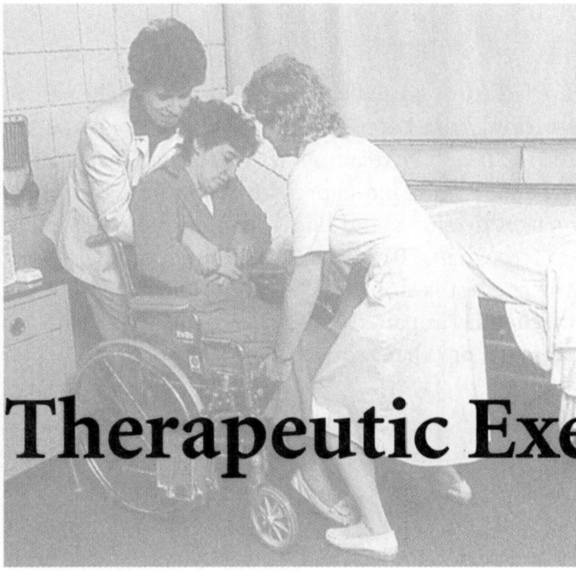

Therapeutic Exercise

CHAPTER OUTLINE

Fitness Assessment
Exercise Prescriptions
Types of Exercise
Nursing Implications

NURSING GUIDELINES

PERFORMING RANGE OF MOTION EXERCISES

SKILLS

SKILL 24–1: PERFORMING RANGE-OF-MOTION EXERCISES
SKILL 24–2: USING A CONTINUOUS PASSIVE MOTION MACHINE

NURSING CARE PLAN

UNILATERAL NEGLECT

KEY TERMS

active exercise
aerobic exercise
ambulatory electrocardiogram
ankylosis
body composition
cardiac ischemia
continuous passive motion machine
exercise
fitness
fitness exercise
isometric exercise
isotonic exercise
maximum heart rate
metabolic energy equivalent
passive exercise
range-of-motion exercises
recovery index
step test
stress electrocardiogram
submaximal fitness test
target heart rate
therapeutic exercise
walk-a-mile test

LEARNING OBJECTIVES

An understanding of the content within this chapter will be evidenced by the student's ability to:

- List at least five benefits of regular exercise.
- Define fitness.
- Identify seven factors that interfere with fitness.
- Name at least two methods of fitness testing.
- Describe how to calculate a person's target heart rate.
- Define metabolic energy equivalent.
- Differentiate fitness exercises from therapeutic exercises.
- Describe the difference between isotonic and isometric exercise.
- Give at least one example of isotonic and isometric exercise.
- Describe the difference between active and passive exercise.
- Discuss how range-of-motion exercises are performed.
- Give two reasons for performing range-of-motion exercises.
- Provide at least two suggestions for helping older adults become or stay physically active.

Exercise (purposeful physical activity) is beneficial to all age groups (Display 24-1), and the health risks of a sedentary life are well documented. This chapter addresses techniques for improving health and maintaining or restoring muscle and joint function by promoting exercise. Exercise must be individualized, so each person's fitness level must be assessed.

Fitness Assessment

Fitness (capacity to exercise) is impaired by factors such as a sedentary lifestyle, health problems, reduced musculoskeletal function, obesity, advanced age, smoking, and high blood pressure. These factors affect the person's stamina and ability to perform exercise and could even result in injury while exercising. Therefore, before beginning an exercise program, a person's fitness level should be assessed. Some assessment techniques include measuring body composition, evaluating trends in vital signs, and undergoing fitness tests.

DISPLAY 24–1

Benefits of Physical Exercise

- Improved cardiopulmonary function
- Reduction of blood pressure
- Increased muscle tone and strength
- Greater physical endurance
- Increased lean mass and weight loss
- Reduction of elevated blood sugar
- Decreased low-density blood lipids
- Improved physical appearance
- Increased bone density
- Regularity of bowel elimination
- Promotion of sleep
- Reduction in tension and depression

BODY COMPOSITION

Body composition (amount of body tissue that is lean versus that which is fat) is determined by anthropometric measurements such as height, weight, body-mass index, skinfold thickness, and mid-arm muscle circumference (see Chap. 14). Inactivity without reduced food intake tends to promote obesity. Overweight or obese people are less fit than their leaner counterparts and need to proceed gradually when initiating an exercise program.

VITAL SIGNS

Vital signs—pulse rate, respiratory rate, and blood pressure—reflect a person's physical status (see Chap. 11). Elevated vital signs at rest are a sign that the person may have life-threatening cardiovascular symptoms during exercise. After a period of modified exercise, the vital signs may be lowered, thus reducing the potential for heart-related complications.

FITNESS TESTS

Fitness tests provide an objective measure of a person's current fitness level and potential to exercise safely. They also help establish safe parameters for the level and length of exercise. One method of fitness testing is a stress electrocardiogram or ambulatory electrocardiogram. Another is a **submaximal fitness test** (exercise test that does not stress a person to exhaustion), such as a step test or walk-a-mile test. Because submaximal tests are less demanding, their validity is subject to doubt.

Stress Electrocardiogram

A **stress electrocardiogram** (test of electrical conduction through the heart during maximal activity) is done in an acute care facility or outpatient clinic (Fig. 24-1). The patient first walks slowly on a flat treadmill. As the test progresses, the speed and incline of the treadmill are increased. The patient's heart rate and rhythm, blood pressure, breathing, and symptoms such as dizziness and chest pain are noted. A pulse oximeter (see Chap. 20) is used to measure peripheral oxygenation. The test is stopped if an abnormal heart rhythm, **cardiac ischemia** (impaired blood flow to the heart), elevated blood pressure, or exhaustion develops.

Ambulatory Electrocardiogram

An **ambulatory electrocardiogram** (continuous recording of heart rate and rhythm during normal activity) requires the patient to wear a device called a Holter monitor for 24 hours. An ambulatory electrocardiogram is a less-taxing version of a stress electrocardiogram. It is used when the person has had prior symptoms or has major health risks that contraindicate a stress electrocardiogram.

Ambulatory electrocardiography helps assess the heart's response to normal activity rather than that imposed during a stress electrocardiogram. It also helps evaluate how a person is responding to cardiac rehabilitation and medical therapy.

The Holter monitor, connected to the chest leads, is attached to a belt or shoulder strap or carried in a pocket (Fig. 24-2). During ambulatory electrocardiography the patient should not shower or swim; a sponge bath is permitted as long as the monitor does not get wet. The patient should also avoid magnets, metal detectors, electric blankets, and high-voltage areas.

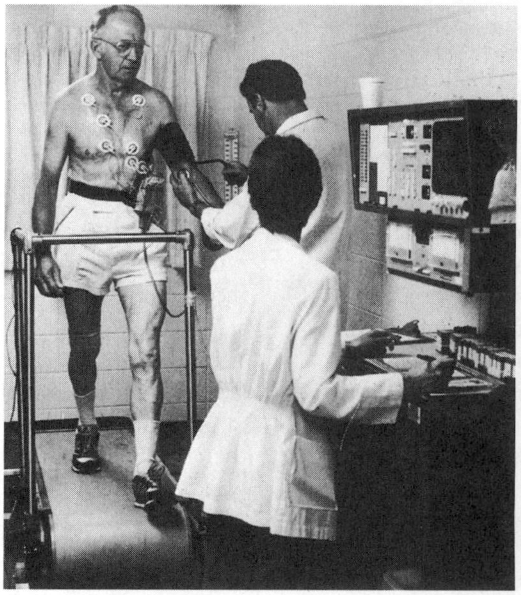

FIGURE 24–1. A stress electrocardiogram in progress. (Courtesy of Borgess Hospital, Kalamazoo, MI.)

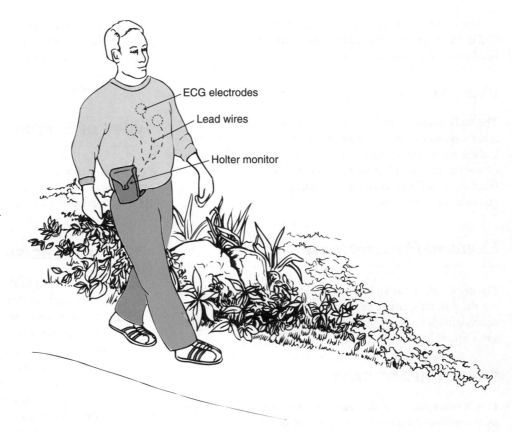

FIGURE 24–2. Ambulatory electrocardiography.

The patient keeps a diary of the time and type of activities performed, when medications are taken, and when symptoms, if any, are experienced. After the test period, the monitor is returned and the electrically recorded information is checked by a computer and the physician. The patient's diary is compared with the electrocardiogram. The assessment results help to determine whether oxygenation to the heart muscle was temporarily impaired during an activity, or whether an abnormal heart rhythm developed. Either of the two indicates that exercise should begin at a very low intensity and for a short duration.

Step Test

There are several variations of the **step test** (type of submaximal fitness test involving a timed stepping activity), including the Harvard Step Test, the Queens College Step Test, and the Chester Step Test. The person being tested steps up and down on a platform of a prescribed height (20″ for men, 16″ for women). The person continues stepping for 3 to 5 minutes at a rate of at least 76 steps per minute. A step up or down is considered one step. The time is shortened when the prescribed rate is no longer sustained or if discomfort develops. A metronome and a stopwatch are used to keep track of the rate and the time.

The **recovery index** (guide for determining a person's fitness level) is calculated by taking a 30-second pulse rate 1, 2, and 3 minutes after the test and using the following formula:

Recovery index = (100 × test duration in seconds) ÷ (2 × total of 3 30-second pulse assessments)

The results are compared with standardized fitness levels (Table 24-1). In addition, a fitter person will show a smaller decline in the heart rate at each assessment. Another fitness indicator is how close the pulse rate at the end of recovery compares with the pretest pulse rate.

TABLE 24–1. **Cardiovascular Endurance Fitness Levels**

Score	Fitness Classification
≥90	Excellent
89–80	Good
79–65	Average
64–56	Below average
≤55	Poor

http://www.mhhe.com/hper/health/personalhealth/labs/cardiovascular/lab3-6.html (accessed 8/20/99) © 1998 McGraw-Hill Companies.

The step test must be used with caution. Personnel certified in cardiopulmonary resuscitation (see Chap. 37) should be available for assistance.

Walk-a-Mile Test

The **walk-a-mile test** (fitness test that measures the time it takes a person to walk a mile) was devised by the American College of Sports Medicine (1995). The person is instructed to walk a mile on a flat surface as fast as possible. The time from start to finish is calculated and interpreted using the guidelines in Table 24-2.

Exercise Prescriptions

The prescription for an exercise program involves determining the person's target heart rate and the metabolic energy equivalents (METs) of particular activities based on the person's fitness level.

TARGET HEART RATE

Target heart rate (goal for heart rate during exercise) is determined by first calculating the person's **maximum heart rate** (highest limit for heart rate during exercise). Maximum heart rate is calculated by subtracting a person's age from 220. Thus, a 20-year-old has a maximum heart rate of 200 beats per minute (bpm), whereas the maximum heart rate for a 50-year-old is 170 bpm. The target heart rate is 60% to 90% of the maximum heart rate (American College of Sports Medicine, 1995). Beginners should not exceed 60%; intermediates can exercise at 70% to 75%; and competitive athletes can tolerate 80% to 90% of their maximum heart rate.

Exercising at the target rate for 15 minutes (excluding the warmup and cooldown periods), three or more times a week strengthens the heart muscle and promotes the use of fat reserves for energy. Exercising beyond the target heart rate reduces endurance by increasing fatigue.

METABOLIC ENERGY EQUIVALENT

Because fitness levels vary, exercises are also prescribed according to their **metabolic energy equivalent** (measure of energy and oxygen consumption during exercise). This is the prescribed amount that a person's cardiovascular system can safely support. Low to vigorous physical activities and their approximate METs are listed in Table 24-3.

TABLE 24–2. **Evaluation Criteria for the Walk-a-Mile Test**

Performance Time for Men	Performance Time for Women	Fitness Level
≥17.5 minutes	≥16.5 minutes	Needs work
≤15 minutes	≤14 minutes	Average
≤11.75 minutes	≤10.25 minutes	Good

Types of Exercise

Exercise is performed to promote fitness or to achieve therapeutic outcomes (Fig. 24-3). The two major types of exercise are fitness exercise and therapeutic exercise.

FITNESS EXERCISE

Fitness exercise (physical activity performed by healthy adults) develops and maintains cardiorespiratory function, muscular strength, and endurance. There are two categories of fitness exercise: isotonic and isometric.

Isotonic exercise (activity that involves movement and work) is exemplified by **aerobic exercise** (rhythmically moving all parts of the body at a moderate to slow speed, without hindering the ability to breathe). In other words, the person is able to talk comfortably if the exercise is within his or her level of fitness. To promote cardiorespiratory conditioning and increase lean muscle mass, isotonic exercise is performed at the person's target heart rate.

TABLE 24–3. **Levels of Physical Activity**

Metabolic Energy Equivalent (MET)	Examples of Activities
1 MET	Sewing Watching television Dressing
1–2 METs	Walking 1 mph on level ground Bowling
2–3 METs	Golfing with a cart Mowing lawn with a power mower
3–4 METs	Playing badminton (doubles) Raking leaves
4–5 METs	Slow swimming Lifting 50 lbs
5–6 METs	Square dancing Shoveling snow
6–7 METs	Water skiing Moving heavy furniture
7–8 METs	Playing basketball Playing noncompetitive handball
8–9 METs	Cross-country skiing Playing contact football
≥10 METs	Running 6 mph or faster

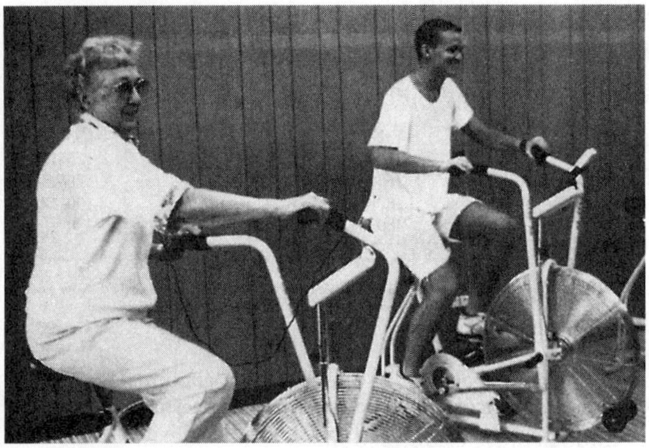

FIGURE 24–3. Stationary cycling. (Courtesy of Ken Timby.)

Isometric exercise (stationary exercises that are generally performed against a resistive force) include body building, weight lifting, and less intense activities such as simply contracting and relaxing muscle groups while sitting or standing. Isometric exercises increase muscle mass, define muscle groups, and increase muscle strength and tone. Although isometric exercises improve the circulation of blood, they do *not* promote cardiorespiratory function. In fact, strenuous isometric exercises elevate the blood pressure temporarily.

Patient Teaching For

A Safe Exercise Program

Teach the patient or family to do the following:

- Seek a pre-exercise fitness evaluation.
- Determine the target heart rate according to fitness level.
- Determine the appropriate level of METs.
- Choose a form of exercise that seems pleasurable and involves as many muscle groups as possible.
- Plan 20-minute exercise periods 3 days per week at a convenient time of day.
- Exercise with a partner for safety and motivation.
- Avoid exercising in extreme weather conditions (high humidity, smog).
- Dress in layers according to the temperature and weather conditions.
- Wear supportive shoes.
- Wear reflective clothing after dark.
- Walk or jog against traffic; cycle in the same direction as traffic.
- Eat complex carbohydrates (pasta, rice, cooked cereal) rather than fasting or eating simple sugars (cookies, chocolate, sweetened drinks) prior to exercising.
- Avoid drinking alcohol: alcohol dilates the blood vessels, promotes heat loss, and interferes with good judgment.
- Warm up for 5 minutes by stretching muscle groups or doing light calisthenics.
- Measure the heart rate two or three times while exercising.
- Slow down if the heart rate exceeds the pre-established target.
- Try to sustain the target heart rate for at least 12 to 15 minutes.
- Never stop exercising abruptly.
- Cool down for at least 5 minutes in a manner similar to the warmup.

THERAPEUTIC EXERCISE

Therapeutic exercise (activity performed by people with health risks or those being treated for an existing health problem) are performed to prevent health-related complications or to restore lost functions (see Performing Leg Exercises in Chap. 27 and Strengthening Pelvic Floor Muscles in Chap. 30). Therapeutic exercise may be isotonic or isometric; isotonic exercises are performed actively or passively.

Active Exercise

Active exercise (therapeutic activity performed independently) is performed after proper instruction. For example, patients who have undergone a mastectomy are taught to exercise the arm on the surgical side by combing their hair, squeezing a soft ball, finger-climbing the vertical surface of a wall, and swinging a rope attached to a doorknob.

Active therapeutic exercise is often limited to a particular part of the body that is in a weakened condition. It is assumed that patients will use their unaffected muscle groups while performing activities of daily living such as bathing and dressing.

Passive Exercise

Passive exercise (therapeutic activity performed with assistance) is provided when a patient cannot move one or more parts of the body. For example, for comatose patients and those paralyzed from a stroke or spinal injury, nurses perform exercises that maintain muscle tone and flexible joints. One form of passive therapeutic exercise that is frequently provided is range-of-motion exercises. Another is delivered with a continuous passive motion machine.

Range-of-Motion Exercises

Range-of-motion (ROM) **exercises** (therapeutic activity in which joints are moved) are performed for the following reasons:

- To assess joint flexibility before initiating an exercise program
- To maintain joint mobility and flexibility in inactive patients
- To prevent **ankylosis** (permanent loss of joint movement)

- To stretch joints before performing more strenuous activities
- To evaluate the patient's response to a therapeutic exercise program

During ROM exercises, unused joints are moved in the positions that the joint normally permits (Table 24-4). Whenever possible, the patient actively exercises as many joints as possible while the nurse assists with those that are compromised.

Nursing Guidelines For

Performing Range-of-Motion Exercises

☑ Use good body mechanics (see Chap. 23).
RATIONALE: Using good body mechanics conserves energy and avoids muscle strain and injury.

☑ Remove pillows and other positioning devices.
RATIONALE: Such items can interfere with the exercises.

☑ Position the patient so the joint can be moved through all its usual positions.
RATIONALE: This positioning makes it easier to perform a comprehensive exercise program.

☑ Follow a systematic, repetitive pattern—such as beginning at the head and moving down.
RATIONALE: A routine prevents overlooking a joint.

☑ Perform similar movements with each extremity.
RATIONALE: Joints are exercised bilaterally.

☑ Support the joint being exercised.
RATIONALE: Support reduces discomfort.

☑ Move each joint until there is resistance but not pain.
RATIONALE: Each joint is exercised to its point of limitation.

☑ Watch for nonverbal communication.
RATIONALE: Nonverbal signs are used to evaluate the patient's response.

☑ Avoid exercising a painful joint.
RATIONALE: Exercising a painful joint can contribute to injury.

☑ Stop if spasticity develops, as manifested by a sudden, continuous muscle contraction.
RATIONALE: Taking a break gives muscles time to relax and recover.

☑ Apply gentle pressure to the muscle or move the spastic limb more slowly.
RATIONALE: These actions relieve spasticity.

☑ Expect the patient's respiratory and heart rates to increase during the exercise, but to return to a resting rate later.
RATIONALE: This is a normal cardiopulmonary response to activity.

☑ Teach the family to perform ROM exercises.
RATIONALE: A regular exercise program improves the potential for regaining function.

TABLE 24–4. **Joint Positions**

Position	Description
Flexion	Bending so as to decrease the angle between two adjoining bones
Extension	Straightening so as to increase the angle between two adjoining bones up to 180°
Hyperextension	Increasing the angle between two adjoining bones more than 180°
Abduction	Moving away from the midline
Adduction	Moving toward the midline
Rotation	Turning from side to side as in an arc
External rotation	Turning outward, away from the midline of the body
Internal rotation	Turning inward, toward the midline of the body
Circumduction	Forming a circle
Pronation	Turning downward
Supination	Turning upward
Plantar flexion	Bending toward the sole of the foot
Dorsiflexion	Bending the foot toward the dorsum or anterior side
Inversion	Turning the sole of the foot toward the midline
Eversion	Turning the sole of the foot away from the midline

ROM exercises are performed whenever caring for inactive patients (Skill 24-1).

Continuous Passive Motion Machine

A **continuous passive motion machine** (electrical device that exercises joints; Fig. 24-4) is used as a supplement or substitute for manual ROM exercise. Machine-assisted ROM is sometimes preferred during the rehabilitation of burn patients and those who have had knee or hip replacement surgery because the degree of joint movement is precisely controlled and can be increased in specific increments throughout recovery.

Besides restoring and increasing joint ROM, the movement created by the machine prevents the pooling of venous blood,

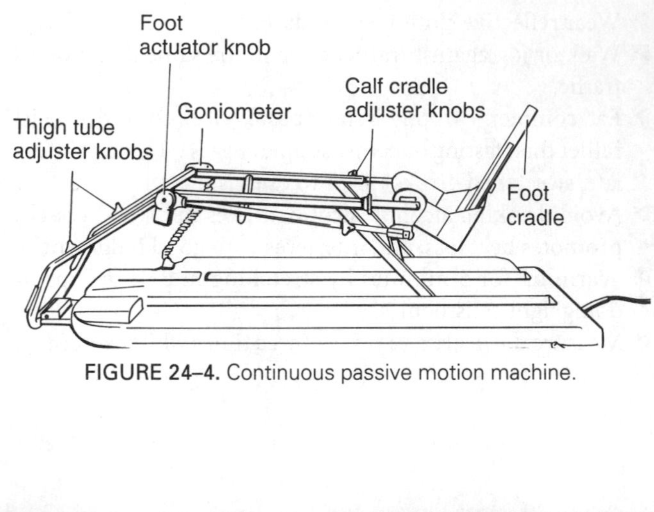

FIGURE 24–4. Continuous passive motion machine.

thus decreasing the risk of blood clots. Also, wound healing is accelerated because the synovial fluid circulates about the joint.

Most machines produce 0° to 110° of motion 2 to 10 times per minute. Initially, the machine is set at very low speeds and degrees of movement—it is common to begin with 5° or 10° of flexion cycling twice a minute, at least six times a day. The settings are increased each day as the patient's tolerance builds. The nurse positions the patient's extremity in the machine and programs the speed and the degree of desired joint flexion according to the physician's exercise prescription (Skill 24-2).

Nursing Implications

Few people exercise sufficiently to promote an optimal level of health. With this in mind, the Department of Health and Human Services established goals and strategies for improving the nation's health (Table 24-5). After evaluating the progress made toward these goals, new objectives for *Healthy People 2010* are set to be issued in January 2000. Nurses can set an example for others in the community by improving their own physical fitness and encouraging others to do so.

For persons with medical disorders, the nurse may identify one or more of the following nursing diagnoses that are treated with activity or an exercise regimen:

- Impaired physical mobility
- Risk for disuse syndrome
- Unilateral neglect
- Risk for delayed surgical recovery
- Activity intolerance

The nursing care plan illustrates how exercise is incorporated into the care of a stroke patient with the nursing diagnosis of Unilateral neglect. The NANDA taxonomy (1999) defines this as "the state in which an individual is perceptually unaware of and inattentive to one side of the body."

During the course of providing nursing care, opportunities arise for teaching patients and their caregivers about techniques that promote activity or reduce the potential for complications that result from inactivity.

TABLE 24–5. **Status of National Physical Activity and Fitness Objectives**

Healthy People 2000 Objective*	Midcourse Progress†
Increase daily participation in physical education in elementary and secondary schools	Data have not been collected for children in elementary and junior high grades.
	There has been a decline in the percentage of students in grades 9–12 who engage in daily physical education at school.
Include more physical activity during physical education classes	Goals have not been met in the proportion of school physical education time spent in being physically active.
Involve children in physical activities that may be readily carried into adulthood	Several trends, such as an increase in the use of computers, indicate a more sedentary lifestyle.
	Schools are devoting fewer financial resources to physical activity instruction, playgrounds, and after-school sports programs.
Increase employer-sponsored physical activities and fitness programs	Worksite fitness programs have increased among places that employ ≥50 people.
Increase community availability and accessibility to physical activity and fitness facilities	Communities with limited resources are investing less in parks, recreation facilities, and staff to maintain and operate them.
	There has been no reduction in the percentage of adults who engage in no leisure time physical activity.
Increase counseling and the provision of exercise prescriptions for patients under the care of a physician	Internists formulate an exercise plan for 25% of the 40% of patients who are questioned about their exercise habits; family practitioners report even lower statistics.
	Nurse practitioners routinely inquire about the exercise habits of 30% of their patients and formulate an exercise plan for 14%.

*Adapted from United States Department of Health and Human Services. Healthy People 2000: national health promotion and disease prevention objectives. Boston, Jones & Bartlett, 1992.

†Adapted from United States Department of Health and Human Services. Healthy People 2000 midcourse review and 1995 revisions. Washington DC, U.S. Public Health Service, 1995. http://odphp.osophs.dhhs.gov/pubs/hp2000/midcrs1.htm, accessed 7/1999.

Nursing Care Plan: Unilateral Neglect

Assessment

Subjective Data

States, "Somebody's arm and leg are in my bed."

Objective Data

76-year-old man previously treated for hypertension. Admitted now for a stroke. Left side of face droops. Unable to fully smile or show teeth. Tongue deviates from midline. Not able to see objects placed on L. side of body. Does not eat food on left side of plate and tray. No movement of L. upper or lower extremities. No response to touch or pain stimuli on L. side. Cannot differentiate between warm or cold on the left, but can do so on right.

Diagnosis

Unilateral neglect related to unawareness of objects in L. visual field secondary to stroke

Plan

Goal

The patient will identify his own L. arm and leg and assist with bathing, exercising, and dressing the L. side of his body by 4/21.

Orders: 4/19

1. Each shift, show the patient three objects on the R. side of the patient's visual field.
2. Locate the same three objects on the L. side of the bed, wall, or room and instruct the patient to turn his head and identify where each is located.
3. Have the patient locate and touch his left arm and leg.
4. Instruct the patient to bathe his left arm in the A.M. and follow with inserting sleeve over left hand and arm; on remaining shifts have patient grasp his left arm and perform range of motion of shoulder, elbow, wrist, and fingers. ________ S. LABADIE, RN

Implementation (Documentation)

4/19 1745 While standing on R. side of bed, patient was shown a pen, flashlight, and watch. Flashlight placed by left hand, watch buckled to left siderail, and pen placed on top sheet. Instructed to turn head to the left and identify relocated items, L. arm, and L. leg. ________ J. PERRY, LPN

Evaluation (Documentation)

1800 Able to scan left side and correctly identify objects and body parts. Able to grasp left hand and extend arm over head. Right elbow flexed and extended; arm adducted. Pronation, supination of hand, flexion and hyperextension of R. wrist and fingers performed by patient five times each. Assisted with abduction of arm and circumduction of shoulder. ________ J. PERRY, LPN

FOCUS ON OLDER ADULTS

- Older adults, especially those who are disabled, need to balance their periods of physical activity with periods of rest.
- Older adults need to increase their intake of noncaffeinated and nonalcoholic beverages before and during physical activity.
- Older adults are encouraged to join organizations and social clubs that promote activities for senior citizens, such as the American Association of Retired Persons (AARP) and programs sponsored by local offices on aging.
- Many shopping malls permit, and even encourage, people to walk through the mall before stores open for business.
- Swimming or exercise in the water creates less stress on the joints and is beneficial for older adults.
- Many physically challenging sports, such as bowling, golfing, walking in marathons, and weight lifting, have competition categories for older adults.
- Precautions, such as wearing safe shoes with nonskid soles, are necessary to prevent falls when older adults are exercising. Complications from falls contribute to morbidity and mortality among people in this age group.
- Exercise in a rocking chair is a safe activity that can be carried out by most older adults.
- Families and caregivers of older adults who are cognitively impaired are encouraged to help older persons participate in physical activities such as walking and ball throwing. If the older adult cannot participate actively in an exercise program, the caregivers can perform range-of-motion exercises at least daily.

KEY CONCEPTS

- Regular exercise has many benefits, including a reduction in blood pressure, blood sugar and blood lipid levels, tension, and depression and increased bone density.
- Fitness refers to a person's capacity to perform physical activities.
- Factors that interfere with fitness include chronic inactivity, concurrent health problems, impaired musculoskeletal function, obesity, advancing age, smoking, and high blood pressure.
- Several approaches are used to determine a person's level of fitness. Two objective methods are a stress electrocardiogram and a submaximal fitness test such as a step test.
- Exercise, regardless of type, should be performed within the person's target heart rate. Target heart rate is calculated by subtracting the person's age from 220, which provides the maximum heart rate, and then multiplying that number by 60% (0.6) to 90% (0.9), based on the person's fitness level.
- Metabolic energy equivalent (MET) is the measure of energy and oxygen consumption that a person's cardiovascular system can safely support. When an exercise prescription is given, exercises are correlated with their MET value.
- Fitness exercises are physical activities that develop and maintain cardiorespiratory function, muscular strength, and endurance in healthy adults. Therapeutic exercise involves physical activities that are designed to prevent health-related complications from an established medical condition or its treatment or to restore lost physical functions.
- Isotonic exercise involves movement and work; an example is aerobic exercise. Isometric exercise refers to stationary activities performed against a resistive force. Examples of isometric exercise are body building and weight lifting.
- Active exercise is performed independently after proper instruction. Passive exercise is performed with the assistance of another person.
- Range-of-motion (ROM) exercise is a form of therapeutic exercise in which joints are moved in the directions permitted by the normal joint. It can be active or passive.
- Two common reasons for performing ROM exercises are to maintain joint mobility and flexibility, especially in inactive patients, and to evaluate the patient's response to a therapeutic exercise program.
- Older adults are encouraged to exercise by walking in shopping malls or joining social groups that include activities such as line dancing or ballroom dancing.

CRITICAL THINKING EXERCISES

- How might you remotivate a friend who began an exercise program and then gradually stopped?
- List at least five excuses people give for not exercising. Offer a counterargument for each.

SUGGESTED READINGS

American College of Sports Medicine. ACSM's guidelines for exercise testing and prescription, 5th ed. Philadelphia, JB Lippincott, 1995.

Artal M, Sherman C. Exercise against depression. Physician and Sports medicine 1998;26(10):55–60.

Cardiovascular Endurance Fitness Levels. http://www.mhhe.com/hper/health/personalhealth/labs/cardiovascular/lab 3-6.html. Updated 1998; accessed 8/99.

Connolly JF. Hazards of immobilizing musculoskeletal injuries: why ice is nice and motion is lotion. Consultant 1998;38(3):602–612.

Dawe D, Moor-Orr R. Low intensity, range-of-motion exercise: invaluable nursing care for elderly patients. Journal of Advanced Nursing. 1995; 21(4):675–681.

Focht BC, Koltyn KF. Influence of resistive exercise of different intensities on state anxiety and blood pressure. Medicine and Science in Sports and Exercise 1999;31(3):456–463.

Francis K, Hopkins S, Feinstein R. Effect of step platform height on stepping efficiency in children. Pediatric Exercise Science 1998;10(4): 337–346.

Handley RT. Standard cardiovascular exercise stress testing: indications, relative indications, contraindications. Physician Assistant 1999;23(4): 37–50.

Health promotion and disease prevention objectives for 2010. Federal Register 62(172), 1997.

Hope A, Kelleher CC, O'Connor M. Lifestyle practices and the health promoting environment of hospital nurses. Journal of Advanced Nursing 1998;28(2):438–447.

Kerr K. Exercise—no easy option. Physiotherapy 1999;85(3):114–115.

Mathews CE, Hall DP, Freedson PS, Pastides H. Classification of cardiorespiratory fitness without exercise testing. Medicine and Science in Sports and Exercise 1999;31(3):486–493.

Mitchell TL, Gibbons LW. Controlling blood lipids: part 1: a practical role for diet and exercise. Physician and Sportsmedicine 1998;26(10): 74–78.

Morris J. The value of continuous passive motion in rehabilitation following total knee replacement. Physiotherapy 1995;81(9):557–562.

NANDA nursing diagnoses: definitions and classification, 1999–2000. Philadelphia, NANDA, 1999.

Shephard RJ. Do work-site exercise and health programs work? Physician and Sportsmedicine 1999;27(2):48–62.

Suni JH, Oja P, Laukkanen RT, et al. Health-related fitness test battery for adults: aspects of reliability. Archives of Physical Medicine and Rehabilitation 1996;77(4):399–405.

Trudeau F, Laurencelle L, Temblay J, et al. Daily primary school physical education effects on physical activity during adult life. Medicine and Science in Sports and Exercise 1999;31(1):111–117.

United States Department of Health and Human Services. Healthy People 2000: national health promotion and disease prevention objectives. Boston, Jones & Bartlett, 1992.

United States Department of Health and Human Services. Healthy People 2000 midcourse review and 1995 revisions. Washington DC, U.S. Public Health Service, 1995.

SKILL 24–1

PERFORMING RANGE-OF-MOTION (ROM) EXERCISES

Suggested Action	Reason for Action
Assessment	
Review the medical record and nursing plan for care.	Determines whether activity problems have been identified and the measures for treating those that exist
Assess the patient's level of activity and joint mobility.	Indicates whether, and the extent to which, joints should be passively exercised
Assess the patient's understanding of the hazards of inactivity and purposes for exercise.	Determines the type and amount of health teaching needed
Planning	
Explain the procedure for performing ROM.	Reduces anxiety and promotes cooperation
Consult with the patient on when ROM exercises may be best performed.	Shows respect for independent decision-making
Suggest performing ROM during a time that requires general activity, such as during bathing.	Demonstrates efficient time management
Perform ROM exercises at least twice a day.	Promotes recovery or maintains functional use
Exercise each joint at least two to five times during each exercise period.	Increases exercise benefits
Implementation	
Wash your hands.	Reduces the potential for transferring microorganisms
Help the patient to a sitting or lying position.	Promotes relaxation and access to the body
Pull the privacy curtains.	Demonstrates respect for modesty
Drape the patient loosely or suggest loose-fitting underwear or shorts.	Avoids exposing the patient
Begin at the head.	Facilitates organization
Support the patient's neck and bring the chin toward the chest and then as far back in the opposite position as possible.	Flexes and hyperextends the neck

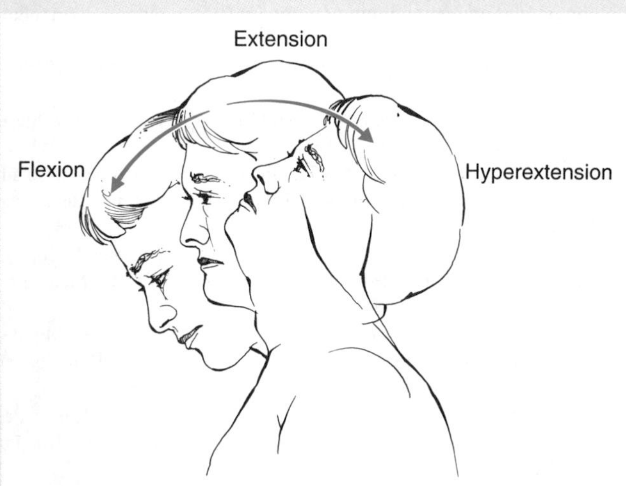

Neck flexion, extension, and hyperextension.

continued

SKILL 24–1

PERFORMING RANGE-OF-MOTION (ROM) EXERCISES *Continued*

Suggested Action	Reason for Action
Place a hand on either side of the head and move the neck from side to side.	Rotates the neck
Turn the head in a circular fashion.	Puts the head and neck through circumduction

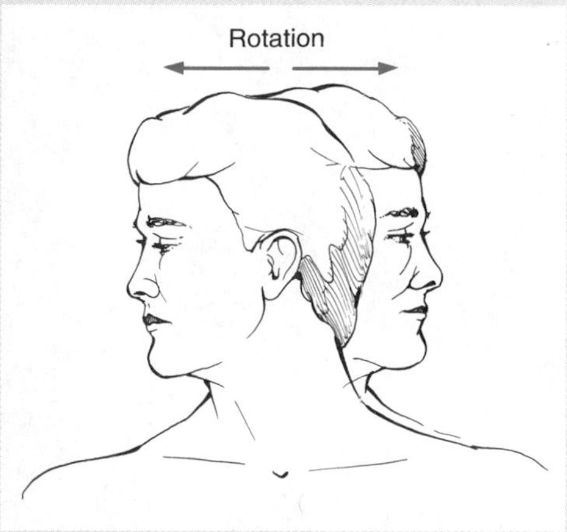

Neck rotation.

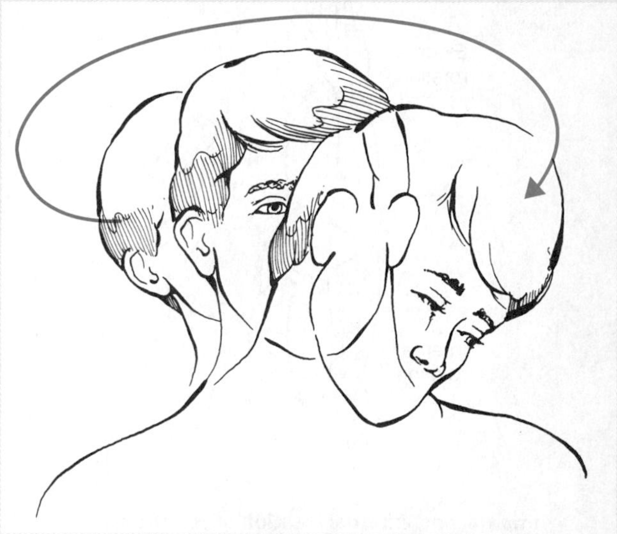

Circumduction of the neck.

Suggested Action	Reason for Action
Support the elbow and wrist while moving the straightened arm above the head and behind the body.	Flexes, extends, then hyperextends the shoulder
Move the straightened arm away from the body and then toward the midline.	Abducts and adducts the shoulder

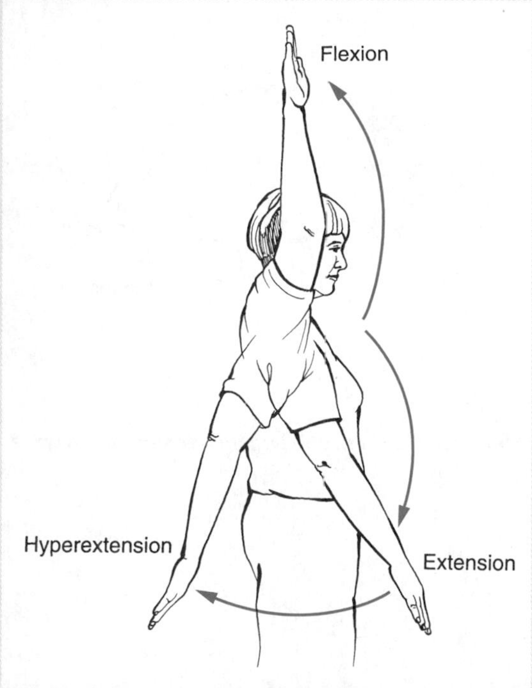

Flexion, extension, and hyperextension of the shoulder.

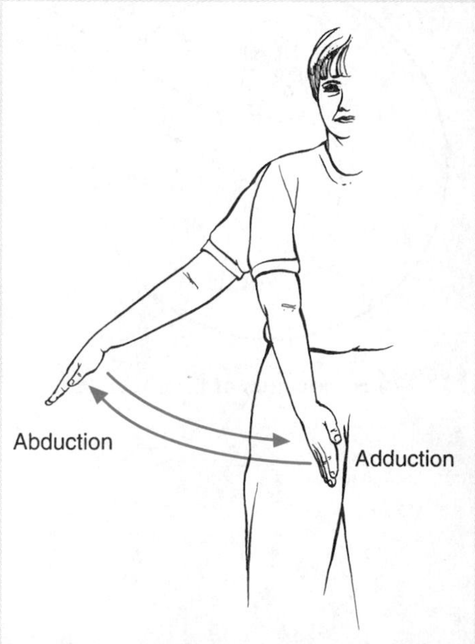

Abduction and adduction of the shoulder.

continued

SKILL 24–1

PERFORMING RANGE-OF-MOTION (ROM) EXERCISES *Continued*

Suggested Action	Reason for Action
Bend the elbow and move the arm so that the palm is upward and then downward.	Produces internal and external rotation of the shoulder

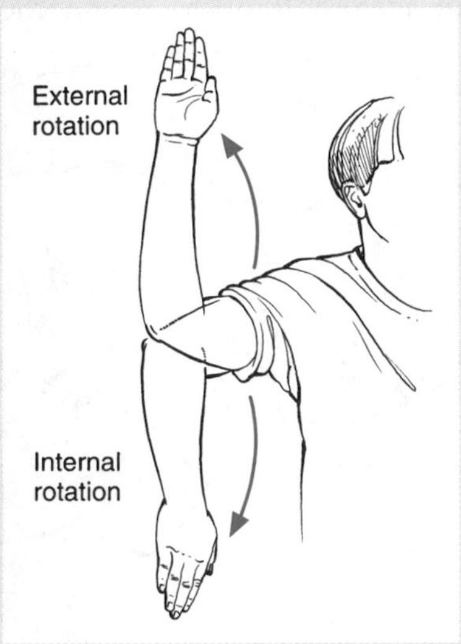

Internal and external rotation of the shoulder.

Suggested Action	Reason for Action
Move the arm in a full circle.	Circumducts the shoulder
Place the arm at the patient's side and bend the forearm toward the shoulder, and then straighten it again.	Flexes and extends the elbow

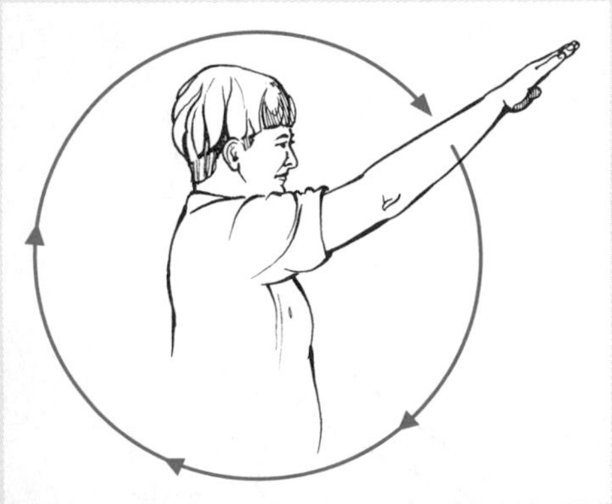

Circumduction of the shoulder.

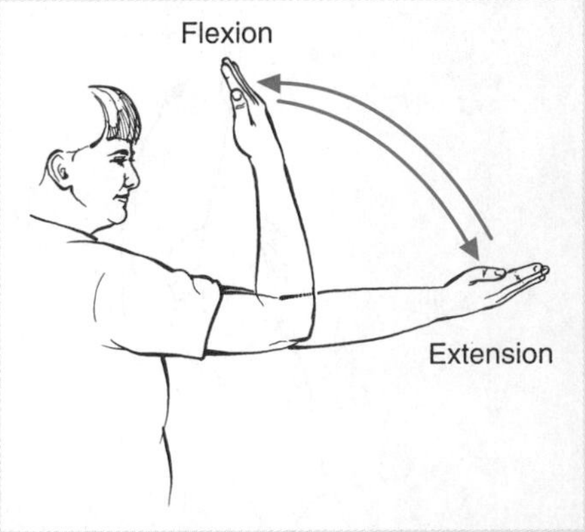

Flexion, extension, and hyperextension of the wrist.

continued

SKILL 24–1

PERFORMING RANGE-OF-MOTION (ROM) EXERCISES *Continued*

Suggested Action	Reason for Action
Bend the wrist backward and then forward.	Moves the wrist from extension to hyperextension and then flexion
Twist the wrist to the right and then left.	Rotates the wrist joint

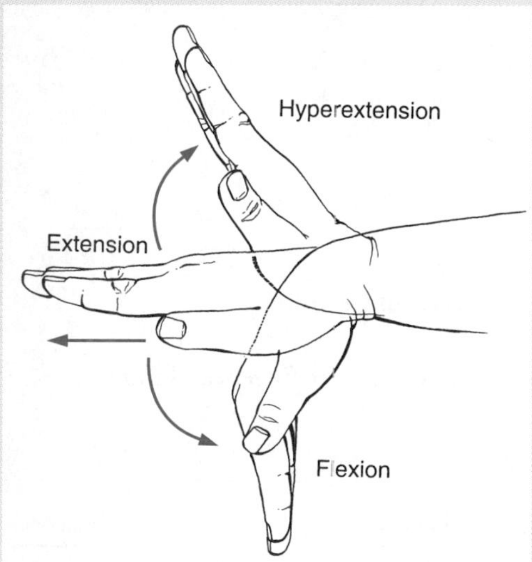

Flexion, extension, and hyperextension of the wrist.

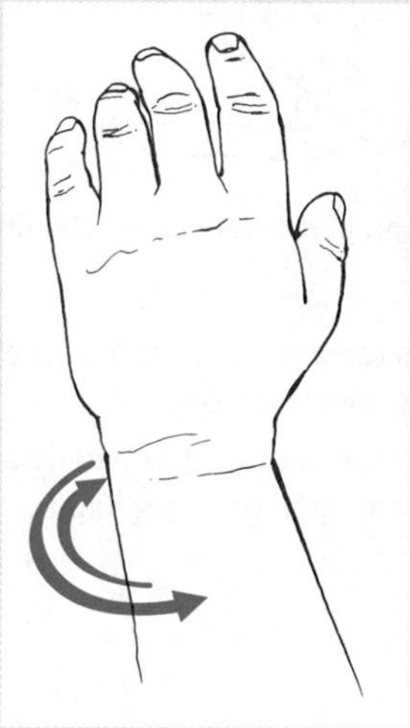

Rotation of the wrist.

Suggested Action	Reason for Action
Bend the thumb side of the hand toward the wrist and then away.	Provides abduction and then adduction of the wrist
Turn the palm upward and then downward.	Supinates and pronates the wrist

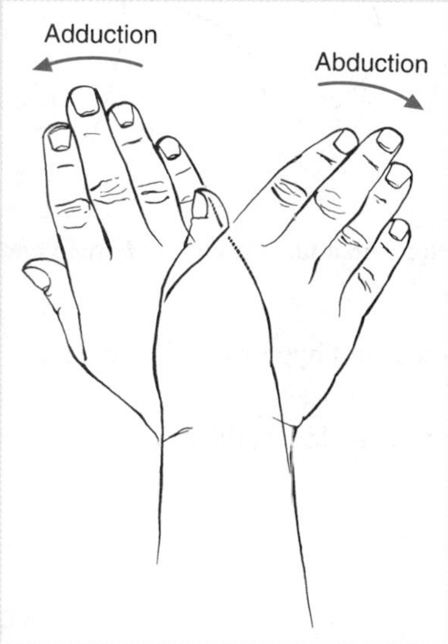

Abduction and adduction of the wrist.

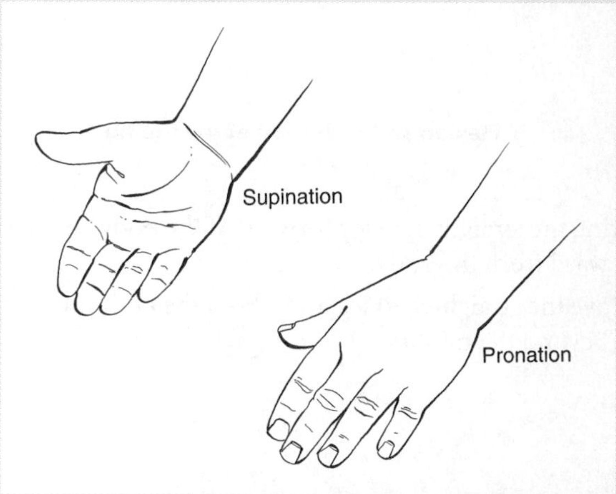

Supination and pronation of the wrist.

continued

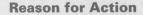

SKILL 24–1

PERFORMING RANGE-OF-MOTION (ROM) EXERCISES *Continued*

Suggested Action	Reason for Action
Open and close the fingers as though making a fist.	Flexes and extends fingers

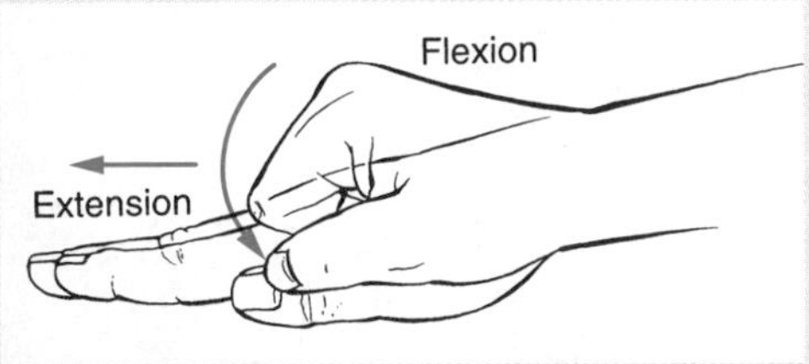

Flexion and extension of the fingers.

Suggested Action	Reason for Action
Bend the thumb toward the center of the palm and then back to its original position.	Flexes and extends the thumb
Spread the fingers and thumb as widely as possible and then bring them back together again.	Abducts and adducts the fingers and thumb

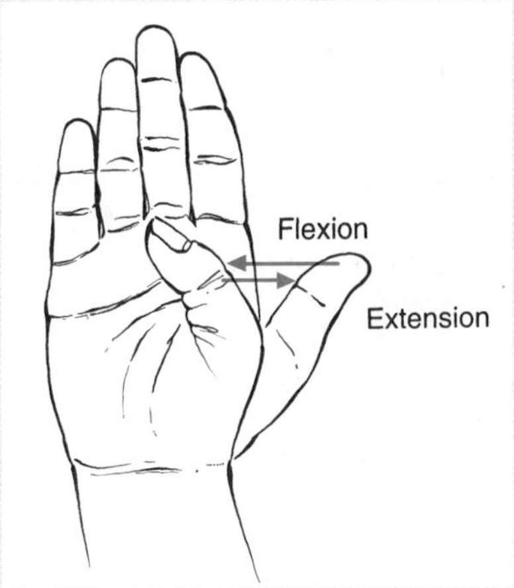

Flexion and extension of the thumb.

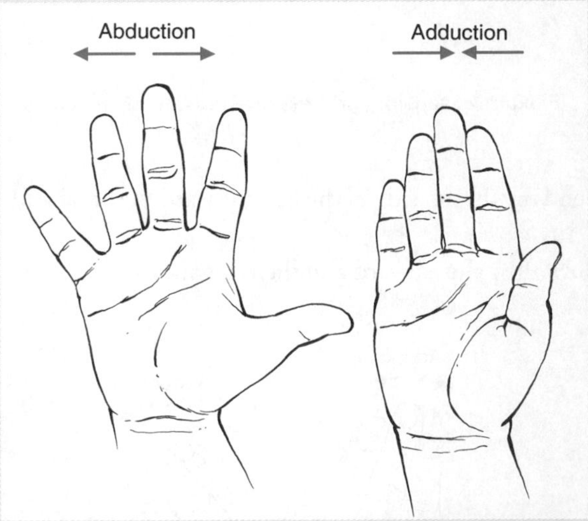

Abduction and adduction of the fingers and thumb.

Suggested Action	Reason for Action
Bring the straightened leg forward of the body and backward from the body.	Flexes, extends, and hyperextends the hip
Move the straightened leg away from the body and back beyond the midline.	Abducts and then adducts the hip

continued

SKILL 24-1

PERFORMING RANGE-OF-MOTION (ROM) EXERCISES *Continued*

Suggested Action	Reason for Action

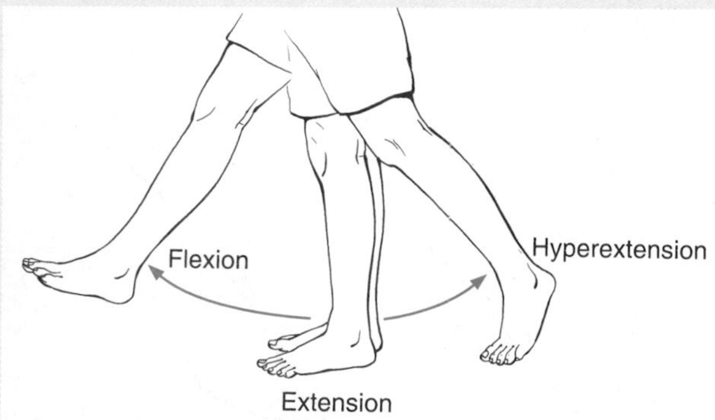

Flexion, extension, and hyperextension of the hip.

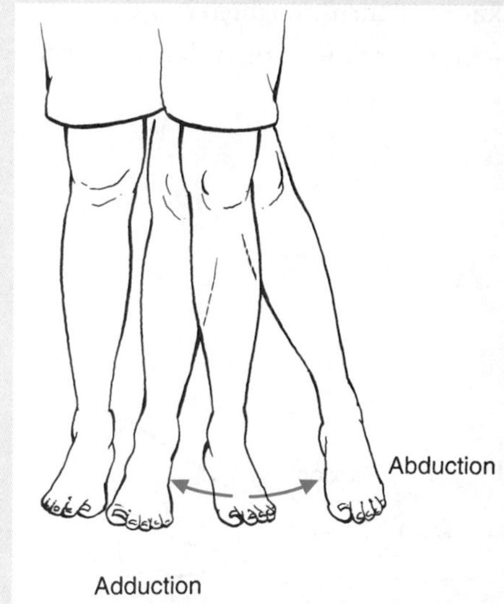

Abduction and adduction of the hip.

Suggested Action	Reason for Action
Turn the leg away from the other leg and then toward it.	Rotates the hip externally and then internally
Turn the leg in a circle	Circumducts the hip

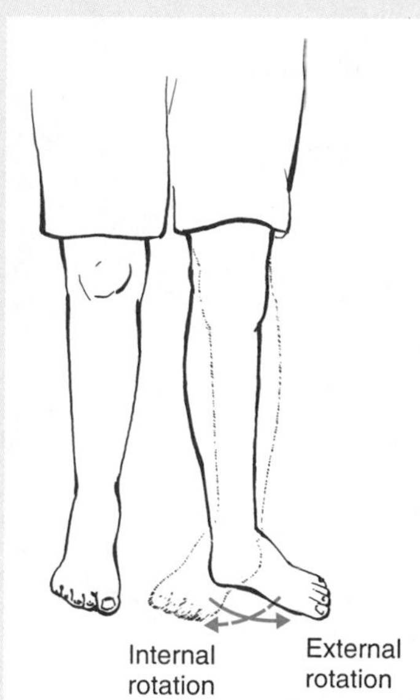

External and internal rotation of the hip.

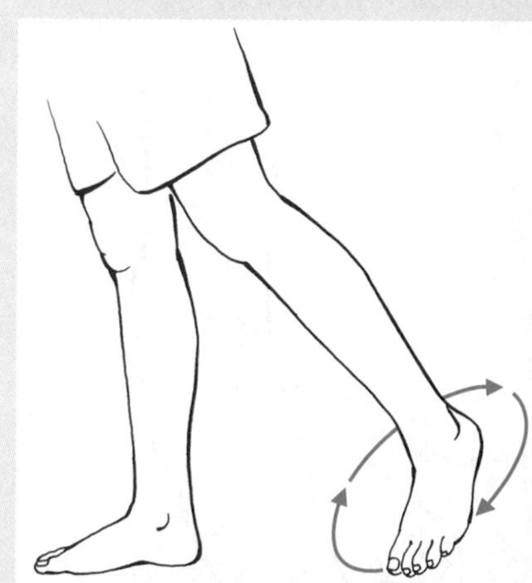

Circumduction of the hip.

continued

SKILL 24–1

PERFORMING RANGE-OF-MOTION (ROM) EXERCISES *Continued*

Suggested Action	Reason for Action
Bend the knee and then straighten it again.	Flexes and extends the knee
Bend the foot toward the ankle and then away from the ankle.	Causes dorsiflexion and plantar flexion

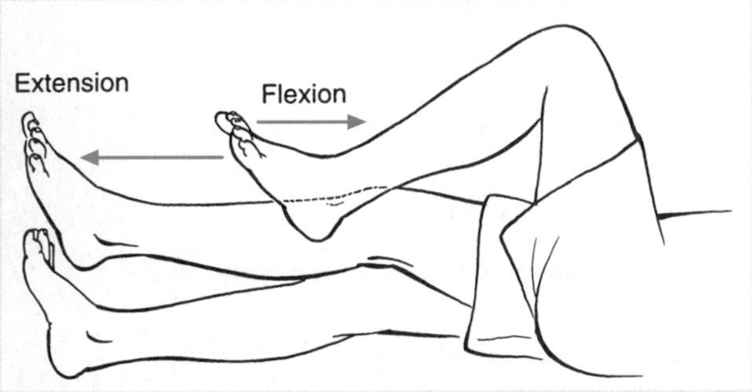

Flexion and extension of the knee.

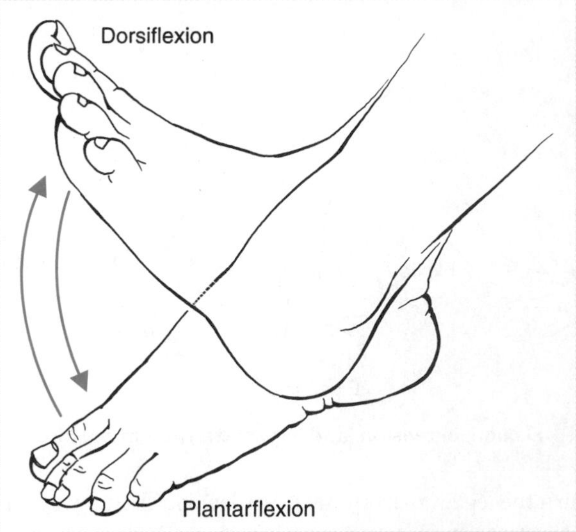

Dorsiflexion and plantar flexion of the foot.

Suggested Action	Reason for Action
Bend the sole of the foot toward the midline and then away from midline.	Inverts and everts the ankle
Bend and then straighten the toes.	Flexes and extends the toes

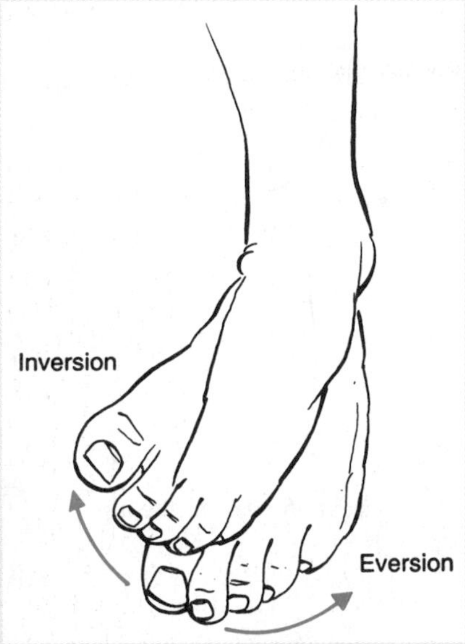

Inversion and eversion of the ankle.

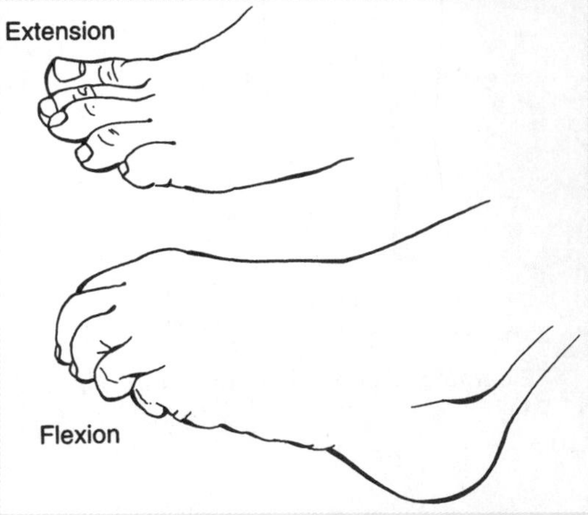

Flexion and extension of the toes.

continued

SKILL 24-1

PERFORMING RANGE-OF-MOTION (ROM) EXERCISES *Continued*

Evaluation

- All joints are exercised to the extent possible

Document

- Performance of exercise regimen
- Response of the patient

SAMPLE DOCUMENTATION

Date and Time Assisted to perform ROM exercises during bath. Actively moves all joints on R. side of body. Joints on L. side passively exercised through full ranges. No resistance or pain experienced. ______________________________ SIGNATURE, TITLE

CRITICAL THINKING

- You are caring for a patient who is paralyzed below the waist from a motor-vehicle accident. For what reasons would you promote active range-of-motion exercises in the patient's upper body?
- The patient with paralysis of his lower extremities is depressed and questions the purpose for performing passive range-of-motion exercises on his lower body. Assuming his paralysis is permanent and he will never walk again, how would you respond?

SKILL 24-2

USING A CONTINUOUS PASSIVE MOTION (CPM) MACHINE

Suggested Action	Reason for Action
Assessment	
Review the medical record and nursing care plan for the amount of joint flexion, cycles per minute, frequency, and duration of exercise.	Determines the exercise prescription for the patient
Explore how much the patient understands about CPM, especially if this is the first time it is being used.	Determines the level and type of health teaching to provide
Assess the quality of peripheral pulses, capillary refill, edema, temperature, sensation, and mobility of the affected extremity.	Provides a baseline of data for future comparisons
Compare assessments with the unaffected extremity.	Provides comparative data
Determine the patient's need for pain-relieving medication before the use of the CPM machine.	Controls pain before it intensifies with exercise
Planning	
Develop a schedule with the patient for when to use the machine as appropriate.	Involves the patient in decision-making
Instruct the patient on techniques for muscle relaxation and pain control such as deep breathing, listening to audiotapes, watching television, or applying an ice bag.	Empowers the patient with techniques for controlling pain

continued

SKILL 24-2

USING A CONTINUOUS PASSIVE MOTION (CPM) MACHINE *Continued*

Suggested Action	Reason for Action
Obtain the CPM machine and secure a length of sheepskin or soft flannel cloth to the horizontal bars to form a cradle (sling) for the calf.	Prepares the machine for supporting the leg
Wash hands.	Reduces the transmission of microorganisms
Don gloves and empty any wound drainage containers; change or reinforce the dressing (see Chap. 28).	Prevents leakage during exercise, when drainage is likely to increase
Implementation	
Explain the purpose, application, and use of the CPM machine.	Reduces anxiety and promotes cooperation
Position the patient flat or slightly elevate the head of the bed.	Promotes comfort during exercise
Place the CPM machine on the bed and position the patient's foot so that it rests against the foot cradle.	Prepares the patient for exercise

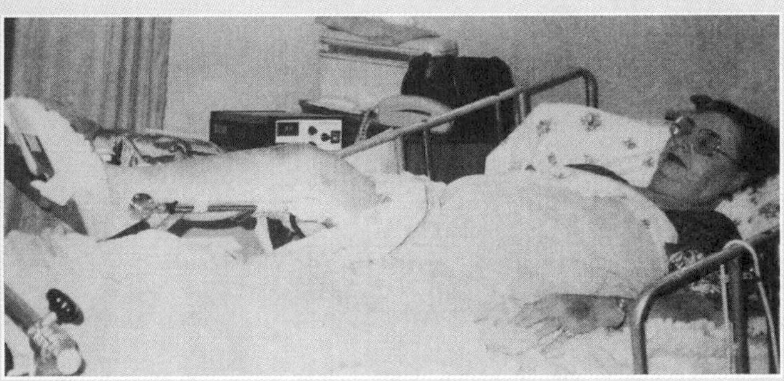

Range of motion of the knee with a continuous passive motion machine. (Courtesy of Ken Timby.)

Suggested Action	Reason for Action
Check that the knee joint corresponds to the foot actuator knob and *goniometer,* a device for measuring range of motion.	Positions the knee correctly
Use Velcro or canvas straps to secure the leg within the fabric cradle of the machine.	Supports and stabilizes leg
Adjust the machine to a lower-than-prescribed rate and degree of flexion.	Provides gradual progression to prescribed parameters
Turn on the machine and observe the patient's response.	Indicates level of tolerance
Readjust the alignment of the leg or position of the machine for optimal comfort.	Demonstrates concern for the patient's well-being
Increase the degree of flexion and cycles per minute gradually until the prescribed levels are reached.	Facilitates adaptation
Turn off the machine with the leg in an extended position at the end of the prescribed period of exercise.	Facilitates lifting the leg from the machine
Release the straps and support the joints beneath the knee and ankle while lifting the leg.	Reduces discomfort
Remove the machine from the bed; encourage active range-of-motion exercises and isometric exercises.	Potentiates effects from CPM

continued

SKILL 24-2

USING A CONTINUOUS PASSIVE MOTION (CPM) MACHINE *Continued*

Evaluation

- CPM applied and used according to exercise prescription.

Document

- Assessment data
- Use of machine
- Current amount of flexion, cycles per minute, and duration
- Tolerance of exercise

SAMPLE DOCUMENTATION

Date and Time Knee incision is dry and intact. Toes on both feet are warm with capillary refill <3 sec. Pedal pulses present and strong bilaterally. CPM machine used for 15 minutes with ROM at 30° of knee flexion for 5 cycles per minute. Discomfort increased from a level 4 before exercise to level 7 during exercise. Pain at a level of 5 after 15 minutes of rest following exercise. ______________________ SIGNATURE, TITLE

CRITICAL THINKING

- List the assessment findings you believe would indicate a positive response to the use of a CPM machine.
- A patient asks that the CPM machine be discontinued after 1 day of use. What reasons could be underlying the request? What nursing measures might be appropriate in response to each of these reasons?

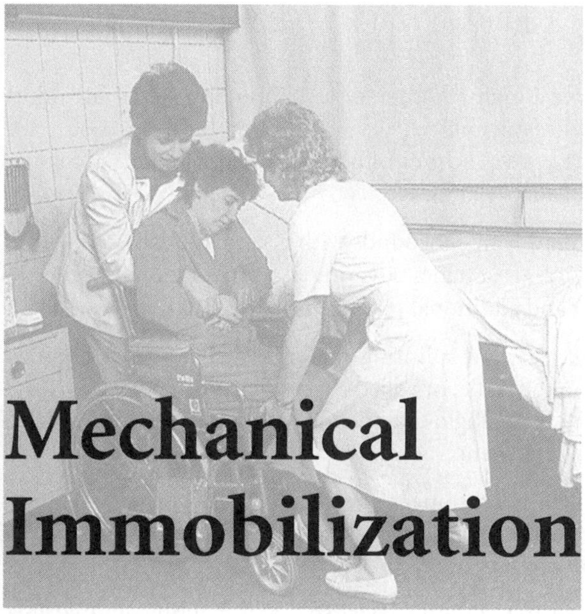

Mechanical Immobilization

CHAPTER 25

CHAPTER OUTLINE

Mechanical Immobilization
Mechanical Immobilizing Devices
Nursing Implications

NURSING GUIDELINES

APPLYING AN EMERGENCY SPLINT
BASIC CAST CARE
THE CARE OF TRACTION PATIENTS

SKILLS

SKILL 25-1: APPLYING AN ARM SLING
SKILL 25-2: ASSISTING WITH A CAST APPLICATION
SKILL 25-3: PROVIDING PIN SITE CARE

NURSING CARE PLAN

RISK FOR PERIPHERAL NEUROVASCULAR DYSFUNCTION

KEY TERMS

bivalved cast
body cast
braces
cast
cervical collar
cylinder cast
external fixator
functional braces
immobilizers
inflatable splints
manual traction
molded splints
orthoses
petals
pin site
prophylactic braces
rehabilitative braces
skeletal traction
skin traction
sling
spica cast
splint
traction
traction splints
windows

LEARNING OBJECTIVES

An understanding of the content within this chapter will be evidenced by the student's ability to:

- List at least three purposes for immobilization.
- Name four types of splints.
- Discuss why slings and braces are used.
- Explain the purpose of a cast.
- Name three types of casts.
- Describe at least five nursing actions that are appropriate when caring for patients with casts.
- Discuss how casts are removed.
- Explain what traction implies.
- List three types of traction.
- Name seven principles that apply to maintaining effective traction.
- Describe the purpose for an external fixator.
- Identify the rationale for performing pin site care.

Some patients are inactive and physically immobile due to an overall debilitating condition. For others, mobility impairment results from trauma or its treatment. Such is the case for patients with **orthoses** (orthopedic devices that support or align a body part and prevent or correct deformities), such as splints, immobilizers, and braces. Other patients have limited mobility when slings, casts, traction, and external fixators are used. Caring for patients who are mechanically immobilized with orthopedic devices requires specialized nursing skills that are described in this chapter.

Mechanical Immobilization

Most patients for whom mechanical immobilization is used have suffered trauma to the musculoskeletal system. These injuries are painful and do not heal as rapidly as those of the skin or soft tissue. They require a period of inactivity to allow new cells to restore the integrity of the damaged structures.

Mechanical immobilization of a body part accomplishes the following:

- Relieves pain and muscle spasm
- Supports and aligns skeletal injuries
- Restricts movement while injuries heal
- Maintains a functional position until healing is complete
- Allows activity while restricting movement of an injured area
- Prevents further structural damage and deformity

Mechanical Immobilizing Devices

Therapeutic benefits are achieved by using a variety of immobilizing devices such as splints, slings, braces, casts, and traction.

SPLINTS

Some conditions are treated with a **splint** (device that immobilizes and protects an injured part of the body). A splint is used before casts or traction are applied, or instead of them.

Emergency Splints

Splints are often applied as a first-aid measure (Fig. 25-1).

Nursing Guidelines For

Applying an Emergency Splint

☑ Avoid changing the position of the injured part, even if it appears grossly deformed.
RATIONALE: Keeping the part in place prevents additional injuries.

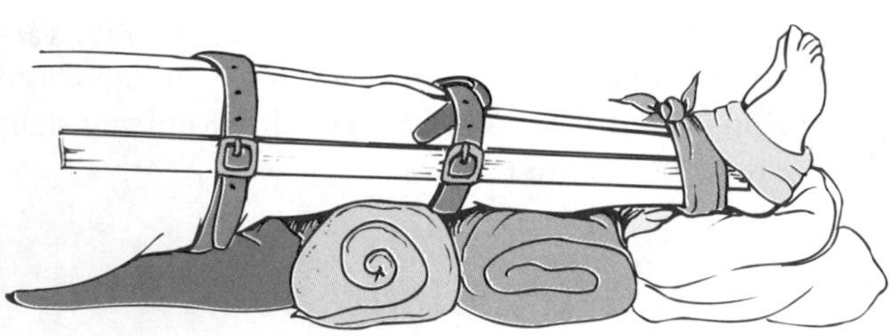

FIGURE 25–1. Emergency first aid splinting immobilizes the injured leg to the uninjured leg with a make-shift splint, such as a board, broom handle, golf club, or the like. Neckties, belts, or scarves keep the splint in place.

☑ Leave a high-top shoe or a ski boot in place if the injury involves an ankle.
RATIONALE: The shoe or boot limits movement and reduces pain and swelling.

☑ Cover any open wounds with clean material.
RATIONALE: Such a covering absorbs blood and prevents dirt and additional pathogens from entering.

☑ Select a rigid splinting material such as a flat board, a broom handle, or rolled-up newspaper.
RATIONALE: Rigid material provides support while restricting movement.

☑ Pad bony prominences with soft material.
RATIONALE: Padding cushions pressure and prevents friction on the skin.

☑ Apply the splinting device so that it spans the injured area, from the joint above the injury to the joint below.
RATIONALE: Such placement immobilizes the injured tissue.

☑ Use an uninjured area of the body adjacent to the injured part as a splint, if no other sturdy material is available.
RATIONALE: The uninjured part can serve as a substitute for an external splint.

☑ Use wide tape or wide strips of fabric to confine the injured part to the splint.
RATIONALE: Securing the body part prevents displacement and reduces the risk of compromising circulation.

☑ Loosen the splint or the material used to attach it if the fingers or toes are pale, blue, or cold.
RATIONALE: Loosening the splint facilitates circulation.

☑ Elevate the immobilized part, if possible, so the lowest point is higher than the heart.
RATIONALE: Elevation reduces swelling and enhances venous return to the heart.

☑ Keep the patient warm and safe.
RATIONALE: Shock is a risk.

☑ Seek assistance in transporting the patient to a health care agency.
RATIONALE: More sophisticated treatment is needed.

Commercial Splints

Commercial splints are more effective than improvised ones. They are available in a variety of designs, depending on the injury. Examples include inflatable splints, traction splints, immobilizers, molded splints, and cervical collars. Inflatable and traction splints are intended for short-term use: they are usually applied just after the injury occurs and are removed shortly after the injury has been assessed more thoroughly. Immobilizers and molded splints are used for longer periods.

Inflatable Splints

Inflatable splints (immobilizing devices that become rigid when filled with air) also are called *pneumatic splints* (Fig. 25-2). Besides limiting motion, they also control bleeding and swelling. The injured body part is inserted into the deflated splint. When air is infused, the splint molds to the contour of the injured part, preventing movement. The splint is filled with air until it can be indented a half-inch (1.3 cm) with the fingertips. The injury should be examined and treated within 30 to 45 minutes after the splint is applied; otherwise, circulation may be affected.

Traction Splints

Traction splints (metal devices that immobilize and pull on muscles that are in a state of contraction) are not as easy to apply as inflatable splints. One example is a *Thomas splint,* which requires special training to avoid causing additional injuries (Fig. 25-3).

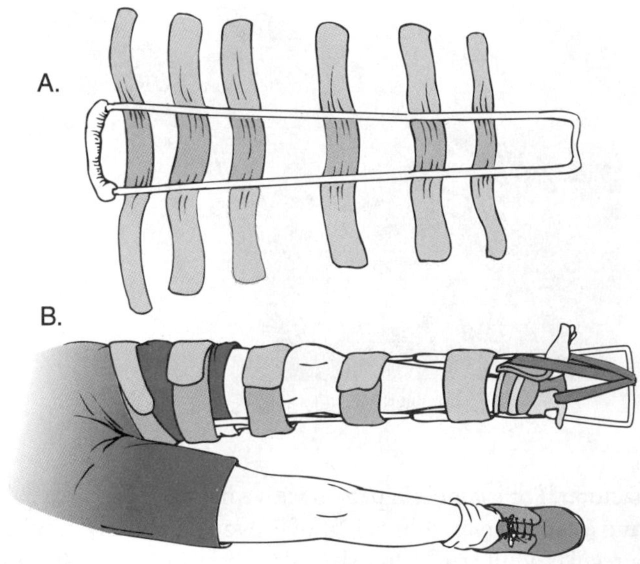

FIGURE 25–3. (*A*) Thomas splint. (*B*) Thomas splint applied to the lower extremity.

Immobilizers

Immobilizers (commercial splints made from cloth and foam) are held in place by adjustable Velcro straps (Fig. 25-4). As their name implies, immobilizers are used to limit motion in the area of a painful but healing injury, such as in the neck and knee. They are removed for brief periods during hygiene and dressing.

Molded Splints

Molded splints (orthotic devices made of rigid materials; Fig. 25-5) are used for chronic injuries or diseases. They provide prolonged support and limit movement to prevent further injury and pain. They maintain the body part in a functional position to prevent contractures and muscle atrophy during immobility.

Cervical Collars

A **cervical collar** (foam or rigid splint around the neck) is used to treat athletic neck injuries and other trauma that results in a neck sprain or strain (Fig. 25-6). A neck strain is sometimes referred to as a whiplash injury. The incidence of whiplash injuries has decreased, primarily for two reasons: improved athletic protective equipment, and shoulder harnesses and neck supports in automobiles.

When the neck injury—which is generally more painful the day after trauma—is mild or moderate, a foam collar, covered with stockinette (a stretchable cotton fabric), is used. It reminds the patient to limit neck and head movements. For more serious injuries, a rigid splint, made from polyurethane, is used to control neck motion and support the head, reducing its load-bearing force on the cervical spine.

To determine the proper collar size, the nurse measures the circumference of the neck and the distance between the shoulder and the chin (Fig. 25-7). The measurements are compared with the size guide suggested by the collar manu-

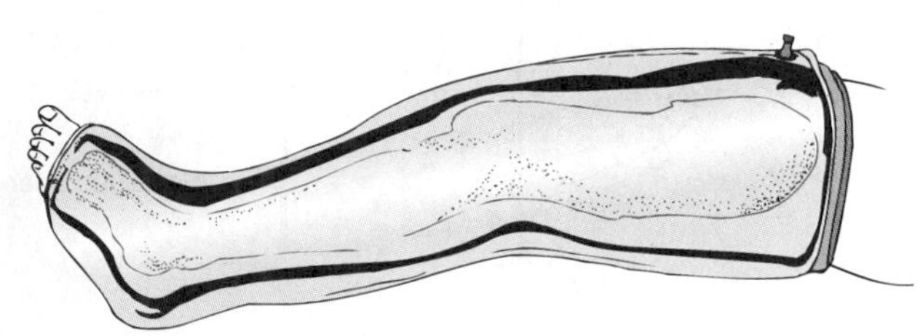

FIGURE 25–2. An inflatable splint.

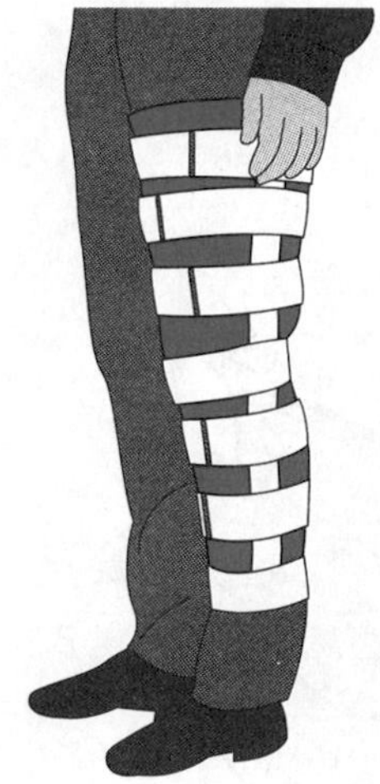

FIGURE 25–4. Leg immobilizer.

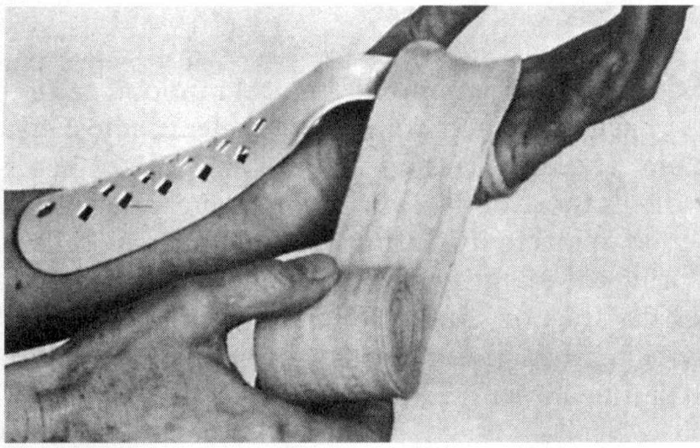

FIGURE 25–5. Molded splint.

facturer. For example, a person with a neck size of 15″ to 20″ and a shoulder-to-chin height of 3″ would probably require a regular adult size. Adult sizes also come in short, tall, and extra-tall sizes. Pediatric collars also are available.

When applying a cervical collar, the head is placed in neutral position (see Chap. 23). The front of the collar is positioned well beneath the chin and slid upward until the chin is well supported. The opening of the collar is centered at the back of the neck. Straps made of Velcro or other materials are used to secure the collar in the desired position. When applied appropriately, the patient can breathe and swallow effortlessly while wearing the collar.

Cervical collars are worn almost continuously, even while sleeping, for 10 days to 2 weeks. They are removed to do gentle range-of-motion neck exercises (see Chap. 24). The sooner exercise is performed (within the patient's pain tolerance), the faster revascularization and recovery take place. Prolonged dependence on the collar for comfort can lead to permanent stiffness in the neck.

During recovery, the nurse assesses the patient's neuromuscular status by having the patient perform movements that correlate with muscular functions controlled by cervical spine and peripheral nerve roots. If neuromuscular function is intact, the patient should be able to:

- Elevate both shoulders
- Flex and extend the elbows and wrists
- Generate a strong hand grip
- Spread the fingers
- Touch the thumb to the little finger on each hand

Any difference in strength or movement on one side or the other is documented and communicated to the physician.

SLINGS

A **sling** (cloth device used to elevate, cradle, and support parts of the body) is commonly applied to the arm (Fig. 25-8), leg, or pelvis after the injury has been immobilized and examined. Although the commercial type of arm sling used by

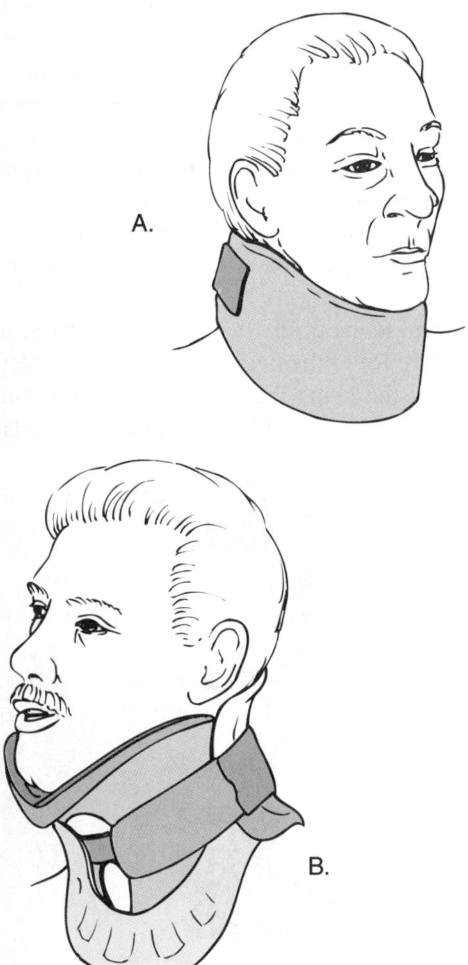

FIGURE 25–6. (*A*) Foam cervical collar. (*B*) Rigid cervical collar.

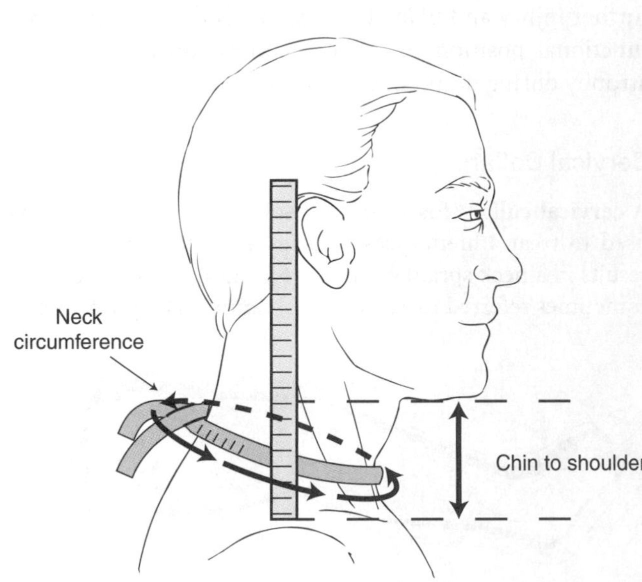

FIGURE 25–7. Vertical and circumferential measurements for cervical collar size.

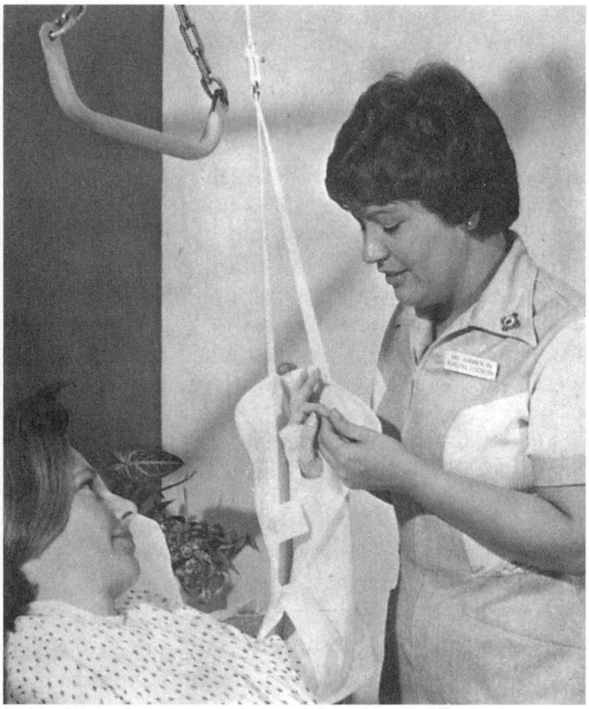
FIGURE 25–8. A sling used for arm suspension.

ambulatory patients is probably the type that comes to mind, a triangular piece of muslin cloth is occasionally used to fashion a sling. To be effective, slings must be properly applied (Skill 25-1).

BRACES

There are three categories of **braces** (custom-made or custom-fitted devices designed to support weakened structures): **prophylactic braces** (those used to prevent or reduce the severity of a joint injury), **rehabilitative braces** (those that allow protected motion of an injured joint that has been treated operatively; Fig. 25-9), and **functional braces** (those that provide stability for an unstable joint).

Because braces are generally worn during active periods, they are made of sturdy materials, such as metal and leather. Leg braces may be incorporated into a shoe. Some back braces are made of cloth with metal staves, or strips, that are sewn within the fabric of the brace. An improperly applied or ill-fitting brace can cause discomfort, deformity, and pressure ulcers.

CASTS

A **cast** (rigid mold about a body part) is used to immobilize an injured structure, usually a fractured (broken) bone, once it has been restored to correct anatomic alignment. Casts are formed using either wetted rolls of plaster of Paris or premoistened rolls of fiberglass (Table 25-1).

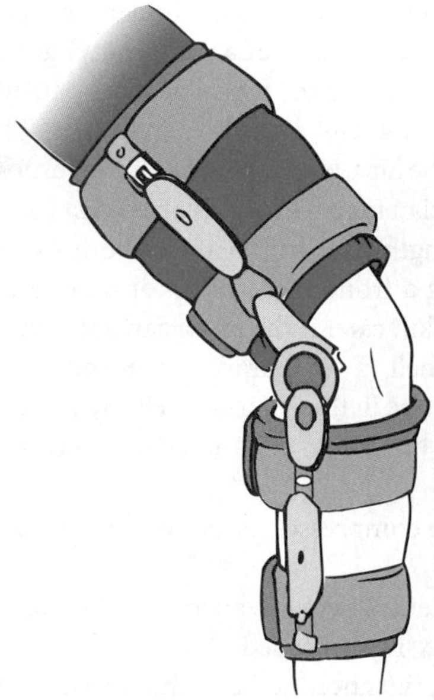
FIGURE 25–9. A rehabilitative brace that ensures appropriate control of knee motion following an operative procedure.

Types of Casts

There are basically three types of casts: cylinder casts, body casts, and spica casts.

A **cylinder cast** (rigid mold that encircles an arm or leg) leaves the toes or fingers exposed. The cast extends from the joints above and below the affected bone. This prevents movement, thereby maintaining correct alignment while healing takes place. As healing progresses, the cast may be trimmed or shortened.

TABLE 25–1. **Cast Materials**

Substance	Advantages	Disadvantages
Plaster of Paris	Inexpensive Easy to apply Low incidence of allergic reactions	Takes 24–48 hours to dry; large casts may take up to 72 hours Weight bearing must be delayed until thoroughly dried Heavy Prone to cracking or crumbling, especially at the edges Softens when wet
Fiberglass	Lightweight Porous Dries in 5–15 minutes Immediate weight bearing allowed Durable Unaffected by water	Expensive Not recommended for severe injuries or those accompanied by excessive swelling Macerates skin if padding becomes wet Cast edges may be sharp and cause skin abrasions

A **body cast** (larger form of a cylinder cast that encircles the trunk of the body instead of an extremity) generally extends from the nipple line to the hips. For some patients with spinal problems, the body cast extends from the back of the head and chin areas to the hips, with modifications for exposing the arms.

The physician may create a **bivalved cast** (one that is cut in two pieces lengthwise) from either a body cast or a cylinder cast. Creating a front and a back for a body cast facilitates bathing and skin care. If the physician approves, the anterior half of the shell is temporarily removed for hygiene; the patient lies prone in the anterior shell when the posterior half is removed. A bivalved cast on an extremity (Fig. 25-10) is created when:

- Swelling compresses tissue and interferes with circulation
- The patient is being weaned from the cast
- A sharp x-ray is needed
- Painful joints need to be immobilized temporarily on a patient with arthritis

A **spica cast** (rigid mold that encircles one or both arms or legs and the chest or trunk) is generally strengthened with a reinforcement bar (Fig. 25-11). When applied to the upper body, the cast is referred to as a *shoulder spica;* one applied to the lower extremities is called a *hip spica.* Spica casts, especially those on the lower extremities, are heavy, hot, and frustrating because they severely restrict activity.

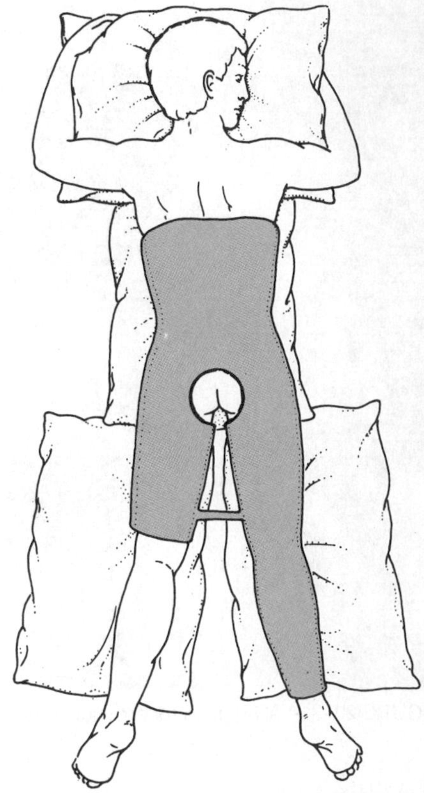

FIGURE 25–11. Hip spica cast. (Timby BK, Scherer JC, Smith N: Introductory medical–surgical nursing, 7th ed, p 1022. Philadelphia, Lippincott Williams & Wilkins, 1999)

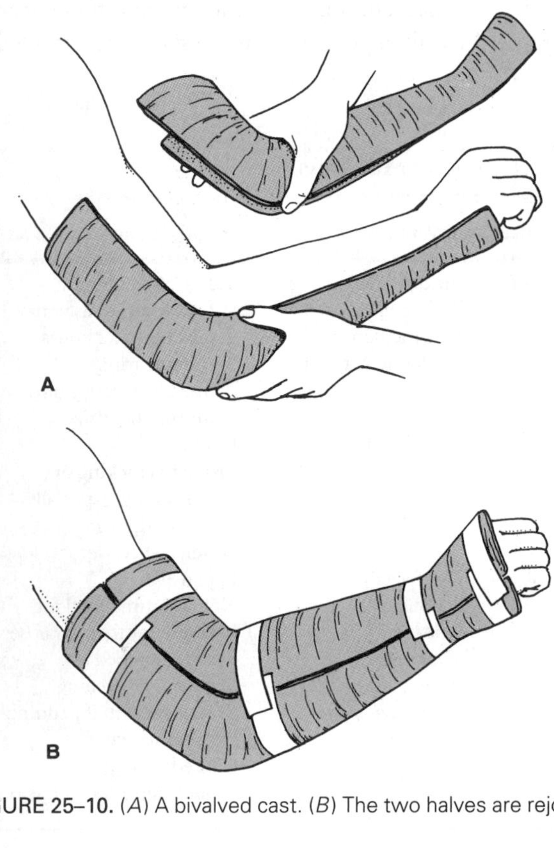

FIGURE 25–10. (*A*) A bivalved cast. (*B*) The two halves are rejoined.

When applied to a lower extremity, the cast is trimmed in the anal and genital areas to allow elimination of urine and stool. Patients with a hip spica cannot sit during elimination, so the nurse protects the cast from soiling using plastic wrap and provides a small bedpan known as a fracture pan.

Cast Application

Cast application generally requires more than one person. The nurse prepares the patient, assembles the cast supplies, and helps the physician during cast application (Skill 25-2). A light-cured fiberglass cast requires exposure to ultraviolet light to harden.

Basic Cast Care

Some patients need extended care after surgery that has included the application of a cast. The nurse is responsible for caring for the cast and making appropriate assessments to prevent complications.

Nursing Guidelines For
Basic Cast Care

- ☑ Leave a freshly applied plaster cast uncovered.
  RATIONALE: Leaving the cast uncovered facilitates assessment and drying.
- ☑ Assess the circulation and sensation in exposed fingers or toes at frequent intervals (Fig. 25-12).
  RATIONALE: The condition of the fingers or toes provides comparative data for identifying neurovascular complications.
- ☑ Monitor the mobility of the fingers (Fig. 25-13) or toes.
  RATIONALE: Mobility status provides data about neuromuscular function.
- ☑ Report significant abnormal findings promptly, especially pain that progressively worsens.
  RATIONALE: Prompt reporting ensures that complications are treated early.
- ☑ Handle a wet plaster cast with the palms of the hand, never the fingers (Fig. 25-14).
  RATIONALE: Fingers can dent the plaster.
- ☑ Elevate the plaster cast on pillows while it is wet.
  RATIONALE: This placement prevents changing the shape of the cast and interfering with the corrected alignment.
- ☑ Remove plaster residue from the skin with a wet washcloth.
  RATIONALE: Plaster flakes, if not removed, can accumulate inside the cast or in the bed.
- ☑ Swab fiberglass resin from the skin with alcohol or acetone.
  RATIONALE: Alcohol and acetone are chemical solvents.
- ☑ Turn the patient frequently while a plaster cast is drying.
  RATIONALE: Turning promotes drying of all surfaces and layers of the cast.

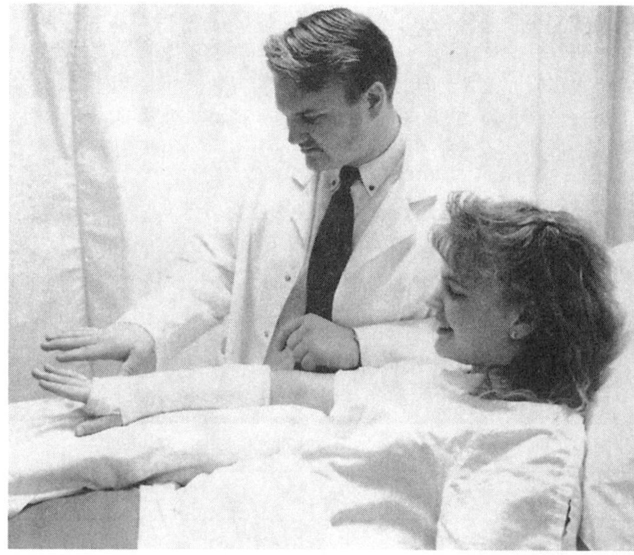

FIGURE 25–13. Checking mobility. (Courtesy of Ken Timby.)

- ☑ Apply ice packs to the cast where surgery has been performed.
  RATIONALE: Ice packs reduce swelling and help control bleeding.
- ☑ Circle areas where blood has seeped through the cast; note the time on the cast.
  RATIONALE: Such actions help evaluate the significance of blood loss.
- ☑ Apply **petals** (strips of adhesive tape) around the edges of the cast wherever there are rough areas or chipping plaster (Fig. 25-15).
  RATIONALE: Petals reinforce the edge of the cast and protect the skin.
- ☑ Caution patients not to insert objects (straws, combs, eating utensils, and the like) within the cast.
  RATIONALE: Such objects could impair the skin if they fell inside.

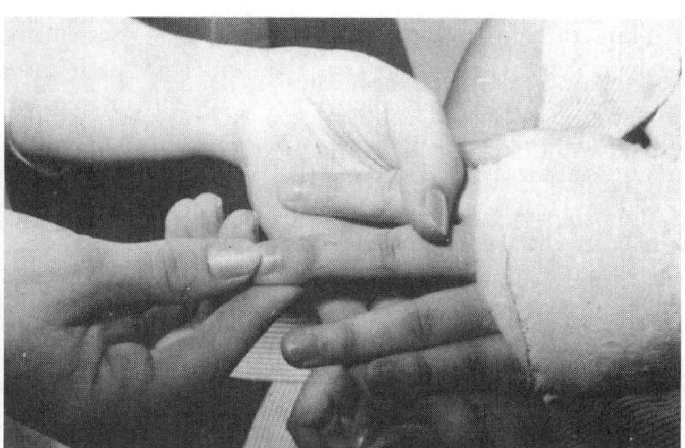

FIGURE 25–12. Assessing capillary refill.

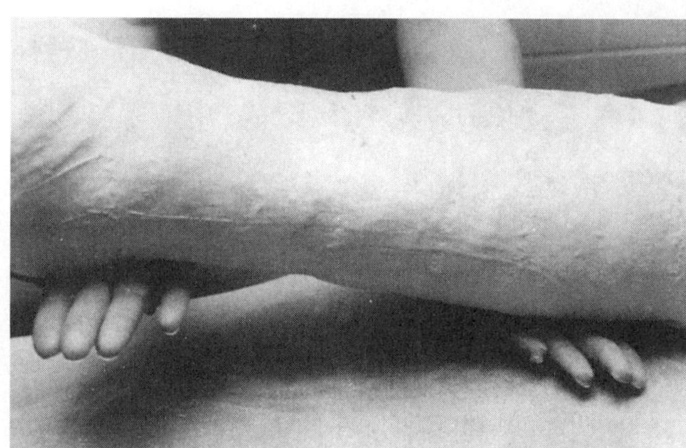

FIGURE 25–14. Support using the palms.

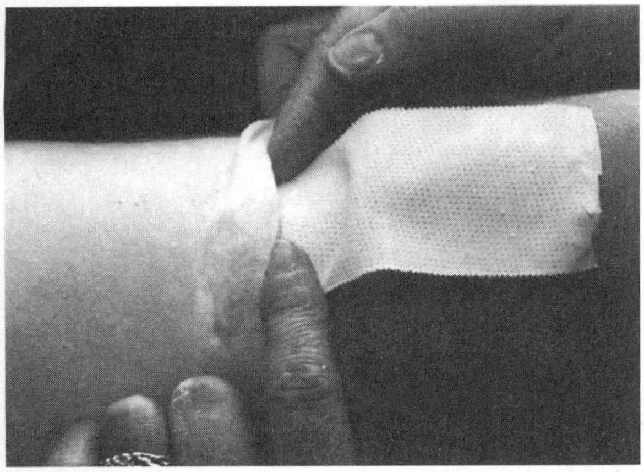

FIGURE 25–15. Applying petals.

☑ Replace **windows** (squares cut from the cast) at their original site (Fig. 25-16).
RATIONALE: Proper window replacement prevents bulging of tissue and subsequent circulatory and skin problems.

☑ Ambulate patients as soon as possible, or have them exercise in bed.
RATIONALE: Movement prevents complications from immobility.

Cast Removal

In most cases, casts are removed when they need to be changed and reapplied, or when the injury has healed sufficiently that the cast is no longer necessary. A cast is removed prematurely if complications develop.

Most casts are removed with an electric cast cutter, an instrument that looks like a circular saw (Fig. 25-17). A cast cutter is a noisy instrument that sounds frightening to patients. There is a natural expectation that an instrument sharp enough to cut a cast is sharp enough to cut skin and tissue. However, when used properly, an electric cast cutter leaves the skin intact.

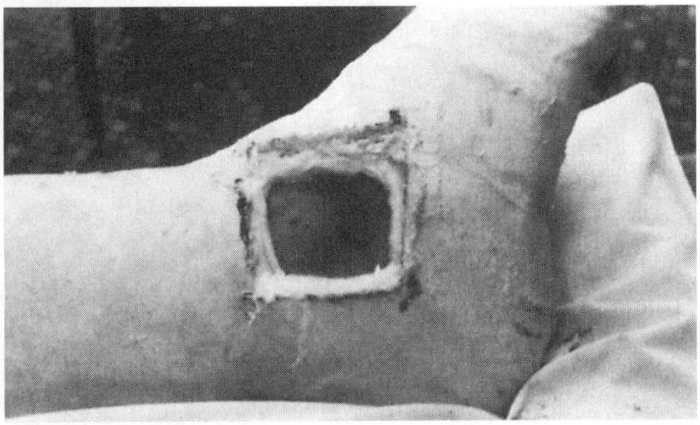

FIGURE 25–16. A cast with a window.

When the cast is removed, the unexercised muscle is usually smaller and weaker. The joints may have a limited range of motion. The skin usually appears pale and waxy and may contain scales or patches of dead skin. The skin is washed as usual with soapy warm water, but the semiattached areas of skin are left in place; they are not forcibly removed. Applying lotion to the skin adds moisture and tends to prevent the rough skin edges from catching on clothing. Eventually the dead skin fragments will slough free.

TRACTION

Traction (pulling effect exerted on a part of the skeletal system) is a treatment measure for musculoskeletal trauma and disorders. Traction is used to:

- Reduce muscle spasms
- Realign bones
- Relieve pain
- Prevent deformities

The pull of the traction is generally offset by the counterpull from the patients's own body weight. Except for traction that is exerted with the hands, the application of traction involves the use of weights that are connected to the patient through a system of ropes, pulleys, slings, and other equipment.

Types of Traction

There are three basic types of traction: manual, skin, and skeletal traction. The categories reflect the manner in which traction is applied.

Manual traction (pulling on the body using a person's hands and muscular strength; Fig. 25-18) is most often used briefly when realigning a broken bone. It is also used when replacing a dislocated bone into its original position within a joint.

Skin traction (pulling effect on the skeletal system by applying devices to the skin) is applied with devices such as a pelvic belt and a cervical halter (Fig. 25-19). Other names for commonly applied forms of skin traction are Buck's traction and Russell's traction (Fig. 25-20).

Skeletal traction (pull exerted directly on the skeletal system by attaching wires, pins, or tongs into or through a bone; Fig. 25-21) is applied continuously for an extended period.

Traction Care

Regardless of the type of traction used, its effectiveness depends on the application of certain principles during patient care (Display 25-1).

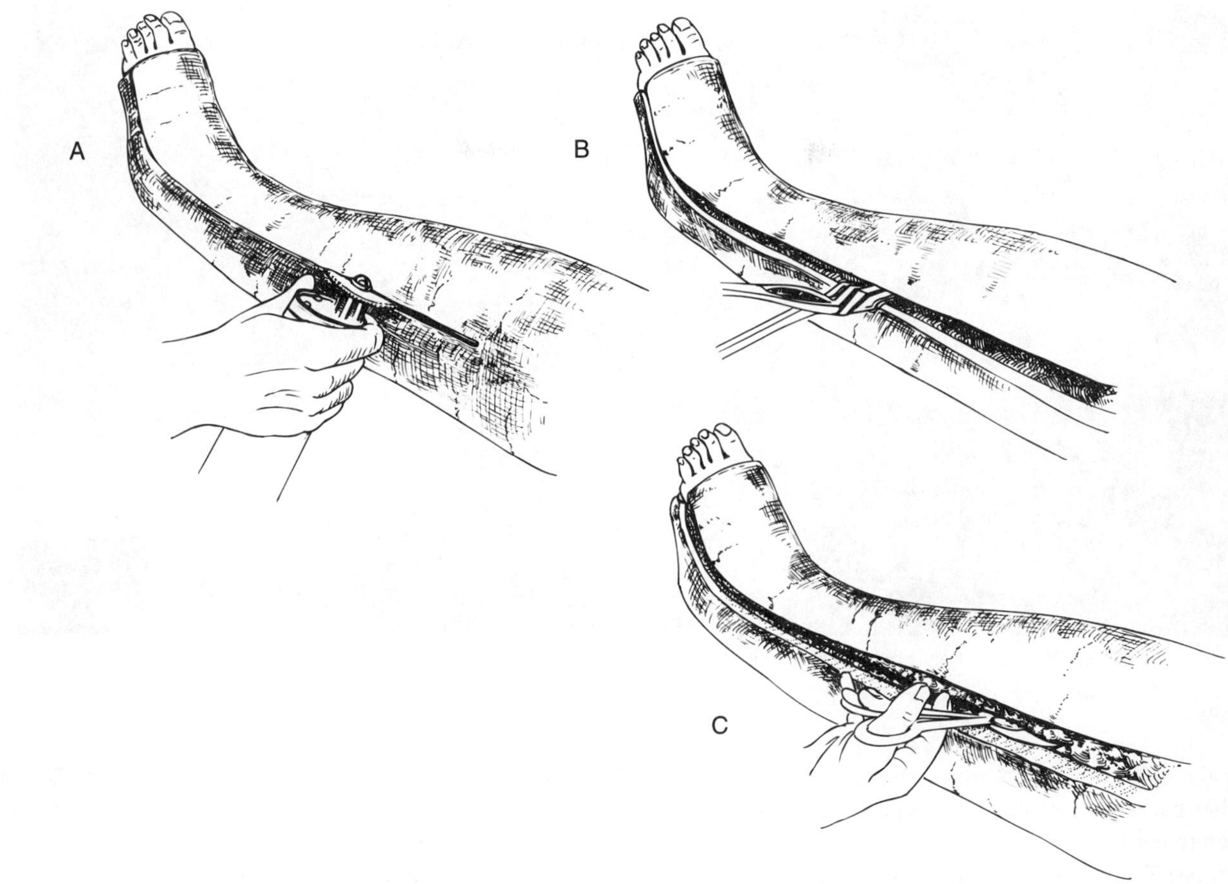

FIGURE 25–17. Cast removal. (*A*) The cast is bivalved with an electric cast cutter. (*B*) The cast is split. (*C*) The padding is manually cut.

Nursing Guidelines For

The Care of Traction Patients

- ☑ Inspect the mechanical equipment used to apply traction.
  RATIONALE: Inspection determines the status of the equipment.
- ☑ Provide a trapeze and an overbed frame if none is present.
  RATIONALE: The trapeze facilitates mobility and self-care.

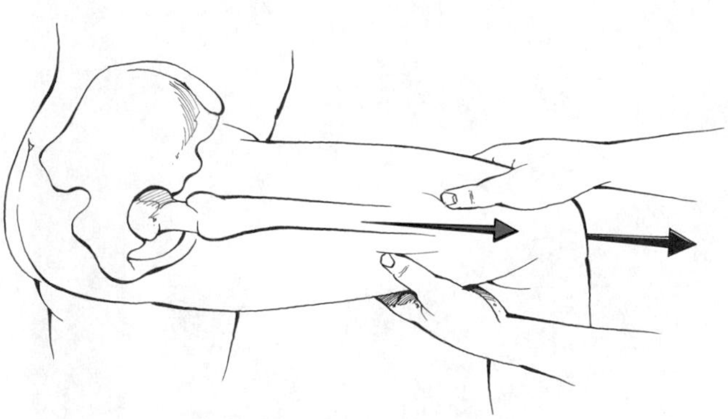

FIGURE 25–18. Manual traction.

- ☑ Position the patient so that the patient's body is in an opposite line with the pull of traction.
  RATIONALE: This is one of the principles for maintaining effective traction.
- ☑ Avoid tucking top sheets, blankets, or bedspreads beneath the mattress.
  RATIONALE: Bed clothes tucked under the mattress would interfere with the pull produced by traction equipment.
- ☑ Keep the traction applied continuously, unless there are medical orders to the contrary.
  RATIONALE: Continuous traction fosters achievement of desired outcomes.
- ☑ Keep the weights from resting on the floor.
  RATIONALE: Keeping the weights above the floor maintains effective traction.
- ☑ Ask the physician to replace fraying ropes or those with knots that interfere with movement through pulleys.
  RATIONALE: Intact equipment maintains effective traction.
- ☑ Limit the patient's positions to those indicated in the medical orders or standards for care.
  RATIONALE: Other positions may alter the pull and counter-pull of effective traction.

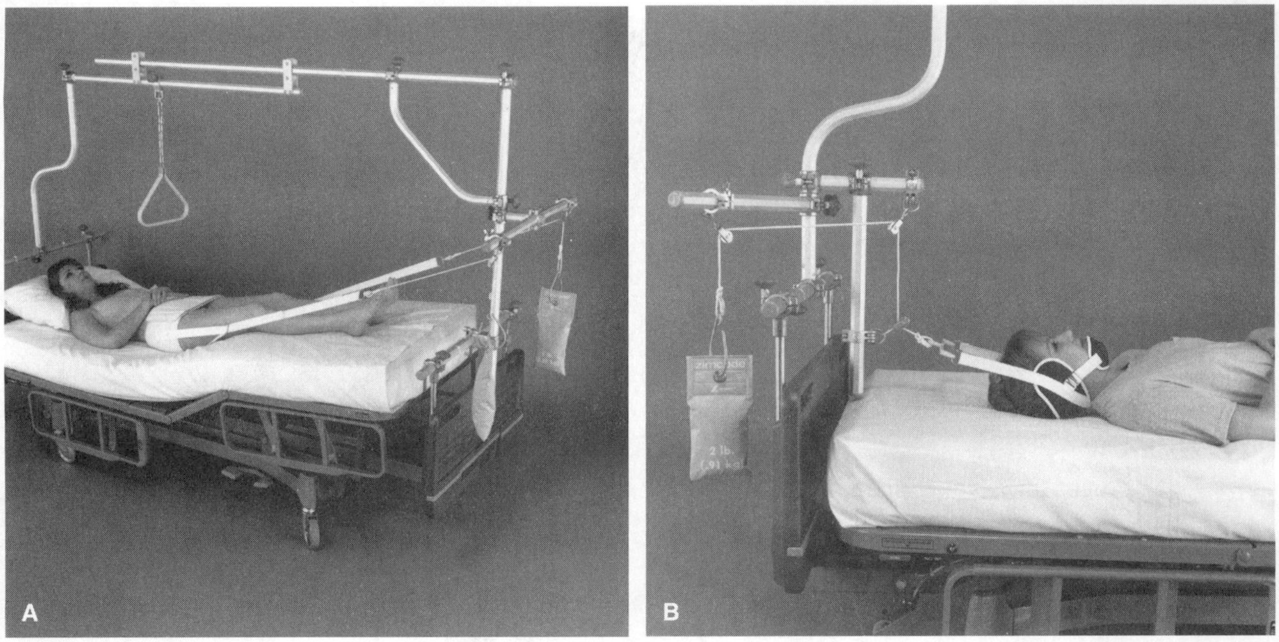

FIGURE 25–19. (*A*) Pelvic belt. (*B*) Cervical halter. (Courtesy of Patient Care Division, Zimmer, Dover, OH.)

- ☑ Bathe the backs of patients who must remain in a supine or other back-lying position by depressing the mattress enough to insert a hand.
  RATIONALE: This action facilitates skin care and hygiene.
- ☑ Make the bed by applying sheets from the bottom of the bed toward the top, rather than side to side.
  RATIONALE: Making the bed in this way maintains the patient in alignment with the traction.
- ☑ Use a pressure-relieving device (see Chaps. 23 and 28) and conscientious skin care if the patient is confined to bed for a prolonged time.
  RATIONALE: Proper care prevents skin breakdown.
- ☑ Do not use a pillow if the patient's head or neck is in traction, unless medical orders indicate otherwise.
  RATIONALE: Using a pillow could disturb the pull and counterpull.

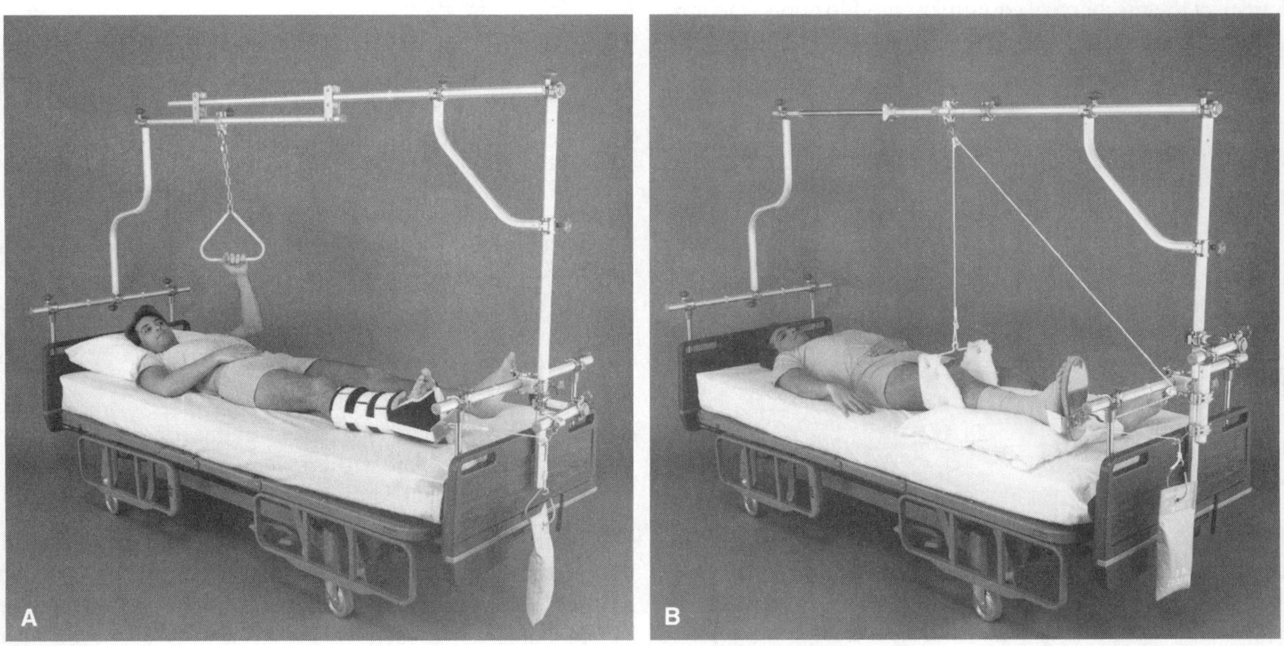

FIGURE 25–20. (*A*) Buck's traction. (*B*) Russell's traction. (Courtesy of Patient Care Division, Zimmer, Dover, OH.)

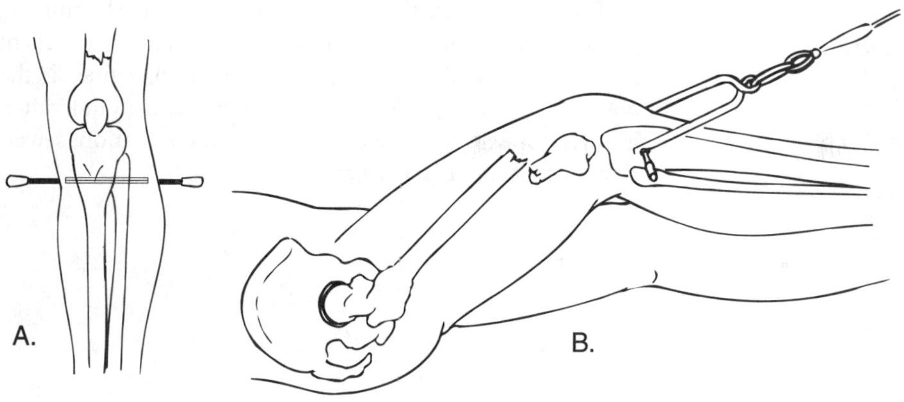

FIGURE 25–21. The application of skeletal traction. (*A*) A pin transects the bone. (*B*) Traction is applied.

☑ Use a small bedpan, called a fracture pan, if elevating the hips alters the line of pull.
RATIONALE: Keeping the hips in the proper position maintains the effectiveness of traction.

☑ Encourage isometric, isotonic, and active range-of-motion exercises.
RATIONALE: Exercise maintains the tone, strength, and flexibility of the musculoskeletal system.

☑ Cleanse the skin around skeletal insertion sites using soap and water or an antimicrobial agent.
RATIONALE: Cleansing reduces the risk for infection.

☑ Cover the tips of protruding metal pins or other sharp traction devices with corks or other protective material.
RATIONALE: Covering these items prevents accidental injury.

☑ Insert padding within slings if they tend to wrinkle.
RATIONALE: Padding helps cushion and distribute pressure, prevents interference with circulation, and reduces the risk for skin breakdown.

☑ Provide diversional activities as often as possible.
RATIONALE: Activities relieve boredom and sensory deprivation.

DISPLAY 25–1

Principles for Maintaining Effective Traction

- Traction must produce a pulling effect on the body.
- Countertraction (counterpull) must be maintained.
- The pull of traction and the counterpull must be in exactly opposite directions.
- Splints and slings must be suspended without interference.
- Ropes must move freely through each pulley.
- The prescribed amount of weight must be applied.
- The weights must hang free.

EXTERNAL FIXATORS

An **external fixator** (metal device inserted into and through one or more bones; Fig. 25-22) is used to stabilize fragments of broken bones during the healing process. Although the area of an injury is immobilized with an external fixator, the patient is encouraged to be active and mobile (see Chap. 26 for information about ambulatory aids).

During recovery, the nurse provides care for the **pin site** (location where pins, wires, or tongs enter or exit the skin). In conjunction with an external fixator and skeletal traction, pin site care is essential for preventing infection. The insertion of pins impairs skin integrity and provides a port of entry for pathogens. Caring for a pin site is described in Skill 25-3.

Nursing Implications

Patients with immobilizing devices such as casts and traction may have one or more of the following nursing diagnoses:
- Pain
- Impaired physical mobility

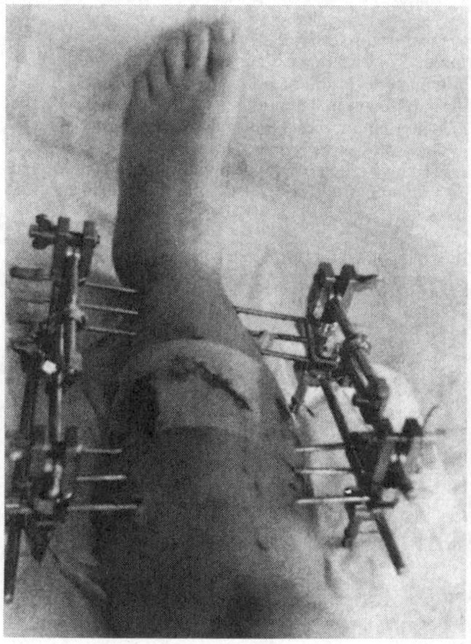

FIGURE 25–22. An external fixator.

- Risk for disuse syndrome
- Risk for peripheral neurovascular dysfunction
- Impaired bed mobility
- Risk for impaired skin integrity
- Risk for altered tissue perfusion
- Self-care deficit: bathing/hygiene

The nursing care plan that follows describes the nursing process as it applies to a patient with a nursing diagnosis of Risk for peripheral neurovascular dysfunction, defined in the NANDA taxonomy (1999) as "a state in which an individual is at risk of experiencing a disruption in circulation, sensation, or motion of an extremity."

Nursing Care Plan

Risk for Peripheral Neurovascular Dysfunction

Assessment

Subjective Data

States, "The cast on my left leg was applied this morning. The pain has been getting worse and worse all day, even though I have been taking the medication the physician prescribed."

Objective Data

Toes on left extremity are cool and swollen in comparison to right extremity. Capillary refill is 3 sec on left, but 2 sec on right. Left pedal pulse diminished but present. Right pedal pulse strong. Reduced sensation between left great toe and left second toe when pressure from sharp point is applied.

Diagnosis

Risk for peripheral neurovascular dysfunction related to mechanical compression of tissue by cast secondary to peripheral edema

Plan

Goal

The patient will experience relief of pain from present rate of 9 to ≤7. Pedal pulses will be equally strong. Capillary refill will be ≤2 seconds bilaterally within 3 hours today (8/20).

Orders: 8/20

1. Elevate casted left leg so that toes are higher than heart.
2. Have patient exercise toes of left foot four times per hour.
3. Apply an ice bag on the cast over the area of injury; empty and refill ice bag every 20 minutes.
4. Monitor circulatory status, sensation including tactile and pain, and mobility of toes in affected extremity every 30 minutes.
5. Report worsening of symptoms to physician immediately. ____________ F. HOLMES, RN

Implementation (Documentation)

8/20 1800 Left leg with cast elevated on 3 pillows. Performing active exercises with toes q 15 min. Ice bag applied to cast over lateral ankle. Rates pain at 10 despite receiving Demerol 75 mg IM 30 minutes ago. ____________ G. BAILEY, LPN

1830 Left pedal pulse detected only by Doppler. Dr. Ewing notified. Given orders to obtain cast cutter for bivalving cast. ____________ G. BAILEY, LPN

Evaluation (Documentation

1900 Cast bivalved by Dr. Ewing. Roller bandage wrapped about separated cast. Capillary refill 2 seconds in toes on both feet. Pedal pulse palpable and equal bilaterally. Rates pain at 9. Affected leg remains elevated with ice bag applied. Doing exercises as directed. ____________ G. BAILEY, LPN

FOCUS ON OLDER ADULTS

- Hip fractures are very common in older adults, especially in postmenopausal women who are not treated for osteoporosis.
- The bones of older adults take longer to heal than those of younger age groups.
- Older adults are mobilized as soon as possible to avoid pressure ulcers and life-threatening complications.
- To promote healing of a musculoskeletal injury, older adults are encouraged to consume a diet rich in protein, calcium, and zinc.
- Older adults who have poor appetites or inadequate oral intake are encouraged to drink liquid supplements that are high in nutrients several times a day. Registered dieticians often are helpful in planning adequate nutritional intake.
- Although musculoskeletal injuries are quite painful, caution is necessary when administering narcotic analgesics to older adults. Although these types of medications are effective in relieving pain, older adults are more susceptible to developing adverse effects, such as constipation, mental changes, and depressed respirations. If narcotic analgesics are necessary, a lower dose may be effective and the length of time between doses may be lengthened.
- Because older adults often have diminished tactile sensation and may be unaware of developing problems with skin pressure, their skin must be checked for redness several times daily.
- When an indwelling catheter is used at the time of orthopedic surgery, the catheter must be removed as soon as possible after the surgery. Older adults are likely to develop incontinence when indwelling catheters are used, and efforts must be made to assist the older adult maintain or regain continence.
- Some fractures, particularly of the upper extremities, are treated nonsurgically with immobilization. Occupational and physical therapists are helpful in assisting older adults regain function and range of motion following any period of immobilization.
- As adults live longer, many are dealing with the pain and loss of function associated with arthritis. Consequently, more and more older adults are choosing to have joint replacement surgery that may involve rehabilitation with various types of mechanical devices.

KEY CONCEPTS

- Immobilization is used to relieve pain and muscle spasm, support and align skeletal injuries, and restrict movement while injuries heal.
- The four types of splints are inflatable splints, traction splints, immobilizers, and molded splints.
- Slings are cloth devices used to elevate and support parts of the body. Braces are custom-made or custom-fitted devices designed to support weakened structures during activity.
- Cast are rigid molds used to immobilize an injured structure that has been restored to correct anatomic alignment. Casts are formed from plaster of Paris or fiberglass.
- Three types of casts are cylinder casts, body casts, and spica casts.
- Appropriate nursing care of patients with casts includes checking circulation, mobility, and sensation in the area of the cast; using the palms of the hands to handle a wet cast; elevating the casted extremity to reduce swelling; circling areas where blood has seeped through; and padding and reinforcing the cast edges to prevent skin breakdown.
- Most casts are removed with an electric cast cutter, an instrument that looks like a circular saw.
- Traction is the application of a pulling effect on a part of the skeletal system.
- The three types of traction are manual traction, skin traction, and skeletal traction.
- To be effective, traction must produce a pulling effect on the body, countertraction must be maintained, the pull of traction and the counterpull must be in exactly opposite directions, splints and slings must be suspended without interference, ropes must move freely through each pulley, the prescribed amount of weight must be applied, and the weights must hang free.
- An external fixator is used to stabilize fragments of broken bones during the healing process.
- Pin site care is essential for preventing infection because the insertion of pins impairs skin integrity and provides a port of entry for pathogens.

CRITICAL THINKING EXERCISES

- Discuss the differences and similarities between caring for patients with casts and those in traction.
- Discuss ways of providing diversion for cast and traction patients who are confined to bed while their injuries heal.
- Identify activities that provide exercise and can be performed in bed by patients with casts or in traction.

SUGGESTED READINGS

Adkins LM. Cast changes: synthetic versus plaster. Pediatric Nursing 1997;23(4):422–427.

Castle R. Unlucky breaks! Be prepared to splint them. First Aider 1998;69(1):4.

DeGeorge P, Dunwooding C. Transfer techniques of the lower extremity with an external fixator. Orthopaedic Nursing 1995;14(6):17–21.

Faria SH. Assessment of immobility hazards. Home Care Provider 1998;3(4):189–191.

Hayes AJ. Fiberglass and its potential health risks related to casting. National Association of Orthopaedic Technologists Journal 1995–1996:4–5.

Huston CJ. Emergency! Cervical spine injury. American Journal of Nursing 1998;98(6):33.

McCarthy L. Safe handling of patients on cervical traction. Nursing Times 1998;94(14):57–59.
Meredith RM, Butcher JD. Emergencies. Field splinting of suspected fractures: preparation, assessment, and application. Physician and Sportsmedicine 1997;25(10):29–39.
Millet S. Care of the orthopaedic patient with traction. Nursing Times 1998;94(22):52–54.
Mollashby A. Immobilization techniques in cervical spine injury: cervical orthoses, skeletal traction, and halo devices. Topics in Emergency Medicine 1997;19(3):26–33.
NANDA nursing diagnoses: definitions and classification, 1999–2000. Philadelphia, NANDA, 1999.
Nichol D. Clinical orthopaedics: understanding the principles of traction. Nursing Standard 1995;9(46):25–28.
Ridgway EM, Byrne DP. To sling or not to sling. OT Practice 1999;5(1):38–42.
Shoemaker M. Living with a leg immobilizer. Nursing 1998;28(8):32hn9.
Sims M, Saleh M. Protocols for the care of external fixator pin sites. Professional Nurse 1996;11(4):261–264.
Wichmann S, Marin DR. Bracing for activity. Physician and Sportsmedicine 1996; 24(9):88–94.

SKILL 25-1

APPLYING AN ARM SLING

Suggested Action	Reason for Action
Assessment	
Check the medical orders.	Collaborates nursing activities with medical treatment
Assess the color, skin temperature, capillary refill time, and amount of edema, and verify the presence of peripheral pulses in the arm that has been injured (don gloves if there is a potential for contact with blood or nonintact skin).	Provides baseline objective data for future comparisons
Ask the patient to describe how the fingers or arm feel and to rate pain, if it is present, on a scale of 1 to 10.	Provides baseline subjective data for future comparisons
Determine if the patient has required an arm sling in the past.	Indicates the level and type of health teaching needed
Planning	
Explain the purpose for the sling.	Adds to the patient's understanding
Obtain a canvas or triangular sling, whichever is available or prescribed for use.	Complies with medical practice
Implementation	
Have the patient sit or lie down.	Promotes comfort and facilitates applying the sling
Position forearm across the patient's chest with the thumb pointing upward.	Flexes the elbow
Avoid more than 90 degrees of flexion, especially if the elbow has been injured.	Facilitates circulation
Canvas Sling	
Slip the flexed arm into the canvas sling so that the elbow fits flush with the corner of the sling.	Encloses the forearm and wrist
Bring the strap around the opposing shoulder and fasten it to the sling.	Provides the means for support
Tighten the strap sufficiently to keep the elbow flexed and the wrist elevated.	Promotes circulation

continued

SKILL 25-1

APPLYING AN ARM SLING *Continued*

Suggested Action	Reason for Action

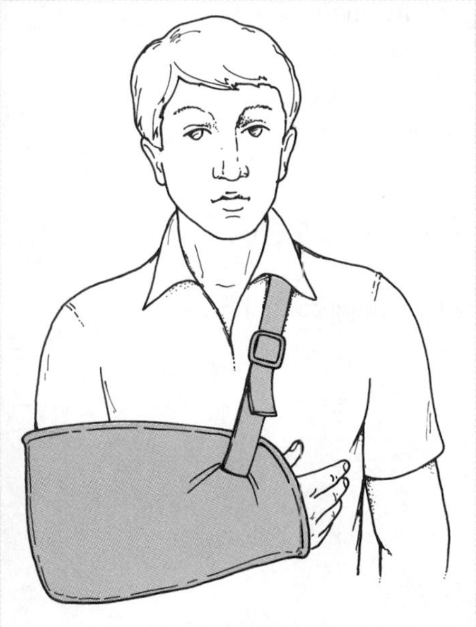

Commercial arm sling.

Triangular Sling

Suggested Action	Reason for Action
Place the longer side of the sling from the shoulder opposite the injured arm to the waist.	Positions the sling where length is needed
Position the apex or point of the triangle under the elbow.	Facilitates making a hammock for the arm
Bring the point at the waist up to join the point at the neck and tie them.	Encloses the injured arm

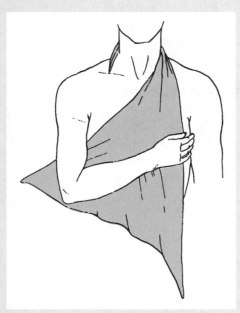

Positioning a triangular sling.

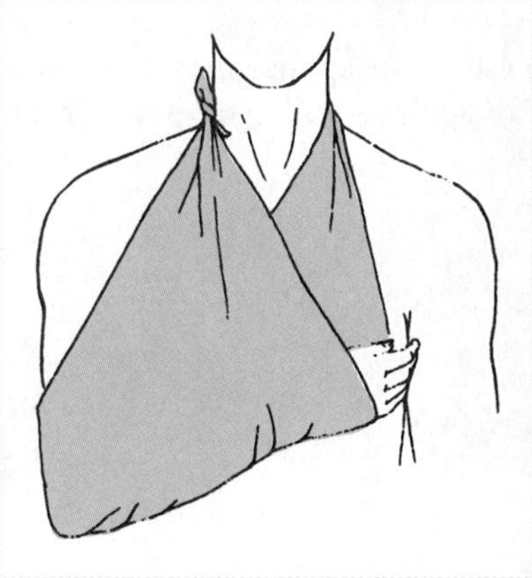

Completed sling.

continued

SKILL 25-1

APPLYING AN ARM SLING *Continued*

Suggested Action	Reason for Action
Position the knot to the side of the neck.	Avoids pressure on the vertebrae
Fold in and secure excess fabric at the elbow; a safety pin may be necessary.	Keeps the elbow enclosed
Inspect the condition of the skin at the neck and the circulation, mobility, and sensation of the fingers at least once per shift.	Provides comparative data
Pad the skin at the neck with soft gauze or towel material if the skin becomes irritated.	Reduces pressure and friction
Tell the patient to report any changes in sensation, especially pain with limited movement or pressure.	Indicates developing complications

Evaluation

- Forearm is supported.
- Wrist is elevated.
- Pain and swelling are reduced.
- Circulation, mobility, and sensation are maintained.

Document

- Baseline and comparative assessment data
- Type of sling applied or used
- To whom significant abnormal assessments were reported
- Outcomes of the verbal report

SAMPLE DOCUMENTATION

Date and Time Fingers on R hand are pale, cool, and swollen. Capillary refill is sluggish, taking 4 sec for color to return. Able to move all fingers. Can discriminate sharp and dull stimuli. No tingling identified. Pain rated at 8 on a scale of 0–10. All above data reported to Dr. Stuckey. Orders received for pain medication and canvas sling. Demerol 75 mg given IM in vastus lateralis. Sling applied. ______________________ SIGNATURE, TITLE

CRITICAL THINKING

- List the advantages and disadvantages of using a commercially made canvas sling and a triangular cloth sling.
- Although slings are applied most often to support injured extremities, discuss possible reasons for applying a sling on an arm paralyzed by a stroke.

SKILL 25-2

ASSISTING WITH A CAST APPLICATION

Suggested Action	Reason for Action
Assessment	
Check the medical orders.	Collaborates nursing activities with medical treatment
Assess the appearance of the skin that will be covered by the cast; also check circulation, mobility, and sensation.	Provides a baseline of data for future comparisons
Ask the patient to describe the location, type, and intensity of pain, if it is present.	Determines whether analgesic medication is needed
Determine what the patient understands about the application of a cast.	Indicates the type of health teaching needed
Check with the physician as to whether a plaster of Paris cast or a fiberglass cast will be applied.	Facilitates assembling appropriate supplies
Planning	
Obtain a signature on a consent for treatment form, if required.	Ensures legal protection
Administer pain medication, if prescribed.	Relieves discomfort
Remove clothing that may not stretch over the cast once it is applied.	Avoids having to cut and destroy clothing
Provide a patient gown.	Preserves dignity and protects clothing
Assemble materials, which may include stockinette, felt padding, cotton batting, rolls of cast material, gloves, and aprons.	Facilitates organization and efficient time management
Anticipate that if the cast is being applied to a lower extremity, the patient may need crutches and instructions on their use (see Chap. 26).	Shows awareness of discharge planning
Have an arm sling available if the cast is being applied to an upper extremity.	Shows awareness of discharge planning
Implementation	
Explain how the cast will be applied. If plaster of Paris is used, be sure to tell the patient that it will feel warm for a period of time.	Reduces anxiety and promotes cooperation
Don gloves and an apron. Provide the physician with the same.	Protects the hands from contact with blood and cast materials
Wash the patient's skin with soap and water and dry well.	Removes dirt, body oil, and some microorganisms
Cover the skin with stockinette, stretchy fabric that comes knitted in a tube.	Protects the skin from direct contact with the cast material
Help the physician apply felt around bony prominences and cotton batting over the stockinette.	Provides a fabric cushion that protects the skin
Open rolls and strips of plaster gauze material. Dip them, one at a time, briefly in water and wring out the excess moisture.	Prepares the cast material for application
If fiberglass material is used, open the foil packets, one at a time.	Reduces the risk of rapidly drying and becoming unfit for use
Support the extremity while the physician wraps the cast material about the arm or leg.	Facilitates going around the injured area

continued

SKILL 25-2

ASSISTING WITH A CAST APPLICATION *Continued*

Suggested Action	Reason for Action
Help to fold back the edges of the stockinette at each end of the cast just before the final layer of cast material is applied.	Forms a smooth, soft edge at the margins of the cast, which may protect the skin from becoming irritated.
Elevate the cast on pillows while it dries.	Prevents flattening due to compression on a hard surface
Dispose of the water in which plaster rolls were soaked in a special sink with a plaster trap.	Prevents clogging of plumbing
Provide verbal and written instructions on cast care.	Facilitates independence and safe self-care

Evaluation

- Skin has been cleaned and protected.
- Cast has been applied and is drying or dried.
- Circulation and sensation are within acceptable parameters.
- Patient can repeat discharge instructions.

Document

- Assessment data
- Type of cast
- Cast material
- Name of physician who applied the cast
- Discharge instructions

SAMPLE DOCUMENTATION

Date and Time Wrist appears swollen but skin is warm, dry, and intact. Capillary refill <3 sec. X-ray Dept. reports a fracture of the wrist. Dr. Roberts notified. Cylinder fiberglass cast applied from middle of hand to above elbow by Dr. Roberts. Assessments remain unchanged after cast application. Casted arm supported in a canvas sling. Standard instructions for cast care provided (see copy attached). Instructed to call Dr. Roberts if pain or swelling increases and make an office appointment in 2 weeks. ______________________ SIGNATURE/TITLE

CRITICAL THINKING

- If you had a choice between having a plaster cast or a fiberglass cast, which would you prefer? Give reasons for your choice.
- Discuss teaching you would provide when discharging a patient who has had a plaster cast applied.

SKILL 25-3

PROVIDING PIN SITE CARE

Suggested Action	Reason for Action
Assessment	
Check the medical orders or standards for care regarding the frequency of pin site care and the preferred cleansing agent.	Demonstrates collaboration with medical treatment
Review the medical record for the trend in the patient's temperature, white blood cell count, reports of pain, and frequency for treating pain.	Uses data that reflects indications of an infection
Inspect the area around the pin insertion site for redness, swelling, increased tenderness, and drainage.	Provides data for current and future comparisons
Examine the pin for signs of bending or shifting.	Identifies potential problems with maintaining traction and desired position
Planning	
Explain the purpose and technique for pin site care to the patient.	Adds to the patient's understanding
Assemble gloves, prescribed cleansing agent (usually hydrogen peroxide or povidone–iodine), and sterile cotton-tipped applicators. Sometimes presaturated swabs are available.	Contributes to organization and efficient time management
Place the bed at a comfortable height.	Prevents back strain
Implementation	
Wash your hands.	Removes transient microorganisms and reduces the transmission of pathogens
Don gloves; clean gloves can be used to hold the stick end of the applicator.	Prevents skin contact with blood or body fluid
Open the package containing cotton-tipped applicators without touching the applicator tips.	Avoids contaminating the point of contact between the applicator tip and the patient's skin
Pour enough cleansing agent to saturate the dry applicators while holding them over a basin or wastebasket.	Prepares applicators for use while maintaining sterility of the applicator tip.
Cleanse the skin at the pin site moving outward in a circular manner.	Prevents moving microorganisms toward the area of open skin.

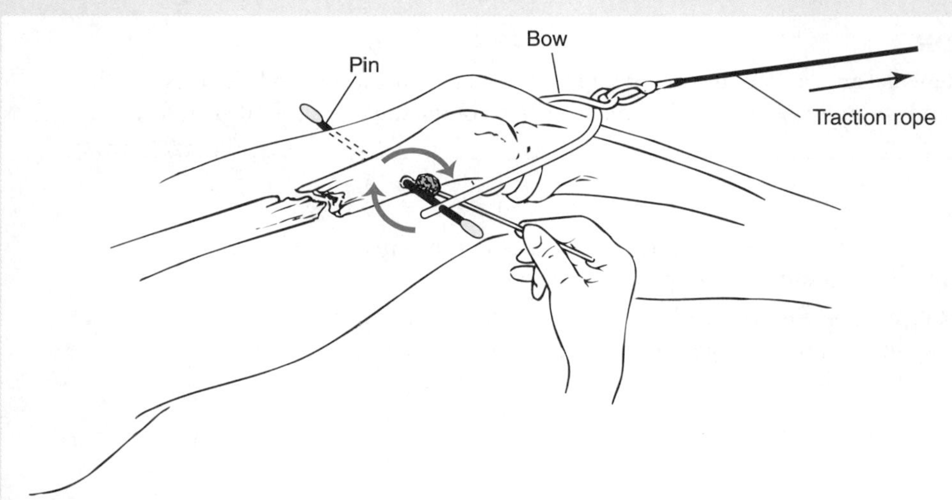

continued

SKILL 25-3

PROVIDING PIN SITE CARE *Continued*

Suggested Action	Reason for Action
Gently remove crusted secretions.	Removes debris that supports the growth of microorganisms
Use a separate applicator for each pin site or if the site needs more than one circular swipe for additional cleansing.	Prevents reintroducing microorganisms into cleaned areas
Avoid applying ointment to pin sites unless prescribed.	Reduces retained moisture at the site and occludes drainage, both of which increase the risk for microbial growth
Check with the physician or infection-control policy about obtaining a wound culture if *purulent drainage* (that which contains pus) is present.	Aids in determining the identity of pathogenic microorganisms and the need to institute infection-control measures such as contact precautions (See Chap. 22)
Teach the patient to not touch the pin sites.	Prevents introducing transient and resident microorganisms into the wound
Discard soiled supplies in an enclosed, lined container; remove gloves; and wash hands.	Demonstrates principles of medical asepsis (See Chap. 21)

Evaluation

- The skin and tissue around the pin site are free of redness, swelling or pain.
- There is no evidence of purulent drainage.
- The patient's temperature and white blood cell count are within normal ranges.

Document

- Date, time, and location of pin site care
- Type of cleansing agent
- Appearance of the pin site and the patient's subjective remarks regarding the presence of tenderness or pain
- Collection of a wound specimen for a culture test, if ordered, and time of its delivery to the laboratory
- To whom abnormal findings were communicated, the content of the reported information, and the response of the caregiver receiving the information

SAMPLE DOCUMENTATION

Date and Time Pin sites on medial and lateral sides of left thigh cleansed with povidone–iodine. Sites appear dry and without evidence of inflammation. No complaints of pain or discomfort.

_______________ SIGNATURE/TITLE

CRITICAL THINKING

- Discuss the information that is reported when a culture and sensitivity test is performed. (Use the information in Chap. 13 as a resource or for purposes of review.)
- If a culture from a specimen taken at the pin site revealed that the pin site was infected with *Staphylococcus aureus,* what nursing actions are required for contact precautions to control the transmission of the pathogen? (Use the information in Chap. 22 as a resource or for purposes of review.)

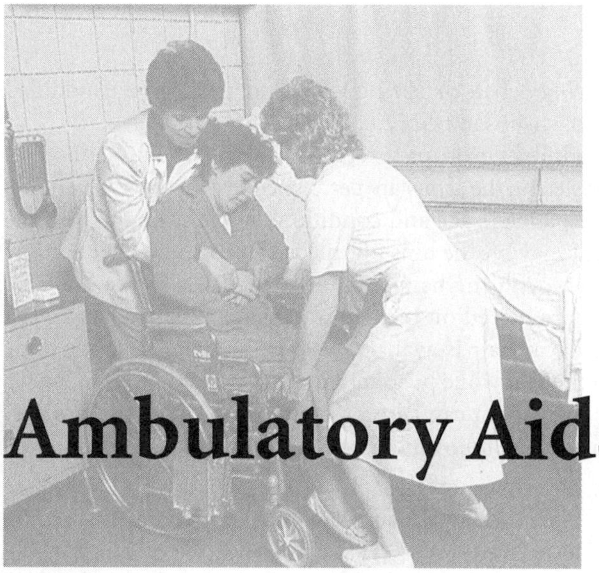

Ambulatory Aids

CHAPTER 26

CHAPTER OUTLINE

Preparing for Ambulation
Assistive Devices
Ambulatory Aids
Prosthetic Limbs
Nursing Implications

NURSING GUIDELINES

ASSISTING PATIENTS TO DANGLE

SKILLS

SKILL 26-1: MEASURING FOR CRUTCHES, CANES, AND WALKERS
SKILL 26-2: ASSISTING WITH CRUTCH-WALKING
SKILL 26-3: APPLYING A LEG PROSTHESIS

NURSING CARE PLAN

IMPAIRED PHYSICAL MOBILITY

KEY TERMS

axillary crutches
cane
crutches
crutch palsy
dangling
forearm crutches
gluteal setting
parallel bars
platform crutches
prosthetic limb
prosthetist
quadriceps setting
strength
tilt table
tone
walker
walking belt

LEARNING OBJECTIVES

An understanding of the content within this chapter will be evidenced by the student's ability to:

- Name four activities that prepare patients for ambulation.
- Give two examples of isometric exercises that tone and strengthen lower extremities.
- Identify one technique for building upper arm strength.
- Explain the reason for dangling patients or using a tilt table.
- Name two devices that are used to assist patients with ambulation.
- Give three examples of ambulatory aids.
- Identify the most stable type of ambulatory aid.
- Describe three characteristics of appropriately fitted crutches.
- Name four types of crutch-walking gaits.
- Explain the purpose of a temporary prosthetic limb.
- Discuss two criteria that must be met before constructing a permanent prosthetic limb.
- Name four components of above-the-knee and below-the-knee prosthetic limbs.
- Describe how a prosthetic limb is applied.
- Discuss age-related changes that affect older adults' gait and ambulation.

Patients with disorders or injuries of the musculoskeletal system and those who are weak or unsteady due to age-related or neurologic problems may have difficulty walking. This chapter provides information on the nursing activities and devices used to promote or enhance mobility.

Preparing for Ambulation

Debilitated patients (those who are frail or weak from prolonged inactivity) require physical conditioning before they can ambulate again. Some techniques for increasing muscular strength and the ability to bear weight include performing isometric exercises with the lower limbs, isotonic exercises with the upper arms, dangling at the bedside, and using a device called a tilt table.

ISOMETRIC EXERCISES

Isometric exercises (see Chap. 24) are used to promote muscle tone and strength. **Tone** (ability of muscles to respond when stimulated) and **strength** (power to perform) are inherent in preserving the ability to maintain mobility. Muscle tone and strength are retained or improved by frequently contracting muscle fibers. Active people maintain these two qualities through their everyday activities, but inactive people and those who have been immobilized in a cast or traction may require focused periods of exercise to re-establish their previous ability to walk. Quadriceps setting and gluteal setting exercises are two types of isometric exercises that promote tone and strength in weightbearing muscles.

Quadriceps setting (isometric exercise in which the quadriceps muscles are alternately tensed and relaxed) is sometimes referred to as "quad setting." The quadriceps muscles (rectus femoris, vastus intermedius, vastus medialis, and vastus lateralis) cover the front and side of the thigh. Together they aid in extending the leg. Exercising the quadriceps muscles, therefore, enables patients to stand and support their body weight.

Gluteal setting (isometric exercise that strengthens and tones the gluteal muscles) contracts and relaxes the gluteal muscles (gluteus maximus, gluteus medius, and gluteus minimus). As a group, the muscles in the buttocks aid in extending, abducting, and rotating the leg—functions that are essential to walking.

Quadriceps and gluteal setting exercises are easily performed in bed or in a chair. They are initiated long before the anticipated time when ambulation will start. Most patients can perform these exercises independently once they have been instructed.

Patient Teaching For

Quadriceps and Gluteal Setting Exercises

Teach the patient to do the following:

- Tighten (contract) the quadriceps muscles by flattening the backs of the knees into the mattress. If that is not possible, place a rolled towel under the knee or heel before attempting to tighten the quadriceps muscles.
- Check to see that the kneecaps move upward. This is an indication that the exercise is being performed correctly.
- Hold the contracted position for a count of five.
- Relax and repeat two or three times each hour.
- Tighten (contract) the gluteal muscles by pinching the cheeks of the buttocks together.
- Hold the contracted position for a count of five.
- Relax and repeat two or three times each hour.

UPPER ARM STRENGTHENING

Upper arm strength is needed by patients who will be using a walker, cane, or crutches. An exercise regimen to strengthen the upper arms typically includes flexion and extension of the arms and wrists, raising and lowering weights with the hands, squeezing a ball or spring grip, and performing modified hand push-ups in bed (Fig. 26-1).

Modified push-ups (exercises in which the upper body is supported on the arms) are performed several ways, depending on the patient's age and condition. While sitting in bed, the patient may lift the hips off the bed by pushing down on the mattress with the hands. If the mattress is soft, a block or books are placed on the bed under the patient's hands. If a sturdy armchair is available, the patient can raise the body from the seat while pushing on the arm rests.

If the patient can lie on the abdomen, push-ups are performed in the following sequence:

1. Flex the elbows.
2. Place the hands, palms down, at approximately shoulder level.
3. Straighten the elbows to lift the head and chest off the bed.

To be effective, push-ups are performed three or four times a day.

DANGLING

Dangling (sitting on the edge of the bed; Fig. 26-2) helps to normalize the blood pressure, which may drop when the patient rises from a reclining position (see the section on postural hypotension in Chap. 11).

Nursing Guidelines For

Assisting Patients to Dangle

- ☑ Perform dangling before ambulating whenever a patient has been inactive for an extended period.
  RATIONALE: Performing dangling before ambulating demonstrates a concern for patient safety.
- ☑ Place the patient in a Fowler's position for a few minutes.
  RATIONALE: The Fowler's position maintains safety should the patient become dizzy or faint.

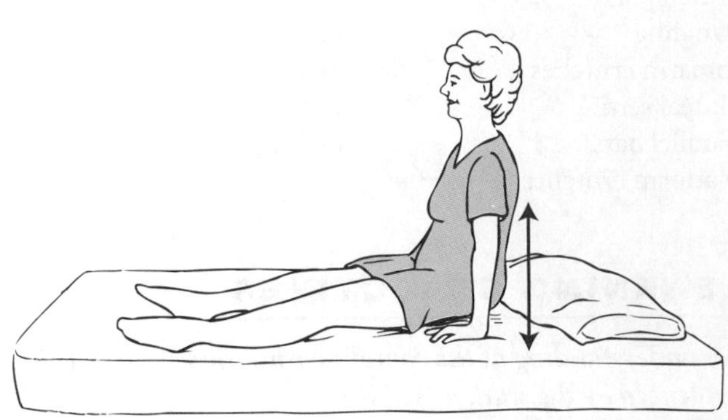

FIGURE 26–1. Modified hand push-ups are performed by extending the elbows and flexing the wrists to lift the buttocks slightly off the mattress.

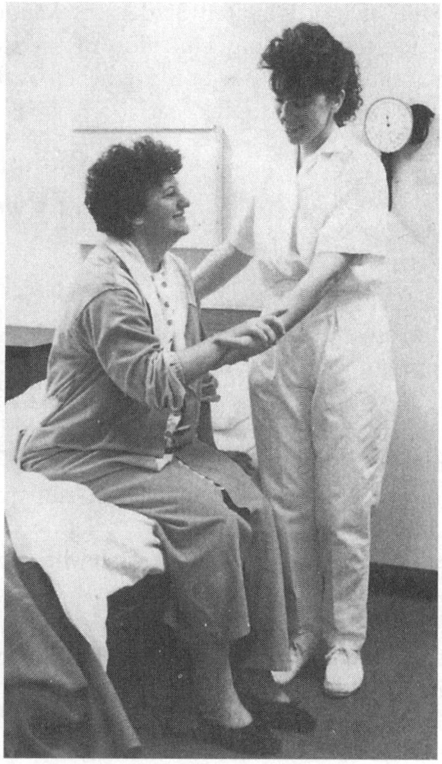

FIGURE 26–2. Dangling. (Courtesy of Ken Timby.)

☑ Lower the height of the bed.
RATIONALE: With a lowered bed, the patient can use the floor for support.

☑ Provide a footstool if the patient's feet do not reach the floor.
RATIONALE: A footstool is an alternative for supporting the feet.

☑ Fold back the top linen.
RATIONALE: Linen can interfere with movement.

☑ Provide the patient with a robe and slippers.
RATIONALE: Providing a robe and slippers maintains warmth and shows respect for the patient's modesty.

☑ Help the patient pivot a quarter of a turn to swing the legs over the side and sit on the edge of the bed.
RATIONALE: This position helps the patient adjust to the sitting position.

☑ Stay with the patient until he or she no longer feels dizzy or light-headed.
RATIONALE: The nurse can provide immediate assistance.

USING A TILT TABLE

A **tilt table** (device that raises the patient from a supine to standing position) helps patients adjust to being upright and bearing weight on their feet. Although the tilt table is usually located in the physical therapy department, nurses often prepare the patient for this type of preambulation therapy and communicate with the therapists about the patient's response.

Just before using a tilt table, the nurse applies elastic stockings (see the section on antiembolism stockings in Chap. 27). These stockings help compress vein walls, thus preventing pooling of blood in the extremities, which may trigger fainting.

After being transferred from the bed or stretcher to the horizontal tilt table, the patient is strapped securely to prevent a fall. The feet are positioned against the foot rest. The entire table is then tilted in increments of 15 to 30 degrees until the patient is in a vertical position. If symptoms develop, the table is lowered or returned to the horizontal position.

Assistive Devices

Even after performing strengthening exercises, some patients still need assistance to ambulate independently. Two devices used to provide support and assistance with walking are parallel bars and a walking belt.

Parallel bars (double row of stationary bars) are used as handrails by patients to gain practice in ambulating. Sometimes the tilt table is positioned just in front of the parallel bars so that the patient can progress from being upright to actually walking again.

A **walking belt** (device used to assist an ambulating patient) has handles at the side and back (Fig. 26-3). If the patient loses balance, the nurse can support him or her and prevent injuries.

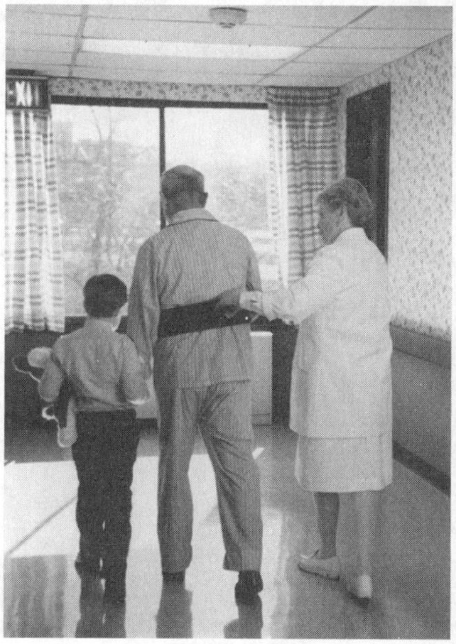

FIGURE 26–3. Using a walking belt. (© 1994 Total Care, Gaithersburg, MD.)

When assisting a patient to ambulate, the nurse walks alongside the patient, holding the handles of the walking belt or the patient's own belt, supporting the patient's arm. The nurse observes for pallor, weakness, or dizziness. If fainting seems likely, the nurse supports the patient by sliding an arm under the axilla and placing a foot to the side, forming a wide base of support. With the patient's weight braced, the nurse balances the patient on a hip until help arrives or slides the patient down the length of the nurse's leg to the floor.

Ambulatory Aids

Three aids are used to help with ambulation: canes, walkers, and crutches.

CANES

A **cane** (hand-held ambulation device) is used by patients who have weakness on one side of their body. Canes are made of wood or aluminum; aluminum ones are more common. Canes have rubber tips to reduce the potential for slipping.

Patients may use different types of canes, depending on their physical deficits. A T-handle cane has a hand grip with a slightly bent shaft, offering the user more stability. A quad cane has four supports at the base and provides even more stability than the other types (Fig. 26-4).

A cane must be the right height for the patient. The cane's handle should be parallel with the patient's hip, providing elbow flexion of approximately 30 degrees. Wooden canes are shortened by removing a portion of the lower end. Aluminum canes are shortened or lengthened by depressing metal buttons in the telescoping shaft.

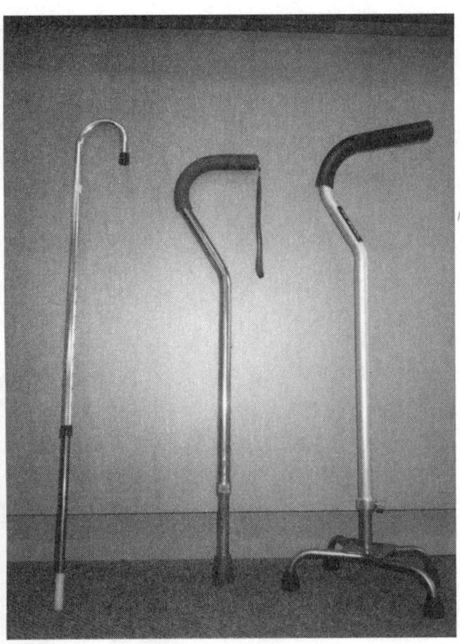

FIGURE 26–4. Straight, T-handle, and quad cane. (Courtesy of Ken Timby.)

Patient Teaching For
Using a Cane

Teach the patient to do the following:

- Place the cane on the stronger side of the body.
- Stand upright with the cane 4″ to 6″ (10 to 15 cm) to the side of the toes.
- Move the cane forward at the same time as the weaker extremity.
- Take the next step with the stronger extremity.
- When Using Stairs
  - Use a stair rail rather than the cane when going up or down stairs, if possible.
  - Take each step up with the stronger leg, followed by the weaker one. Reverse the pattern for descending the stairs.
  - If there is no stair rail, advance the cane just before rising or descending with the weaker leg.
- When Sitting
  - Back up to the chair until the seat is against the back of the legs.
  - Rest the cane close by.
  - Grip the arm rests with both hands.
  - Sit down.
- When Getting Up From a Chair
  - Grip the arm rests while holding the cane in the stronger hand.
  - Advance the stronger leg.
  - Lean forward.
  - Push with both arms against the arm rests.
  - Stand until balanced and any symptoms of dizziness pass.

When patients are beginning to use a cane, the nurse assists by applying a walking belt and standing toward the back of the patient's stronger side.

WALKERS

A **walker** (most stable form of ambulatory aid) is used by patients who require considerable support and assistance with balance. Patients who are beginning to ambulate after prolonged bed rest or after hip surgery often use a walker initially.

Standard walkers are constructed of curved aluminum bars that form a three-sided enclosure, with four legs for support. Some have front wheels (Fig. 26-5) or a seat. Other

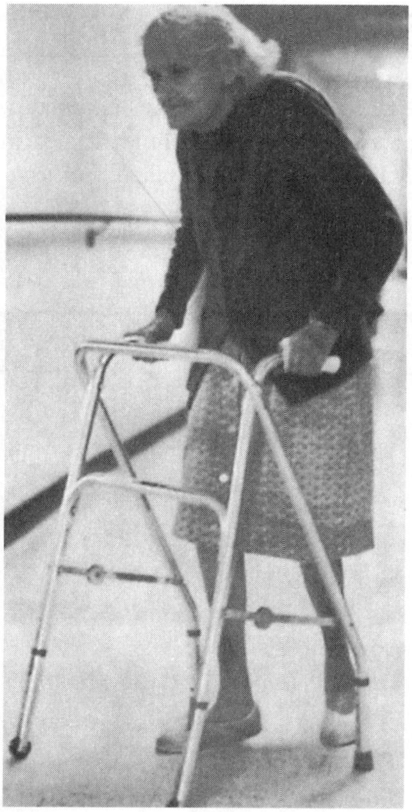

FIGURE 26–5. Using a walker with wheels.

adaptations are made for patients who have compromised use of one or both arms or those who must use stairs. The height of a walker is adjusted, as for canes.

When using a walker, patients are instructed to:

- Stand within the walker.
- Hold on to the walker at the padded hand grips.
- Pick up the walker and advance it 6″ to 8″ (15 to 20 cm).
- Take a step forward.
- Support the body weight on the hand grips when moving the weaker leg (for patients with partial or nonweightbearing on one leg).

When the patient with a walker wants to sit down, the technique is similar to that with a cane, with one exception. When the legs are at the front of the chair seat, the patient grips an arm rest with one arm while using the other hand on the walker and the stronger leg for support. The patient releases the grip on the walker while using the free hand to grasp the opposite arm rest and lower himself or herself into the chair. To rise, the patient moves to the edge of the chair and repositions the walker. After pushing up on the arm rests with both arms until the body weight is centered, one hand is used to grasp the walker, then the other.

CRUTCHES

Crutches (ambulatory aid generally used in pairs) are constructed of wood or aluminum. Because the use of crutches requires a great deal of upper arm strength and balance, they are not commonly used by older adults or weak patients.

The three basic types of crutches are axillary, forearm, and platform crutches (Fig. 26-6). **Axillary crutches** (standard type of crutches) have a bar that fits beneath the axilla; this is the most familiar type. Patients who need brief, temporary assistance with ambulation are likely to use axillary crutches. **Forearm crutches** (crutches that have an arm cuff but no axillary bar) include Lofstrand and Canadian crutches. Forearm crutches are generally used by experienced patients who need permanent assistance with walking. **Platform crutches** (crutches that support the forearm) are used by patients who cannot bear weight with their hands and wrists. Many patients with arthritis use them. Sometimes a patient uses one axillary crutch and one platform crutch—for example, when one arm is broken.

Once the type of ambulatory aid is medically prescribed, the patient is measured (Skill 26-1).

CRUTCH-WALKING GAITS

The term *gait* refers to one's manner of walking. A crutch-walking gait is the walking pattern used when ambulating with crutches, but some of the same gaits are used with a walker or cane.

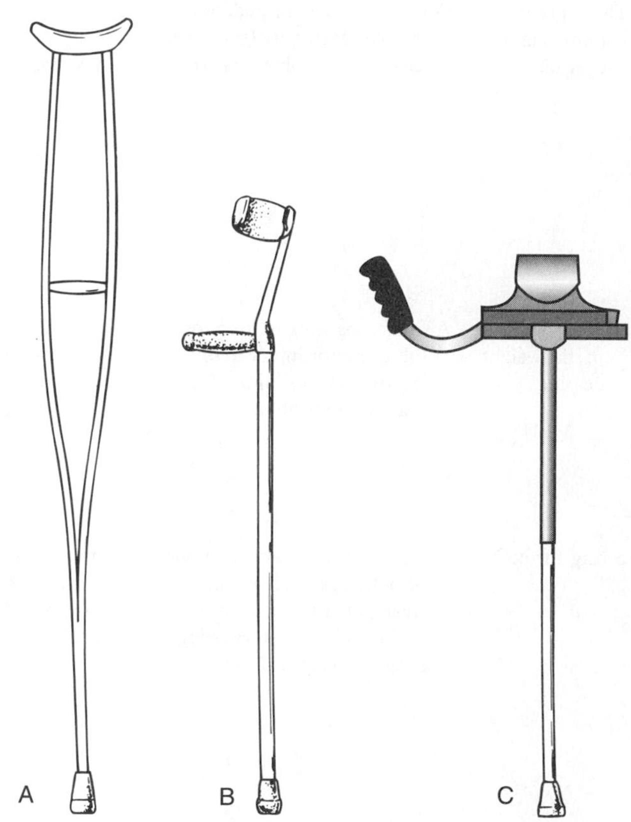

FIGURE 26–6. Three types of crutches: (*A*) axillary, (*B*) forearm, and (*C*) platform.

There are four types of crutch-walking gaits: four-point gait, three-point gait (non-weightbearing or partial weight-bearing), two-point gait, and swing-through gait (Table 26-1). The word *point* refers to the sum of the crutches and legs used when performing the gait. Nurses are responsible for assisting patients who are learning to walk with crutches (Skill 26-2).

Prosthetic Limbs

Some patients with leg amputations ambulate without the assistance of crutches or other ambulatory aids, instead using a **prosthetic limb** (substitute for an arm or leg). The design

TABLE 26–1. **Crutch-Walking Gaits**

Gait	Indications for Use	Gait Pattern	Illustration
Four-point	Bilateral weakness or disability such as arthritis or cerebral palsy	One crutch, opposite foot, other crutch, remaining foot	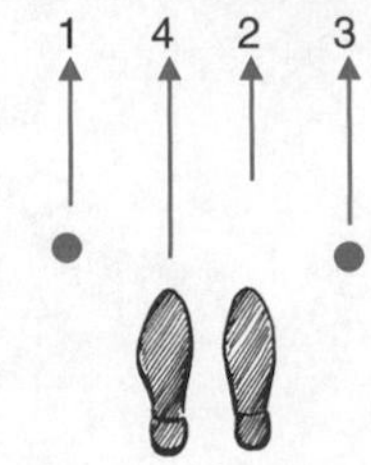
Two-point	Same as for four-point, but patients have more strength, coordination, and balance	One crutch and opposite foot moved in unison, followed by the remaining pair	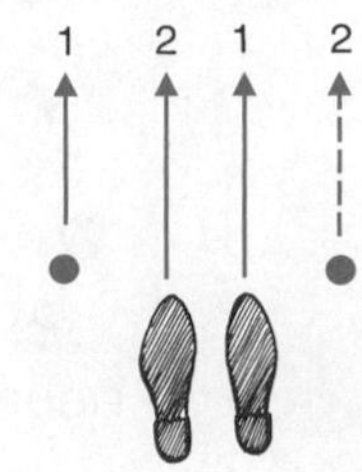
Three-point non-weight-bearing	One amputated, injured, or disabled extremity (fractured leg or severe ankle sprain)	Both crutches move forward followed by the weight-bearing leg	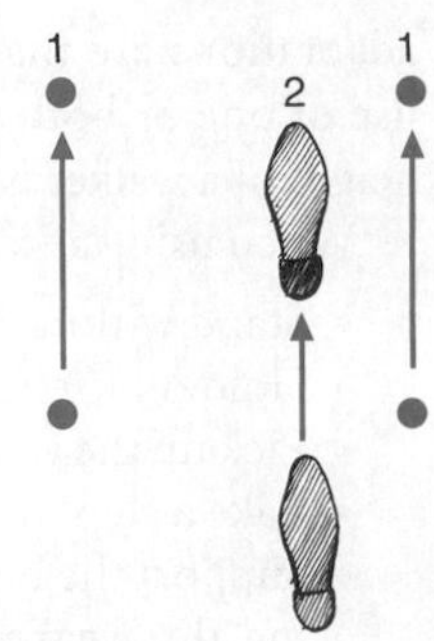
Three-point partial weight-bearing	Amputee learning to use prosthesis, minor injury to one leg, or previous injury showing signs of healing	Both crutches are advanced with weaker leg; stronger leg is placed parallel to weaker leg	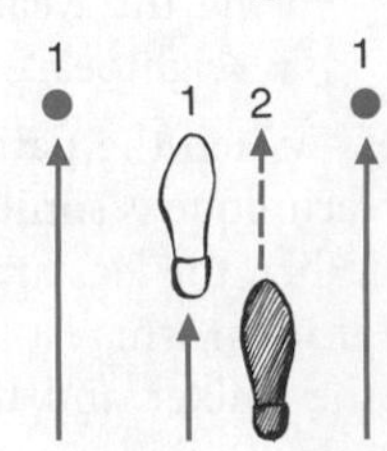
Swing-through	Injury or disorder affecting one or both legs, such as a paralyzed patient with leg braces or an amputee before being fitted with a prosthesis	Both crutches are moved forward; one or both legs are advanced beyond the crutches.	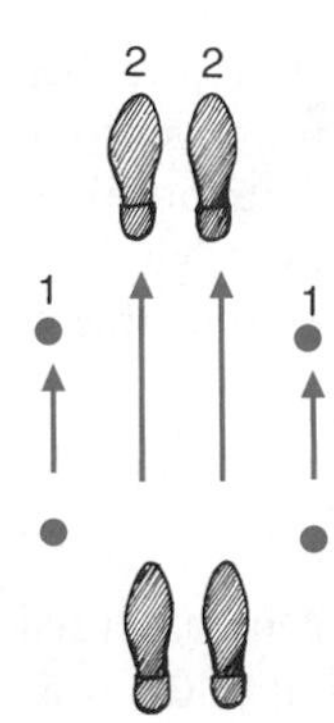 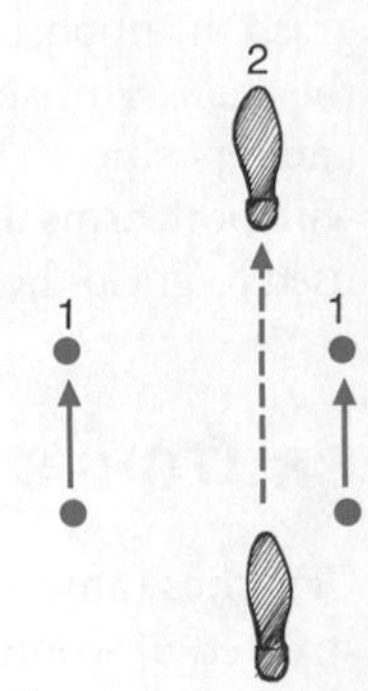

of a prosthetic limb varies depending on whether the lower extremity is amputated at the foot (Symes amputation), below-the-knee (BK amputation), or above-the-knee (AK amputation), or whether the entire leg and a portion of the hip (hemipelvectomy) is removed.

TEMPORARY PROSTHETIC LIMB

In most cases, patients return from surgery with a temporary prosthetic limb. It consists of a walking pylon, a lightweight tube, attached to a plaster shell on the stump and a rigid foot (Fig. 26-7). A belt keeps the temporary prosthesis in place. The belt is loosened while the patient is in bed and is tightened during ambulation. The temporary prosthesis facilitates early ambulation and promotes an intact body image immediately after surgery. It also helps control stump swelling.

The nurse is responsible for ensuring that the incision heals and that no complications, such as joint contractures or infection, develop. Complications delay rehabilitation. Contractures interfere with limb and prosthetic alignment, which ultimately affects the patient's ability to walk.

PERMANENT PROSTHETIC COMPONENTS

Construction of a permanent prosthesis is delayed for several weeks or months until the wound heals and the stump size is relatively stable. The permanent prosthesis is custom-made to conform to the stump and to meet the patient's needs.

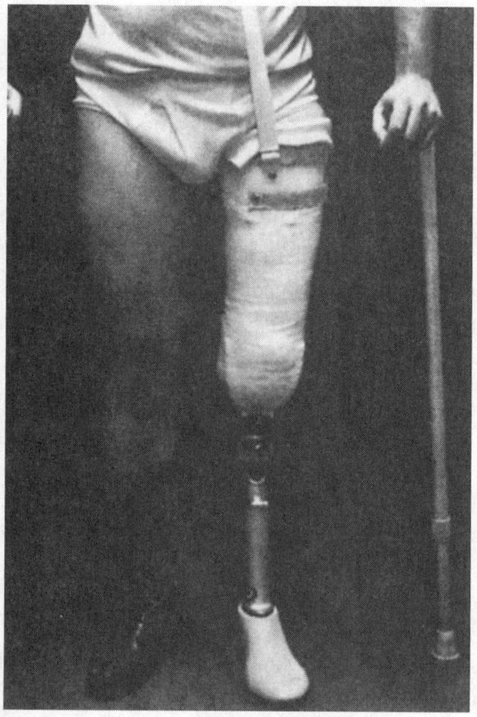

FIGURE 26–7. Example of a temporary prosthetic limb. (Timby BK, Scherer JC, Smith NE. Introductory medical-surgical nursing, 7th ed. Philadelphia. Lippincott Williams and Wilkins, 1999.)

Permanent prostheses for BK amputees include a socket, a shank, and an ankle/foot system (Fig. 26-8). AK prostheses also include a knee system to replace the knee joint.

The socket, a molded cone, holds the stump and enables the amputee to move the prosthesis. It is held in place by suction or by a leather belt, also referred to as a sling. Many patients wear one or more socks over the stump as a layer between the skin and the socket. Stump socks, made of wool or cotton, come in a variety of thicknesses to accommodate slight changes in stump size. Tube socks are not an appropriate substitute. Despite the expense, stump socks must be replaced whenever holes develop or they become worn: a darned stump sock can cause skin breakdown as a result of friction within the socket. Some amputees also wear a nylon sheath beneath the stump sock to wick perspiration from the skin toward the sock and reduce friction on the skin.

For AK amputees, the prosthetic knee system allows flexion and extension to accommodate sitting and a natural gait while walking. The knee system connects the socket to the shank of the prosthesis.

The shank is usually shaped like a natural lower leg. It transfers the body weight to the walking surface. The shank is painted to resemble the patient's skin color.

There are two basic types of ankle/foot systems: those that have one or more moving artificial joints (articulated systems) and those that do not. Although articulated systems allow more motion, the nonarticulated type has a cushion in the heel that permits compression during walking. The patient wears a sock and shoe on the prosthetic foot. The patient can vary his or her shoes, but all should be of similar height to ensure alignment of the prosthesis and a near-normal gait pattern.

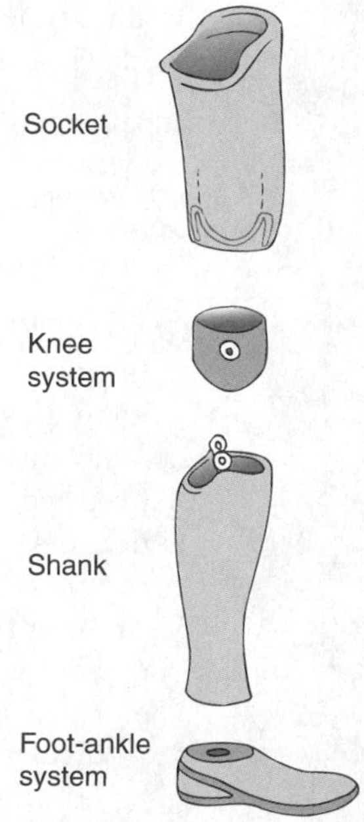

FIGURE 26–8. Components of a permanent prosthetic limb; a prosthesis for a BK amputation does not contain a knee system.

PATIENT CARE

Nurses are responsible for managing the care of the stump and ensuring that the prosthesis is maintained (Skill 26-3).

AMBULATION WITH A LIMB PROSTHESIS

Ambulation with a prosthesis requires strength and endurance. The more natural joints that are preserved, the more natural the gait appears and the more easily it is performed. To ensure as normal a gait as possible, patients are taught to stand erect and look ahead when walking. The feet are kept close together and each step is taken without hiking the hip unnaturally to swing the artificial limb forward. If a cane is used, it is held in the hand opposite the prosthetic limb. When going up or down stairs, curbs, or hills, the unaffected leg is moved first, followed by the one with the prosthesis.

A sturdier modified prosthesis can be used by amputees who wish to participate in strenuous activities such as snow skiing.

Nursing Implications

Many nursing diagnoses are possible for patients who need to use an ambulatory aid. Applicable nursing diagnoses include:

- Impaired physical mobility
- Risk for disuse syndrome
- Unilateral neglect
- Risk for trauma
- Risk for peripheral neurovascular dysfunction
- Risk for activity intolerance

The nursing care plan demonstrates how a care plan is devised for a patient with the nursing diagnosis of Impaired physical mobility, defined in the NANDA taxonomy (1999) as "a limitation in independent, purposeful physical movement of the body or of one or more extremities." This diagnosis can be used for patients who are completely independent; those who require help from another person for assistance, supervision, or teaching; those who require help from another person for assistance and a device; or those who are totally dependent (NANDA, 1999).

Nursing Care Plan

Impaired Physical Mobility

Assessment

Subjective Data

States, "I wish I could just get up and move around. My hip hurts and I feel so scared about walking."

Objective Data

70-year-old man admitted for a L. total hip replacement done on 2/7. Must maintain limited flexion of operative hip and continuous abduction of operative leg. Scheduled for physical therapy instruction on performing a three-point partial weightbearing gait 2/10.

Diagnosis

Impaired physical mobility related to restricted positioning, limited weightbearing, pain, and fear

Plan

Goal

The patient will ambulate 6 feet with the assistance of a walker by 2/10.

Orders: 2/9

1. Instruct and supervise dorsiflexion, plantar flexion, and quad-setting exercises of both legs q 1 h while awake.
2. Maintain abduction wedge between legs to keep knees apart at all times while in bed.
3. Keep bed flat or with slight elevation (30°–45°) of head.
4. Encourage use of patient-controlled analgesia (PCA) pump at frequent intervals to control pain.
5. Transfer from bed to standing position at the bedside, following these directions:
   a. Slide affected L. leg to edge of bed; remove abduction wedge.
   b. Have patient use trapeze or elbows and hands to slide buttocks and legs perpendicular to bed. Remind to avoid leaning forward and praise efforts at moving.
   c. Lower unaffected R. foot to floor and help with lowering affected L. foot, keeping knees apart. Dangle at bedside for approximately 5 minutes.

continued

Nursing Care Plan

Impaired Physical Mobility Continued

d. Apply safety belt around waist.
e. Brace feet and pull forward on belt.
f. Stand at bedside, putting only partial weight on L. leg.
g. Reverse actions for returning to bed. ________________ D. FENTON, RN

Implementation (Documentation)

2/9 0730 Positioned from back to R. side with abduction wedge between legs. ________________ F. CLINTON, LPN

0930 Positioned on back with head of bed raised 45° for breakfast. Active isotonic and isometric (quad-setting) exercises done. Assisted with bathing legs and back. Complaining of sharp, throbbing pain in L. hip. Encouraged to use PCA pump. Pain reduced after administration of morphine by PCA pump. ________________ F. CLINTON, LPN

1000 Assisted to transfer out of bed and stand at bedside following procedure outlined in written plan of care. ________________ F. CLINTON, LPN

Evaluation (Documentation)

1030 Follows directions well when transferring from bed. Needs frequent reminding to lean backward. Alternated full weightbearing on R. leg with partial weightbearing on L. States, "That was easier than I imagined." Assisted back to bed, keeping knees apart and hips slightly flexed. Abduction splint reapplied. ________________ F. CLINTON, LPN

FOCUS ON OLDER ADULTS

- Some older adults have limited or unsteady mobility because of age-related postural changes. Older adults tend to acquire flexion of the spine as they get older, which alters their center of gravity.
- Older adults tend to compensate for skeletal changes by flexing their hips and knees to accommodate for the shift in their center of gravity.
- Older adults often develop a swaying or shuffling gait because of postural changes.
- If an unusual gait is noted, the patient's feet are checked because some problems may be caused by corns, calluses, bunions, and ingrown or very long toenails. In these situations, a referral for podiatry care is warranted.
- Walking belts, also called gait belts, are an important safety device for older adults who need assistance with transferring, even if they are not ambulatory.
- Before discharging an older adult who will be using an ambulatory aid, an evaluation of the home's safety is recommended. Permission should be gained from the older adult to remove scatter rugs (or replace them with secure mats), to make sure there are no electric cords in passageways, and to evaluate for adequate lighting. Also, furniture needs to be rearranged to allow for adequate passageways, and outside entrances should have railings or grab bars.
- Older adults who require ambulatory aids may also have difficulty getting on and off toilet seats; an elevated toilet seat and grab bars improve the person's ability to transfer safely and independently.
- A home evaluation by a physical or occupational therapist is helpful in assessing and recommending adaptations and devices to improve safety, mobility, and independent function. This service may be covered by the older adult's health insurance plan.
- Assessment of an older adult's attitude toward the use of assistive devices is important because attitudes are likely to influence the acceptability of using recommended aids. If an older adult refuses to use an aid because it signifies dependence and loss of vitality to him or her, the nurse can emphasize that the purpose of assistive devices is to promote safety and independence and to prevent a decline in function.
- Older adults who have difficulty going up and down stairs may consider rearranging their homes so all necessary furnishings are on one level. A bedside commode decreases the number of trips up and down stairs if the bathroom is not on the same level as the bedrooms or living area.
- A ramp helps older adults enter and leave their residence more conveniently and safely when they are using an ambulatory aid.
- Older adults sometimes use a "stop-stop" pattern when using an ambulatory aid—that is, they take one step, then stop, and repeat again. If that is the case, a smooth, progressive cadence should be encouraged.
- Some older adults develop the habit of picking up and carrying a walker rather than having it make contact with the floor. In these situations the person may benefit from another type of walker, such as a walker with wheels or a three-wheeled walker. A physical therapist can assess the situation and recommend an appropriate walker.
- Rubber tips and handgrips on ambulatory aids should be kept clean and replaced when they are worn. Worn or dirty tips and handgrips contribute to falls and unsafe mobility.

KEY CONCEPTS

- Activities that help prepare patients for ambulation include performing isometric exercises with the lower limbs, strengthening the upper arms, dangling at the bedside, and using a tilt table.
- Two isometric exercises that tone and strengthen the lower extremities are quadriceps setting and gluteal setting.
- The upper arms are strengthened by a regimen of flexing and extending the arms and wrists, raising and lowering weights with the hands, squeezing a ball or spring grip, and performing modified hand push-ups while in a bed or chair.
- Patients dangle or are placed on a tilt table to normalize their blood pressure and help them adjust to being upright.
- Parallel bars and walking belts are devices used to assist patients with ambulation.
- Three types of ambulatory aids are canes, walkers, and crutches.
- Walkers are the most stable form of ambulatory aid. Straight canes are the least stable.
- Crutches should permit the patient to stand upright with the shoulders relaxed, provide space for two fingers between the axilla and the axillary bar, and facilitate approximately 30 degrees of elbow flexion and slight hyperextension of the wrist.
- A temporary prosthesis facilitates early ambulation, promotes an intact body image, and controls stump swelling immediately after surgery.
- The permanent prosthesis is constructed when the surgical wound heals and the stump size is relatively stable.
- Components of permanent prostheses for BK amputees are a socket, a shank, and an ankle/foot system; AK prostheses also include a knee system.
- To apply a prosthetic limb, the patient covers the stump with an optional nylon sheath, over which one or more stump socks are applied. A nylon stocking is used to ease the sock-covered stump into the socket and is eventually removed. The patient pumps the stump within the socket to expel air and create a vacuum seal. If the socket has supportive belts or slings, they are fastened when the stump is well seated in the socket.
- Older adults tend to acquire flexion of the spine as they get older; this may alter their center of gravity. They tend to compensate by flexing their hips and knees when walking and may have a swaying or shuffling gait.

CRITICAL THINKING EXERCISES

- If you needed to use an ambulatory aid, which type would you prefer, and why? Which type would be least appealing to you, and why?
- Discuss stereotypes of people who use ambulatory aids.

SUGGESTED READINGS

Burger H, Marincek C, Isakov E. Mobility of persons after traumatic lower limb amputation. Disability and Rehabilitation 1997;19(7):272–277.

Campbell BA. Vasovagal syncope and head upright tilt table testing. Critical Care Nursing Quarterly 1994;17(3):27–34.

Canes and crutches. Postgraduate Medicine 1998;104(2):187–188.

Canes, walkers and crutches: don't let choosing one throw you off balance. Mayo Clinic Health Letter 1999;17(1):4.

Cherniack EP, Caprio D, Fischer AA, Tuckman J. A novel device for walking training in elderly patients. Physiotherapy 1999;85(3):144–148.

Finkel J, Fernie G, Cleghorn W. A guideline for the design of a four-wheeled walker. Assistive Technology 1997;9(2):116–129.

Fisher K, Hanapal R. Body image and patients with amputations: does the prosthesis maintain the balance? International Journal of Rehabilitation Research 1998;21(4):355–363.

Foley MP, Prax B, Crowell R, Boone T. Effects of assistive devices on cardiorespiratory demands in older adults. Physical Therapy 1996;76(12): 1113–1119.

Gabauer E. Walkers often interfere with carrying things. Home Health Focus 1996;3(6):43.

Kumor R, Roe MC, Scremin OU. Methods for estimating the proper length of a cane. Archives of Physical Medicine and Rehabilitation 1995;76(12): 173–1175.

Lilja M, Oberg T. Proper time for definitive transtibial prosthetic fitting. Journal of Psychosocial Oncology 1997;9(2):90–95.

Lu C, Yu B, Basford JR, Johnson ME, An K. Influences of cane length on the stability of stroke patients. Journal of Rehabilitation Research and Development 1997;34(1):91–100.

Mann WC, Granger C, Hummen D, Tomita M, Charvat B. An analysis of problems with canes encountered by elderly persons. Physical and Occupational Therapy in Geriatrics 1995;13(1):25–49.

Muilenberg Al, Wilson AB Jr. A manual for above-knee amputees. Topping, VA, 1996. http://www.oandp.com/manuals/index.htm, accessed 8/26/99.

Muilenberg Al, Wilson AB Jr. A Manual for Below-Knee Amputees. Topping, VA, 1996. http://www.oandp.com/manuals/index.htm, accessed 8/26/99.

NANDA nursing diagnoses: definitions and classification, 1999–2000. Philadelphia: NANDA, 1999.

Nichols PH. Cane or walker: which is better for your patient? RN 1997; 60(7):65.

Pippin K, Fernie GR. Designing devices that are acceptable to the frail elderly: a new understanding based upon how older people perceive a walker. Technology and Disability 1997;7(1):93–102.

Raikin S, Froimson MI. Bilateral brachial plexus compressive neuropathy (crutch palsy). Journal of Orthopaedic Trauma 1997;11(2):136–138.

Stewart KB, Murry HC. How to use crutches correctly. Nursing 1997; 27(5):32hn20–22.

Stewart KB, Murry HC. How to use a walker correctly. Nursing 1998; 28(9):32hn22–23.

Walkers & riders. Consumer Reports 1998;63(1):26–29.

Yeltzer EA. Helping the patient through the experience of amputation. Orthopedic Nursing 1996;15:45.

SKILL 26–1

MEASURING FOR CRUTCHES, CANES, AND WALKERS

Suggested Action	Reason for Action
Assessment	
Check the medical orders.	Collaborates nursing activities with medical treatment
Determine the type of ambulatory aid the patient will use.	Indicates the type of measurements needed
Check agency policy about personnel responsible for measuring and dispensing ambulatory aids.	Complies with agency procedures; inpatients are sometimes referred to personnel in the physical therapy department.
Determine the strength of the patient's arm and leg muscles.	Indicates the patient's potential for weightbearing; weakness suggests a need to measure the patient in bed or for further collaboration with the physician concerning muscle strengthening.
Planning	
Obtain a long tape measure.	Facilitates measuring patients with a range of heights
Assist the patient with donning socks and walking shoes, if the patient can stand for the measurement.	Aids in more accurate measurement that accommodates added height of the heel
Implementation	
Axillary Crutches	
Assist the patient who can support his or her body weight to a standing position at the bedside with supportive shoes.	Positions the patient in a posture for actual use of crutches
Measure from the anterior skinfold of the axilla to approximately 6″ to 8″ (15 to 20 cm) diagonally from the foot.	Approximates the length required for appropriate use

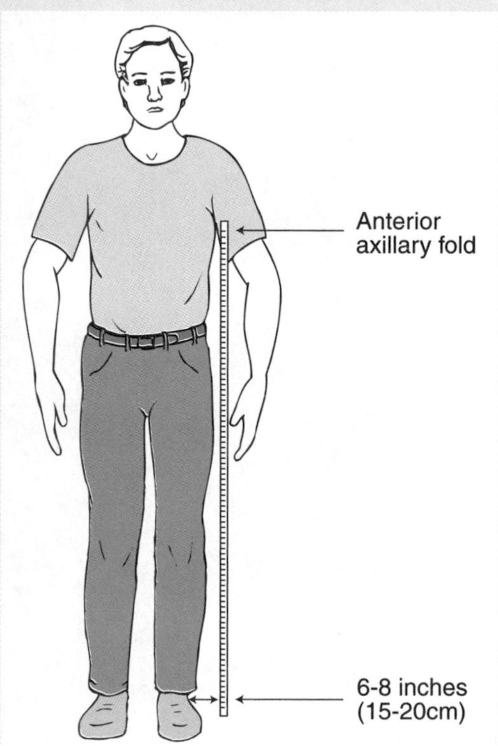

Measuring for crutches in a standing position.

continued

SKILL 26-1

MEASURING FOR CRUTCHES, CANES, AND WALKERS *Continued*

Suggested Action	Reason for Action
Place a patient who is weak in a supine position.	Simulates the patient's height in a standing position
Measure the distance from the anterior skinfold of the axilla to heel and add 2″ (5 cm), or subtract 16″ (40 cm) from the patient's height.	Accommodates for the added height of the heel

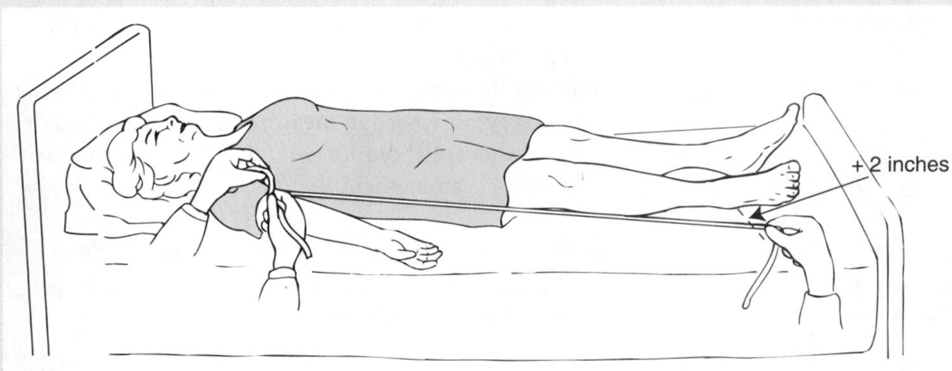

Measuring for crutches in a supine position.

Suggested Action	Reason for Action
Adjust the hand grips so there is 30° of elbow flexion and 15° of wrist hyperextension when patient grasps the handgrips standing upright.	Ensures the potential for extending the elbow and supporting body weight

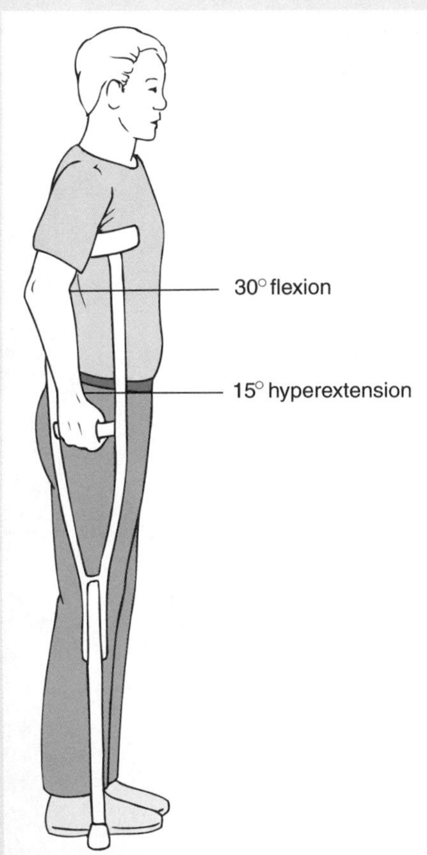

Appropriate position for handgrips.

continued

SKILL 26–1

MEASURING FOR CRUTCHES, CANES, AND WALKERS *Continued*

Suggested Action	Reason for Action
Lengthen or shorten axillary crutches by removing wing nuts and replacing metal screws in the appropriate hole in the stem of the crutch; adjust hand grips in the same way.	Customizes the length of the crutches according to the height of the patient
Forearm Crutches	
Stand the patient in shoes with the elbows flexed so the crease of the wrist is at the hip.	Simulates appropriate posture when using forearm crutches
Measure the forearm from 3″ below the elbow, then add the distance between the wrist and floor.	Adjusts total length to accommodate for elbow and wrist flexion

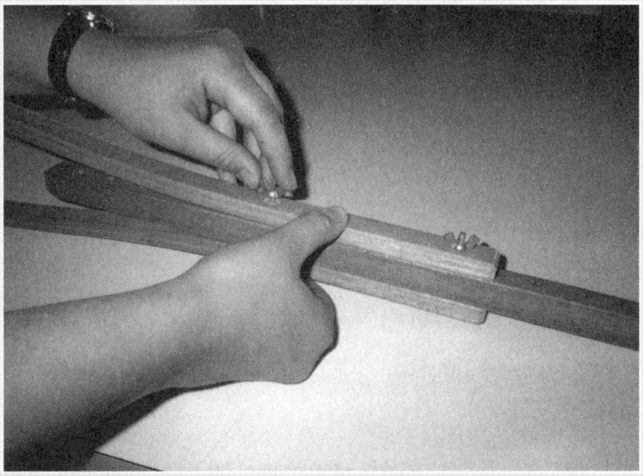

Adjusting crutch length. (Courtesy of Ken Timby.)

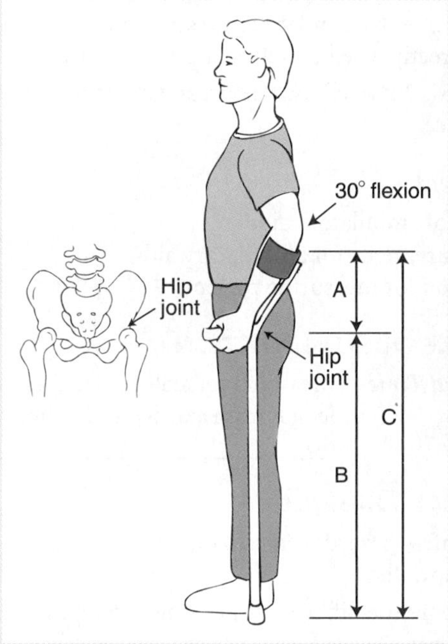

Measuring forearm crutches. Total length C = sum of A (3 inches below elbow to wrist) + B (wrist to floor).

Suggested Action	Reason for Action
Adjust the length of the forearm crutches by telescoping them up or down.	Customizes the final fit
Canes	
Have the patient stand erect in shoes that are most often worn for ambulating	Incorporates the height of the patient's shoes
Instruct the patient to avoid leaning forward or elevating the shoulders.	Ensures accurate measurement
Measure from the wrist to the floor.	Determines the appropriate length of the cane
Adjust the length of cane to provide 30° elbow flexion with the hand on the grip.	Customizes the final height of the cane

continued

SKILL 26–1

MEASURING FOR CRUTCHES, CANES, AND WALKERS *Continued*

Suggested Action	Reason for Action
Walkers	
Have the patient stand while wearing supportive shoes.	Accommodates for the added height of shoes
Measure from the mid-buttocks to the floor.	Facilitates the approximate height of the walker
Adjust the legs of the walker to provide approximately 30° of elbow flexion.	Customizes the final fit of the walker

Evaluation

- The patient stands upright with the shoulders relaxed.
- With axillary crutches, there is space for two fingers between the axilla and axillary bar to prevent **crutch palsy** (weakened forearm, wrist, and hand muscles from nerve impairment secondary to pressure on the brachial plexus of nerves in the axilla) from incorrectly fitted crutches or poor posture.
- There is 30° of elbow flexion and slight hyperextension of the wrist when standing in place.

Document

- Type of ambulatory aid
- Measurements for ambulatory aid
- Method for measuring patient

SAMPLE DOCUMENTATION

Date and Time Measured for axillary crutches. Approximate length of crutches is 53″ (132.5 cm) based on length from axillary fold to heel (51″) while in a supine position and the addition of 2″.
_______________ R. WOOD, LPN

CRITICAL THINKING

- List safety hazards that can occur if ambulatory aids are not measured and adjusted appropriately.
- Compare the differences in using two types of ambulatory aids, such as crutches and a walker.

SKILL 26–2

ASSISTING WITH CRUTCH-WALKING

Suggested Action	Reason for Action
Assessment	
Review the medical orders for the type of activity and crutch-walking gait.	Reflects the implementation of the medical treatment
Read any previous nursing documentation regarding the patient's efforts at crutch-walking.	Provides evaluative data and indicates need to simulate or modify nursing interventions
Observe the condition of the patient's axillae and palms.	Provides objective data concerning the weightbearing effects on the upper body

continued

SKILL 26–2

ASSISTING WITH CRUTCH-WALKING *Continued*

Suggested Action	Reason for Action
Ask the patient if there is any muscle or joint pain, or tingling or numbness in the fingers.	Provides subjective data concerning the effects of crutch-walking and possible nerve irritation
Inspect the conditions of the axillary pads and rubber crutch tips.	Demonstrates concern for safety
Planning	
Consult with the patient about the preferred time for ambulation.	Shows respect for individual decision-making
Assist the patient to don clothes or a robe and supportive shoes or slippers with nonskid soles.	Demonstrates concern for modesty and safety
Apply a walking belt if the patient is weak or inexperienced in the use of crutches.	Demonstrates concern for safety
Clear a pathway where the patient will ambulate.	Demonstrates concern for safety
Review the technique for performing the prescribed crutch-walking gait.	Reinforces prior learning
Implementation	
Wash your hands.	Reduces the transmission of microorganisms
Help the patient to a standing position.	Prepares the patient for ambulation
Offer the crutches and observe that they are placed 4″ to 8″ (10–20 cm) to the side of the feet.	Forms a triangle for good balance
Remind the patient to stand straight with the shoulders relaxed.	Reduces muscle strain
Position yourself to the side and slightly behind the patient on the weaker side.	Facilitates assistance without causing interference

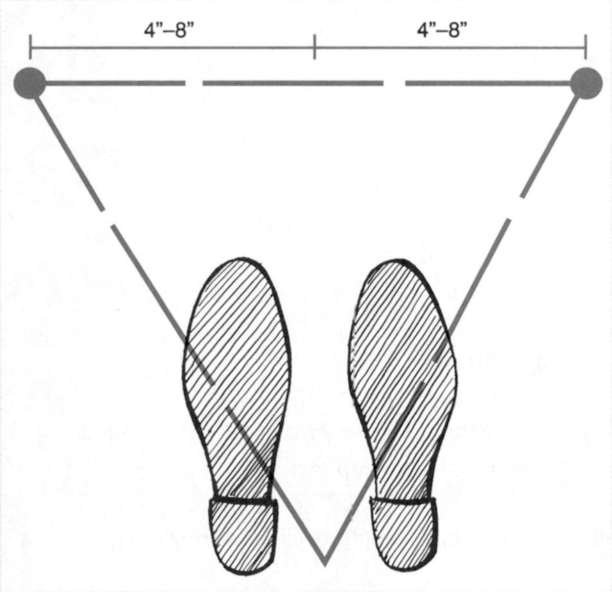

A tripod of support.

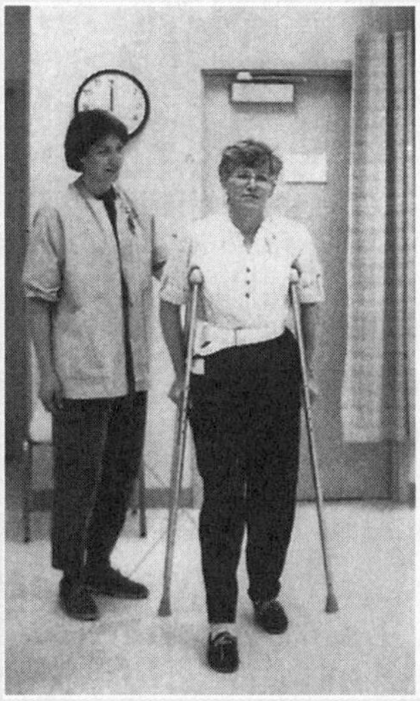

Positioning for assistance. (Courtesy of Ken Timby.)

continued

SKILL 26–2

ASSISTING WITH CRUTCH-WALKING *Continued*

Suggested Action	Reason for Action
Take hold of the walking belt.	Helps steady or support the patient
Instruct the patient to advance the crutches, lean forward, put some weight on the hand grips, and move one or both feet, depending on the prescribed gait.	Promotes walking
Remind the patient to slow down if there is evidence of fatigue or intolerance to the activity.	Demonstrates concern for the patient's well-being
For Sitting	
Recommend backing up to the seat of the chair.	Promotes a position for sitting
Have patient place both crutches in the hand on the same side as the weaker leg.	Frees the opposite hand
While using the hand grips on the crutches for support, have the patient grasp one arm rest with the free hand.	Reduces the potential for falling

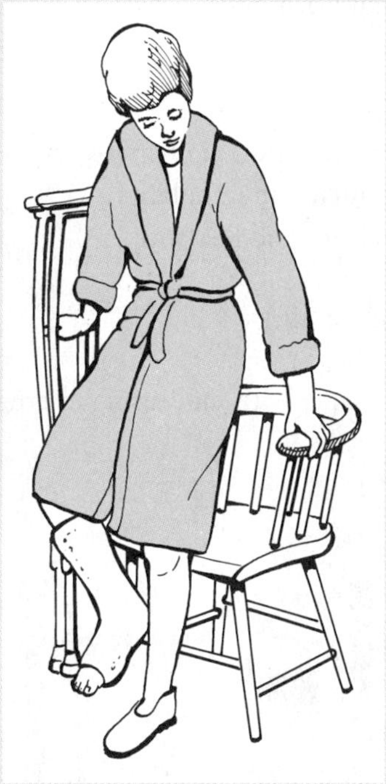

Sitting down.

Suggested Action	Reason for Action
When balanced, tell the patient to lower himself or herself into the seat of the chair.	Facilitates sitting
To get up, help the patient to the edge of the chair.	Facilitates using the stronger muscles of the thighs
Instruct the patient to hold the crutches upright on the weaker side, balancing them with one hand.	Positions crutches for support
Tell the patient to position the weaker leg forward of the body and the stronger leg toward the base of the chair.	Helps to distribute weight over the stronger leg
Tell the patient to push on the hand grips and arm rest, lean forward, and press down with the stronger leg.	Raises the patient from the chair

continued

SKILL 26-2

ASSISTING WITH CRUTCH-WALKING *Continued*

Suggested Action	Reason for Action
To Climb Stairs	
Have patient use a handrail on the stronger side of the body, if possible.	Balances needed support
Have the patient transfer both crutches to the hand opposite the handrail.	Frees one hand for grasping the handrail for support
Tell the patient to push down on the handrail and step up with the good leg.	Uses the stronger muscles for bearing weight

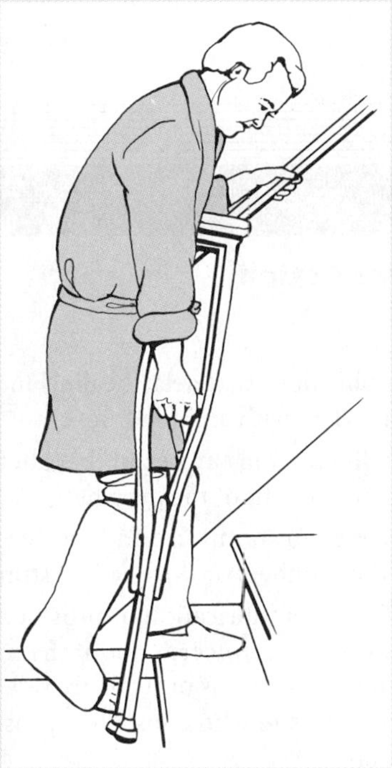

Climbing stairs.

Suggested Action	Reason for Action
Follow by raising the weaker leg.	Brings both legs to the same stair
Remind the patient that when going down the stairs, the weaker leg is advanced first with the support of the crutches or handrail; then the stronger leg is moved.	Enables safe descent

Evaluation

- Crutches fit appropriately.
- Patient performs crutch-walking gait correctly.
- No fatigue or other symptoms develop.
- Patient remains free of injury.

Document

- Distance ambulated
- Gait used
- Response of the patient

continued

SKILL 26-2

ASSISTING WITH CRUTCH-WALKING *Continued*

SAMPLE DOCUMENTATION

Date and Time Ambulated length of hospital corridor (approx. 100 feet) using crutches and a three-point non-weightbearing gait. No breathlessness noted. States upper arms "ache" and attributes discomfort to "muscle strain" from previous day's ambulation efforts. Refuses medication for muscle discomfort. ______________________ SIGNATURE, TITLE

CRITICAL THINKING

- List safety hazards as they relate to crutch-walking and suggestions for preventing them.

SKILL 26-3

APPLYING A LEG PROSTHESIS

Suggested Action	Reason for Action
Assessment	
Inspect the stump for evidence of bleeding, wound drainage, skin abrasions, blisters, and edema.	Detects complications that delay healing and rehabilitation, or interfere with ambulation
Weigh the patient at regular intervals.	Helps detect fluctuations in weight that alter the size of the stump and the fit of the prosthesis
Observe the ease or difficulty of inserting the stump within the socket.	Indicates changes in stump size and the need to add or decrease the numbers or thickness of stump socks
Examine the joint connections in the prosthetic limb.	Determines whether lubrication or prosthetic maintenance is necessary; concerns about the mechanical features of the prosthesis or its fit are referred to a **prosthetist** (person who constructs prostheses) immediately.
Inspect the shoe on the prosthetic limb for signs of wear or moisture.	Establishes whether heels or the entire shoe need to be replaced or dried.
Planning	
Cleanse the skin on the stump each evening, not in the morning.	Allows sufficient time for the skin to be moisture-free
Rinse the soap from the stump and dry it well.	Avoids skin impairment and irritation
Encourage the patient to lie supine or prone periodically during the day.	Promotes venous circulation, reduces stump edema, and avoids joint contractures
Instruct the patient to avoid crossing the legs or keeping the natural knee flexed for a prolonged period.	Prevents circulatory problems
Wash the socket each evening with water and mild soap.	Removes soil and perspiration
Dry the socket well before application.	Prevents skin breakdown
Use a small brush to clean the valve on a prosthesis with a suction socket.	Removes dust and facilitates the formation of a vacuum
Keep a supply of clean stump socks to facilitate a daily change, and a nylon sheath if one is used.	Promotes cleanliness and comfort

continued

SKILL 26-3

APPLYING A LEG PROSTHESIS *Continued*

Suggested Action	Reason for Action
Store clean wool stump socks for several days before use.	Allows the restoration of wool fiber resiliency
Wash a nylon sheath in soapy lukewarm water, rinse well, and stretch it lengthwise before air drying; never remove water by twisting the sheath.	Maintains shape and integrity
Advise the patient with a new prosthesis to wear it for short periods initially and then increase the wearing time each day.	Prevents overexertion and impaired skin integrity
Implementation	
Cover the prosthetic foot with the stocking and shoe of choice.	Coordinates apparel and helps to conceal the appearance of the prosthetic limb
Apply the nylon sheath, if used, and the appropriate number or ply of stump socks.	Promotes comfort and fit of the stump within the prosthesis
Place a nylon stocking over the stump sock, allowing a long portion of the toe to extend from the base of the stump.	Helps to slide the stump within the socket
Stand and position the prosthetic limb next to the residual limb.	Facilitates application
Pull the toe of the nylon stocking through the valve at the base of the socket.	Locates the stump well within the lower area of the socket

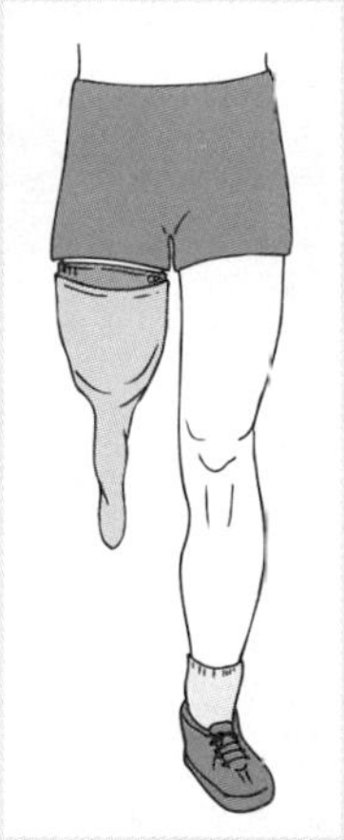

A nylon stocking covers the stump sock.

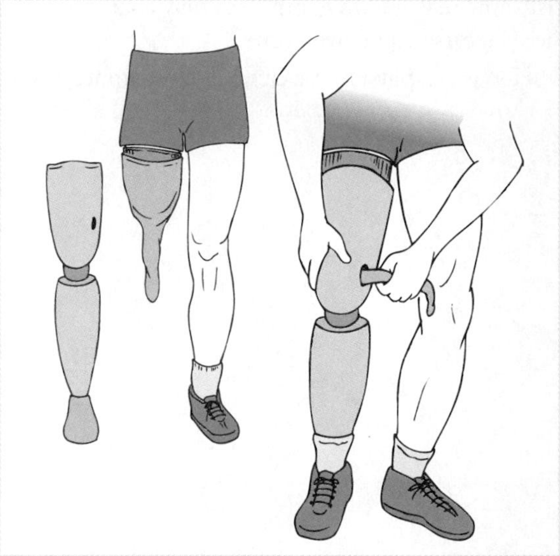

The nylon is pulled through the valve hole on the socket of the prosthesis.

Suggested Action	Reason for Action
Pump the stump up and down as the nylon stocking is completely removed.	Expels air and creates a vacuum that keeps the prosthesis attached to the stump
Replace the plug within the valve opening.	Ensures retention of vacuum suction
Fasten all slings if other than a suction-socket type of prosthesis is used.	Secures the prosthesis to the stump

continued

SKILL 26-3

APPLYING A LEG PROSTHESIS *Continued*

Evaluation

- Stump size is unchanged.
- Skin is intact.
- Circulation is adequate based on similar skin color in the stump and remaining limb.
- Joints above the amputation have full range of motion.
- Prosthesis is mechanically sound.
- Patient ambulates without discomfort or injury.

Document

- Care and condition of the stump
- Care of stump socks
- Care and condition of the prosthesis
- Level of patient performance in stump care and application of the prosthesis
- Patient's performance in ambulation

SAMPLE DOCUMENTATION

Date and Time Stump washed and dried by patient. No evidence of skin breakdown. Soiled stump socks exchanged with spouse for supply of clean socks. Inside of prosthetic socket cleaned and dried. Patient observed while independently donning prosthesis. Procedure completed accurately and appropriately. Ambulated for approximately 15 minutes without loss of balance or other difficulties. ______________________ SIGNATURE, TITLE

CRITICAL THINKING

- List some reasons why amputees may abandon rehabilitation and prosthesis use; discuss how these factors can be overcome.
- Discuss ways that a nurse can help an amputee overcome an impaired body image.

UNIT EIGHT

THE SURGICAL PATIENT

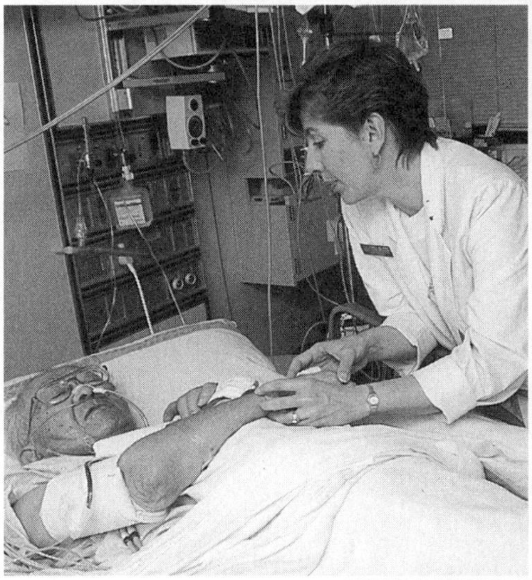

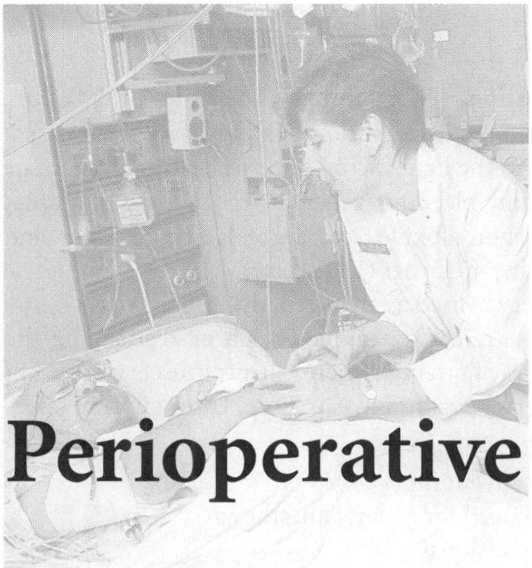

CHAPTER 27

Perioperative Care

CHAPTER OUTLINE

Preoperative Period
Intraoperative Period
Postoperative Period
Nursing Implications

NURSING GUIDELINES

PROVIDING IMMEDIATE POSTOPERATIVE CARE

SKILLS

SKILL 27-1: APPLYING ANTIEMBOLISM STOCKINGS
SKILL 27-2: PERFORMING PRESURGICAL SKIN PREPARATION
SKILL 27-3: APPLYING A PNEUMATIC COMPRESSION DEVICE

NURSING CARE PLAN

BODY IMAGE DISTURBANCE

KEY TERMS

anesthesiologist
anesthetist
antiembolism stockings
atelectasis
autologous transfusion
depilatory agent
directed donors
discharge instructions
emboli
forced coughing
informed consent
inpatient surgery
intraoperative period
microabrasions
outpatient surgery
perioperative care
plume
pneumatic compression device
pneumonia
postanesthesia care unit
postoperative care
postoperative period
preoperative checklist
preoperative period
receiving room
surgical waiting area
thrombophlebitis
thrombus

LEARNING OBJECTIVES

An understanding of the content within this chapter will be evidenced by the student's ability to:

- Define perioperative care.
- Name three components of perioperative care.
- Differentiate inpatient from outpatient surgery.
- List at least four advantages of laser surgery.
- Discuss two methods for donating blood before surgery.
- Identify four major nursing tasks conducted during the immediate preoperative period.
- Name three topic to address in preoperative teaching.
- Explain the purpose of antiembolism stockings.
- Name three methods for removing hair when preparing the skin before surgery.
- List at least five items that are verified on the preoperative checklist.
- Name three parts of the surgical department used during the intraoperative period.
- Describe the focus of nursing care during the immediate postoperative period.
- Discuss the purpose of a pneumatic compression device.
- Give four examples of common postoperative complications.
- Describe at least two items of information included in discharge instructions for postsurgical patients.
- Discuss at least two ways in which the surgical care of older adults differs from that of other age groups.

Perioperative care (care that patients receive before, during, and after surgery) is unique. This chapter discusses the general responsibilities nurses assume when caring for patients during the preoperative, intraoperative, and postoperative periods.

Preoperative Period

The **preoperative period** (time that starts when patients are informed that surgery is necessary and ends when they are transported to the operating room) can be short or long. One of the major factors affecting the length of the preoperative period is the urgency with which the surgery must be performed (Table 27-1). The trend today is to keep the perioperative period as short as possible.

INPATIENT SURGERY

Inpatient surgery (operative procedures performed on patients who are admitted to the hospital and expected to remain at least overnight) is planned for patients who will require nursing care for more than 1 day after surgery. All except the sickest of patients are usually admitted the morning of the scheduled surgery.

Many people who have inpatient surgery undergo prior laboratory and diagnostic tests. Some have met with an **anesthesiologist** (physician who administers chemical agents that temporarily eliminate sensation and pain; Table 27-2) or an **anesthetist** (nurse specialist who administers anesthesia under the direction of a physician). Most will have received preoperative instructions from either the surgeon's office nurse or a hospital nurse.

OUTPATIENT SURGERY

Outpatient surgery (operative procedures performed on patients who return home on the same day) also is called *ambulatory surgery* or *same-day surgery*. It is generally reserved for patients who are in an optimal state of health and whose course is expected to be uneventful. Advantages and disadvantages of outpatient surgery are listed in Table 27-3.

Laser Surgery

The use of outpatient surgery has increased greatly, partly due to advances in laser surgery. The acronym *laser* stands for *l*ight *a*mplification by the *s*timulated *e*mission of *r*adiation. Lasers convert a solid, gas, or liquid into light. When focused, the energy from the light is converted to heat, causing tissue to vaporize and bleeding vessels to coagulate. Examples include the carbon dioxide laser, argon laser, ruby laser, and yttrium-aluminum-garnet (YAG) laser.

Laser surgery is used as an alternative to many previously conventional surgical techniques, such as reattaching the retina and revascularizing ischemic heart muscle (instead of coronary artery bypass graft surgery). Laser surgery offers advantages such as:

- Cost effectiveness
- Reduced need for general anesthesia
- Smaller incisions
- Minimal blood loss
- Reduced swelling
- Less pain
- Decreased incidence of wound infections
- Reduced scarring
- Less time recuperating

Laser technology requires unique safety precautions, such as eye protection, fire and heat protection, and vapor protection.

Depending on the type of laser used, everyone—including the patient—wears goggles. In some cases, prescription glasses with side shields, but not contact lenses, are allowed.

Because lasers produce heat, fire and electrical safety are paramount. Volatile substances such as alcohol and acetone are not used around lasers. Surgical instruments are coated black to avoid absorbing scattered light. Sometimes even the patient's teeth are covered with plastic or a rubber mouth guard to shield metal fillings. For the same reason, no jewelry is allowed.

When a laser is used, it releases **plume** (substance composed of vaporized tissue, carbon dioxide, and water) that may contain intact cells. Plume is accompanied by smoke, an offensive odor, and (for some) burning and itching eyes. The latter effects are not hazardous and can usually be reduced with the use of smoke evacuators. The greater concern involves the consequences of inhaling plume. Inhaled plume may contain viruses in the airborne cells that could theoretically transmit HIV. Although no cases of this have been documented, high-efficiency respirator masks (see Chap. 22) are

TABLE 27–1. **Types of Surgery According to Their Urgency**

Type	Description	Example
Optional	Surgery is performed at the request of the patient.	Surgery for cosmetic purposes
Elective	Surgery is planned at the convenience of the patient. Failure to have the surgery does not result in catastrophe.	Surgery for the removal of a superficial cyst
Required	Surgery is necessary and should be done relatively promptly.	Surgery for the removal of a cataract
Urgent	Surgery is required promptly, within a day or two if at all possible.	Surgery for the removal of a malignant tumor
Emergency	Surgery is required immediately for survival.	Surgery to relieve an intestinal obstruction

TABLE 27–2. **Types of Anesthesia**

Type	Description
General Anesthesia	Eliminates all sensation and consciousness or memory for the event
Inhalants	Includes gas or volatile liquids
Injectables	Are given intravenously
Regional Anesthesia	Blocks sensation in an area, but consciousness is unaffected
Spinal (includes epidural)	Eliminates sensation in lower extremities, lower abdomen, pelvis
Local	Blocks sensation in a circumscribed area of skin and subcutaneous tissue
Topical	Inhibits sensation in epithelial tissues such as skin and mucous membranes where directly applied

better than conventional surgical masks for reducing the risk of infection transmission.

INFORMED CONSENT

Regardless of whether surgery is performed conventionally or with a laser, patients are commonly fearful and anxious. Patients often have a multitude of questions and preconceived ideas about what surgery involves. Some of these questions may be answered when the physician provides information for **informed consent** (permission a patient gives after having the risks, benefits, and alternatives explained; see Chap. 13). A signed form, witnessed by a nurse, is evidence that consent has been obtained (Fig. 27-1).

PREOPERATIVE BLOOD DONATION

The low risk of acquiring HIV from a blood transfusion is sometimes discussed during the preoperative period. Although publicly donated blood is tested for several pathogens, the potential for acquiring a bloodborne disease still exists. Therefore, some surgical patients donate their own blood before surgery. Predonated blood is held on reserve should they need a blood transfusion during or after surgery. Receiving one's own blood is called an **autologous transfusion** (self-donated blood). Autologous transfusions also are prepared by salvaging blood that is lost during or immediately after surgery. The salvaged blood is suctioned, cleaned, and filtered from drainage collection devices.

Patients who do not meet the time or health requirements for self-donation may select **directed donors** (blood donors chosen from among the patient's relatives and friends). The patient's siblings should not donate blood for the patient, because doing so would rule them out as future organ or tissue donors for the patient. Antigens in the transfused blood would sensitize the recipient, increasing the risk of organ or tissue rejection. Also, a male sexual partner of a woman in her reproductive years should not be a directed donor for her to avoid possible antibody reactions against a fetus in a future pregnancy.

Most authorities believe that receiving blood from directed donors is no safer than receiving blood from public donors. Although predonation of blood is common in the United States, the criteria for autologous and directed donors (Table 27-4) vary among regions and hospitals. Because directed donors must meet the same requirements as public donors, if the blood is not used by the intended recipient, it is released into the public pool and can be given to someone else.

IMMEDIATE PREOPERATIVE CARE

Although some presurgical activities take place weeks in advance, others cannot be performed until just before surgery. During the immediate preoperative period—the few hours before the procedure—several major tasks must be completed: conducting a nursing assessment, providing preoperative teaching, preparing the skin, and completing the surgical checklist.

TABLE 27–3. **Advantages and Disadvantages of Outpatient Surgery**

Advantages	Disadvantages
Lowers the surgical costs because of the reduced use of hospital services	Reduces the time for establishing a nurse–patient relationship
Reduces the time spent away from home, school, or place of employment	Requires intensive preoperative teaching in a short amount of time
Interferes less with the patient's usual daily routine	Reduces the opportunity for reinforcement of teaching and for answering questions
Provides the potential for more rest and sleep before and after surgery	Allows for fewer delays in assessing and preparing a patient once he or she arrives for surgery
Allows more opportunity for family contact and support	Requires that care of the patient after discharge be carried out by unskilled people

THREE RIVERS AREA HOSPITAL
THREE RIVERS, MICHIGAN 49093

AUTHORIZATION FOR MEDICAL
AND/OR
SURGICAL TREATMENT

Date July 18 20 00 Time 2:30 a.m. (p.m.)

I, the undersigned, a patient in Three Rivers Area Hospital, hereby authorize Dr. Robert Morrison, M.D. (and whomever he may designate as his assistant) to administer such treatment as is necessary, and to perform the following operation Exploratory Laparotomy and Appendectomy.
(Name of operation and/or procedure)
and such additional operations or procedures as are considered therapeutically necessary on the basis of findings during the course of said operation, with the following exception, None.

I also consent to the administration of such anesthetics as are necessary, with the exception of None.
(None, spinal anesthesia, or other)

I hereby certify that I have read and fully understand the above AUTHORIZATION FOR MEDICAL and/or SURGICAL TREATMENT, the reasons why the above named surgery is considered necessary, its advantages and possible complications, if any, as well as possible alternative modes of treatments, which were explained to me by Dr. Morrison.

I also certify that no guarantee or assurance has been made as to the results that may be obtained.

Gary Holmes
(Patient or nearest relative)

Judi Ebbert, RN
(Witness)

(Relationship)

I hereby certify that I have explained to Gary Holmes (a patient at Three Rivers Area Hospital), the reasons why the above named surgery is considered necessary, its advantages and possible complications, if any, as well as possible alternative modes of treatment.

Robert Morrison, M.D.
(Surgeon signature)

7-18-00
(Date)

FIGURE 27–1. Surgical consent form.

Nursing Assessment

Nurses share with physicians the responsibility for assessing preoperative patients. Certain surgical risk factors increase the likelihood of perioperative complications:

- Extremes of age
- Dehydration
- Malnutrition
- Obesity
- Smoking
- Diabetes
- Cardiopulmonary disease
- Drug and alcohol abuse
- Bleeding tendencies
- Low hemoglobin and red cells
- Pregnancy

Some problems, such as an unexplained elevation in temperature, abnormal laboratory data, current infectious disease, or significant deviations in vital signs, are cause for postponing or canceling the surgery.

TABLE 27–4. **Criteria for Autologous and Directed Blood Donation**

Autologous Donation	Directed Donation
To Bank One's Own Blood, the Donor Must:	**To Be a Directed Donor, the Person Must:**
Have a physician's recommendation	Be at least 17 years of age
Have a hematocrit within safe range	Meet all the criteria of a public donor
Be free of infection at time of donation	Have the same blood type as the potential recipient or one that is compatible
Meet the blood collection center's minimum weight requirement	Not have received a blood transfusion within the last 6 months
Donate 40 to 3 days before the anticipated date of use	Donate 20 to 3 days before the anticipated use
Donate no more frequently than every 3 to 5 days; once per week is preferred	Be free from bloodborne pathogens and high-risk behaviors
Assume responsibility for costs above the usual processing fees even if blood is not used	
Be advised that his or her blood will be discarded if unused	

Preoperative Teaching

Before patients are sent to surgery, they are given instructions on how to perform deep breathing, coughing, and leg exercises.

Deep Breathing

Deep breathing, a form of controlled ventilation that opens and fills small air passages in the lungs (see Chap. 20), is especially advantageous for patients who received general anesthesia or who breathe shallowly after surgery due to pain. Deep breathing reduces the postoperative risk for respiratory complications such as **atelectasis** (airless, collapsed lung areas) and **pneumonia** (lung infection), both of which can lead to hypoxemia.

The nurse should practice deep breathing with patients before they undergo surgery (Fig. 27-2). Deep breathing involves inhaling deeply using the abdominal muscles, holding the breath for several seconds, and exhaling slowly. Pursing the lips may extend the period of exhalation.

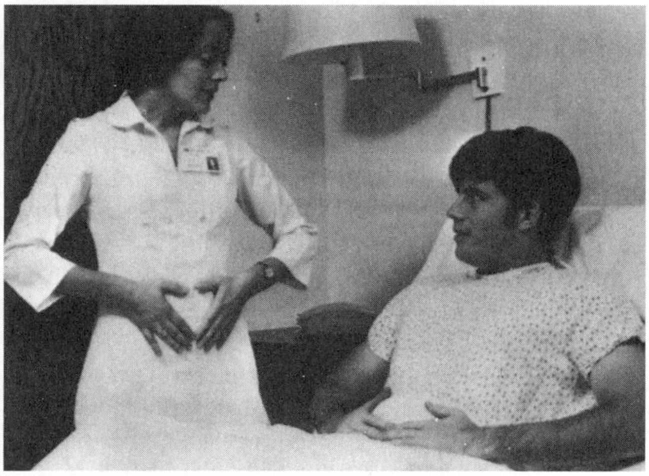

FIGURE 27–2. Teaching deep breathing.

Incentive spirometers (see Chap. 20) also are used to promote deep breathing.

Coughing

Impaired ventilation is often accompanied by thickened respiratory secretions. Coughing is a natural method for clearing secretions from the airways. Deep breathing alone is sometimes sufficient to produce a natural cough. Although **forced coughing** (coughing that is purposely produced) may not be necessary for all postoperative patients, it is important to prepare patients for the possibility. Forced coughing is most appropriate for patients who have diminished or moist lung sounds or who raise thick sputum. However, all patients need to be prepared for the possibility and receive instructions about the technique.

Patient Teaching For

Performing Forced Coughing

Teach the patient to do the following:

- Sit upright.
- Take a slow, deep breath through the nose.
- Make the lower abdomen rise as much as possible.
- Lean slightly forward.
- Exhale slowly through the mouth.
- Pull the abdomen inward.
- Repeat, but this time cough three times in a row while exhaling.

Coughing is painful for patients with abdominal or chest incisions. The discomfort can be reduced by administering pain medication about a half-hour before coughing or by splinting the incision during coughing. Splinting is accomplished by pressing on the incision with both hands, by pressing on a pillow placed over the incision, or by wrapping a bath blanket around the patient (Fig. 27-3).

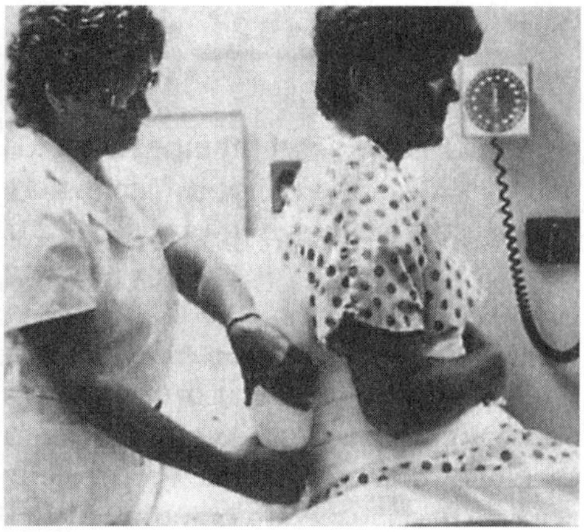

FIGURE 27–3. Using a bath blanket to splint. (Courtesy of Ken Timby.)

Leg Exercises

Leg exercises help promote circulation and reduce the risk of forming a **thrombus** (stationary blood clot) in the veins. Blood clots form when venous circulation is sluggish and when the fluid component of blood is reduced—both situations that occur in surgical patients.

Surgical patients have reduced circulatory volume because of preoperative restriction of food and fluids and because of blood loss during surgery. Also, blood tends to pool in the lower extremities because of the stationary position during surgery and patients' reluctance to move about afterward. With the use of leg exercises, efforts to reduce circulatory complications can begin as soon as the patient recovers from anesthesia.

Patient Teaching For

Performing Leg Exercises

Teach the patient to do the following:

- Sit with the head slightly raised.
- Bend one knee. Raise and hold the leg above the mattress for a few seconds (Fig. 27-4).
- Straighten the raised leg.
- Lower the leg gradually back to the bed.
- Do the same with the other leg.
- Rest both legs on the bed.
- Point the toes toward the mattress and then toward the head.
- Move both feet in clockwise and then counterclockwise circles.
- Repeat the exercises five times at least every 2 hours while awake.

Antiembolism stockings (elastic stockings) are knee-high or thigh-high elastic stockings. They are sometimes called TED (thromboembolic disorder) hose. Antiembolism stockings help prevent the development of thrombi and **emboli** (mobile blood clots) by compressing superficial veins and capillaries, redirecting more blood to larger and deeper veins, where it flows more effectively toward the heart. Intermittent pneumatic compression devices (discussed later in this chapter) are used for the same purpose but are applied postoperatively.

Antiembolism stockings must fit the patient properly and must be applied correctly (Skill 27-1). Stockings that become dirty are laundered, during which time a second pair is used.

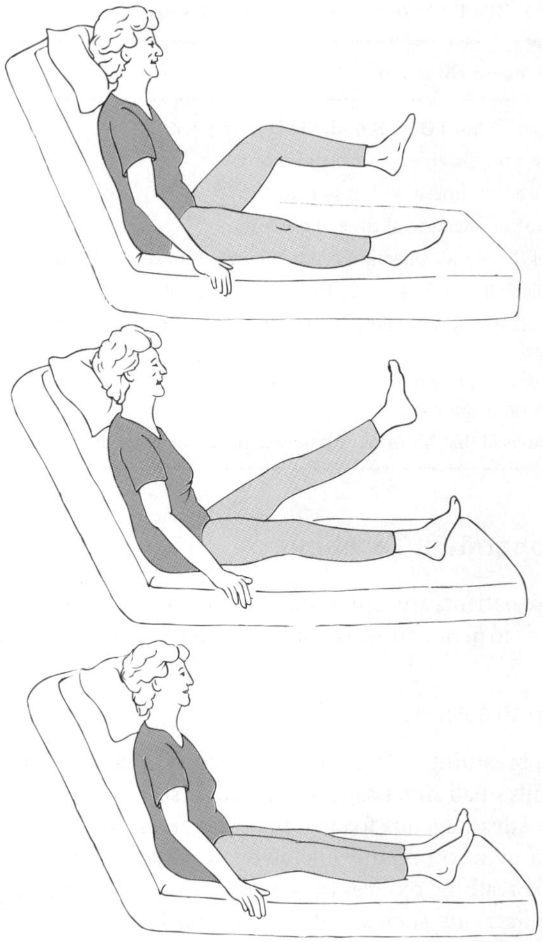
A.

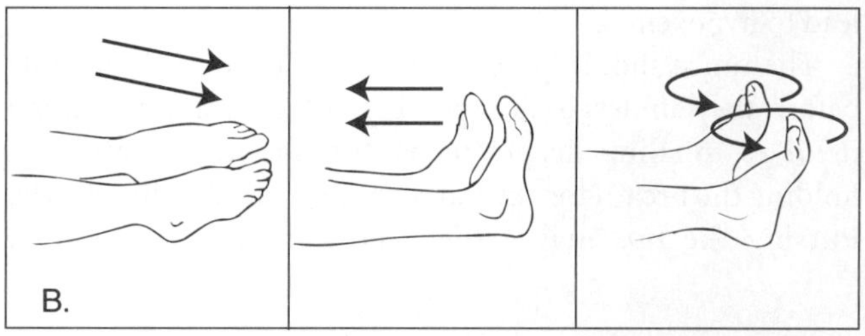
B.

FIGURE 27–4. Components of leg exercises: (*A*) exercising the lower legs; (*B*) exercising the feet.

If washed by hand, the stockings are laid flat to dry to prevent loss of their elasticity.

Skin Preparation

Skin preparation involves removing hair and cleansing the skin, because hair and skin are reservoirs for microorganisms (Skill 27-2). By reducing their presence, postoperative wound infections may be avoided. Shaving causes **microabrasions** (tiny cuts that provide an entrance for microorganisms). For this reason, many institutions use electric clippers for hair removal unless otherwise specified by the surgeon.

In some cases, patients are instructed to shower with an antimicrobial soap or agent before coming for surgery. Some authorities believe that simply washing the skin and hair is sufficient for preventing infections. Although the research is limited to statistically small numbers of patients, infection rates among patients whose hair is clean do not differ significantly from those whose body hair is removed.

Preoperative Checklist

A **preoperative checklist** (form that identifies the status of essential presurgical activities) is completed before surgery. The nurse verifies the following:

- The history and physical examination have been documented.
- The name of the procedure on the surgical consent form matches that scheduled in the operating room.
- The surgical consent form has been signed and witnessed.
- All laboratory test results have been returned and reported if abnormal.
- The patient is wearing an identification bracelet.
- Allergies have been identified.
- The patient has had nothing by mouth (NPO, *nil per os*) since midnight or the correct number of hours.
- Skin preparation has been completed.
- Vital signs have been assessed and recorded.

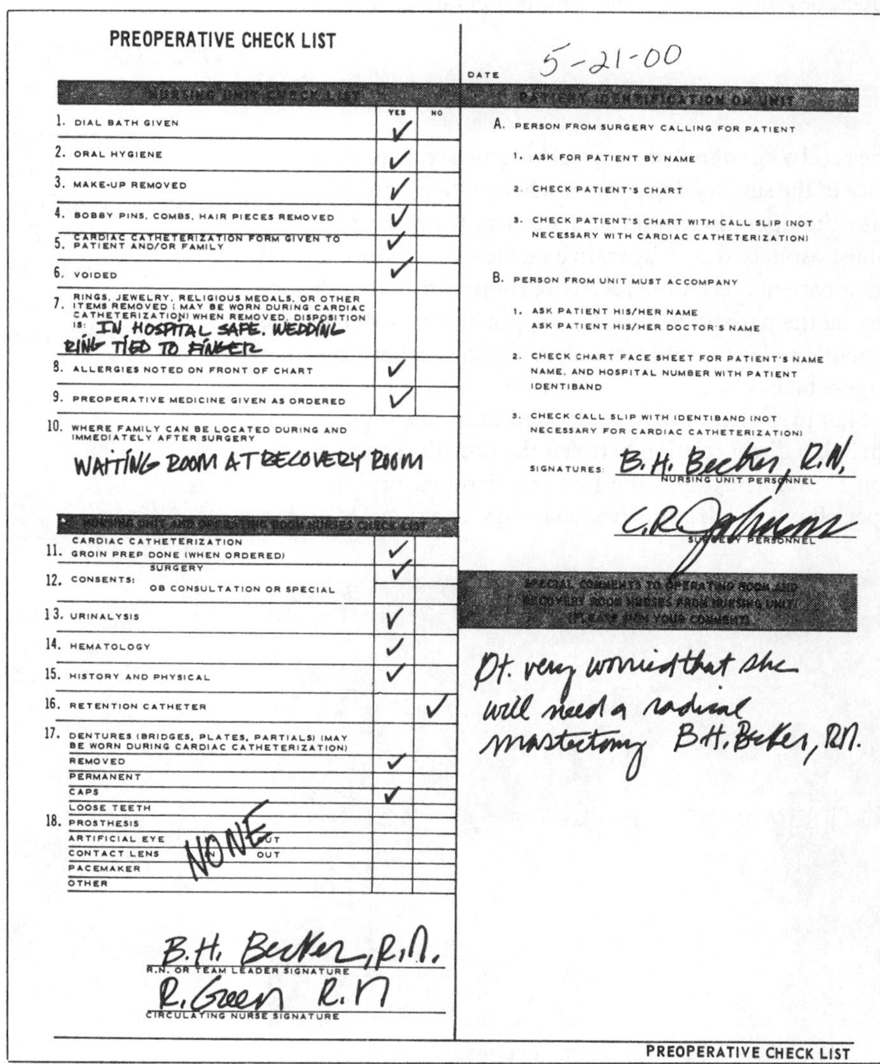
PREOPERATIVE CHECK LIST

DATE 5-21-00

NURSING UNIT CHECK LIST

	YES	NO
1. DIAL BATH GIVEN	✓	
2. ORAL HYGIENE	✓	
3. MAKE-UP REMOVED	✓	
4. BOBBY PINS, COMBS, HAIR PIECES REMOVED	✓	
5. CARDIAC CATHETERIZATION FORM GIVEN TO PATIENT AND/OR FAMILY	✓	
6. VOIDED	✓	
7. RINGS, JEWELRY, RELIGIOUS MEDALS, OR OTHER ITEMS REMOVED (MAY BE WORN DURING CARDIAC CATHETERIZATION) WHEN REMOVED, DISPOSITION IS: IN HOSPITAL SAFE. WEDDING RING TIED TO FINGER		
8. ALLERGIES NOTED ON FRONT OF CHART	✓	
9. PREOPERATIVE MEDICINE GIVEN AS ORDERED	✓	

10. WHERE FAMILY CAN BE LOCATED DURING AND IMMEDIATELY AFTER SURGERY
WAITING ROOM AT RECOVERY ROOM

NURSING UNIT AND OPERATING ROOM NURSES CHECK LIST

	YES	NO
11. CARDIAC CATHETERIZATION GROIN PREP DONE (WHEN ORDERED)	✓	
12. CONSENTS: SURGERY	✓	
OB CONSULTATION OR SPECIAL		
13. URINALYSIS	✓	
14. HEMATOLOGY	✓	
15. HISTORY AND PHYSICAL	✓	
16. RETENTION CATHETER		✓
17. DENTURES (BRIDGES, PLATES, PARTIALS) (MAY BE WORN DURING CARDIAC CATHETERIZATION)		
REMOVED	✓	
PERMANENT		
CAPS	✓	
LOOSE TEETH		
18. PROSTHESIS		
ARTIFICIAL EYE IN OUT		
CONTACT LENS IN OUT		
PACEMAKER		
OTHER		

NONE

B.H. Becker, R.N.
R.N. OR TEAM LEADER SIGNATURE
R. Green R.N.
CIRCULATING NURSE SIGNATURE

PATIENT IDENTIFICATION ON UNIT

A. PERSON FROM SURGERY CALLING FOR PATIENT
1. ASK FOR PATIENT BY NAME
2. CHECK PATIENT'S CHART
3. CHECK PATIENT'S CHART WITH CALL SLIP (NOT NECESSARY WITH CARDIAC CATHETERIZATION)

B. PERSON FROM UNIT MUST ACCOMPANY
1. ASK PATIENT HIS/HER NAME
ASK PATIENT HIS/HER DOCTOR'S NAME
2. CHECK CHART FACE SHEET FOR PATIENT'S NAME NAME, AND HOSPITAL NUMBER WITH PATIENT IDENTIBAND
3. CHECK CALL SLIP WITH IDENTIBAND (NOT NECESSARY FOR CARDIAC CATHETERIZATION)

SIGNATURES: B.H. Becker, R.N.
NURSING UNIT PERSONNEL
C.R. Johnson
SURGERY PERSONNEL

SPECIAL COMMENTS TO OPERATING ROOM AND RECOVERY ROOM NURSES FROM NURSING UNIT (PLEASE SIGN YOUR COMMENTS)

Pt. very worried that she will need a radical mastectomy B.H. Becker, RN.

PREOPERATIVE CHECK LIST

FIGURE 27–5. Preoperative checklist.

- Nail polish, glasses, contact lenses, and hairpins have been removed.
- Jewelry has been removed, or the wedding ring has been secured.
- Dentures have been removed.
- The patient is wearing only a hospital gown and hair cover.
- The patient has urinated.
- The prescribed preoperative medication has been given (Fig. 27-5).

The nurse is responsible for completing and signing the checklist. Operating room personnel review it when they arrive to transport the patient. Surgery may be delayed if the checklist is incomplete.

Intraoperative Period

The **intraoperative period** (time during which the patient undergoes surgery) takes place in the operating suite.

RECEIVING ROOM

The **receiving room** (presurgical holding area; Fig. 27-6) is a place in the surgery department where patients are observed until the operating room and surgical team are ready. In some hospitals, the preoperative medication is administered when patients reach the receiving room rather than before leaving the patient care unit. This practice coordinates the patient's sedation more closely with the actual time that surgery takes place.

Skin preparation may be delayed until this time as well. There is a direct relation between the time the skin preparation is performed and the rate of microbial proliferation, especially when it has involved shaving with a razor. Microbes tend to grow vigorously in the plasma-rich environment of abraded skin.

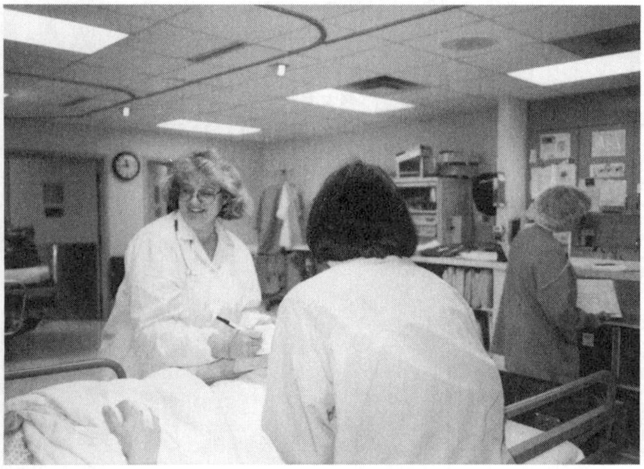

FIGURE 27–6. Receiving room. (Courtesy of Ken Timby.)

OPERATING ROOM

Eventually, patients are taken to the operating room, where their care and safety are in the hands of a team of experts, including physicians and nurses.

SURGICAL WAITING AREA

The **surgical waiting area** (room where family and friends await information about the patient) is staffed by volunteers who provide comfort, support, and news about how the patient's surgery is progressing. Many agencies provide food and beverages, coffee, public telephones, television, and magazines in this area. Often, the surgeon comes here immediately after the procedure to communicate with the family.

Postoperative Period

The **postoperative period** (time that begins after the operative procedure is completed and ends when the patient is discharged) is initiated when the patient is transported to an area to recover from the anesthesia. The **postanesthesia care unit** (PACU; area in the surgical department where patients are intensively monitored) is also known as the *postanesthesia reacting* (PAR) room or the *recovery room* (Fig. 27-7). Nurses

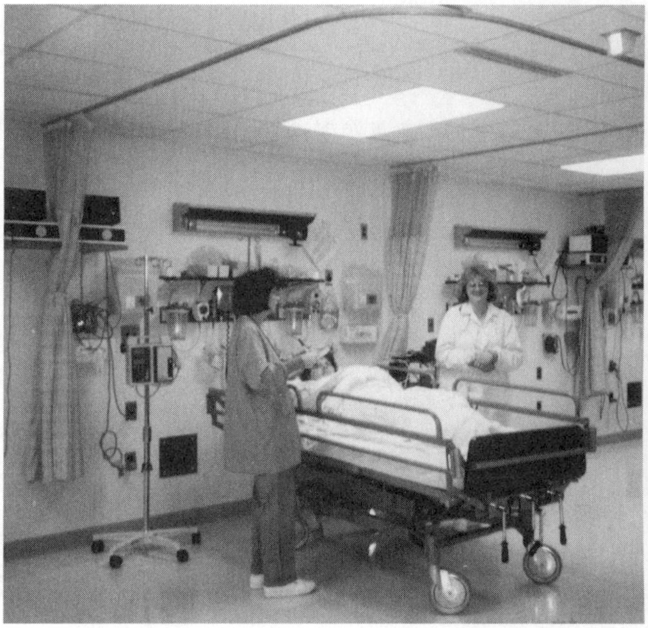

FIGURE 27–7. Postanesthesia care unit. (Courtesy of Ken Timby.)

in the PACU ensure the safe recovery of surgical patients from anesthesia. During this time, nurses on the general patient unit prepare for the patient's return.

The focus of **postoperative care** (nursing care after surgery) is different during the immediate postoperative period than it is later, when patients are more stable.

IMMEDIATE POSTOPERATIVE CARE

The immediate postoperative period refers to the first 24 hours after surgery. During this time, nurses prepare the room for the patient's return and monitor the patient for potential complications.

Preparing the Room

The top bed linen is folded toward the foot or side of the bed. The bed is placed in high position to facilitate transferring the patient from the stretcher. Often, additional blankets are kept ready for use because some patients feel cold after being quiet and inactive.

Bedside supplies and equipment that facilitate patient care are assembled. Some items that may be needed include oxygen equipment (see Chap. 20), a pole or electronic infusion device for continuing the administration of intravenous fluids (see Chap. 15), an emesis basin if the patient vomits, paper tissues, and a device for collecting and measuring urine (see Chap. 30). Suction canisters may be necessary for patients who have gastric tubes (see Chap. 29).

Monitoring for Complications

Postoperative patients are at risk for many complications (Table 27-5), some of which are more likely to occur soon after surgery. A safe postoperative recovery is facilitated by making frequent focused assessments of the patient and equipment.

Nursing Guidelines For

Providing Immediate Postoperative Care

- ☑ Obtain a summary report from a PACU nurse.
  RATIONALE: This report provides current assessment data concerning the patient's progress.
- ☑ Check the postoperative medical orders on the chart.
  RATIONALE: The medical orders provide instructions for individualized care.
- ☑ Assist PACU personnel to transfer the patient to bed.
  RATIONALE: The patient should be continuously observed.
- ☑ Observe the patient's respiratory pattern and auscultate the lungs.
  RATIONALE: Maintaining breathing is a priority for care.
- ☑ Check oxygen saturation using a pulse oximeter if the patient seems hypoxic (see Chap. 20).
  RATIONALE: An oximeter indicates the quality of internal respiration.
- ☑ Administer oxygen if the oxygen saturation is less than 90%, or if prescribed by the physician.
  RATIONALE: Oxygen administration increases the amount of oxygen available for binding with hemoglobin and for becoming dissolved in the plasma.
- ☑ Note the patient's level of consciousness and response to stimulation.
  RATIONALE: The level of consciousness and response to stimulation indicate the patient's neurologic status.
- ☑ Orient the patient and instruct him or her to take several deep breaths, as taught preoperatively.
  RATIONALE: Deep breathing improves ventilation and gas exchange.
- ☑ Check vital signs.
  RATIONALE: Vital signs provide data for assessing the patient's current general condition.
- ☑ Repeat vital sign assessments at least every 15 minutes until they are stable; then take them every hour to every 4 hours, depending on the patient's condition or medical orders.
  RATIONALE: Repeat assessment of vital signs provides comparative data.
- ☑ Check the incisional area and the dressing for drainage.
  RATIONALE: Provides data concerning the status of the wound and blood loss.
- ☑ Inspect all tubes, insertion sites, and connections.
  RATIONALE: For optimal outcomes, the equipment must function properly.
- ☑ Check the type of intravenous fluid, the rate of administration, and the volume that remains.
  RATIONALE: Provides data regarding fluid therapy.
- ☑ Monitor urination; report failure to void within 8 hours of surgery.
  RATIONALE: Failure to void indicates urinary retention.
- ☑ Auscultate bowel sounds.
  RATIONALE: Provides data concerning bowel motility.
- ☑ Assess the patient's level of pain and its location and characteristics.
  RATIONALE: Pain indicates the need for analgesia.

TABLE 27–5. **Postoperative Complications**

Complication	Description	Treatment
Airway occlusion	Obstruction of throat	Tilt head and lift chin. Insert an artificial airway.
Hemorrhage	Severe, rapid blood loss	Control bleeding. Administer intravenous fluid. Replace blood.
Shock	Inadequate blood flow	Place in modified Trendelenburg position. 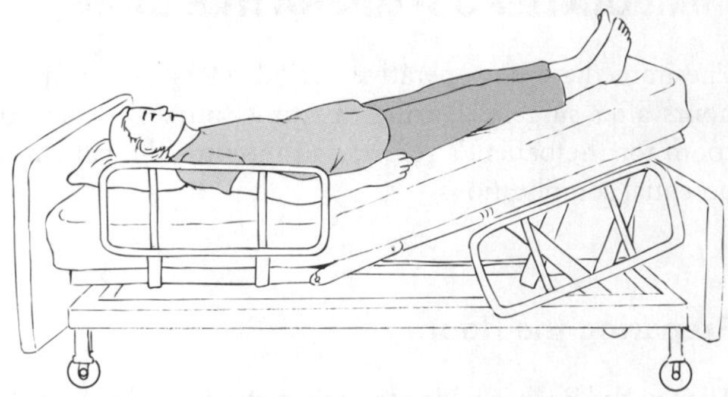 **Modified Trendelenburg position.** Replace fluids. Administer oxygen. Give emergency drugs.
Pulmonary embolus	Obstruction of circulation through the lung due to a wedged blood clot that began as a thrombus	Give oxygen. Administer anticoagulant drugs.
Hypoxemia	Inadequate oxygenation of blood	Give oxygen.
Adynamic ileus	Lack of bowel motility	Treat cause. Give nothing by mouth. Insert a nasogastric tube and connect to suction. Administer intravenous fluid.
Urinary retention	Inability to void	Insert a catheter.
Wound infection	Proliferation of pathogens at or beneath the incision	Cleanse with antimicrobial agents. Open and drain incision. Administer antibiotics.
Dehiscence	Separation of incision	Reinforce wound edges. Apply a binder.
Evisceration	Protrusion of abdominal organs through separated wound	Cover with wet dressing. Reapproximate wound.

☑ Administer analgesic drugs according to prescribed medical orders, if it is safe to do so.
RATIONALE: Analgesic drugs relieve pain.

☑ Remind the patient to perform leg exercises or apply antiembolism stockings.
RATIONALE: Leg exercises and antiembolism stockings promote circulation.

☑ Use a side-lying position if the patient is lethargic or unresponsive.
RATIONALE: This position helps keep the airway open.

☑ Raise the siderails unless providing direct care.
RATIONALE: Keeping the siderails up ensures safety.

☑ Fasten the signal device within the patient's reach.
RATIONALE: The signal device is a way for the patient to communicate and obtain assistance.

CONTINUING POSTOPERATIVE CARE

After surgery, the patient needs to resume eating and to demonstrate adequate elimination, circulation, and wound healing.

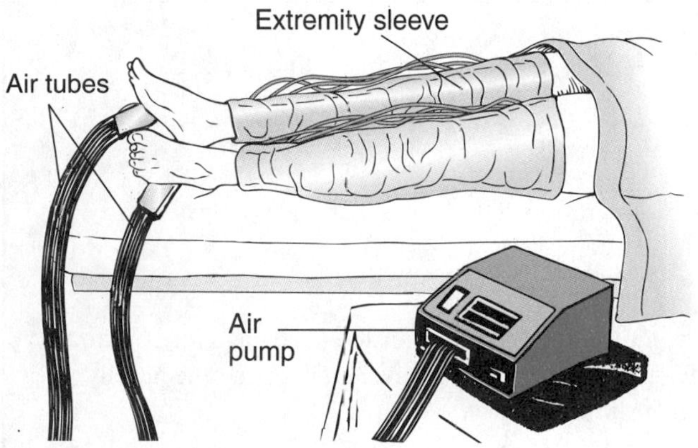

FIGURE 27–8. Pneumatic compression device.

Food and Oral Fluids

Food and oral fluids are withheld until patients are awake and free of nausea and vomiting, and bowel sounds are active. Postoperative patients usually progress from a clear liquid diet to a surgical soft diet, unless complications develop. Fluid intake and output are monitored to ensure patients are adequately hydrated.

Venous Circulation

Surgical patients should ambulate as soon as possible to reduce the potential for pulmonary and vascular complications. However, after some surgical procedures, antiembolism stockings, leg exercises, ambulation, and elevation of the lower extremities may not be enough to reduce swelling of the lower extremities and the potential for thrombus formation.

For patients who have the potential for impaired circulation in one or both extremities, a **pneumatic compression device** (machine that promotes circulation of venous blood and relocation of excess fluid into the lymphatic vessels) may be medically prescribed. Various companies make pneumatic compression devices, but they all consist of an extremity sleeve with tubes that connect to an electrical air pump (Fig. 27-8). The device compresses the sleeved extremity either intermittently or sequentially from distal to proximal areas. Most cycle on for a few seconds and then cycle off for a longer period. Depending on the manufacturer, pumps may cycle one to four times per minute. The nurse is responsible for applying this device (Skill 27-3).

Other measures to prevent thrombi include drinking plenty of fluids, avoiding long periods of sitting, keeping the legs uncrossed (especially at the knees), and changing position frequently.

Wound Management

The condition of the wound and the characteristics of drainage are assessed at least once each shift. Dressings are reinforced or changed if they become soiled or saturated. Eventually, sutures or staples are removed (see Chap. 28). Most inpatients are discharged within 3 to 5 days of surgery to continue their recuperation at home.

Discharge Instructions

Discharge instructions (directions for managing self-care and medical follow-up) are provided by the nurse before the patient leaves. Common areas addressed when discharging both inpatients and outpatients who have undergone surgery include:

- How to care for the incision site
- Signs of complications to report
- What drugs to use for relieving pain
- How to self-administer prescribed drugs
- When presurgical activity can be resumed
- If and how much weight can be lifted
- Which foods to consume or avoid
- When and where to return for a medical appointment

Information should be given both verbally and in written form.

Nursing Implications

Surgical patients offer unique patient care problems. Applicable nursing diagnoses include:

- Knowledge deficit
- Fear
- Acute pain
- Impaired skin integrity
- Risk for infection
- Risk for fluid volume deficit
- Ineffective breathing patterns
- Ineffective airway clearance
- Risk for impaired gas exchange
- Body image disturbance
- Risk for ineffective management of therapeutic regimen

The nursing care plan shows how the nursing process is used to identify and resolve a diagnosis of Body image disturbance, defined in the NANDA taxonomy as "confusion in (the) mental image of one's physical self." This diagnosis is especially pertinent to patients who have had their appearance altered as a result of surgery.

Nursing Care Plan

Body Image Disturbance

Assessment

Subjective Data

States, "I hate myself for agreeing to this operation. This 'thing' fills up, it bulges, and smells. No one will ever want to come near me again."

Objective Data

31-year-old woman with prior history of ulcerative colitis admitted 4 days ago for colectomy with ileostomy. Asks that room freshener be sprayed frequently. Applies perfume heavily. Positions herself more than 5 feet from visitors.

Diagnosis

Body image disturbance related to fear of rejection based on altered elimination

Plan

Goal

The patient will demonstrate acceptance and less self-consciousness about ostomy by interacting with a visitor within 3 feet by 10/9.

Orders: 10/5

1. Spend at least 15 minutes with patient midmorning, midafternoon, and early evening without performing direct care to communicate acceptance. During interaction:
   a. Sit within 3 feet to show by example that closeness is not a problem.
   b. Empathize with the patient; agree that this change is difficult to accept.
   c. Offer to contact another person with an ostomy through the United Ostomy Association to share mutual feelings and experiences while still in the hospital.
   d. Offer referral to an enterostomal nurse therapist for suggestions on odor-control techniques.
2. During ostomy teaching sessions and care of the stoma, implement the following:
   a. Avoid facial expressions that may communicate disgust or repulsion with the care of the ileostomy.
   b. Use terminology such as "your stoma" (avoiding any depersonalized or pet names) to promote the concept that the stoma is not a separate entity but rather part of her natural body. ______ N. NUNN, RN

Implementation (Documentation)

10/5 1330 Interacted socially for approx. 15 min. Sat within 3 feet. Patient moved her own chair away to provide more distance. Reinforced that adjusting to an ostomy is difficult. Explained the purpose of the United Ostomy Association and gave booklet, "So You Have . . . Or Will Have An Ostomy." Offered to contact another person with an ostomy or the enterostomal therapist. ______ G. ORSINI, LPN

Evaluation (Documentation)

10/6 1030 Demonstrated stoma care. Used the term "your ostomy" and "your appliance" during teaching session. Pt. used the term "Mt. Vesuvius" when referring to stoma. Page marker noted in ostomy booklet, indicating that reading has begun. States, "I don't know if talking with someone else will help. Not everyone has friends like mine." ______ G. ORSINI, LPN

FOCUS ON OLDER ADULTS

- Because older adults who undergo surgery are likely to have several chronic medical problems as well as the surgical problem, their pre- and postoperative care is more complex.
- Older adults accounted for 38% of all hospital stays and 48% of all days of care in hospitals in 1995 (American Association of Retired Persons (AARP) and Administration on Aging, U.S. Department of Health and Human Services, 1997).
- The average length of hospital stay was 6.8 days for patients age 65 years and older, and 4.5 days for patients under the age of 65 years in 1995 (American Association of Retired Persons (AARP) and Administration on Aging, U.S. Department of Health and Human Services, 1997).
- Older adults are likely to be sensory deprived if eyeglasses and hearing aids are removed prior to surgery, possibly interfering with communication and contributing to confusion and changes in mental status. Older adults also are likely to be self-conscious when dentures are removed before surgery. Collaboration with operating room personnel regarding the removal of dentures, eyeglasses, and hearing aids is helpful to ensure their use as much as or as long as possible.
- The period of fluid restriction before surgery may be shortened for older adults to reduce their risk for dehydration and hypotension.
- Older adults are likely to need instructions about which of their usual medications should be taken or discontinued preoperatively. Many older adults are on anticoagulation therapy—including self-therapy with low-dose aspirin—and may need to have this addressed as a preoperative consideration. Similarly, chronic use of aspirin by patients who have inflammatory conditions increases the risk of bleeding and needs to be evaluated preoperatively. Surgical patients also need instructions about resuming medications that were discontinued at the time of surgery.
- The cardiac status of older adults is monitored carefully after surgery because they may not be able to tolerate or eliminate intravenous fluids that are given at standard rates. Similarly, rates of intravenous fluids may need to be adjusted for older adults, especially if their renal or cardiac status is compromised.
- Older adults who have been on bed rest even for a day or two may benefit from physical therapy to help them regain mobility, especially if their mobility was even slightly compromised prior to the surgery.
- Wound healing in older adults is much slower because of age-related skin changes and impaired circulation and oxygenation. Poor hydration and nutrition further interfere with wound healing. A registered dietitian can recommend nutritional interventions to improve wound healing.
- If older adults develop postoperative infections, the manifestations are likely to be more subtle or delayed. Because older adults are likely to have a lower "normal" temperature, it is imperative to document the person's normal baseline temperature so that deviations from the normal can be assessed. A change in mental status is an early indicator of infection in older adults.
- If an indwelling catheter is inserted prior to surgery, it is best to remove it as soon as possible to prevent incontinence and urinary tract infections.
- Well before discharge, it is important to assess the extent of the older adult's support system regarding the ability to provide assistance after the patient's discharge.
- Older adults may require care in an extended care or skilled nursing facility, or they may qualify for skilled home care at the time of a surgical discharge if they are unable to manage their postoperative care independently.

KEY CONCEPTS

- Perioperative care refers to the nursing care that patients receive before, during, and after surgery.
- Perioperative care spans the preoperative, intraoperative, and postoperative periods.
- Inpatient surgery is performed on patients who remain in the hospital at least overnight. Outpatient surgery is performed on patients who return home the same day.
- Laser surgery, which can be performed on an outpatient basis, offers several advantages: it is cost effective, requires smaller incisions, results in minimal blood loss, and produces less pain.
- Some patients choose to donate their own blood before surgery or ask specific donors to do so.
- Four major tasks that must be completed during the immediate preoperative period are conducting a nursing assessment, providing preoperative teaching, preparing the skin, and completing the surgical checklist.
- Preoperative patients are taught how to perform deep breathing, coughing, and leg exercises.
- Antiembolism stockings are worn by surgical patients to prevent the development of thrombi and emboli.
- During preoperative skin preparation, hair can be removed with electric clippers, depilatory agents, or a safety razor, depending on agency policy and medical orders.
- On the preoperative checklist, the nurse verifies that the history and physical examination have been completed, the name of the procedure matches the one scheduled, the surgical consent form has been signed and witnessed, the patient is wearing an identification bracelet, and all laboratory test results have been returned and reported if abnormal.
- The receiving room, the operating room, and the surgical waiting room are three areas in the surgical department that are used during the intraoperative period.
- During the immediate postoperative care, nurses focus on preparing the patient's room and monitoring for complications.
- Common postoperative complications are airway obstruction, hemorrhage, pulmonary embolus, and shock.
- During recovery, a pneumatic compression device may be prescribed to promote circulation of venous blood and relocation of excess fluid into the lymphatic vessels.

- Discharge instructions for surgical patients include the following: how to care for the incisional site, signs of complications to report, and how to self-administer prescription drugs.
- Older adults have unique surgical needs and problems. For example, the period of fluid restriction before surgery may be shortened for older adults to reduce their risk for dehydration and hypotension. Also, the cardiac status of older adults must be monitored carefully after surgery because they may not be able to circulate or eliminate intravenous fluids given at standard rates.

CRITICAL THINKING EXERCISES

- You assess a postoperative patient and obtain the following data: blood pressure 102/64, pulse rate 90, respirations 32 and shallow, responds when shaken, experiencing nausea. What finding is most serious at this time, and what nursing actions are appropriate?
- A preoperative patient who is a Native American wants you to attach a dream catcher, a circular object with a woven web, to the IV pole. How would you respond to the patient's request?

SUGGESTED READINGS

ACE bandages cheaper than SCD, just as effective. Laparoscopic Surgery Update 1999;7(2):18–19.

American Association of Retired Persons (AARP) and Administration on Aging, U.S. Department of Health and Human Services. A Profile of Older Americans: 1997. Washington, D.C.: AARP, 1997.

Chesny M. Preadmission testing today. Today's Surgical Nurse 1999; 21(3):30–33.

Despite reported safety of the blood supply, many people prefer to store their own blood for transfusions. Research Activities 1999 (Dec):6.

Hube RF, Cohen PZ, Sotereanos NG, et al. Postoperative complications of lower extremity surgical procedures in older patients. Topics in Emergency Medicine 1998;20(1):55–62.

Jester R, Williams S. Preoperative fasting: putting research into practice. Nursing Standard 1999;13(39):33–35.

Lee ST, Liljas B, Churchill WH, et al. Perceptions and preferences of autologous blood donors. Transfusion 1998;28(8):757–763.

Leionen T, Leino-Kilpi H. Research in perioperative nursing care. Journal of Clinical Nursing 1999;8(2):123–138.

NANDA nursing diagnoses: definitions and classification, 1999–2000. Philadelphia: NANDA, 1999.

Oeltjen AM, Sandtrach PJ. Autologous transfusion techniques. Journal of Intravenous Nursing 1997;20(6):305–310.

Parker CB, Minick P, Kee CC. Clinical decision-making processes in perioperative nursing. AORN Journal 1999;70(1):45–50.

Patton CM. Preoperative nursing assessment of the adult patient. Seminars in Perioperative Nursing 1999;8(1):42–47.

Ramos R, Salem BI, de Pawlikowski MP, et al. The efficacy of pneumatic compression stockings in the prevention of pulmonary embolism after cardiac surgery. Chest 1996;109(1):82–85.

Rudoslovich N. Providing safe blood with autologous transfusion. Nursing and Allied Healthweek 1996;1(22):12–16.

Shuldham C. A review of the impact of pre-operative education on recovery from surgery. International Journal of Nursing Studies 1999;36(2): 171–177.

Sliney DH, Mainster MA. Ophthalmic laser safety: tissue interactions, hazards, and protection. Ophthalmology Clinics of North America 1998; 11(2):157–164.

Stewart-Rose J. Deep vein thrombosis: the risk. Journal of Orthopaedic Nursing 1998;2(3):130–131.

Thomas S. Graduated compression and the prevention of deep vein thrombosis. Journal of Wound Care 1999;8(1):41–43.

Thompson J. Compression stockings. AORN Journal 1995;62(6):939–940.

Wilburn S. Is the air in your hospital making you sick? American Journal of Nursing 1999;99(7):71.

Williams GD. Preoperative assessment and health history interview. Nursing Clinics of North America 1997;32(2):395–416.

SKILL 27–1

APPLYING ANTIEMBOLISM STOCKINGS

Suggested Action	Reason for Action
Assessment	
Review the medical orders and nursing plan for care.	Directs patient care
Assess the circulation of the toes and integrity of the skin.	Provides a baseline of data for future comparison
Check *Homans' sign* by dorsiflexing the foot and noting if pain is experienced in the calf. Report a positive finding.	Indicates the possibility of **thrombophlebitis** (inflammation of a vein due to the presence of a thrombus)
Measure the patient's leg from the flat of the heel to the bend of the knee or to midthigh.	Determines the length needed for knee-high or thigh-high stockings
Measure the calf or thigh circumference.	Determines the size needed
Assess the patient's understanding of the purpose and use of elastic stockings.	Determines the type and amount of health teaching needed
Check the fit of stockings that are currently being worn.	Identifies the potential complications from tight, loose, or wrinkled stockings
Planning	
Obtain the correct size of stockings before surgery or as soon as possible after they are ordered.	Facilitates early preventive treatment
Plan to remove the stockings for 20 minutes once each shift or at least twice a day and then reapply them.	Allows for assessment and hygiene
Elevate the legs for at least 15 minutes before applying the stockings, if the patient has been sitting or standing for a period of time.	Promotes venous circulation and avoids trapping venous blood in the lower extremities
Implementation	
Wash and dry the feet.	Removes dirt, skin oil, and some microorganisms
Apply corn starch or talcum powder if desired.	Reduces friction when applying the stockings
Avoid massaging the legs.	Prevents dislodging a thrombus if one is present
Turn the stockings inside out.	Facilitates threading the stockings over the foot and leg

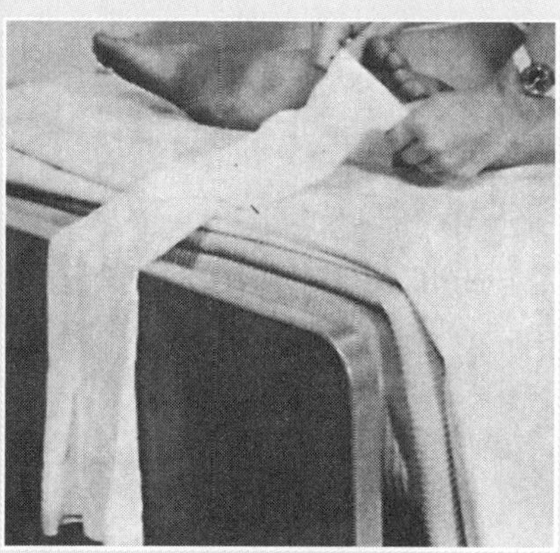

Antiembolism stocking turned inside out.

continued

SKILL 27–1

APPLYING ANTIEMBOLISM STOCKINGS *Continued*

Suggested Action	Reason for Action
Insert the toes and pull the stocking upward a few inches until it covers the foot.	Reduces bunching and bulkiness
Gather the remaining length of stocking and pull it upward a few inches at a time.	Eases application and avoids forming wrinkles

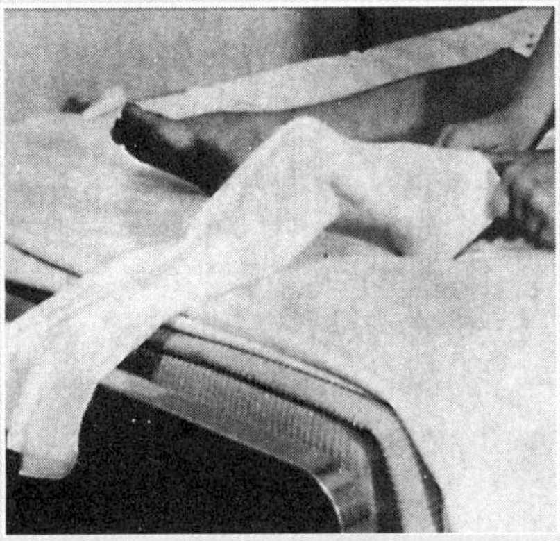

Inserting foot.

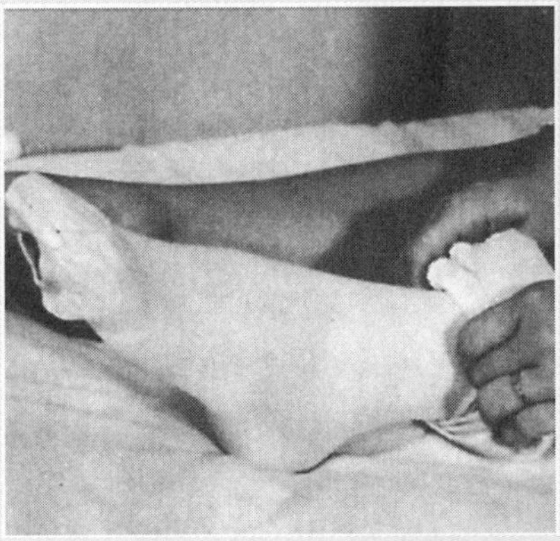

Pulling stocking upward.

Evaluation

- Skin remains intact and circulation is adequate.
- No calf pain on dorsiflexion of the foot.
- Stockings are removed and reapplied at least b.i.d.

Document

- Assessment findings
- Removal and reapplication of elastic stockings
- To whom abnormal assessment findings have been reported, and the outcome of the communication

SAMPLE DOCUMENTATION

Date and Time Toes are warm. Blood returns to nailbeds within 3 seconds of compression. Skin over legs is smooth and intact. Homans' sign is negative. TED hose applied after bathing.

________________________ SIGNATURE, TITLE

CRITICAL THINKING

- Discuss reasons why surgical patients are not as active and mobile as nonsurgical patients.
- List examples when it would be appropriate to apply antiembolism stockings for nonsurgical patients.

SKILL 27-2

PERFORMING PRESURGICAL SKIN PREPARATION

Suggested Action	Reason for Action
Assessment	
Consult the preoperative medical orders or a guide for surgical skin preparation.	Indicates the location and extent of skin preparation according to the planned surgical procedure

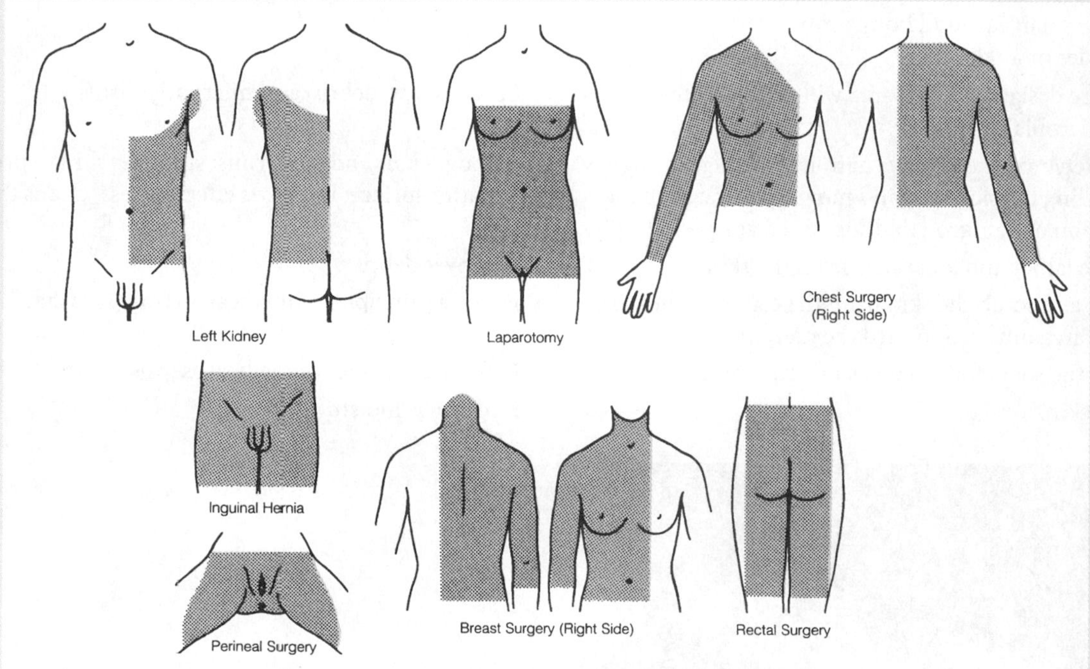

Guide for surgical skin preparation.

Suggested Action	Reason for Action
Assess the condition of the skin, looking especially for skin lesions.	Indicates areas that may bleed if irritated or provide a reservoir of microorganisms
Explore how much the patient understands about the purpose and extent of skin preparation.	Helps identify the extent and level of health teaching needed
Planning	
Arrange to perform the skin preparation shortly before the patient is scheduled for surgery.	Reduces the interim time during which microorganisms will recolonize the skin
Explain the procedure.	Reduces anxiety and promotes cooperation
Provide an opportunity for the patient to don a hospital gown.	Protects personal clothing and provides access for care
Obtain a skin preparation kit, towels, bath blanket, gloves, hair removal items, if ordered, and source of water.	Provides essential supplies
Implementation	
Wash your hands and don clean gloves.	Reduces the transmission of microorganisms
Provide privacy.	Shows respect for dignity
Position the patient so the area to be prepared is accessible.	Facilitates performing the procedure
Drape the patient with a bath blanket.	Maintains dignity as well as warmth

continued

SKILL 27–2

PERFORMING PRESURGICAL SKIN PREPARATION *Continued*

Suggested Action	Reason for Action
Protect the bed with towels or an absorbent pad.	Collects moisture
Use electric hair clippers to remove hair from the designated area.	Prevents microabrasions
If policy permits, use a **depilatory agent** (chemical that removes hair) around bony prominences like the knuckles or ankle.	Removes hair where clippers or razors may be ineffective
Lather the designated skin area with soap or other antimicrobial agent.	Loosens dirt, debris, and microorganisms
Use a safety razor to remove hair, if that is agency policy, by pulling the skin taut and moving the razor in the direction of hair growth. Rinse the razor periodically.	Removes hair and epidermis; stretches skin to produce a flatter surface; increases effectiveness; cleans the blade
Rinse the lather and loose hair from the skin.	Removes debris
Relather and scrub the skin from the center of the designated area outward toward the margins.	Follows principles of medical asepsis (see Chap. 21)
Remove the soap, following a similar pattern.	Follows principles of medical asepsis
Dry the skin.	Eliminates moisture

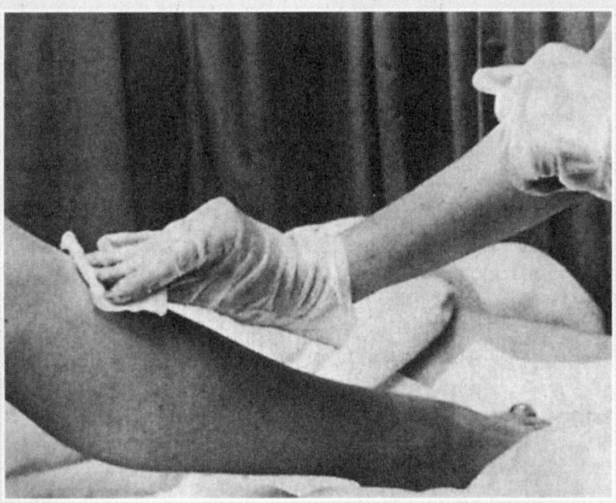

Drying the skin.

Suggested Action	Reason for Action
Discard the razor, if one was used, in a biohazard container.	Reduces the potential for injury and transmission of bloodborne viruses
Deposit the wet towels and bath blanket in a laundry hamper.	Restores comfort and orderliness
Place the used supplies in a waste receptacle.	Confines sources of infectious disease transmission
Remove gloves and wash hands.	Reduces the transmission of microorganisms

Evaluation

- Skin has been prepared according to policy and medical orders.
- Skin remains essentially intact.

continued

SKILL 27-2

PERFORMING PRESURGICAL SKIN PREPARATION *Continued*

Document

- Assessment findings
- Technique used
- Area prepared

SAMPLE DOCUMENTATION

Date and Time Skin areas for laparotomy procedure cleansed with Betadine and shaved. Skin is intact. No evidence of bleeding. ________________________________ SIGNATURE, TITLE

CRITICAL THINKING

- Correlate the potential for transmitting an infection using a razor for presurgical skin preparation with the chain of infection discussed in Chapter 21.

SKILL 27-3

APPLYING A PNEUMATIC COMPRESSION DEVICE

Suggested Action	Reason for Action
Assessment	
Review the medical orders and nursing plan for care.	Directs patient care
Determine whether the device will be applied to one or both extremities.	Gives direction for gathering assessment data and applying the device
Assess the circulation of the toes and integrity of the skin.	Provides a baseline of data for future comparison
Check Homans' sign (see Skill 27-1) and report if it is positive.	Indicates a possible thrombophlebitis; if positive, it is a contraindication for use of a pneumatic compression device
Measure the calf circumference and assess for pitting edema in extremities.	Provides a baseline of data for future comparisons
Palpate the pedal pulses.	Validates arterial blood flow to the foot if present and strong
Assess the patient's understanding of the purpose and use of a pneumatic compression device.	Determines the type and amount of health teaching needed
Planning	
Obtain the extremity sleeves, electric air pump, and accompanying air tubes.	Facilitates expeditious implementation of the medical order
Assist the patient with any elimination needs.	Avoids having to disconnect the equipment shortly after the device is applied
Arrange supplies the patient may need within his or her reach, including the signal device.	Promotes independence yet ensures that the patient can call for assistance
Help the patient to a position of comfort, such as a supine or low Fowler's position.	Fosters rest and relaxation

continued

SKILL 27-3

APPLYING A PNEUMATIC COMPRESSION DEVICE *Continued*

Suggested Action	Reason for Action
Implementation	
Wrap the extremity sleeve snugly about the calf of the leg.	Positions the sleeve where compression is desired
Secure the sleeve once it encircles the leg; most are secured with Velcro.	Ensures that the sleeve will remain in the applied position
Secure the air pump to the bottom of the bed or a stable surface.	Protects the device from damage and prevents injury to staff or visitors
Attach the air tubes to the ports that extend from the stocking and to the adapter within the air pump.	Provides a channel through which air is delivered to the extremity sleeve
Check that the air tubes are unkinked and not compressed under the patient or the wheels of the bed.	Ensures the unobstructed delivery of air
Plug the air pump into an electrical outlet.	Delivers power to the air pump motor
Set the pressure on the air pump to the amount prescribed (most medical orders range from 35 to 55 mmHg, with a common average of 40 mmHg).	Provides intermittent compression at an appropriate pressure to promote venous circulation
Turn the power switch on and observe that the function lights illuminate during compression and turn off between compressions.	Indicates that the machine is operational

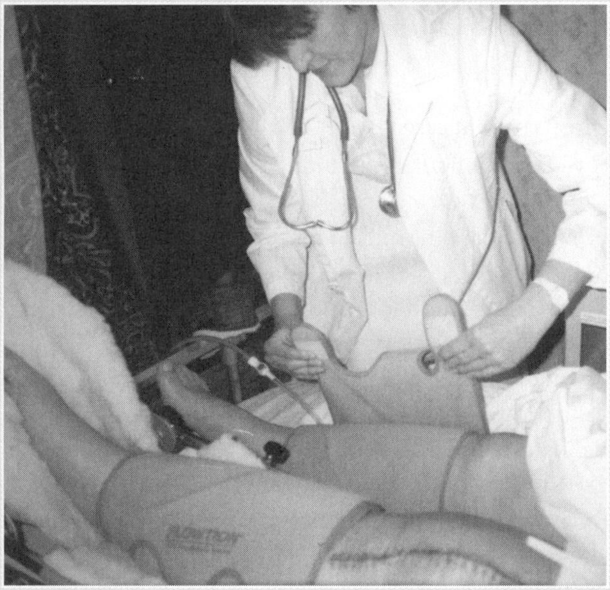

Applying the extremity sleeve. (Courtesy of Ken Timby.)

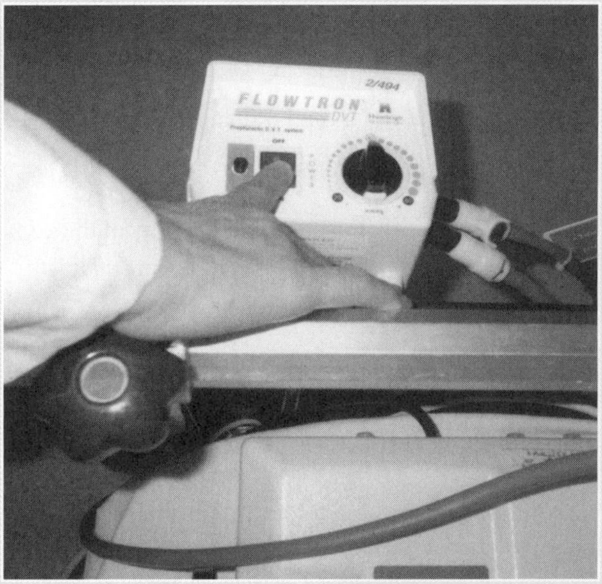

Turning on the air pump. (Courtesy of Ken Timby.)

Suggested Action	Reason for Action
Assess the patient's circulatory status and comfort every 2 to 4 hours throughout the therapeutic treatment, which is continuous for some patients.	Focuses assessment on signs that indicate adverse effects
Remove the extremity sleeve before ambulation or other out-of-bed activities.	Allows freedom of movement from the tether of the air tubes and pump
Discontinue the compressions if serious impairment of circulation and sensation, tingling or numbness, or leg pain occurs.	Helps avoid serious complications

continued

SKILL 27-3

APPLYING A PNEUMATIC COMPRESSION DEVICE *Continued*

Suggested Action	Reason for Action
Remove the extremity sleeve and assess calf size and circulation to distal areas of the extremity at least once per day.	Provides comparative data with which to evaluate the therapeutic response
Apply elastic stockings and reinforce the need to perform leg exercises every hour when the machine is not in use.	Promotes venous circulation
Place equipment in a safe area where it is available for the next use.	Demonstrates regard for safety and efficient time management

Evaluation

- Calf size is reduced or does not increase in diameter.
- Homans' sign is negative.
- Skin in lower extremity is intact, warm, and appropriate color for ethnicity.
- Capillary refill is <2 to 3 seconds.
- Pedal pulses are present and strong

Document

- Assessment findings before and after application
- Extremity to which device was applied
- Pressure setting and duration of application
- To whom abnormal assessment findings have been reported and the outcome of the communication

SAMPLE DOCUMENTATION

Date and Time R. calf measures 18″ (45 cm). L. calf is 20″ (50 cm). Toes are warm. Blood returns to nailbeds within 3 seconds of compression. Skin over legs is pink, warm, and intact. Homans' sign is negative bilaterally. Pneumatic compression device applied to calves of both legs and set at a pressure of 40 mmHg. ______________________ SIGNATURE, TITLE

Date and Time Pneumatic compression device removed after 2 hrs. of use to facilitate bathing and reapplied at 40 mmHg. ______________________ SIGNATURE, TITLE

CRITICAL THINKING

- Compare the use of TED hose with a pneumatic compression device; list advantages and disadvantages for each.

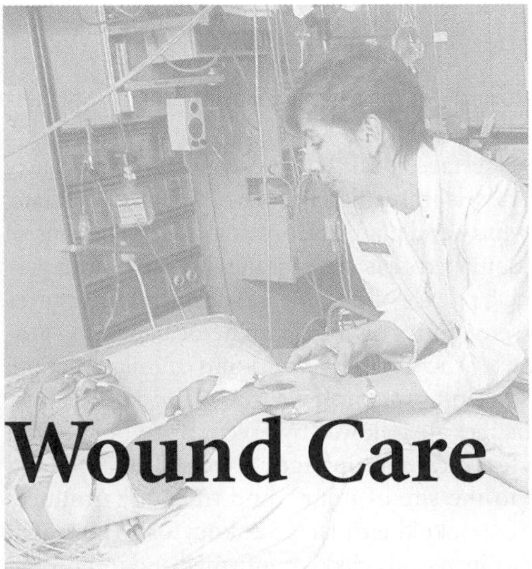

CHAPTER 28

Wound Care

CHAPTER OUTLINE

Wounds
Wound Repair
Wound Healing
Wound Management
Pressure Ulcers
Nursing Implications

NURSING GUIDELINES

PERFORMING AN EYE IRRIGATION
PREVENTING PRESSURE ULCERS

SKILLS

SKILL 28-1: CHANGING A GAUZE DRESSING
SKILL 28-2: IRRIGATING A WOUND
SKILL 28-3: PROVIDING A SITZ BATH

NURSING CARE PLAN

IMPAIRED SKIN INTEGRITY

KEY TERMS

aquathermia pad
bandage
binder
capillary action
closed wound
collagen
compresses
debridement
douche
drains
dressing
first-intention healing
granulation tissue
hydrotherapy
inflammation
irrigation
leukocytes
leukocytosis
macrophages
Montgomery straps
necrotic tissue
open wound
pack
phagocytosis
pressure ulcer
proliferation
purulent drainage
regeneration
remodeling
resolution
scar formation
second-intention healing
sepsis
serous drainage
shearing force
sitz bath
skin tear
soak
staples
sutures
therapeutic baths
third-intention healing
trauma
wound

LEARNING OBJECTIVES

An understanding of the content within this chapter will be evidenced by the student's ability to:

- Define the term "wound."
- Name three phases of wound repair.
- Identify five signs and symptoms classically associated with the inflammatory response.
- Discuss the purpose of phagocytosis, including the two types of cells involved with this activity.
- Name three ways in which the integrity of a wound is restored.
- Explain first-, second-, and third-intention healing.
- Name two types of wounds.
- State at least three purposes for using a dressing.
- Explain the rationale for keeping wounds moist.
- Describe two types of drains, including the purpose of each.
- Name the two major methods for securing surgical wounds together until they heal.
- Explain three reasons for using a bandage or binder.
- Discuss the purpose for using one type of binder.
- Give examples of four methods used to remove nonliving tissue from a wound.
- List three structures that are commonly irrigated.
- State two uses each for applying heat and for applying cold.
- Identify at least four methods for applying heat and cold.
- List at least five risk factors for developing pressure ulcers.
- Discuss three techniques for preventing pressure ulcers.

The body has a remarkable ability to recover when tissue is injured. This chapter discusses several types of tissue injury, including those caused by surgical incisions and prolonged pressure. Nursing interventions to support the healing process and actions to prevent tissue injury are also addressed.

Wounds

A **wound** (damaged skin or soft tissue) occurs as a result of **trauma** (general term referring to injury). Tissue trauma occurs, for example, from cuts, blows, poor circulation, strong chemicals, and excessive heat or cold. The trauma produces two basic types of wounds: open and closed (Table 28-1).

An **open wound** (one in which the surface of the skin or mucous membrane is no longer intact) may be caused accidentally or intentionally, as when a surgeon incises the tissue. A **closed wound** (one in which there is no opening in the skin or mucous membrane) occurs more often from blunt trauma or pressure.

Wound Repair

Regardless of the type of wound, the body immediately attempts to repair the injury and heal the wound. The process of wound repair proceeds in three sequential phases: inflammation, proliferation, and remodeling.

INFLAMMATION

Inflammation (physiologic defense that occurs immediately after tissue injury) lasts about 2 to 5 days. Its purposes are to limit the local damage, remove injured cells and debris, and prepare the wound for healing. Inflammation progresses through several stages (Fig. 28-1).

TABLE 28–1. **Types of Wounds**

Wound Types	Description
Open Wounds	
Incision	A clean separation of skin and tissue with smooth, even edges
Laceration	A separation of skin and tissue in which the edges are torn and irregular
Abrasion	A wound in which the surface layers of skin are scraped away
Avulsion	Stripping away of large areas of skin and underlying tissue, leaving cartilage and bone exposed
Ulceration	A shallow crater in which skin or mucous membrane is missing
Puncture	An opening of skin, underlying tissue, or mucous membrane caused by a narrow, sharp, pointed object
Closed Wounds	
Contusion	Injury to soft tissue underlying the skin from the force of contact with a hard object, sometimes called a bruise

During the first stage, local changes occur. When an injury occurs, blood vessels immediately constrict, but later dilate, in the zone of injury and platelets form a loose clot to control bleeding. The damaged cells' membranes become more permeable, causing a release of plasma and chemical substances that transmit a sensation of discomfort. The local response produces the characteristic signs and symptoms of inflammation: *swelling, redness, warmth, pain*, and *decreased function.*

The local changes are followed by a second wave of defense when **leukocytes** and **macrophages** (types of white blood cells) migrate to the site of injury, and the body produces more and more to take their place. **Leukocytosis** (increased production of white blood cells) is confirmed and monitored by counting the number and type of white blood cells in a sample of the patient's blood. The laboratory test is called a white blood cell count and differential. A rise in white blood cells, particularly neutrophils and monocytes, suggests that an inflammatory and, in some cases, an infectious process is occurring.

Neutrophils and monocytes, specific kinds of white blood cells, are primarily responsible for the **phagocytosis** (process of consuming substances) of pathogens, coagulated blood, and cellular debris. Collectively, they clean the area of injury and prepare the site for wound healing.

PROLIFERATION

Proliferation (period during which new cells fill and seal a wound) occurs from 2 days to 3 weeks after the inflammatory phase. It is characterized by the appearance of **granulation tissue** (combination of new blood vessels, fibroblasts, and epithelial cells), which is bright pink to red because of the extensive projections of capillaries in the area.

Granulation tissue grows from the wound margin toward the center. It is fragile and easily disrupted by physical or chemical means. As more and more fibroblasts produce **collagen** (protein substance that is tough and inelastic), the adhesive strength of the wound increases. Toward the end of the proliferative phase, the new blood vessels degenerate, causing the previously pink color to disappear.

Generally, the integrity of the skin and damaged tissue is restored by **resolution** (process by which damaged cells recover and re-establish their normal function), **regeneration** (cell duplication), or **scar formation** (replacement of damaged cells with fibrous tissue). Fibrous scar tissue acts as a nonfunctioning patch. The extent of scar tissue that forms depends on the magnitude of tissue damage and the manner of wound healing, which is discussed later in this chapter.

REMODELING

Remodeling (period during which the wound undergoes changes and maturation) follows the proliferative phase and

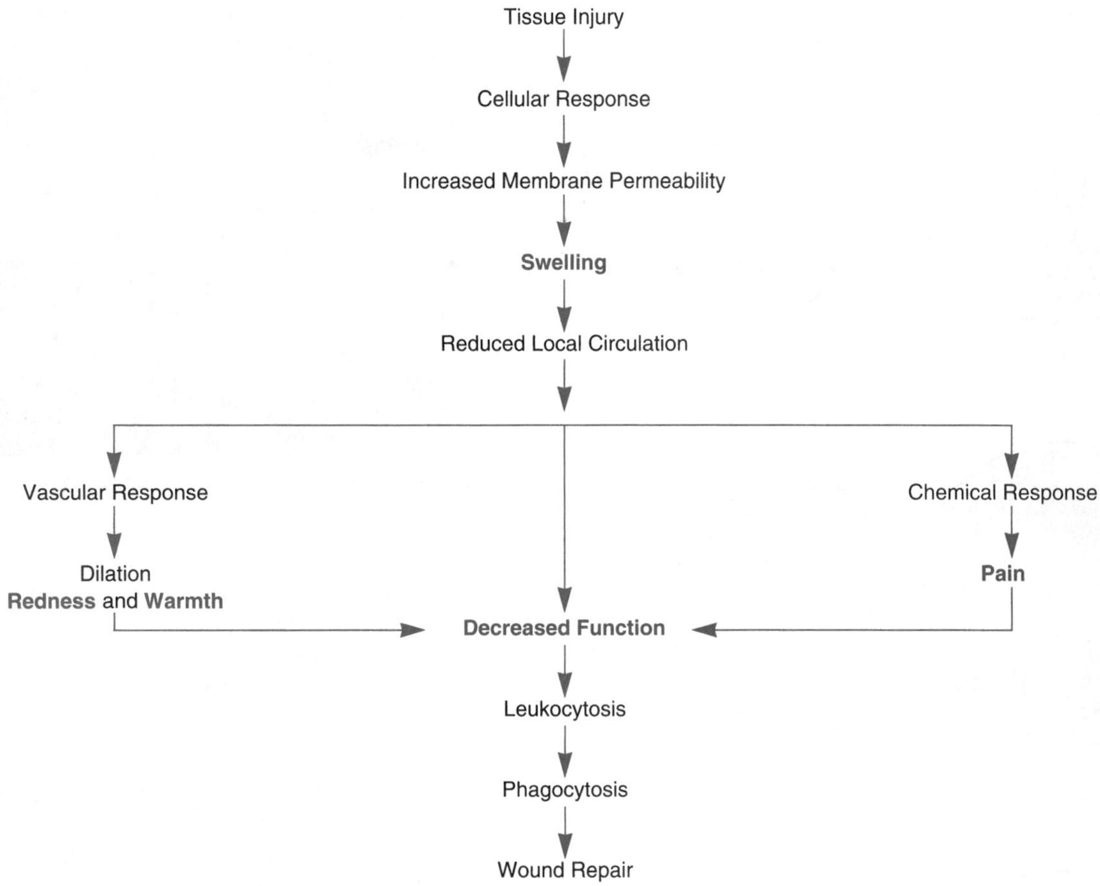

FIGURE 28–1. The inflammatory response.

may last 6 months to 2 years (Porth, 1998). During this time, the wound contracts and the scar shrinks.

Wound Healing

Wound healing is affected by a number of factors, including:

- Type of wound injury
- Expanse or depth of wound
- Quality of circulation
- Amount of wound debris
- Presence of infection
- Status of the patient's health

The speed with which wound repair takes place and the extent of scar tissue that forms depend on whether the wound heals by first, second, or third intention (Fig. 28-2).

First-intention healing (reparative process when wound edges are directly next to one another) is also called healing by primary intention. Because the space between the wound is so narrow, only a small amount of scar tissue forms. Most surgical wounds that are closely approximated heal by first intention.

Second-intention healing (reparative process when the wound edges are widely separated) is more time-consuming and complex. Because the margins of the wound are not in direct contact, additional time is needed for the granulation tissue to extend across the expanse of the wound. Generally, a conspicuous scar results. Healing by second intention is prolonged when the wound contains body fluid or other wound debris. Wound care must be performed cautiously to avoid disrupting the granulation tissue and retarding the healing process.

Third-intention healing (reparative process when the wound edges are widely separated and are later brought together with some type of closure material) results in a broad, deep scar. Generally a wound that heals by third intention is deep and likely to contain extensive drainage and tissue debris. To speed healing, the wound may contain drainage devices or may be packed with absorbent gauze (Fig. 28-3).

Wound Management

Wound management involves techniques that promote wound healing. Surgical wounds occur as a result of incising tissue with a laser (see Chap. 27) or an instrument called a scalpel. The primary goal of surgical or open wound management is to reapproximate the tissue to restore its integrity.

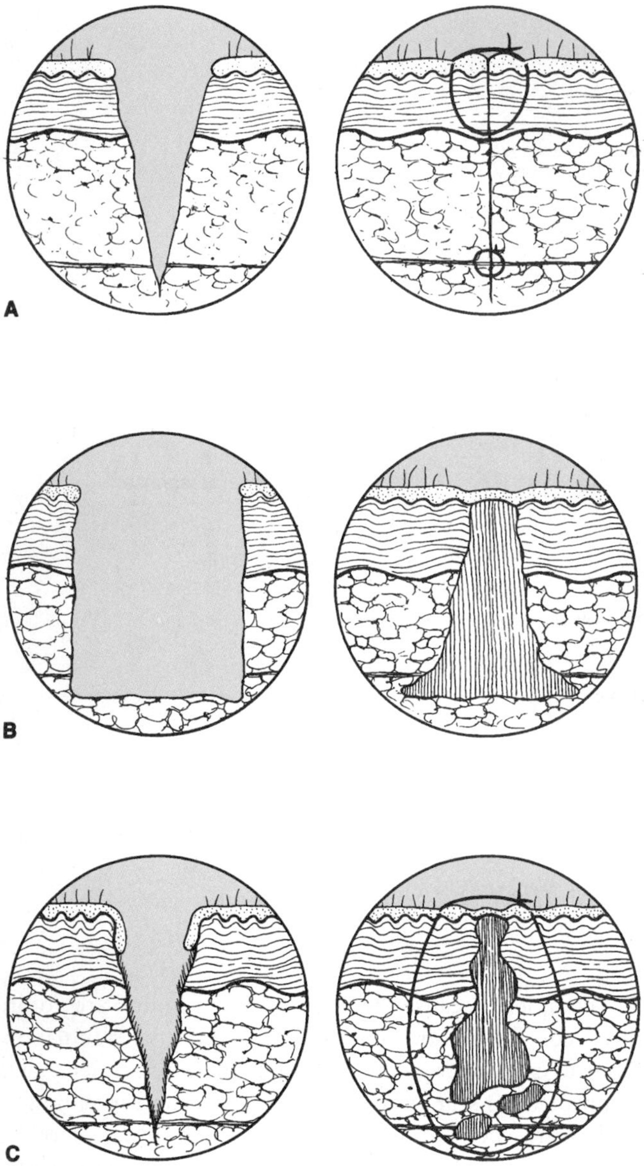

FIGURE 28–2. (*A*) First intention healing (*B*) Second intention healing (*C*) Third intention healing.

For a **pressure ulcer** (wound caused by capillary compression that is prolonged and sufficient to impair circulation to the skin and underlying tissue), the primary goal is prevention. Once a pressure ulcer forms, however, the nurse implements measures to reduce the size of the wound and to restore skin and tissue integrity.

Wound management involves using dressings, caring for drains, removing sutures or staples, applying bandages and binders, and administering irrigations.

DRESSINGS

A **dressing** (cover over a wound) may serve one or more purposes, such as:

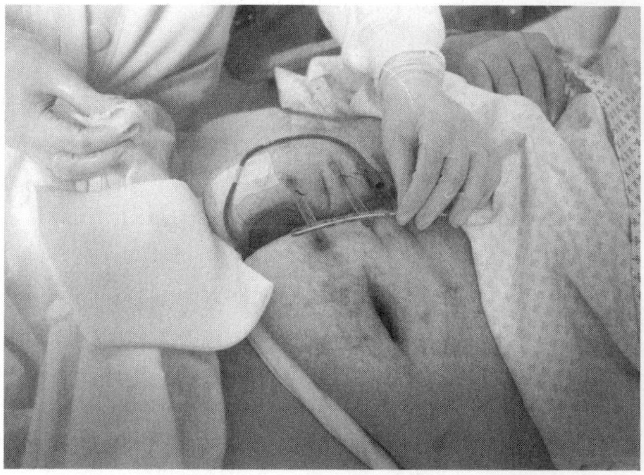

FIGURE 28–3. Example of third intention healing. (Courtesy of Ken Timby.)

- Keeping the wound clean
- Absorbing drainage
- Controlling bleeding
- Protecting the wound from injury
- Holding medication in place
- Maintaining a moist environment

There are several different types of dressings, depending on the purpose for their use. The most common wound coverings are gauze, transparent, and hydrocolloid dressings. All dressing materials come in a variety of sizes.

Gauze Dressings

Gauze dressings are made of woven cloth fibers. Their highly absorbent nature makes them ideal for covering fresh wounds that are likely to bleed or those that exude drainage. Unfortunately, gauze dressings cover the wound and interfere with wound assessment. Unless ointment is used on the wound or the gauze is lubricated with an ointment such as petroleum, granulation tissue may adhere to the gauze fibers.

Gauze dressings are usually secured with tape. If gauze dressings need frequent changing, **Montgomery straps** (strips of tape with eyelets) may be used (Fig. 28-4). Another method

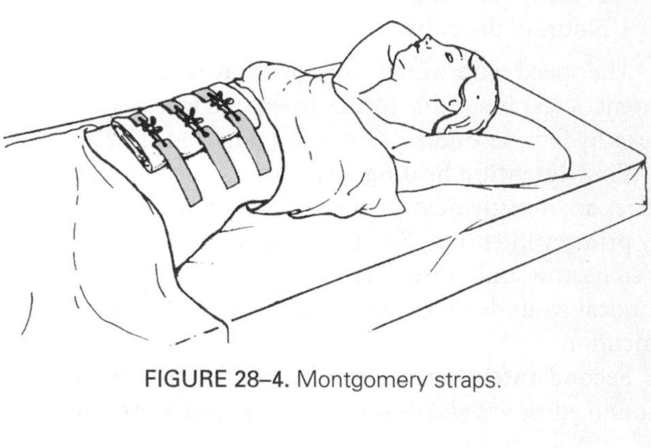

FIGURE 28–4. Montgomery straps.

may be necessary if the patient is allergic to tape (see the section about bandages and binders later in this chapter).

Transparent Dressings

Transparent dressings such as Op-Site are clear wound coverings. One of their chief advantages is that they allow the nurse to assess the wound without removing the dressing. In addition, they are less bulky than gauze dressings and do not require tape because they consist of a single sheet of adhesive material (Fig. 28-5). They are commonly used to cover peripheral and central IV insertion sites. Transparent dressings are not absorbent, so if wound drainage accumulates, the dressing tends to loosen. Once the dressing is no longer intact, many of its original purposes are defeated.

Hydrocolloid Dressings

Hydrocolloid dressings such as DuoDerm are self-adhesive, opaque, air- and water-occlusive wound coverings (Fig. 28-6). They keep wounds moist; a moist wound heals more quickly because new cells grow more rapidly in a wet environment. If the dressing remains intact, it can be left in place for up to a week. The occlusive nature of hydrocolloid dressings also repels other body substances, such as urine or stool.

Dressing Changes

Dressings are changed when the wound requires assessment or care and when the dressing becomes loose or saturated with drainage. In some cases, the physician may choose to assume total responsibility for changing the dressing—at least for the first time. However, the dressing is *reinforced* (additional absorbent layers are applied) if it becomes moist. Reinforcing a dressing prevents wicking microorganisms toward the wound (see Chap. 21).

Because most surgical wounds are covered with gauze dressings, this example is used when describing the technique for changing a dressing in Skill 28-1. When other types of dressings are used, nurses can modify the dressing technique by following the manufacturer's directions.

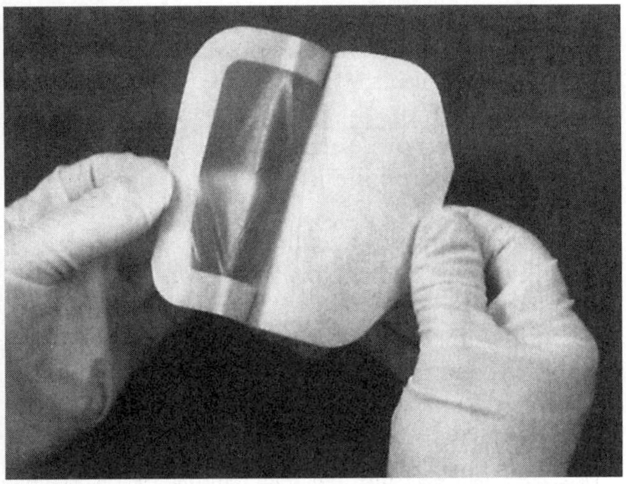

FIGURE 28–5. Transparent dressing. (Courtesy of Ken Timby.)

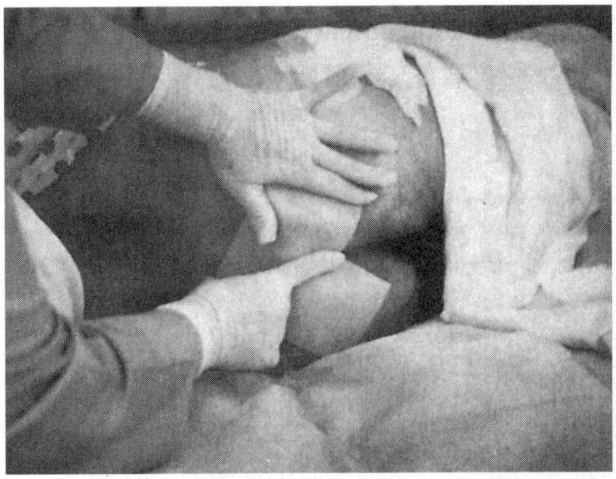

FIGURE 28–6. Hydrocolloid dressing. (Courtesy of E. R. Squibb & Sons, Inc., Princeton, NJ.)

DRAINS

Drains (tubes that provide a means for removing blood and drainage from a wound) promote wound healing by removing fluid and cellular debris. Although some drains are placed directly within a wound, the current trend is to insert them so that they exit from a separate location beside the wound. This approach keeps the wound margins approximated and avoids a direct entry site for pathogens. The physician may choose to use an open or closed drain.

Open Drains

Open drains are flat, flexible tubes that provide a pathway for drainage toward the dressing. The drainage takes place passively by gravity and **capillary action** (movement of a liquid at the point of contact with a solid). Sometimes a safety pin or long clip is attached to the drain as it extends from the wound. This prevents the drain from slipping within the tissue. As the drainage decreases, the physician may instruct the nurse to shorten the drain, enabling the wound to heal from the inside toward the outside of the wound. To shorten a drain, it is pulled from the wound for the specified length. The safety pin or clip is then repositioned near the wound to prevent the drain from sliding back into the wound (Fig. 28-7).

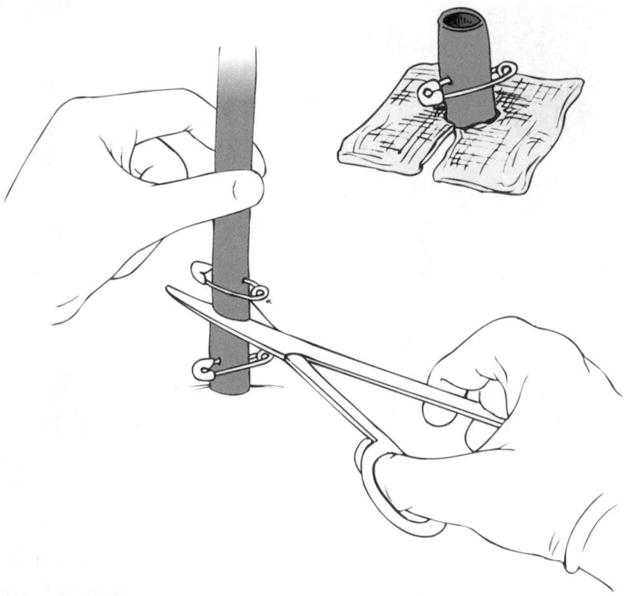

FIGURE 28–7. An open drain is pulled from the wound, and the excess portion is cut. A drain sponge is placed around the drain, and the wound is covered with a gauze dressing.

Closed Drains

Closed drains are tubes that terminate in a receptacle. Some examples of closed drainage systems are a Hemovac and Jackson-Pratt (JP) drain (Fig. 28-8). Closed drains are more efficient than open drains because they pull fluid by creating a vacuum or negative pressure. This is done by opening the vent on the receptacle, squeezing the drainage collection chamber, and then capping the vent.

When caring for a wound with a drain, the insertion site is cleansed in a circular manner. After cleansing, a precut drain gauze, which is open to its center, is placed around the base of the drain. An open drain may require additional layers of gauze because the drainage does not collect in a receptacle.

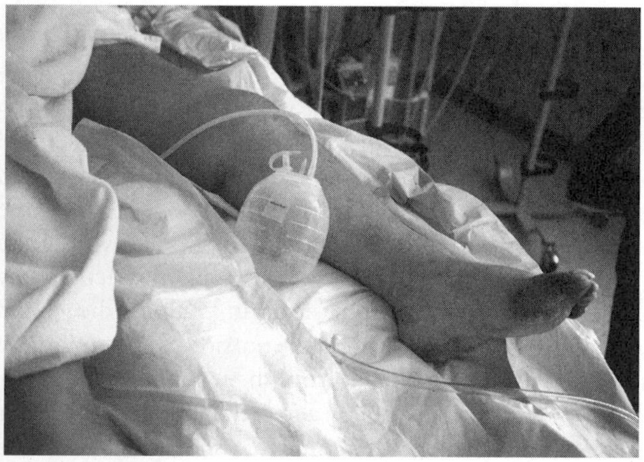

FIGURE 28–8. Jackson-Pratt (closed) drain. (Courtesy of Ken Timby.)

SUTURES AND STAPLES

Sutures (knotted ties that hold an incision together) are generally constructed from silk or synthetic materials such as nylon. **Staples** (wide metal clips) perform a similar function. Staples do not encircle a wound like sutures; instead, they form a bridge that holds the two wound margins together. Staples are advantageous because they do not compress the tissue should the wound swell.

Sutures and staples are left in place until the wound has healed sufficiently to prevent reopening. Depending on the location of the incision, this may be a few days to as long as 2 weeks.

The nurse may be directed by the physician to remove sutures and staples (Fig. 28-9), sometimes half on one day and the other half on another. A weak incision is temporarily held together afterwards with adhesive *Steri-strips*, also known as *butterflies* because of their winged appearance. Sometimes Steri-Strips are used instead of sutures or staples to close superficial lacerations.

BANDAGES AND BINDERS

A **bandage** (strip or roll of cloth) is wrapped around a body part. One example is an Ace bandage. A **binder** (type of bandage) is generally applied to a particular part of the body, such as the abdomen or breast. Bandages and binders are made from gauze, muslin, elastic rolls, and stockinette (see Chap. 25).

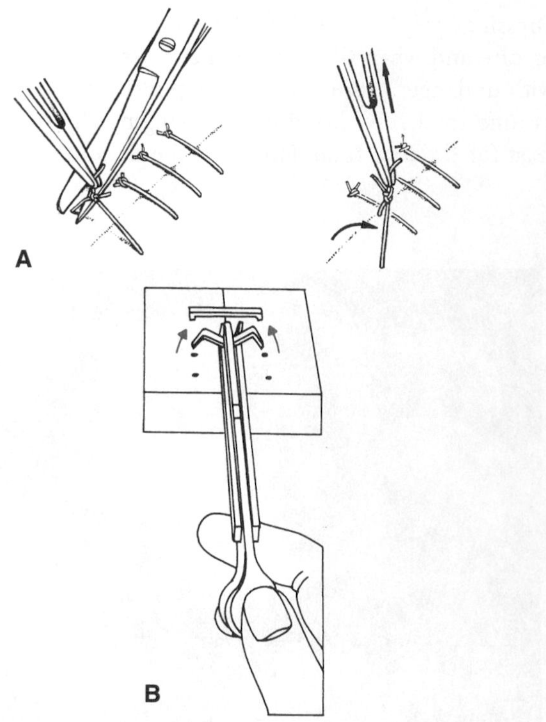

FIGURE 28–9. (*A*) Technique for suture removal. (*B*) Technique for staple removal.

Bandages and binders serve various purposes, including:

- Holding dressings in place, especially when tape cannot be used or the dressing is extremely large
- Supporting the area around a wound or injury to reduce pain
- Limiting movement in the wound area to promote healing

Roller Bandage Application

Most bandages are prepared in rolls of varying widths. The end is held in one hand while the roll is passed around the part being bandaged.

Several principles are followed when applying a roller bandage:

- Elevate and support the limb.
- Wrap from a distal to proximal direction.
- Avoid gaps between each turn of the bandage.
- Exert equal, but not excessive, tension with each turn.
- Keep the bandage free of wrinkles.
- Secure the end of the roller bandage with metal clips.
- Check the color and sensation of exposed fingers or toes often.
- Remove the bandage for hygiene and replace at least twice a day.

Six basic techniques are used for wrapping a roller bandage (Fig. 28-10): circular turn, spiral turn, spiral-reverse turn, figure-of-eight turn, spica turn, and recurrent turn.

A *circular turn* is used to anchor and secure a bandage where it starts and ends. It simply involves holding the free end of the rolled material in one hand and wrapping it about the area, bringing it back to the starting point.

A *spiral turn* partly overlaps a previous turn. The amount of overlapping varies from half to three fourths of the width of the bandage. Spiral turns are used when wrapping a cylindrical part of the body, such as the arms and legs.

A *spiral-reverse turn* is a modification of a spiral turn. The roll is reversed or turned downward halfway through the turn.

A *figure-of-eight turn* is best when bandaging a joint such as the elbow or knee. This pattern is made by making oblique turns that alternately ascend and descend, simulating the number eight.

A *spica turn* is a variation of the figure-of-eight pattern. It differs in that the wrap includes a portion of the trunk or chest (see spica cast, Chap. 25).

A *recurrent turn* is made by passing the roll back and forth over the tip of a body part. Once several recurrent turns are made, the bandage is anchored by completing the application with another basic turn, such as the figure-of-eight. A recurrent turn is especially beneficial when wrapping the stump of an amputated limb or the head.

Binder Application

Binders are not used as commonly as bandages. Many have been replaced by more modern or convenient commercial devices. For example, brassieres have largely replaced breast binders. Sometimes after rectal or vaginal surgery, nurses apply a T-binder, which, as the name implies, looks like the letter T (Fig. 28-11). T-binders are used for securing a dressing to the anus or perineum or within the groin. To apply a T-binder, the crossbar of the T is fastened about the waist. Then the single or double tails are passed between the legs and pinned to the belt. Adhesive sanitary napkins worn inside underwear briefs are an alternative to a T-binder for stabilizing absorbent materials.

DEBRIDEMENT

Most wounds heal rapidly with conventional care. However, some wounds require **debridement** (removal of dead tissue) to promote healing. There are four methods for debriding a wound: sharp, enzymatic, autolytic, and mechanical.

Sharp Debridement

Sharp debridement is performed by removing **necrotic tissue** (nonliving tissue) from the healthy areas of a wound with sterile scissors and other instruments. This method is preferred if the wound is infected because it helps the wound heal quickly and well. The procedure is done at the bedside, or in the operating room if the wound is extensive. Sharp debridement is painful, and the wound may bleed afterward.

Enzymatic Debridement

Enzymatic debridement involves the use of topical substances that break down and liquefy wound debris. A dressing is used to keep the enzyme in contact with the wound and help absorb the drainage. This form of debridement is appropriate for uninfected wounds or for patients who cannot tolerate sharp debridement.

Autolytic Debridement

Autolytic debridement, or self-dissolution, is a painless, natural physiologic process that allows the body's enzymes to soften, liquefy, and release devitalized tissue. It is used when a wound is small and free of infection. The main disadvantage to autolysis is the prolonged time it takes to achieve desired results. To accelerate autolysis, the wound is kept moist with an occlusive or semi-occlusive dressing. Because removal of tissue debris is slow, the nurse monitors the patient closely for signs of wound infection.

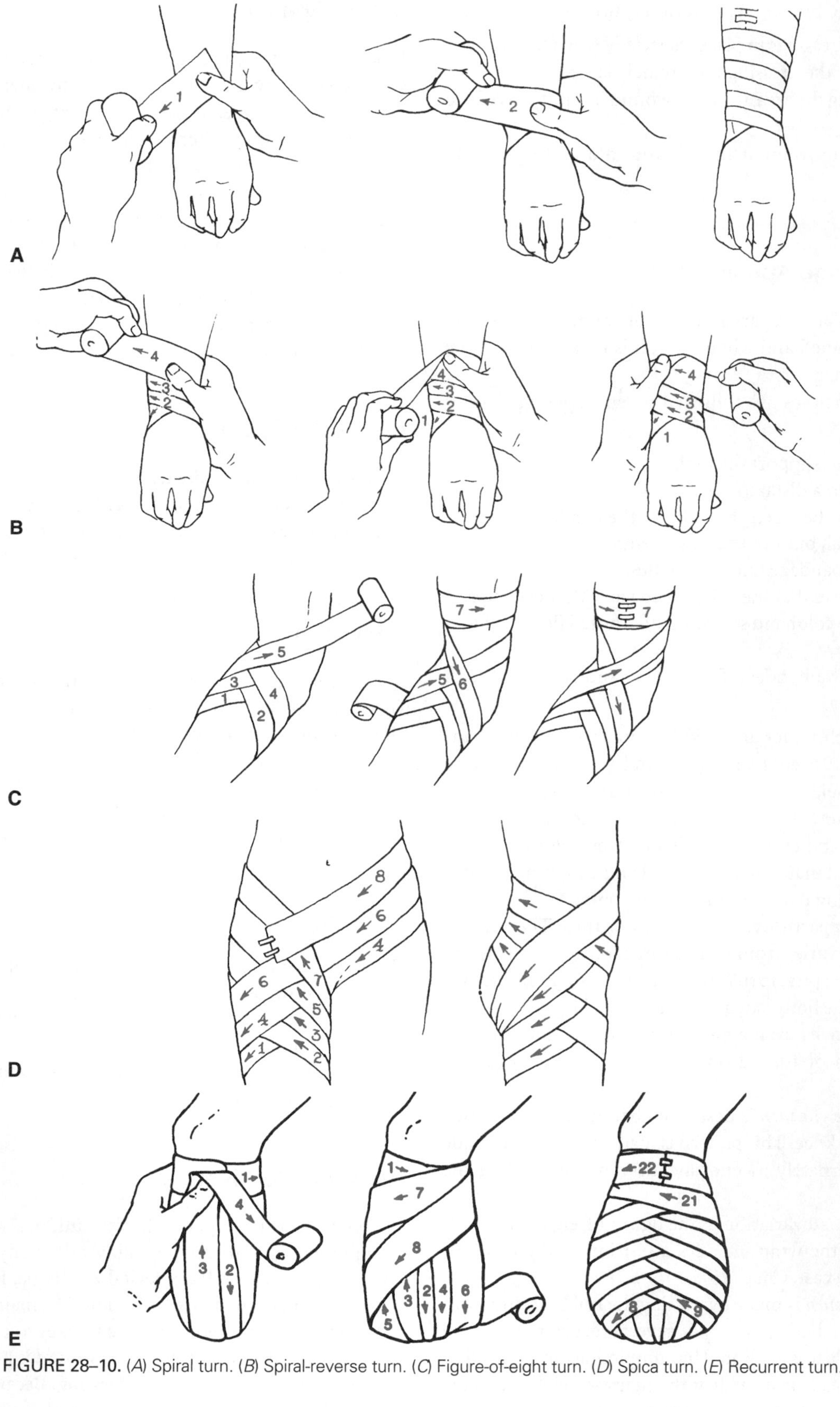

FIGURE 28–10. (*A*) Spiral turn. (*B*) Spiral-reverse turn. (*C*) Figure-of-eight turn. (*D*) Spica turn. (*E*) Recurrent turn.

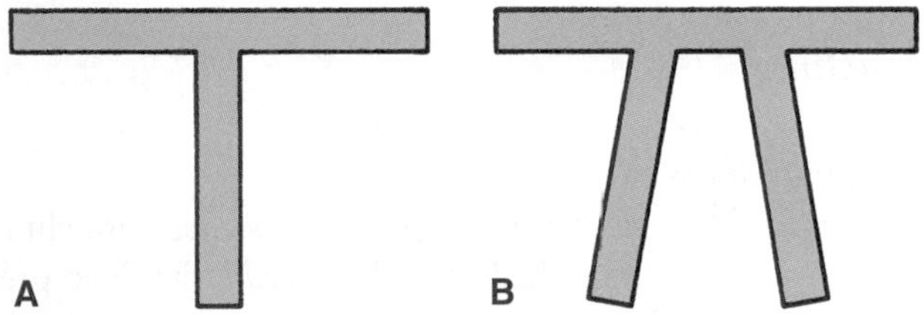

FIGURE 28–11. (*A*) Single T-binder. (*B*) Double T-binder.

Mechanical Debridement

Mechanical debridement involves physical removal of debris. One technique is the application of wet-to-dry dressings. The wound is packed with moist gauze that is removed about 4 to 6 hours later, when the gauze is dry or nearly dry. Dead tissue adheres to the meshwork of the gauze and is removed when the dressing is changed. The procedure is often painful, and healthy granulation tissue is sometimes disrupted or removed in the process.

Another approach to mechanical removal of wound debris is **hydrotherapy** (therapeutic use of water). The body part where the wound is located is submerged in a whirlpool tank. The agitation of the water, which contains an antiseptic, softens the dead tissue. Loose debris that remains attached is removed afterward by sharp debridement.

A third method for mechanically removing wound debris is an **irrigation** (technique for flushing debris). An irrigation is used when caring for a wound and also when cleaning an area of the body such as the eye, ear, and vagina.

Wound Irrigation

Wound irrigation (Skill 28-2) is generally carried out just before applying a new dressing. This technique is best used when granulation tissue has formed. Surface debris should be removed gently without disturbing the healthy proliferating cells.

Eye Irrigation

An eye irrigation is used to flush a toxic chemical from one or both eyes or to displace dried mucus or other drainage that accumulates from inflamed or infected eye structures.

Nursing Guidelines For

An Eye Irrigation

- ☑ Assemble supplies: bulb syringe, irrigating solution, gauze squares, gloves and other standard precaution apparel, absorbent pads, and at least one towel.
  RATIONALE: Assembling the equipment ahead of time ensures organization and efficient time management.
- ☑ Warm the solution to approximately body temperature by placing the container in warm water, except when administering emergency first aid.
  RATIONALE: A warm solution is more comfortable for the patient.
- ☑ Position the patient with the head tilted slightly toward the side.
  RATIONALE: This position facilitates drainage.
- ☑ Place absorbent material in the area of the shoulder.
  RATIONALE: Use of absorbent material prevents saturating the patient's gown and bed linen.
- ☑ Give the patient an emesis basin to hold beneath the cheek.
  RATIONALE: The basin can be used to collect the irrigating solution.
- ☑ Wash hands and don gloves.
  RATIONALE: Handwashing and glove use reduce the transmission of microorganisms.
- ☑ Open and prepare supplies.
  RATIONALE: This enables the nurse to perform the irrigation efficiently.
- ☑ Wipe a moistened gauze square from the nasal corner of the eye toward the temple; use additional gauze squares, one at a time, as needed.
  RATIONALE: This removes gross debris.
- ☑ Separate the eyelids widely with the fingers of one hand.
  RATIONALE: This action widens the exposed surface area.
- ☑ Direct the solution onto the conjunctiva, holding the syringe or irrigating device about 1″ (2.5 cm) above the eye (Fig. 28-12).
  RATIONALE: Holding the syringe away from the eye prevents injury to the cornea.
- ☑ Instruct the patient to blink periodically.
  RATIONALE: Blinking distributes solution under the eyelids and about the eye.

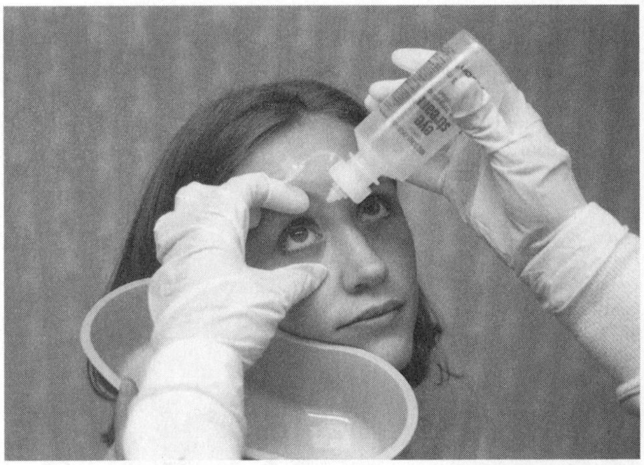

FIGURE 28–12. Eye irrigation. (Courtesy of Ken Timby.)

☑ Continue irrigating until debris is removed.
RATIONALE: This accomplishes the desired result.

☑ Dry the face and replace wet gown or linen.
RATIONALE: These actions make the patient comfortable.

☑ Dispose of soiled materials and gloves; wash hands.
RATIONALE: Getting rid of used materials and washing hands reduce the transmission of microorganisms.

☑ Record assessment data, specifics of the procedure, and outcome.
RATIONALE: Documentation is used to record the nursing care provided and the patient's response.

Ear Irrigation

An ear irrigation removes debris from the ear. An ear irrigation is contraindicated if the tympanic membrane (eardrum) is perforated. Performing a gross inspection of the ear is important if a foreign body is suspected, because a bean, pea, or other dehydrated substance can swell if the ear is irrigated, causing it to become even more tightly fixed. Solid objects may require removal with an instrument.

If an ear irrigation is not contraindicated, it is performed much like an eye irrigation, except that the solution is directed toward the roof of the auditory canal (Fig. 28-13). Also, the nurse takes care to avoid occluding the ear canal with the tip of the syringe, because the pressure of the trapped solution could rupture the eardrum. After the irrigation, a cotton ball is placed *loosely* within the ear to absorb drainage but not to obstruct its flow.

Vaginal Irrigation

A vaginal irrigation, also known as a **douche** (procedure for cleansing the vaginal canal), is sometimes necessary to treat an infection.

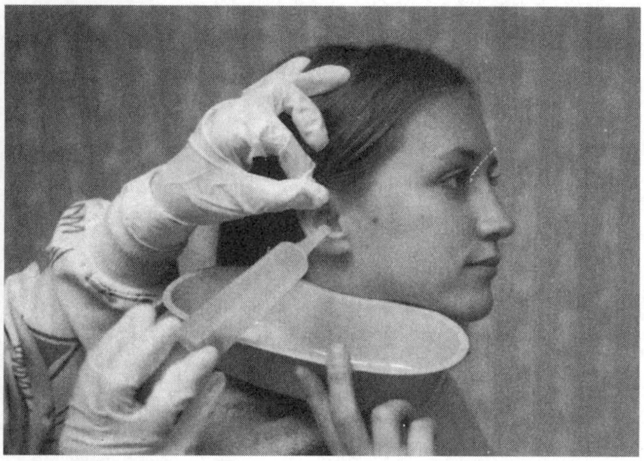

FIGURE 28–13. Ear irrigation. (Courtesy of Ken Timby.)

Patient Teaching About
Douching

Teach the patient to do the following:
- Do not douche as a routine practice, because douching removes microbes, called *Döderlein bacilli*, that help prevent vaginal infections.
- Do not douche 24 to 48 hours before a Pap test (see Chap. 13). Douching may wash away diagnostic cells.
- Consult a physician about symptoms such as itching, burning, or drainage rather than attempting self-diagnosis.
- Find out from the physician whether sexual partners also need to be treated with medications to avoid reinfection.
- Buy douching equipment from a drugstore; prefilled disposable containers are available.
- Warm the solution to a comfortable temperature (no more than 110°F (43.3°C).
- Clamp the tubing (on reusable equipment), and fill the reservoir bag.
- Undress and lie down in the bathtub.
- Suspend the douche bag (if used) about 18″ to 24″ (45–60 cm) above the hips.
- Insert the lubricated tip of the nozzle or the prefilled container downward and backward within the vagina about the distance of a tampon.
- Unclamp the tubing and rotate the nozzle as the fluid is instilled.
- Contract the perineal muscles as though trying to stop urinating, and then relax the muscles. Repeat the exercise four or five times while douching.
- Sit up to facilitate drainage, or shower afterward.
- Use a sanitary napkin or perineal pad to absorb residual drainage.

HEAT AND COLD APPLICATIONS

Heat and cold have various therapeutic uses (Display 28-1), and there are several ways each can be used. An ice bag, collar, chemical pack, compresses, and aquathermia pad can be used. Heat also is applied with soaks, moist packs, and therapeutic baths.

DISPLAY 28–1

Common Uses for Heat and Cold Applications

Uses for Heat	*Uses for Cold*
• Provides warmth	• Reduces fevers
• Promotes circulation	• Prevents swelling
• Speeds healing	• Controls bleeding
• Relieves muscle spasm	• Relieves pain
• Reduces pain	• Numbs sensation

The terms "hot" and "cold" are subject to wide interpretation. Table 28-2 correlates common terms with temperature ranges. Because injuries can occur when the skin is exposed to extremes of temperature, the nurse assesses the temperature of the application and frequently monitors the condition of the skin. Direct contact between the heating or cooling device and the skin is avoided. Hot and cold applications are used cautiously in children younger than 2 years, older adults, patients with diabetes, and patients who are comatose or neurologically impaired.

Ice Bag and Ice Collar

Ice bags and ice collars are containers into which crushed ice or small ice cubes are placed. Ice collars are usually applied after tonsil removal. Ice bags are applied to any small injury that is in the process of swelling. Although ice bags are available commercially, they can also be improvised. A rubber or plastic glove, a plastic bag with a zipper closure, or a bag of small frozen vegetables, such as peas, can be used. Patient instruction minimizes the risk for injury.

Patient Teaching For:

Using an Ice Bag

Teach the patient or family to do the following:

- Test the ice bag for leaks.
- Fill it half to two-thirds full of crushed ice or small cubes so it can be easily molded to the injured area.
- Eliminate as much air from the bag as possible.
- Pour water over the ice to provide slight melting. This tends to smooth the sharp edges from frozen ice crystals.
- Cover the ice bag with a layer of cloth before placing it on the body.
- Leave the ice bag in place no more than 20 to 30 minutes. Allow the skin and tissue to recover for at least a half-hour before reapplying.
- If the skin becomes mottled or numb, remove the ice bag; it is too cold.

TABLE 28–2. **Temperature Ranges for Applications of Heat and Cold**

Level of Heat or Cold	Temperature Range
Very hot	40.5°C to 46.1°C (105°F–115°F)
Hot	36.6°C to 40.5°C (98°F–105°F)
Warm and neutral	33.8°C to 36.6°C (93°F–98°F)
Tepid	26.6°C to 33.8°C (80°F–93°F)
Cool	18.3°C to 26.6°C (65°F–80°F)
Cold	10°C to 18.3°C (50°F–65°F)
Very cold	Below 10°C (below 50°F)

Chemical Packs

Commercial cold packs are struck or crushed to activate the chemicals inside, causing them to become cool. This type of cold pack is generally included in most first-aid kits. They can be used only once. Gel packs, designed for cold or hot application, are reusable (Fig. 28-14). They are stored in the freezer until needed or heated in a microwave.

Compresses

Compresses (moist, warm or cool cloths) are applied to the skin. The compress is soaked in tap water or medicated solution at the appropriate temperature, excess moisture is wrung out, and the compress is applied to the skin. To maintain the moisture and temperature, a piece of plastic or plastic wrap is used to cover the compress and the area is secured in a towel. As the compress material cools, it is removed, rewarmed, and reapplied if necessary.

If the skin is not intact, as in the case of a draining wound, gloves must be worn when applying a compress. Aseptic technique should be used when applying compresses to an open wound.

Aquathermia Pad

An **aquathermia pad** (electrical heating or cooling device) is sometimes called a *K-pad*. It resembles a mat, but it contains hollow channels through which heated or cooled distilled water circulates (Fig. 28-15). An aquathermia pad is used alone or as a cover over a compress. A thermostat is used to

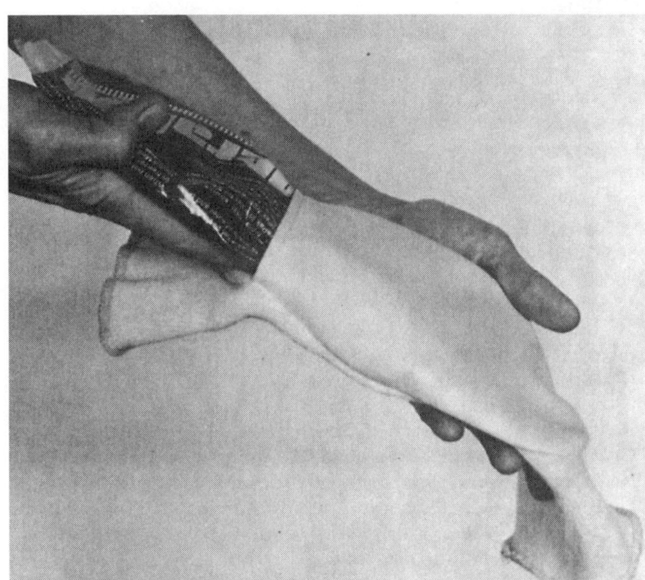

FIGURE 28–14. Commercial cold pack. (Courtesy of HydroMed Products, Inc., Dallas, TX.)

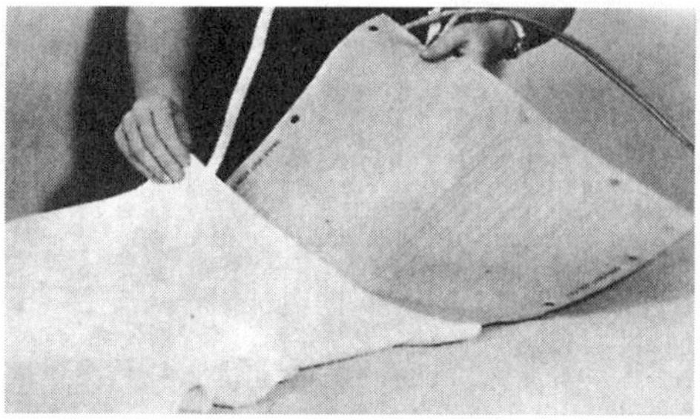

FIGURE 28–15. Aquathermia pad (K-pad).

keep the temperature of the water at the specified setting. As with other forms of hot and cold therapeutic devices, the skin is assessed frequently and the device is removed periodically.

Before placing the patient on the pad or wrapping it about a part of the body, the pad is covered to help prevent thermal skin damage. A roller bandage may help hold it in place. The electrical unit is positioned slightly higher than the patient to promote gravity circulation of the fluid.

Larger styles are used to warm patients with hypothermia or to cool those with heat stroke. Because these patients have dangerously altered body temperatures, the nurse must monitor vital signs continuously.

Soaks and Moist Packs

A **soak** (procedure in which a part of the body is submerged in fluid) is a technique for providing warmth or applying a medicated solution. A **pack** (commercial device for applying moist heat) can also be used (Fig. 28-16). Moist heat is more comforting and therapeutic than dry heat.

A soak usually lasts 15 to 20 minutes. The temperature of the fluid is kept as constant as possible, which requires frequent emptying and refilling of the basin. The newly added water should not be too hot; overly hot water causes discomfort or tissue damage.

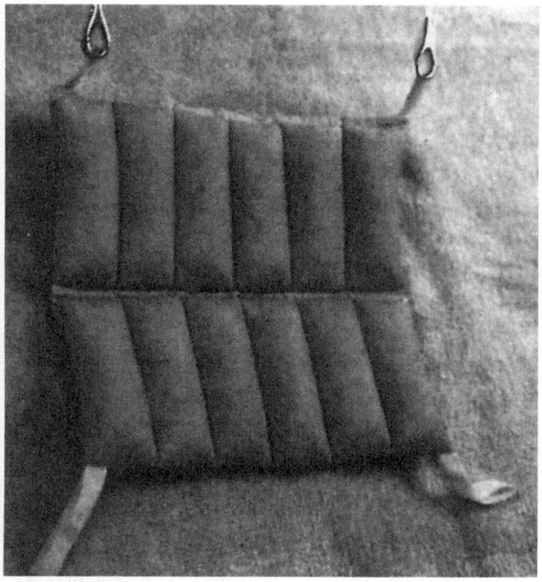

FIGURE 28–16. Hot pack. (Courtesy of Ken Timby.)

Packs differ from soaks in two major ways: the duration of the application is usually longer, and the initial application of heat is generally more intense. Packs are usually applied at temperatures as warm as the patient can tolerate. Because of the potential for causing burns, a pack is never used on a patient who is unresponsive or paralyzed and cannot perceive temperatures. The nurse must make frequent assessments and remove the pack if there is any likelihood of a thermal injury.

Therapeutic Baths

Therapeutic baths (those performed for other than hygiene purposes) can be used to reduce a high fever or apply medicated substances to the skin to treat skin disorders or discomfort. Examples are baths to which sodium bicarbonate (baking soda), cornstarch, or oatmeal paste are added.

The most common type of therapeutic bath is a **sitz bath** (soak of the perianal area). A sitz bath is used to reduce swelling and inflammation and to promote healing of wounds after a *hemorrhoidectomy* (surgical removal of engorged veins inside and outside the anal sphincter) or an *episiotomy* (incision that facilitates vaginal birth). Some health care agencies have special tubs for administering sitz baths, but most patients are provided with disposable equipment (Skill 28-3).

Pressure Ulcers

Pressure ulcers, also referred to as *decubitus ulcers*, most often appear over bony prominences of the sacrum, hips, and heels. They can also develop in other locations such as the elbows, the shoulder blades, the back of the head, and places where pressure is unrelieved because of infrequent movement (Fig. 28-17). The tissue in these areas is particularly vulnerable because body fat, which acts as a pressure-absorbing cushion, is minimal. Consequently, the tissue is compressed between the bony mass and a rigid surface such as a chair or bed. If the compression reduces the pressure in local capillaries to less than 32 mmHg for 1 to 2 hours without intermittent relief, the cells die from lack of oxygen and nutrition.

STAGES OF PRESSURE ULCERS

Pressure ulcers are grouped into four stages according to the extent of tissue injury (Fig. 28-18). Care and healing depend on the stage of injury. Without aggressive nursing care, early-

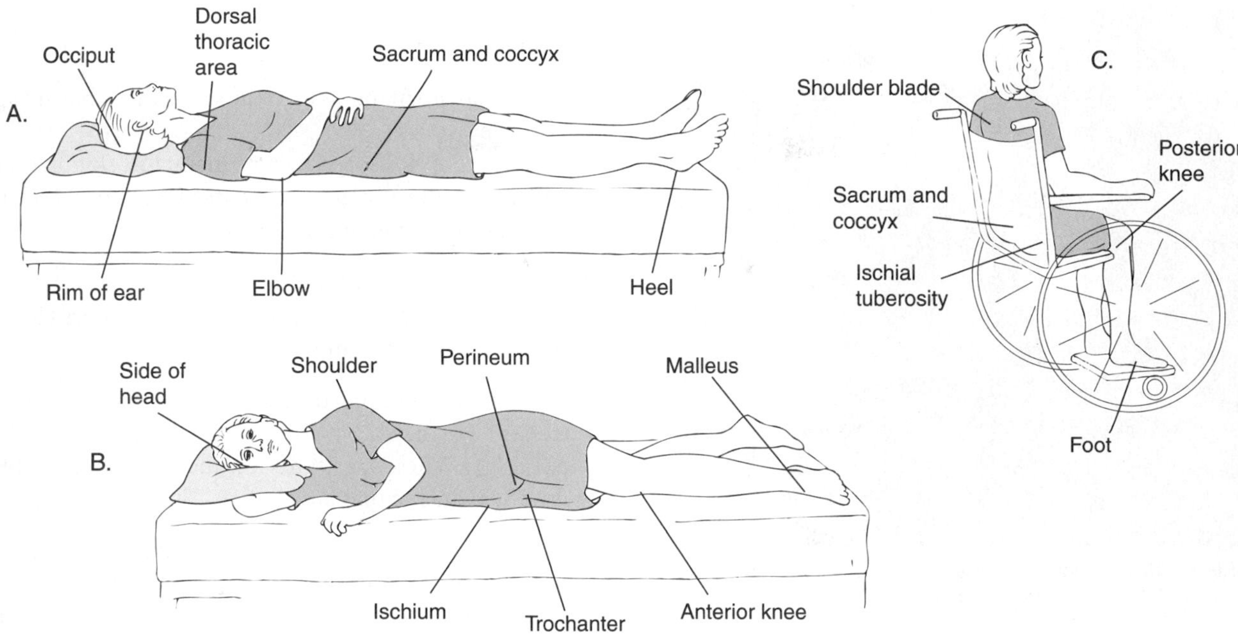

FIGURE 28–17. Locations where pressure ulcers commonly form: (*A*) supine position, (*B*) side-lying position, (*C*) sitting position.

stage pressure ulcers can easily progress to much more serious ones.

Stage I is characterized by intact but reddened skin. The hallmark of cellular damage is skin that remains red and fails to resume its normal color when pressure is relieved.

A stage II pressure ulcer is red and accompanied by blistering or a **skin tear** (shallow break in the skin). Impairment of the skin may lead to colonization and infection of the wound.

A stage III pressure ulcer has a shallow skin crater that extends to the subcutaneous tissue. It may be accompanied by **serous drainage** (leaking plasma) or **purulent drainage** (white or greenish fluid) caused by a wound infection. The area is relatively painless despite the severity of the ulcer.

Stage IV pressure ulcers are life-threatening. The tissue is deeply ulcerated, exposing muscle and bone (Fig. 28-19). The dead or infected tissue may produce a foul odor. The infection easily spreads throughout the body, causing **sepsis** (potentially fatal systemic infection).

PREVENTION OF PRESSURE ULCERS

The first step in prevention is to identify patients with risk factors for pressure ulcers (Display 28-2). The second step is to implement measures that reduce conditions under which pressure ulcers are likely to form.

Nursing Guidelines For

Preventing Pressure Ulcers

- Change the bedridden patient's position frequently. Remind a patient sitting in a chair to stand and move about hourly or at least to shift his or her weight every 15 minutes while sitting.
  RATIONALE: Changing positions relieves pressure and restores circulation.
- Lift rather than drag the patient during repositioning.
  RATIONALE: Dragging causes friction, which abrades the skin and damages underlying blood vessels.

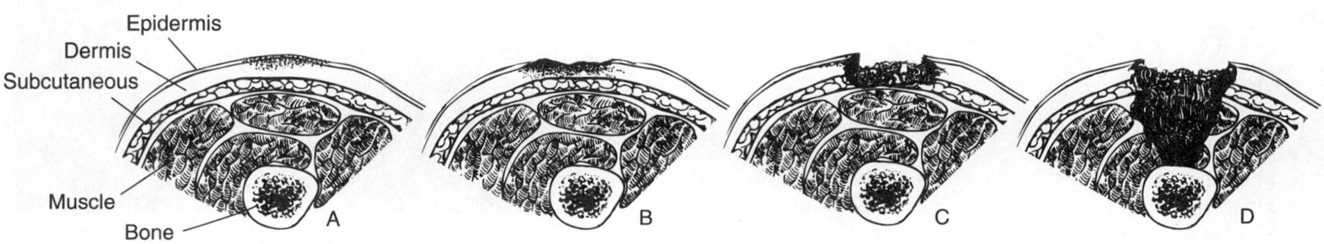

FIGURE 28–18. Pressure sore stages: (*A*) Stage I, (*B*) Stage II, (*C*) Stage III, (*D*) Stage IV.

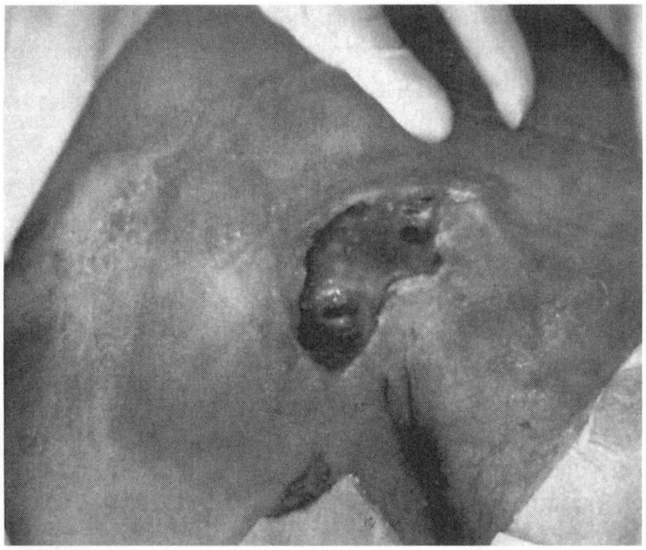

FIGURE 28–19. Example of stage IV pressure sore. (Courtesy of E. R. Squibb & Sons, Inc., Princeton, NJ.)

☑ Avoid using plastic-covered pillows when positioning patients.
RATIONALE: Plastic prevents evaporation of perspiration because it is nonporous. It also raises skin temperature, further contributing to the growth of microorganisms.

☑ Use positioning devices such as pillows to keep two parts of the body from direct contact with each other.
RATIONALE: Such devices absorb perspiration, reduce localized heat, and avoid compression of tissue between two body parts.

☑ Use the lateral oblique position (see Chap. 23) rather than the conventional lateral position for side-lying.
RATIONALE: The lateral oblique position reduces the potential for pressure on vulnerable bony prominences more effectively.

☑ Massage bony prominences only if the skin blanches with pressure relief.
RATIONALE: Massage improves circulation to normal tissue but causes further damage to areas where pressure ulcers—even those that are stage I—are already established.

☑ Keep the skin clean and dry, especially when patients cannot control their bladder or bowel function.
RATIONALE: Cleansing removes substances that chemically injure the skin.

☑ Use a moisturizing skin cleanser rather than soap, if possible.
RATIONALE: A nonsoap cleanser maintains skin hydration and avoids altering the skin's natural acidity, which protects it from bacterial colonization.

☑ Rinse and dry the skin well.
RATIONALE: Cleansing and then drying removes chemical residues and surface moisture.

☑ Use pressure-relieving devices such as special beds or mattresses (see Chap. 23).
RATIONALE: These special devices maintain capillary blood flow by reducing pressure.

☑ Pad body areas such as the heels, ankles, and elbows, which are vulnerable to friction and pressure (Fig. 28-20).
RATIONALE: Padding prevents friction and adds a cushioning layer over the bony prominence.

☑ Use seat cushions such as a commercial gel-filled pad when patients sit for extended periods.
RATIONALE: These cushions distribute pressure over a wider area, relieving direct pressure on the coccyx.

☑ Keep the head of the bed elevated no more than 30 degrees.
RATIONALE: Sliding down in bed can produce **shearing force** (effect that moves layers of tissue in opposite directions).

☑ Provide a balanced diet and adequate fluid intake.
RATIONALE: Adequate nutrition maintains and restores cells and keeps tissues hydrated.

DISPLAY 28–2

Risk Factors for Developing Pressure Ulcers

- Inactivity
- Immobility
- Malnutrition
- Emaciation
- Diaphoresis
- Incontinence
- Vascular disease
- Localized edema
- Dehydration
- Sedation

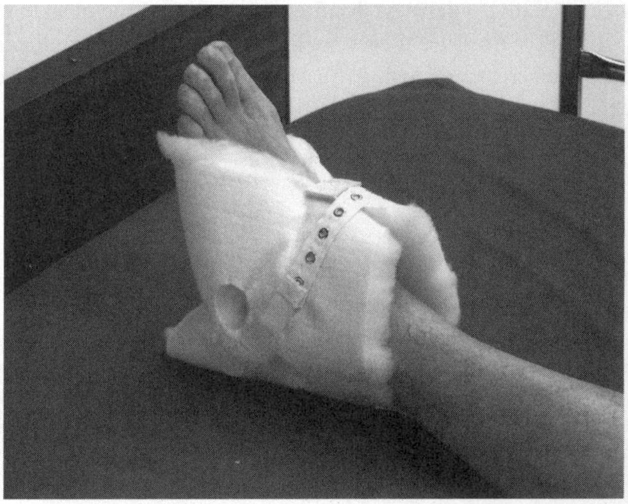

FIGURE 28–20. Heel and ankle protection. (Courtesy of J.T. Posey Company, Arcadia, CA.)

Nursing Implications

Patients with a surgical wound, pressure ulcer, or other type of tissue injury are likely to have one or more of the following nursing diagnoses:

- Pain
- Impaired skin integrity
- Impaired tissue integrity
- Risk for infection
- Altered tissue perfusion

The nursing care plan shows how the nursing process is used to care for a patient with Impaired tissue integrity, defined in the 1999 NANDA taxonomy as "a state in which an individual experiences damage to mucous membrane, corneal, integumentary, or subcutaneous tissue."

Nursing Care Plan

Impaired Tissue Integrity

Assessment

Subjective Data

States, "I have no feeling below my upper back and chest."

Objective Data

18-year old man with spinal cord injury at the C7 (7th cervical vertebrae) level 2 years ago after an auto accident in which he was not wearing a seat belt and was thrown from the car. Admitted for treatment of a pressure ulcer over the coccyx that has not responded to home treatment. The skin over the coccyx is open and measures 2″ × 3″ × 1/2″. Approximately 2″ of intact skin around the sore remains red and warm even after pressure is relieved. Tissue within the ulcer is gray with a yellow base. Elbows and heels are reddened but skin is intact. Wears an external catheter. Bowel elimination is regulated with the use of a suppository q 2 days.

Diagnosis

Impaired tissue integrity related to unrelieved pressure secondary to immobility (stage III pressure ulcer over coccyx and stage I over bilateral heels and elbows)

Plan

Goal

The coccygeal pressure ulcer will develop an 1/8″ margin of granulation tissue around the circumference of the wound by 8/30. The elbows and heels will blanch with pressure relief by 8/18.

Orders: 8/15

1. Reposition q 2 h until an air-fluidized bed can be obtained.
2. Avoid the supine and Fowler's position as much as possible.
3. After bathing, spray heels and elbows with Bard Barrier Film.
4. Until results of wound culture are obtained, care for the open wound as follows:
   - Mix antimicrobial solution with water and cleanse wound.
   - Rinse with normal saline.
   - Pack the wound loosely with a continuous strip of gauze moistened with normal saline.
   - Cover with an abdominal (ABD) pad.
   - Repeat above routine q 4 h as the packing becomes dry.
5. If wound culture is negative for pathogens:
   - Eliminate wet-to-dry dressing.
   - Clean, dry, and cover wound with transparent dressing (Op-Site) and leave in place for 5 days.
   - If drainage collects, pierce Op-Site and aspirate fluid from underneath. Seal opened area with a small reinforcement of Op-Site over punctured area.
6. Measure open pressure sore q 3 days (8/18, 8/21, etc.) during day shift.

______ R. ROSEN, RN

Implementation (Documentation)

8/16 1700 Turned q 2 h alternating side to side using a 30° lateral position with slight elevation of the upper body. ______ A FOX, LPN

continued

Nursing Care Plan — *Impaired Tissue Integrity* Continued

Evaluation (Documentation)

2000 Dressing and packing removed. Wound cleansed with antimicrobial solution and rinsed with saline. Repacked with saline-moistened gauze and covered with ABD secured with paper tape. ________________ A. FOX, LPN

2045 Removed packing contains white debris. Tissue within wound looks pink with slight bleeding. Wet-to-dry dressing drying more rapidly with Clinitron bed therapy. Will change in 3 h and evaluate again. Evidence of skin coating on elbows and heels. Areas still appear red over bony prominences. States, "I really like this bed. I wasn't sleeping much at night with all that turning going on." Advised that fluid intake must be increased to compensate for increased evaporation from skin due to blowing air from bed. Placed on I & O.
________________ A. FOX, LPN

FOCUS ON OLDER ADULTS

- Because regeneration of healthy skin takes twice as long for an 80-year-old person as for a 30-year-old person, wound healing is delayed in older adults.
- Age-related changes that affect wound healing include diminished collagen and blood supply and decreased quality of elastin. These age-related changes are compounded by long-term exposure to ultraviolet rays from the sun.
- Because the dermal layer of skin becomes thinner and the amount of subcutaneous tissue decreases with age, older adults are much more susceptible to the development of pressure ulcers and shear-type injuries. Special care must be taken when moving older adults to avoid friction on the skin.
- Diminished immune response due to a reduction in T cells predisposes older adults to wound infections.
- Signs of inflammation may be more subtle in older adults.
- Older adults who have diabetes or any other condition that interferes with circulation are more susceptible to delayed wound healing and wound infections.
- Impaired tactile sensation or sensory nerve problems due to diabetes or any other factor increases the risk for thermal skin injury. Older adults who have problems with the ability to sense temperatures need to take special precautions, such as using a thermometer to ensure that bath water is less than 100°F (38°C) to avoid burns or injury.
- Although there are many other possible reasons, compliance with a medical treatment regimen is a problem for many older adults who are economically limited. Another possible reason is that cultural factors or health beliefs conflict with discharge instructions.
- Some factors that interfere with adequate nutrition in older adults, thus impairing wound healing, are depression, poor appetite, cognitive impairments, and physical or economic barriers that interfere with the ability to obtain or prepare food. Attempts must be made to address these factors by using registered dietitians, who can suggest appropriate nutritional interventions, and by making referrals to community resources such as home-delivered meals or homemaker/home health aide services.
- Use of absorbent undergarments by incontinent older adults may contribute to skin breakdown because the garments may not allow for air circulation, and they may not be changed immediately when they are wet.
- If urinary incontinence interferes significantly with wound healing, an indwelling catheter may be necessary. However, it should be removed as soon as feasible, and efforts must be made to restore continence.
- Older adults whose mobility is diminished require aggressive skin care to prevent pressure ulcers. The elbows, heels, coccyx, shoulder blades, and hips are especially vulnerable. Special precautions include heel and elbow protectors, pressure relief pads and mattresses, and a strict routine of changing position every 2 hours.

KEY CONCEPTS

- A wound is damaged skin or soft tissue.
- Wound repair involves three sequential phases: inflammation, proliferation, and remodeling.
- Signs and symptoms classically associated with inflammation are swelling, redness, warmth, pain, and decreased function.
- Wounds heal by first, second, or third intention.
- The integrity of damaged skin and tissue is restored by resolution, regeneration, or scar formation.
- Two common types of wounds that require special care are pressure ulcers and surgical wounds.
- Some of the purposes for covering a wound with a dressing are keeping it clean, absorbing drainage, and controlling bleeding.

- A moist wound heals more quickly because new cells grow more rapidly in a wet environment.
- Open or closed drains are placed in or near a wound to provide a means for removing blood and drainage.
- The edges of an incision are generally held together with sutures or staples.
- A bandage or binder helps to hold a dressing in place, especially when tape cannot be used or the dressing is extremely large; to support the wound to reduce pain; or to limit movement to promote healing.
- A T-binder is used for securing a dressing to the anus, perineum, or groin.
- Four methods used to debride nonliving tissue from a wound are sharp debridement, enzymatic debridement, autolytic debridement, and mechanical debridement. A wound irrigation is an example of mechanical debridement.
- An irrigation is used to flush debris from a wound or body area, such as the eye, ear, and vagina.
- Heat is applied to promote circulation and speed healing; cold is used to prevent swelling and control bleeding.
- Methods for applying heat or cold include ice bags, compresses, soaks, and therapeutic baths.
- Five factors that place patients at risk for developing pressure ulcers are inactivity, immobility, malnutrition, dehydration, and incontinence.
- Techniques for preventing pressure ulcers include changing patients' positions every 1 to 2 hours, keeping the skin clean and dry, and preventing friction and shearing force on the skin.

CRITICAL THINKING EXERCISES

- You are assigned to care for a patient with a stage III pressure ulcer, one with an abdominal incision, and one with a peripheral intravenous infusion site. Describe the wound care appropriate for each.
- A 75-year-old patient is admitted from a nursing home to have surgery to repair a fractured hip. Discuss the factors that may threaten wound healing in this patient.

SUGGESTED READINGS

Baranoski S. Wound dressings: challenging decisions. Home Healthcare Nurse 1999;17(1):19–26.

Barr JE, Cuzzell J. Wound care clinical pathway: a conceptual model. Ostomy/Wound Management 1996;42(7):18–26.

Booth L. Ear syringing. Practice Nurse 1998;16(9):580–581.

Calvin M. Cutaneous wound repair. Wounds: A Compendium of Clinical Research and Practice 1998;10(1):12–32.

Cooper DM. Wound healing: new understandings. Nurse Practitioner Forum 1999;10(2):74–86.

Davis P. The pressure is on: preventing pressure sores. Journal of Orthopaedic Nursing 1999;3(Suppl. 1):46–52.

Dickerson P, Purdue GF, Hunt JL. Traumatic wound care. Dermatology Nursing 1999;11(1):53–63.

Ennis D. Reducing the risk of surgical site infection. Nursing 1999; 29(6):32hn1–5.

Fishman TD. Lessons in managing lower-extremity wounds. Nursing 1998; 28(10):50–51.

Kiernan M. The process of granulation and its role in wound healing. Community Nurse 1999;5(5):47–48.

Lindholm C, Bersten A, Berglund E. Chronic wounds and nursing care. Journal of Wound Care 1999;8(1):5–10.

Maklebust J. Treating pressure ulcers in the home. Home Healthcare Nurse 1999;17(5):307–316.

Marsden J. Ocular burns. Emergency Nurse 1999;6(10):20–24.

McCullough JM. The role of physiotherapy in managing patients with wounds. Journal of Wound Care 1998;7(5):241–244.

Mong CL. Wet, dry, or damp? Journal of Wound Care Nursing 1997; 24(4):19.

Mosher BA, Cuddingan J, Thomas DR, Boudreau DM. Outcomes of 4 methods of debridement using a decision analysis methodology. Advances in Wound Care: The Journal for Prevention and Healing 1999;12(Suppl. 2):12–21.

NANDA nursing diagnoses: definitions and classification, 1999–2000. Philadelphia, NANDA, 1999.

Netscher D, Clamon J, Fincher L, Thompson R. Surgical repair of pressure ulcers. Plastic Surgical Nursing 1996;6(4):225–239.

Pieper B, Templin TN, Dobal M, Jacox A. Wound prevalence, types, and treatments in home care. Advances in Wound Care: The Journal for Prevention and Healing 1999;12(3):117–126.

Pontieri-Lewis V. Principles for selecting the right wound dressing. MedSurg Nursing 1999;8(4):267–270.

Porth CM. Pathophysiology: concepts of altered health states, 5th ed. Philadelphia, Lippincott Williams & Wilkins, 1998.

Reed MJ, Weksler ME. Wound repair in older patients: preventing problems and managing the healing. Geriatrics 1998;53(5):88–90.

Shaw MM. Pressure ulcers in older persons: a preventive approach. Wound Repair and Regeneration 1996;4(3):316–320.

Smith I. Eye care: irrigation of the eye. Nursing Times 1998;94(40, insert):p. 2p.

Stone CM. Preventing cerumen impaction in nursing facility residents. Journal of Gerontological Nursing 1999;25(5):43–45.

Tong A. Back to basics: wound care, part 1. Nursing Times 1999;1(1):17–21.

SKILL 28–1

CHANGING A GAUZE DRESSING

Suggested Action	Reason for Action
Assessment	
Inspect the current dressing for drainage, integrity, and type of dressing supplies used.	Provides assessments indicating a need to change the dressing and supplies that may be needed
Check the medical orders for a directive to change the dressing.	Shows collaboration with the prescribed medical treatment
Determine if the patient has allergies to tape or antimicrobial wound agents.	Helps determine dressing supplies to use
Assess the patient's level and characteristics of pain.	Determines if analgesia will be beneficial before changing the dressing
Planning	
Explain the need and technique for changing the dressing.	Relieves anxiety and promotes cooperation
Consult the patient on a preferred time for the dressing change if there is no immediate need for it.	Empowers the patient to participate in decision making
Give pain medication, if needed, 15 to 30 minutes before the dressing change.	Allows time for absorption and effectiveness
Gather the necessary supplies, which are likely to include a paper bag for the soiled dressing, clean and sterile gloves, individually packaged gauze dressings, tape, and, in some cases, an antimicrobial agent such as povidone-iodine swabs for wound cleansing.	Facilitates organization and efficient time management
Implementation	
Wash your hands.	Reduces the transmission of microorganisms
Pull the privacy curtain.	Shows respect for the patient's dignity
Position the patient to allow access to the dressing.	Facilitates comfort and dexterity
Drape the patient to expose the area of the wound.	Ensures modesty but facilitates care
Loosen the tape securing the dressing; pull the tape toward the wound.	Facilitates removal without separating the healing wound
Don at least one glove and lift the dressing from the wound.	Provides a barrier against contact with blood and body substances

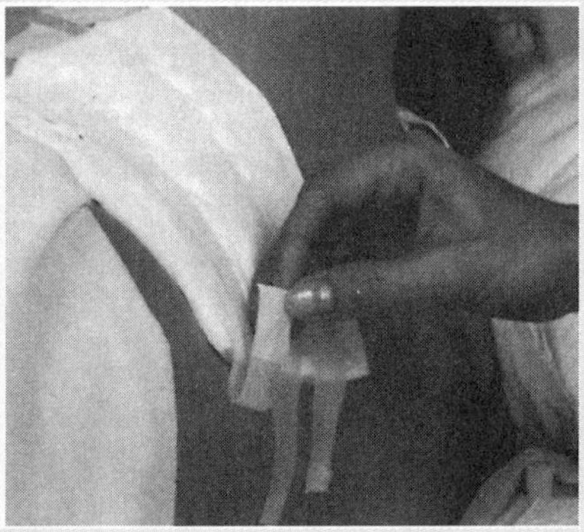

Loosen the tape.

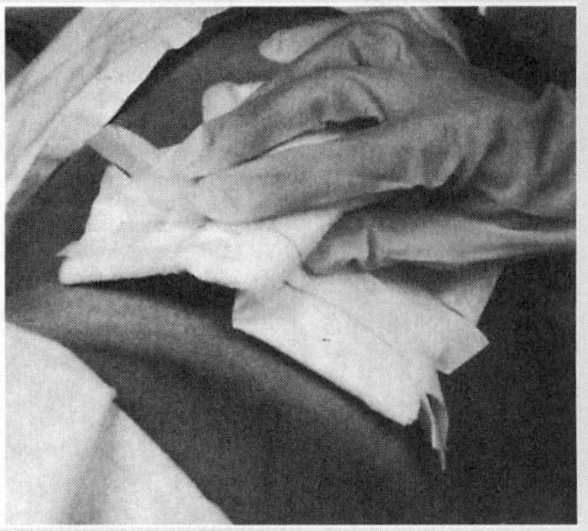

Remove the dressing.

continued

SKILL 28–1

CHANGING A GAUZE DRESSING *Continued*

Suggested Action	Reason for Action
Moisten the gauze with sterile normal saline, if it adheres to the wound.	Prevents disrupting granulation tissue
Discard the soiled dressing in a paper bag or other receptacle along with the glove(s).	Confines sources of pathogens
Wash your hands again.	Removes transient microorganisms
Tear several long strips of tape and fold the ends over, forming tabs.	Facilitates handling tape later when wearing gloves and eases tape removal during the next dressing change

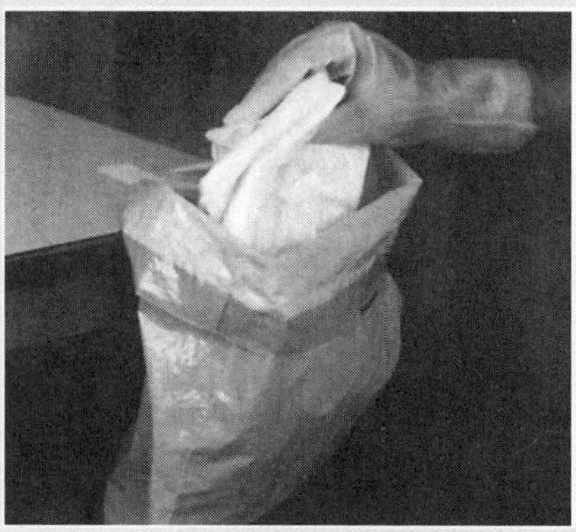

Dispose of the dressing

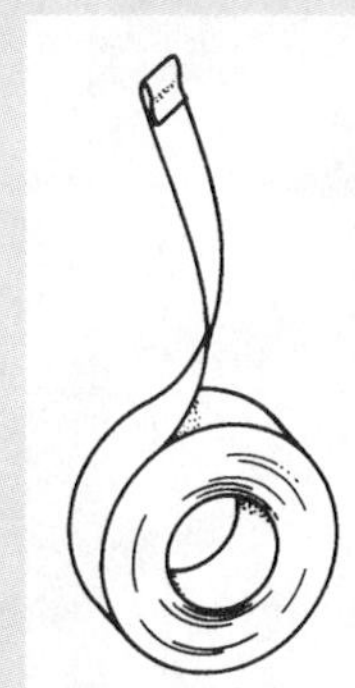

Form tabs on the ends of the tape.

Suggested Action	Reason for Action
Open sterile supplies, using the inside wrapper of one of the gauze dressings as a sterile field, if needed.	Ensures aseptic technique
Don sterile gloves.	Ensures sterility
Inspect the wound.	Provides data for description and comparison
Cleanse the wound with the antimicrobial agent.	Remove drainage and microorganisms
Use a technique that prevents transferring microorganisms back to a cleaned area.	Supports principles of medical asepsis

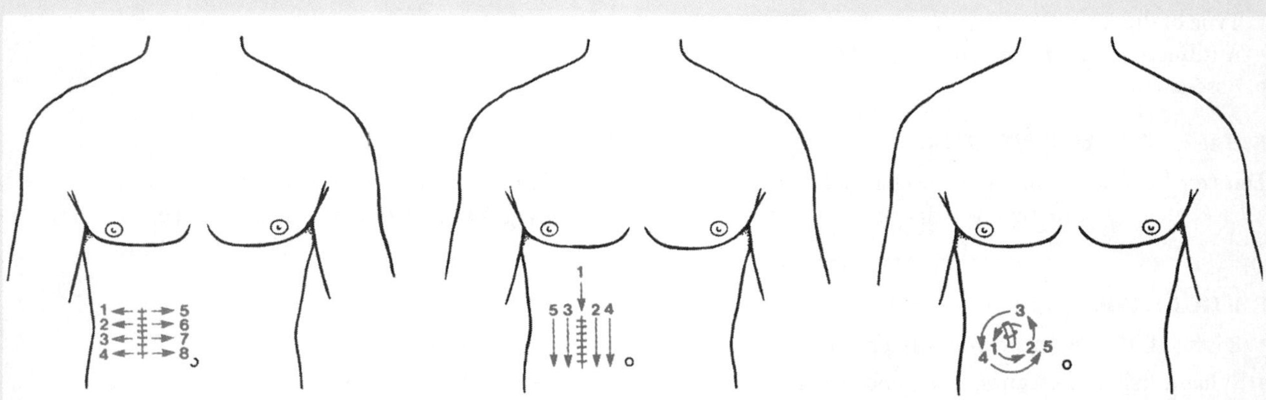

Wound cleansing techniques.

continued

SKILL 28–1

CHANGING A GAUZE DRESSING *Continued*

Suggested Action	Reason for Action
Use a single swab or small gauze square for each stroke.	Prevents transferring microorganisms to clean areas
Allow the antimicrobial agent to dry.	Ensures that the tape will stay secured when applied
Cover the wound with the gauze dressing.	Protects the wound
Secure the dressing with tape in the opposite direction of the incision or across a joint. Place a strip of tape at each end of the dressing and in the middle if needed.	Prevents loosening with activity; holds the dressing in place without exposing the wound or incision.

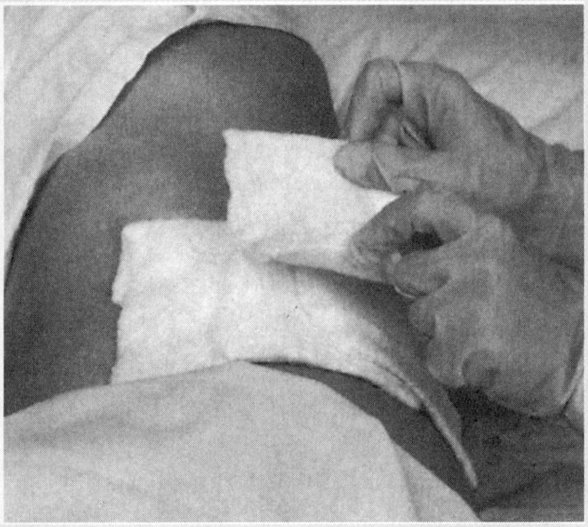

Apply the dressing.

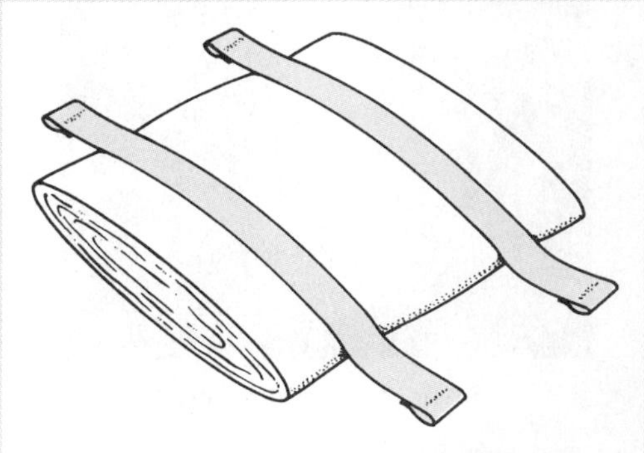

Position the tape.

Suggested Action	Reason for Action
Remove and discard gloves.	Confines sources of microorganisms

Evaluation

- Dressing covers the entire wound.
- Dressing is secure, dry, and intact.

Document

- Type of dressing
- Antimicrobial agent used for cleansing
- Assessment data

SAMPLE DOCUMENTATION

Date and Time Gauze dressing changed over abdominal wound. Wound cleansed with povidone–iodine. Incision is well approximated with sutures. No drainage, swelling, or tenderness observed.

_______________________________ SIGNATURE, TITLE

CRITICAL THINKING

- Discuss the signs and symptoms a person would exhibit if a wound is infected.
- What nursing interventions are appropriate when caring for a patient with an infected wound?

SKILL 28-2

IRRIGATING A WOUND

Suggested Action	Reason for Action
Assessment	
Check the medical orders for a directive to irrigate the wound.	Shows collaboration with the prescribed medical treatment
Determine how much the patient understands about the procedure.	Indicates the level of health teaching needed
Planning	
Plan to irrigate the wound at the same time that the dressing requires changing.	Makes efficient use of time
Gather the equipment required, which is likely to include a container of solution, basin, bulb or asepto syringe, gloves, and absorbent material, including a towel to dry the skin.	Facilitates organization
Bring supplies for changing the dressing.	Makes efficient use of time
Consider additional items for standard precautions such as goggles or face shield, and cover apron or gown.	Follows infection control guidelines when there is a potential for being splashed with blood or body substances
Implementation	
Wash your hands.	Reduces the transmission of microorganisms
Pull the privacy curtain.	Shows respect for the patient's dignity
Drape the patient to expose the area of the wound.	Ensures modesty but facilitates care
Follow earlier directions for removing the dressing.	Provides access to the wound
Wash your hands.	Reduces the transmission of microorganisms
Position the patient to facilitate filling the cavity with solution.	Ensures contact between the solution and all areas of the wound
Pad the bed with absorbent material and place an emesis basin adjacent to and below the wound.	Reduces the potential for saturating the bed linen
Open and prepare supplies following principles of surgical asepsis.	Confines and controls the transmission of microorganisms
Don gloves and other standard precautions apparel.	Reduces the potential for contact with blood and body substances
Fill the syringe with solution and instill it into the wound without touching the wound directly.	Dilutes and loosens debris
Hold the emesis basin close to the patient's body to catch the solution as it drains from the wound.	Collects and contains irrigating solution
Repeat the process until the draining solution seems clear.	Indicates that debris has been evacuated
Tilt the patient toward the basin.	Drains remaining solution from the wound
Dry the skin.	Facilitates applying a dressing
Dispose of the drained solution, soiled equipment, and linen.	Reduces the potential for transmitting microorganisms
Remove gloves, wash hands, and prepare to change the dressing.	Provides for absorption of residual solution and coverage of the wound

continued

SKILL 28–2

IRRIGATING A WOUND *Continued*

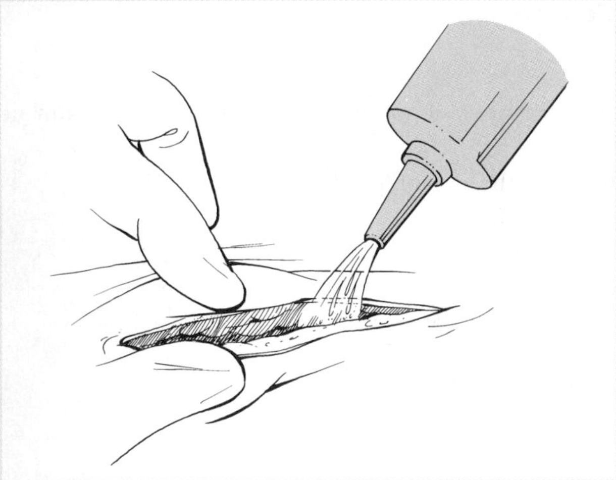

Instill the irrigant.

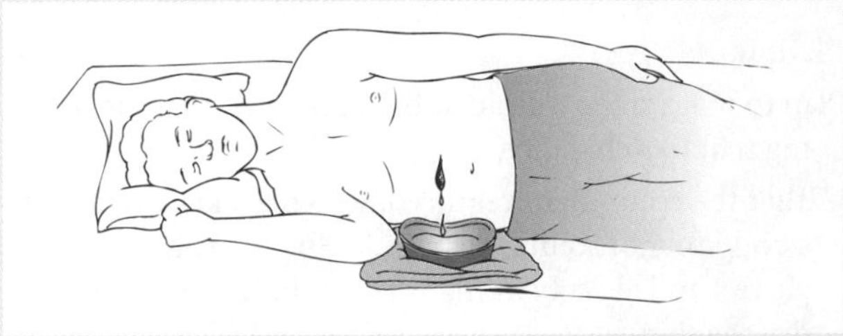

Position the patient to drain the irrigant.

Evaluation

- Irrigation solution shows evidence of debris removal.
- Wound shows evidence of healing.

Document

- Assessment data
- Type and amount of solution
- Outcome of procedure

SAMPLE DOCUMENTATION

Date and Time Dressing removed. Moderate amount of purulent drainage on soiled dressing. Wound is separated 3″. Approximately 300 mL of sterile NSS instilled within wound. Drained solution is cloudy with particles of debris. ______________________ SIGNATURE, TITLE

CRITICAL THINKING

- Discuss methods for debriding a wound other than with wound irrigation.
- List advantages and disadvantages of one other method of wound debridement.

SKILL 28-3

PROVIDING A SITZ BATH

Suggested Action	Reason for Action
Assessment	
Check the medical orders for a directive to administer a sitz bath.	Shows collaboration with the prescribed medical treatment
Determine how much the patient understands about the procedure.	Indicates the level of health teaching needed
Assess the condition of the rectal or perineal wound and the patient's level of pain.	Provides baseline data for future comparisons; indicates if pain medication is needed
Planning	
Explain the procedure.	Relieves anxiety and promotes cooperation
Ask if the patient prefers the sitz bath before or after routine hygiene.	Involves the patient in the decision-making process
Obtain disposable equipment unless specially installed tubs are available.	Facilitates organization and efficient time management
Assemble other supplies, such as a bath blanket and towels.	Prepares for maintaining warmth and provides a means for drying the skin
Inspect and clean the bathroom area or the tub room.	Supports principles of medical asepsis
Place the basin inside the rim of the raised toilet seat.	Allows submerging of the rectum and perineum

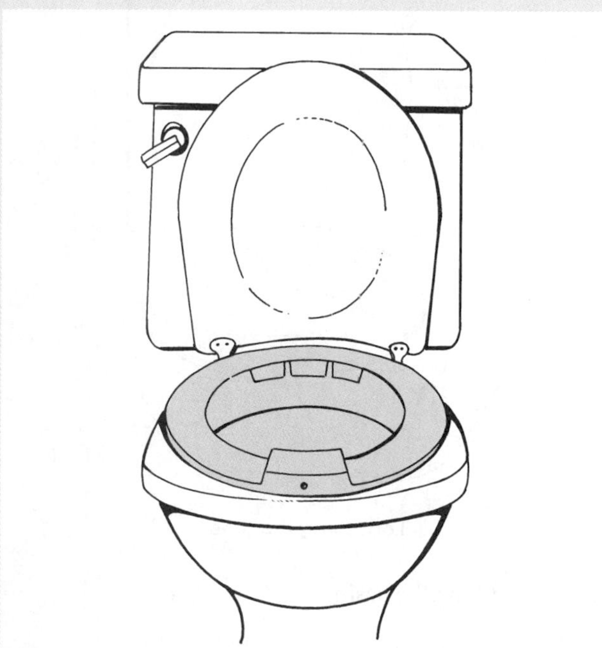

Position the sitz bath basin.

Suggested Action	Reason for Action
Implementation	
Wash your hands.	Reduces the transmission of microorganisms
Help the patient don a robe and slippers.	Maintains warmth, safety, and comfort
Help the patient ambulate to the location where the sitz bath will be administered.	Demonstrates concern for safety

continued

SKILL 28–3

PROVIDING A SITZ BATH *Continued*

Suggested Action	Reason for Action
Shut the door to the bathroom or tub room.	Provides privacy
Clamp the tubing attached to the water bag.	Prevents loss of fluid
Fill the container with warm water, no hotter than 110°F (43.3°C).	Provides comfort without danger of burning the skin
Hang the bag above the toilet seat.	Facilitates gravity flow
Insert the tubing from the bag into the front of the basin.	Provides a means for filling the basin

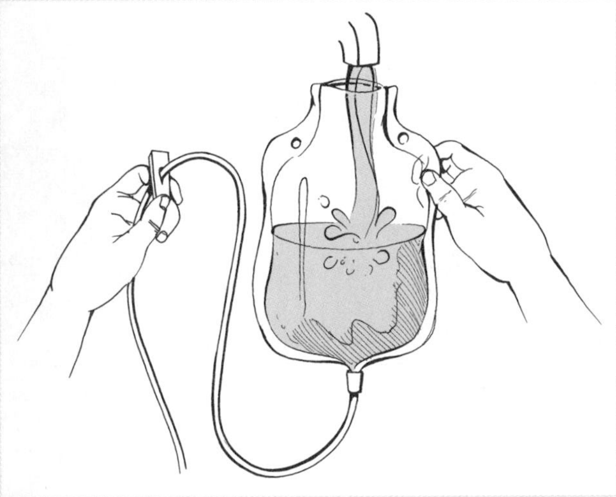

Fill the solution container.

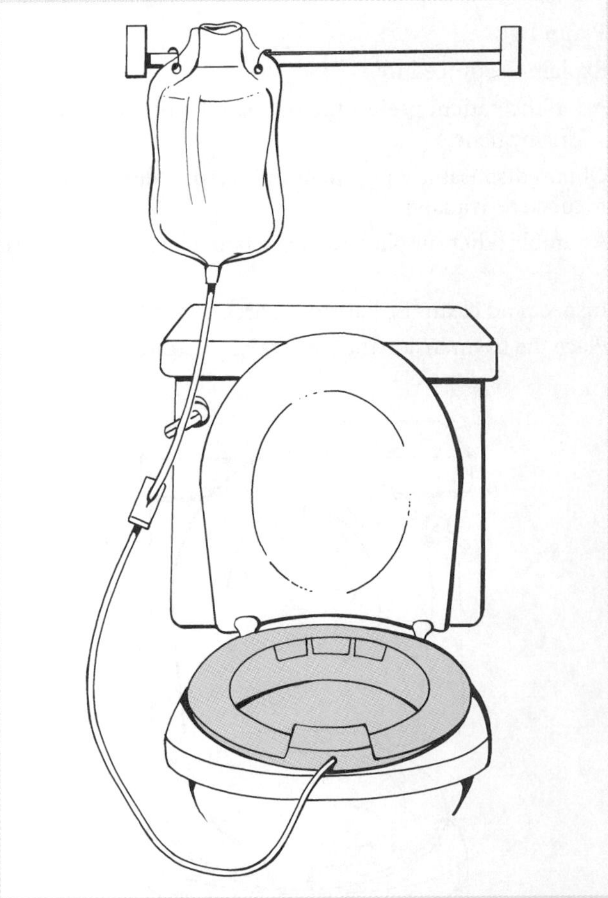

Loosening the tape.

Suggested Action	Reason for Action
Help the patient sit on the basin and unclamp the tubing.	Facilitates filling the basin
Cover the patient's shoulders with a bath blanket if the patient feels chilled.	Promotes comfort
Instruct the patient on how to signal for assistance.	Ensures safety
Leave the patient alone, but recheck at frequent intervals to add more warm water to the reservoir bag.	Provides sustained application of warm water
Help the patient pat the skin dry after soaking for 20 to 30 minutes.	Restores comfort

continued

SKILL 28-3

PROVIDING A SITZ BATH *Continued*

Suggested Action	Reason for Action
Assist the patient back to bed.	Ensures safety in case the patient feels dizzy from hypotension caused by peripheral vasodilation.
Don gloves and clean the disposable equipment and bath area.	Supports principles of medical asepsis and infection control
Replace the sitz bath equipment in the patient's bedside cabinet or leave it in the patient's private bathroom.	Reduces costs by reusing disposable equipment

Evaluation

- Sitz bath is administered according to policy or standards of care.
- Safety is maintained.
- Patient reports symptoms relieved.

Document

- Procedure
- Response of the patient
- Assessment data

SAMPLE DOCUMENTATION

Date and Time Sitz bath provided over 30 minutes. States, "I always feel so good after this treatment." Perineum is slightly swollen. Margins of episiotomy are approximated. Continues to have moderate bloody vaginal drainage. ______________________________ SIGNATURE, TITLE

CRITICAL THINKING

- What advantages are there in using disposable equipment for administering a sitz bath?
- What assessment findings suggest that a sitz bath is providing a therapeutic effect?

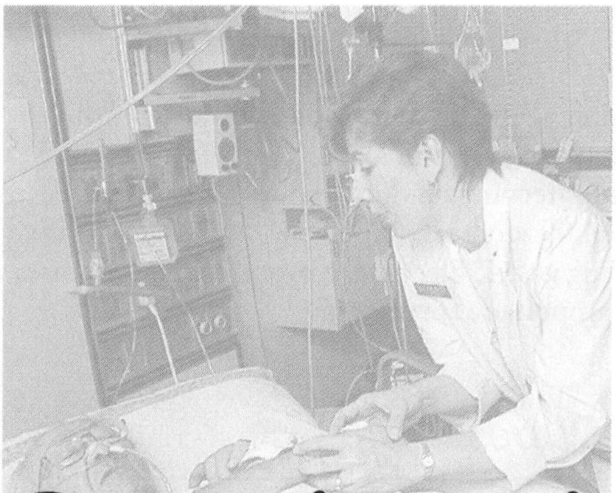

CHAPTER 29

Gastrointestinal Intubation

CHAPTER OUTLINE

Intubation
Types of Tubes
Nasogastric Tube Management
Nasointestinal Tube Management
Transabdominal Tube Management
Tube Feedings
Intestinal Decompression
Nursing Implications

NURSING GUIDELINES

ASSESSING THE pH OF ASPIRATED FLUID
INSERTING A NASOINTESTINAL FEEDING TUBE
MANAGING A GASTROSTOMY
CHECKING GASTRIC RESIDUAL
CLEARING AN OBSTRUCTED FEEDING TUBE
INSERTING AN INTESTINAL DECOMPRESSION TUBE

SKILLS

SKILL 29-1: INSERTING A NASOGASTRIC TUBE
SKILL 29-2: IRRIGATING A NASOGASTRIC TUBE
SKILL 29-3: REMOVING A NASOGASTRIC TUBE
SKILL 29-4: ADMINISTERING TUBE FEEDINGS

NURSING CARE PLAN

RISK FOR ASPIRATION

KEY TERMS

bolus feeding
continuous feeding
cyclic feeding
decompression
dumping syndrome
enteral nutrition
gastric reflux
gastric residual
gastrostomy tube (G-tube)
gavage
intermittent feeding
intestinal decompression
intubation
jejunostomy tube (J-tube)
lavage
lumen
nasogastric tube
nasointestinal intubation
nasointestinal tubes
NEX measurement
orogastric intubation
orogastric tube
ostomy
percutaneous endoscopic gastrostomy (PEG) tube
percutaneous endoscopic jejunostomy (PEJ) tube
stylet
sump tubes
tamponade
transabdominal tubes

LEARNING OBJECTIVES

An understanding of the content within this chapter will be evidenced by the student's ability to:

- Define intubation.
- List six purposes for gastrointestinal intubation.
- Identify four general types of gastrointestinal tubes.
- Name at least four assessments that are necessary before inserting a tube nasally.
- Explain the purpose for and how to obtain a NEX measurement.
- Describe three techniques for checking distal placement in the stomach.
- Discuss three ways that nasointestinal feeding tubes or their insertion differ from their gastric counterparts.
- Name two common problems associated with transabdominal tubes.
- Define enteral nutrition.
- Name four schedules for administering tube feedings.
- Explain the purpose for assessing gastric residual.
- Name five nursing activities involved in managing the care of patients who are being tube-fed.
- List four items of information that should be included in the written instructions for patients administering their own tube feedings.
- Name two nursing responsibilities for assisting with the insertion of a tungsten-weighted intestinal decompression tube.

Patients, especially those undergoing abdominal or gastrointestinal (GI) surgery, may require some type of tube placed within their stomach or intestine. Problems associated with surgery or conditions affecting the GI tract, such as impaired peristalsis, vomiting, or gas accumulation, are reduced or eliminated when a gastric or intestinal tube is used. Tubes also are used to provide nourishment for patients who cannot eat. This chapter discusses the multiple uses for gastric and intestinal tubes and the nursing guidelines and skills for managing patient care.

Intubation

Intubation (placement of a tube into a structure of the body), in this chapter, refers to the insertion of a tube into the stomach or intestine by way of the mouth or nose. **Orogastric intubation** (insertion of a tube through the mouth into the stomach), **nasogastric intubation** (insertion of a tube through the nose into the stomach; Fig. 29-1), and **nasointestinal intubation** (insertion of a tube through the nose to the intestine) are performed to remove gas or fluids or to administer liquid nourishment.

A tube may also be inserted within an **ostomy** (surgically created opening). The anatomic site of the ostomy is identified by a prefix; for instance, a gastrostomy is an artificial opening into the stomach.

Gastric or intestinal tubes are used for a variety of reasons, including:

- Performing a **gavage** (providing nourishment)
- Administering oral medications that cannot be swallowed
- Obtaining a sample of secretions for diagnostic testing
- Performing a **lavage** (removing substances from the stomach, typically poisons)
- Promoting **decompression** (removing gas and secretions from the stomach or bowel)
- Controlling gastric bleeding, a process called compression or **tamponade** (pressure)

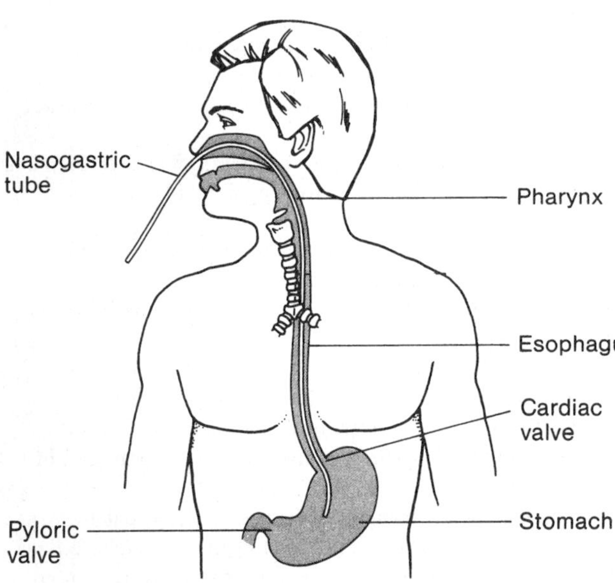

FIGURE 29–1. Nasogastric intubation pathway.

Types of Tubes

Although all gastric and intestinal tubes have a proximal and distal end, their size, construction, and composition vary according to their use (Table 29-1). The outside diameter of most tubes is measured using the French scale, indicated by a number followed by the letter "F." Each number on the French scale equals approximately 0.33 mm. The larger the number, the larger the diameter of the tube.

Tubes can be identified according to the location of their insertion (mouth, nose, or abdomen) or the location of their distal end (stomach [gastric] or intestinal).

OROGASTRIC TUBE

An **orogastric tube** (tube inserted at the mouth into the stomach), such as an Ewald tube, is used in an emergency to remove toxic substances that have been ingested. The diameter of the tube is large enough to remove pill fragments and stomach debris. Because of its size, the tube is introduced through the mouth rather than the nose.

NASOGASTRIC TUBES

A **nasogastric tube** (tube placed through the nose and advanced to the stomach) is smaller in diameter than an orogastric tube but larger and shorter than a nasointestinal tube. Some have more than one **lumen** (channel) within the tube.

A Levin tube (Fig. 29-2*A*), a commonly used, single-lumen gastric tube, has multiple uses, one of which is decompression. Gastric **sump tubes** (double-lumen tubes) are used almost exclusively to remove fluid and gas from the stomach (see Fig. 29-2*B*). The second lumen serves as a vent. The use of sump tubes decreases the possibility that the stomach wall will adhere to and obstruct the drainage openings when suction is applied.

Because nasogastric tubes remain in place for several days or more, many patients complain of nose and throat discomfort. If the tube's diameter is too large or pressure from the tube is prolonged, tissue irritation or breakdown may occur. Further, gastric tubes tend to dilate the esophageal sphincter, a circular muscle between the esophagus and the stomach. The stretched opening may allow **gastric reflux** (reverse flow of gastric contents), especially when the tube is used to administer liquid formula. If gastric reflux occurs, the liquid could enter the airway and interfere with respiratory function.

TABLE 29–1. **Types of Gastrointestinal Tubes**

Tube	Purpose	Characteristics
Orogastric		
Ewald	Lavage	• Large diameter: 36–40 F • Single lumen • Multiple distal openings for drainage
Nasogastric		
Levin	Lavage Gavage Decompression Diagnostics	• Usual adult size 14–18 F • Single lumen • 42″–50″ (107–127 cm) long • Multiple drain openings
Salem sump	Decompression	• Same diameter as Levin • Double lumen • Pig-tail vent • 48″ (122 cm) long • Marked at increments to indicate depth of insertion • Radiopaque
Sengstaken-Blakemore	Compression Drainage	• Usual diameter: 20 F • 36″ (90 cm) long • Triple lumen; two lead to balloons in the esophagus and stomach and the third is for removing gastric drainage; a fourth lumen may be used to remove pharyngeal secretions
Nasointestinal		
Keofeed	Gavage	• Small diameter: 8 F • 36″ (90 cm) long • Polyurethane or silicone • Weighted tip • Extremely flexible and may require the use of a stylet during insertion • Radiopaque • Bonded lubricant that becomes activated with moisture
Maxter	Intestinal decompression	• Usual size: 18 F • 100″ (250 cm) long • Double lumen • Tungsten-weighted tip • Graduated marks every 10″ (25 cm)
Transabdominal		
Gastrostomy	Gavage; may be used for decompression while the patient is fed through a jejunostomy tube	• Sizes 12–24 F for adults • Rubber or silicone • Some may have additional side ports for balloon inflation to maintain placement • May be capped or plugged between feedings • Radiopaque
Jejunostomy	Gavage	• Sizes 5–14 F for adults • Silicone or polyurethane • Radiopaque

NASOINTESTINAL TUBES

Nasointestinal tubes (tubes inserted through the nose for distal placement below the stomach) are longer than their gastric counterparts. The added length permits them to be placed in the small bowel. They are used to provide nourishment or to remove gas and liquid drainage from the small intestine.

Feeding Tubes

Nasointestinal tubes used for nutrition, such as a Keofeed tube, are usually small in diameter and made of a flexible substance such as polyurethane or silicone. Their narrow width and softer composition allow them to remain in the same nostril for 4 weeks or longer. In addition, gastric

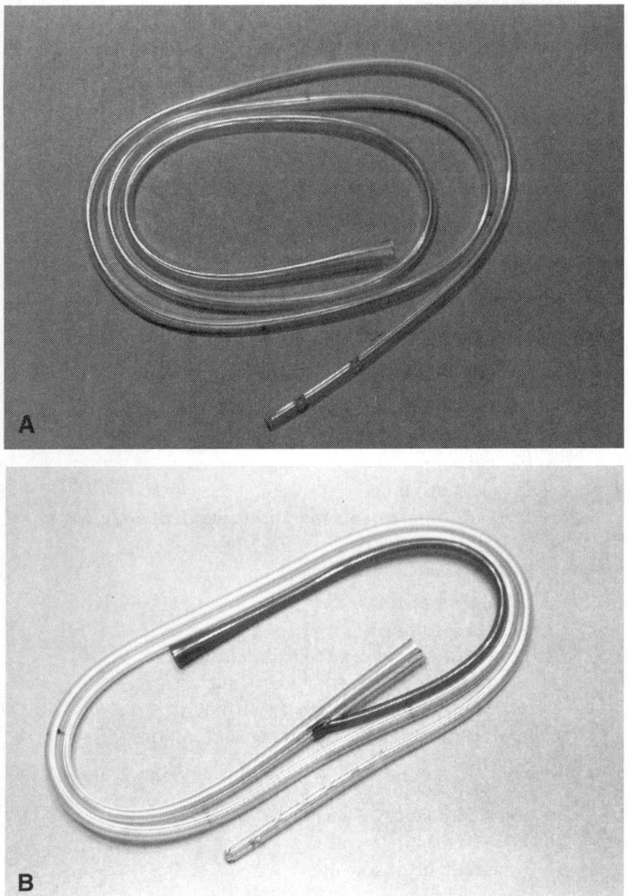

FIGURE 29–2. Nasogastric tubes. (*A*) Levin tube. (Courtesy of Ken Timby.) (*B*) Vented Salem sump tube. (Courtesy of Ken Timby.)

reflux is less likely because they deliver liquid nutrition beyond the stomach.

Narrow tubes are not problem-free. They tend to curl during insertion because they are so flexible. Therefore, some are supplied with a **stylet** (metal guidewire) that helps straighten and support the tube during insertion. Almost all have a weighted tip that helps them descend past the stomach. Checking the placement of the distal end is more difficult, and these tubes become obstructed more easily.

Despite the problems associated with maintenance, small-diameter tubes are preferred for their comfort. They are ideal for providing a continuous infusion of nourishment.

Intestinal Decompression Tube

Intestinal decompression (removal of gas and intestinal contents) is performed when a patient has a partial or complete bowel obstruction. A tube used for intestinal decompression has a double lumen and a weighted tip (Fig. 29-3). One lumen is used to suction the intestinal contents, while the other acts as a vent to reduce suction-induced trauma to intestinal tissue. The weighted tip and peristalsis, if present, propel the tube beyond the stomach and into the intestine. The progress of the radiopaque tip through the GI tract is monitored by x-ray.

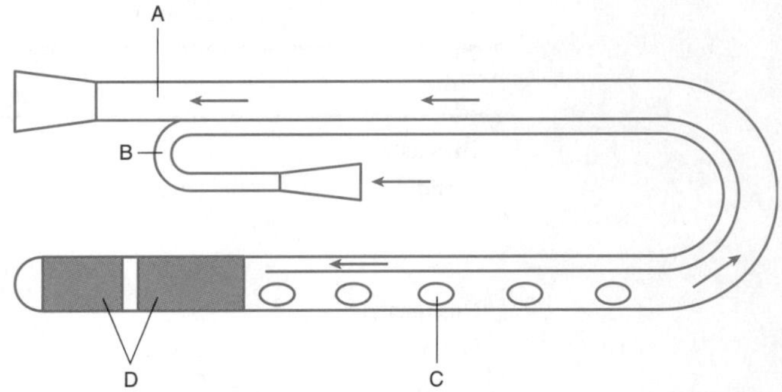

FIGURE 29–3. Intestinal decompression tube. (*A*) Suction lumen. (*B*) Vent lumen. (*C*) Openings for suction. (*D*) Radiopaque tungsten tip.

At one time, intestinal tubes, such as the Cantor tube and the Miller-Abbott tube, were weighted with mercury. However, because of the hazards of mercury, both to the patient and to the environment, mercury-weighted tubes are rarely used today. Instead, intestinal tubes are now weighted with tungsten—for instance, the Maxter tube (see Table 29-1).

TRANSABDOMINAL TUBES

Transabdominal tubes (tubes placed through the abdominal wall) provide access to various areas of the GI tract. Two examples are a **gastrostomy tube** or G-tube (transabdominal tube located within the stomach) and a **jejunostomy tube** or J-tube (transabdominal tube that leads to the jejunum of the small intestine).

A gastrostomy tube is placed surgically or with the use of an endoscope. A surgically inserted G-tube resembles a long rubber catheter sutured to the abdomen. A **percutaneous endoscopic gastrostomy** (PEG) **tube** (transabdominal tube inserted under endoscopic guidance) is anchored with internal and external crossbars called bumpers (Fig. 29-4*A*). A **percutaneous endoscopic jejunostomy** (PEJ) **tube** (tube that is passed through a PEG tube into the jejunum) is small in diameter so it can be inserted through the larger PEG tube (see Fig. 29-4*B*).

Transabdominal tubes are used instead of nasogastric or nasointestinal tubes when patients require an alternative to oral feeding for more than a month.

Nasogastric Tube Management

Nasogastric tubes are usually inserted by nurses. Nursing responsibilities include keeping the tube patent (or unob-

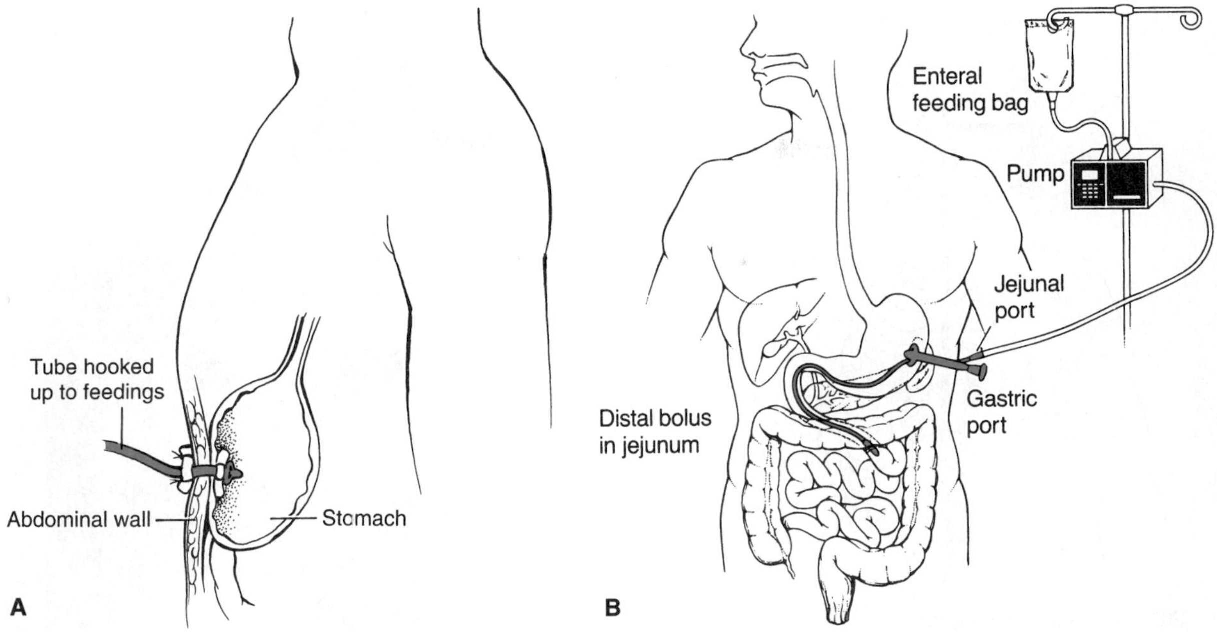

FIGURE 29–4. Transabdominal tubes. (*A*) Percutaneous endoscopic gastrostomy (PEG) tube. (*B*) Percutaneous endoscopic jejunostomy (PEJ) tube. (Courtesy of IVAC Corporation, San Diego, CA.)

structed), implementing the prescribed use, and removing the tube when it has accomplished its therapeutic purpose.

INSERTION

The task of inserting a nasogastric tube involves preparing the patient, conducting preintubation assessments, and placing the tube.

Patient Preparation

Most patients are anxious about having to swallow a tube. Suggesting that the diameter of the tube is smaller than most pieces of food may foster a positive outcome. Anxiety may be further reduced by explaining the procedure and giving instructions on how the patient can assist while the tube is being passed. One of the most important ways to support patients is to provide them with some means of control. A signal such as raising the hand should be established to indicate that the patient needs a pause during the tube's passage.

Assessment

Before insertion, the nurse conducts a focused assessment that includes the patient's:

- Level of consciousness
- Weight
- Bowel sounds
- Abdominal distention
- Integrity of nasal and oral mucosa
- Ability to swallow, cough, and gag
- Presence of nausea and vomiting

The findings of this assessment serve as a baseline for future comparisons and may suggest a need to modify the procedure or the equipment used. The main goal of the assessment is to determine which nostril is best to use when inserting the tube and the length to which the tube will be inserted.

Nasal Inspection

After the patient clears nasal debris by blowing into a paper tissue, each nostril is inspected for size, shape, and patency. The patient should exhale while each nostril in turn is occluded. The presence of nasal polyps (small growths of tissue), a deviated septum (nasal cartilage deflected from the midline of the nose), or a narrow nasal passage excludes a nostril for placement.

Tube Measurement

Some tubes are already marked to indicate the approximate length at which the distal tip will be located within the stomach. However, these markings may not correlate exactly with the patient's anatomy. Therefore, before a tube is inserted, the nurse obtains the patient's **NEX measurement** (length from ***n***ose to ***e***arlobe to the ***x***iphoid process [tip of the sternum]; Fig. 29-5) and marks the tube appropriately.

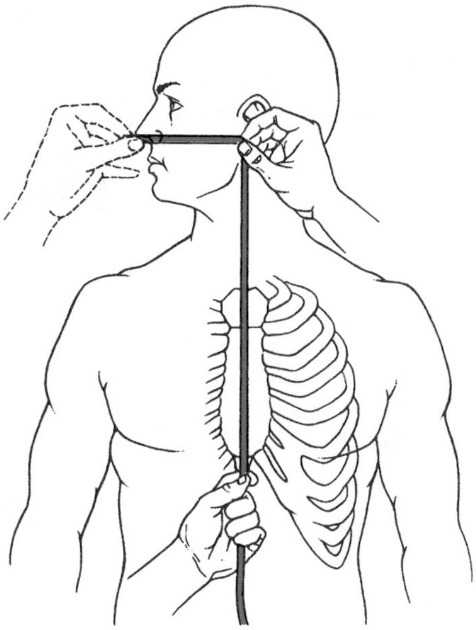

FIGURE 29–5. Obtaining the NEX measurement.

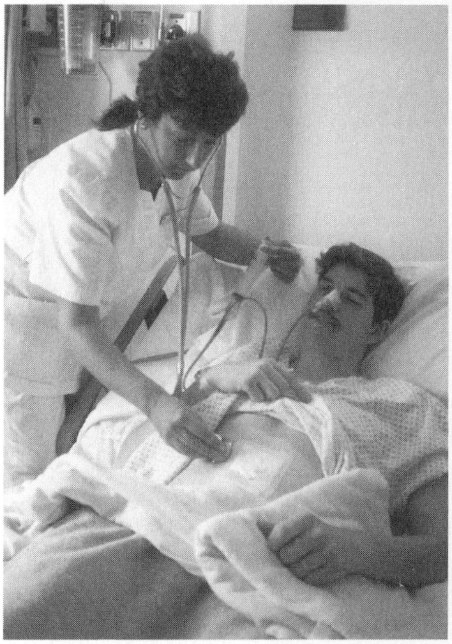

FIGURE 29–6. Checking distal placement. (Courtesy of Ken Timby.)

The first mark on the tube is made at the measured distance from the nose to the earlobe. It indicates the distance to the nasal pharynx, a location that places the tip at the back of the throat but above where the gag reflex is stimulated. A second mark is made at the point where the tube reaches the xiphoid process, indicating the depth required to reach the stomach.

Placement

When inserting a nasogastric tube, the nurse's primary concerns are to cause as little discomfort as possible, to preserve the integrity of the nasal tissue, and to locate the tube within the stomach, not in the respiratory passages.

Checking Placement

Once the tube is at its final mark, the location within the stomach must be verified. The physical assessment methods used to determine the distal location of a nasogastric tube are:

- Aspirating fluid: If aspirated fluid appears clear, brownish-yellow, or green, the nurse can presume that its source is the stomach.
- Auscultating the abdomen: The nurse instills 10 mL or more of air while listening with a stethoscope over the abdomen (Fig. 29-6). If a swooshing sound is heard, the nurse can infer that it was caused by the air entering the stomach. Belching often indicates that the tip is still in the esophagus.
- Testing the pH of aspirated liquid: The first two techniques provide only presumptive signs that the tube is in the stomach, but testing pH provides confirmation of acidic gastric contents. Other than obtaining an abdominal x-ray, the pH test is the most accurate technique for checking tube placement.

Nursing Guidelines For

Assessing the pH of Aspirated Fluid

☑ Don gloves.
RATIONALE: Reduces the transmission of microorganisms

☑ Aspirate a small volume of fluid from the tube with a clean syringe.
RATIONALE: Ensures valid test results

☑ Drop a sample of gastric fluid onto an indicator strip.
RATIONALE: Initiates a chemical reaction on contact and saturation

☑ Compare the color on the test strip with the color guide on the container of reagent strips (Fig. 29-7).
RATIONALE: The color of the test strip changes according to the hydrogen ion concentration of the liquid. Stomach fluid usually has a pH of 1 to 3—very acid on the pH scale. If the pH is 5 or 6, the patient may be receiving medications to decrease gastric acidity, or the fluid may be from the duodenum. A pH of 7 or greater indicates that the tube is in the respiratory tract.

Once stomach placement is confirmed (using two methods is best), the tube is secured to avoid upward or downward migration (Fig. 29-8). The tube is then ready to use for its intended purpose.

The steps to follow when inserting a nasogastric tube are outlined in Skill 29-1.

USE AND MAINTENANCE

Nasogastric tubes are connected to suction for gastric decompression or are used for tube feeding.

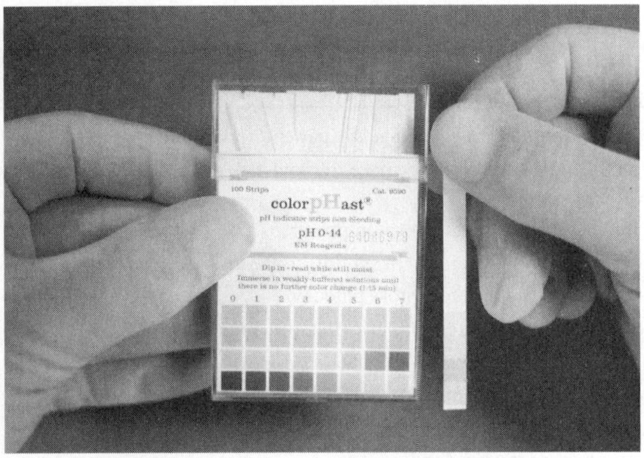

FIGURE 29–7. Checking pH. (Courtesy of Ken Timby.)

Gastric Decompression

Suction is either continuous or intermittent. The use of continuous suctioning with an unvented tube can cause the tube to adhere to the stomach mucosa, causing localized irritation and interfering with drainage. Using a vented tube or intermittent suction prevents or minimizes these effects.

The tube is connected to a wall outlet or a portable suction machine. The suction setting is prescribed by the physician or indicated in the agency's standards for care. Usually low pressure (40 to 60 mm Hg) is used.

The tube is plugged during ambulation or after instilling medications (see Chap. 32).

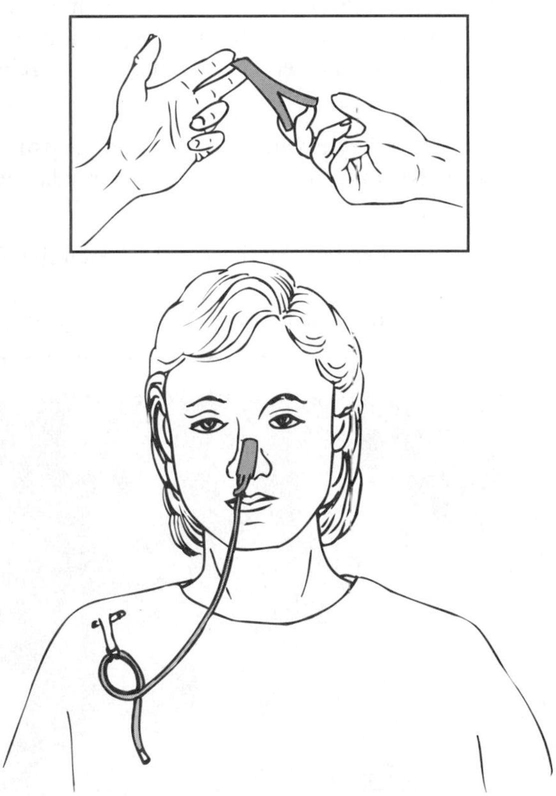

FIGURE 29–8. Technique for securing a nasal tube.

Promoting Patency

Even with intermittent suctioning, the tube may become obstructed. Tube patency is promoted by giving ice chips or occasional sips of water to a patient who is otherwise NPO. The fluid helps dilute the gastric secretions. However, both must be given sparingly because water is hypotonic and draws electrolytes into the gastric fluid. Because the diluted fluid is ultimately removed, giving the patient liberal amounts of water can deplete serum electrolytes (see Chap. 15).

Restoring Patency

The nurse assesses tube patency frequently by monitoring the volume and characteristics of drainage and observing for signs and symptoms suggesting an obstruction (nausea, vomiting, and abdominal distention). Inspection of the equipment helps identify possible causes for the assessment findings (Table 29-2). Once the cause is identified, it can be resolved with a variety of simple nursing interventions. Sometimes the nasogastric tube must be irrigated to maintain or restore patency (Skill 29-2). A medical order must be obtained before attempting an irrigation.

Enteral Nutrition

Enteral nutrition (nourishment provided via the stomach or small intestine rather than by the oral route) is delivered by tube feeding. Although a nasogastric tube can be used, it is more likely that liquid formula will be administered through a nasointestinal or transabdominal tube.

REMOVAL

A nasogastric tube is removed (Skill 29-3) when the patient's condition improves, when the tube becomes hopelessly obstructed, or according to the agency's standards for maintaining the integrity of the nasal mucosa. Unobstructed larger-diameter tubes are usually removed and changed at least every 2 to 4 weeks for adults. Small-diameter, flexible tubes are removed and changed every 6 weeks to 3 months, depending on agency policy. Tubes used for pediatric patients are changed more frequently.

Before permanent removal, some physicians prescribe a trial period during which the tube is clamped and the patient is allowed to consume oral fluids. Remaining asymptomatic is a good indication that the patient no longer requires intubation. If symptoms develop, the tube is already in place and can be easily reconnected to suction. This practice avoids subjecting the patient to the discomfort associated with tube replacement.

Nasointestinal Tube Management

Nasointestinal tubes that are used for enteral feeding are inserted by nurses.

TABLE 29–2. **Troubleshooting a Poorly Draining Nasogastric Tube**

Possible Causes	Solutions
Drainage holes are adhering to the gastric mucosal wall	Turn the suction off momentarily. Change the patient's position.
Tube is displaced above the cardiac sphincter	If measured mark is not at the tip of the nose, remove tape, advance the tube, check placement, and resecure.
Portable suction machine is disconnected or turned off	Replace plug into electrical outlet or turn on power.
Drainage container is filled beyond capacity	Empty and record amount of drainage in suction container.
The vent is acting as a siphon	Instill a bolus of air into the vent to restore patency.
The vent is capped or plugged	Remove cap and restore port to atmospheric pressure.
The tubing is kinked or disconnected	Straighten tubing or reconnect to suction machine.
Inadequate suction	Check that pressure is 40 to 60 mm Hg.
Loose cover on suction container	Resecure the lid to the container.
Solid particle or thick mucus obstructs lumen	Increase suction pressure momentarily. Obtain and implement a medical order for an irrigation.

INSERTION

The techniques for patient preparation, positioning, and advancement of a nasointestinal tube are similar to those for nasogastric tubes. However, some modifications are necessary because nasointestinal tubes are constructed differently.

To estimate the length of tube required for intestinal placement, the nurse determines the NEX measurement and adds 9 inches (23 cm). The additional measurement is also marked on the tubing.

Nursing Guidelines For

Inserting a Nasointestinal Feeding Tube

☑ Follow the manufacturer's suggestions for activating the lubricant that is bonded to the tube. Two common techniques are to instill water through the tube and to immerse the tip in water.
RATIONALE: Transforms the dry bond to a gelatinous consistency

☑ Secure the stylet within the tube.
RATIONALE: Stiffens the tube and facilitates insertion

☑ Insert the tube to the second mark.
RATIONALE: Places the tube in the presumed area of the stomach

☑ Aspirate fluid using a 50-mL syringe (Fig. 29-9) and test its pH.
RATIONALE: Provides data for determining gastric placement

☑ Loop the tubing and tape it temporarily to the cheek, if the test for placement suggests that the tip is in the stomach.
RATIONALE: Provides slack so the tube can descend into the small intestine

☑ Ambulate or position the patient on his or her right side for at least an hour, or the time specified in agency policy.
RATIONALE: Allows the tube to move by gravity through the pyloric valve

☑ Secure the tube at the nose when the third measured mark is at the nasal tip.
RATIONALE: Prevents the tube from migrating further than the desired distance

☑ Verify placement by x-ray, especially in unconscious patients or those with a depressed gag reflex.
RATIONALE: Provides confirmation of the distal location

☑ Remove the stylet using gentle traction (Fig. 29-10), or follow the manufacturer's suggestions.
RATIONALE: Opens the lumen to allow instillation of water and liquid nourishment

☑ Store the stylet in a clean wrapper at the patient's bedside.
RATIONALE: Avoids charging the patient for a new tube should the current one need to be removed and reintroduced

☑ Never reinsert the stylet while the tube is in the patient.
RATIONALE: Prevents trauma to the patient and damage to the tube

☑ Measure and record the length of tubing extending from the nose.
RATIONALE: Provides data for reassessing distal placement.

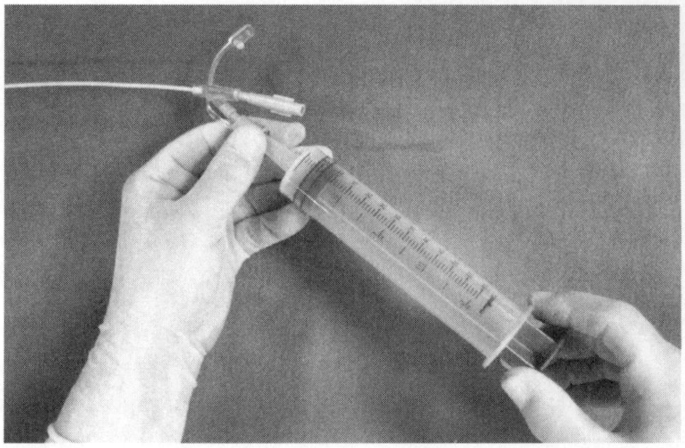

FIGURE 29–9. Aspirating to assess pH. (Courtesy of Ken Timby.)

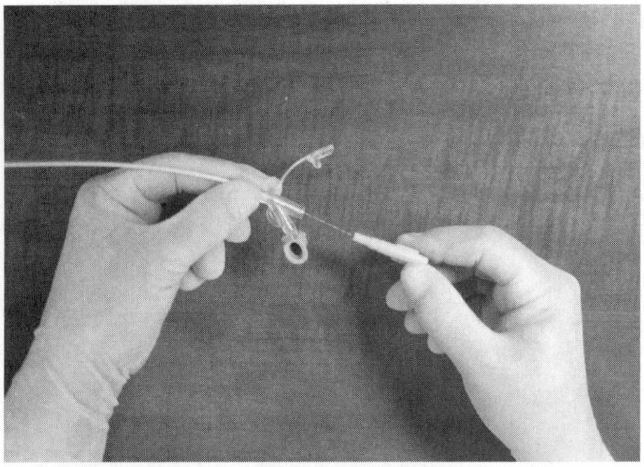

FIGURE 29–10. Removing stylet. (Courtesy of Ken Timby.)

CHECKING TUBE PLACEMENT

Tube placement is always initially verified with an x-ray because checking placement by auscultating air may be inconclusive. Because the tube's diameter is smaller, there may be a less pronounced escape of air from its tip. Aspiration of stomach contents from small-diameter tubes is not always possible because the negative pressure that is created causes the tube to collapse on itself.

Checking placement on a frequent basis is essential. However, repeated x-rays to assess tube placement are expensive, impractical, and potentially harmful. By modifying the aspiration technique after an initial x-ray, it may be possible to verify the tube's distal placement. The modification involves using a large-volume (50-mL) rather than a small-volume (3- to 5-mL) syringe to obtain a sample of fluid. The larger syringe creates less negative pressure during aspiration and therefore provides enough fluid to test the pH 90% of the time.

Transabdominal Tube Management

Transabdominal tubes, such as gastrostomy and jejunostomy tubes, are inserted by the physician, but nurses are responsible for assessing and caring for the tube and its insertion site. Conscientious care is required because gastrostomy tubes may leak (Display 29-1) and cause skin breakdown.

DISPLAY 29–1

Causes of Gastrostomy Leaks

- Disconnection between the feeding delivery tube and G-tube
- Clamped G-tube while tube feeding is infusing
- Mismatch between the size of the G-tube and stoma
- Increased abdominal pressure from formula accumulation, retching, sneezing, coughing
- Underinflation of the balloon beneath the skin
- Less-than-optimal stoma or stomal location

Nursing Guidelines For

Managing a Gastrostomy

☑ Wash hands and don gloves.
RATIONALE: Reduces the transmission of microorganisms

☑ Assess and replace the gauze dressing over a new gastrostomy if it becomes moist; slight bleeding or clear serous drainage from the wound is normal for a few weeks after the procedure.
RATIONALE: Reduces the conditions that support growth of microorganisms and maceration of the skin

☑ Remove and discontinue the dressing after the first 24 hours unless the physician orders otherwise.
RATIONALE: Facilitates assessment

☑ Inspect the skin around the tube daily.
RATIONALE: Provides assessment data about the status of wound repair

☑ Make sure that the sutures holding a surgically placed tube are intact.
RATIONALE: Prevents tube migration

☑ Report any redness or tissue maceration.
RATIONALE: Indicates evidence of early skin impairment

☑ Apply a skin barrier ointment such as zinc oxide, karaya gum wafer, hydrocolloid dressing, or ostomy pouch if the skin appears irritated (see section on Ostomy Care, Chap. 31).
RATIONALE: Protects the skin and promotes healing

☑ Press down on the skin at the base of the tube (Fig. 29-11*A*). If the patient has a PEG tube, compress the arms of the external bumper together and lift them about 1 inch (2.5 cm) (see Fig. 29-11*B*).
RATIONALE: Aids in assessing for drainage, which normally disappears by the end of the first week

☑ Clean the skin with half-strength hydrogen peroxide or 0.9% saline. After a week's time, using soap and water is sufficient. Dry the skin well using air or a blow dryer on a cool or low heat setting.
RATIONALE: Removes secretions and reduces the presence of microorganisms

☑ Rotate the direction of the external bumper 90° or other external retaining device at least once a day.
RATIONALE: Relieves pressure; maintains skin integrity

☑ Slide the external bumper down so it is flush with the skin.
RATIONALE: Restabilizes the tube

☑ Avoid placing any type of dressing material under the arms of the external bumper.
RATIONALE: Avoids creating pressure on the internal bumper and causing damage to the tissue

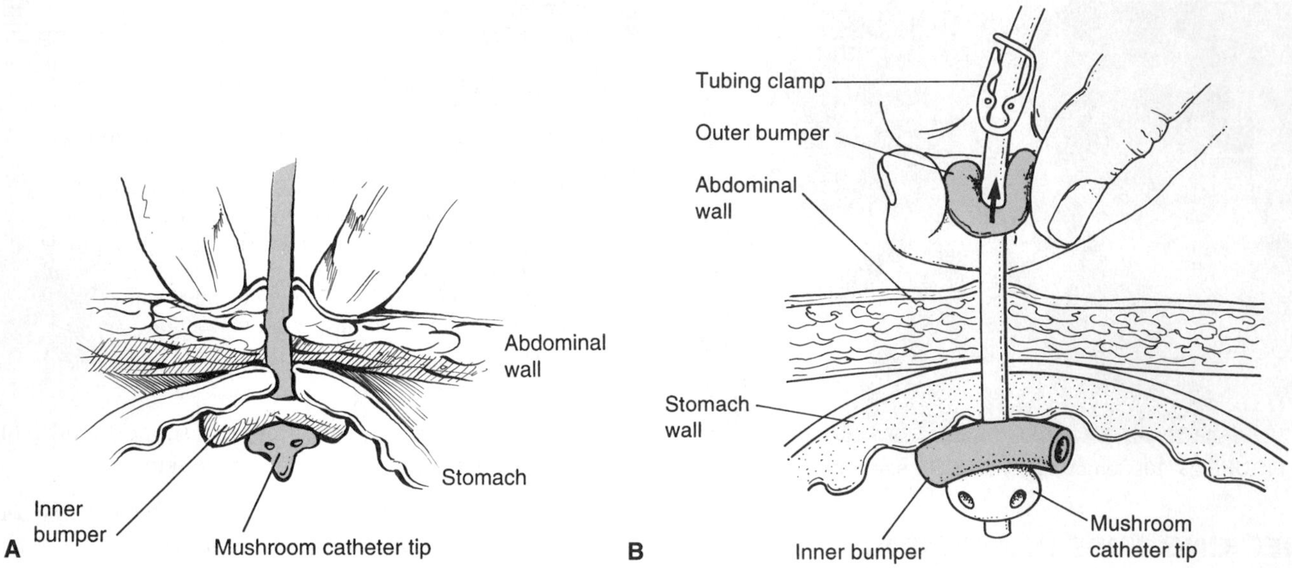

FIGURE 29–11. Inspection. (*A*) Inspecting for drainage. (*B*) Inspecting the skin.

- ☑ Replace the water in the balloon weekly using a Luer-tip (not Luer-lok) syringe.
  RATIONALE: Keeps the balloon fully inflated and prevents tube migration
- ☑ Tape the gastrostomy tube to the abdomen or secure it with an abdominal binder or commercial tube stabilizer.
  RATIONALE: Maintains the tube's position
- ☑ Make sure the tube is not kinked or the skin stretched.
  RATIONALE: Ensures tube patency and skin integrity
- ☑ Insert a Foley catheter (see Chap. 30), if the patient is not sensitive to latex, 2 to 5 inches (5 to 10 cm) within the opening, and inflate the balloon if the tube comes out.
  RATIONALE: Maintains temporary access to the stomach and, if done within 3 hours of accidental extubation, prevents the site from closing
- ☑ Use the gastrostomy tube in a manner similar to the way a nasogastric tube is used for administering feedings.
  RATIONALE: Provides nourishment

Tube Feedings

It is always best to provide nutrition by the oral route. However, if oral feedings are impossible or jeopardize the patient's safety, nourishment is provided enterally or parenterally (see Total Parenteral Nutrition, Chap. 15). Tube feedings are used when patients have an intact stomach or intestinal function but are unconscious, have undergone extensive mouth surgery, have difficulty swallowing, or have esophageal or gastric disorders.

BENEFITS AND RISKS

Tube feedings are delivered through a nasogastric, nasointestinal, or transabdominal tube. Each has its advantages and disadvantages (Table 29-3).

Instilling nutritional formulas into the stomach uses the body's natural reservoir for food. It also reduces the potential for enteritis (inflammation of the intestine) because the chemicals in the stomach tend to destroy microorganisms. However, gastric feedings create a greater potential for gastric reflux because of their volume and temporary retention within the stomach.

Although tubes placed within the intestine reduce the risk of gastric reflux, they do not eliminate it. Additional problems are associated with intestinal tube feedings. For example, **dumping syndrome** (cluster of symptoms from the rapid deposition of calorie-dense nourishment into the small intestine) may occur with an intestinally placed tube. The symptoms, which include weakness, dizziness, sweating, and nausea, are the result of fluid shifts from the circulating blood to the intestine and low blood sugar caused by a surge of insulin. Diarrhea may also result from administering hypertonic formula solutions.

FORMULA CONSIDERATIONS

In addition to the type of tube and the access site, the type of formula is also individualized, based on the patient's nutritional needs (Table 29-4). Factors include the patient's weight, nutritional status, and concurrent medical conditions and the projected length of therapy. The feeding schedule also affects the choice of formula: calories may need to be concentrated if the patient is being fed several times a day rather

TABLE 29–3. **Comparison of Feeding Tubes**

Tube	Advantages	Disadvantages
Nasogastric	Low incidence of obstruction Accommodates crushed medications Facilitates bolus or intermittent feedings Easy to check distal placement and gastric residual	Can damage nasal and pharyngeal mucosa from pressure or friction Dilates esophageal sphincter, potentiating gastric reflux Potential for aspiration Requires frequent replacement to ensure integrity of nasal tissue
Nasointestinal	Easy to insert Comfortable Only slight dilation of esophageal sphincter Reduced danger for aspiration Can remain in place for 4 weeks or longer	Requires x-ray to verify placement Becomes obstructed easily Best used for continuous feeding
Gastrostomy	No nasal tube Easily concealed Accommodates long-term use Infrequent tube replacement Patient can be taught self-care	Must wait 24 hours to use after initial placement May leak and cause skin breakdown Increased incidence of infection Requires skin care at tube site Can migrate or become dislodged if tube is not secured Gastric overfill and aspiration possible
Jejunostomy	Same as gastrostomy Reduced potential for reflux and aspiration	Same as gastrostomy

than on a continuous basis. Most formulas provide 0.5 to 2.0 kcal/mL of formula.

TUBE-FEEDING SCHEDULES

Tube feedings may be administered on bolus, intermittent, cyclic, or continuous schedules.

Bolus Feedings

A **bolus feeding** (instillation of liquid nourishment four to six times a day in less than 30 minutes) usually involves 250 to 400 mL of formula. This schedule is the least desirable because it distends the stomach rapidly, causing gastric discomfort and increased risk of reflux.

Bolus feedings mimic, to some extent, the natural filling and emptying of the stomach. Some patients experience dis-

TABLE 29–4. **Tube-Feeding Formulas**

Type of Liquid Nutrition	Examples	Use
Isotonic balanced	Osmolite Isocal	Meets total nutritional needs or supplements oral nutrition without altering water distribution
Balanced	Ensure Nutren 1.0 Resource Sustacal 8.8	Meets total nutritional needs or supplements oral nutrition
High-calorie	Ensure Plus Comply Resource Plus Nutren 1.5	Meets needs of patients who require more than usual caloric intake
High-nitrogen	Ensure HN Promote Magnacal Attain	Furnishes more protein than other formulas
High-fiber	Jevity Ensure with Fiber Compleat Modified Ultracal	Provides nutrition and decreases constipation or diarrhea
Partially hydrolyzed	Alitraq Criticare HN TraumaCal Impact Vivonex Plus	Supplies elemental nutrients for people with malabsorption syndromes or impaired GI function

comfort from the rapid delivery of this quantity of fluid. Patients who are unconscious or who have delayed gastric emptying are at greater risk for regurgitation, vomiting, and aspiration when this method of administration is used.

Intermittent Feedings

An **intermittent feeding** (gradual instillation of liquid nourishment four to six times a day) is administered over 30 to 60 minutes, the time most people spend eating a meal. The usual volume is 250 to 400 mL. Intermittent feedings are generally given by gravity drip from a suspended container or with a feeding pump. Gradual filling of the stomach at a slower rate reduces the bloated feeling experienced with bolus feedings. The container that holds the formula is cleaned thoroughly after each feeding to reduce the growth of microorganisms. Tube-feeding administration sets are replaced every 24 hours regardless of the feeding schedule.

Cyclic Feedings

A **cyclic feeding** (continuous instillation of liquid nourishment for 8 to 12 hours) is followed by a 16- to 12-hour pause. This routine is often used to wean patients from tube feedings while continuing to maintain an adequate amount of nutrition. The tube feeding is given during the late evening and during sleep. During the day, patients eat some food orally. As the patient's oral intake increases, the volume and duration of the tube feeding are gradually decreased.

Continuous Feedings

A **continuous feeding** (instillation of liquid nutrition without interruption) is administered at a rate of approximately 1.5 mL/minute. A feeding pump is used to regulate the instillation. Because only a small amount of fluid is being instilled at any one time, the formula does not need to be held in the reservoir of the stomach; it can be delivered directly into the small intestine. Instilling small amounts of fluid beyond the stomach reduces the risk of vomiting and aspiration. Continuous feeding creates some inconvenience, though, because the pump must go wherever the patient does.

PATIENT ASSESSMENT

The following daily assessments are standard for almost every patient who receives tube feedings: weight, fluid intake and output, bowel sounds, lung sounds, temperature, condition of the nasal and oral mucous membranes, breathing pattern, gastric complaints, abdominal distention, vomiting, bowel elimination patterns, and skin condition at the site of a transabdominal tube. Once tube feedings have been initiated, it is also necessary to assess the patient's gastric residual on a routine basis.

Gastric Residual

Gastric residual (volume of liquid within the stomach) is measured to determine whether the rate or volume of feeding exceeds the patient's physiologic capacity. Overfilling the stomach can cause gastric reflux, regurgitation, vomiting, aspiration, and pneumonia. As a rule of thumb, the gastric residual should be no more than 100 mL, or no more than 20% of the previous hour's tube-feeding volume (Smeltzer & Bare, 2000).

Nursing Guidelines For

Checking Gastric Residual

- ☑ Stop the infusion of tube-feeding formula.
  RATIONALE: Facilitates assessment
- ☑ Aspirate fluid from the feeding tube using a 50-mL syringe.
  RATIONALE: Allows collection of a large volume of fluid
- ☑ Continue aspirating until no more fluid is obtained.
  RATIONALE: Ensures an accurate assessment
- ☑ Measure the aspirated fluid and record the amount.
  RATIONALE: Provides objective data for evaluation
- ☑ Reinstill the aspirated fluid.
  RATIONALE: Returns partially digested nutrients and electrolytes to the patient
- ☑ Postpone tube feeding and report residual amounts that exceed agency guidelines or those established by the physician.
  RATIONALE: Reduces the risk of aspiration
- ☑ Check gastric residual again in 30 minutes.
  RATIONALE: Allows time for part of the stomach contents to empty into the small intestine
- ☑ Provide or resume tube feeding if the gastric residual is within an acceptable range.
  RATIONALE: Prevents overfeeding.

Skill 29-4 describes the technique for administering tube feedings.

NURSING MANAGEMENT

Caring for patients with feeding tubes generally involves maintaining tube patency, clearing any obstructions, providing adequate hydration, dealing with common formula-related problems, and preparing patients for home care.

Maintaining Tube Patency

Feeding tubes, especially those smaller than 12 F, are prone to obstructions. Common causes of obstruction are using formulas with large-molecule nutrients, refeeding partially digested gastric residual, administering formula at a rate less than 50 mL/hour, and instilling crushed or hydrophilic (water-absorbing) medications into the tube. To maintain patency, it is best to flush feeding tubes with 30 to 60 mL of water immediately before and after administering a feeding or medications, every 4 hours if the patient is being continuously fed, and after refeeding the gastric residual.

Although tap water is effective as a flush solution, cranberry juice and carbonated beverages may be used. Formula tends to curdle when it comes in contact with cranberry juice, which detracts from the efficacy of this approach.

Clearing an Obstruction

If an obstruction occurs, the physician is consulted. Occasionally it is possible to clear the tube with a solution of meat tenderizer or pancreatic enzyme, but both require written medical orders.

Nursing Guidelines For

Clearing an Obstructed Feeding Tube

- ☑ Select a syringe with a capacity of at least 50 mL.
  RATIONALE: Reduces negative pressure during aspiration, which could lead to collapse of the tube walls
- ☑ Aspirate as much as possible from the feeding tube.
  RATIONALE: Clears the path above the obstructing debris
- ☑ Instill 5 mL of the selected solution.
  RATIONALE: Allows direct contact between the irrigating solution and the debris
- ☑ Clamp the tube and wait 15 minutes.
  RATIONALE: Gives the substance in solution time to have a physical effect on the obstructing debris
- ☑ Aspirate or flush the tube with water.
  RATIONALE: Uses negative pressure or positive pressure to restore patency
- ☑ Repeat if necessary.
  RATIONALE: Promotes patency.

When an obstruction cannot be cleared, the tube should be removed and another inserted rather than compromising nutrition by the delay.

Providing Adequate Hydration

Although tube feedings are approximately 80% water, patients usually require more hydration. Adults require 30 mL of water per kilogram of weight, or 1 mL/kcal, on a daily basis.

To determine whether a patient's hydration needs are being met, the amount of water is identified on the label of commercial formula. This plus the total volume of flush solution can be added and compared with the recommended amount. If there is a significant deficit, the plan of care is revised to provide either an increase in the volume or, preferably, the frequency of flushing the tube. If the fluid volume is excessive, the urine output and lung sounds are monitored to determine whether the patient can excrete comparable amounts (see Chap. 15).

Dealing With Miscellaneous Problems

Several common or potential problems are experienced by patients who require enteral feeding. Many are associated with tube-feeding formulas or the mechanical effects of the tubes themselves (Table 29-5). Problems are reported promptly, and changes are made in the plan of care.

Preparing for Home Care

Because of shortened lengths of stay in hospitals, some patients who continue to need tube feedings are discharged to care for themselves at home. Before the procedure is demonstrated, a written instruction sheet is provided that includes:

- Ways to obtain equipment and formula
- The amount and schedule for each feeding and flush, using household measurements
- Guidelines for delaying a feeding
- Special instructions for skin, nose, or stomal care, including frequency and types of products to use
- Problems to report, such as weight loss, reduced urination, weakness, diarrhea, nausea and vomiting, and breathing difficulties
- Names and phone numbers of people to call if questions arise
- Date, time, and place for continued medical follow-up

Depending on the patient's self-confidence and competence in self-administering tube feedings, often a referral is made to a home health agency for postdischarge nursing support.

Intestinal Decompression

Most nasogastric, nasointestinal, and transabdominal tubes are used for enteral feeding or gastric decompression.

TABLE 29–5. **Common Tube-Feeding Problems**

Problem	Common Causes	Solutions
Diarrhea	Highly concentrated formula	Dilute initial tube feeding to ¼ to ½ strength.
	Rapid administration	Start at 25 mL/hour and increase rate by 25 mL q 12 h.
	Bacterial contamination	Wash hands. Change formula bag and tubing q 24 h. Hang no more than 4 hours' worth of formula. Refrigerate unused formula.
	Lactose intolerance	Consult with the physician on using a milk-free formula.
	Inadequate protein content	Raise serum albumin levels with total parenteral nutrition solutions containing supplemental protein, or administer albumin intravenously.
	Medication side effects	Consult with the physician about adjusting drug therapy or administering an antidiarrheal.
Nausea and vomiting	Rapid feeding	Instill bolus and intermittent feedings by gravity.
	Overfeeding	Delay feeding until gastric residual is less than 100 mL or less than 20% of hourly volume. Maintain sitting position for at least 30 minutes after feeding. Consult with the physician about ordering medication that facilitates gastric emptying. Administer continuous feedings. Instill feedings within the small intestine.
	Air in stomach	Keep tubing filled with formula or water.
	Medication side effects	Consult with the physician about adjusting drug therapy or administering drugs to control symptoms.
Aspiration	Incorrect tube placement	Check placement before instilling liquids.
	Vomiting	Keep head elevated at least 30° during feedings and for ½ hour afterwards. Keep cuffed tracheostomy and endotracheal tubes inflated. Refer to measures for controlling vomiting.
Constipation	Lack of fiber	Change formula.
	Dehydration	Increase supplemental water. Consult with the physician on giving a laxative, enema, or suppository.
Elevated blood sugar	Calorie-concentrated formula	Instill diluted formula and gradually increase concentration. Administer insulin according to medical orders.
Weight loss	Inadequate calories	Increase calories in formula. Increase rate or frequency of feedings.
Elevated electrolytes	Dehydration	Increase supplemental water.
Dry oral and nasal mucous membranes	Mouth breathing Dried nasal mucus	Provide frequent oral and nasal hygiene
Middle ear inflammation	Narrowing or obstruction of eustachian tube from presence of tube in pharynx	Turn from side to side q 2 h. Insert a small-diameter feeding tube.
Sore throat	Pressure and irritation from tube	Use a small-diameter feeding tube.
Plugged feeding tube	Instilling crushed or powdered medications through the tube	Use liquid medications. Dilute crushed drugs. Flush the tubing liberally after drug administration.
	Formula coagulation from drug–food interactions	Flush tubing with water before and after drug administration. Follow agency policy for alternative flush solutions such as carbonated beverages or solutions of meat tenderizer.
	Kinked tube	Maintain neck in neutral position or change position frequently.
	Large molecules in formula	Dilute formula. Flush tubing at least q 4 h. Use a larger-diameter feeding tube.
Dumping syndrome	Rapid and large instillation of highly concentrated formula into the intestine	Administer small, continuous volume. Adjust glucose content of formula.

However, sometimes patients require intestinal decompression, which is performed with a tungsten-weighted tube (see Table 29-1). Intestinal decompression sometimes makes it possible to avoid surgery.

TUBE INSERTION

A nasointestinal decompression tube is inserted in the same manner as a nasogastric tube, and the nurse then promotes and monitors its passage into the intestine. In the presence of peristalsis, the weight of the tungsten propels the tip of the tube beyond the stomach. Openings through the distal end provide channels through which the intestinal contents are suctioned. An intestinal decompression tube is generally left in place until the intestinal lumen is patent or surgical treatment is instituted.

Nursing Guidelines

Inserting an Intestinal Decompression Tube

- ☑ Assemble all the necessary equipment as needed for any nasally inserted tube.
  RATIONALE: Ensures organization and efficient time management
- ☑ Follow the techniques in Skill 29-1 for inserting a nasogastric tube.
  RATIONALE: Involves the same principles during initial insertion
- ☑ Thread the excess tubing through a sling of folded gauze taped to the forehead (Fig. 29-12) once gastric placement is confirmed.
  RATIONALE: Supports the tube as it advances
- ☑ Ambulate the patient, if possible.
  RATIONALE: Helps the tube move through the pyloric valve into the small intestine

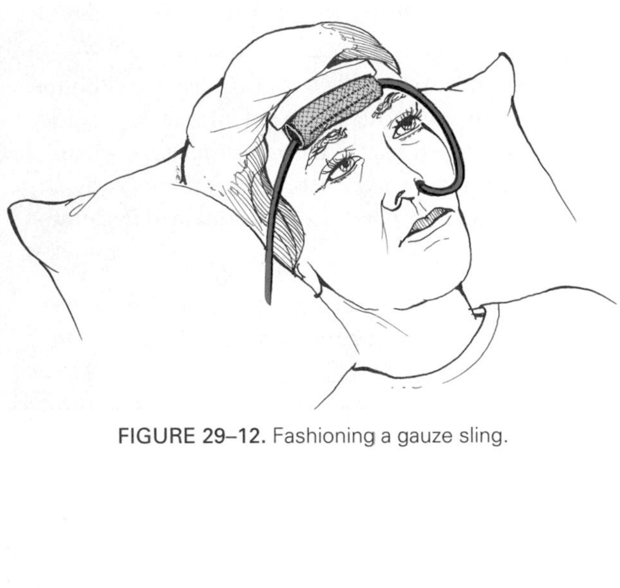

FIGURE 29–12. Fashioning a gauze sling.

- ☑ When the radiograph indicates that the intestinal tube has advanced beyond the stomach, position the patient on the right side for 2 hours, then on the back in a Fowler's position for 2 hours, then on the left side for 2 hours.
  RATIONALE: Uses gravity and positioning to promote movement through intestinal curves
- ☑ Follow agency policy or the physician's instructions for manually advancing the tube several inches each hour.
  RATIONALE: Supplements natural peristaltic advancement
- ☑ Observe the graduated marks on the tube.
  RATIONALE: Provides a means for monitoring the tube's progression and approximate anatomic location
- ☑ Request x-ray confirmation when the tube has reached the prescribed distance.
  RATIONALE: Provides objective evidence to verify the terminal location of the distal tip
- ☑ Secure the tube to the nose once its distal location has been confirmed.
  RATIONALE: Stabilizes the tube and prevents further migration
- ☑ Coil the excess tubing and attach it to the patient's hospital gown.
  RATIONALE: Prevents accidental extubation
- ☑ Connect the proximal end to a wall or portable suction source.
  RATIONALE: Produces negative pressure to pull substances from the intestine.

REMOVAL

Once the intestinal decompression tube has served its purpose, the nurse begins the process of removing it. An intestinal decompression tube is removed slowly because removal is in a reverse direction through the curves of the intestine and the valves of the lower and upper ends of the stomach.

First, the tube is disconnected from the suction source. Next, the tape that secures the tube to the face is removed and the tube is withdrawn 6 to 10 inches (15 to 25 cm) at 10-minute intervals. When the last 18 inches (45 cm) remains, the tube is pulled gently from the nose. Afterward, nasal and oral hygiene measures are provided.

Nursing Implications

Depending on the data collected during patient care, one or more of the following nursing diagnoses may be identified:

- Altered nutrition: less than body requirements
- Self-care deficit: feeding

- Impaired swallowing
- Risk for aspiration
- Altered oral mucous membranes
- Diarrhea
- Constipation

The accompanying nursing care plan is a model for managing the care of a patient with a large gastric residual, defined by NANDA (1999) as "the state in which an individual is at risk for entry of gastrointestinal secretions, oropharyngeal secretions, or solids or fluids into tracheobronchial passages."

Nursing Care Plan

Risk for Aspiration

Assessment

Subjective Data

None obtained; patient is unresponsive.

Objective Data

35-year-old with head trauma after motor vehicle accident. Opens eyes, but makes no verbal response. Moves away when painful stimulus is applied. #16 nasogastric tube in L. naris. Tube placement verified by instilling air and auscultating over stomach. Gastric residual measures 150 mL 4 hours after previous bolus feeding of 400 mL.

Diagnosis

Risk for aspiration related to slow gastric emptying

Plan

Goal

Gastric residual will be less than 100 mL within 1 hour of feeding schedule.

Orders: 8/22

1. Keep cuff of endotracheal tube inflated.
2. Maintain head elevation at no less than 30° at all times.
3. Monitor bowel sounds; report if absent or less than five sounds per minute.
4. Measure gastric residual before all tube feedings.
5. Refeed gastric residual and follow with 30 mL tap water flush.
6. Postpone tube feeding for 1 hour if gastric residual measures ≥100 mL.
7. Report gastric residual volume to physician if ≥100 mL after delaying feeding for 1 hour and reassess.
8. Maintain suction machine at the bedside. ______ J. RHAMES, RN

Implementation (Documentation)

8/23 0800 Bowel sounds present and active in all quadrants. Endotracheal tube cuff remains inflated. Head is elevated 30°. Gastric residual measures 150 mL. Residual reinstilled followed with 30 mL flush with tap water. Tube feeding postponed. ______ A. PETRY, LPN

0900 Gastric residual measures 100 mL after 1-hour delay of tube feeding. Volume of gastric residual reported to Dr. Burns. Orders received for metaclopramide and replacement of nasogastric tube with a small nasointestinal tube when residual measures 50 mL, and resume tube feeding on a continuous basis once tube is in intestine (see physician's orders). Head maintained in elevated position at 60°. ______ A. PETRY, LPN

Evaluation (Documentation)

1030 Gastric residual measures 50 mL. Nasogastric tube replaced with 8 F Keofeed tube. Placement verified by x-ray. Tube feeding resumed at 100 mL/hr with feeding pump as ordered. ______ A. PETRY, LPN

FOCUS ON OLDER ADULTS

- An age-related reduction in the number of laryngeal nerve endings contributes to diminished efficiency of the gag reflex. Other conditions that depress the gag reflex include neurologic disorders such as dementia and strokes and repeated insertion and removal of dentures.
- Because older adults are at increased risk for fluid and electrolyte disturbances, they develop hyperglycemia (elevated blood glucose levels) more rapidly than other adults when tube feedings are administered.
- It is best to check an older patient's capillary blood glucose level every 4 hours until the patient's blood sugar is within normal range for 48 hours while receiving full-strength concentrations of tube-feeding formulas.
- Monitor older adults for agitation or confusion, which may possibly cause the patient to pull out the feeding tube inadvertently. Also, a change in mental status is an early indicator of a fluid or electrolyte imbalance.
- Patients who have or are at risk for pressure sores benefit from formulas that are fortified with additional zinc, protein, and other nutrients.
- Older adults tend to tolerate small, continuous feedings better than other tube feeding schedules.
- When teaching an older adult or older caregiver how to manage a gastrostomy tube or administer tube feedings at home, the teaching plan should allow more time for processing the information and include several practice sessions. A referral for skilled nursing, usually covered by most health insurance plans, may be appropriate for ongoing teaching and assessment for patients being discharged with tube feedings.
- In home and long-term care settings, the services of a registered dietician may be helpful in ongoing assessment of tube feedings.
- For older adults living on a fixed income, the dietician can suggest ways of preparing less costly home-blenderized formulas that meet the nutritional needs of the patient.
- The long-term use of tube feedings in older adults with dementia or other chronic declining conditions entails many ethical considerations. In 1992, the American Nurses Association (ANA) published a position statement that advance directives indicating a wish to avoid artificial nutrition and hydration should be followed. Nurses, especially those working in home care and long-term care settings, need up-to-date knowledge about ethical and legal issues related to the use of tube feedings (see Chap. 3).

KEY CONCEPTS

- Intubation refers to the insertion of a tube into a structure of the body.
- GI intubation is used for providing nourishment; administering medications; obtaining diagnostic samples; removing poisons, gas, and secretions; and controlling bleeding.
- Four types of tubes may be used for intubating the GI system: orogastric, nasogastric, nasointestinal, and transabdominal.
- Common assessments performed before inserting a tube nasally include determining the patient's level of consciousness, the characteristics and location of bowel sounds, the structure and integrity of the nose, and the patient's ability to swallow, cough, and gag.
- An NEX measurement, which helps to determine how far to insert a tube for stomach placement, is the distance from the nose to the earlobe and then to the xiphoid process.
- Stomach placement is checked by aspirating gastric fluid, auscultating the abdomen as a bolus of air is instilled, and testing the pH of aspirated fluid.
- Nasointestinal feeding tubes differ from their nasogastric counterparts in that they are longer, narrower, and more flexible; their lubricant is bonded to the tube; they are frequently inserted with a stylet; and an x-ray is used to confirm their placement.
- Although transabdominal feeding tubes can be used for long periods, they are prone to leaking and causing skin impairment.
- Enteral nutrition refers to nourishing patients by means of the stomach or small intestine rather than the oral route.
- Four common schedules for administering tube feedings are bolus, intermittent, cyclic, and continuous.
- Gastric residual is checked to determine whether the rate or volume of feeding exceeds the patient's physiologic capacity.
- Caring for patients with feeding tubes involves maintaining tube patency, clearing any obstructions, providing adequate hydration, dealing with common formula-related problems, and preparing patients for home care.
- Before discharge, patients who will administer their own tube feedings at home are provided with written instructions on ways to obtain equipment and formula, the amount and schedule for each feeding, guidelines for delaying a feeding, and skin or nose care.
- When assisting with the insertion of a tungsten-weighted tube, nurses are responsible for promoting and monitoring its movement into the intestine.

CRITICAL THINKING EXERCISES

- Describe the similarities and differences between inserting a tube for gastric decompression and one for intestinal decompression.
- What questions would be important to ask if a patient receiving tube feedings at home calls to report the onset of diarrhea?

SUGGESTED READINGS

American Nurses Association. Position statement: Foregoing nutrition and hydration. Task Force on the Nurse's Role in End-of-Life Decisions. American Nurses Association, April 2, 1992.

Bass DJ, Forman LP, Abrams SE, Hsueh AM. The effect of dietary fiber in tube-fed elderly patients. Journal of Gerontological Nursing 1996; 22(10):37–44.

Bliss DZ, Lehmann S. Tube feeding: immune-boosting formulas. RN 1999; 62(8):26–28.

Clevenger FW, Rodriguez DJ. Techniques and procedures. Decision-making for enteral feeding administration: the why behind the where and how. Nutrition in Clinical Practice 1995;10(3):104–113.

Hall JC, Krupp KB, Heximer B. Troubleshooting G-tubes: balloon deflation problems. RN 1996;59(7):25–28.

Hanlon MD. Techniques and procedures. Preplacement marking for optimal gastrostomy and jejunostomy tube site locations to decrease complications and promote self-care. Nutrition in Clinical Practice 1998;13(4):167–171.

Heximer B. Teaching case. Pressure necrosis: implications and interventions for PEG tubes. Nutrition in Clinical Practice 1997;12(6):256–258.

Lawrence V. Clinicians' forum. A dressing technique to stabilize percutaneous tubes. Home Healthcare Nurse 1997;15(7):501–503.

Loan T, Kearney P, Magnuson B, Williams S. Enteral feeding in the home environment. Home Healthcare Nurse 1997;15(8):531–538.

Lord LM. Enteral access devices. Nursing Clinics of North America 1997; 32(4):685–704.

Lord LM, Lipp J, Stull S. Adult tube feeding formulas. MedSurg Nursing 1996;5(6):407–432.

McConnell EA. Clinical do's & don'ts. Maintaining a feeding tube exit site. Nursing 1996;26(12):61.

NANDA nursing diagnoses: definitions and classification, 1999–2000. Philadelphia, NANDA, 1999.

Northover RC. Tube talk . . . gastrostomy tube. Nursing 1996;26(11):9.

O'Brien B, Davis S, Erwin-Toth P. G-tube site care: a practical guide. RN 1999;62(2):52–56.

Pendlebury J. Skills update: feeding by PEG—percutaneous endoscopic gastrostomy. Community Nurse 1997;3(4):11–12.

Smeltzer SC, Bare BG. Medical-surgical nursing. 9th ed. Philadelphia: Lippincott, 2000.

Taylor LJ, Faria SH. Practice teaching. Caring for the patient with a gastrostomy/jejunostomy tube. Home Care Provider 1997;221–224.

White S. Percutaneous endoscope gastrostomy (PEG). Nursing Standard 1998;12(28):41–48.

SKILL 29-1

INSERTING A NASOGASTRIC TUBE

Suggested Action	Reason for Action
Assessment	
Check that a medical order has been written.	Ensures that care is within the legal scope of practice
Determine the purpose for the nasogastric tube.	Facilitates evaluation of outcomes
Identify the patient.	Ensures that the procedure will be performed on the correct patient
Assess how much the patient understands about the procedure.	Indicates the need for and level of health teaching
Inspect the nose after the patient blows into a paper tissue.	Provides data that will determine which naris to use
Unwrap and uncoil the tube.	Straightens tube and releases bends from product packaging

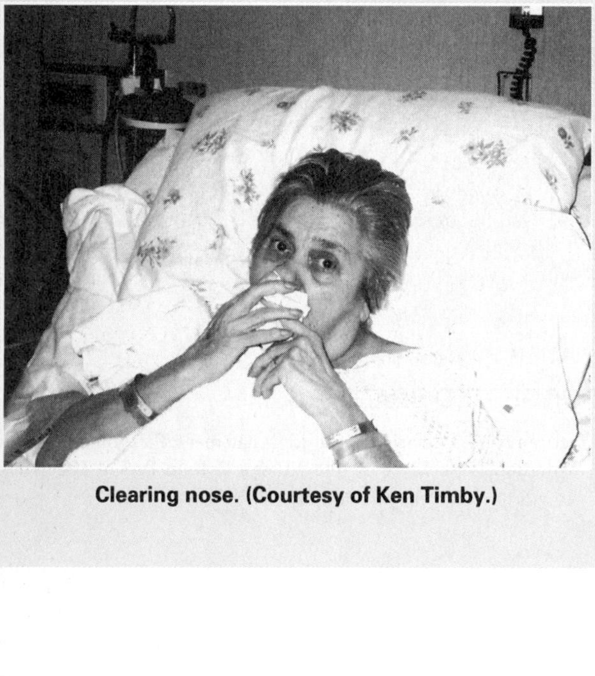

Clearing nose. (Courtesy of Ken Timby.)

continued

SKILL 29-1

INSERTING A NASOGASTRIC TUBE *Continued*

Suggested Action	Reason for Action
Obtain the NEX measurements.	Determines length for insertion
Mark the tube at the NE (nose-to-ear) and NX (nose-to-xiphoid) measurements.	Provides a guide during insertion

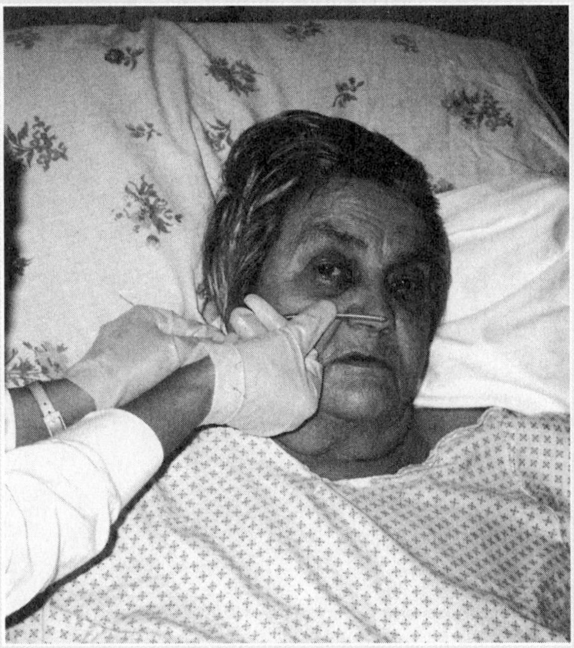

Measuring the tube. (Courtesy of Ken Timby.)

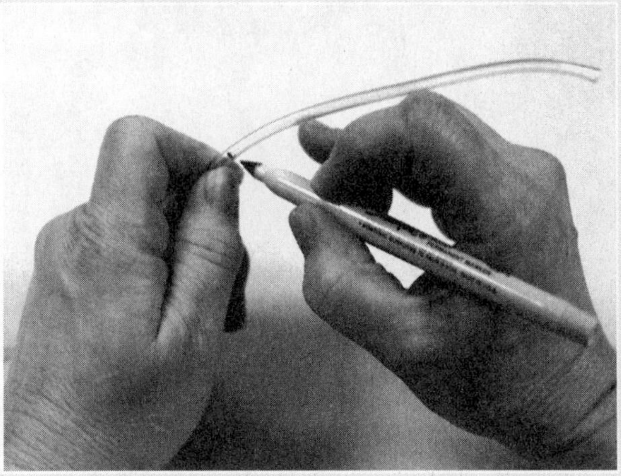

Marking the tube. (Courtesy of Ken Timby.)

Suggested Action	Reason for Action
Planning	
If a plastic tube feels rigid, place it in warm water or flush the tube with warm water.	Promotes flexibility
Assemble the following equipment, in addition to the tube: water, straw, towel, lubricant, tissues, tape, emesis basin, flashlight, stethoscope, clean gloves, 50-mL syringe.	Contributes to organization and efficient time management
Place a suction machine at the bedside if the patient is unresponsive or has difficulty swallowing.	Provides a method for clearing the patient's airway of vomitus
Remove dentures.	Avoids choking should they become loose or displaced
Establish a hand signal for pausing.	Relieves anxiety by providing the patient with some locus for control
Implementation	
Wash your hands.	Reduces the transmission of microorganisms
Pull the privacy curtain.	Demonstrates respect for dignity
Assist the patient to sit in semi-Fowler's or high-Fowler's position and hyperextend the neck as if in a sniffing position.	Ensures visualization of nasal passageway to facilitate inserting the tube
Protect the patient, bedclothing, and linen with a towel.	Avoids linen changes

continued

SKILL 29–1

INSERTING A NASOGASTRIC TUBE *Continued*

Suggested Action	Reason for Action
Don gloves.	Reduces the transmission of microorganisms
Lubricate the tube with water-soluble gel over 6 to 8 inches (15–20 cm) at the distal tip.	Reduces friction and tissue trauma
Insert the tube into the nostril while pointing the tip backward and downward.	Follows the normal contour of the nasal passage

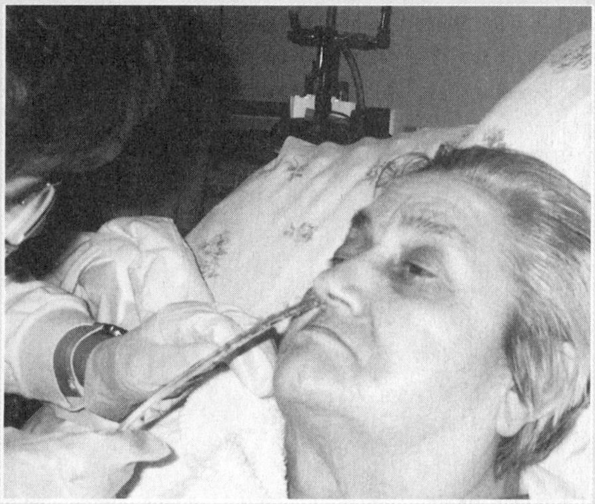

Inserting the tube. (Courtesy of Ken Timby.)

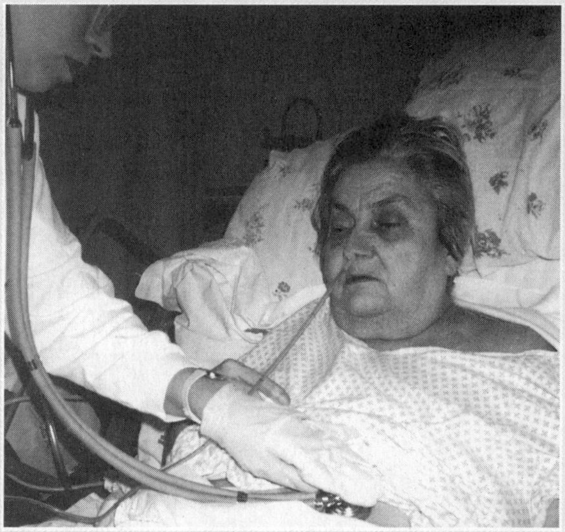

Assessing placement. (Courtesy of Ken Timby.)

Suggested Action	Reason for Action
Do not force the tube. Relubricate the tube or rotate it if there is resistance.	Prevents trauma
Stop when the first mark on the tube is at the tip of the nose.	Places the tip above the area where the gag reflex may be stimulated
Use a flashlight to inspect the back of the throat.	Confirms that the tube has been maneuvered around the nasal curve
Instruct the patient to lower his or her chin to the chest and swallow sips of water.	Narrows the trachea and opens the esophagus; helps advance the tube
Advance the tube 3 to 5 inches (7.5–12.5 cm) each time the patient swallows.	Coordinates insertion; reduces the potential for gagging or vomiting
Pause if the patient gives the preestablished signal.	Demonstrates respect and cooperation
Discontinue the procedure and raise the tube to the first mark if there are signs of distress such as gasping, coughing, a bluish skin color, or the inability to speak or hum.	Indicates that the tube is possibly in the airway
Assess placement when the second mark is reached.	Provides data on distal placement
Withdraw the tube to the first mark and reattempt insertion if the assessment findings are inconclusive, or consult with the physician about obtaining an x-ray.	Ensures safety
Proceed to secure the tube if data indicate the tube is in the stomach.	Prevents tube migration
Connect the tube to suction or clamp it while awaiting further orders.	Promotes gastric decompression or potential use

continued

SKILL 29–1

INSERTING A NASOGASTRIC TUBE *Continued*

Suggested Action	Reason for Action
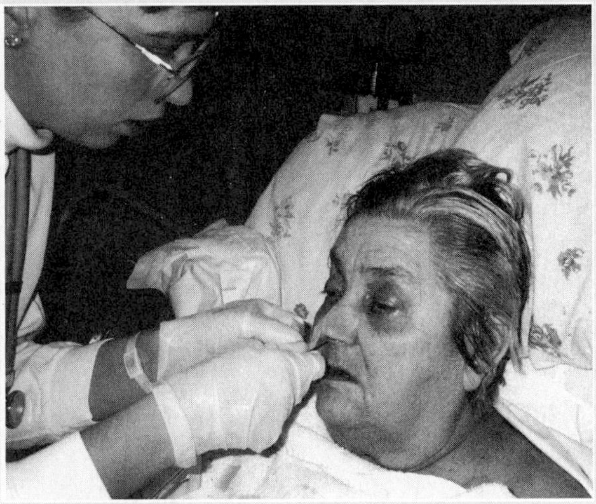 Securing the tube. (Courtesy of Ken Timby.)	
Remove gloves and wash your hands.	Reduces the transmission of microorganisms
Position the patient with a minimum head elevation of 30°.	Prevents gastric reflux
Remove equipment from the bedside.	Restores orderliness and supports principles of medical asepsis
Measure and record the volume of drainage at least every 8 hours.	Provides data for evaluating fluid balance

Evaluation

- Distal placement within the stomach is confirmed
- Patient exhibits no evidence of respiratory distress
- Patient can speak or hum
- Lung sounds are present and clear bilaterally
- No bleeding or pain is noted in area of nasal mucosa

Document

- Type of tube
- Outcomes of the procedure
- Method for determining placement
- Description of drainage
- Type and amount of suction, if the tube is used for decompression

SAMPLE DOCUMENTATION

Date and Time 16 F Salem sump tube inserted without difficulty. Placement verified by aspirating gastric secretions, which are yellowish-green and reveal a pH of 3 when tested. Salem sump tube secured to nose and connected to low, intermittent wall suction. Positioned with head of bed elevated 30°. ______________________ SIGNATURE, TITLE

CRITICAL THINKING

- Discuss the consequences of inserting a nasogastric tube into the respiratory passages.
- Describe skin and nasal hygiene measures that are appropriate when caring for a patient with a nasogastric tube.

SKILL 29-2

IRRIGATING A NASOGASTRIC TUBE

Suggested Action	Reason for Action
Assessment	
Monitor the patient's symptoms, volume and rate of drainage, and evidence of abdominal distention.	Provides data for future comparisons
Check that a medical order has been written, if that is the agency's policy.	Complies with the legal scope of nursing practice
Identify the patient.	Ensures that the procedure will be performed on the correct patient
Assess how much the patient understands about the procedure.	Provides an opportunity for patient teaching
Planning	
Assemble the following equipment: Asepto or irrigating syringe, irrigating fluid (isotonic saline solution), container, clean towel or pad, clean gloves, cover or plug for end of tube.	Contributes to organization and efficient time management
Turn off the suction.	Facilitates implementation
Implementation	
Pull the privacy curtain.	Demonstrates respect for dignity
Wash your hands.	Reduces the transmission of microorganisms
Place a clean pad or towel beneath where the tube will be separated.	Avoids changing bed linen and protects the patient from soiling
Don clean gloves.	Complies with standard precautions
Disconnect the nasogastric tube from the suction tubing and apply cover or insert plug to suction tubing.	Keeps connection area clean
Check the distal placement of the tube.	Ensures safety
Fill irrigating syringe with 30 to 60 mL of normal saline solution.	Provides an adequate quantity of isotonic solution to clear tubing
Insert the tip of the syringe within the proximal end of the tube and allow the solution to flow in by gravity, or apply gentle pressure.	Dilutes and mobilizes debris
Aspirate after the fluid has been instilled.	Removes substances that may impair future drainage
Reconnect the tube to the source of suction.	Resumes therapeutic management
Observe the characteristics of the aspirated solution; measure and discard.	Provides data for evaluating the effectiveness of the procedure
Monitor for the flow of drainage through the suction tubing.	Provides evidence that patency is being maintained
Remove gloves and wash hands.	Reduces the transmission of microorganisms
Record the volume of instilled and drained fluid on the bedside intake and output sheet.	Provides accurate data for determining fluid balance

continued

SKILL 29-2

IRRIGATING A NASOGASTRIC TUBE *Continued*

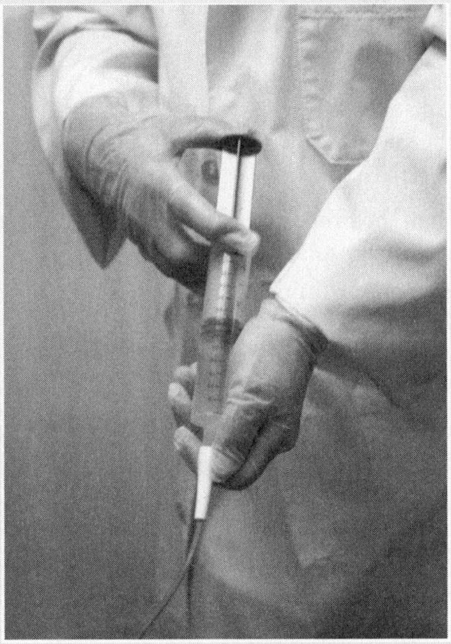

Instilling irrigation solution. (Courtesy of Ken Timby.)

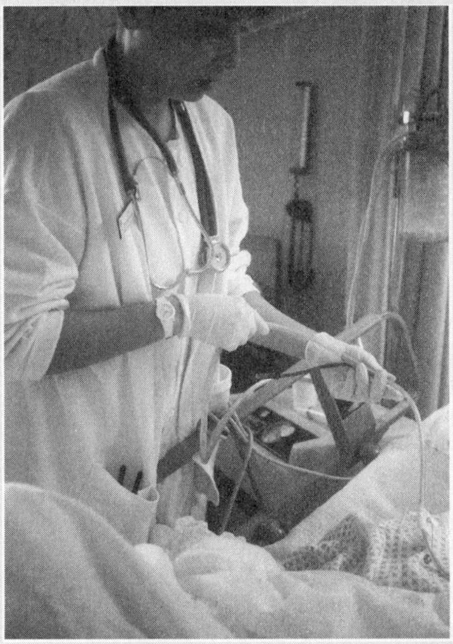

Monitoring drainage. (Courtesy of Ken Timby.)

Evaluation

- Drainage is restored
- Nausea and vomiting are relieved
- Abdominal distention is reduced

Document

- Volume and type of fluid instilled
- Appearance and volume of returned drainage
- Response of patient

SAMPLE DOCUMENTATION

Date and Time Salem sump tube irrigated with 60 mL of normal saline. Solution instilled with slight pressure. 100 mL of solution returned with several large mucus particles. Reconnected to low, intermittent suction. Draining well at the present time. Abdomen is soft. No vomiting.

____ SIGNATURE, TITLE

CRITICAL THINKING

- Discuss reasons why a nasogastric tube may become obstructed.
- Explain the reason for using an isotonic saline solution for irrigating a nasogastric tube rather than a solution that is hypotonic or hypertonic.

SKILL 29-3

REMOVING A NASOGASTRIC TUBE

Suggested Action	Reason for Action
Assessment	
Assess bowel sounds, condition of mouth and nasal mucosa, level of consciousness, and gag reflex.	Provides data for future comparisons and may affect the manner in which the procedure is performed
Check that a medical order has been written.	Complies with the legal scope of nursing practice
Identify the patient.	Ensures that the procedure will be performed on the correct patient
Assess how much the patient understands about the procedure.	Provides an opportunity for patient teaching
Planning	
Assemble the following equipment: towel, emesis basin, applicator sticks, oral hygiene equipment, clean gloves.	Contributes to organization and efficient time management
Implementation	
Pull the privacy curtain.	Demonstrates respect for dignity
Wash your hands.	Reduces the transmission of microorganisms
Place the patient in a sitting position, if alert, or in a lateral position if not.	Prevents aspiration of stomach contents
Cover the chest with a clean towel and place the emesis basin and tissues within easy reach.	Prepares for possible vomiting and protects the patient from soiling
Remove the tape securing the tube to the patient's nose.	Facilitates pulling the tube from the stomach
Don clean gloves.	Complies with standard precautions
Turn off the suction.	Prepares for removal
Instill a bolus of air into the lumen that drains gastric secretions.	Prevents residual fluid from leaking as the tube is withdrawn
Clamp, plug, or pinch the tube.	Prevents fluid from leaking as the tube is withdrawn

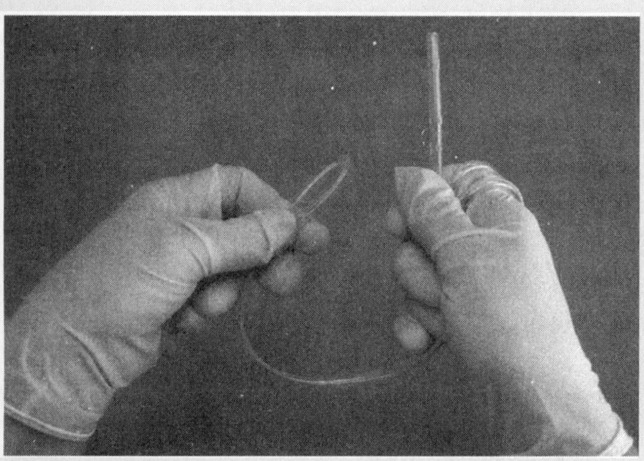

Occluding the tube. (Courtesy of Ken Timby.)

Suggested Action	Reason for Action
Instruct the patient to take a deep breath and hold it just before removing the nasogastric tube.	Reduces the risk for aspirating gastric fluid
Remove the tube from the patient's nose gently and slowly.	Lessens the potential for trauma

continued

SKILL 29-3

REMOVING A NASOGASTRIC TUBE *Continued*

Suggested Action	Reason for Action
Enclose the tube within the towel or glove and discard the tube in a covered container.	Provides a transmission barrier against microorganisms

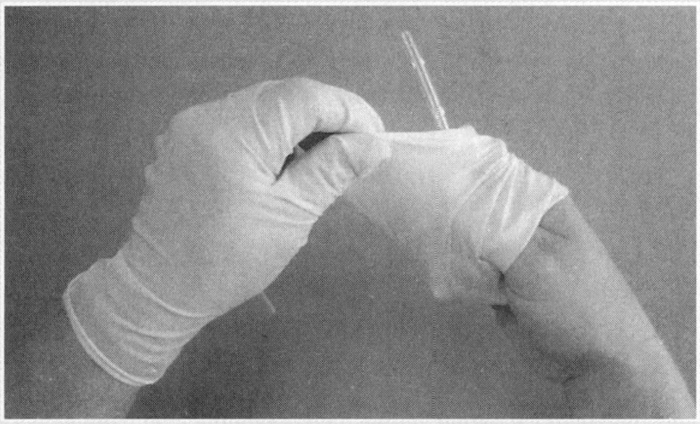

Enclosing the tube. (Courtesy of Ken Timby.)

Suggested Action	Reason for Action
Empty, measure, and record the drainage in the suction container.	Provides data for evaluating the patient's fluid status
Remove gloves and wash hands.	Reduces the transmission of microorganisms
Offer an opportunity for oral hygiene.	Removes disagreeable tastes from the patient's mouth
Encourage the patient to clear the nose of mucus and debris with paper tissues or cotton applicators.	Promotes integrity of nasal tissue
Discard disposable equipment; rinse and return portable suction equipment.	Preserves cleanliness and orderliness in the patient's unit; demonstrates accountability for equipment

Evaluation

- Tube is removed
- Patient resumes eating and taking fluids
- Patient experiences no nausea or vomiting
- Airway remains clear
- Nasal mucosa is moist and intact

Document

- Type of tube removed
- Response of patient
- Appearance and volume of drainage
- Appearance of nose and nasopharynx

SAMPLE DOCUMENTATION

Date and Time Salem sump tube removed. Brief period of retching during removal. Total of 75 mL clear green drainage emptied from suction container. Oral care provided. L. naris swabbed with applicator lubricated with petroleum jelly. Mucosa is red but intact.

________________________ SIGNATURE, TITLE

CRITICAL THINKING

- If the patient who has just had a nasogastric tube removed wants something to eat, what nursing actions are appropriate to take?
- List assessment data that are appropriate to monitor after the removal of a nasogastric tube.

SKILL 29-4

ADMINISTERING TUBE FEEDINGS

Suggested Action	Reason for Action
Bolus Feeding	
Assessment	
Check the medical order for the type of nourishment, volume, and schedule to follow.	Complies with the legal scope of nursing practice
Check the date and identifying information on the container of tube-feeding formula.	Ensures accurate administration and avoids using outdated formula
Identify the patient.	Ensures that the procedure will be performed on the correct patient
Distinguish the tubing for gastric or intestinal feeding from tubing being used to instill intravenous solutions.	Prevents administering nutritional formula into the vascular system
Assess bowel sounds.	Provides data indicating safety for instilling liquids through the tube
Measure gastric residual if a 12 F or larger tube is in place.	Determines if the stomach has the capacity to manage the next instillation of formula; aspiration of fluid may be impossible with small-lumen tubes

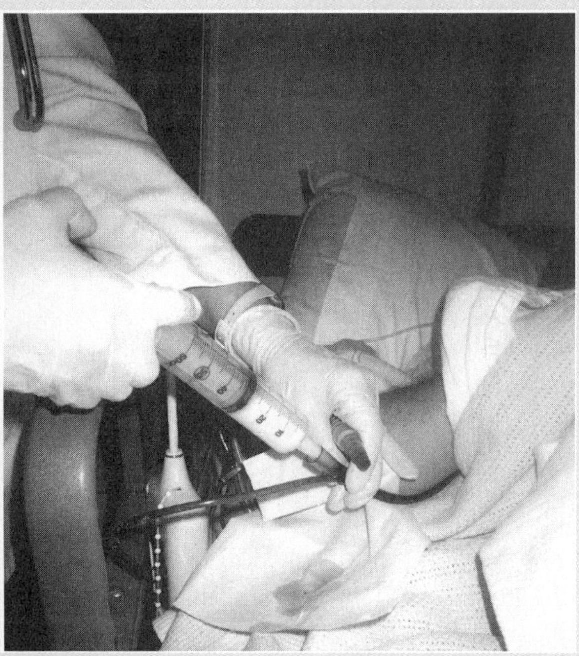

Measuring gastric residual. (Courtesy of Ken Timby.)

Suggested Action	Reason for Action
Measure capillary blood glucose or glucose in the urine.	Provides data indicating response to caloric intake
Assess how much the patient understands about the procedure.	Provides an opportunity for patient teaching
Planning	
Replace any unused formula every 24 hours.	Reduces the potential for bacterial growth
Wait and recheck gastric residual in ½ hour if it exceeds 100 mL.	Avoids overfilling the stomach

continued

SKILL 29-4

ADMINISTERING TUBE FEEDINGS *Continued*

Suggested Action	Reason for Action
Assemble the following equipment: Asepto syringe, formula, tap water.	Contributes to organization and efficient time management
Warm refrigerated nourishment to room temperature in a basin of warm water.	Prevents chilling and abdominal cramping
Implementation	
Wash your hands.	Reduces the transmission of microorganisms
Place the patient in a 30° to 90° sitting position.	Prevents regurgitation
Refeed gastric residual by gravity flow.	Returns predigested nutrients without excessive pressure
Pinch the tube just before all the residual has instilled.	Prevents air from entering the tube
Add fresh formula to the syringe and adjust the height to allow a slow but gradual instillation.	Provides nourishment
Continue filling the syringe before it becomes empty.	Prevents air from entering the tube
If a gastrostomy tube is being used, tilt the barrel of the syringe during the feeding.	Permits air displacement from the stomach

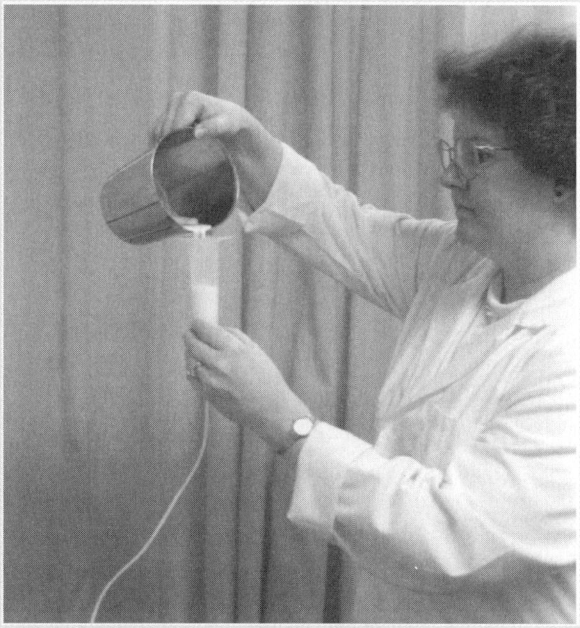

Administering a bolus feeding. (Courtesy of Ken Timby.)

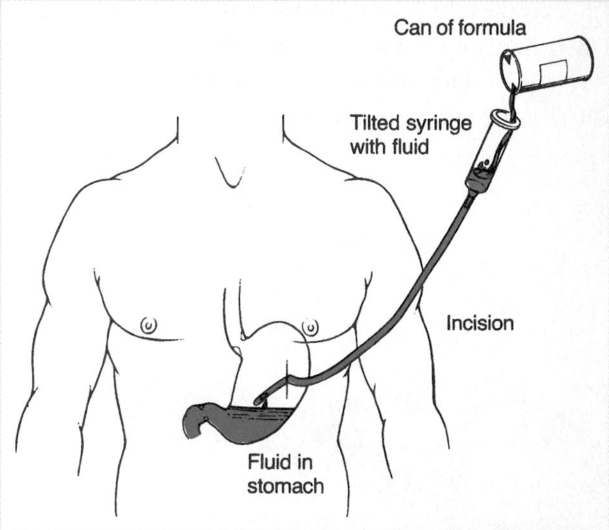

Bolus feeding through a gastrostomy tube.

Suggested Action	Reason for Action
Flush the tubing with at least 30 to 60 mL of water after each feeding, or follow agency policy for suggested amounts.	Ensures that all nourishment has entered the stomach; prevents fermentation and coagulation of formula in the tube; provides water for fluid balance
Plug or clamp the tube as the water leaves the syringe.	Prevents air from entering the tubing; maintains patency
Keep the head of the bed elevated for at least 30 to 60 minutes after a feeding.	Prevents gastric reflux
Wash and dry the feeding equipment. Return items to the bedside.	Supports principles of medical asepsis

continued

SKILL 29–4

ADMINISTERING TUBE FEEDINGS *Continued*

Suggested Action	Reason for Action
Record the volume of formula and water administered on the bedside intake and output record.	Provides accurate data for assessing fluid balance and caloric value of nourishment
Provide oral hygiene at least twice daily.	Removes microorganisms and promotes comfort and hygiene of patient
INTERMITTENT FEEDING	
Assessment	
Follow the previous sequence for assessment.	Principles remain the same
Planning	
In addition to those activities listed for bolus feeding:	
Replace unused formula, feeding containers, and tubing every 24 hours.	Reduces the potential for bacterial growth
Implementation	
Fill the feeding container with room-temperature formula.	Prevents administration of cold formula, which can cause cramping; room-temperature formula will be instilled before supporting bacterial growth
Purge the air from the tube by gradually opening the clamp on the tubing.	Prevents instilling air
Connect the tubing to the nasogastric or nasoenteral tube.	Provides access to formula
Open the clamp and regulate the drip rate according to the physician's order or agency policy.	Supports safe administration of liquid nourishment
Check at 10-minute intervals.	Ensures early identification of infusion problems

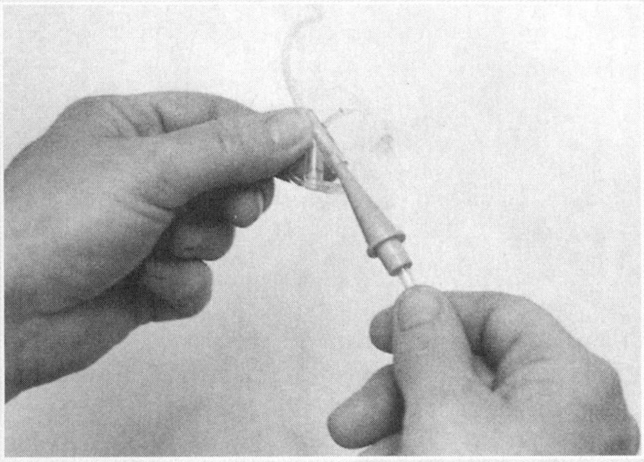

Connecting the tubing. (Courtesy of Ken Timby.)

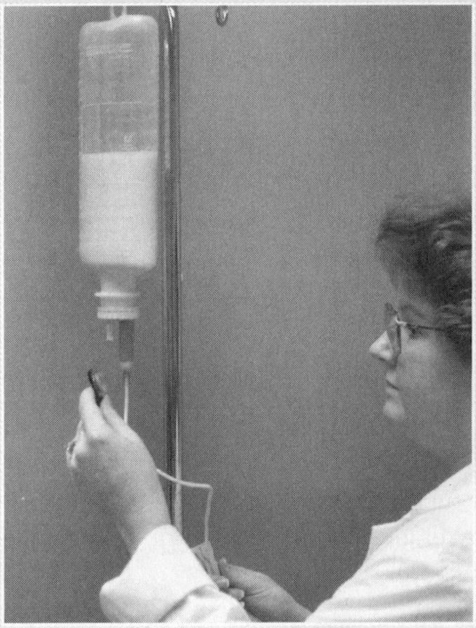

Checking the rate of flow. (Courtesy of Ken Timby.)

Suggested Action	Reason for Action
Flush the tubing with water after the formula has infused.	Clears the tubing of formula, prevents obstruction, and provides water for fluid balance

continued

SKILL 29-4

ADMINISTERING TUBE FEEDINGS *Continued*

Suggested Action	Reason for Action
Pinch the feeding tube just as the last volume of water is administered.	Prevents air from entering the tube
Clamp or plug the feeding tube.	Prevents leaking
Record the volume of formula and water instilled.	Provides accurate data for assessing fluid balance and caloric value of nourishment
Follow recommendations for postprocedural care as described with bolus feeding.	Principles for care remain the same
CONTINUOUS FEEDING	
Assessment	
In addition to previously described assessments:	Principles remain the same
Check the gastric residual every 4 hours.	Ensures a routine pattern for assessment to accommodate the schedule of continuous feedings; prevents inadvertent overfeeding
Planning	
In addition to previously described planning activities:	
Obtain equipment for regulating continuous infusion, such as a tube-feeding pump.	Aids accurate administration and sounds an alarm if the infusion is interrupted
Replace unused formula, feeding containers, and tubing every 24 hours.	Reduces the potential for bacterial growth
Attach a time tape to a feeding container.	Facilitates periodic assessment

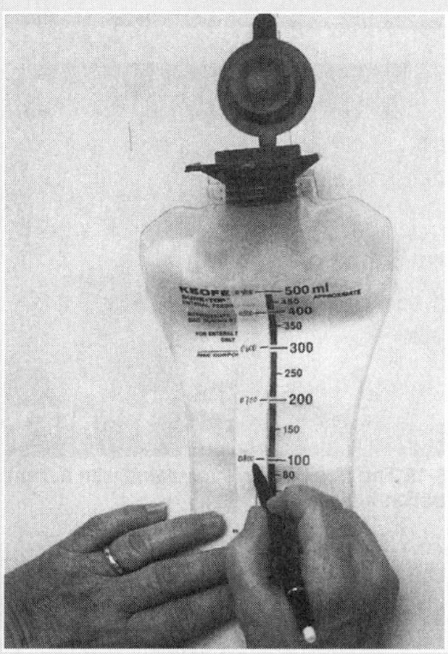

Attaching a time strip. (Courtesy of Ken Timby.)

Suggested Action	Reason for Action
Implementation	
Flush the new feeding container with water.	Reduces surface tension within the tube and enhances the passage of large protein molecules.

continued

SKILL 29-4

ADMINISTERING TUBE FEEDINGS *Continued*

Suggested Action	Reason for Action
Fill the feeding container with no more than 4 hours' worth of refrigerated formula. *Exception:* Commercially prepared, sterilized containers of formula or formula that is kept iced while infusing may hang for longer periods.	Prevents growth of bacteria; cold formula will be warmed by body heat when infused at a slow rate
Purge the tubing of air.	Prevents distention of the stomach or intestine
Thread the tubing within the feeding pump according to the manufacturer's directions.	Ensures correct mechanical operation of equipment and accurate administration to the patient

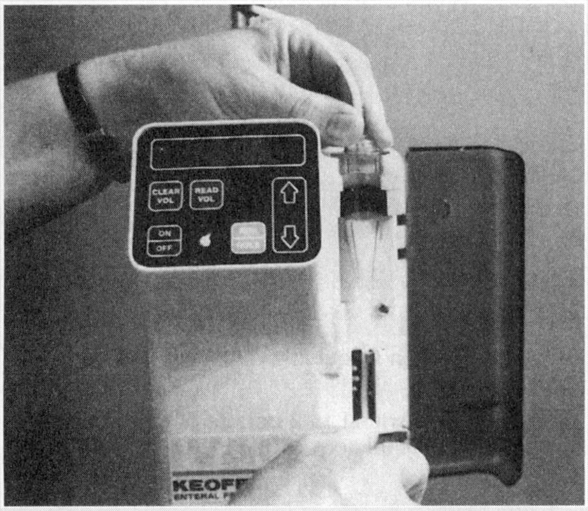

Preparing the pump. (Courtesy of Ken Timby.)

Suggested Action	Reason for Action
Connect the tubing from the feeding pump to the patient's feeding tube.	Provides access to formula
Set the prescribed rate on the feeding pump.	Complies with medical order
Open the clamp on the feeding tube and start the pump.	Initiates infusion
Keep the patient's head elevated at all times.	Prevents reflux and aspiration
Flush the tubing with 30 to 60 mL of water, or more, every 4 hours after checking and refeeding gastric residual, and after administering medications.	Promotes patency and contributes to the patient's fluid balance
Record the instilled volume of formula and water.	Provides accurate data for assessing fluid balance and caloric value of nourishment
Follow recommendations for postprocedural care as described with bolus feeding.	Principles for care remain the same

continued

SKILL 29-4

ADMINISTERING TUBE FEEDINGS *Continued*

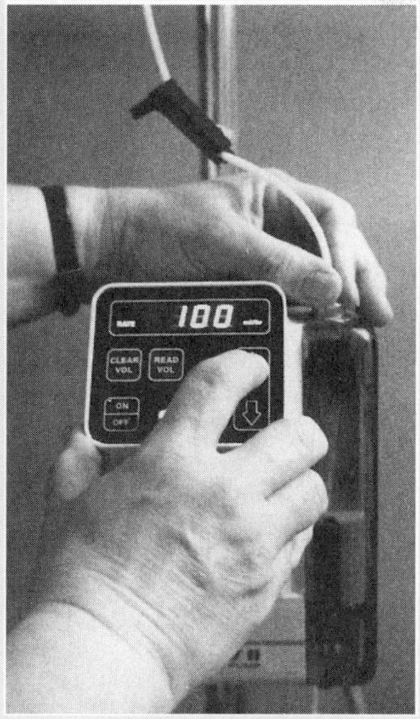

Programming the pump. (Courtesy of Ken Timby.)

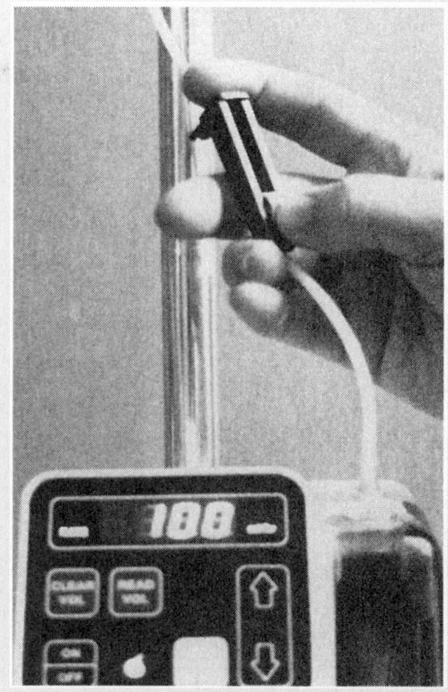

Releasing the clamp. (Courtesy of Ken Timby.)

Evaluation

- Patient receives prescribed volume of formula according to established feeding schedule
- Weight remains stable or patient reaches target weight
- Lungs remain clear
- Bowel elimination is within normal parameters for patient
- Patient demonstrates a daily fluid intake between 2,000 and 3,000 mL, unless intake is otherwise restricted

Document

- Volume of gastric residual and actions taken if excessive
- Type and volume of formula
- Rate of infusion, if continuous
- Volume of water used for flushes
- Response of patient; if symptomatic, describe actions taken and results

SAMPLE DOCUMENTATION

Date and Time 50 mL of gastric residual. Residual reinstilled and tube flushed with 60 mL of tap water. 480 mL of Enrich with Fiber placed in tube-feeding bag. Formula infusing at 120 mL/hr. No diarrhea or gastric complaints at this time. ____________________ SIGNATURE, TITLE

CRITICAL THINKING

- If a patient's nutritional needs are met entirely with tube feedings, what effects might that have on the person physically, emotionally, and socially?
- Which schedule for tube feedings do you feel is best, and which is the least desirable? Support your answers with rationales.

UNIT NINE

PROMOTING ELIMINATION

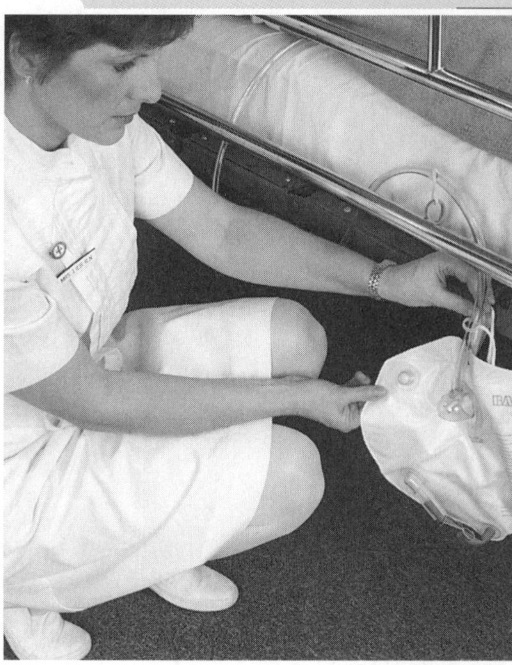

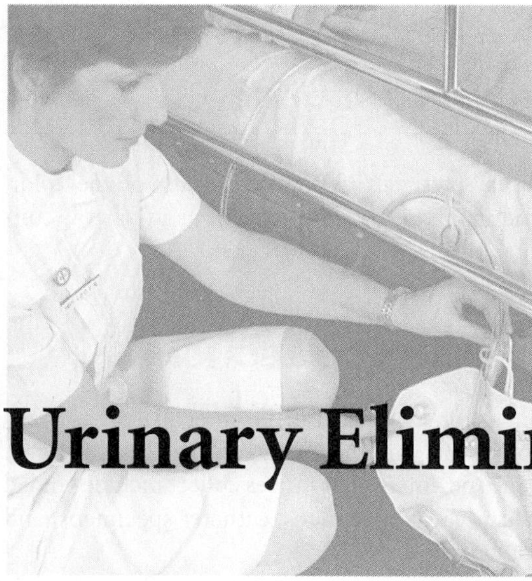

CHAPTER 30

Urinary Elimination

CHAPTER OUTLINE

NURSING GUIDELINES

SKILLS

NURSING CARE PLAN

KEY TERMS

anuria
bedpan
catheter care
catheter irrigation
catheterization
clean-catch specimen
closed drainage system
commode
continence training
continuous irrigation
Credé's maneuver
cutaneous triggering
dysuria
external catheter
fenestrated drape
frequency
incontinence
Kegel exercises
nocturia
oliguria
peristomal skin
polyuria
residual urine
retention catheter
stasis
straight catheter
24-hour specimen
urgency
urinal
urinary diversion
urinary elimination
urinary retention
urine
urostomy
voided specimen
voiding reflex

LEARNING OBJECTIVES

An understanding of the content within this chapter will be evidenced by the student's ability to:

- Identify the collective functions of the urinary system.
- Name at least five factors that affect urination.
- List three physical characteristics of urine.
- Name four types of urine specimens that nurses commonly collect.
- List six abnormal urinary elimination patterns.
- Identify three alternative devices for urinary elimination.
- Define continence training.
- Name three types of urinary catheters.
- Describe two principles that apply to using a closed drainage system.
- Explain why catheter care is important in the nursing management of patients with retention catheters.
- Discuss the purpose for irrigating a catheter.
- Identify three ways of irrigating a catheter.
- Define urinary diversion.
- Discuss factors that contribute to impaired skin integrity in patients with a urostomy.
- Describe two age-related changes in the older adult that may affect urinary elimination.

This chapter reviews the process of urinary elimination and describes nursing skills for assessing and maintaining urinary elimination.

Urinary Elimination

The urinary system (Fig. 30-1) consists of the kidneys, ureters, bladder, and urethra. These major components, along with some accessory structures, such as the ring-shaped muscles called the internal and external sphincters, work together to produce **urine** (fluid within the bladder), collect it, and excrete it from the body.

Urinary elimination (the process of releasing excess fluid and metabolic wastes), or urination, occurs when urine is excreted. Under normal conditions, approximately 1,500 to 3,000 mL of urine is eliminated each day. If urinary elimination is impaired, the consequences can be life-threatening.

Urination takes place several times each day. The need to urinate becomes apparent when the bladder distends with approximately 150 to 300 mL of urine (Bullock & Henze, 2000). This distention causes an increase in fluid pressure, stimulating stretch receptors in the bladder wall and creating a desire to empty it of urine.

Patterns of urinary elimination depend on physiologic, emotional, and social factors, such as the degree of neuromuscular development and integrity of the spinal cord; the volume of fluid intake and the amount of fluid losses, including those from other sources; the amount and type of food consumed; and the person's circadian rhythm, habits, opportunities for urination, and anxiety.

General measures to promote urination include providing privacy, assuming a natural position for urination (sitting for women, standing for men), maintaining an adequate fluid intake, and using stimuli such as running water from a tap to initiate voiding.

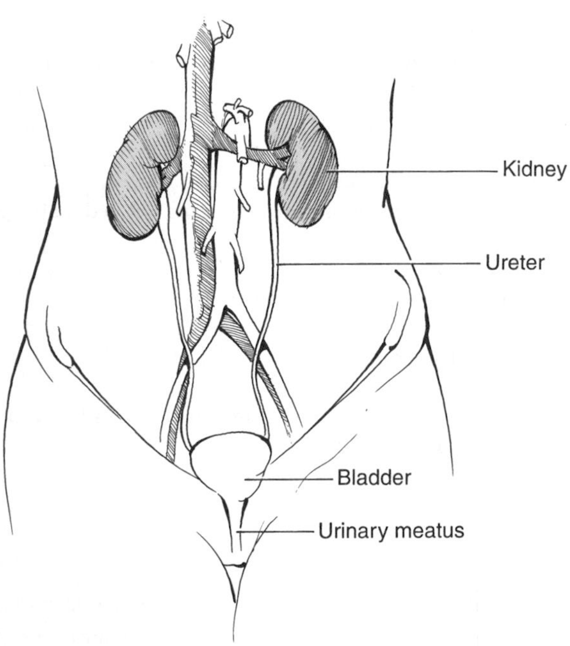

FIGURE 30–1. Major structures of the urinary system.

Characteristics of Urine

The physical characteristics of urine include its volume, color, clarity, and odor. There are wide variations in what is considered normal (Table 30-1).

URINE SPECIMEN COLLECTION

Urine specimens, or samples of urine, are collected to identify the microscopic or chemical constituents of urine. Common urine specimens that nurses collect include voided specimens, clean-catch specimens, catheter specimens, and 24-hour specimens.

Voided Specimens

A **voided specimen** (sample of urine that has been freshly urinated) is collected in a clean collection container. The first voided specimen of the day is preferred because it is most likely to contain a substantial amount of urinary substances that have accumulated during the night. However, the specimen can be voided and collected at any time it is needed.

The sample of urine is transferred into a specimen container and delivered to the laboratory for testing and analysis. If the specimen cannot be examined in less than 1 hour after collection, it is labeled and refrigerated.

Clean-Catch Specimens

A **clean-catch specimen** (voided sample of urine that is considered sterile) is sometimes called a *midstream specimen* because of the manner in which it is collected. To avoid contaminating the voided sample with microorganisms or substances other than those present in the urine, the external structures through which urine passes are cleansed—the urinary meatus, the opening to the urethra, and the tissues surrounding it. The urine is collected after the initial stream of urine has been released.

Clean-catch specimens are preferred to randomly voided specimens. This method of collection is also preferable when a urine specimen is needed during a woman's menstrual period. As soon as the specimen is collected, it is labeled and taken to the laboratory. A clean-catch urine specimen is refrigerated if the analysis will be delayed more than 1 hour.

Recent research (Leisure et al., 1993; Prandoni et al., 1996; Winslow, 1993) suggests that collecting a specimen in midstream without prior cleansing provides results as reliable as those in which cleansing was performed. Nurses should follow their agency's policy until the standard procedure is revised.

When a clean-catch specimen is needed, patients who can do so are instructed on the collection technique.

TABLE 30–1. **Characteristics of Urine**

Characteristic	Normal	Abnormal	Common Causes of Variations
Volume	500–3,000 mL/day 1,200 mL/day average	<400 mL/day	Low fluid intake Excess fluid loss Kidney dysfunction
		>3,000 mL/day	High fluid intake Diuretic medication Endocrine diseases
Color	Light yellow	Dark amber Brown Reddish-brown Orange, green, blue	Dehydration Liver/gallbladder disease Blood Water-soluble dyes
Clarity	Transparent	Cloudy	Infection Stasis
Odor	Faintly aromatic	Foul Strong Pungent	Infection Dehydration Certain foods

Patient Teaching For

Collecting a Clean-Catch Specimen

Teach the female patient to do the following:

- Wash your hands.
- Remove the lid from the specimen container.
- Rest the lid upside down on its outer surface, taking care not to touch the inside areas.
- Sit on the toilet and spread your legs.
- Separate your labia with your fingers.
- Cleanse each side of the urinary meatus with a separate antiseptic swab, wiping from front to back toward the vagina.
- Use the final clean, moistened swab to wipe directly down the center of the separated tissue.
- Begin to urinate.
- After a small amount of urine has been released into the toilet, catch a sample of urine in the specimen container.
- Take care not to touch the mouth of the specimen container to your skin.
- Place the specimen container nearby on a flat surface.
- Release your fingers and continue voiding normally.
- Wash your hands.
- Cover the specimen container with the lid.

The male patient should follow the same steps as for a woman but should perform the following cleansing routine:

- Retract your foreskin, if you are uncircumcised, or cleanse in a circular direction around the tip of the penis toward its base using a premoistened antiseptic swab.
- Repeat with another swab.
- Continue retracting the foreskin while initiating the first release of urine and until the midstream specimen has been collected.

Catheter Specimens

A urine specimen can be collected under sterile conditions using a catheter, but this is usually done when patients are catheterized for other reasons, such as to control incontinence in an unconscious patient. For patients who are already catheterized, a sample can be aspirated through the lumen of a latex catheter or from a self-sealing port (Fig. 30-2).

24-Hour Specimens

A **24-hour specimen** (collection of all the urine produced in a full 24-hour period) is collected, labeled, and delivered to the laboratory for analysis. Because the contents in urine decompose over time, the collected urine is placed in a container with a chemical preservative, or the container is placed in a basin of ice or a refrigerator.

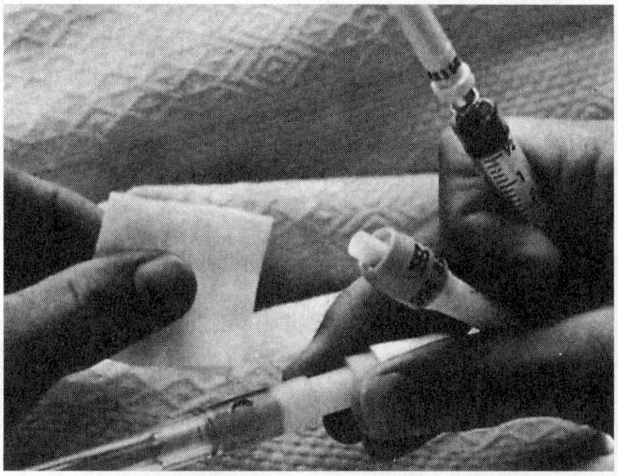

FIGURE 30–2. Location for collecting a catheter specimen.

To establish the 24-hour collection period accurately, the patient is instructed to urinate just before starting the test, and the urine is discarded. All urine voided thereafter becomes a part of the collected specimen. Exactly 24 hours after the test was initiated, the patient is asked to void once again. After the final urination, the specimen is labeled and taken to the laboratory.

ABNORMAL URINE CHARACTERISTICS

Laboratory analysis is a valuable diagnostic tool for identifying abnormal characteristics of urine. There are specific terms that describe particular abnormal characteristics of urine and urination. Many terms use the suffix *-uria*, which refers to urine or urination. For example:

- Hematuria: urine containing blood
- Pyuria: urine containing pus
- Proteinuria: urine containing plasma proteins
- Albuminuria: urine containing albumin, a plasma protein
- Glycosuria: urine containing glucose
- Ketonuria: urine containing ketones

Abnormal Urinary Elimination Patterns

Analyzing assessment data may indicate that some patients have abnormal urinary elimination patterns. Some common problems include anuria, oliguria, polyuria, nocturia, dysuria, and incontinence.

ANURIA

Anuria (absence of urine, or a volume of 100 mL or less in 24 hours) indicates that the kidneys are not forming sufficient urine. In this case, the term "urinary suppression" is used. In urinary suppression the bladder is empty, and therefore the patient feels no urge to urinate. This distinguishes anuria from **urinary retention** (condition in which urine is produced but is not released from the bladder). Urinary retention is identified by a progressively distending bladder.

OLIGURIA

Oliguria (urine output of less than 400 mL per 24 hours) indicates that an inadequate amount of urine is being eliminated. Sometimes oliguria is a sign that the bladder is being only partially emptied at the time of voiding. **Residual urine** (more than 50 mL of urine that remains in the bladder after voiding) can support the growth of microorganisms, leading to an infection. Also, when there is urinary **stasis** (lack of movement), dissolved substances such as calcium can precipitate, causing urinary stones to form.

POLYURIA

Polyuria (greater than normal urinary volume) may occur without any reasonable explanation. Ordinarily, urine output is nearly equal to fluid intake. When this is not the case, the excessive urination may result from a disorder. Common disorders associated with polyuria include *diabetes mellitus*, an endocrine disorder caused by insufficient insulin, and *diabetes insipidus*, an endocrine disease caused by insufficient antidiuretic hormone.

NOCTURIA

Nocturia (nighttime urination) is unusual because the rate of urine production is normally reduced at night. Consequently, nocturia suggests an underlying medical problem. An enlarging prostate gland is commonly associated with nocturia. The gland, which encircles the urethra in men, interferes with complete bladder emptying if it increases in size. As a result, the man senses the need to urinate more frequently, including during the usual hours of sleep.

DYSURIA

Dysuria (difficult or uncomfortable voiding) is a common symptom of trauma to the urethra or a bladder infection. Dysuria is often accompanied by **frequency** (need to urinate often) and **urgency** (strong feeling that urine must be eliminated quickly).

INCONTINENCE

Incontinence (inability to control either urinary or bowel elimination) is abnormal after a person is toilet-trained. The term "urinary incontinence" should not be used indiscriminately: anyone may be incontinent if his or her need for assistance goes unnoticed. Once the bladder becomes extremely distended, spontaneous urination may be more of a personnel problem than a patient problem.

Assisting Patients With Urinary Elimination

Stable patients who can ambulate and are stable are assisted to the bathroom to use the toilet. Patients who are weak or unable to walk to the bathroom may need a commode. Patients who are confined to bed use a urinal or bedpan.

COMMODE

A **commode** (chair with an opening in the seat under which a receptacle is placed) is located beside or near the bed. It is used for eliminating urine or stool. Immediately afterward, the waste container is removed, emptied, cleaned, and replaced.

URINAL

A **urinal** (cylindrical container for collecting urine) is more easily used by male patients. When given to the patient, the urinal should be empty; otherwise, the bed linen may become wet and soiled. If the patient needs help placing the urinal:

- Pull the privacy curtain.
- Don gloves.
- Ask the patient to spread his legs.
- Hold the urinal by its handle.
- Direct the urinal at an angle between the patient's legs so that the bottom rests on the bed (Fig. 30-3).
- Lift the penis and place it well within the urinal.

After use, the urinal is promptly emptied. The volume of urine is measured and recorded if the patient's intake and output are being monitored (see Chap. 15). Patients are always offered an opportunity to wash their hands after voiding.

USING A BEDPAN

A **bedpan** (seatlike container for elimination) is used to collect urine or stool. Most are made of plastic and are several inches deep. A *fracture pan*, a modified version of a conventional bedpan, is flat on the sitting end rather than rounded (Fig. 30-4). A fracture pan is used by patients with musculoskeletal disorders who cannot elevate their hips and sit on a bedpan in the usual manner. When a patient who is confined to bed feels the need to eliminate, a bedpan is placed under the buttocks (Skill 30-1).

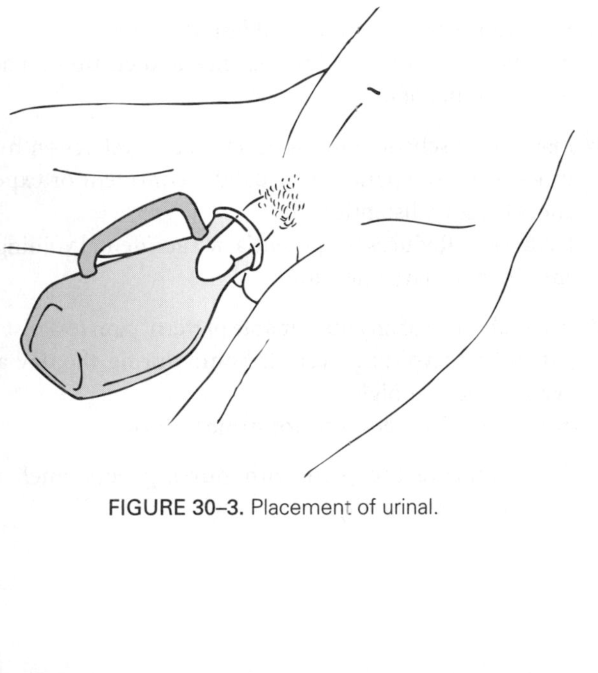

FIGURE 30–3. Placement of urinal.

Managing Incontinence

Urinary incontinence, depending on its type, may be permanent or temporary. The six types of urinary incontinence are stress, urge, reflex, functional, overflow, and total (Table 30-2).

The management of incontinence is complex because there are so many variations. Treatment is further complicated by the fact that some patients have more than one type of incontinence—for example, stress incontinence is often accompanied by urge incontinence.

Some forms of incontinence respond to simple measures such as modifying clothing to make elimination easier. Other forms improve only with a more regimented approach, like continence training. Inserting a retention catheter is the least desirable approach to managing incontinence because it is the leading cause of urinary tract infections (Marchiondo, 1998).

CONTINENCE TRAINING

Continence training (process of restoring control of urination) involves teaching the patient to restrain from urinating until an appropriate time and place. Continence training is sometimes referred to as *bladder retraining*, but this term is inaccurate because the various techniques used involve mechanisms other than those unique to the bladder.

Continence training primarily benefits patients who have the cognitive ability and desire to participate in a rehabilitation program. This includes patients with lower body paralysis who wish to facilitate urination without the use of urinary drainage devices such as catheters. Patients who are not can-

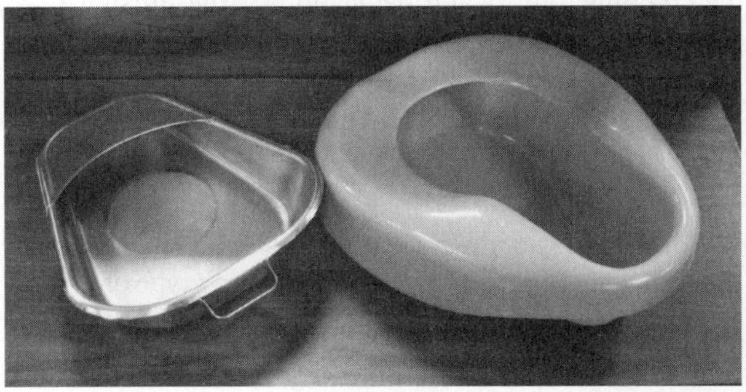

FIGURE 30–4. Two types of bedpans: fracture pan (*left*) and conventional bedpan (*right*). (Courtesy of Ken Timby.

TABLE 30–2. **Types of Incontinence**

Type	Description	Example	Common Causes	Nursing Approach
Stress	The loss of small amounts of urine during situations when intraabdominal pressure rises	Dribbling is associated with sneezing, coughing, lifting, laughing, or rising from a bed or chair	Loss of perineal and sphincter muscle tone secondary to childbirth, menopausal atrophy, prolapsed uterus, or obesity	Pelvic floor muscle strengthening Weight reduction
Urge	Need to void perceived frequently, with short-lived ability to sustain control of the flow	Voiding commences when there is a delay in accessing a restroom	Bladder irritation secondary to infection; loss of bladder tone due to recent continuous drainage with an indwelling catheter	Maintain fluid intake of at least 2,000mL/day Omit bladder irritants, such as caffeine or alcohol Administer diuretics in the morning
Reflex	Spontaneous loss of urine when the bladder is stretched with urine, but without prior perception of a need to void	Automatic release of urine that cannot be controlled by the person	Damage to motor and sensory tracts in the lower spinal cord secondary to trauma, tumor, or other neurologic conditions	Cutaneous triggering Straight intermittent catheterization
Functional	Control over urination lost because of inaccessibility of a toilet or a compromised ability to use one	Voiding occurs while attempting to overcome barriers such as doorways, transferring from a wheelchair, manipulating clothing, acquiring assistance, or making needs known	Impaired mobility, impaired cognition, physical restraints, inability to communicate	Modify clothing Facilitate access to a toilet, commode, or urinal Assist to a toilet according to a preplanned schedule
Total	Loss of urine without any identifiable pattern or warning	The person passes urine without any ability or effort to control	Altered consciousness secondary to a head injury, loss of sphincter tone secondary to prostatectomy, anatomic leak through a urethral/vaginal fistula	Absorbent undergarments External catheter Indwelling catheter
Overflow	Urine leakage because the bladder is not completely emptied; bladder distended with retained urine	The person voids small amounts frequently, or urine leaks around a catheter	Overstretched bladder or weakened muscle tone secondary to obstruction of the urethra by debris within a catheter, an enlarged prostate, distended bowel, or postoperative bladder spasms	Hydration Adequate bowel elimination Maintain patency of catheter Perform Credé's maneuver

didates for continence training require alternative methods, such as absorbent undergarments.

Continence training is often a slow process that requires the combined effort and dedication of the nursing team, patient, and family.

Nursing Guidelines For

Providing Continence Training

☑ Compile a log of the patient's elimination patterns.
RATIONALE: Aids in analyzing the patient's type of incontinence and planning rehabilitation

☑ Set realistic, specific, short-term goals with the patient.
RATIONALE: Prevents self-defeating consequences and promotes patient control

☑ Discourage strict limitation of liquid intake.
RATIONALE: Maintains fluid balance and ensures an adequate volume of urine

☑ Plan a trial schedule for voiding that correlates with the times when the patient is usually incontinent or experiences bladder distention.
RATIONALE: Reduces the potential for accidental voiding or sustained urinary retention

☑ In the absence of any identifiable pattern, plan to assist the patient with voiding every 2 hours during the day and every 4 hours at night.
RATIONALE: Provides time for urine to form

☑ Communicate the plan with nursing personnel, the patient, and the family.

RATIONALE: Promotes continuity of care and dedication to reaching goals

☑ Assist the patient to a toilet or commode; position the patient on a bedpan, or place a urinal just before the scheduled time for trial voiding.
RATIONALE: Readies the patient for releasing urine

☑ Simulate the sound of urination, such as by running water from the faucet.
RATIONALE: Stimulates relaxation of the sphincter muscles, allowing the release of urine

☑ Suggest performing **Credé's maneuver** (the act of bending forward and applying hand pressure over the bladder; Fig. 30-5).
RATIONALE: Increases abdominal pressure to overcome the resistance of the internal sphincter muscle

☑ Instruct paralyzed patients to identify any sensation that precedes voiding, such as a chill, a muscular spasm, restlessness, or a spontaneous erection.
RATIONALE: Provides a cue for anticipating urination

☑ Suggest that paralyzed patients with reflex incontinence use **cutaneous triggering** (lightly massaging or tapping the skin above the pubic area).
RATIONALE: Initiates urination in patients who have retained a **voiding reflex** (spontaneous relaxation of the urinary sphincter in response to physical stimulation)

☑ Teach patients with stress incontinence to perform **Kegel exercises** (isometric exercises to improve the ability to retain urine within the bladder; Display 30-1).
RATIONALE: Strengthens and tones the pubococcygeal and levator ani muscles used voluntarily to hold back urine and intestinal gas or stool

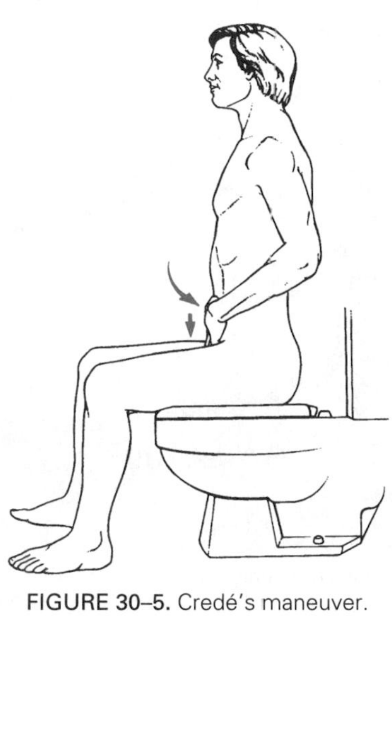
FIGURE 30–5. Credé's maneuver.

DISPLAY 30–1

Technique for Performing Kegel Exercises

- Tighten the internal muscles used to prevent urination or interrupt urination once it has begun
- Keep the muscles contracted for at least 10 seconds
- Relax the muscles for the same period of time
- Repeat the pattern of contraction and relaxation 10 to 25 times
- Perform the exercise regimen three or four times a day for 2 weeks to 1 month

☑ Assist patients with urge incontinence to walk slowly and concentrate on holding their urine when nearing the toilet.
RATIONALE: Reverses previous mental conditioning in which the urge to urinate becomes stronger and more overpowering close to the toilet

Catheterization

Catheterization (act of applying or inserting a hollow tube), in this case, refers to using a device inside the bladder or externally about the urinary meatus. A urinary catheter is used for various reasons, including:

- Keeping incontinent patients dry (however, catheterization is a last resort, used only when all other continence measures have been exhausted)
- Relieving bladder distention when patients cannot void
- Assessing fluid balance accurately
- Keeping the bladder from becoming distended during procedures such as surgery
- Measuring the residual urine
- Obtaining sterile urine specimens
- Instilling medication within the bladder

TYPES OF CATHETERS

There are three common types of catheters: external catheters, straight catheters, and retention catheters. Most catheters are made of latex. For patients who are sensitive or allergic to latex, latex-free catheters are used.

External Catheters

An **external catheter** (urine-collecting device applied to the skin) is not inserted within the bladder; instead, it surrounds the urinary meatus. Examples of external catheters are a con-

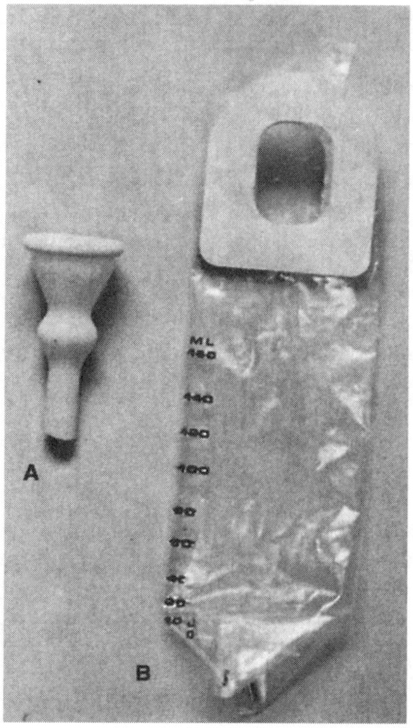

FIGURE 30–6. External urine collection devices: (*A*) Condom catheter; (*B*) "U" or urinary bag. (Courtesy of Ken Timby.)

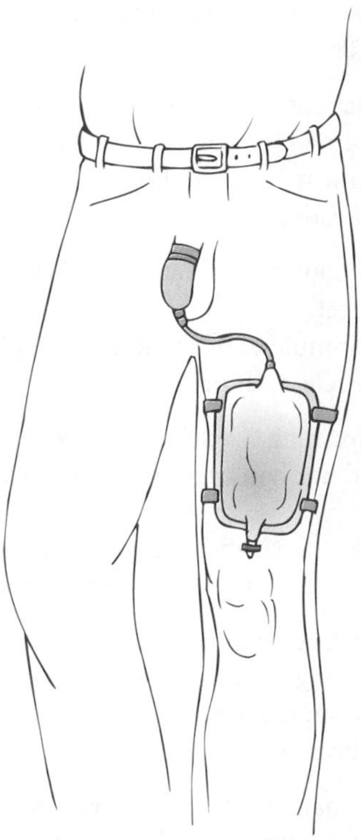

FIGURE 30–7. A leg bag collects urine from a catheter but is concealed under clothing.

dom catheter and a urinary bag or U-bag (Fig. 30-6). External catheters are more effective for male patients.

Condom catheters are helpful for patients being cared for at home because they are easy to apply. A condom catheter has a flexible sheath that is unrolled over the penis. The narrow end is connected to tubing that serves as a channel for draining urine. The drainage tube is attached to a leg bag (Fig. 30-7) or connected to a larger urine-collection device.

There are three potential problems involved in the use of condom catheters. First, the sheath may be applied too tightly, restricting blood flow to the skin and tissues of the penis. Second, moisture tends to accumulate beneath the sheath, leading to skin breakdown. Third, condom catheters frequently leak. These problems can be avoided by applying the catheter correctly and managing care appropriately (Skill 30-2).

A urinary bag is more often used for collecting urine specimens from infants. It is attached by means of an adhesive backing to the skin surrounding the genitals. Urine collects in the self-contained bag. Once enough urine is collected, the bag is removed.

Straight Catheters

A **straight catheter** (urine drainage tube that is inserted but not left in place) is used to drain urine temporarily or obtain a sterile urine specimen (Fig. 30-8).

Retention Catheters

A **retention catheter** (urinary tube that is left in place for a period of time) is also called an indwelling catheter (see Fig. 30-8). The most common type of retention catheter is a Foley catheter.

Unlike straight catheters, retention catheters are secured with a balloon that is inflated once the distal tip is within the bladder. Both straight and retention catheters are available in various diameters, sized according to the French scale (see Chap. 29). For adults, sizes 14, 16, and 18 F urinary catheters are commonly used.

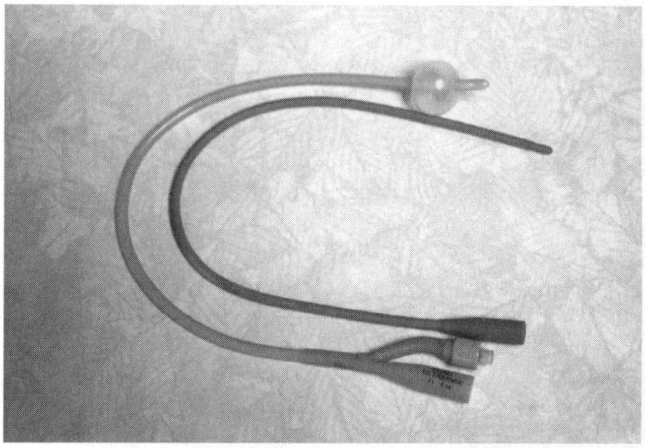

FIGURE 30–8. Types of urinary catheters: retention (Foley) catheter with balloon and straight catheter. (Courtesy of Ken Timby.)

INSERTING A CATHETER

The techniques for inserting straight and retention catheters are similar, although the steps for inflating the retention balloon do not apply to a straight catheter. When a straight or a retention catheter is inserted in a health agency, sterile technique is used. In the home, clean technique is used because most patients have adapted to the organisms in their own environment.

Because of anatomic differences, the techniques for insertion are different in men and women and are described in Skills 30-3 and 30-4.

CONNECTING A CLOSED DRAINAGE SYSTEM

A **closed drainage system** (device used to collect urine from a catheter) consists of a calibrated bag, which can be opened at the bottom, tubing of sufficient length to accommodate for turning and positioning patients, and a hanger from which to suspend the bag from the bed (Fig. 30-9). Excess tubing is coiled on the bed, but the section from the bed to the collection bag is kept vertical. Dependent loops in the tubing interfere with gravity flow. Care is also taken to avoid compressing the tubing, which can obstruct drainage. Placing the tubing over the patient's thigh is acceptable.

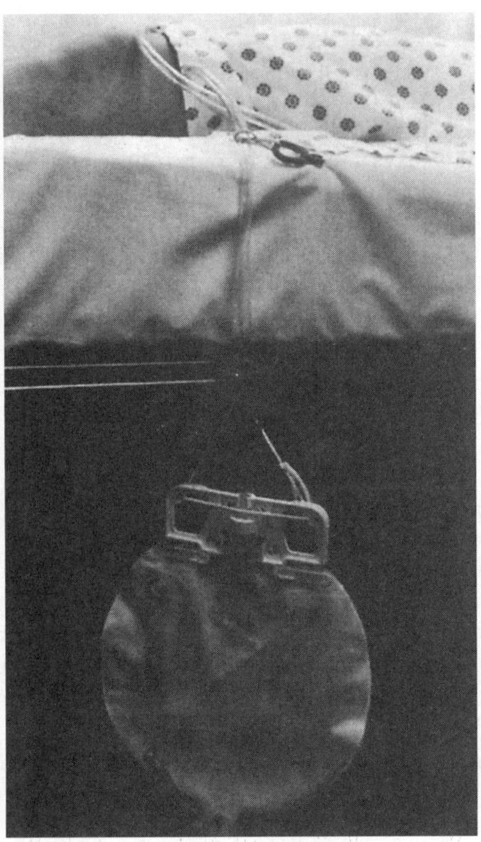

FIGURE 30–9. Closed urine drainage system.

The drainage system is always positioned lower than the bladder to avoid backflow of urine. When the patient is being transported in a wheelchair, the drainage bag is suspended from the chair below the level of the bladder. When the patient is ambulating, the drainage bag is secured to the lower part of an IV pole or carried by hand (Fig. 30-10).

To reduce the potential for the drainage system becoming a reservoir of pathogens, the entire drainage system is replaced whenever the catheter is changed and at least every 2 weeks in patients with a urinary tract infection.

PROVIDING CATHETER CARE

A retention catheter keeps the meatus slightly dilated, providing pathogens with a direct pathway to the bladder, where an infection could develop. "Catheters left in place for more than a few weeks become encrusted or obstructed, and lead to infection. In addition, bacteria that adhere to the urinary catheter develop a complex biologic structure, which protects them from antibiotics" (Marchiondo, 1998, p. 38).

Catheter care (hygiene measures used to keep the meatus and adjacent area of the catheter clean) helps deter the growth and spread of colonizing pathogens. The nursing guidelines given here describe the technique for providing catheter care. Nurses must follow agency policy for using antiseptic and antimicrobial agents, because the use of these substances is not standard among all physicians or agencies.

Nursing Guidelines For

Providing Catheter Care

- ☑ Cleanse the meatus and a nearby section of the catheter at least once a day.
  RATIONALE: Reduces the number of colonizing microorganisms
- ☑ Gather clean gloves, soap, water, washcloth, towel, and a disposable pad.
  RATIONALE: Facilitates organization and efficient time management
- ☑ Place a disposable pad beneath the hips of a female patient and beneath the penis of a male patient.
  RATIONALE: Prevents bed linen from becoming wet or soiled
- ☑ Don clean gloves and wash the meatus, the catheter where it meets the meatus, the genitalia, and the perineum (in that order) with warm, soapy water. Rinse and dry. Follow agency policy for using antiseptic or antimicrobial agents.
  RATIONALE: Removes gross secretions and transient microorganisms while following principles of asepsis
- ☑ Remove soiled materials and gloves, and wash hands.
  RATIONALE: Removes colonizing microorganisms

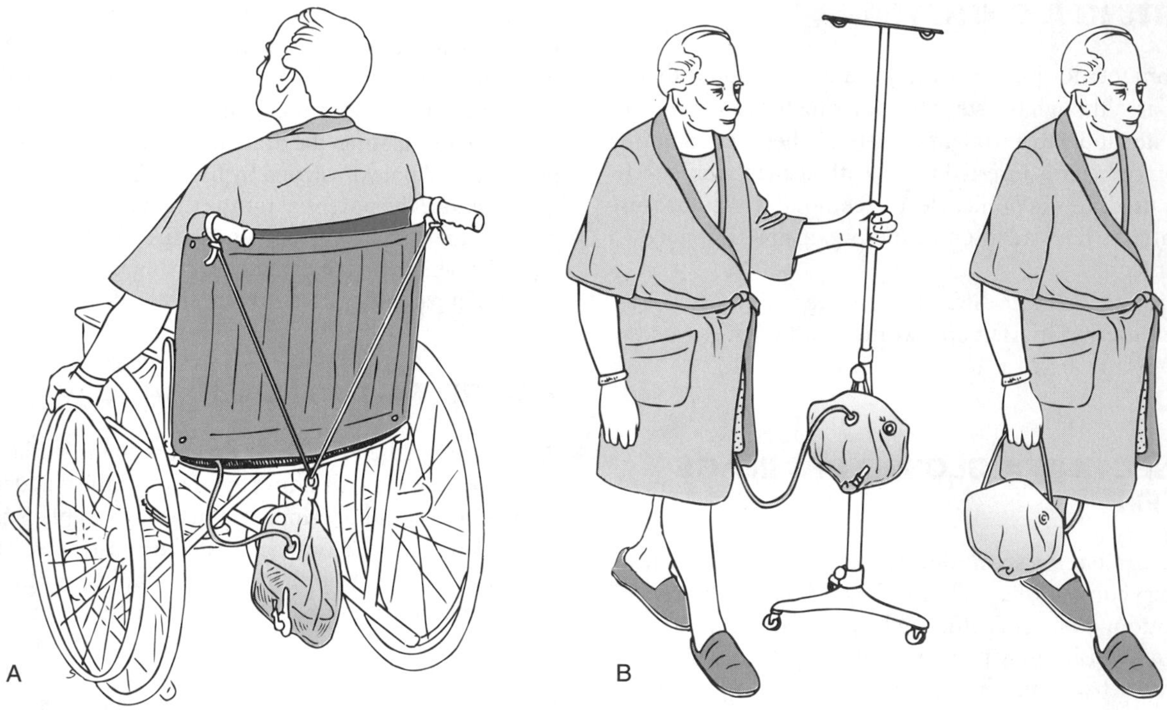

FIGURE 30–10. Techniques for suspending a drainage system below the bladder: (*A*) wheelchair patient; (*B*) ambulating patient with and without an IV pole.

CATHETER IRRIGATION

A **catheter irrigation** (flushing the lumen of a catheter) is a technique for restoring or maintaining catheter patency. However, a catheter that drains well does not need irrigating. Providing a generous oral fluid intake is usually sufficient to produce dilute urine, thus keeping the catheter from becoming obstructed with small shreds of mucus or tissue debris. However, there are times when the catheter may need to be irrigated, such as after a surgical procedure that results in bloody urine.

Depending on the type of indwelling catheter, catheters are irrigated periodically using an open system or closed system, or continuously through a three-way catheter.

Using an Open System

An open system is one in which the retention catheter is separated from the drainage tubing to insert the tip of an irrigating syringe. Opening the system creates the potential for infection because it provides an opportunity for pathogens to enter the exposed connection. Consequently, it is the least desirable of the three methods; nonetheless, it is the one most commonly used (Skill 30-5).

Using a Closed System

A closed system is irrigated without separating the catheter from the drainage tubing. To do so, the catheter or drainage tubing must have a self-sealing port. After cleansing the port with an alcohol swab, the port is pierced with an 18- or 19-gauge, 1.5-inch needle (see Chap. 34). The needle is attached to a 50-mL syringe containing sterile irrigation solution. The tubing is pinched or clamped beneath the port, and the solution is instilled. The tubing is released for drainage. The volume of irrigant is recorded as fluid intake or subtracted from the urine output to maintain an accurate intake and output record.

Continuous Irrigation

A **continuous irrigation** (ongoing instillation of solution) instills irrigating solution into a catheter by gravity over a period of days (Fig. 30-11). Continuous irrigations are used to keep a catheter patent after prostate or other urologic surgery in which blood clots and tissue debris collect within the bladder.

A three-way catheter is necessary to provide a continuous irrigation. The catheter has three lumens or channels within the catheter, each leading to a separate port.

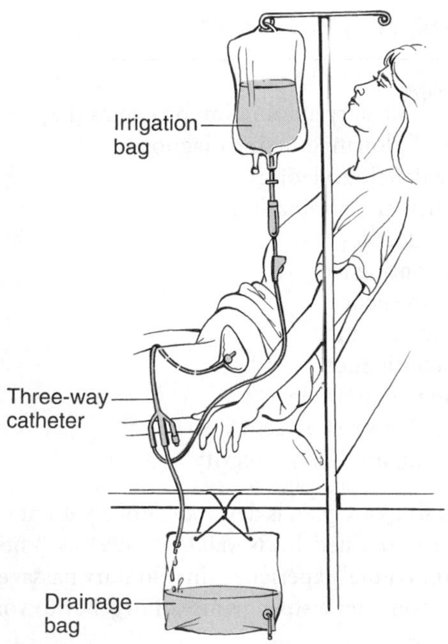

FIGURE 30–11. Bladder irrigation using a three-way catheter.

The steps involved in providing a continuous irrigation are as follows:

- Hang the sterile irrigating solution from an IV pole.
- Purge the air from the tubing.
- Connect the tubing to the catheter port for irrigation.
- Regulate the rate of infusion according to the medical order.
- Monitor the appearance of the urine and volume of urinary drainage.

INDWELLING CATHETER REMOVAL

A catheter is removed when it needs to be replaced or when its use is being discontinued. The best time to remove a catheter is in the morning so there is more opportunity to address any urination difficulties without depriving a patient of sleep.

Nursing Guidelines For

Removing a Foley Catheter

- ☑ Wash your hands and don clean gloves.
  RATIONALE: Follows standard precautions
- ☑ Empty the balloon by aspirating the fluid with a syringe.
  RATIONALE: Ensures that all the fluid has been withdrawn
- ☑ Gently pull the catheter near the point where it exits from the meatus.
  RATIONALE: Facilitates withdrawal
- ☑ Inspect the catheter and discard if it appears to be intact.
  RATIONALE: Ensures safety
- ☑ Clean the urinary meatus.
  RATIONALE: Promotes comfort and hygiene
- ☑ Monitor the patient's voiding, especially for the next 8 to 10 hours; measure the volume of each voiding.
  RATIONALE: Determines whether normal elimination is occurring, as well as the characteristics of the urine

Urinary Diversions

A **urinary diversion** (procedure in which one or both ureters are surgically implanted elsewhere) is created for various life-threatening conditions. The ureter(s) may be brought to and through the skin of the abdomen (Fig. 30-12) or implanted within the bowel (called an ileal conduit). A **urostomy** (urinary diversion that discharges urine from an opening on the abdomen) is the focus of this discussion.

Care for an ostomy, a surgically created opening, is discussed in more detail in Chapter 31 because those formed for

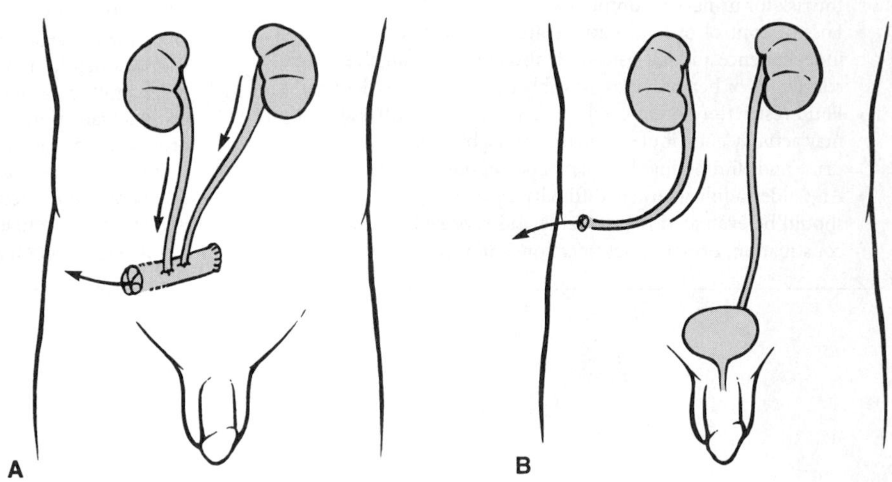

FIGURE 30–12. Examples of urinary diversions. (*A*) Ileal conduit. (*B*) Cutaneous ureterostomy. (Smeltzer SC, Bare BG: Brunner and Suddarth's textbook of medical-surgical nursing, 8th ed, p 1218. Philadelphia, JB Lippincott, 1996)

bowel elimination are more common. Chapter 31 also provides a detailed description of an ostomy appliance, the device used for collecting stool or urine, and the manner in which it is applied and removed from the skin.

Caring for a urostomy and changing a urinary appliance are more challenging than the care of intestinal stomas. Urine drains continuously from a urostomy, increasing the risk for skin breakdown. In addition, because moisture and the weight of the collected urine tend to loosen the appliance from the skin, a urinary appliance may need to be changed more frequently. When changing the appliance, it may help to place a tampon within the stoma to absorb urine temporarily while the skin is cleansed and prepared for another appliance.

It is often difficult to maintain the integrity of the **peristomal skin** (skin around the stoma) because of the frequent appliance changes and the ammonia in urine. Skin barrier products are used, and sometimes antibiotic or steroid ointment is applied.

Nursing Implications

Patients with urinary elimination problems may have one or more of the following nursing diagnoses:

- Self-care deficit: toileting
- Altered urinary elimination
- Risk for infection
- Stress incontinence
- Urge incontinence
- Reflex incontinence
- Total incontinence
- Functional incontinence
- Situational low self-esteem
- Risk for impaired skin integrity

The nursing care plan is developed for a patient with Urge incontinence, defined by NANDA (1999) as "the state in which an individual experiences involuntary passage of urine occurring soon after a strong sense of urgency to void."

FOCUS ON OLDER ADULTS

- Older adults are likely to experience urinary urgency and frequency because of normal physiologic changes, such as diminished bladder capacity and degenerative changes in the cerebral cortex. Subsequently, when they perceive the urge to void, they need to access or use a bathroom as soon as possible.
- Age-related changes, such as diminished bladder capacity and relaxation of the pelvic floor muscles, increase the risk of incontinence.
- Older adults are more likely to have chronic residual urine (excessive amounts of urine in the bladder after urinating), increasing the risk for developing urinary tract infections.
- Enlargement of the prostate, a common problem among older men, can totally obstruct urinary outflow and make catheterization difficult or impossible. Sometimes a catheter is inserted into the bladder through the abdominal wall when it cannot be inserted into a narrowed urethra.
- Diuretic therapy commonly prescribed for older adults can increase the risk for urinary incontinence.
- Loss of control over urination often threatens an older adult's independence and self-esteem. It also may cause an older adult to restrict his or her activities, possibly contributing to depression.
- Fluid restriction, often used in an attempt to control urination, may actually contribute to incontinence by causing concentrated urine and eliminating the normal perception of a full bladder.
- Any older adult who has difficulty controlling his or her urine should be evaluated for treatable and reversible causes, such as constipation, urinary tract infection, and medication side effects.
- Older adults need encouragement to discuss urinary incontinence with a knowledgeable, nonjudgmental health care provider. If they understand that urinary incontinence is a condition that frequently responds to treatment, they are more likely to seek professional help.
- Many resources are available to assist older adults in evaluating and treating incontinence. For example, some health care facilities offer special incontinence clinics and physical therapy departments to teach pelvic muscle exercises. Nurses can encourage older adults to take advantage of these kinds of resources rather than accepting incontinence as an inevitable condition that compromises their quality of life.
- In institutional settings, older adults may become incontinent because they do not have the assistance needed to get to a commode or toilet in a timely manner. Also, if absorbent products are used, these are likely to interfere with the person's independence in toileting. Incontinence products are never used primarily for staff convenience in institutional settings.
- When efforts to restore continence are unsuccessful, nurses can encourage older adults to verbalize their feelings and identify interventions helpful in maintaining dignity, ultimately enabling the older adult to participate in meaningful activities.
- Careful evaluation is necessary regarding the selection of absorbent products because many products are available. Cost and effectiveness of each product are factors to consider.
- The National Association for Continence (800-252-3337; *http://www.nafc.org*) is an excellent source of information for products, resources, and continence programs.

Nursing Care Plan

Urge Incontinence

Assessment

Subjective Data

States, "I hope when this catheter comes out I don't wet myself again. I'd like to go home without wearing a leg bag or being connected to a drainage bag."

Objective Data

75-year-old woman admitted to long-term care facility for rehabilitation after repair of a fractured hip. Fracture occurred as a result of tripping on way to bathroom because of feeling an urgent need to void. Has had an indwelling catheter with continuous drainage for 4 weeks.

Diagnosis

Urge incontinence related to reduced bladder capacity secondary to continuous urine drainage from an indwelling catheter

Plan

Goal

The patient will be able to wait at least 3 hours between voidings without experiencing incontinence by 6/12.

Orders: 6/2

1. Remove the catheter and maintain a 3-day log of:
   - Time of each urination
   - Volume per voiding
   - Episodes of incontinence
   - Cause of incontinence
2. Instruct patient to use call light to summon assistance when feeling need to void.
3. Maintain a total intake of approximately 2,500 mL/day, divided in the following amounts:
   - 1,200 mL on day shift
   - 1,200 mL on evening shift
   - 100 mL during the night
4. When there is an urge to void, help patient to:
   - Breathe deeply while waiting longer to void
   - Sing a song
   - Tell a story about her family as a distraction technique while proceeding to the toilet at a safe pace
5. Praise every urinary elimination that occurs without incontinence.

____________________ F. WISNIECKI, RN

Implementation (Documentation)

6/2 1000 Instructed to drink approximately one glass of fluid per hour. Explained the 3-day assessment log. Explored distraction techniques to avoid incontinence while increasing bladder capacity. ____________ N. ZAK, LPN

Evaluation (Documentation)

2000 Feeling a need to void at approximately 2-hour intervals (see log for specifics). Has had two episodes of dribbling while getting onto toilet. Sings "Amazing Grace" as a distraction technique. States, "I was so hoping this wouldn't happen; I'm determined to avoid that catheter again." Praised for the two successful voidings without incontinence. Drinking fluids at scheduled intervals.

____________________ S. BURKE, LPN

KEY CONCEPTS

- The urinary system is composed of the kidneys, ureters, bladder, and urethra. Collectively, they serve to produce urine, collect it, and excrete it from the body.
- Various factors affect urination, such as a person's neuromuscular development, the integrity of the spinal cord, the volume of fluid intake, fluid losses from other sources, and the amount and type of food consumed.
- The physical characteristics of urine include its volume, color, clarity, and odor.
- Nurses often collect voided urine specimens, clean-catch urine specimens, catheter specimens, and 24-hour urine specimens.
- Common abnormal patterns of urinary elimination include anuria, oliguria, polyuria, nocturia, dysuria, and incontinence.
- Other than a conventional toilet, urine may be eliminated in a commode, urinal, or bedpan.
- Continence training is the process used to restore the ability to empty the bladder at an appropriate time and place.
- The three general types of catheters are external catheters, straight catheters, and retention catheters.
- When using a closed drainage system, it is important to avoid dependent loops in the tubing, and the collection bag must be kept below the level of the bladder.
- Catheter care is important because it helps to deter the growth and spread of colonizing pathogens.
- Catheters are irrigated to keep them patent, or free-flowing. They may be irrigated using an open or closed system, or continuously by way of a three-way catheter.
- A urinary diversion is a procedure in which one or both ureters are surgically implanted elsewhere.
- Skin impairment is a common problem in patients with a urostomy because they require frequent appliance changes, and the contact of urine with the skin causes skin irritation.
- Older adults tend to have diminished bladder capacity and relaxation of pelvic floor muscles.

CRITICAL THINKING EXERCISES

- An older adult patient confides that she would like to participate in activities outside her home, but she is worried her problem with incontinence will be noticed. What response might help this patient? What suggestions could you offer?
- A resident in a nursing home who has had a retention catheter for the last 6 months says, "I'd do anything if I didn't have to have this catheter." What suggestions would be appropriate at this time?

SUGGESTED READINGS

Agency for Health Care Policy and Research. Clinical practice guidelines: managing acute and chronic incontinence. Washington DC, United States Department of Health and Human Services, 1996.

Bullock BL, Henze R. Focus on pathophysiology. Philadelphia, Lippincott, 2000.

Dest V. Don't use this outdated catheterization technique. RN 1998;61(7):66.

DiBattiste J, Bradley M, Pupiales M. Uses of a Kock pouch: essentials of ostomy care. American Journal of Nursing 1997;97(12):17.

Evans E. Indwelling catheter care: dispelling the misconceptions. Geriatric Nursing: American Journal of Care for the Aging 1999;20(2):85–89.

Gerard L, Sueppel C. Lubrication technique for male catheterization. Urologic Nursing 1997;17(4):156–158.

Hardyck C, Petrinovich L. Reducing urinary tract infections in catheterized patients. Ostomy/Wound Management 1998;44(12):36–43.

Hiser V. Nursing interventions for urinary incontinence in home health. Journal of Wound, Ostomy, and Continence Nursing 1999;26(3):142–160.

Leisure MK, Dudley SM, Donowitz LG. Does a clean-catch urine sample reduce bacterial contamination? New England Journal of Medicine 1993;328:289.

Marchiondo K. A new look at urinary tract infection. American Journal of Nursing 1998;98(3):34–39.

McConnell EA. Maintaining a closed urinary drainage system. Nursing 1997;27(10):22.

NANDA nursing diagnoses: definitions and classification, 1999–2000. Philadelphia, NANDA, 1999.

National Association for Continence. *http://www.nafc.org*

Newman DK. Managing indwelling urethral catheters. Ostomy/Wound Management 1998;44(12):26–32.

Prandoni D, Boone MH, Larson E, Blane CG, Fitzpatrick H. Assessment of urine collection technique for microbial culture. American Journal of Infection Control 1996;24(3):219–221.

Prieto-Fingerhut T, Banovac K, Lynne CM. A study comparing sterile and nonsterile urethral catheterization in patients with spinal cord injury. Rehabilitation Nursing 1997;22(6):299–302.

Russell B. Nosocomial infections. American Journal of Nursing 1999; 99(6):24J–24P.

Ritter J. Using invasive medical devices safely: guide to infection control. Nursing 1998;28(5):32hn12–32hn16.

Sienty MK, Dawson N. Preventing urosepsis from indwelling urinary catheters. American Journal of Nursing 1999;99(1):24C–24H.

Steed CJ. Common infections acquired in the hospital: the nurse's role in prevention. Nursing Clinics of North America 1999;34(2):443–461.

Warren JW. Catheter-associated urinary tract infections. Infectious Disease Clinics of North America 1997;11(3):609–622.

Watt E, Lillibridge J. Time of day urinary catheters are removed: a study of current practices. Urologic Nursing 1998;18(1):23–25.

Weber EM, McDowell BJ, Engberg S, Brodak I, Donovan N. Protocol for indwelling bladder catheter removal in the homebound older adult. Home Healthcare Nurse 1998;16(9):603–611.

Winslow EH. Myth of the clean catch. American Journal of Nursing 1993;93(8):20.

SKILL 30–1

PLACING AND REMOVING A BEDPAN

Suggested Action	Reason for Action
Assessment	
Ask the patient if he or she feels the need to void.	Anticipates elimination needs
Palpate the lower abdomen for signs of bladder distention.	Indicates bladder fullness
Determine if there is a need to use a fracture pan or if there are any restrictions in turning or lifting.	Prevents further injury
Planning	
Gather needed supplies such as clean gloves, the bedpan, toilet tissue, and a disposable pad.	Promotes organization and efficient time management
Warm the bedpan by running warm water over it, especially if it is made of metal.	Demonstrates a concern for the patient's comfort
Implementation	
Wash your hands and don clean gloves.	Reduces the transmission of microorganisms
Place the adjustable bed in high position.	Promotes use of good body mechanics
Close the door and pull the privacy curtains.	Demonstrates concern for the patient's right to privacy and dignity
Raise the top linen enough to determine the location of the patient's hips and buttocks.	Prevents unnecessary exposure
Instruct the patient to bend the knees and press down with the feet.	Helps in elevating the hips
Place a disposable pad over the bottom sheets, if necessary.	Protects bed linen from becoming wet and soiled
Slip the bedpan beneath the patient's buttocks.	Ensures proper placement
Or, roll the patient to the side and position the bedpan.	Reduces work effort and the potential for a work-related injury; aids in placement if patient cannot lift buttocks

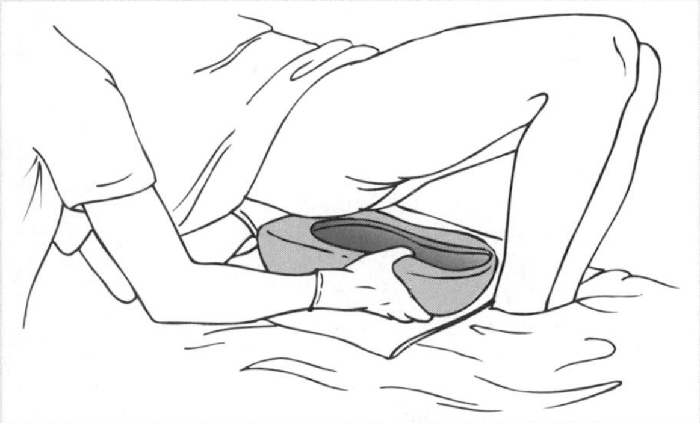

Placing a bedpan from a sitting position.

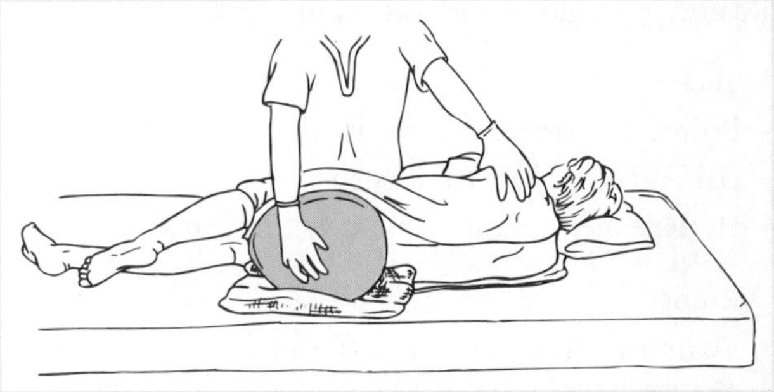

Placing a bedpan from a side-lying position.

Suggested Action	Reason for Action
Raise the head of the bed.	Simulates the natural position for elimination
Ensure that the toilet tissue is within the patient's reach.	Provides supplies for hygiene
Identify the location of the signal device and leave the patient, if it is safe to do so.	Respects privacy yet provides a mechanism for communicating a need for assistance

continued

SKILL 30–1

PLACING AND REMOVING A BEDPAN *Continued*

Suggested Action	Reason for Action

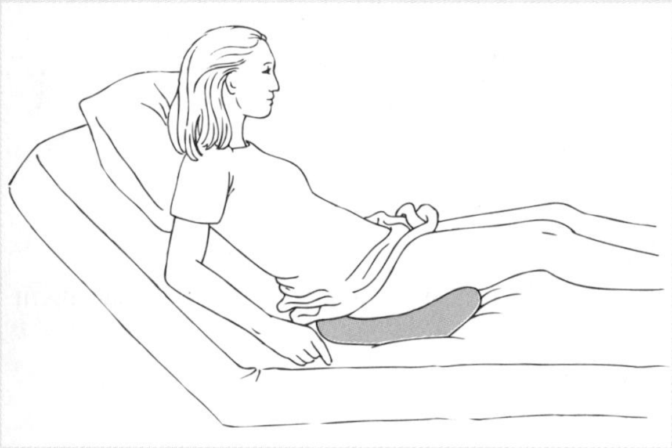

Position for elimination.

Suggested Action	Reason for Action
Return and remove the bedpan.	Prevents discomfort
Assist with removing residue of urine from the skin, if necessary.	Prevents offensive odors and skin irritation
Wrap the gloved hand with toilet tissue and wipe from the meatus toward the anal area.	Supports principles of medical asepsis
Place soiled tissue in the bedpan.	Contains soiled tissue until the time of disposal
Help the patient to a position of comfort.	Ensures the patient's well-being
Provide supplies for handwashing.	Removes residue of urine and colonizing microorganisms
Measure the volume of urine if the patient's intake and output are being monitored.	Ensures accurate data collection
Save a sample of urine if it appears abnormal in any way.	Facilitates laboratory examination or further assessment
Empty the urine into a toilet and flush.	Facilitates disposal
Clean the bedpan and replace it in a place that is separate from clean supplies.	Supports principles of asepsis
Remove your gloves and wash your hands.	Removes colonizing microorganisms

Evaluation

- Bedpan is positioned without injury
- Urine and stool are eliminated
- Hygiene measures are accurately performed

Document

- Volume of urine eliminated (for monitoring intake and output)
- Appearance and other characteristics of the urine

SAMPLE DOCUMENTATION

Date and Time Assisted to use the bedpan. Voided 300 mL of clear, amber urine without difficulty.
________________________________ SIGNATURE, TITLE

CRITICAL THINKING

- Discuss how a patient might feel about using a bedpan for elimination.
- Describe measures that may reduce a patient's concerns when a bedpan is required.

SKILL 30-2

APPLYING A CONDOM CATHETER

Suggested Action	Reason for Action
Assessment	
Assess the penis for swelling or skin breakdown.	Provides data for future comparison or provides a basis for using some other method for urine collection
Determine how much the patient understands about the application and use of an external catheter.	Provides an opportunity for health teaching
Verify the willingness of the patient to use a condom catheter.	Respects the patient's right to participate in making decisions
Check the patient's medical record to determine if the patient has a latex allergy.	Maintains patient safety and prevents possible allergic reaction
Planning	
Gather supplies such as soap, water, towel, condom catheter, drainage tubing, collection device, and clean gloves. Some devices come packaged with an adhesive strip or Velcro device for securing the catheter.	Promotes organization and efficient time management
Provide privacy.	Demonstrates respect for dignity
Place the patient in a supine position and cover him with a bath blanket.	Facilitates application of the catheter and maintains privacy
Implementation	
Wash your hands and don clean gloves.	Reduces the transmission of microorganisms and follows standard precautions
Wash and dry the penis well.	Promotes skin integrity
Wind the adhesive strip in an upward spiral about the penis.	Reduces the potential for restricting blood flow
Roll the wider end of the condom toward the narrow tip.	Facilitates application to the penis

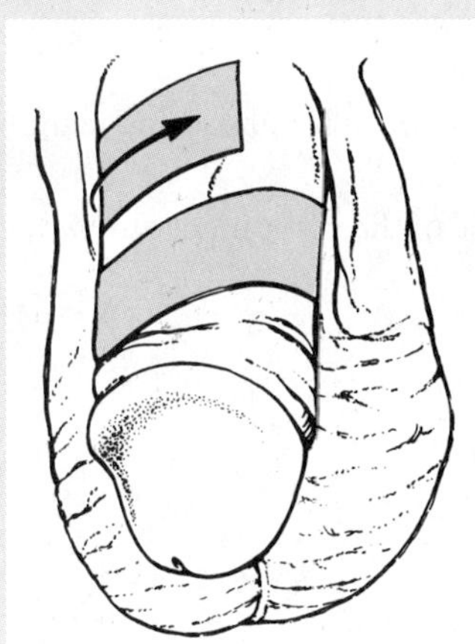

Applying adhesive strip in a spiral.

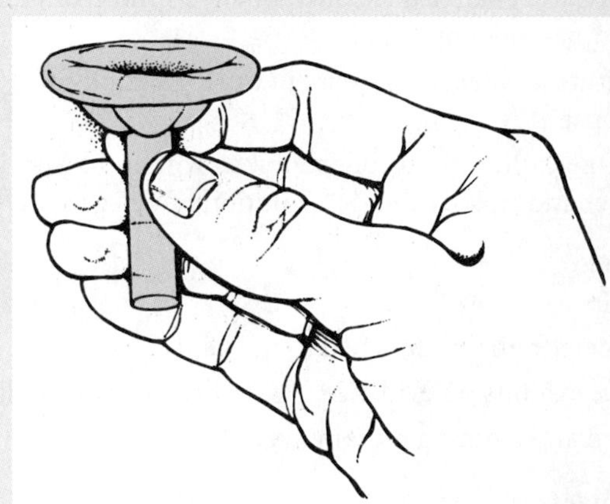

A rolled condom sheath.

Hold approximately 1 to 2 inches (2.5–5 cm) of the lower sheath below the tip of the penis and unroll the sheath upward.	Leaves space below the urethra to prevent irritation of the meatus

continued

SKILL 30–2

APPLYING A CONDOM CATHETER *Continued*

Suggested Action	Reason for Action

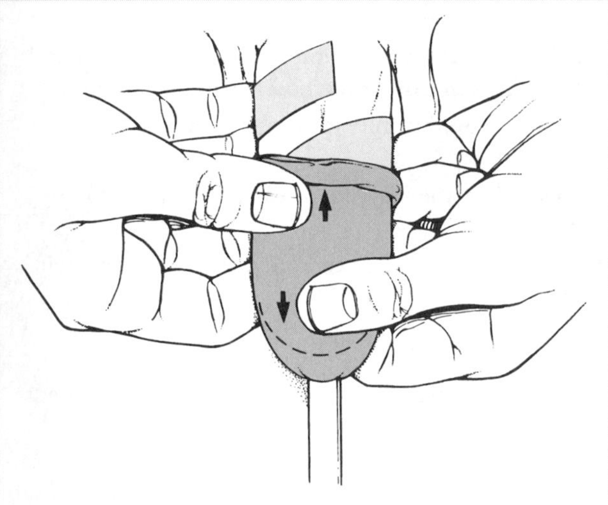

Leaving space at the meatus.

Suggested Action	Reason for Action
Secure the upper end of the unrolled sheath to the skin firmly with a second strip of adhesive or a Velcro strap, but not so tight as to interfere with circulation.	Ensures that the catheter will remain in place
Connect the drainage tip to a drainage bag.	Allows for urine drainage and collection
Keep the penis in a downward position.	Promotes urinary drainage
Assess the penis at least every 2 hours.	Ensures prompt attention to signs of impaired circulation
Check that the catheter has not become twisted.	Maintains catheter patency
Empty the leg bag, if one is used, as it becomes partially filled with urine.	Ensures that the catheter will not be pulled from the penis by the weight of the collected urine
Remove and change the catheter daily or more often if it becomes loose or tight.	Maintains skin integrity
Substitute a waterproof garment during periods of nonuse.	Provides a mechanism for absorbing urine
Wash the catheter and collection bag with mild soap and water and rinse with a 1 : 7 solution of vinegar and water.	Extends the use of the equipment and reduces offensive odors

Evaluation

- Catheter remains attached to the penis
- Penis exhibits no evidence of skin breakdown, swelling, or impaired circulation
- Linen and clothing remain dry.

Document

- Preapplication assessment data
- Hygiene measures performed
- Time of catheter application
- Content of teaching
- Postapplication assessment data

continued

SKILL 30-2

APPLYING A CONDOM CATHETER *Continued*

SAMPLE DOCUMENTATION

Date and Time Penis washed with soap and water. Penile skin is intact. No discoloration or lesions noted. Condom catheter applied and connected to a leg bag. Instructed to report any swelling or local discomfort. ________________________ SIGNATURE, TITLE

CRITICAL THINKING

- Discuss assessments that indicate common problems associated with the use of a condom catheter.
- Describe nursing measures that prevent or resolve physical problems associated with condom catheters.

SKILL 30-3

INSERTING A FOLEY CATHETER IN A FEMALE PATIENT

Suggested Action	Reason for Action
Assessment	
Check the patient's record to verify that a medical order has been written.	Demonstrates the legal scope of nursing; catheterization is not an independent measure
Inspect the medical record to determine if the patient has a latex allergy.	Determines if it is safe to use a latex catheter or a need to select one that is latex-free
Determine the type of catheter that has been prescribed.	Ensures selection of appropriate catheter
Review the patient's record for documentation of genitourinary problems.	Provides data by which to modify the procedure or equipment
Assess the age, size, and mobility of the patient.	Influences the size of the catheter and the need for additional assistance
Assess the time of the last voiding.	Indicates how full the bladder may be
Determine how much the patient understands about catheterization.	Provides an opportunity for health teaching
Familiarize yourself with the anatomic landmarks.	Facilitates insertion in the appropriate location
Planning	
Gather supplies, which include a catheterization kit, bath blanket, and additional light, if necessary.	Promotes organization and efficient time management
Implementation	
Close the door and pull the privacy curtain.	Demonstrates concern for the patient's dignity
Raise the bed to a high position.	Prevents back strain
Cover the patient with a bath blanket and pull the top linen to the bottom of the bed.	Avoids unnecessary exposure
Position an additional light at the bottom of the bed or ask an assistant to hold a flashlight.	Ensures good visualization
Use the corners of the bath blanket to cover each leg.	Provides warmth and maintains modesty

continued

SKILL 30-3

INSERTING A FOLEY CATHETER IN A FEMALE PATIENT *Continued*

Suggested Action	Reason for Action
Place the patient in a dorsal recumbent position with the feet about 2 feet apart.	Provides access to the female urinary system

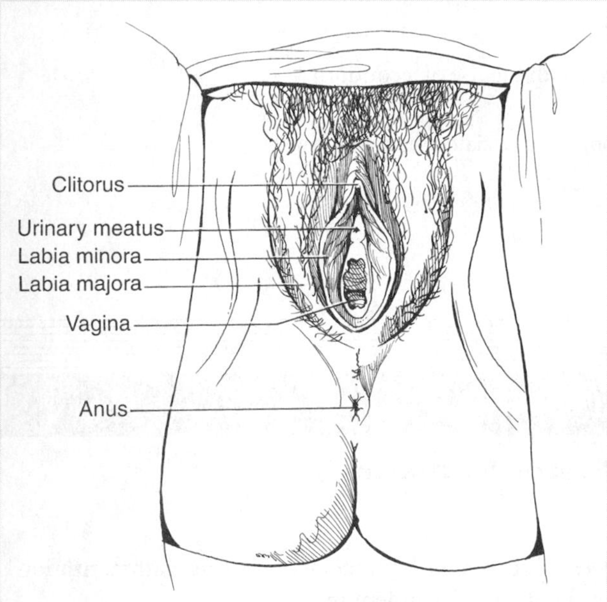

Female anatomic landmarks.

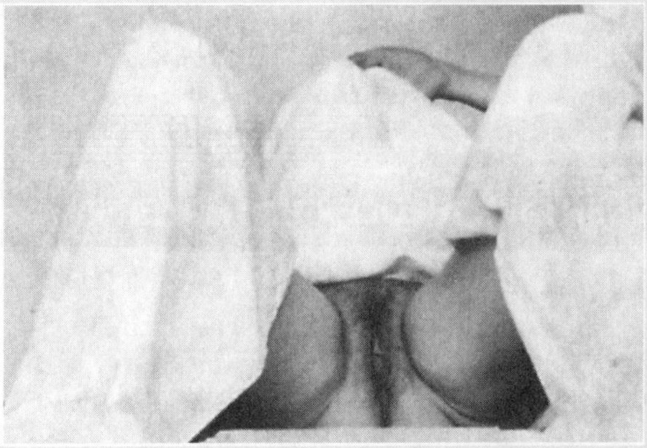

Draped and placed in dorsal recumbent position.

Suggested Action	Reason for Action
Use a lateral or Sims' position for patients who have difficulty maintaining a dorsal recumbent position.	Provides access to the female urinary system, but neither is the preferred position
If the patient is soiled, don gloves, wash the patient, remove gloves, and rewash your hands.	Supports principles of asepsis
Remove the wrapper from the catheterization kit and position it nearby.	Provides a receptacle for collecting soiled supplies
Unwrap the sterile cover to maintain the sterility of the supplies inside (see Chap. 21).	Prevents contamination and the potential for infection
Remove and don the packaged sterile gloves (see Chap. 21).	Facilitates handling the remaining equipment without transferring microorganisms
Remove the sterile towel from the kit and place it beneath the patient's hips.	Provides a sterile field
Open and pour the packet of antiseptic solution (Betadine) over the cotton balls.	Prepares sterile supplies before contaminating one of two hands later in the procedure
Test the balloon on the catheter by instilling fluid from the prefilled syringe; then aspirate the fluid back within the syringe.	Determines if the balloon is intact or defective
Spread lubricant on the tip of the catheter.	Facilitates insertion
Place the catheterization tray on top of the sterile towel between the patient's legs.	Promotes access to supplies and reduces the potential for contamination
Pick up a moistened cotton ball with the sterile forceps and wipe one side of the labia majora from an anterior to posterior direction.	Cleanses outer skin before cleansing deeper areas of tissue

continued

SKILL 30-3

INSERTING A FOLEY CATHETER IN A FEMALE PATIENT *Continued*

Suggested Action	Reason for Action
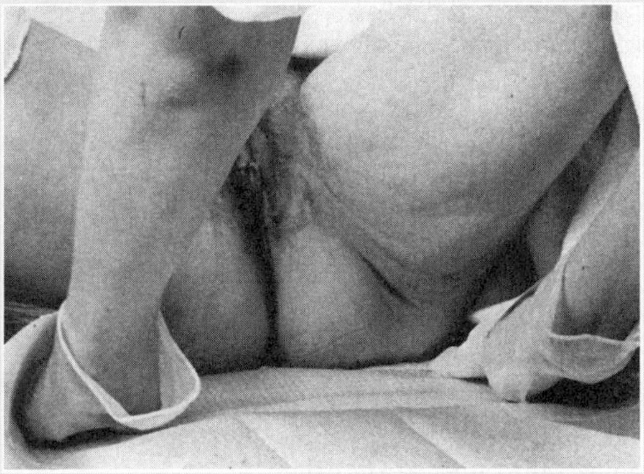 Placing a sterile towel.	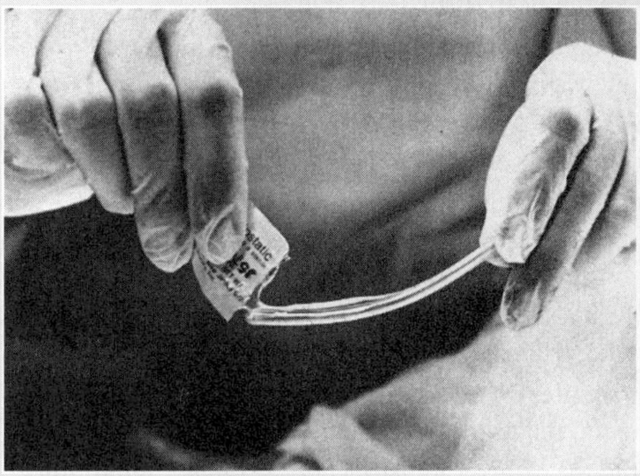 Lubricating the catheter.
Discard the soiled cotton ball in the outer wrapper of the catheterization kit; repeat cleansing the other side of the labia majora.	Completes bilateral cleansing
Separate the labia majora and minora with the thumb and fingers of the nondominant hand, exposing the urinary meatus.	Facilitates visualization of anatomic landmarks and prevents contaminating the catheter during insertion
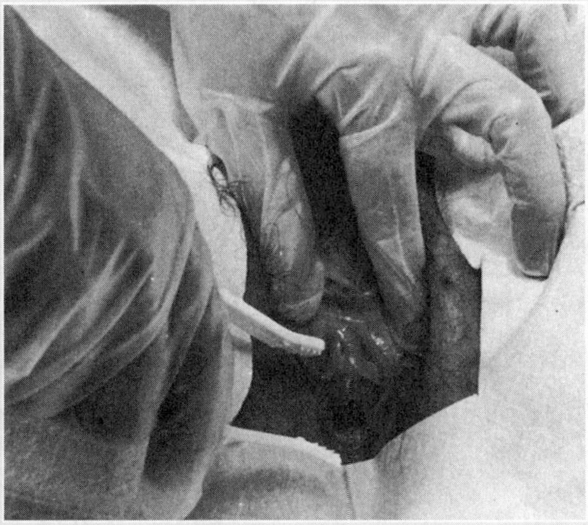 Separating the labia.	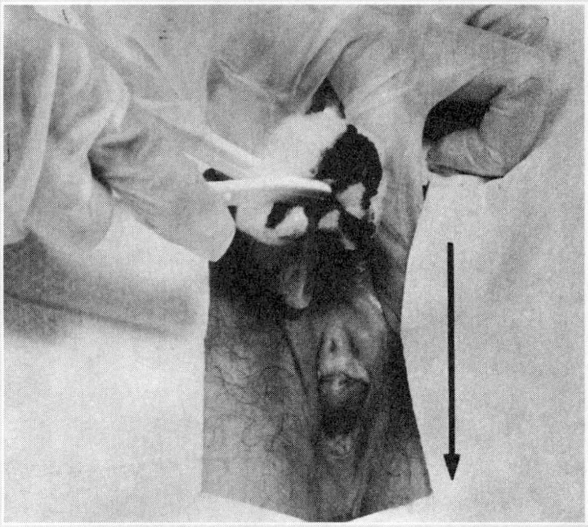 Wiping from above the meatus downward.
Consider the hand separating the labia to be contaminated.	Avoids transferring microorganisms to sterile equipment and supplies
Clean each side of the labia minora with a separate cotton ball while continuing to retract the tissue with the nondominant hand.	Removes colonizing microorganisms
Use the last cotton ball to wipe centrally, starting above the meatus down toward the vagina.	Completes the cleaning of external structures
Discard the forceps with the last cotton ball into the wrapper for contaminated supplies.	Follows principles of asepsis

continued

SKILL 30-3

INSERTING A FOLEY CATHETER IN A FEMALE PATIENT *Continued*

Suggested Action	Reason for Action
Keep the clean tissue separated.	Prevents recontamination
Pick up the catheter, holding it approximately 3 to 4 inches (7.5–10 cm) from its tip.	Facilitates control during insertion
Insert the tip of the catheter into the meatus approximately 2 to 3 inches (5–7.5 cm) or until urine begins to flow.	Locates the tip beyond the length of the female urethra, which is approximately 1.5 to 2.5 inches (4–6.5 cm)
Recheck anatomic landmarks if there is no evidence of urine; remove an incorrectly placed catheter and repeat, using another sterile catheter.	Indicates one of two possibilities: either the bladder is empty or the catheter has been placed within the vagina by mistake; ensures sterility of equipment
Advance the catheter another ½ to 1 inch (1.3–2.5 cm) after urine begins to flow.	Ensures that the catheter is well within the bladder, where the balloon can be safely inserted
Direct the end of the catheter so that it drains into the equipment tray or specimen container.	Avoids wetting the linen
Hold the catheter in place with the fingers and thumb that were separating the labia.	Stabilizes the catheter externally
Pick up the prefilled syringe with the sterile, dominant hand, insert it into the opening to the balloon, and instill the fluid.	Stabilizes the catheter internally
Withdraw the fluid from the balloon if the patient describes feeling pain or discomfort, advance the catheter a little more, and try again.	Prevents internal injury
Tug gently on the catheter after the balloon has been filled.	Tests whether the catheter is well anchored within the bladder
Connect the catheter to a urine collection bag.	Provides a means of assessing the urine and its volume
Wipe the meatus and labia of any residual lubricant.	Demonstrates concern for the patient's comfort
Secure the catheter to the leg with tape or other commercial device.	Prevents pulling on the balloon within the catheter

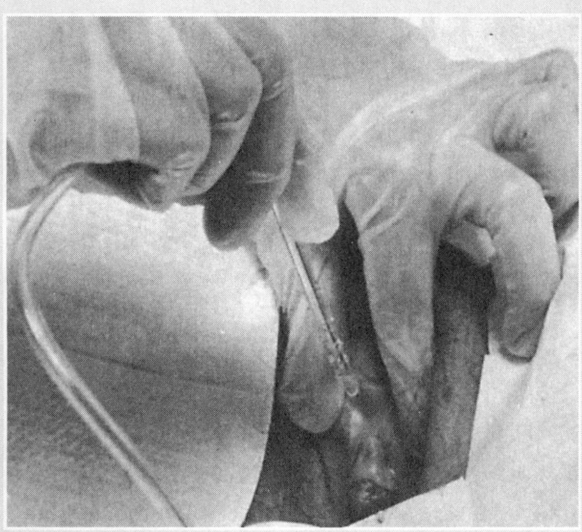

Preparing to insert the catheter.

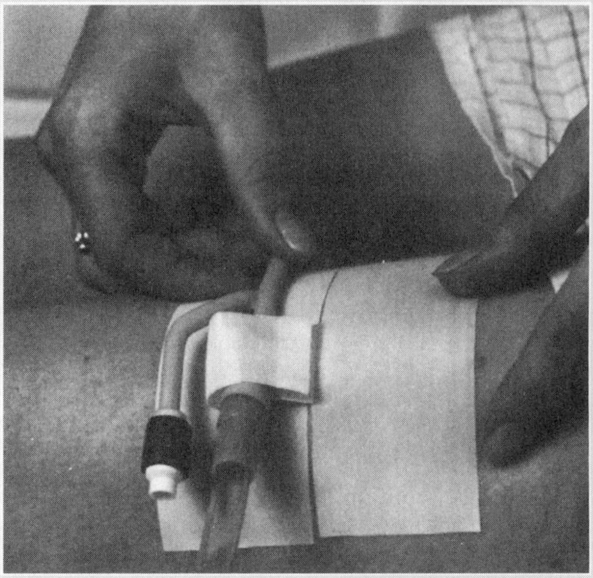

Securing the catheter to the thigh. (Courtesy of the MC Johnson Company, Inc., Leominster, MA.)

continued

SKILL 30-3

INSERTING A FOLEY CATHETER IN A FEMALE PATIENT *Continued*

Suggested Action	Reason for Action
Hang the collection bag below the level of the bladder; coil excess tubing on the mattress.	Ensures gravity drainage
Discard the catheterization tray and wrapper with soiled supplies.	Follows principles of asepsis
Remove your gloves and wash your hands.	Removes colonizing microorganisms
Remove the drape, restore the top sheets, make the patient comfortable, and lower the bed.	Restores comfort and safety

Evaluation

- Catheter is inserted under aseptic conditions
- Urine is draining from the catheter
- Patient exhibits no evidence of discomfort during or after insertion

Document

- Preassessment data
- Size and type of catheter
- Amount and appearance of urine
- Patient's response

SAMPLE DOCUMENTATION

Date and Time Unable to void in past 8 hours. Bladder feels distended. Dr. Peter notified. 18 F Foley catheter inserted per order and connected to gravity drainage. 550 mL of urine drained from bladder at this time. Urine appears light amber. No discomfort reported.

_______________________________ SIGNATURE, TITLE

CRITICAL THINKING

- Discuss an appropriate action to take if a catheter is initially inserted within the vagina.
- Discuss factors that predispose a female with a Foley catheter to develop a urinary tract infection.

SKILL 30-4

INSERTING A FOLEY CATHETER IN A MALE PATIENT

Suggested Action	Reason for Action
Assessment	
Check the patient's record to verify that a medical order has been written.	Demonstrates the legal scope of nursing; catheterization is not an independent measure
Inspect the medical record to determine if the patient has a latex allergy.	Determines if it is safe to use a latex catheter or to select one that is latex-free
Determine the type of catheter that has been prescribed.	Ensures selection of the appropriate catheter

continued

SKILL 30–4

INSERTING A FOLEY CATHETER IN A MALE PATIENT *Continued*

Suggested Action	Reason for Action
Review the patient's record for documentation of genitourinary problems.	Provides data by which to modify the procedure or equipment
Assess the age, size, and mobility of the patient.	Influences the size of the catheter and the need for additional assistance
Assess the time of the last voiding.	Indicates how full the bladder may be
Determine how much the patient understands about catheterization.	Provides an opportunity for health teaching
Familiarize yourself with the anatomic landmarks.	Facilitates insertion

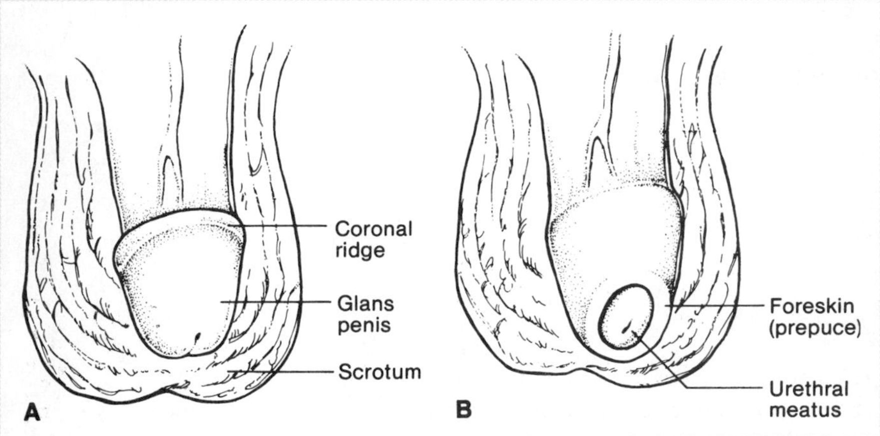

Male anatomic landmarks. (*A*) Circumcised. (*B*) Uncircumcised. (Fuller J, Schuller-Ayers J. Health assessment: A nursing approach, 3rd ed, p. 570. Philadelphia, Lippincott Williams & Wilkins, 1999)

Planning

Suggested Action	Reason for Action
Gather supplies, which include a catheterization kit, bath blanket, and additional light.	Promotes organization and efficient time management

Implementation

Suggested Action	Reason for Action
Close the door and pull the privacy curtain.	Demonstrates concern for the patient's dignity
Raise the bed to a high position.	Prevents back strain
Place the patient in a supine position.	Provides access to the male urinary system
Cover the patient's upper body with a bath blanket, and lower the top linen to expose just the penis.	Provides minimal exposure
Position an additional light at the bottom of the bed or ask an assistant to hold a flashlight.	Ensures good visualization
If the patient is soiled, don gloves, wash the patient, remove gloves, and rewash your hands.	Supports principles of asepsis
Remove the wrapper from the catheterization kit and position it nearby.	Provides a receptacle for collecting soiled supplies
Unwrap the sterile inner cover so as to maintain the sterility of the supplies inside (see Chap. 21).	Prevents contamination and the potential for infection
Remove and don the packaged sterile gloves (see Chap. 21).	Facilitates handling the remaining equipment without transferring microorganisms

continued

SKILL 30-4

INSERTING A FOLEY CATHETER IN A MALE PATIENT *Continued*

Suggested Action	Reason for Action
Place the **fenestrated drape** (one with an open circle in its center) over the patient's penis without touching the upper surface of the drape.	Provides a sterile field
Open and pour the packet of antiseptic solution (Betadine) over the cotton balls.	Prepares sterile supplies before contaminating one of two hands later in the procedure
Test the balloon on the catheter by instilling fluid from the prefilled syringe; then aspirate the fluid back within the syringe.	Determines if the balloon is intact or defective
Place the catheterization tray on top of the sterile drape over the patient's thighs.	Promotes ease of access to supplies and reduces the potential for contamination
Lift the penis at its base with the nondominant hand; retract the foreskin, if the patient is uncircumcised.	Promotes visualization and support during catheter insertion
Consider the gloved hand holding the penis to be contaminated.	Avoids transferring microorganisms to sterile equipment and supplies
Pick up a moistened cotton ball with the sterile forceps and wipe the penis in a circular manner from the meatus toward the base; repeat using a different cotton ball each time.	Moves microorganisms away from the meatus

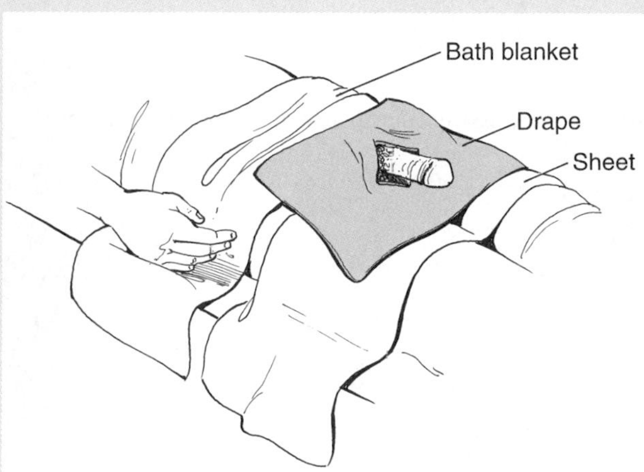

Placing a fenestrated drape.

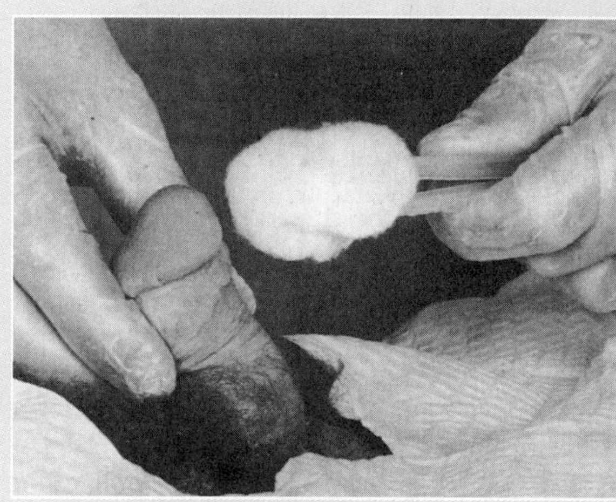

Cleaning the penis.

Suggested Action	Reason for Action
Discard the forceps with the last cotton ball into the wrapper for contaminated supplies.	Follows principles of asepsis
Apply gentle traction to the penis by pulling it straight up with the nondominant gloved hand.	Straightens the urethra
Instill the contents of a prefilled syringe containing lubricant directly through the meatus into the urethra.	Avoids trauma to the urethra caused by insufficient lubrication; this technique replaces the traditional practice of lubricating the outer surface of the catheter, which resulted in its accumulation at the meatus only (Gerard & Sueppel, 1997)

continued

SKILL 30-4

INSERTING A FOLEY CATHETER IN A MALE PATIENT *Continued*

Suggested Action	Reason for Action

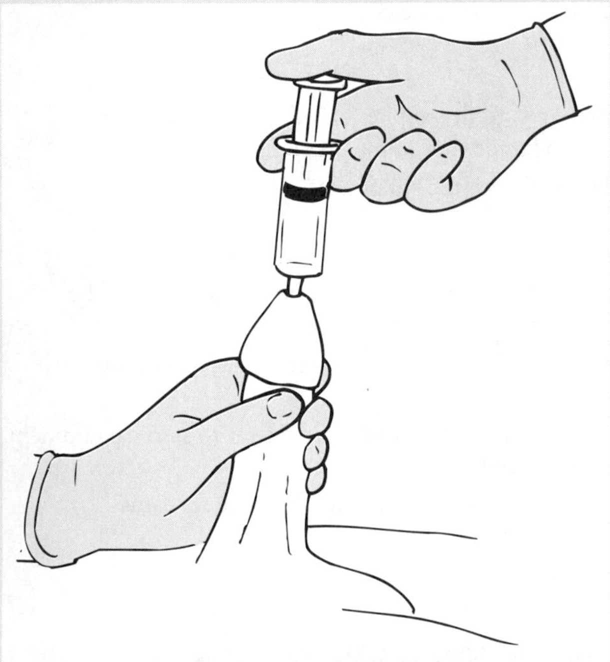

Instilling lubricant.

Insert, but never force the catheter; rather, rotate the catheter, apply more traction to the penis, encourage the patient to breathe deeply, or angle the penis toward the toes.

Adjusts for passing the catheter beyond the prostate gland

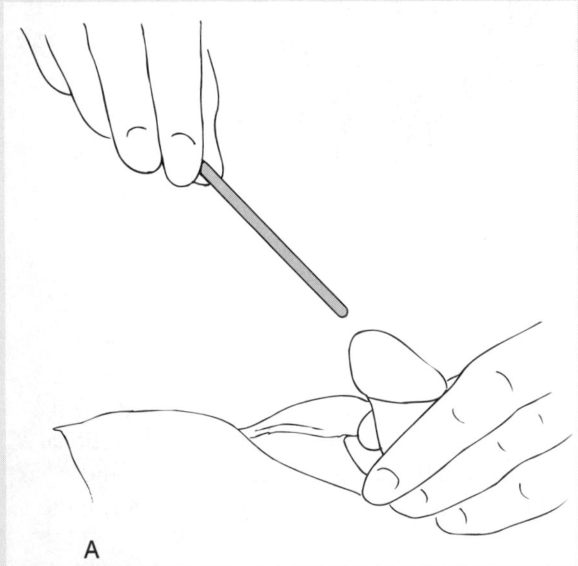

A. Preparing to insert the catheter.

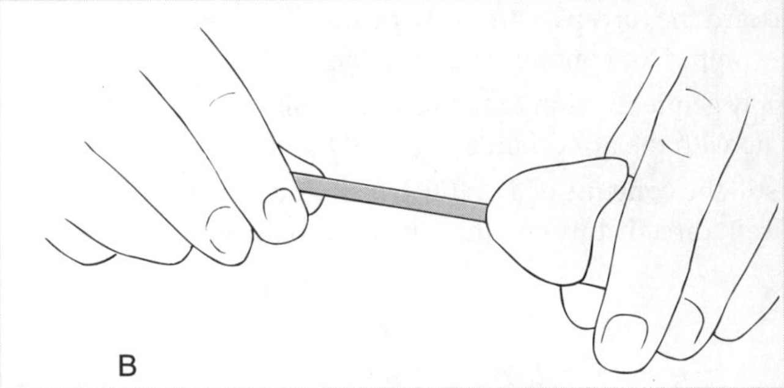

B. Angling the penis downward.

continued

SKILL 30-4

INSERTING A FOLEY CATHETER IN A MALE PATIENT *Continued*

Suggested Action	Reason for Action
Continue insertion until only the inflation and drainage ports are exposed and urine flows.	Locates the tip beyond the length of the male urethra

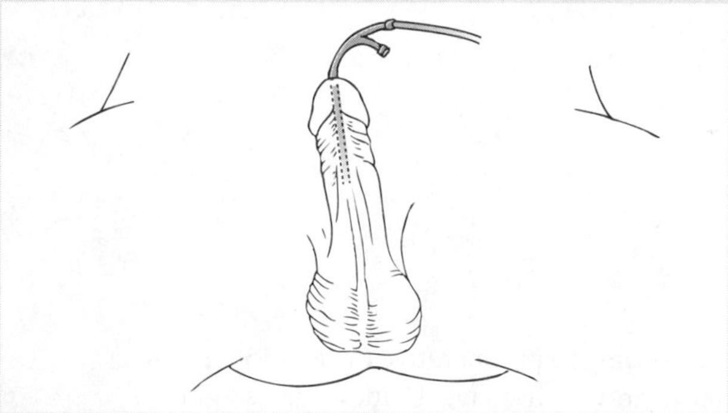

Catheter insertion.

Suggested Action	Reason for Action
Pick up the prefilled syringe with the sterile, dominant hand, insert it into the opening to the balloon, and instill the fluid.	Stabilizes the catheter internally
Withdraw the fluid from the balloon if the patient describes feeling pain or discomfort, advance the catheter a little more, and try again.	Prevents internal injury
Tug gently on the catheter after the balloon has been filled.	Tests whether the catheter is well anchored within the bladder
Connect the catheter to a urine collection bag.	Provides a means of assessing the urine and its volume
Wipe the meatus and penis of any residual lubricant.	Demonstrates concern for the patient's comfort
Secure the catheter to the leg or abdomen with tape or other commercial device.	Prevents pulling on the balloon within the catheter

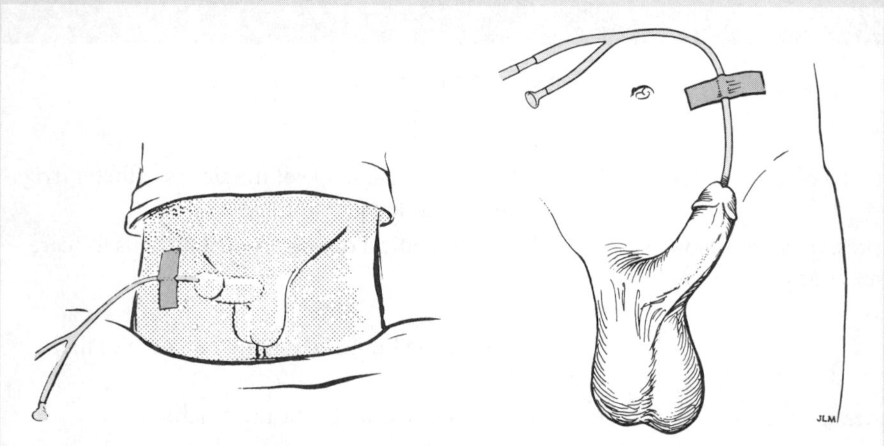

Methods for securing a catheter.

Suggested Action	Reason for Action
Hang the collection bag below the level of the bladder; coil excess tubing on the mattress.	Ensures gravity drainage
Discard the catheterization tray and wrapper with soiled supplies.	Follows principles of asepsis
Remove your gloves and wash your hands.	Removes colonizing microorganisms
Remove the drape, restore the top sheets, make the patient comfortable, and lower the bed.	Restores comfort and safety

continued

SKILL 30-4

INSERTING A FOLEY CATHETER IN A MALE PATIENT *Continued*

Evaluation

- Catheter is inserted under aseptic conditions
- Urine is draining from the catheter
- Patient demonstrates no evidence of discomfort during or after insertion

Document

- Preassessment data
- Size and type of catheter
- Amount and appearance of urine
- Patient's response

SAMPLE DOCUMENTATION

Date and Time #16 F Foley catheter inserted before surgery according to preoperative orders. 350 mL of urine obtained before connecting the catheter to gravity drainage. Urine appears light yellow and clear. ______________________ SIGNATURE, TITLE

CRITICAL THINKING

- Discuss possible explanations for why urine may not flow when a catheter is inserted.
- Describe the consequences of inflating the catheter's balloon before determining that the catheter is draining urine.

SKILL 30-5

IRRIGATING A FOLEY CATHETER

Suggested Action	Reason for Action
Assessment	
Check the patient's record to verify that a medical order has been written.	Demonstrates the legal scope of nursing; a catheter irrigation is not an independent measure
Verify the type of irrigating solution prescribed, or follow the standard for practice, which usually advises sterile normal saline solution.	Complies with medical directives or standards for care
Assess the urine characteristics.	Provides a baseline for assessing the outcome of the procedure
Determine how much the patient understands about a catheter irrigation.	Provides an opportunity for health teaching
Planning	
Gather the equipment and supplies that are needed. They include an irrigation kit, a flask of sterile irrigating solution, alcohol swabs, and a sterile cap for the tip of the drainage tubing.	Promotes organization and efficient time management

continued

SKILL 30-5

IRRIGATING A FOLEY CATHETER *Continued*

Suggested Action	Reason for Action
Implementation	
Wash hands.	Follows principles of asepsis and standards of practice
Raise the height of the bed.	Reduces back strain
Pull the privacy curtain	Demonstrates concern for the patient's dignity
Remove the container for the irrigating solution from the irrigation set and add 100 to 200 mL of solution.	Avoids contaminating and wasting all the solution in the flask
Don gloves kept at the bedside or within the irrigation kit.	Complies with standard precautions
Remove the cap on the tip of the irrigating syringe found in the irrigation kit. Fill the syringe with 30 to 60 mL of solution, and loosely replace the cap.	Maintains sterility but eases the cap's removal

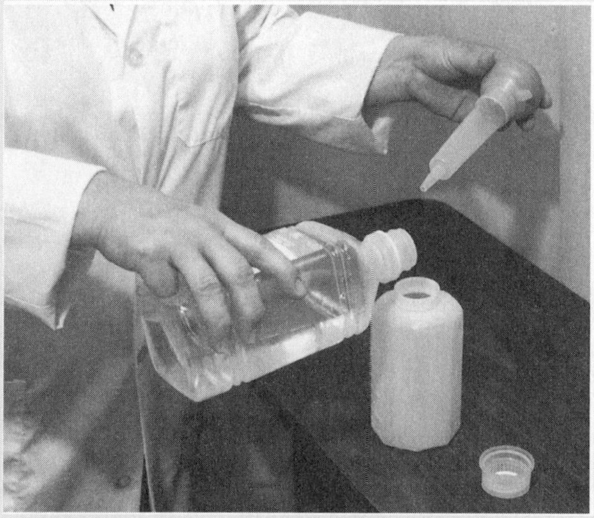

Preparing irrigation solution. (Courtesy of Ken Timby.)

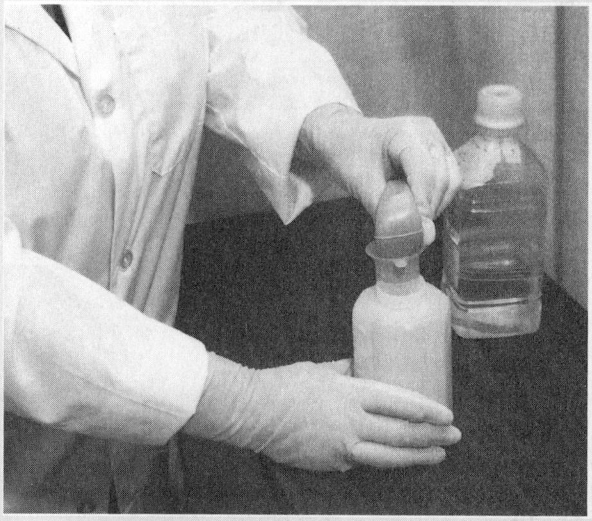

Filling the irrigation syringe. (Courtesy of Ken Timby.)

Suggested Action	Reason for Action
Place the drainage basin from the irrigation kit nearby.	Facilitates collecting the drainage of irrigating solution and urine
Clean the area where the catheter and drainage tubing connect with an alcohol swab.	Removes gross debris and colonizing microorganisms
Separate the two tubes and place a cap on the exposed end of the drainage tube.	Prevents contamination
While holding the catheter with one hand, insert the syringe into the catheter with the other hand.	Maintains sterility
Gently instill the solution.	Clears the catheter of debris and dilutes particles within the bladder
Pinch the catheter and remove the syringe.	Prevents leaking
Replace the tip of the syringe loosely within its cap or place it tip down in the drainage basin of the irrigation kit.	Maintains sterility
Direct the end of the catheter over the drainage basin and unpinch the tubing.	Facilitates gravity drainage

continued

SKILL 30-5

IRRIGATING A FOLEY CATHETER *Continued*

Suggested Action	Reason for Action

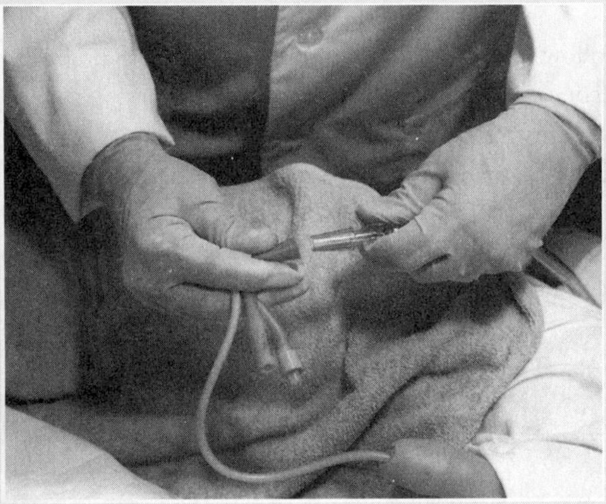

Capping the drainage tubing to ensure sterility. (Courtesy of Ken Timby.)

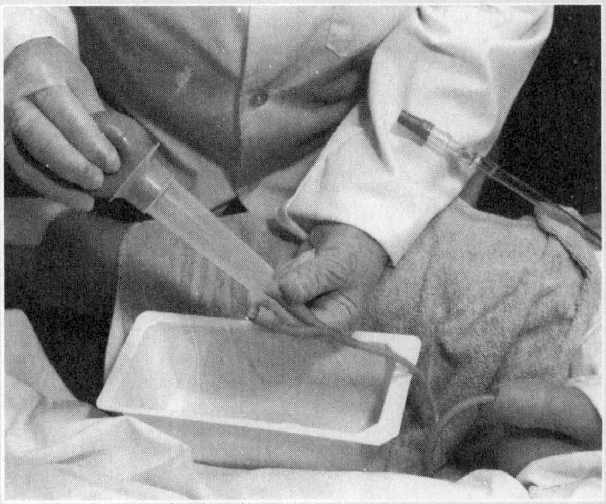

Instilling irrigation solution. (Courtesy of Ken Timby.)

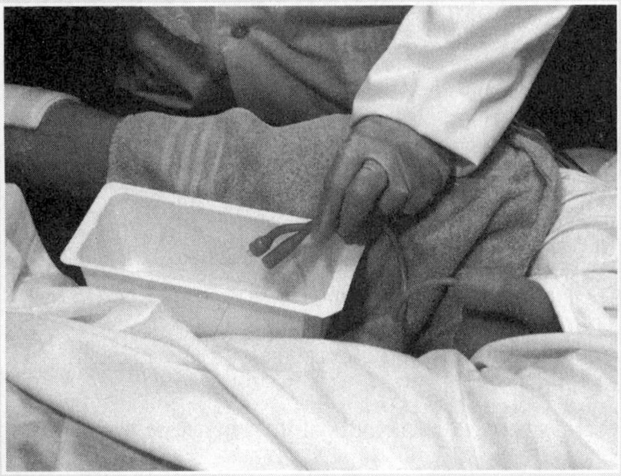

Draining the irrigation solution. (Courtesy of Ken Timby.)

Suggested Action	Reason for Action
Repeat the instillation and drainage if the urine appears to contain an appreciable amount of debris.	Promotes patency
Remove the cap on the drainage tubing and reconnect it to the catheter.	Reestablishes a closed system
Measure the amount of drained fluid. Record the volume of instilled solution as fluid intake and the drained volume as output.	Maintains accurate assessment data
Discard or protect the sterility of the irrigating equipment, which may be reused for the next 24 hours as long as it is not contaminated.	Complies with principles of infection control

continued

SKILL 30–5

IRRIGATING A FOLEY CATHETER *Continued*

Evaluation

- The prescribed amount and type of solution are instilled
- Principles of asepsis have been maintained
- Urine continues to drain well through the catheter
- Patient reports no discomfort

Document

- Preassessment data
- Volume, type of solution
- Volume and appearance of drainage

SAMPLE DOCUMENTATION

Date and Time Urine appears amber with some evidence of white particles. 60 mL of sterile normal saline solution instilled into catheter. 120 mL drainage returned. Urine appears to have less sediment. Catheter remains patent. ______________________ SIGNATURE, TITLE

CRITICAL THINKING

- Discuss what actions might be appropriate if the irrigation was unsuccessful in promoting catheter patency.
- List advantages and disadvantages of the three methods for catheter irrigation (using an open system, using a closed system, and using a continuous irrigation).

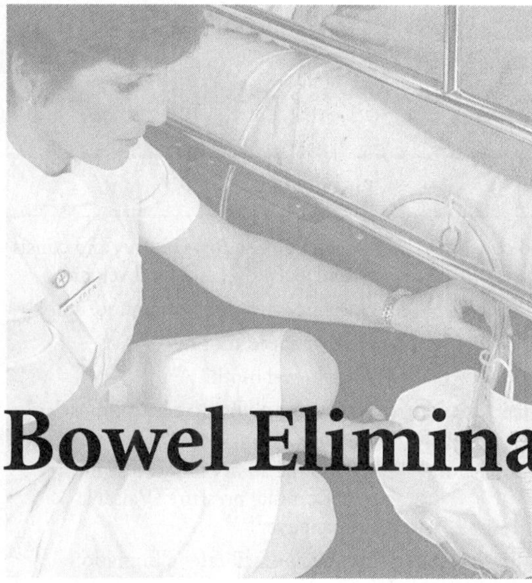

CHAPTER 31

Bowel Elimination

CHAPTER OUTLINE

NURSING GUIDELINES

TESTING STOOL FOR OCCULT BLOOD
REMOVING A FECAL IMPACTION
ADMINISTERING A HYPERTONIC ENEMA SOLUTION

SKILLS

SKILL 31-1: INSERTING A RECTAL TUBE
SKILL 31-2: INSERTING A RECTAL SUPPOSITORY
SKILL 31-3: ADMINISTERING A CLEANSING ENEMA
SKILL 31-4: CHANGING AN OSTOMY APPLIANCE
SKILL 31-5: IRRIGATING A COLOSTOMY

NURSING CARE PLAN

CONSTIPATION

KEY TERMS

anal sphincters
appliance
colostomy
constipation
continent ostomy
defecation
diarrhea
enema
excoriation
fecal impaction
fecal incontinence
feces
flatulence
flatus
gastrocolic reflex
ileostomy
ostomy
peristalsis
retention enema
stoma
suppository
Valsalva maneuver

LEARNING OBJECTIVES

An understanding of the content within this chapter will be evidenced by the student's ability to:

- Describe the process of defecation.
- Name two components of a bowel elimination assessment.
- List five common alterations in bowel elimination.
- Name four types of constipation.
- Identify measures for treating constipation within the scope of nursing practice.
- Identify two interventions for promoting bowel elimination when it does not occur naturally.
- Name two categories of enema administration.
- List at least three common solutions used in a cleansing enema.
- Explain the purpose of an oil retention enema.
- Name four nursing activities involved in ostomy care.

This chapter reviews briefly the process of intestinal elimination and discusses measures to help promote it. Nursing skills that may assist patients with alterations in bowel elimination are also described.

Bowel Elimination

Defecation (bowel elimination) is the act of expelling **feces** (stool) from the body. To do so, all the structures of the gastrointestinal tract, especially the components of the large intestine (also referred to as the *bowel* or *colon*), must function in a coordinated manner (Fig. 31-1). In the large intestine, a remarkable volume of water is removed from the remnants of digestion, causing the bowel's contents to become a consolidated mass of residue before being eliminated.

DEFECATION

Defecation is facilitated by **peristalsis** (rhythmic contractions of intestinal smooth muscle). Peristalsis moves fiber, water,

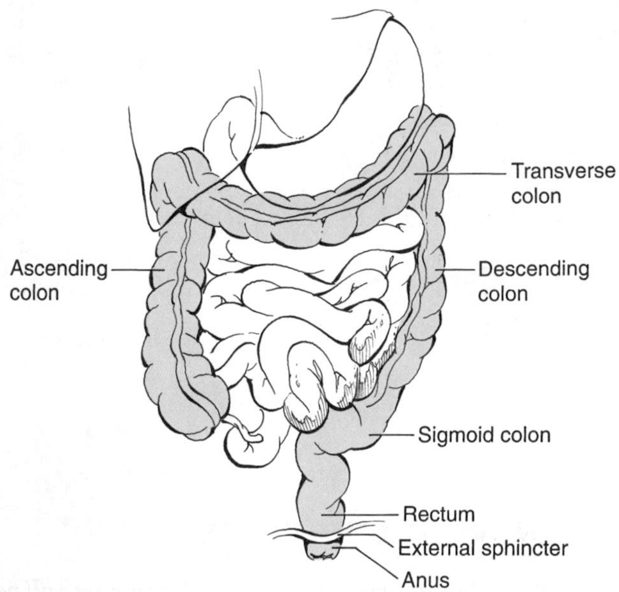

FIGURE 31–1. The large intestine.

and nutritional wastes along the ascending, transverse, descending, and sigmoid colon toward the rectum. Peristalsis becomes even more active during eating; this is termed the **gastrocolic reflex** (increased peristaltic activity).

The gastrocolic reflex usually precedes defecation. Its accelerated wavelike movements, sometimes perceived as slight abdominal cramping, propel stool forward, packing it within the rectum. As the rectum distends, there is an urge to defecate. Stool is eventually released when the **anal sphincters** (ring-shaped bands of muscles) relax. The process is facilitated by performing the **Valsalva maneuver** (closing the glottis and contracting the pelvic and abdominal muscles to increase abdominal pressure). Several factors, including dietary, physical, social, and emotional factors, can influence the bowel's mechanical function (Table 31-1).

TABLE 31–1. **Common Factors Affecting Bowel Elimination**

Factor	Effect
Types of food consumed	Affects color, odor, volume, and consistency of stool, and fecal velocity
Fluid intake	Influences moisture content of stool
Drugs	Slow or speed motility
Emotions	Alter bowel motility
Neuromuscular function	Affects the ability to control muscles about the rectum
Abdominal muscle tone	Affects the ability to increase intra-abdominal pressure (Valsalva maneuver)
Opportunity for defecation	Inhibits or facilitates elimination

Assessment of Bowel Elimination

A comprehensive assessment includes collecting data about the patient's elimination patterns, or bowel habits, and the actual characteristics of the feces.

ELIMINATION PATTERNS

Because various elimination patterns can still be normal, it is essential to determine the patient's usual patterns, including the frequency of elimination, the effort required to expel the stool, and what elimination aids, if any, are used.

STOOL CHARACTERISTICS

Objective data is obtained by inspecting the stool or having the patient describe its appearance. Information that is particularly diagnostic includes the stool color, odor, consistency, shape, and unusual components (Table 31-2).

Whenever stool appears abnormal, a sample is saved in a covered container for the physician's inspection. In some instances, the nurse may independently perform screening

TABLE 31–2. **Characteristics of Stool**

Characteristic	Normal	Abnormal
Color	Brown	Black Clay-colored (tan) Yellow Green
Odor	Aromatic	Foul
Consistency	Soft, formed	Soft, bulky Hard, dry Watery Paste-like
Shape	Round, full	Absent Flat Pencil-shaped Stone-like
Components	Undigested fiber	Worms Blood Pus Mucus

tests on stool samples, such as those that determine the presence of blood.

Nursing Guidelines For
Testing Stool for Occult Blood

- ☑ Collect stool within a toilet liner or bedpan.
  RATIONALE: Prevents mixing stool with water or urine
- ☑ Don gloves and use an applicator stick to collect the specimen.
  RATIONALE: Reduces the transmission of microorganisms
- ☑ Take a sample from the center area of the stool.
  RATIONALE: Provides more diagnostic findings because the sample is not superficially tainted with blood from local tissue
- ☑ Apply a thin smear of stool onto the test area supplied with the screening kit.
  RATIONALE: Ensures thorough contact with the chemical reagent
- ☑ Cover the entire test space.
  RATIONALE: Ensures more accurate findings
- ☑ Place two drops of chemical reagent onto the test space.
  RATIONALE: Promotes a chemical reaction
- ☑ Wait 60 seconds.
  RATIONALE: Allows time for chemical interaction with the stool
- ☑ Observe for a blue color.
  RATIONALE: Indicates blood is present

The results, which can be falsely positive, are then reported to the physician, who may order more extensive laboratory or diagnostic tests.

By analyzing the assessment findings, the nurse may help the physician diagnose a medical problem or use the conclusions to identify alterations within the scope of nursing management.

Common Alterations in Bowel Elimination

Patients often have temporary or chronic problems with bowel elimination and intestinal function such as constipation, fecal impaction, flatulence, diarrhea, and fecal incontinence. If these conditions are a component of a serious disorder, they are addressed by collaborative efforts between nurses and physicians. However, alterations within the scope of nursing practice may be treated independently.

CONSTIPATION

Constipation (elimination problem characterized by dry, hard stool that is not easily passed) is accompanied by a variety of signs and symptoms, such as:

- Complaints of abdominal fullness or bloating
- Abdominal distention
- Complaints of rectal fullness or pressure
- Pain on defecation
- Decrease in frequency of bowel movements
- Inability to pass stool
- Changes in stool characteristics, such as oozing liquid stool or hard small stool

Infrequent elimination of stool does not necessarily indicate that a person is constipated. Some people may be constipated even though they have a daily bowel movement, whereas others who defecate irregularly may have normal bowel function.

Among Americans and people from other affluent countries, the incidence of constipation tends to be high. Many authorities attribute this to diets that lack adequate fiber (such as raw fruits and vegetables, whole grains, seeds, and nuts). Fiber, which becomes undigested cellulose, attracts water, resulting in the formation of bulkier stool that is more quickly and easily eliminated.

Some researchers speculate that a shortened transit time—the time between when food is eaten and when it is eliminated—protects against serious medical disorders. They argue that the longer stool is retained, the more contact with and absorption of toxic substances takes place.

Types of Constipation

Constipation may be classified into one of four distinct types (primary, secondary, iatrogenic, and pseudoconstipation), primarily based on the underlying cause.

Primary Constipation

Primary or simple constipation, which is well within the treatment domain of nurses, occurs as a result of lifestyle factors such as inactivity, inadequate intake of fiber, insufficient fluid intake, or ignoring the urge to defecate.

Secondary Constipation

Secondary constipation is a consequence of a pathologic disorder such as a partial bowel obstruction. It usually resolves when the primary cause is treated.

Iatrogenic Constipation

Iatrogenic constipation occurs as a consequence of other medical treatment. For example, prolonged use of narcotic analgesia tends to cause constipation. These and other drugs slow peristalsis, delaying transit time. The longer the stool remains in the colon, the drier it becomes, making it more difficult to pass.

Pseudoconstipation

"Pseudoconstipation," which the North American Nursing Diagnosis Association (NANDA, 1999) refers to as perceived constipation, is a term used when patients believe themselves to be constipated even though they are not. Pseudoconstipation may occur in people who are extremely concerned about having a daily bowel movement. In their zeal for regularity, they often overuse or abuse laxatives, suppositories, and enemas. Such self-treatment may ultimately *cause* rather than treat constipation. Chronic purging eventually weakens the tone of the bowel; consequently, bowel elimination is less likely to occur unless it is artificially stimulated.

FECAL IMPACTION

Fecal impaction (condition in which it is impossible to pass feces voluntarily) occurs when a large, hardened mass of stool interferes with defecation. Fecal impactions may be the result of unrelieved constipation, retained barium from an intestinal x-ray, dehydration, and muscle weakness.

Patients with a fecal impaction usually report a frequent desire to defecate, but an inability to do so. Rectal pain may occur as a result of the unsuccessful efforts to evacuate the lower bowel. Some patients with an impaction pass liquid stool, which may be misinterpreted as diarrhea. However, the liquid stool is caused by the forceful muscular contractions of peristalsis in higher bowel areas, where the stool is still fluid. These contractions send the liquid around the margins of the impacted stool, but this passage of liquid stool does not relieve the initial condition.

To determine whether fecal impaction is present, it may be necessary to insert a lubricated, gloved finger into the rectum. If the rectum is filled with a mass of stool, the nurse implements measures for its removal. Sometimes enemas, first oil retention and then cleansing, are administered. These therapeutic measures are discussed later in this chapter. Another intervention is to remove the stool digitally.

Nursing Guidelines For
Removing a Fecal Impaction

☑ Wash your hands.
RATIONALE: Reduces the transmission of microorganisms

☑ Provide privacy.
RATIONALE: Demonstrates respect for the patient's dignity

☑ Place the patient in a Sims' position (see Chap. 13).
RATIONALE: Facilitates access to the rectum

☑ Cover the patient with a drape and place a disposable pad under the patient's hips.
RATIONALE: Prevents soiling

☑ Place a bedpan conveniently on the bed.
RATIONALE: Provides a container for removed stool

☑ Don clean gloves.
RATIONALE: Reduces the transmission of microorganisms

☑ Lubricate the forefinger of your dominant hand.
RATIONALE: Eases insertion within the rectum

☑ Insert your lubricated finger within the rectum to the level of the hardened mass.
RATIONALE: Facilitates digital manipulation of the stool

☑ Move your finger about slowly and carefully to break up the mass of stool.
RATIONALE: Facilitates removal or voluntary passage

☑ Withdraw segments of the stool (Fig. 31-2) and deposit them in the bedpan.
RATIONALE: Reduces the internal mass of stool

☑ Provide periods of rest, but continue until the mass has been removed or sufficiently reduced.
RATIONALE: Restores patency to the lower bowel

☑ Clean the patient's rectal area; dispose of the stool and soiled gloves; wash your hands.
RATIONALE: Supports principles of medical asepsis

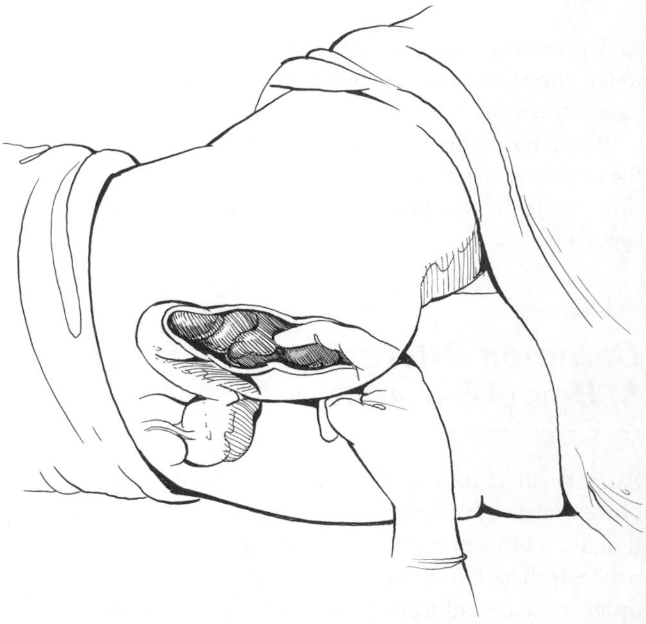

FIGURE 31–2. Removing impacted stool.

FLATULENCE

Flatulence or **flatus** (excessive accumulation of intestinal gas) is caused by swallowing air while eating or by sluggish peristalsis. It also may be caused by the gas that forms as a byproduct of bacterial fermentation in the bowel. Vegetables such as cabbage, cucumbers, and onions are commonly known for producing gas. Beans are other gas-formers. They create intestinal gas because humans lack an enzyme to completely digest their particular form of complex carbohydrate.

Regardless of its cause, flatus may be expelled rectally, thus reducing intestinal accumulation and distention. However, sometimes this is not sufficient to eliminate the cramping pain or other symptoms. When patients are extremely uncomfortable, and ambulating does not eliminate the flatus, a rectal tube may be inserted to help the gas escape (Skill 31-1).

DIARRHEA

Diarrhea (urgent passage of watery stool) commonly is accompanied by abdominal cramping. Simple diarrhea usually begins suddenly and lasts only a short period. Other associated signs and symptoms include nausea and vomiting and the presence of blood or mucus in the stools.

Usually diarrhea is a means of eliminating an irritating substance, such as tainted food or intestinal pathogens. However, diarrhea may also result from emotional stress, dietary indiscretions, laxative abuse, or bowel disorders.

Simple diarrhea may be relieved by resting the bowel temporarily. This means the person can drink clear liquids but should avoid solid foods for 12 to 24 hours. When eating is resumed, it is best to start with bland foods and those that are low in residue, such as bananas, applesauce, and cottage cheese. If the diarrhea is not relieved within 24 hours, it may be best to consult a physician.

FECAL INCONTINENCE

Fecal incontinence (inability to control the elimination of stool) does not necessarily imply that the stool is loose or watery, although that may be the case. In many cases of incontinence, bowel function is normal, but the incontinence results from neurologic changes that impair muscle activity, sensation, or thought processes. Even a fecal impaction may be an underlying cause of incontinence. Incontinence may also occur when a person cannot reach a toilet in time to eliminate, such as after taking a harsh laxative.

Chronic fecal incontinence can be devastating socially and emotionally. These patients and their families require much support, understanding, and teaching.

Patient Guidelines For
Managing Fecal Incontinence

Teach the patient to do the following:
- Eat regularly and nutritiously.
- Monitor the pattern of incontinence to determine whether it occurs at a similar time each day.
- Sit on the toilet or bedside commode before the time elimination tends to occur.
- Consult the physician about inserting a suppository or administering an enema every 2 to 3 days to establish a pattern for bowel elimination.
- Use moisture-proof undergarments and absorbent pads to protect clothing and bed linen.

Teach caregivers to do the following:
- Do not imply, verbally or nonverbally, that the patient is to blame for the incontinence or that cleaning him or her is disgusting.
- Avoid anything that connotes diapering, to preserve the patient's dignity and self-esteem.

Measures to Promote Bowel Elimination

Two interventions—inserting suppositories and administering enemas—are commonly used to promote elimination when it does not occur naturally or when the bowel must be cleansed for other purposes, such as preparation for surgery and endoscopic or x-ray examinations.

INSERTING A RECTAL SUPPOSITORY

A **suppository** (oval or cone-shaped mass that melts at body temperature) is inserted into a body cavity such as the rectum. The most common reason for inserting a suppository is to deliver a drug that will promote the expulsion of feces.

Medications released from the suppository can have a local or systemic effect. Depending on the drug, local effects may include softening and lubricating dry stool, irritating the wall of the rectum and anal canal to stimulate smooth muscle contraction, or liberating carbon dioxide, thus increasing rectal distention and the urge to defecate. Occasionally drugs are administered in suppository form to achieve a systemic effect. This route is chosen when patients have difficulty retaining or absorbing oral medications because of chronic vomiting or an impaired ability to swallow.

Administering a suppository is a form of medication administration (Skill 31-2). For additional principles, refer to Chapters 32 and 33.

ADMINISTERING AN ENEMA

An **enema** (introduction of a solution into the rectum; Skill 31-3) is given to:

- Cleanse the lower bowel (most common reason)
- Soften feces
- Expel flatus
- Soothe irritated mucous membranes
- Outline the colon during diagnostic x-rays
- Treat worm and parasite infestations

Cleansing Enemas

Cleansing enemas use different types of solution to remove feces from the rectum (Table 31-3). Defecation usually occurs within 5 to 15 minutes after administration.

Large-volume cleansing enemas may create discomfort because they distend the lower bowel. They must be cautiously administered to patients with intestinal disorders such as colitis (inflammation of the colon) because they may rupture the bowel or cause other secondary complications.

Tap Water and Normal Saline Enemas

Tap water and normal saline solutions may be preferred for their nonirritating effects, especially for patients with rectal diseases or those being prepared for rectal examinations. Tap water and normal saline appear to have about the same degree of effectiveness for cleansing the bowel.

Tap water, because it is hypotonic, can be absorbed through the bowel. Consequently, if several enemas are administered in succession, fluid and electrolyte imbalances may occur (see Chap. 15). Therefore, to ensure patient safety, if stool continues to be expelled after the administration of three enemas, the physician is consulted before administering any more.

Soap Solution Enemas

A soap solution enema is a mixture of water and soap. Many disposable enema kits contain an envelope of soap that is mixed with up to a quart (1,000 mL) of water. If these soap packets are not available, a comparable mixture would be 1 mL of mild liquid soap per 200 mL of solution, or a 1:200 ratio. Therefore, to prepare a volume of 1,000 mL, 5 mL of soap would be added.

Soap causes chemical irritation of the mucous membranes. Adding too much soap or using strong soap can potentiate the irritating effect.

TABLE 31–3. **Types of Cleansing Enema Solutions**

Solution	Amount	Mechanism of Action
Tap water	500–1,000 mL	Distends rectum, moistens stool
Normal saline	500–1,000 mL	Distends rectum, moistens stool
Soap and water	500–1,000 mL	Distends rectum, moistens stool, irritates local tissue
Hypertonic saline	120 mL	Irritates local tissue
Mineral, olive, or cottonseed oil	120–180 mL	Lubricates and softens stool

Hypertonic Saline Enemas

A hypertonic saline (sodium phosphate) enema draws fluid from body tissues into the bowel. This increases the fluid volume in the intestine beyond what was originally instilled. The concentrated solution also acts as a local irritant on the mucous membranes.

Hypertonic enema solutions are available in commercially prepared, disposable containers holding approximately 4 oz (120 mL) of solution (Fig. 31-3). The container, which has a lubricated tip, substitutes for enema equipment and tubing.

Nursing Guidelines For

Administering a Hypertonic Enema Solution

- ☑ Warm the container of solution by placing it in a basin or sink of warm water, if it is cold.
  RATIONALE: Promotes comfort
- ☑ Assist the patient to a Sims' position, or use a knee-chest position (see Chap. 13).
  RATIONALE: Promotes gravity distribution of the solution
- ☑ Wash hands and don gloves.
  RATIONALE: Reduces the transmission of microorganisms
- ☑ Remove the cover from the lubricated tip.
  RATIONALE: Facilitates administration
- ☑ Cover the tip with additional lubricant.
  RATIONALE: Eases insertion
- ☑ Invert the container.
  RATIONALE: Causes air in the container to rise toward the upper end
- ☑ Insert the full length of the tip within the rectum.
  RATIONALE: Places the tip at a level that promotes effectiveness
- ☑ Apply gentle, steady pressure on the solution container for 1 to 2 minutes, or until the solution has been completely administered.
  RATIONALE: Instills a steady stream of solution
- ☑ Compress the container as the solution instills.
  RATIONALE: Provides positive pressure rather than gravity to instill fluid
- ☑ Encourage the patient to retain the solution for 5 to 15 minutes.
  RATIONALE: Promotes effectiveness

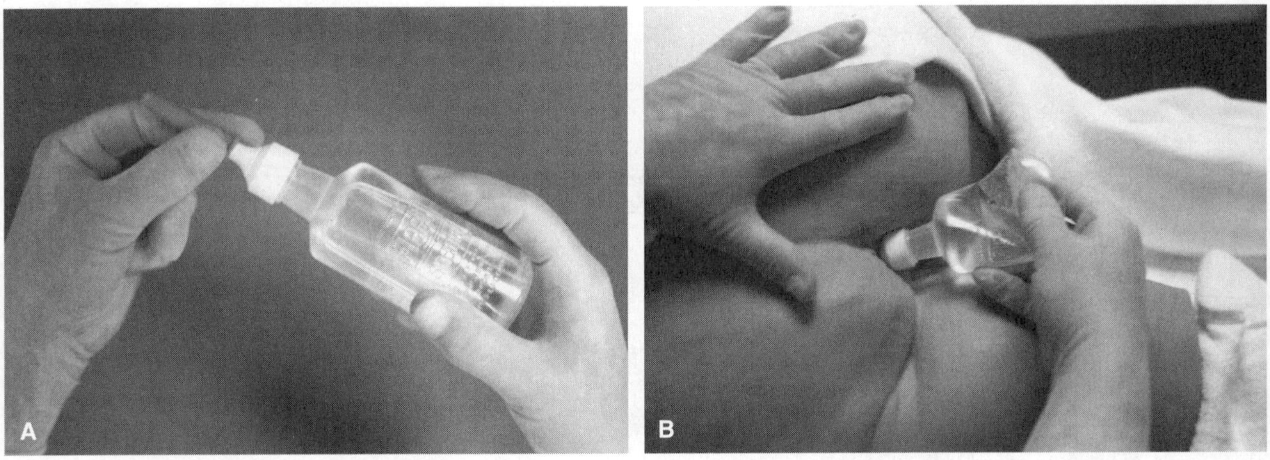

FIGURE 31–3. Hypertonic enema administration. (*A*) Solution container. (*B*) Compressing enema container. (Courtesy of Ken Timby.)

☑ Clean the patient, and position for comfort.
RATIONALE: Demonstrates concern for the patient's well-being

☑ Discard the container, remove gloves, and wash hands.
RATIONALE: Follows principles of medical asepsis

In many health agencies and in the home, commercially prepared disposable administration sets have become the method of choice for cleansing the bowel. Their smaller volume makes them less fatiguing and distressing than large-volume enemas, and they can be easily self-administered.

Retention Enemas

A **retention enema** (enema solution held within the large intestine for a specified period of time) usually is retained for at least 30 minutes; some retention enemas are not expelled at all. One type of retention enema is called an *oil retention enema* because the fluid instilled is mineral, cottonseed, or olive oil. Oils are used to lubricate and soften the stool so it can be expelled more easily.

The oil may come in a prefilled container similar to those that contain hypertonic saline. If disposable equipment is not available, a 14F to 22F tube is lubricated and inserted in the rectum. A small funnel or large syringe is attached to the tube, and approximately 100 to 200 mL of warmed oil is instilled slowly to avoid stimulating an urge to defecate. Premature defecation defeats the purpose of retaining the oil.

Ostomy Care

A patient with an **ostomy** (surgically created opening to the bowel or other structure; see Chap. 30) requires additional care for promoting bowel elimination. Two examples of ostomies are **ileostomy** (surgically created opening to the ileum) and **colostomy** (surgically created opening to a portion of the colon; Fig. 31-4). Materials enter and exit through a **stoma** (entrance to the opening).

Most persons with an ostomy, also called *ostomates,* wear an **appliance** (bag or collection device over the stoma) to collect stool. Depending on the type and location of the ostomy, patient care may involve providing peristomal care, applying an appliance, draining a continent ileostomy, and, for patients with a colostomy, administering irrigations through the stoma.

PROVIDING PERISTOMAL CARE

Preventing skin breakdown is a major challenge in ostomy care. Enzymes in stool can quickly cause **excoriation** (chemical injury of skin). The integrity of the skin can be preserved by washing the stoma and surrounding skin with mild soap and water and patting it dry. Skin barrier substances such as *karaya,* a plant substance that becomes gelatinous when moistened, and commercial skin preparations can be applied around the stoma.

APPLYING AN OSTOMY APPLIANCE

A variety of appliances are available, but all consist of a pouch for collecting stool and a faceplate, or disk, that attaches to the abdomen. The stoma protrudes through an opening in the center of the appliance (Fig. 31-5). The pouch fastens into position when it is pressed over the circular support on the faceplate. Some patients prefer a type that is also fastened to an elastic belt worn around the waist. The belt helps support the weight of the fecal material and prevents the faceplate from being pulled away from the abdomen. The pouch is emptied by releasing the clamp at the bottom.

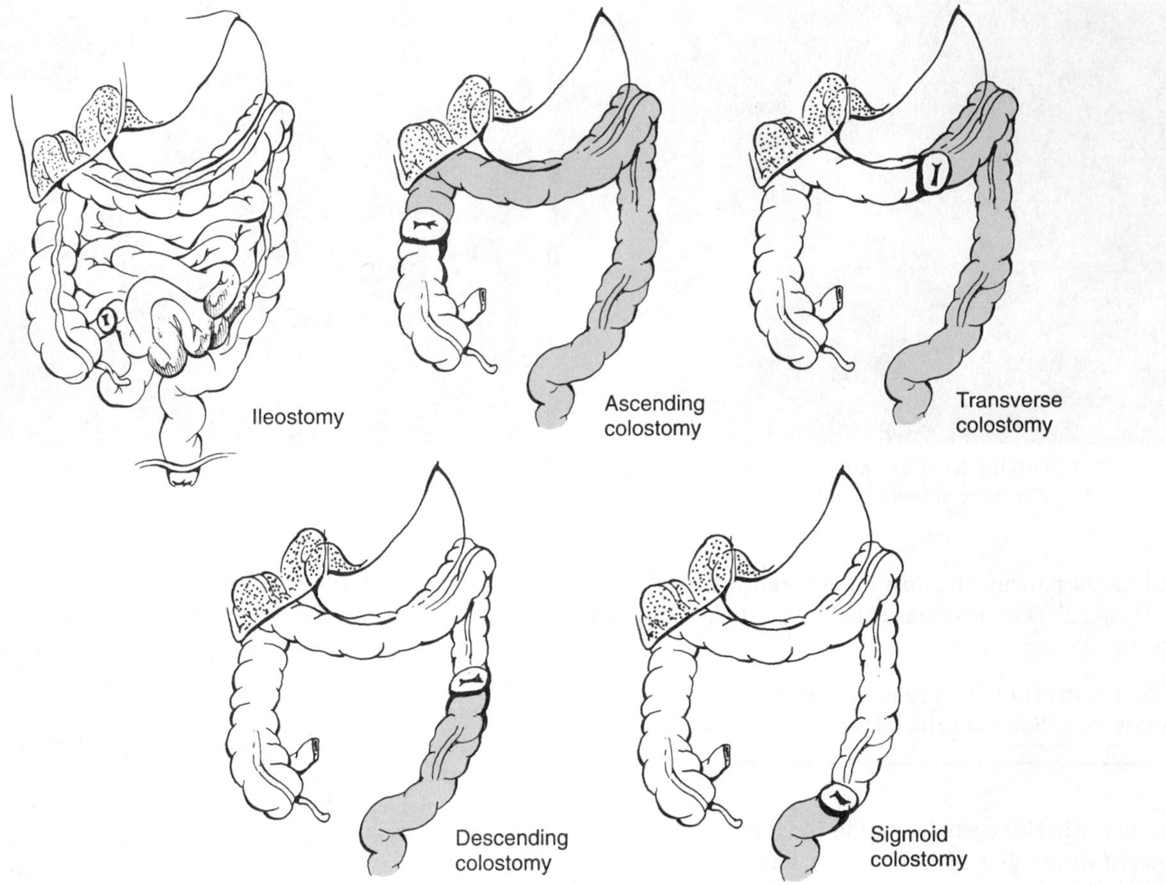

FIGURE 31–4. Locations of intestinal ostomies.

The faceplate is usually left in place for 3 to 5 days unless it becomes loose or causes skin discomfort. Pouches may be emptied and rinsed, or detached and replaced periodically. The pouch should be emptied when it is one-third to one-half full; otherwise, it may become too heavy and pull the faceplate from the skin. Although there are variations in the design of the equipment, almost all types of appliances are changed in a similar manner (Skill 31-4).

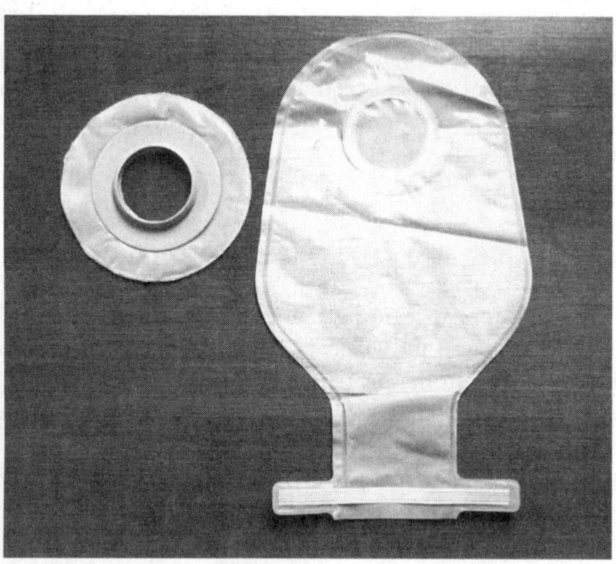

FIGURE 31–5. An ostomy appliance: faceplate and pouch. (Courtesy of Ken Timby.)

DRAINING A CONTINENT ILEOSTOMY

A **continent ostomy** (surgically created opening in which the drainage of liquid stool or urine is controlled by siphoning it from an internal reservoir) is also referred to as a *Kock pouch,* after the surgeon who developed the technique.

With this type of ostomy, no appliance is needed. However, the patient must drain the accumulating liquid stool or urine about every 4 to 6 hours. A gravity drainage system can be used at night.

Patient Teaching Guidelines For
Draining a Continent Ileostomy

Teach the patient or family to do the following:

- Assume a sitting position.
- Insert a lubricated 22F to 28F catheter into the stoma.
- Expect resistance after the tube has been inserted approximately 2 inches; this is the location of the valve that controls the retention of liquid stool or urine.

- Gently advance the catheter through the valve at the end of exhalation, while coughing, or while bearing down as if to pass stool.
- Lower the external end of the catheter at least 12 inches below the stoma.
- Direct the end of the catheter into a container or toilet as stool or urine begins to flow.
- Allow at least 5 to 10 minutes for complete emptying.
- Remove the catheter and clean it with warm soapy water.
- Place the clean catheter in a sealable plastic bag until its next use.
- Cover the stoma with a gauze square or a large bandage.
- If the catheter becomes plugged with stool or mucus:
  - Bear down as if to have a bowel movement.
  - Rotate the catheter tip inside the stoma.
  - Milk the catheter.
  - If these are not successful, remove the catheter, rinse it, and try again.
  - Notify the physician if these efforts do not result in drainage.
- Never wait longer than 6 hours without obtaining drainage.

IRRIGATING A COLOSTOMY

Patients with a colostomy whose stool is more solid sometimes require an instillation of fluid to promote elimination. A colostomy irrigation involves instilling solution through the stoma into the colon, a process similar to administering an enema (Skill 31-5). The purpose of this irrigation is to remove formed stool and in some cases to regulate the timing of bowel movements. With regulation, a patient with a sigmoid colostomy may not need to wear an appliance.

Nursing Implications

While assessing and caring for patients with altered bowel elimination, the nurse may identify one or more of the following nursing diagnoses:

- Constipation
- Risk for constipation
- Perceived constipation
- Diarrhea
- Bowel incontinence
- Toileting self-care deficit
- Situational low self-esteem

The nursing care plan reflects the nursing process as it applies to a patient with Constipation. Constipation is defined by NANDA (1999) as "a decrease in a person's normal frequency of defecation accompanied by difficult or incomplete passage of stool and/or passage of excessively hard, dry stool."

Nursing Care Plan

Constipation

Assessment

Subjective Data

States, "I've got a problem with constipation. I haven't had a bowel movement in 4 days even though I've felt like I need to pass stool. I sit and strain but I only pass a small amount of hard stool. I used to have a problem now and then when I was a kid; but since I'm living alone it's getting to be very frequent. Maybe it's because I don't eat regularly and when I do, it's a lot of convenience food."

Objective Data

21-year-old man recovering from a fractured ankle that occurred when he tripped on an area rug in his apartment yesterday. Plaster cast on L. leg that extends from toes to midcalf. Abdomen tympanic during percussion. Bowel sounds are hypoactive in all four quadrants.

Diagnosis

Constipation related to inadequate dietary habits

Plan

Goal

The patient will have a bowel movement within 24 hours and list three ways to improve the regularity of bowel elimination by 10/25.

Orders: 10/24

1. Give oil retention enema as ordered for prn administration.
2. Give prescribed laxative at HS if no bowel movement has occurred.

continued

Nursing Care Plan — Constipation *Continued*

3. Encourage drinking at least 8 to 10 glasses of fluid per day; avoid carbonated beverages.
4. Instruct about high-fiber foods and inform that daily consumption should consist of at least four servings. ______ A. ZIMMERMAN, RN

Implementation (Documentation)

10/24 1300 Instructed to drink at least 5 more glasses of fluids today and 8 to 10 thereafter. Explained that soft drinks increase intestinal gas. Given paper and pencil to record his current eating pattern, food likes and dislikes. ______ M. HASS, LPN

1330 200 mL oil retention enema administered. Instructed to remain in bed and retain solution for at least 30 minutes or longer if possible. ______ M. HASS, LPN

Evaluation (Documentation)

1400 Helped to bathroom using crutches and three-point non–weight-bearing gait. Passed a moderate amount of hard stool. Blood observed on stool and toilet paper. States, "It took a lot of straining but I feel much better now." ______ M. HASS, LPN

1400 Reviewed dietary list. Noted the following: does not eat breakfast, usually eats lunch at fast-food establishment near campus, fixes frozen meals in evening, snacks on chips. ______ M. HASS, LPN

1445 Recommended eating breakfast and waiting at home a little while for urge to eliminate. Include whole grain bread/toast, cereal, fresh fruits, fruit juices, salads, and nuts or seeds as additions to diet for at least four servings each day. States, "I guess I could eat an apple or carrots between classes. I used to eat shredded wheat for breakfast. They sell salads where I eat lunch. I didn't realize soda pop could add to the bloating I've been feeling. Maybe I'll have to start shopping and eating a little differently from now on." ______ M. HASS, LPN

KEY CONCEPTS

- Defecation, the elimination of stool, occurs when peristalsis moves fecal waste toward the rectum and the rectum distends, creating an urge to relax the anal sphincters; this releases stool.
- Two components of a bowel elimination assessment include assessing elimination patterns and stool characteristics.
- Constipation, fecal impaction, flatulence, diarrhea, and fecal incontinence are common alterations in bowel elimination.
- There are four types of constipation: primary constipation (which can be treated independently by nurses), secondary constipation, iatrogenic constipation, and pseudoconstipation.
- When bowel elimination does not occur naturally, defecation can be promoted by inserting a rectal suppository or administering an enema.
- Cleansing enemas and oil retention enemas are two categories of enemas.
- Cleansing enemas are administered by instilling tap water, normal saline, soap and water, and other solutions.
- Oil retention enemas are given to lubricate and soften dry stool.
- When caring for patients with intestinal ostomies, nursing activities are likely to include providing peristomal care, applying an ostomy appliance, draining a continent ileostomy, and irrigating a colostomy.

CRITICAL THINKING EXERCISES

- Develop a list of suggestions designed to promote healthy bowel elimination.
- Formulate suggestions for promoting bowel continence among older adults with impaired cognition, such as those with Alzheimer's disease.

FOCUS ON OLDER ADULTS

- Age-related changes, such as loss of elasticity in intestinal wall and slower motility throughout the gastrointestinal tract, predispose older adults to constipation. However, these changes alone do not cause constipation. Other factors, such as adverse medication effects, diminished physical activity, and inadequate intake of fluid and fiber, contribute to its development.
- Nurses can discuss constipation with older adults to identify any health beliefs and behaviors that contribute to it.
- Older adults are likely to implement various home remedies for promoting bowel elimination, such as drinking prune juice or hot water in the morning. As long as the health beliefs are not harmful—and in some cases, they are helpful—the older adult may continue the practice.
- Older adults may be receptive to instructions about eating bran cereal or adding bran to casseroles or muffins as a means to increase fiber intake and also as a healthier alternative to using laxatives to maintain bowel elimination.
- Health education regarding constipation includes the following points: (1) adults should identify their own patterns of bowel regularity, which can range from 3 times a day to 3 times a week; (2) daily exercise, high-fiber foods, and 8 to 10 glasses of liquid a day (unless contraindicated) contribute to good bowel elimination; (3) if medication is needed to promote bowel regularity, a bulk-forming agent is a better choice than laxatives or enemas; and (4) the older adult is encouraged to respond to the urge to defecate as soon as possible.
- Older adults who live alone may rely on commercially prepared meals that are easy to heat and eat. This consumption pattern increases the risk of constipation because the older adult is less likely to have adequate amounts of fiber and fresh fruits and vegetables.
- Some older adults become very bowel-conscious and overuse laxatives or have a long-standing habit of laxative abuse. To develop healthy bowel elimination habits, using bulk-forming products containing psyllium or polycarbophil, which are more effective and less irritating than types of laxatives, is encouraged. Examples of these agents include Metamucil (Procter & Gamble, Cincinnati, OH) and FiberCon (Lederle Laboratories, Pearl River, NY).
- Older adults who use mineral oil for preventing or relieving constipation need to be informed that prolonged use interferes with absorption of fat-soluble vitamins (A, D, E, and K).
- The incidence of colorectal cancer increases with age. One of the early signs is a change in bowel elimination patterns and stool characteristics. Therefore, older adults are advised to have regular endoscopic bowel examinations after the age of 50 years. Any change in bowel elimination that does not respond to simple dietary or lifestyle changes requires further investigation.
- Diarrhea can easily lead to dehydration and electrolyte imbalances (especially hypokalemia) in older adults, who tend to have less body fluid reserve than younger people.
- Because many older adults have benign lesions such as hemorrhoids or polyps in their lower bowel, removing an impaction must be done gently to prevent bleeding and tissue trauma.
- Musculoskeletal disorders, such as arthritis of the hands, may interfere with an older adult's ability to care for an ostomy appliance or perform colostomy irrigations. An occupational therapist or an enterostomal therapist (a nurse who is certified in caring for ostomies and related skin problems) can offer suggestions for promoting self-care.

SUGGESTED READINGS

Aron S, Carrateta R, Prazeres SM, et al. Self-perceptions about having an ostomy: a postoperative analysis. Ostomy/Wound Management 1999; 45(4):46–48.

Bisanz A. Managing bowel elimination problems in patients with cancer. Oncology Nursing Forum 1997;24(4):679–688.

Black P. Practical stoma care. Nursing Standard 1997;11(47):49–55.

Carabajal B. Practical points in the care of patients recovering from a colostomy. Journal of Perianesthesia Nursing 1997;12(3):188–190.

Clayton HA, Boudreau L, Rodman R, et al. Development of an ostomy competency. Medsurg Nursing 1997;6(5):256–269.

Cohen MR. Suppository mix-up: Don't be foiled. Nursing 1995;25(5):13.

Colostomies and their management. Nursing Standard 1996;11(8):49–55.

House JG, Stiens SA. Pharmacologically initiated defecation for persons with spinal cord injury: Effectiveness of three agents. Archives of Physical Medicine and Rehabilitation 1997;78(10):1062–1065.

Kaufman MW, Todd D. Postoperative care of the Kock continent ileostomy. Journal of Wound and Ostomy Care Nursing 1995;22(2):105–108.

Lovejoy L, Bussey C, Sherer AP. The path to a clinical pathway: Collaborative care for the patient with an ostomy. Journal of Wound and Ostomy Care Nursing 1997;24(4):200–218.

Moppett S, Parker M. Practical procedures for nurses: Insertion of a suppository. Nursing Times 1999;95(23):insert 2.

NANDA nursing diagnoses: definitions and classification, 1999–2000. Philadelphia, NANDA, 1999.

Northouse LL, Schafer JA, Tipton J, et al. The concerns of patients and spouses after the diagnosis of colon cancer: A qualitative analysis. Journal of Wound and Ostomy Care Nursing 1999;26(1):8–17.

Roberts DJ. The pursuit of colostomy continence. Journal of Wound and Ostomy Care Nursing 1997;24(2):92–97.

Ross DG. Altered bowel elimination patterns among hospitalized elderly and middle-aged persons: Quantitative results. Orthopedic Nursing 1995; 14(1):25–31.

Schmelzer M, Wright KB. Enema administration techniques used by experienced registered nurses. Gastroenterology Nursing 1996;19(5):171–175.

Tolch M. Four steps to teaching ostomy care. Nursing 1997;27(6):32hn9–10.

Vaccari J. Sudden colostomy problems call for a thorough history. RN 1998;61(12):67–68.

Vaccari JA. Making it easy for patients to clean colostomy pouches. RN 1998;61(12):9–10.

Winney J. Constipation and the role of nurses in assessment, management, and health promotion. Elderly Care 1998;10(4):26–31.

SKILL 31–1

INSERTING A RECTAL TUBE

Suggested Action	Reason for Action
Assessment	
Check the medical orders.	Collaborates nursing activities with medical treatment
Inspect the abdomen, auscultate bowel sounds, and gently palpate for distention and fullness.	Provides baseline data for future comparisons
Determine how much the patient understands about the procedure.	Provides an opportunity for health teaching
Planning	
Obtain a 22F to 32F catheter and lubricant.	Ensures proper size and easy insertion
Implementation	
Wash your hands and don gloves.	Reduces the transmission of microorganisms
Pull the privacy curtain.	Demonstrates respect for the patient's dignity
Place the patient in a Sims' position.	Facilitates access to the rectum
Lubricate the tip of the tube generously.	Eases insertion
Separate the buttocks well so that the anus is in plain view.	Helps visualize insertion location
Insert the tube 4 to 6 inches (10–15 cm) in an adult.	Places the distal tip above the sphincter muscles, stimulates peristalsis, and prevents displacement of the tube

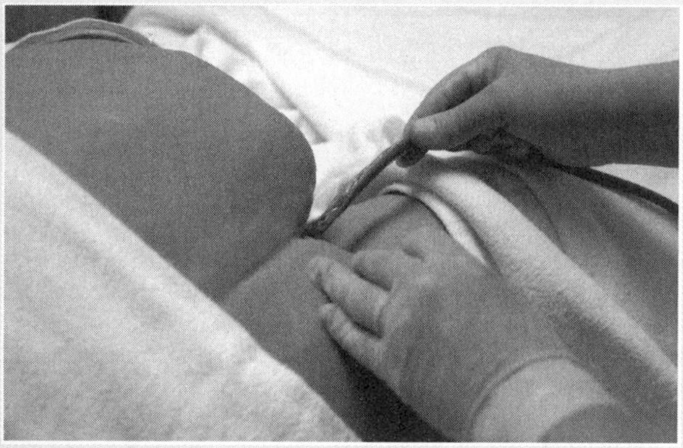

Preparing for insertion. (Courtesy of Ken Timby.)

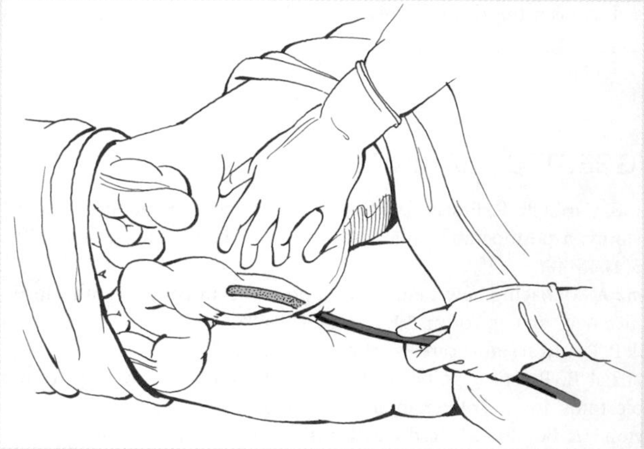

Inserting rectal tube.

Suggested Action	Reason for Action
Enclose the free end of the tube within a clean, soft washcloth or gauze square.	Provides a means for absorbing stool should it drain from the tube
Tape the tube to the buttocks or inner thigh.	Allows the patient to ambulate or change positions without tube displacement
Leave the rectal tube in place no longer than 20 minutes.	Reduces the risk of impairing the sphincters
Reinsert the tube every 3 to 4 hours if discomfort returns.	Reinstitutes therapeutic management

Evaluation

- Patient states symptoms are relieved.
- Patient reports no ill effects.

continued

SKILL 31–1

INSERTING A RECTAL TUBE *Continued*

Document

- Assessment data
- Intervention
- Length of time tube was in place
- Patient response

SAMPLE DOCUMENTATION

Date and Time Abdomen round, firm, and tympanic. Bowel sounds present in all four quadrants, but difficult to hear because of distention. States, "I can't hardly stand the pain any more." Ambulated without relief. 26F straight catheter inserted into rectum for 20 minutes. Flatus expelled during tube insertion. Abdomen softer. _____________ SIGNATURE, TITLE

CRITICAL THINKING

- Discuss measures to include in a teaching plan that would help patients reduce or eliminate intestinal gas.

SKILL 31–2

INSERTING A RECTAL SUPPOSITORY

Suggested Action	Reason for Action
Assessment	
Check the medical orders.	Collaborates nursing activities with medical treatment
Compare the medication administration record (MAR) with the written medical order.	Ensures accuracy
Read and compare the label on the suppository with the MAR at least three times—before, during, and after preparing the drug.	Prevents errors
Determine how much the patient understands about the purpose and technique for administering a suppository.	Provides an opportunity for health teaching
Planning	
Prepare to administer the suppository according to the time prescribed by the physician.	Complies with medical orders
Obtain clean gloves and lubricant.	Facilitates insertion
Implementation	
Read the name on the patient's identification band.	Prevents errors
Pull the privacy curtain.	Demonstrates respect for the patient's modesty and dignity
Place the patient in a Sims' position.	Facilitates access to the rectum
Drape the patient to expose only the buttocks.	Ensures modesty and dignity
Wash hands and don gloves.	Reduces the transmission of microorganisms

continued

SKILL 31–2

INSERTING A RECTAL SUPPOSITORY *Continued*

Suggested Action	Reason for Action
Lubricate the suppository and index finger of the dominant hand and separate the buttocks so that the anus is in plain view.	Reduces friction and tissue trauma and enhances visualization
Instruct the patient to take several slow, deep breaths. Introduce the suppository, tapered end first, beyond the internal sphincter, about the distance of the finger.	Promotes muscle relaxation and places the suppository in the best location for achieving a local effect

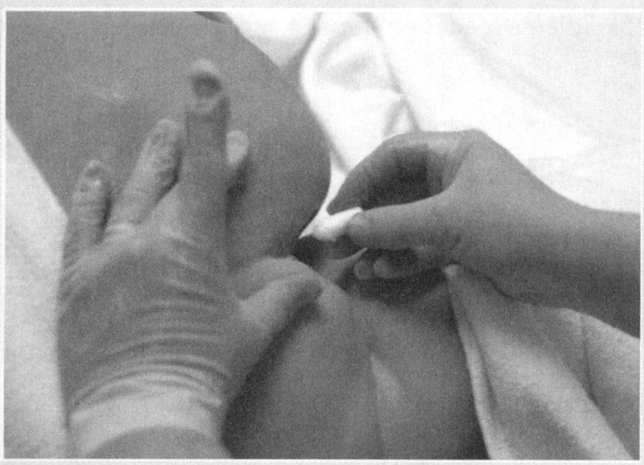

Lubricated suppository and insertion finger. (Courtesy of Ken Timby.)

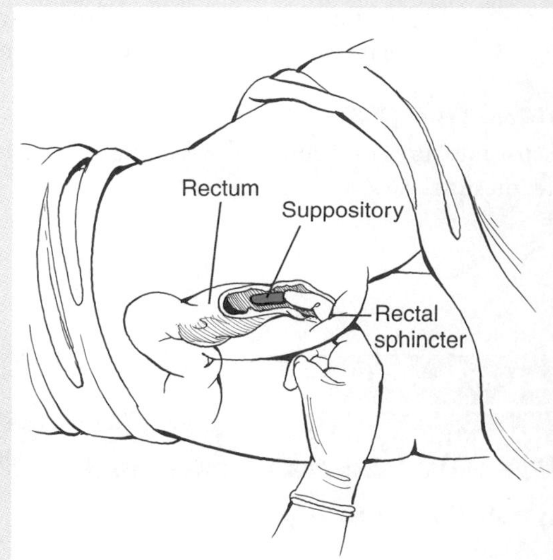

Inserting suppository.

Suggested Action	Reason for Action
Avoid placing the suppository within stool.	Reduces effectiveness
Wipe the excess lubricant from around the anus with a paper tissue.	Promotes comfort
Tell the patient to try to retain the suppository for at least 15 minutes.	Enhances effectiveness
Suggest contracting the gluteal muscles if there is a premature urge to expel the suppository.	Tightens the anal sphincters
Ask the patient to wait to flush the toilet until the stool has been inspected.	Provides an opportunity for evaluating the drug's effectiveness
Remove your gloves and wash your hands.	Reduces the transmission of microorganisms

Evaluation

- Patient retains suppository for 15 minutes.
- Bowel elimination occurs.

Document

- Drug, dose, route, and time (see Chap. 32)
- Outcome of drug administration

continued

SKILL 31–2

INSERTING A RECTAL SUPPOSITORY *Continued*

SAMPLE DOCUMENTATION

Date and Time Biscodyl (Dulcolax) suppository inserted within rectum. Lg. brown formed stool expelled.
______________________________ SIGNATURE, TITLE

CRITICAL THINKING

- Discuss actions that are appropriate if you feel a mass of stool when inserting a suppository.

SKILL 31–3

ADMINISTERING A CLEANSING ENEMA

Suggested Action	Reason for Action
Assessment	
Check the medical orders for the type of enema and prescribed solution.	Collaborates nursing activities with medical treatment
Check the date of the patient's last bowel movement.	Helps determine the need to check for an impaction or the basis for realistic expected outcomes
Auscultate bowel sounds.	Establishes the status of peristalsis
Determine how much the patient understands about the procedure.	Provides an opportunity for health teaching
Planning	
Plan the location where the patient will expel the enema solution and stool.	Determines if a bedpan is necessary
Obtain appropriate equipment, including an enema set, solution, absorbent pad, lubricant, bath blanket, and gloves.	Facilitates organization and efficient time management
Plan to perform the procedure according to the time specified by the physician or when it is most appropriate during patient care.	Demonstrates collaboration and participation of the patient in decision-making
Prepare the solution and equipment in the utility room.	Provides access to supplies
Warm the solution to approximately 105°F to 110°F (40°C–43°C).	Promotes comfort and safety
Clamp the tubing on the enema set.	Prevents loss of fluid
Fill the container with the specified solution.	Provides the mechanism for cleansing the bowel
Implementation	
Pull the privacy curtain.	Demonstrates respect for the patient's dignity
Place the patient in a Sims' position.	Facilitates access to the rectum
Drape the patient, exposing the buttocks, and place a waterproof pad under the hips.	Preserves modesty and protects bed linen
Wash your hands and don gloves.	Reduces the transmission of microorganisms

continued

SKILL 31-3

ADMINISTERING A CLEANSING ENEMA *Continued*

Suggested Action	Reason for Action
Place (or hang) the solution container so that it is 12 to 20 inches (30–50 cm) above the level of the patient's anus.	Facilitates gravity flow
Open the clamp and fill the tubing with solution. Reclamp.	Purges air from the tubing

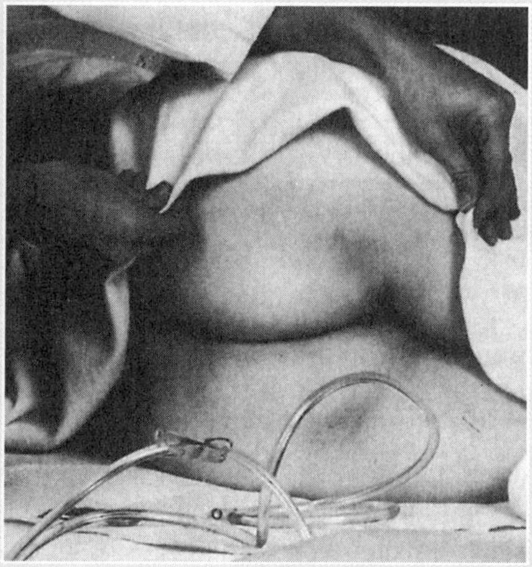

Draping for an enema.

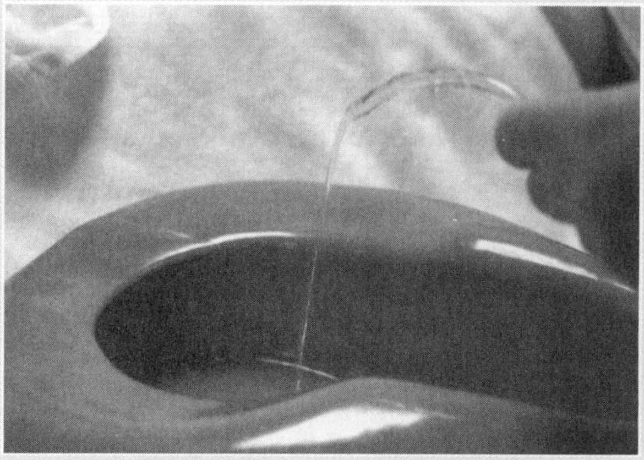

Purging air. (Courtesy of Ken Timby.)

Suggested Action	Reason for Action
Lubricate the tip of the tube generously.	Eases insertion
Separate the buttocks well so that the anus is in plain view.	Helps visualize insertion
Insert the tube 3 to 4 inches (7–10 cm) in an adult.	Places the distal tip above the sphincters
Direct the tubing at an angle pointing toward the umbilicus.	Follows the contour of the rectum

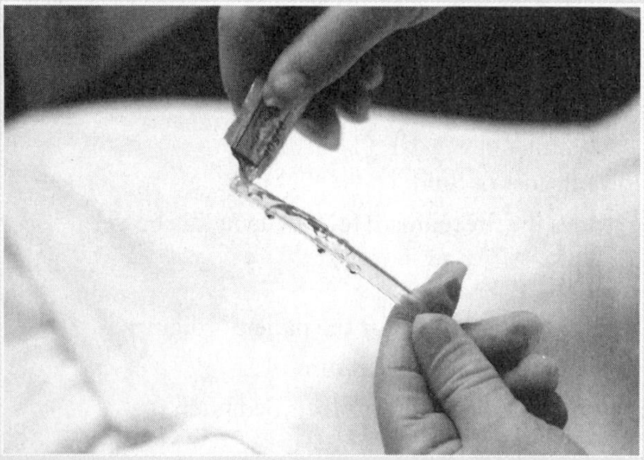

Lubricating tube. (Courtesy of Ken Timby.)

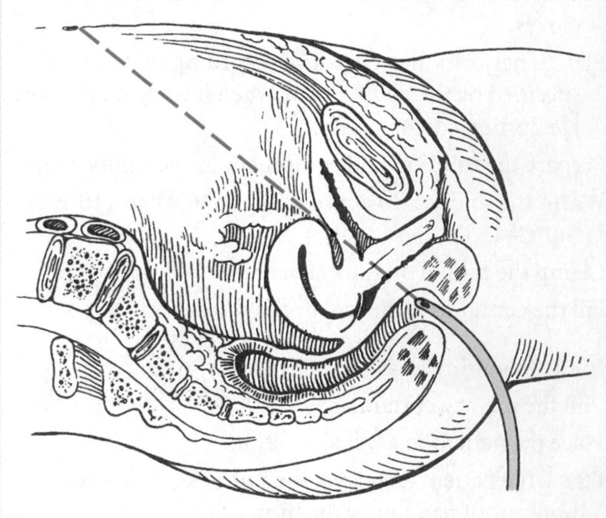

Direction for tube insertion.

continued

SKILL 31-3

ADMINISTERING A CLEANSING ENEMA *Continued*

Suggested Action	Reason for Action
Hold the tube in place with one hand.	Avoids displacement

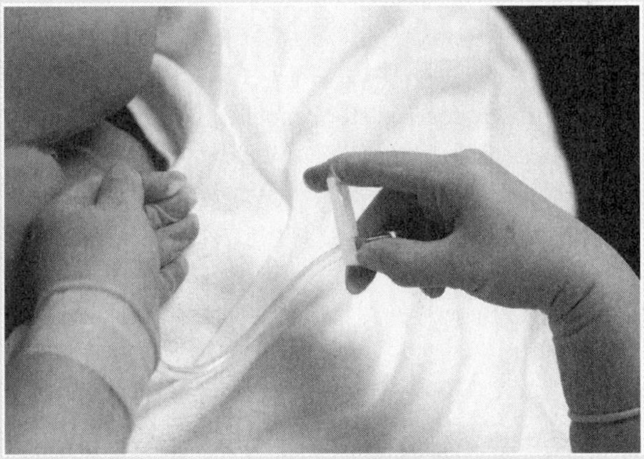

Holding the tube in place. (Courtesy of Ken Timby.)

Suggested Action	Reason for Action
Release the clamp.	Promotes instillation
Instill the solution gradually over 5 to 10 minutes.	Fills the rectum
Clamp the tube for a brief period while the patient takes deep breaths and contracts the anal sphincters if cramping occurs.	Avoids further stimulation
Resume instillation when cramping is relieved.	Facilitates effectiveness
Clamp and remove the tubing after sufficient solution has been instilled or the patient states that he or she is unable to retain more.	Completes the procedure
Encourage the patient to retain the solution for 5 to 15 minutes.	Promotes effectiveness
Hold the enema tubing in one hand and pull a glove over the inserting end of the tubing.	Prevents direct contact
Remove and discard the remaining glove and dispose of the enema equipment.	Follows principles of medical asepsis
Assist the patient to sit while eliminating the solution and stool.	Aids defecation
Examine the expelled solution.	Provides data for evaluating the effectiveness of the procedure
Clean and dry the patient and help to a position of comfort.	Demonstrates concern for well-being

Evaluation

- Sufficient amount of solution is instilled.
- Comparable amount of solution is expelled.
- Patient eliminates stool.

continued

SKILL 31–3

ADMINISTERING A CLEANSING ENEMA *Continued*

Document

- Type of enema solution
- Volume instilled
- Outcome of procedure

SAMPLE DOCUMENTATION

Date and Time 1,000 mL tap water enema administered. Lg. amt of brown, formed stool expelled.

____ SIGNATURE, TITLE

CRITICAL THINKING

- List measures for preventing constipation.
- Identify consequences of self-administering enemas on a regular basis.

SKILL 31–4

CHANGING AN OSTOMY APPLIANCE

Suggested Action	Reason for Action
Assessment	
Inspect the faceplate, pouch, and peristomal skin.	Determines the necessity for changing the appliance and provides data about the condition of the stoma and surrounding skin
Determine how much the patient understands about stomal care and changing an ostomy appliance.	Provides an opportunity for health teaching; prepares the patient for assuming self-care
Planning	
Obtain replacement equipment, supplies for removing the adhesive, such as the manufacturer's recommended solvent if appropriate, and products for skin care.	Facilitates organization and efficient time management
Plan to replace the appliance immediately if the patient has localized symptoms.	Prevents complications
Schedule an appliance change for an asymptomatic patient before a meal and before a bath or shower.	Coincides with a time when the gastrocolic reflex is less active and prevents repeating hygiene
Empty the pouch just before the appliance will be changed.	Prevents soiling
Implementation	
Pull the privacy curtain.	Demonstrates respect for the patient's dignity
Place the patient in a supine or dorsal recumbent position.	Facilitates access to the stoma
Wash your hands and don gloves.	Reduces the transmission of microorganisms
Unfasten the pouch and discard it in a lined receptacle or waterproof container.	Facilitates access to the faceplate
Gently peel the faceplate from the skin.	Prevents skin trauma

continued

SKILL 31-4

CHANGING AN OSTOMY APPLIANCE *Continued*

Suggested Action	Reason for Action
Wash the stoma and peristomal area with water or mild soapy water using a soft washcloth or gauze square.	Cleans mucus and stool from the skin and stoma
Suggest that the patient shower or bathe at this time.	Provides an opportunity for daily hygiene and will not affect the exposed stoma
After bathing or in lieu of bathing, pat the peristomal skin dry.	Promotes potential for adhesion when the faceplate is applied
Measure the stoma using a stomal guide.	Determines the size of the stomal opening in the faceplate

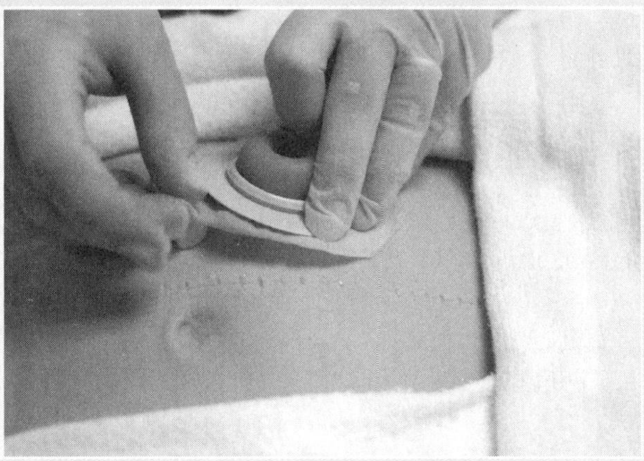

Removing faceplate. (Courtesy of Ken Timby.)

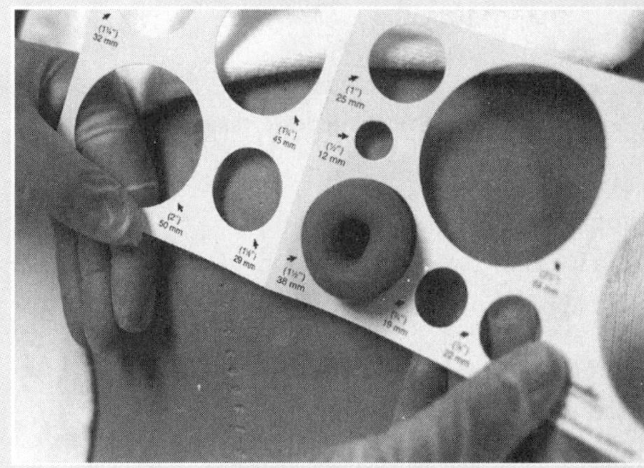

Measuring the stoma. (Courtesy of Ken Timby.)

Suggested Action	Reason for Action
Trim the opening in the faceplate to the measured diameter plus approximately ⅛ to ¼ inch larger.	Avoids pinching of or pressure on the stoma and causing circulatory impairment
Attach a new pouch to the ring of the faceplate.	Avoids pushing it into place after the faceplate has been applied
Fold and clamp the bottom of the pouch.	Seals the pouch so leaking will not occur

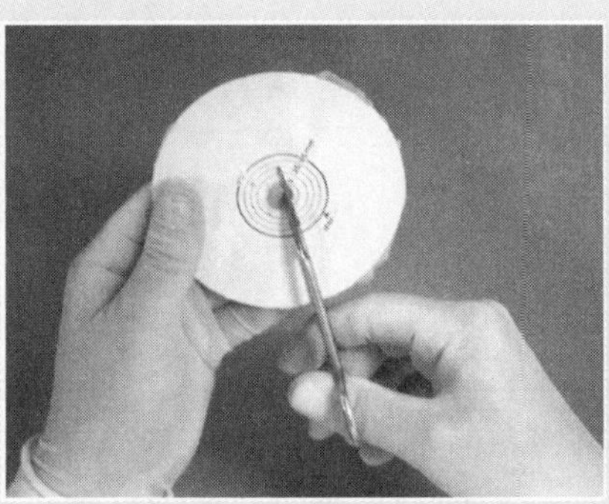

Trimming the stomal opening. (Courtesy of Ken Timby.)

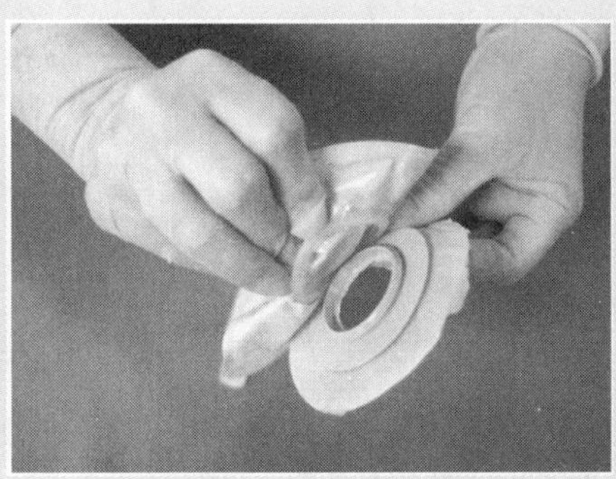

Attaching the pouch. (Courtesy of Ken Timby.)

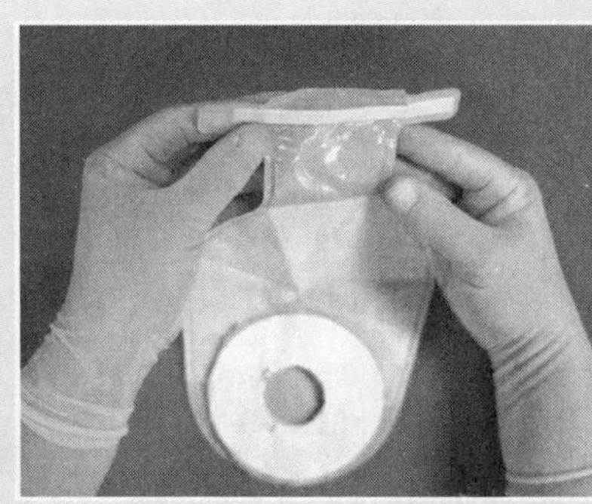

Sealing the pouch. (Courtesy of Ken Timby.)

Suggested Action	Reason for Action
Peel the backing from the adhesive on the faceplate.	Prepares the appliance for application
Have the patient stand or lie flat.	Keeps the skin taut and avoids wrinkles
Position the opening over the stoma and press into place from the center outward.	Prevents air gaps and skin wrinkles

continued

SKILL 31-4

CHANGING AN OSTOMY APPLIANCE *Continued*

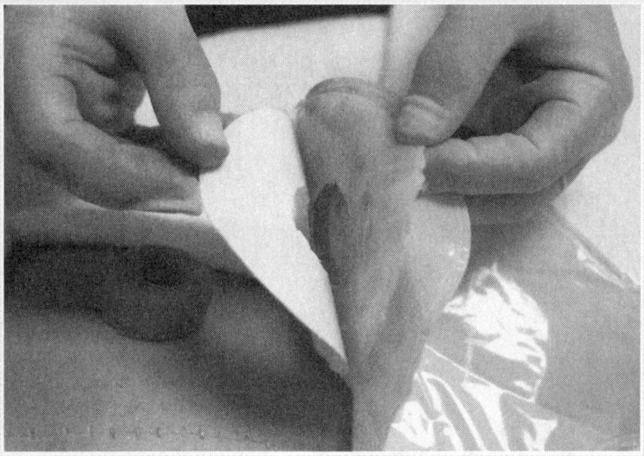

Removing adhesive backing. (Courtesy of Ken Timby.)

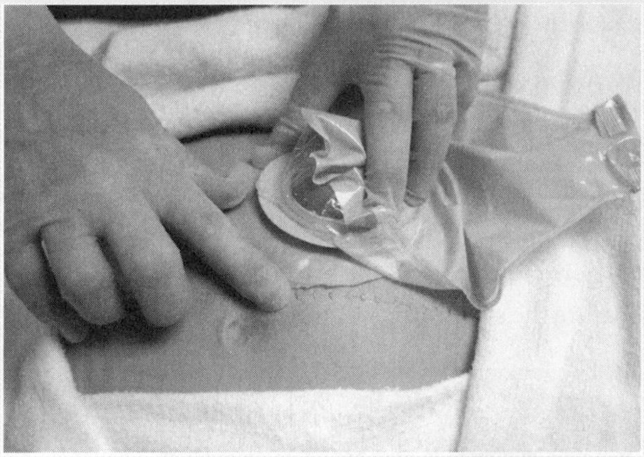

Attaching appliance. (Courtesy of Ken Timby.)

Evaluation

- Stoma appears pink and moist.
- Skin is clean, dry, and intact with no evidence of redness, irritation, or excoriation.
- New appliance adheres to the skin without wrinkles or gaps.

Document

- Assessment data
- Peristomal care
- Application of new appliance

SAMPLE DOCUMENTATION

Date and Time Ostomy appliance removed. Stoma and peristomal skin cleansed with soapy water and patted dry. Stoma is pink and moist. Peristomal skin is intact and painless. New appliance applied over stoma. ______________________________ SIGNATURE, TITLE

CRITICAL THINKING

- Discuss the various ways an ostomy affects the lives of patients who have one.

SKILL 31-5

IRRIGATING A COLOSTOMY

Suggested Action	Reason for Action
Assessment	
Check the medical orders to verify that a written order exists and the type of solution to use.	Collaborates nursing activities with medical treatment
Determine how much the patient understands about a colostomy irrigation.	Provides an opportunity for health teaching; prepares the patient for assuming self-care

continued

SKILL 31-5

IRRIGATING A COLOSTOMY *Continued*

Suggested Action	Reason for Action
Planning	
Obtain an irrigating bag and sleeve, lubricant, and belt. A bedpan will be needed if the patient is confined to bed.	Promotes organization and efficient time management
Prepare the irrigating bag with solution in the same way as an enema set is prepared (see Skill 31-3).	Provides the mechanism for cleansing the bowel
Unclamp the tubing and fill it with solution.	Purges air from the tubing
Implementation	
Place the patient in a sitting position in bed, in a chair in front or beside the toilet, or on the toilet itself.	Facilitates collecting drainage
Place absorbent pads or towels on the patient's lap.	Prevents soiling of linen or clothing
Hang the container approximately 12 inches (30 cm) above the stoma.	Facilitates gravity flow
Wash your hands and don gloves.	Reduces the transmission of microorganisms
Empty and remove the pouch from the faceplate, if one is worn.	Provides access to the stoma
Secure the sleeve over the stoma and fasten it about the patient with an elastic belt.	Provides a pathway for drainage

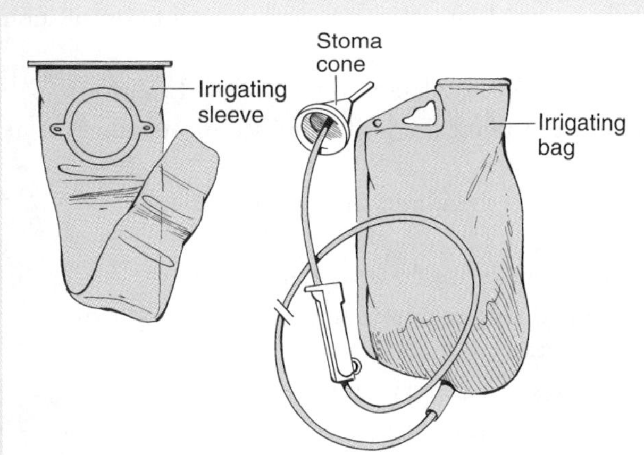

Irrigating sleeve and bag.

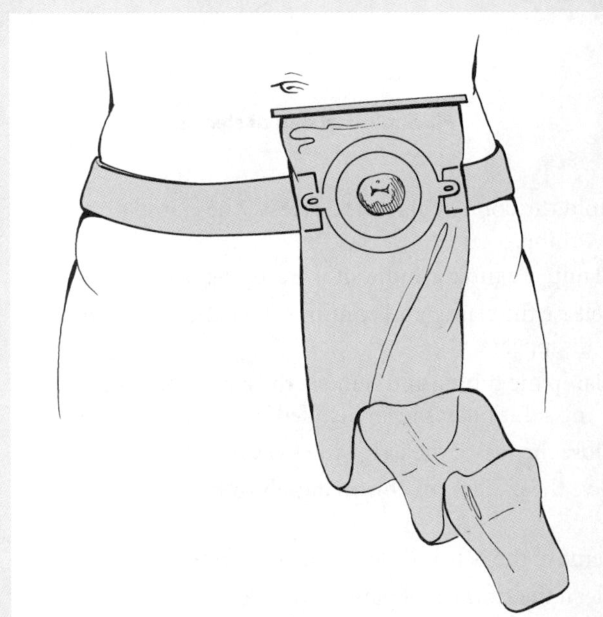

Positioning irrigation sleeve.

Suggested Action	Reason for Action
Place the lower end of the sleeve into the toilet, commode, or a bedpan.	Collects drainage
Lubricate the cone at the end of the irrigating bag.	Facilitates insertion
Open the top of the irrigating sleeve.	Provides access to the stoma
Insert the cone into the stoma.	Dilates the stoma and provides a means for instilling fluid

continued

SKILL 31–5

IRRIGATING A COLOSTOMY *Continued*

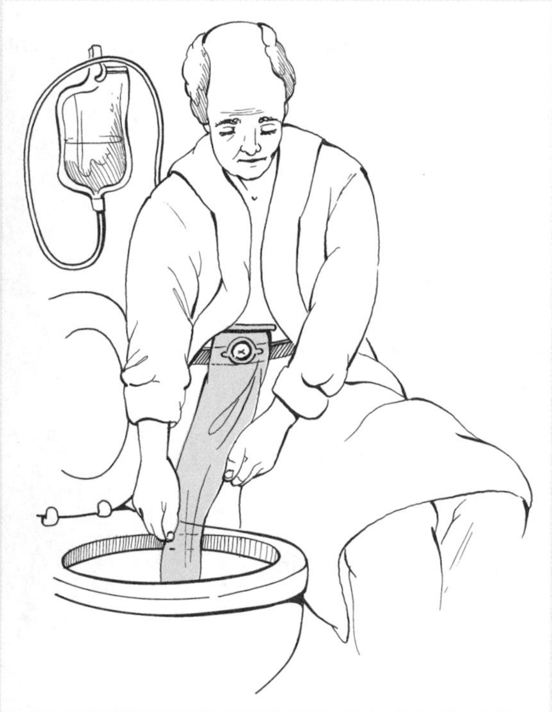

Placing distal end of sleeve.

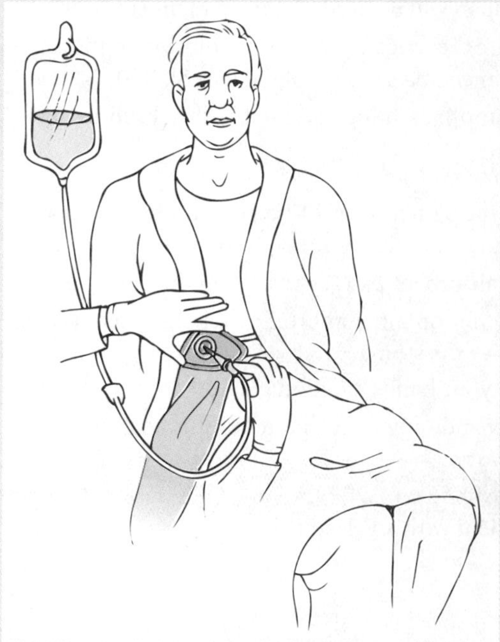

Inserting irrigation cone.

Suggested Action	Reason for Action
Hold the cone in place and release the clamp on the tubing.	Prevents expulsion of the cone and initiates the instillation
Clamp the tubing and wait if cramping occurs.	Interrupts the instillation while the bowel adjusts
Release the clamp and continue once the discomfort disappears.	Resumes instilling fluid without discomfort to the patient
Clamp the tubing and remove the cone when the irrigating solution has been instilled.	Discontinues the administration of solution
Close the top of the irrigating sleeve.	Keeps drainage in a downward direction
Give the patient reading materials or hygiene supplies.	Provides diversion or uses time for other productive activities
Remove the belt and sleeve when draining has stopped.	Eliminates unnecessary equipment
Clean the stoma and pat it dry.	Maintains tissue integrity
If an appliance is worn, place a clean pouch over the stoma, or cover the stoma temporarily with a gauze square.	Collects fecal drainage

Evaluation

- Sufficient amount of solution is instilled.
- Comparable amount of solution is expelled.
- Stool is eliminated.

continued

SKILL 31-5

IRRIGATING A COLOSTOMY *Continued*

Document

- Type of irrigation solution
- Volume instilled
- Outcome of procedure

SAMPLE DOCUMENTATION

Date and Time Colostomy irrigated with 500 mL of tap water. Instilled without difficulty. Mod. amt. of semiformed stool expelled with solution. Stoma cleansed with soapy water and dried. Covered with a gauze square. ________________________ SIGNATURE, TITLE

CRITICAL THINKING

- Discuss possible nursing actions if the irrigation solution will not instill or drain as expected.

UNIT TEN

MEDICATION ADMINISTRATION

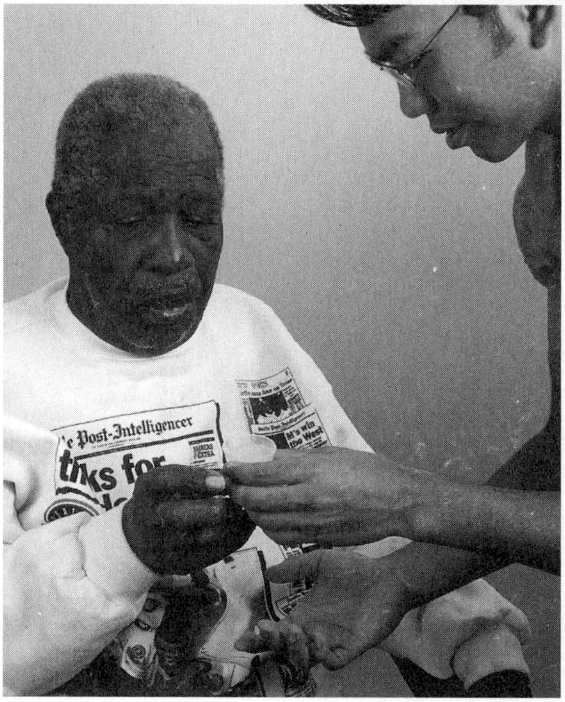

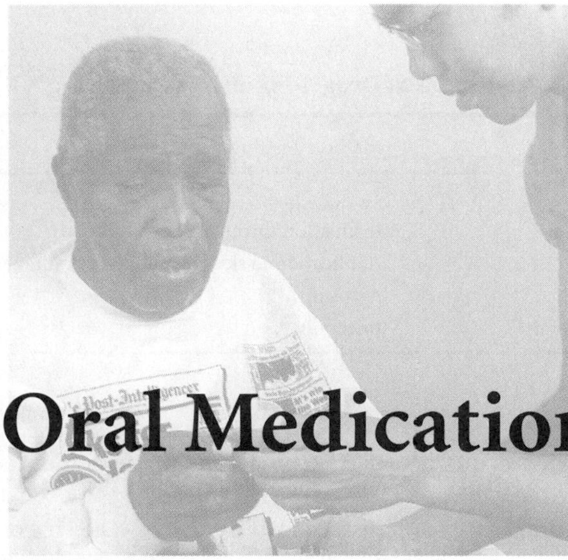

CHAPTER 32

Oral Medications

CHAPTER OUTLINE

Medication Orders
Medication Administration Record
Methods of Supplying Medications
Medication Administration
Nursing Implications

NURSING GUIDELINES

TAKING TELEPHONE ORDERS
PREPARING MEDICATIONS SAFELY
PREPARING MEDICATIONS FOR ENTERAL TUBE ADMINISTRATION

SKILLS

SKILL 32-1: ADMINISTERING ORAL MEDICATIONS
SKILL 32-2: ADMINISTERING MEDICATIONS THROUGH AN ENTERAL TUBE

NURSING CARE PLAN

NONCOMPLIANCE

KEY TERMS

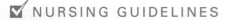

dose
enteric-coated tablet
generic name
individual supply
medication administration record
medication order
medications
oral route
over-the-counter medication
polypharmacy
route of administration
scored tablet
stock supply
sustained release
trade name
unit dose

LEARNING OBJECTIVES

An understanding of the content within this chapter will be evidenced by the student's ability to:

- Describe a medication.
- Name seven components of a drug order.
- Explain the difference between trade and generic drug names.
- Name four common routes for administration.
- Describe the oral route.
- Name two general forms of medications that are administered by the oral route.
- Explain the purpose of a medication record.
- Name three ways that drugs are supplied.
- Discuss two nursing responsibilities that apply to the administration of narcotics.
- Name the five rights of medication administration.
- Give the formula for calculating a drug dose.
- Discuss at least one guideline that applies to the safe administration of medications.
- Discuss one point to stress when teaching patients about taking medications.
- Explain the circumstances when oral medications are given by an enteral tube.
- Identify one common problem associated with administering medications through an enteral tube.
- Describe three actions that are appropriate if a medication error occurs.

Among one of the nurse's most important responsibilities is the administration of **medications** (chemical substances that change body function). (In this chapter, the terms "medications" and "drugs" are used synonymously.) This chapter emphasizes the safe preparation and administration of medications, particularly those given by the oral route. Information on specific drugs can be found in pharmacology texts or drug reference manuals.

Medication Orders

A **medication order** (drug name and directions for its administration) is usually written by a physician or dentist. Other persons, such as a physician's assistant or advanced practice nurse, if legally designated by state statutes, also can write medication orders. Medication orders written on the patient's medical record are used here for the purposes of discussion.

TABLE 32–1. **Routes of Drug Administration**

Route	Method of Administration
Oral	Swallowing Instillation through an enteral tube
Topical	Application to skin or mucous membrane
Inhalant	Aerosol
Parenteral	Injection

COMPONENTS OF A MEDICATION ORDER

All medication orders must have seven components:

1. Patient's name
2. Date and time the order is written
3. Drug name
4. Dose to be administered
5. Route of administration
6. Frequency of administration
7. Signature of the person ordering the drug

If any one of these components is absent, the drug is withheld until the missing information is obtained. Medication errors are serious. *A questionable medication order is never implemented until after consulting with the person who has written the order.*

Drug Name

Each drug has a **trade name** (name used by the pharmaceutical company that makes the drug). A trade name is sometimes called a brand or proprietary name. Drugs also have a **generic name** (chemical name that is not protected by a company's trademark). For example, Demerol is a trade name used by Winthrop Pharmaceuticals for the generically named drug meperidine hydrochloride.

Drug Dose

The **dose** (amount of drug to be administered) is prescribed using the metric system or, sometimes, the apothecary system of measurement. For home use, metric and apothecary doses are sometimes converted to household measurements that are more easily interpreted by nonprofessionals.

Route of Administration

The **route of administration** (manner in which the drug is given) may be the oral, topical, inhalant, or parenteral route (Table 32-1). Topical and inhalant routes of administration are discussed in Chapter 33; parenteral administration is described in Chapters 34 and 35.

The **oral route** (administration of drugs by swallowing or instillation through an enteral tube) allows drug absorption through the gastrointestinal tract. The oral route is the most common route for medication administration because it is safer, more economical, and more comfortable than others. Medications administered by the oral route come in both solid and liquid forms.

Solid medications include tablets and capsules. One solid drug form is a **scored tablet** (manufactured with a groove in the center), which is convenient when only part of a tablet is needed. Another solid drug form is an **enteric-coated tablet** (drug covered with a substance that dissolves beyond the stomach). Enteric-coated tablets are never cut, crushed, or chewed because when the integrity of the coating is impaired, the drug is released too soon. Some capsules also contain beads or pellets of drugs for **sustained release** (drug that dissolves at timed intervals). Sustained-release capsules are never opened or crushed: doing so affects the rate of drug absorption.

Liquid forms of oral drugs include syrups, elixirs, and suspensions. Liquid medications are measured and administered in calibrated cups, droppers, or syringes or with a dosing spoon (Fig. 32-1).

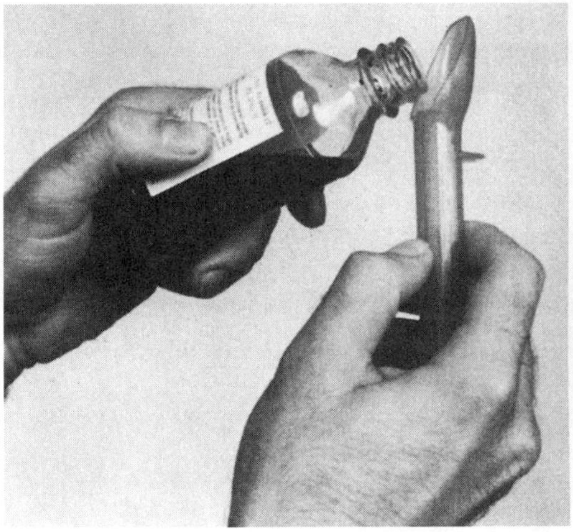

FIGURE 32–1. A dosing spoon.

Frequency of Administration

The frequency of drug administration refers to how often and how regularly the medication is to be administered. The frequency of administration is written using standard abbreviations that have their origin in Latin words. Some common words used in medication administration are:

- Stat—Immediately
- q.d.—Every day
- q.o.d—Every other day
- b.i.d.—Twice a day
- t.i.d.—Three times a day
- q.i.d.—Four times a day
- q.h.—Hourly
- q4h—Every 4 hours

Chapter 9 and Appendix A list other common abbreviations.

When the medication order is implemented, the drug administration is scheduled according to the prescribed frequency. Drug administrations are scheduled according to a predetermined timetable set by the health agency. The hours of administration may vary from one agency to another. For example, if a physician orders a q.i.d. (four times a day) administration of a medication, it may be scheduled for administration at 8 a.m., noon, 4 p.m., and 8 p.m., or 10 a.m., 2 p.m., 6 p.m., and 10 p.m., or 6 a.m., noon, 6 p.m., and midnight.

VERBAL ORDERS

Verbal orders are instructions for patient care that are given during a face-to-face conversation or by telephone. Verbal instructions are more likely to result in misinterpretation than those that are written. If the prescriber is physically present, it is appropriate to ask tactfully that the order be handwritten. In the absence of the prescriber, it is sometimes necessary to obtain verbal orders by telephone.

Nursing Guidelines For

Taking Telephone Orders

☑ Have a second nurse listen simultaneously on an extension.
RATIONALE: Provides a witness to the communication

☑ Record the drug order directly on the patient's record.
RATIONALE: Avoids errors in memory

☑ Repeat the written information back to the prescriber.
RATIONALE: Clarifies understanding

☑ Make sure the order includes the essential components of a drug order.
RATIONALE: Complies with standards for care

☑ Clarify any drug names that sound similar, such as Feldene and Seldane, Nicobid and Nitro-Bid.
RATIONALE: Avoids medication errors

☑ Spell or repeat numbers that could be misinterpreted, such as 15 (one, five) and 50 (five, zero)
RATIONALE: Avoids medication errors

☑ Use the abbreviation "T.O." at the end of the order.
RATIONALE: Indicates the order is a telephone order

☑ Write the prescriber's name, and cosign with your name and title.
RATIONALE: Complies with legal standards and demonstrates accountability for the communication

DOCUMENTATION IN THE MEDICATION ADMINISTRATION RECORD

Once the medication order is obtained, the order is transcribed to the **medication administration record** (MAR; agency form used to document drug administration). Use of the MAR ensures the timely and safe administration of medications. Some use a form on which the drug order is transcribed by hand; others use a computer-generated form (Fig. 32-2). Regardless of the type used, all MARs provide a space for documenting when a drug is administered, along with a place for the signature, title, and initials of each nurse who administers a medication. The current MAR is usually kept separate from the patient's medical record, but it eventually becomes a permanent part of it.

Methods of Supplying Medications

After the medication order is transcribed to the MAR, the drug is requested from the pharmacy. Drugs are supplied, or dispensed, in three major ways. An **individual supply** (container of prescribed drug with enough of the drug for several days or weeks) is generally provided to long-term care facilities such as nursing homes (Fig. 32-3). A **unit dose supply** (self-contained packet that holds one tablet or capsule) is most common in acute care hospitals where drugs are stocked for individual patients several times in one day (Fig. 32-4). A **stock supply** (stored drugs) is kept on the nursing unit for use in an emergency or so that a drug can be administered without delay.

Some facilities use automated medication-dispensing systems. These systems usually contain frequently used medications for that unit, any as-needed (PRN) medications, controlled drugs, and emergency medications. The nurse accesses the system by using a password and then selects the appropriate choice from a computerized menu. This type of system automatically keeps a record of medications used.

MEDICATION ADMINISTRATION RECORD

PAGE 1

PHARMACY/CHART

SHIFT	FULL NAME/TITLE	INITIAL
0701 - 1500		
0701 - 1500		
0701 - 1500		
1501 - 2300		
1501 - 2300		
1501 - 2300		
2301 - 0700		
2301 - 0700		

01/02/00 00010 7
TESTDP DON'T DISC AGE: 041
00000000107 DEMPSEY. JAMES
ACCT #: 000000108 ADMIT DATE 12/31/99
DIAG.: ASTHMA-EXACERBATED BY PNEUMONIA
ALL: CODEINE TETRACYCLINE

	1501 01/02/00 THRU 1500 DATE 01/03/00	1501-2300	2301-0700	0701-1500	COMMENTS
1	(01016) 01/01/00 1800 SOLU-CORTEF 100 MG/2ML-HYDROCORT DOSE: 100 MG. IP Q6H IP RATE = 500 MG. OVER 1 MIN. ABBOTT	1800	0000 0600	1200	
2	(03090) 12/31/99 0900 ACETAMINOPHEN EXTRA ST.CAP DOSE: 1 PO Q DAY TYLENOL			0900	
3	(04841) 01/01/00 0900 TENORMIN TAB. 50 MG. DOSE: 50 MG. PO Q DAY			0900	
4	(03096) 01/01/00 0900 LANOXIN (DIGOXIN) TAB. 0.25 MG. DOSE: 0.25 MG. PO Q DAY			0900	
5	(00543) 01/01/00 1800 BRETHINE AMP. 1 MG./ML. 1 ML. DOSE: 0.25MG SC Q6H (TERBUTALINE)	1800	0000 0600	1200	
6					
7					
8					
9					
10					
11					
12					
13					

TESTDP DON'T DIS 00000000107 DEMPSEY. JAMES THRU 1500 01/03/00

FIGURE 32–2. A computer-generated medication administration record (MAR).

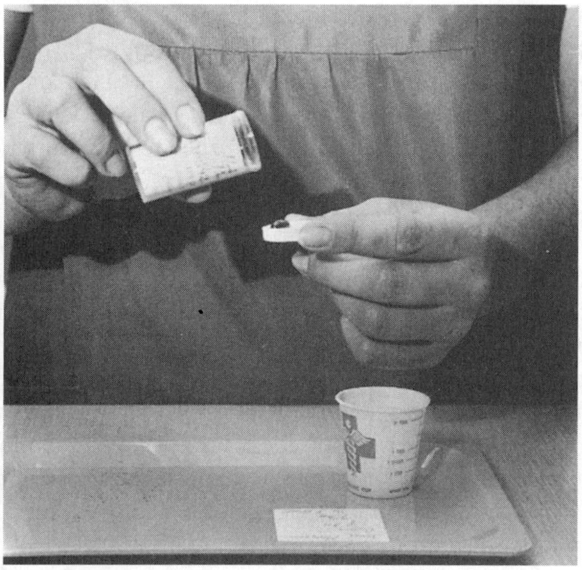

FIGURE 32–3. Medication from an individual supply.

STORING MEDICATIONS

In each health agency, there is one area where drugs are stored. Some agencies keep medications in a mobile cart; others store them in a separate room. Each patient has a separate drawer or cubicle in which his or her prescribed medications are kept. Regardless of their location, medications are kept locked up until they are administered.

ACCOUNTING FOR NARCOTICS

Narcotics are controlled substances, meaning that there are federal laws regulating their possession and administration. In health agencies, narcotics are kept in a double-locked drawer, box, or room on the nursing unit. Because narcotics are usually delivered by stock supply, nurses are responsible for an accurate account of their use. A record is kept of each narcotic that is used from the stock supply.

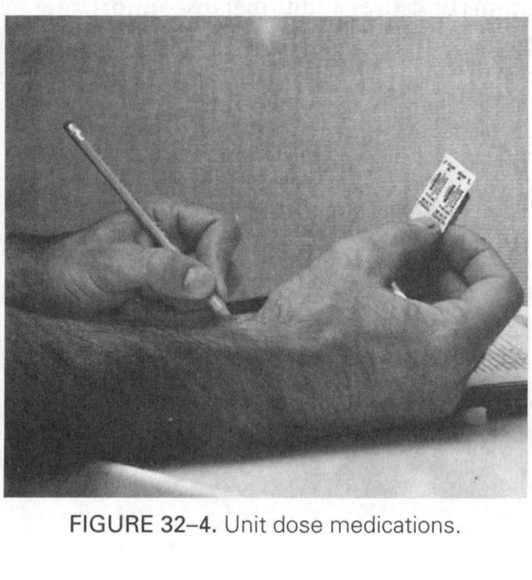

FIGURE 32–4. Unit dose medications.

Narcotics are counted at each change of shift. One nurse counts the number in the supply while another checks the record of their administration. Both counts must agree. Inconsistencies are accounted for as soon as possible.

Medication Administration

Safety is the main concern in medication administration. By taking various precautions before, during, and after the administration of medications, the potential for making medication errors is reduced. Some of the precautions include ensuring the five rights of medication administration, calculating drug dosages accurately, preparing medications carefully, and recording their administration.

APPLYING THE FIVE RIGHTS

To ensure that medication errors do not occur, nurses follow the five rights of medication administration (Fig. 32-5). Some nurses have added a sixth right, the right to refuse. Every rational adult patient has the right to refuse medication. If this happens, the nurse identifies the reason why the drug was not administered, circles the scheduled time on the MAR, and reports the situation to the prescriber.

CALCULATING DOSAGES

One of the major nursing responsibilities, and one of the five rights, is preparing the dose accurately. Preparing an accurate dose sometimes requires the nurse to convert doses into the metric, apothecary, and household equivalents. Once the pre-

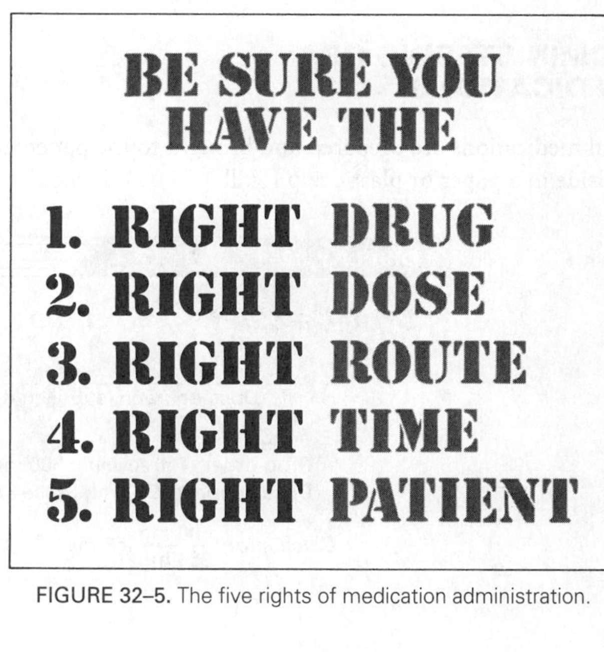

BE SURE YOU
HAVE THE
1. RIGHT DRUG
2. RIGHT DOSE
3. RIGHT ROUTE
4. RIGHT TIME
5. RIGHT PATIENT

FIGURE 32–5. The five rights of medication administration.

scribed and supplied amounts are in the same measurements and system of measurement, the quantity for administration can be easily calculated using a standard formula (Display 32-1).

Nursing Guidelines For

Preparing Medications Safely

- Prepare medications under well-lighted conditions.
  RATIONALE: Improves the ability to read labels accurately
- Work alone, without interruptions and distractions.
  RATIONALE: Promotes concentration
- Check the label of the drug container three times: (1) when reaching for the medication, (2) just before placing the medication into an administration cup, and (3) when returning the medication to the patient's drawer.
  RATIONALE: Ensures attention to important information
- Avoid using medications from containers with a missing or obliterated label.
  RATIONALE: Eliminates speculating on the drug name or dose
- Return medications with dubious or obscured labels to the pharmacy.
  RATIONALE: Facilitates replacement or new labeling
- Never transfer medications from one container to another.
  RATIONALE: Avoids mismatching contents
- Check the expiration dates on liquid medications.
  RATIONALE: Ensures administration at desired potency
- Inspect the medication and reject any that appears to be decomposing.
  RATIONALE: Promotes appropriate absorption

ADMINISTERING ORAL MEDICATIONS

Oral medications are prepared and brought to the patient's bedside in a paper or plastic cup (Skill 32-1). Only medications that the nurse has personally prepared are administered to patients; *never administer medications prepared by another nurse.* Once at the bedside, it also is important to remain with the patient while medications are taken. If the patient is not on the unit, the medications are returned to the medication cart or room. Leaving medications unattended may result in their loss or accidental ingestion by another patient.

Many opportunities exist for patient teaching when administering medications. Teaching is especially important before discharge, because the patient is often given prescriptions for oral medications. This opportunity for health teaching helps to ensure that patients administer their own medications safely and remain compliant. Compliance means that the patient follows instructions for medication administration. Even patients who purchase **over-the-counter medications** (nonprescription drugs) may benefit from instruction about medications.

Patient Teaching Guidelines For

Taking Medications

Teach the patient and family to do the following:

- Inform the prescriber of all other drugs that are currently prescribed or being taken.
- Have prescriptions filled at the same pharmacy so that the pharmacist can spot any potential drug interactions.
- Ask for a new prescription to be filled only partially. This provides an opportunity to evaluate the drug's effect and side effects before purchasing the full amount.
- Read and follow label directions carefully.
- Take prescription medication for the full time that it has been prescribed.
- Check with the prescriber before combining nonprescription drugs with prescription drugs.
- Dispose of old prescription drugs and outdated over-the-counter medications; they tend to disintegrate or change in potency.
- Consult with the prescriber if a drug does not relieve symptoms or causes additional discomfort.
- Ask the prescriber or pharmacist if it is appropriate to take specific medications with food or on an empty stomach.

DISPLAY 32–1

Drug Calculation Formula

$$\frac{D}{H} \times Q - \frac{\textit{Desired}\text{ dose}}{\text{Dose on }\textit{hand}\text{ (supplied dose)}} \times \textit{Quantity} = \text{Amount to administer}$$

Example

Drug order: Tetracycline 500 mg (*desired dose*) by mouth q.i.d.
Dose supplied: 250 mg (*dose on hand*) per 5 mL (*quantity*)

Calculation: $\frac{500\text{ mg}}{250\text{ mg}} \times 5\text{ mL} = 10\text{ mL}$

- Drink a liberal amount of water or other fluids each day so that drugs can be absorbed and eliminated appropriately.
- Do not take drugs prescribed for someone else, even if your symptoms are similar.
- Wear a Medic-Alert tag if prescription drugs are taken on a regular and long-term basis.
- Use a pill organizer if you have trouble remembering whether you took a medication (Fig. 32-6).

ADMINISTERING ORAL MEDICATIONS BY ENTERAL TUBE

Oral medications can be instilled by enteral tube when they cannot be swallowed (Skill 32-2). Because the lumen of a tube is smaller than the esophagus, special techniques may be required to avoid obstructing the tube.

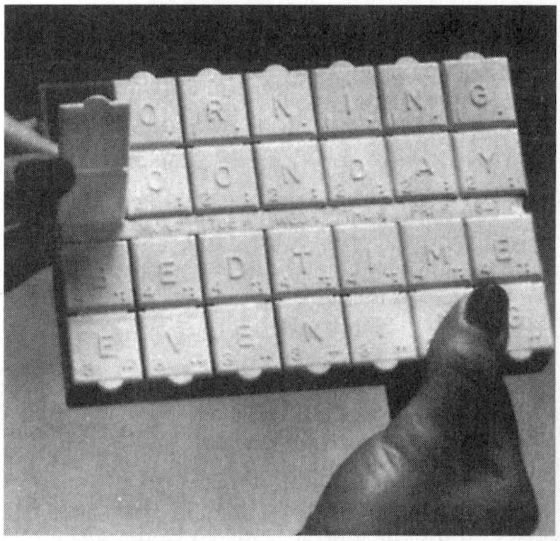

FIGURE 32–6. A pill organizer. (Courtesy of Apex Medical Corporation, Bloomington, MN.)

Nursing Guidelines For

Preparing Medications for Enteral Tube Administration

- Use the liquid form of the drug whenever possible.
  RATIONALE: Promotes tube patency
- Add 15 to 60 mL of water to liquid medications that are thick.
  RATIONALE: Dilutes the medication and facilitates instillation
- Pulverize tablets, except those that are enteric-coated.
  RATIONALE: Creates small granules that may instill more readily
- Open the shell of a capsule to release the powdered drug.
  RATIONALE: Facilitates mixing into a liquid form
- Avoid crushing sustained-release pellets.
  RATIONALE: Ensures their sequential rate of absorption
- Mix each drug separately with at least 15 to 30 mL of water.
  RATIONALE: Provides a medium and dilute volume for administration
- Use warm water when mixing powdered drugs.
  RATIONALE: Promotes dissolving the solid form
- Pierce the end of a sealed gelatin capsule and squeeze out the liquid medication, or aspirate it with a needle and syringe.
  RATIONALE: Facilitates access to the medication
- As an alternative, soak a soft gelatin capsule in 15 to 30 mL of warm water for approximately 1 hour.
  RATIONALE: Dissolves the gelatin seal
- Avoid administering bulk-forming laxatives through an enteral tube.
  RATIONALE: Reduces the potential for obstructing the tube
- Interrupt a tube feeding for 15 to 30 minutes before and after the administration of a drug that should be given on an empty stomach.
  RATIONALE: Facilitates the drug's therapeutic action or its absorption

Slightly different techniques are used for administering medications through an enteral tube that is being used for decompression and one being used for nourishment.

Medications may be given through gastric tubes used for decompression (e.g., suctioning; see Chap. 29). After drug administration, the tube is clamped or plugged for at least a half-hour. This allows adequate absorption and prevents removing the drug before it leaves the stomach.

Medications can be given while a patient is receiving tube feedings, but the medications are instilled separately—that is, they are not added to the formula. This is done for two reasons. First, some drugs may physically interact with the components in the formula, causing it to curdle or otherwise change its consistency. Also, a slow infusion would alter the drug's dose and rate of absorption.

DOCUMENTATION

Medication administration is documented on the MAR, the patient's chart, or both as soon as possible. Timely documentation prevents medication errors: if the dose is not recorded, another nurse may assume that the patient has not received the medication and may give a second dose. Documentation also demonstrates that the medication order has been implemented.

If a medication is withheld, its omission is documented according to agency policy. This is commonly done by circling the time of administration and initialing the entry. The reason for the omission may be documented in a comment section on the MAR or elsewhere in the patient's medical record.

MEDICATION ERRORS

Medication errors do happen. When they do, nurses have an ethical and legal responsibility to report them so that the patient's safety is maintained.

As soon as an error is recognized, the patient's condition is checked and the mistake is reported to the prescriber and the supervising nurse immediately. Health care agencies have a form for reporting medication errors called an incident sheet or accident sheet (see Chap. 3). The incident sheet is not a part of the patient's permanent record, nor is any reference made in the chart to the fact that an incident sheet has been completed.

Nursing Implications

Whenever nursing care involves the administration of medications, one or more of the following nursing diagnoses may be applicable:

- Knowledge deficit
- Risk for aspiration
- Ineffective management of therapeutic regimen
- Altered health maintenance
- Noncompliance

The nursing care plan shows how the steps in the nursing process are followed to manage the care of a patient with the nursing diagnosis of Noncompliance, defined by NANDA (1999) as

> . . . the extent to which a person's and/or caregiver's behavior coincides or fails to coincide with a health-promoting or therapeutic plan agreed upon by the person (and/or family, and/or community) and health care professional. In the presence of an agreed-upon, health-promoting or therapeutic plan, person's or caregiver's behavior may be fully, partially, or nonadherent and may lead to clinically effective, partially effective, or ineffective outcomes.

Nursing Care Plan

Noncompliance

Assessment

Subjective Data

States, "I didn't get my prescription refilled. I wasn't having any chest pain and I didn't think I needed to take my pills anymore. My sister and I figured the surgery fixed my heart."

Objective Data

63-year-old man admitted for chest pain and dyspnea. Lives with widowed sister who remains employed. Was discharged 6 weeks ago after coronary bypass surgery. Was to continue taking a beta-blocker (Tenormin 50 mg PO daily) and a diuretic (Lasix 20 mg PO q.o.d.). Abruptly stopped taking both medications 1 week ago. Pulse rate is 94 at rest and BP is 178/94 in R arm while sitting.

Diagnosis

Noncompliance related to inaccurate health belief

Plan

Goal

The patient will explain the consequences that can occur if medications are not taken by 3/7.

Orders: 3/5

1. Explain the following at separate times during the next 2 days:
   - The purpose for reducing myocardial oxygen consumption
   - The benefit for lowering blood pressure
   - The advantage of reducing blood volume
   - The therapeutic actions of Tenormin and Lasix
2. Have patient rephrase explanations in his own words and note his level of understanding; clarify any misunderstanding immediately.
3. Go over schedule of medication administration on 3/7 with patient and again with patient and his sister before discharge.
4. Advise the patient to discuss any deviations in medication schedule or dosage with his physician. ____________ M. Mohney, RN

continued

Nursing Care Plan — Noncompliance *Continued*

Implementation (Documentation)	3/5	0930	Chest pain relieved by sublingual nitroglycerin administered 30 minutes earlier. Has voided 700 mL of urine in past hour after IV Lasix. Resting comfortably. Pulse = 90 bpm, BP 156/90 R arm in semi-Fowler's position. ______ B. VIANNY, LPN
		1000	Explained that the nitroglycerin dilates blood vessels and eases the work of the heart. Used the analogy of blowing air through a very narrow straw vs. a very wide one. Informed that one of the actions of Tenormin is to reduce blood pressure and therefore reduce the work of the heart and its need for oxygen. ______ B. VIANNY, LPN
Evaluation (Documentation)		1015	Could paraphrase explanation correctly. States, "I know people take nitroglycerin for chest pain, but I didn't know how it helped relieve it. I'd rather take a pill once a day and prevent chest pain than have to take a pill to get rid of it." ______ B. VIANNY, LPN

FOCUS ON OLDER ADULTS

- Several age-related changes can influence the way medications act in older adults: diminished kidney and liver function increase the concentration of many medications; increased proportions of body water and fat and decreased proportion of lean tissue affect the concentration of some medications; lower albumin levels in the blood increase the amount of active drug components for medications that are protein-bound; and alterations in the gastric acidity alter the absorption of some medications. The degree to which medications are influenced by these age-related changes is highly influenced by the chemical properties of the medication. For example, only medications that are excreted through the kidneys are influenced by age-related changes in the urinary system.
- **Polypharmacy** (administration of multiple medications to the same person) in older adults increases the risk for drug interactions and adverse medication reactions. Thus, older adults who are taking more than one medication are more likely than younger adults to develop mental changes as an early and common sign of adverse medications effects. In fact, medications are the most common physiologic cause of mental changes in older adults. Therefore, any change in the mental status of an older adult must be reported.
- Older adults who have had cerebrovascular accidents (strokes) or who are experiencing middle and later stages of dementia often have an impaired ability to swallow. Speech therapists are helpful in evaluating swallowing difficulties (dysphagia) and recommending safe and effective methods of administering oral medications.
- Mixing oral medications with a small amount of soft food (such as applesauce) facilitates administration. Before altering oral medications, however, the pharmacist must be contacted to determine if there are any contraindications to crushing and mixing the medications.
- If an older adult has any difficulty comprehending information about medication routines, a second responsible person must be included in the discharge instructions to ensure the patient's safety. A referral for skilled nursing visits is appropriate for homebound older adults who need additional instructions about medication routines after discharge.
- Glasses or hearing aids, if needed by the older adult, should be worn to ensure the best conditions for teaching. Also, appropriate environmental surroundings, such as adequate non-glare lighting and little if any background noise, are important.
- Having the older adult repeat information after providing instructions on medications is a means of evaluating his or her comprehension. Verbal instructions are reinforced with simple written instructions. Use a copy machine to enlarge instructions for patients with visual impairments or difficulties. Written instructions are particularly important for patients with hearing impairments and those who have difficulty remembering or comprehending information.
- If the medication regimen is complex, the prescribing practitioner may be able to simplify it if asked. In some instances, a longer-acting medication can be used to decrease the frequency of administration or the number of pills the patient must take at one time.
- Older adults who have insurance coverage for payment of prescriptions may find it easier and more economical to have the prescriptions filled at 3-month intervals. It also may be more economical to purchase the prescriptions by mail if this option is provided by the insurance carrier.
- As a cost-saving measure, older adults are encouraged to question the primary care provider about prescribing generic forms of the medication.
- If manual dexterity or strength problems are evident, older adults may request that the pharmacist use non-childproof caps on their prescription containers.
- Older adults who are visually impaired benefit from suggestions on how to identify medication containers other than by reading the labels. Suggestions include using rubber bands or textured materials on certain containers or using bright colors to mark the labels. Many simple-to-use medication management systems are available. Often a family member is helpful in setting up weekly medication management systems. For example, a family member may set out the medications in specially designed containers on a weekly basis. While providing a mechanism for others to monitor patterns and adherence to the regimen, this method is especially important when working with older adults who have memory impairments.

KEY CONCEPTS

- A medication is a chemical substance that changes body function.
- A complete drug order contains the date and time of the order, the name of the patient, the name of the drug, its dose, route, and frequency of administration, and the signature or name of the writer.
- A drug's trade name is the name used by the manufacturer of the drug. The drug's generic name is a chemical name that is not protected by a company's trademark.
- Common routes of medication administration are the oral, topical, inhalant, and parenteral routes.
- The oral route is used to administer drugs that are intended for absorption in the gastrointestinal tract. Oral medications can be instilled by enteral tube when they cannot be swallowed.
- A medication administration record (MAR) is a form used to document drug administration to ensure the timely and safe administration of medications.
- Methods of supplying drugs to nursing units include an individual supply, a supply of unit dose packets, and a stock supply.
- Nurses are responsible for keeping the supply of narcotic medications locked and maintaining an accurate record of their use.
- The five rights involve making sure that the right patient receives the right drug, in the right dose, at the right time, and by the right route.
- Once drug doses are converted to the same system of measurement and the same measurement within that system, the amount to be administered can be calculated by dividing the desired dose by the dose on hand and then multiplying it by the quantity of the supply.
- The nurse should check the drug label three times before administering the medication.
- When teaching patients about taking medications, advise them to inform each health care provider of all prescription and nonprescription drugs currently being taken.
- A common problem when administering drugs through an enteral tube is maintaining the tube's patency.
- If a medication error occurs, nurses must report the error to the prescriber and supervisor, check the patient, and document the situation on an incident report or accident sheet.
- Because older adults have age-related changes in digestion, metabolism, and elimination, they are observed closely for adverse reactions to medications.

CRITICAL THINKING EXERCISES

- While you are administering medications to a patient, the patient says, "I've never taken that little yellow pill before." What actions would be appropriate to take next?
- A patient who lives alone says, "You have to be a genius to keep all these pills straight." How could you help this patient organize his medication regimen?

SUGGESTED READINGS

Advice, p.r.n. Off label route: On whose say-so? Nursing 1999;29(1):18–20.

Ahmed DS, Hamrah PM. Med errors: Right drug, wrong dose. American Journal of Nursing 1999;99(1):12.

Ahmed DS, Hamrah PM. Med errors: Similar name, different diagnosis. American Journal of Nursing 1999;99(5):12.

Belknap DC, Seifert CF, Perterman M. Administration of medications through enteral feeding catheters. American Journal of Critical Care 1997;6(5):382–392.

Cohen MR. Medication errors. Nursing 1999;29(9):12.

Cook DH, Farwell A. Solving the compliance conundrum. Nursing 1999; 29(8):64hh1–2.

DeBrew JK, Barba BE, Tesh S. Assessing medication knowledge and practices of older adults. Home Healthcare Nurse 1998;16(10):686–692.

Eager R, van Carrapiett D, Tate KE, et al. Managers' forum. Double-checking medications. Journal of Emergency Nursing 1998;24(6):586–587.

Fahey-Walsh J. RSVP . . . administering medications prepared by other registered nurses. Nurse to Nurse 1997;8(3):18.

Hayes KS. Adding medications in the emergency department: Effect on knowledge of medications in older adults. Journal of Emergency Nursing 1999;25(3):178–182.

Karch AM, Karch FE. Med errors. What did you say? I can't quite understand your spoken order. American Journal of Nursing 1999;99(8):12.

McGann E. Medication compliance in adults with asthma. American Journal of Nursing 1999;99(3):45–46.

McMahan SR, Rimsza ME, Bay RC. Parents can dose liquid medication accurately. Pediatrics 1997;100(3):330–333.

Medication error: Directions, please. Nursing 1999;29(3):30.

Medication error: Knowing your rights. Nursing 1998;28(12):20.

Morris MR. Legally speaking. Preventing med errors. RN 1999;62(9):69–73.

NANDA nursing diagnoses: Definitions and classification, 1999–2000. Philadelphia, NANDA, 1999.

Osborne J, Blais K, Hayes JS. Nurses' perceptions: When is it a medication error? Journal of Nursing Administration 1999;29(4):33–38.

Pharmacy group issues warning on drug errors. Healthcare Risk Management 1998;20(10):130–131.

Provide tools for medication compliance: Calendars, hands-on instruction boost confidence. Patient Education Management 1998;5(11):1p, 14.

Ryan AA. Medication compliance and older people: A review of the literature. International Journal of Nursing Studies 1999;36(2):153–162.

Schmieding NJ, Waldman RC. Nasogastric tube feeding and medication administration: A survey of nursing practices. Gastroenterology Nursing 1997;20(4):118–124.

Sullivan GH. Advice of counsel. Who is to blame when a med error occurs? RN 1999;62(7):68.

Wendt DA. Evaluation of medication management interventions for the elderly. Home Healthcare Nurse 1998;16(9):612–617.

Williams RD. Medication and older adults. Healthline 1998;17(5):8.

SKILL 32-1

ADMINISTERING ORAL MEDICATIONS

Suggested Action	Reason for Action
Assessment	
Compare the medication administration record (MAR) with the written medical order.	Prevents medication errors
Review the patient's drug, allergy, and medical history.	Avoids potential complications
Consult a current drug reference concerning the drug's action, side effects, contraindications, and administration information.	Ensures appropriate administration based on a thorough knowledge base
Planning	
Plan to administer medications within a half-hour to an hour of the time they are scheduled.	Demonstrates timely administration and compliance with the medical order
Allow sufficient time to prepare the medications in a location where there are minimal distractions.	Promotes safe preparation of drugs
Make sure that there is a sufficient supply of paper and plastic medications cups.	Facilitates organization and efficient time management
Chill oily medications.	Reduces their unpleasant odor and improves palatability
Implementation	
Wash your hands.	Removes colonizing microorganisms
Read and compare the label on the drug with the MAR at least three times—before, during, and after preparing the drug.	Ensures that the *right drug* is given at the *right time* by the *right route*

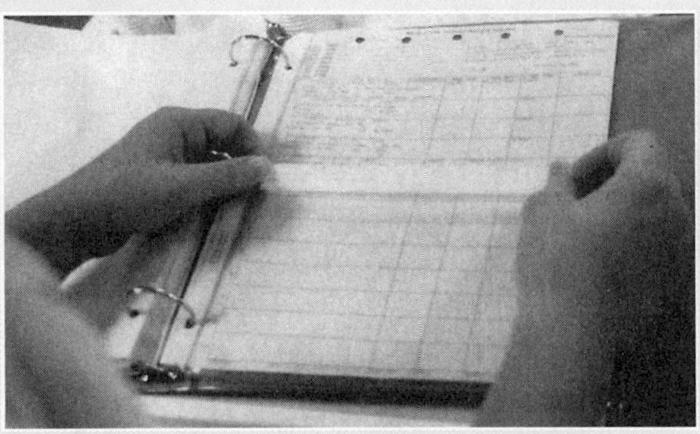

Checking the MAR. (Courtesy of Ken Timby.)

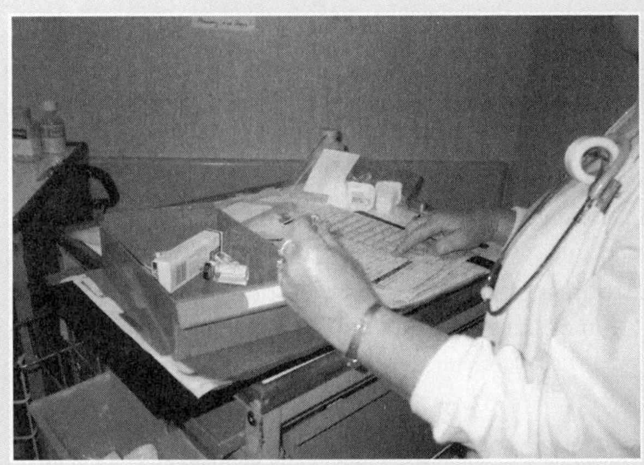

Comparing the drug label and MAR. (Courtesy of Ken Timby.)

Suggested Action	Reason for Action
Calculate doses.	Complies with the medical order and ensures that the *right dose* is given
Place medications or unit dose packets within a paper or plastic cup without touching the medication itself.	Supports principles of asepsis
Keep drugs that require special assessments or administration techniques in a separate cup.	Helps identify drugs that require special nursing actions
Pour liquids with drug label toward the palm of hand.	Prevents liquid from running onto the label
Hold the cup for liquid medications at eye level when pouring.	Facilitates accurate measurement

continued

SKILL 32–1

ADMINISTERING ORAL MEDICATIONS *Continued*

Suggested Action	Reason for Action
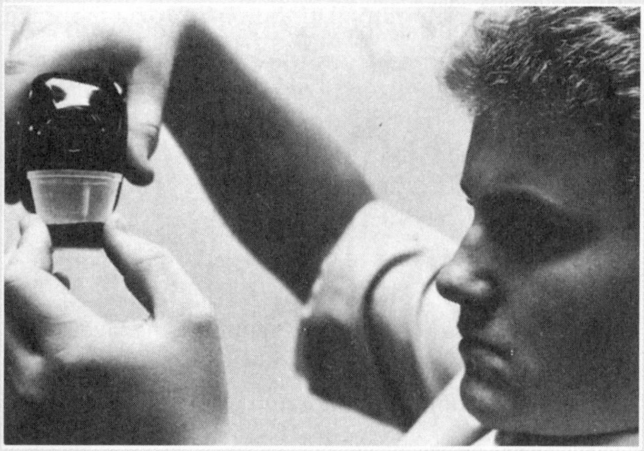 Pouring liquid medication. (Courtesy of Ken Timby.)	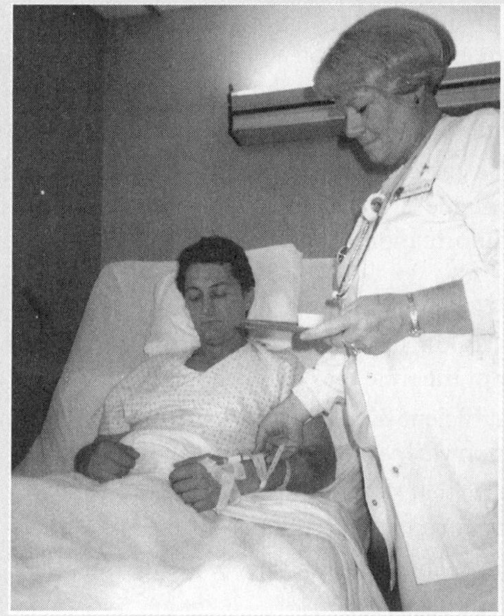 Checking the identification band. (Courtesy of Ken Timby.)
Prepare a supply of soft-textured food such as applesauce or pudding, according to the patient's individual needs.	Facilitates administration for patients with impaired swallowing
Help the patient to a sitting position.	Facilitates swallowing and prevents aspiration
Identify the patient by checking the wristband or asking the patient's name.	Ensures that medications are given to the *right patient*
Prepare fresh water in a glass with or without a straw.	Facilitates swallowing the medication
Offer water before giving solid forms of oral medications.	Moistens mucous membranes and prevents medication from sticking
Advise patients to take medications one at a time or in amounts they can easily swallow.	Prevents choking
Encourage patients to keep their head in a neutral position or one of slight flexion, rather than hyperextending the neck.	Protects the airway

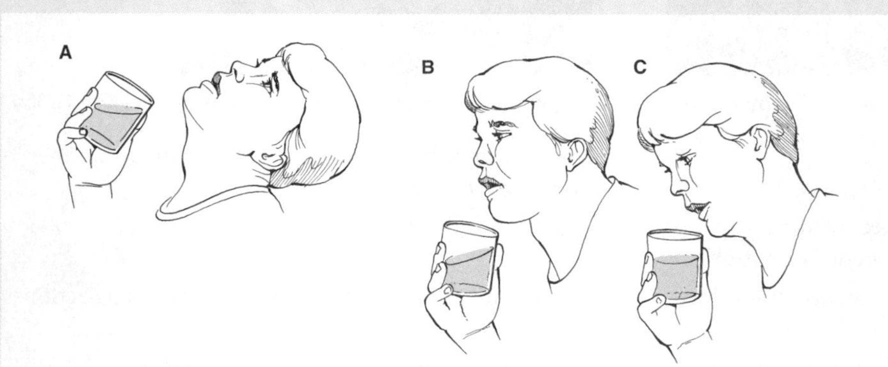

(*A*) Inappropriate neck position; (*B*) and (*C*) appropriate neck positions.

Suggested Action	Reason for Action
Remain with patients until their medications are swallowed.	Ensures appropriate administration

continued

SKILL 32–1

ADMINISTERING ORAL MEDICATIONS *Continued*

Suggested Action	Reason for Action
Restore the patient to a position of comfort and safety.	Shows concern for the patient's well-being
Record the volume of fluid consumed on the intake and output record.	Demonstrates responsibility for accurate fluid assessment
Record the administration of the medication.	Prevents medication errors
Assess the patient in 30 minutes for desired and undesired drug effects.	Aids in evaluating the patient's response and effect of drug therapy

Evaluation

- The five rights are upheld.
- Patient experiences no choking or aspiration.
- Patient exhibits a therapeutic response to the medication.
- Patient demonstrates minimal or absent side effects.

Document

- Preassessment data, if indicated
- Date, time, drug, dose, route, signature, title, and initials (usually on the MAR)
- Evidence of patient's response, if it can be determined

SAMPLE DOCUMENTATION

Date and Time Temp. 103.8°F. Tylenol tabs ii given by mouth for relief of fever. Fever reduced to 103°F 30 minutes later. ______________________ SIGNATURE, TITLE

CRITICAL THINKING

- Discuss actions that would be appropriate if a patient could not swallow medications prescribed by the oral route.
- What actions would you take if you found an oral tablet on the floor while caring for a patient?

SKILL 32–2

ADMINISTERING MEDICATIONS THROUGH AN ENTERAL TUBE

Suggested Action	Reason for Action
Assessment	
Check the medication administration record (MAR) and compare the information with the written medical order.	Prevents medication errors
Review the patient's drug, allergy, and medical history.	Avoids potential complications
Consult a current drug reference concerning the drug's action, side effects, contraindications, and administration information.	Ensures appropriate administration based on a thorough knowledge base

continued

SKILL 32-2

ADMINISTERING MEDICATIONS THROUGH AN ENTERAL TUBE *Continued*

Suggested Action	Reason for Action
Verify the location of the tube by auscultating instilled air or aspirating secretions.	Ensures airway protection and proper placement
Compare the length of the external tube with its measurement at the time of insertion.	Determines if the tube has migrated
Inspect the patient's mouth and throat.	Determines if the tube has been displaced and coiled at the back of the throat
Planning	
Plan to administer medications within a half-hour to an hour of the time they are scheduled.	Demonstrates timely administration and compliance with the medical order
Separate and clamp or plug a feeding tube for 15 to 30 minutes if the drug will interact with food.	Ensures that the stomach will be relatively empty
Allow sufficient time to prepare the medications in a location where there are minimal distractions.	Promotes safe preparation of drugs
Make sure that there is a sufficient supply of plastic medication cups.	Facilitates organization and efficient time management
Implementation	
Wash your hands.	Removes colonizing microorganisms
Read and compare the label on the drug with the MAR at least three times—before, during, and after preparing the drug.	Ensures that the *right drug* is given at the *right time* by the *right route*
Prepare each drug separately.	Prevents potential physical changes when some drugs are combined
Take the cups containing diluted medications to the bedside with water for flushing, a 30- to 50-mL syringe, a towel or disposable pad, and clean gloves.	Facilitates instillation
Identify the patient by checking the wristband or asking the patient's name.	Ensures that medications are given to the *right patient*
Help the patient into a Fowler's position.	Prevents gastric reflux
Don clean gloves.	Prevents contact with body fluids
Insert the syringe into the tube and instill 15 to 30 mL of water by gravity.	Flushes and reduces the surface tension of the tube
Add the diluted medication to the syringe as it becomes nearly empty.	Prevents instilling air
Apply gentle pressure with the plunger or bulb of a syringe if the medication fails to instill easily.	Provides positive pressure
Flush with at least 5 mL of water between each instillation of medication and as much as 30 mL after all the medications have been instilled.	Prevents drug interactions and obstruction of the tube; fully instills all of the prescribed drug
Pinch the tube as the syringe empties.	Prevents distending the abdomen with air; maintains patency of the tube
Clamp or plug the tube for 30 minutes before reconnecting a tube to suction.	Prevents removing the medication after it has been instilled

continued

SKILL 32-2

ADMINISTERING MEDICATIONS THROUGH AN ENTERAL TUBE *Continued*

Suggested Action	Reason for Action

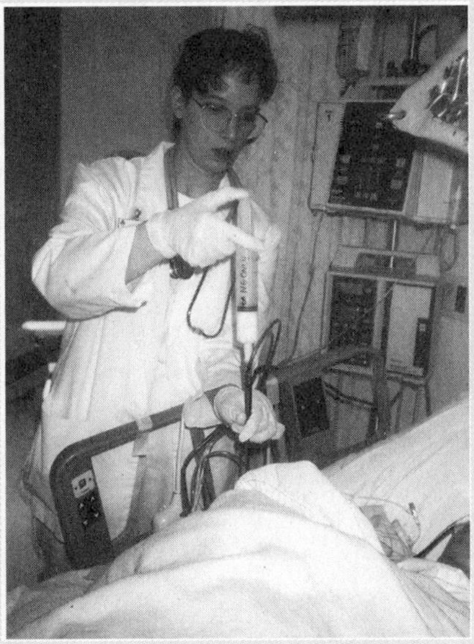

Instilling medication. (Courtesy of Ken Timby.)

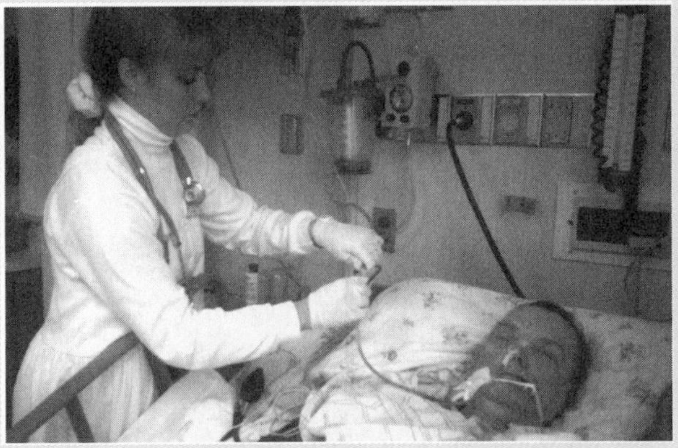

Plugging a gastric tube. (Courtesy of Ken Timby.)

Suggested Action	Reason for Action
Connect a tube used for nourishment immediately if the medication and formula will not interact.	Facilitates the primary purpose of the enteral tube
Keep the head of the bed elevated for at least 30 minutes.	Reduces the potential for aspiration

Evaluation

- Tube placement is verified.
- The five rights are upheld.
- Medications instill freely and are flushed afterward.
- Patient experiences no abdominal distention, nausea, vomiting, or other undesirable effects.
- Tube remains patent.

Document

- Preadministration assessment data
- Medication administration on the MAR
- Volume of fluid instilled with the medication as well as for flushing the tube on the bedside intake and output record
- Response of the patient

SAMPLE DOCUMENTATION

Date and Time Placement of NG tube verified by auscultation. No evidence of tube migration. Medications administered (see MAR) per NG tube. Flushed with 30 mL after instilling medications. Tube clamped at this time. No evidence of nausea or distention.

________________________ SIGNATURE, TITLE

CRITICAL THINKING

- Explain the reason for administering medications through the tube rather than having the patient swallow them.

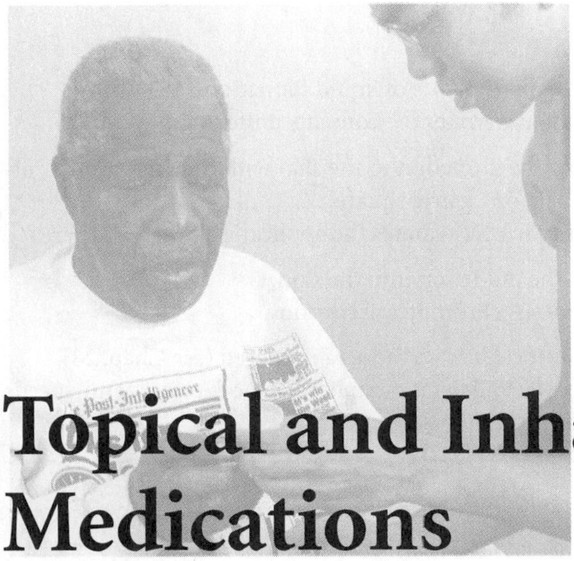

CHAPTER 33

Topical and Inhalant Medications

CHAPTER OUTLINE

NURSING GUIDELINES

APPLYING AN INUNCTION
APPLYING NITROGLYCERIN PASTE

SKILLS

SKILL 33-1: INSTILLING EYE MEDICATIONS
SKILL 33-2: ADMINISTERING NASAL MEDICATIONS

NURSING CARE PLAN

IMPAIRED GAS EXCHANGE

KEY TERMS

aerosol	paste
buccal application	rebound effect
cutaneous application	skin patches
inhalant route	spacer
inhalers	sublingual application
inunction	topical route
metered-dose inhaler	turbo-inhaler
ophthalmic application	transdermal application
otic application	

LEARNING OBJECTIVES

An understanding of the content within this chapter will be evidenced by the student's ability to:

- Explain how topical medications are administered.
- Give at least five examples of where topical medications are commonly applied.
- Give three examples of an inunction.
- Name two forms of drugs applied by the transdermal route.
- Discuss at least two principles that are followed when applying a skin patch.
- Describe where eye medications are applied.
- Explain how the administration of ear medications differs for adults and children.
- Explain the rebound effect that occurs with the administration of nasal decongestants.
- Describe the difference between sublingual and buccal administration.
- Explain why inhalation is a good route for medication administration.
- Describe the mechanism for creating an aerosol.
- Name two types of inhalers.
- Name a device that can maximize the absorption of an inhaled medication.

Drugs are administered by routes other than the oral route. This chapter describes the techniques used to administer drugs by the topical and inhalant routes.

Topical Route

Drugs applied by the **topical route** (method of drug administration in which medications are applied to the skin or mucous membranes) can be applied externally or internally (Table 33-1). Topically applied drugs may have a local or systemic effect. However, many are administered to achieve a direct effect on the tissue to which they are applied.

CUTANEOUS APPLICATIONS

Cutaneous applications (drugs that are rubbed into or placed in contact with the skin) include inunctions, pastes, and patches.

TABLE 33–1. **Common Routes of Topical Administration**

Routes	Location of Application	Vehicles
Cutaneous	To the skin	Ointment Cream Lotion Patch Paste
Sublingual	Under the tongue	Tablet Sprays
Buccal	Between the cheek and gum	Lozenge Tablet
Vaginal	In the vagina	Douche Suppository
Rectal	In the rectum	Irrigation Suppository
Otic	In the ear	Drops Irrigation
Ophthalmic	In the eye	Drops Ointment
Nasal	In the nose	Spray Drops

Inunction Application

An **inunction** (medication that is incorporated into an agent, such as an ointment, oil, lotion, or cream) is administered by rubbing the agent into the skin. Alert patients may self-administer an inunction after they have been instructed. In that situation, the nurse teaches proper application techniques and checks that the medication has been applied appropriately as often as it has been prescribed. For patients who cannot perform their own skin applications, the nurse does so.

Nursing Guidelines For

Applying an Inunction

☑ Wash your hands.
RATIONALE: Removes colonizing microorganisms

☑ Check the identity of the patient.
RATIONALE: Prevents administering medication to the wrong patient

☑ Don clean gloves if your skin or that of the patient is not intact.
RATIONALE: Provides a barrier to pathogens

☑ Cleanse the area of application with soap and water.
RATIONALE: Promotes absorption

☑ Warm the inunction, if it will be applied to a sensitive area of the skin, by holding it temporarily in your hands or placing the sealed container in warm water.
RATIONALE: Promotes comfort

☑ Shake the contents of liquid inunctions.
RATIONALE: Mixes the contents uniformly

☑ Apply the inunction to the skin with the fingertips, a cotton ball, or a gauze square.
RATIONALE: Distributes the application over a wide area

☑ Rub the inunction into the skin.
RATIONALE: Promotes absorption

☑ Apply local heat to the area if desired (see Chap. 28).
RATIONALE: Dilates peripheral blood vessels and speeds absorption

Transdermal Applications

Drugs incorporated into patches or paste are administered as a **transdermal application** (method of applying a drug on the skin and allowing it to become passively absorbed). After the application, the drug migrates through the skin and is eventually absorbed into the bloodstream.

Skin Patches

Skin patches (drugs that are bonded to an adhesive bandage; Fig. 33-1) are applied to the skin. Several drugs are now prepared in patch form, including nitroglycerin (used to dilate the coronary arteries), scopolamine (used to relieve motion sickness), and estrogen (hormone used to treat menopausal symptoms).

Skin patches are applied to any skin area where there is adequate circulation. Most patches are applied to the upper body in places such as the chest, shoulders, and upper arms. Small patches can be applied behind the ear. Each time a new

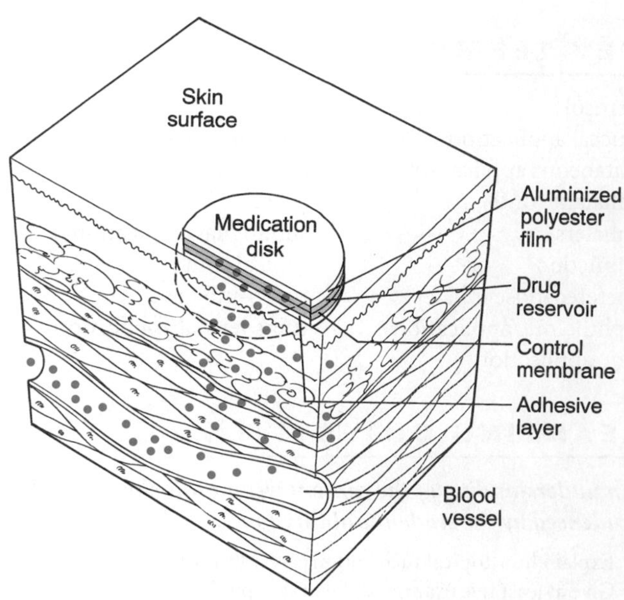

FIGURE 33–1. Pathway for absorption from a transdermal skin patch.

patch is applied, it is placed in a slightly different location. It may help adhesion to clip extremely hairy skin areas.

After the patch is applied, it may take approximately 30 minutes for the drug to reach a therapeutic level. Thereafter, however, the patch provides a continuous supply of medication. In fact, the drug may still be active for up to 30 minutes after the patch is removed. It is always best to date and initial a patch so that others can determine when it was applied.

Drug Paste

A **paste** (vehicle that contains a drug within a thick base) is applied to the skin but is not rubbed in. Nitroglycerin can be applied as a paste. Although sometimes the product is referred to as an ointment, the term is a misnomer because the skin is not massaged once the drug is applied.

Nursing Guidelines For

Applying Nitroglycerin Paste

- ☑ Wash your hands.
  RATIONALE: Removes colonizing microorganisms
- ☑ Check the identity of the patient.
  RATIONALE: Prevents administering medication to the wrong patient
- ☑ Squeeze a ribbon of paste from the tube onto an application paper (Fig. 33-2).
  RATIONALE: Complies with the medication order, which usually specifies the dose in inches
- ☑ Fold the paper or use a wooden applicator to spread the paste over approximately a 2.25 × 3.5-inch (5.6 × 8.8-cm) area of the paper.
  RATIONALE: Facilitates distributing the drug over a wider area for quicker absorption
- ☑ Do not touch the paste with your bare fingers.
  RATIONALE: Prevents potential self-absorption of the drug
- ☑ Place the application paper on a clean, nonhairy area of skin.
  RATIONALE: Facilitates drug absorption
- ☑ Cover the paper with a square of plastic kitchen wrap, or tape all the edges of the paper to the skin.
  RATIONALE: Seals the drug between the paper and the skin
- ☑ Remove one application before applying another, and remove any residue remaining on the skin.
  RATIONALE: Prevents excessive drug levels
- ☑ Rotate the sites where the medication is placed.
  RATIONALE: Reduces the potential for skin irritation

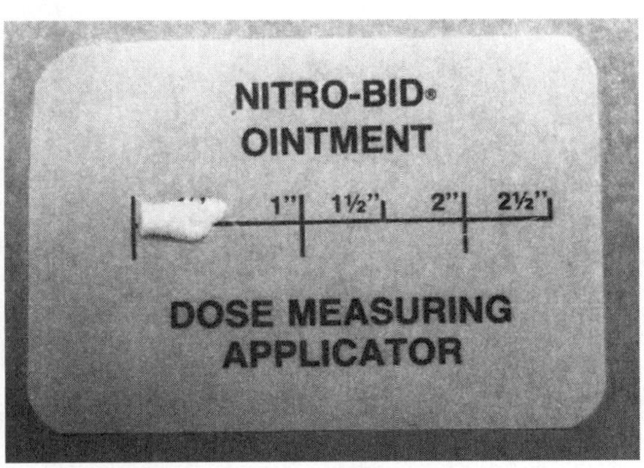

FIGURE 33–2. Paste and applicator paper. (Courtesy of Ken Timby.)

OPHTHALMIC APPLICATIONS

An **ophthalmic application** (method of applying drugs onto the mucous membrane of one or both eyes) is described in Skill 33-1. The mucous membrane of the eyes is called the *conjunctiva.* It lines the inner eyelids and the anterior surface of the *sclera* (Fig. 33-3).

Ophthalmic medications are supplied in liquid form and instilled as drops, or as ointments that are applied along the lower lid margin. Blinking, rather than rubbing, distributes the drug over the surface of the eye.

The eye is a delicate structure and is susceptible to infection and injury, just like any other tissue. Therefore, care is taken to keep the applicator tip of the medication container sterile.

OTIC APPLICATIONS

An **otic application** (drug instilled in the outer portion of the ear) is usually administered to moisten impacted cerumen or instill medications to treat a local bacterial or fungal infection.

When ear medication is instilled, the ear is first manipulated to straighten the auditory canal. The technique varies depending on whether the patient is a young child (ear is pulled down and back) or an adult (ear is pulled up and back) (see Chap. 12).

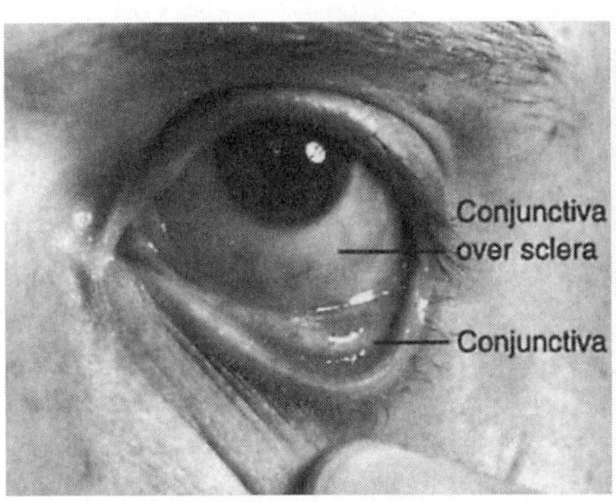

FIGURE 33–3. Ophthalmic application sites. (Fuller J, Schuller-Ayers J. Health assessment: A nursing approach, 3rd ed. Philadelphia, Lippincott Williams & Wilkins, 1999).

With the head tilted away from the nurse, the prescribed number of drops of medication are instilled within the ear. The patient remains in this position briefly as the solution travels toward the eardrum. A small cotton ball can be placed *loosely* in the ear to absorb excess medication. The nurse should wait at least 15 minutes before instilling medication in the opposite ear, if necessary.

NASAL APPLICATIONS

Topical medications may be dropped or sprayed within the nose (Skill 33-2). Proper instillation is important to avoid displacing the medication into nearby structures such as the back of the throat. Adults often self-administer their own nasal medications, but sometimes nurses must assist older adults and children.

Patients who use over-the-counter decongestant nasal sprays should be warned that if they are used too frequently or if more than the recommended amount is administered, a **rebound effect** (swelling of the nasal mucosa within a short time of drug administration) can occur. Rebound effect can be avoided by following label directions or by using nasal sprays containing only normal saline solution.

SUBLINGUAL AND BUCCAL APPLICATIONS

A tablet given by **sublingual application** (drug placed under the tongue) is left to dissolve slowly and to become absorbed by the rich blood supply in the area. Some drugs in spray or liquid form also are administered sublingually. A **buccal application** (drug placed against the mucous membranes of the inner cheek) is another method of drug administration. When buccal or sublingual administrations are given, patients are instructed not to chew or swallow the medication. Eating and smoking also are contraindicated during the brief time that it takes for the medication to dissolve.

VAGINAL APPLICATIONS

Topical vaginal applications are most often used to treat local infections. Vaginal infections are common and usually result from colonization of the vaginal tissue by microorganisms, such as yeasts, that are abundant in the stool. The microorganisms usually become transferred at the time of bowel elimination if the patient wipes the rectal area toward the vagina rather than away from it. Symptoms of a yeast infection include intense vaginal itching and a white, cheese-like vaginal discharge.

Several drugs useful in the treatment of vaginal yeast infections are available over the counter in suppository, tablet, or cream form. Early and appropriate self-treatment restores the normal integrity to the tissue. It may be helpful to provide patients with instructions on how to administer vaginal medications for their most effective action.

Patient Teaching Guidelines For

Administering Medications Vaginally

Tell the patient to do the following:

- Obtain a form of medication based on personal preference; all come with a vaginal applicator (Fig 33-4A).
- Plan to instill the medication before going to bed so that it can be retained for a prolonged period.
- Empty your bladder just before inserting the medication.
- Place the drug in the applicator.
- Lubricate the applicator tip with a water-soluble lubricant such as K-Y Jelly.
- Lie down, bend your knees, and spread your legs.
- Separate the labia and insert the applicator into the vagina to the length recommended in the package directions, usually 2 to 4 inches (5 to 10 cm) (Fig. 33-4B).
- Depress the plunger to insert the medication.
- Remove the applicator and place it on a clean tissue. Discard the applicator if it is disposable. Wash a reusable applicator when you wash your hands.

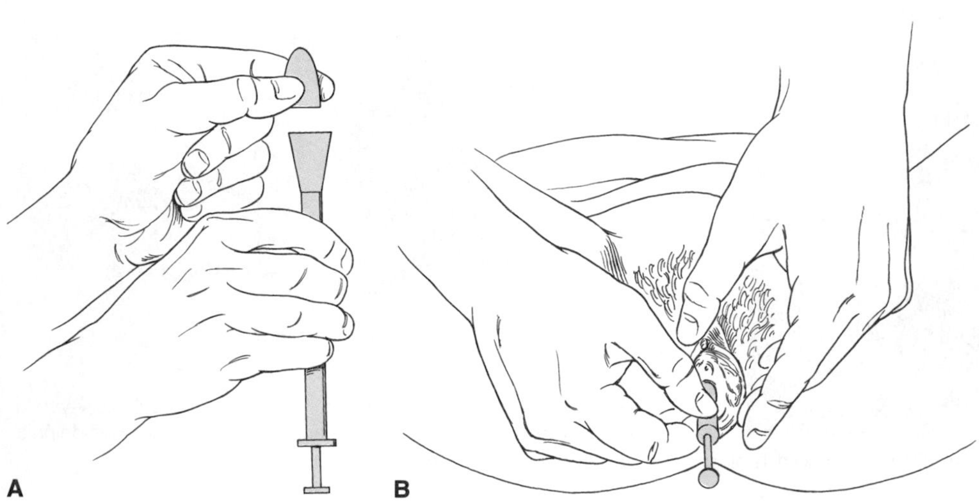

FIGURE 33–4. Vaginal medication. (*A*) Example of a vaginal applicator. (*B*) Vaginal insertion.

- Apply a sanitary pad if you prefer.
- Remain recumbent for at least 10 to 30 minutes.
- Consult a physician if symptoms persist.

If the patient cannot self-administer vaginal medication, the nurse wears gloves to avoid contact with secretions. After the gloves are removed, handwashing is critical. The same advice holds true for rectal applications.

RECTAL APPLICATIONS

Drugs that are administered rectally are usually in the form of suppositories (see Chap. 31), but creams and ointments may also be prescribed. The technique for using a rectal applicator is similar to that for using a vaginal applicator.

Inhalant Route

The **inhalant route** (drug administration to the lower airways) is an effective method for medication administration because the lungs provide an extensive area from which the drug may be absorbed quickly into the circulatory system. To distribute the medication to the distal areas of the airways, liquid medication is converted to an aerosol.

An **aerosol** (mist) results after a liquid drug is forced through a narrow channel using pressurized air or an inert gas. Examples of common household aerosol products are hairspray and furniture polish. A simple method of administering aerosolized medications is via an inhaler.

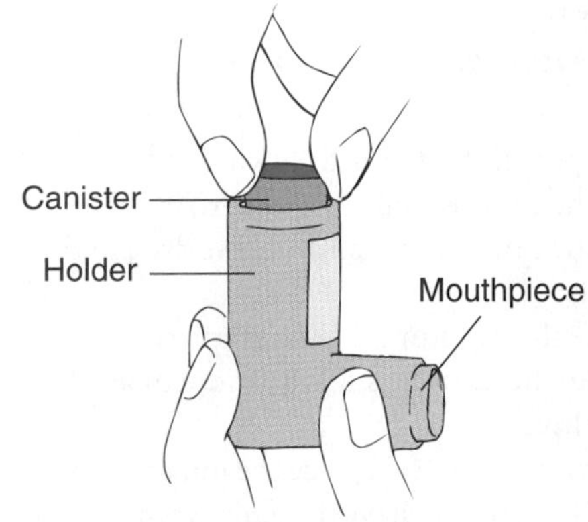

FIGURE 33–5. Parts of an inhaler.

INHALERS

Inhalers (hand-held devices for delivering medication into the respiratory passages) consist of a canister that contains the medication and a holder with a mouthpiece through which the aerosol is inhaled (Fig. 33-5).

There are two types of inhalers. A **turbo-inhaler** (propeller-driven device) spins and suspends a finely powdered medication. The propellers are activated during inhalation. A **metered-dose inhaler** (canister that contains medication under pressure) is much more common. The inhaler is placed into a holder containing a mouthpiece, and when the container is compressed, a measured volume (metered dose) of aerosolized drug is released.

Patients who use metered-dose inhalers do not always use them correctly. As a result, much of the medication may be swallowed rather than inhaled, and the patient's respiratory symptoms may not be relieved.

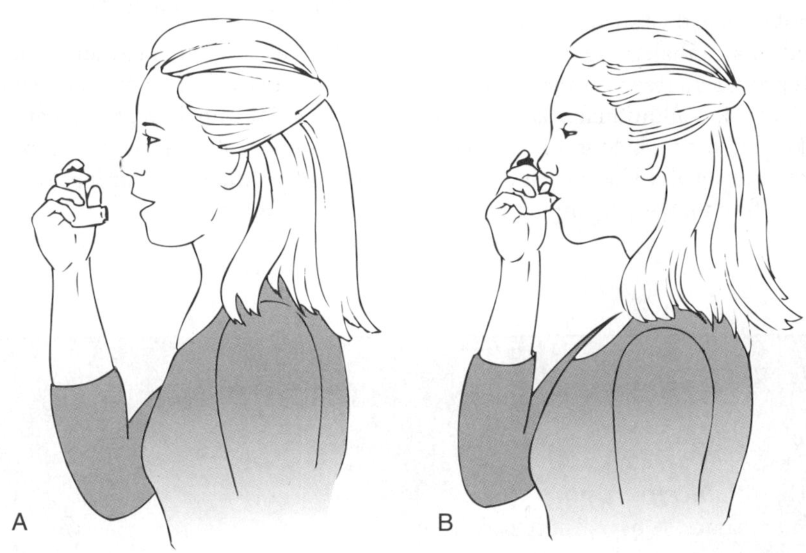

FIGURE 33–6. Using a metered dose inhaler. (*A*) Holding the inhaler 1 to 2 inches away. (*B*) Holding the inhaler in the mouth.

Patient Teaching Guidelines For
Using a Metered-Dose Inhaler

Teach the patient to do the following:
- Insert the canister into the holder.
- Shake the canister to distribute the drug in the pressurized chamber.
- Remove the cap from the mouthpiece.
- Tilt your head back slightly and exhale slowly through pursed lips.
- Open your mouth and place the inhaler 1 to 2 inches away (Fig. 33-6*A*). If you have difficulty with this method, place the inhaler in your mouth and close your lips around the mouthpiece (Fig. 33-6*B*).
- Press down on the canister once to release the medication.
- As the medication is released, breathe in slowly through your mouth for approximately 3 to 5 seconds.
- Hold your breath for 10 seconds to let the medication reach your lungs.
- Exhale slowly through pursed lips.
- Wait 1 full minute before doing another inhalation if more than one is ordered.
- Clean the inhaler (holder and mouthpiece) daily by rinsing it in warm water and weekly with mild soap and water. Allow the inhaler to air-dry. Have another inhaler available to use while the one is drying.

Some patients find that the inhaled drug leaves an unpleasant aftertaste. Gargling with salt water may diminish this. Drug residue may accumulate in the mouthpiece, so the mouthpiece should be rinsed in warm water after use.

Spacers

Some patients have problems coordinating their breathing with inhaler use and do not receive the full dose of aerosol. A **spacer** (chamber attached to an inhaler; Fig. 33-7) may be helpful in this situation. It provides a reservoir for the aerosol medication, so as the patient takes additional breaths, he or she continues to inhale the medication held in the reservoir. This tends to maximize drug absorption because it prevents drug loss. Some patients also find that by prolonging the time over which the drug is inhaled, side effects such as tachycardia or tremulousness are reduced.

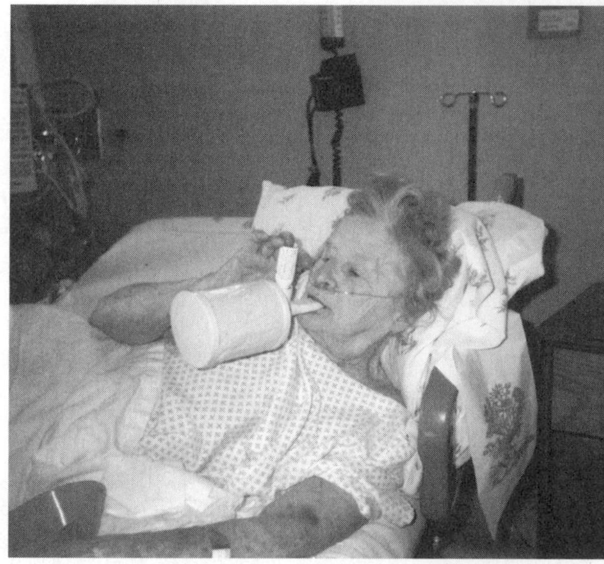
FIGURE 33–7. A spacer and inhaler. (Courtesy of Ken Timby.)

Nursing Implications

When administering topical or inhalant drugs, nurses often assess and take steps to maintain the integrity of the skin and mucous membranes. Health teaching may be important to prevent improper self-administration. Applicable nursing diagnoses may include:
- Knowledge deficit
- Ineffective management of therapeutic regimen
- Impaired gas exchange
- Impaired skin integrity
- Impaired tissue integrity

The nursing care plan shows how the steps of the nursing process are used when managing the care of a patient with the diagnosis of Impaired gas exchange, defined in the NANDA taxonomy (1999) as a "excess or deficit oxygenation and/or carbon dioxide elimination at the alveolar-capillary membrane."

Nursing Care Plan
Impaired Gas Exchange

Assessment

Subjective Data
States, "I have trouble breathing even though I use my inhaler when my chest starts getting tight."

continued

Nursing Care Plan: *Impaired Gas Exchange* Continued

Objective Data

Patient is a 56-year-old man who smoked two packs of cigarettes a day for the last 30 years. Chronic emphysema recently aggravated by pneumonia. Given a prescription 2 days ago for albuterol (Ventolin) to be administered by a metered-dose inhaler. Appears to exhale quickly rather than retaining the inhaled aerosol for a brief time. Skin pale and complaining of shortness of breath. SpO_2 89%.

Diagnosis

Impaired gas exchange related to improper technique using metered-dose inhaler and underlying lung disease

Plan

Goal

The patient's ventilations will maintain an SpO_2 of no less than 90% with appropriate use of an inhaler.

Orders: 8/02

1. Redemonstrate the correct use of a metered-dose inhaler.
2. Observe patient's technique at least four times after demonstration.
3. Monitor SpO_2 with pulse oximeter before and after use of metered-dose inhaler.

D. FORTIS, RN

Implementation (Documentation)

8/02 1000 Short of breath. Sitting up to breathe. Lung sounds are diminished bilaterally. SpO_2 @ 88% per pulse oximeter. Shown how to use metered-dose inhaler. Having difficulty inhaling with mouthpiece 1 to 2 inches away from mouth. Advised to enclose the mouthpiece within the lips. Coached to hold the inhaled breath for several seconds. J. BENTHIN, LPN

Evaluation (Documentation)

1030 Observed to perform technique appropriately with each of two puffs from the inhaler. SpO_2 90% within 15 minutes of using the inhaler.

J. BENTHIN, LPN

FOCUS ON OLDER ADULTS

- Some older adults have difficulty instilling eye medications independently. Devices are available that can diminish the frequency of instillation or facilitate the administration. For example, one type of medication for glaucoma is inserted inside the lower eyelid, needing only to be replaced every 7 days. Sight Centers, which provide assistive devices for people who are visually impaired, are a good resource for other devices that facilitate the instillation of eye drops.
- Some older adults take two or more types of eye medications once or several times daily. If the tops of the eye medications are not color-coded, ways of color coding the containers to help distinguish the different medications can be suggested.
- Older adults often require complex medication regimens for glaucoma, involving the instillation of one or more types of drops up to four times daily. Recently, longer-acting medications have been developed that may be useful in decreasing the frequency of the medication routines. The older adult is encouraged to collaborate with the prescribing practitioner on ways to simplify the routine.
- When more than one eye medication is prescribed, it is common to have to wait 5 minutes between the instillation of eye drops. Older adults can use a simple timer to help them keep track of time, serving as a reminder when the time period has elapsed.
- Eye medications can have adverse systemic effects and interact with other medications.
- The onset of drug action may be atypical when topical medications are administered to older adults because they tend to have less subcutaneous fat. The lack of subcutaneous tissue causes topical medications to be absorbed more rapidly than in a younger adult.
- Some older adults have difficulty reaching areas of the body to which some topical drugs are applied. For example, arthritis may interfere with applying medication within the vagina or rectum or to skin lesions on the lower extremities.
- The mechanics of inhaling and compressing the inhaler simultaneously may be awkward for some older adults. Spacer devices help compensate for less-than-optimal administration techniques.
- Sometimes two inhalers containing different drugs are prescribed. During teaching sessions, stressing how and when each is used is important. Providing simple written instructions, including illustrations, with each medication is also helpful.
- Monitoring heart rate and blood pressure of older adults who use inhaled bronchodilators is important because these medications commonly cause tachycardia and hypertension. Either or both of these effects increase the risks for complications, especially in older adults with underlying cardiovascular disease.

KEY CONCEPTS

- Topical medications are applied to the skin or mucous membranes.
- Common locations for topical medications are the skin, eye, ear, nose, vagina, rectum, and mouth.
- An inunction is a medication that is incorporated into a vehicle, or transporting agent, such as an ointment, oil, lotion, or cream.
- Skin patches and applications of paste are two methods for administering medications by the transdermal route.
- Skin patches can be applied to any skin area where there is adequate circulation. Each time a new patch is applied, it is placed in a slightly different location.
- Eye medications are applied onto the mucous membrane, or conjunctiva, of the eye, which lines the inner eyelids and the anterior surface of the sclera.
- The way the ear is manipulated to straighten the auditory canal is the major difference in the technique for administering ear medications to adults and children.
- The rebound effect is a phenomenon characterized by rapid swelling of the nasal mucosa. It is likely to occur when more than the recommended amount of nasal decongestant is chronically administered, or if the drug is administered too frequently.
- For sublingual administration, the drug is placed under the tongue. For buccal administration, the medication is placed in contact with the mucous membrane of the cheek.
- The inhalant route is used for medication administration because the lungs provide an extensive area of tissue from which drugs may be absorbed.
- To create an aerosol, liquid medication is forced through a narrow channel under high pressure.
- Drug are commonly inhaled using turbo-inhalers or metered-dose inhalers. A turbo-inhaler delivers a burst of fine powder at the time of inhalation. A metered-dose inhaler releases a measured volume of aerosolized drug when its canister is compressed.
- A spacer provides a reservoir for aerosol medication, which can then be inhaled beyond the time of the initial breath.

CRITICAL THINKING EXERCISES

- Before Mr. Rumsey, who has had a heart attack, is discharged, he says, "You nurses always put my nitroglycerin patches on my back. How can I do that when I have to do it myself?" How would you respond?
- How might you help Mrs. Fuller, who is legally blind and lives alone, identify two different containers of eye medication?

SUGGESTED READINGS

Abley C. Teaching elderly patients how to use inhalers. Journal of Advanced Nursing 1997;25(4):699–708.

Cohen MR. Medication errors. Soundalike ophthalmics: Eye-opening error. Nursing 1995;25(4):15.

Connolly MJ. Inhaler technique of elderly patients: Comparison of metered-dose inhalers and large volume spacer devices. Age and Ageing 1995; 24(3):190–192.

Dehand R, Fink J. Dry powder inhalers. Respiratory Care 1999;44(8): 940–951.

Doody J. Intranasal corticosteroids in allergic rhinitis: Ensuring patient compliance. Physician Assistant 1996;20(2):59–66.

Duvall B, Kershner RM. Fundamentals in focus. Journal of Ophthalmic Nursing & Technology 1998;17(4):151–158.

Gandham SB. New topical medications in the treatment of glaucoma. Journal of Ophthalmic Nursing & Technology 1997;16(6):290–291.

Gift AG. Applications in research. Proper use of metered-dose inhalers. Perspectives in Respiratory Nursing 1997;8(1):5.

Hannemann LA. What is new in asthma: New drug powder inhalers. Journal of Pediatric Health Care 1999;13(4):159–165.

Haworth J. Asthma control and morbidity: A comparison of inhaler devices. Nursing Standard 1996;11(1):31–34.

Hays H, Woodroffe MA. Use of transdermal fentanyl for chronic pain. Home Healthcare Consultant 1998;5(3):23–30.

McConnell EA. Applying transdermal ointments. Nursing 1998;28(10):30.

McConnell EA. Using transdermal medication patches. Nursing 1997; 27(7):18.

NANDA nursing diagnoses: Definitions and classification, 1999–2000. Philadelphia, NANDA, 1999.

Rokosky JM. Misuse of metered-dose inhalers: Helping patients get it right. Home Healthcare Nurse 1997;15(1):13–24.

SKILL 33-1

INSTILLING EYE MEDICATIONS

Suggested Action	Reason for Action
Assessment	
Compare the medication administration record (MAR) with the written medical order.	Prevents medication errors
Review the patient's drug, allergy, and medical history.	Avoids potential complications
Consult a current drug reference concerning the drug's action, side effects, contraindications, and administration information.	Ensures appropriate administration based on a thorough knowledge base
Planning	
Plan to administer medications within a half-hour to an hour of the time they are scheduled.	Demonstrates timely administration and compliance with the medical order
Allow sufficient time to prepare the medications in a location where there are minimal distractions.	Promotes safe preparation of drugs
Warm eye drops and ointments by holding them between the hands if they have not been stored at room temperature.	Promotes comfort
Read and compare the label on the drug with the MAR at least three times—before, during, and after preparing the drug.	Ensures that the *right drug* is given at the *right time* by the *right route*
Implementation	
Wash your hands.	Removes colonizing microorganisms
Identify the patient by checking the wristband or asking the patient's name.	Ensures that medications are given to the *right patient*
Position the patient supine or sitting with the head tilted back and slightly to the side into which the medication will be instilled.	Prevents the drug from passing into the nasolacrimal duct or from being blinked onto the cheek
Don clean gloves.	Acts as a barrier to pathogens in body fluids
Clean the lids and lashes if they contain debris. Use a cotton ball or tissue that has been moistened with water.	Promotes comfort and maximizes the potential for absorption
Wipe the eye from the corner by the nose, called the *inner canthus,* toward the *outer canthus,* the corner of the eye near the temple.	Moves debris away from the nasolacrimal duct
Instruct the patient to look toward the ceiling.	Prevents looking directly at the applicator, which usually causes a blinking reflex as it comes close to the eye
Make a pouch in the lower lid by pulling the skin over the bony orbit downward.	Provides a natural reservoir for depositing liquid medication
Move the container of medication from below the patient's line of vision or from the side of the eye.	Prevents a blink reflex
Steady the container above the location for instillation without touching the surface of the eye.	Prevents injury
Instill the prescribed number of drops into the appropriate eye within the conjunctival pouch.	Complies with the medical order by administering the *right dose*

continued

SKILL 33-1

INSTILLING EYE MEDICATIONS *Continued*

Suggested Action	Reason for Action
If ointment is used, squeeze a ribbon onto the lower lid margin.	Applies the ointment to the conjunctiva

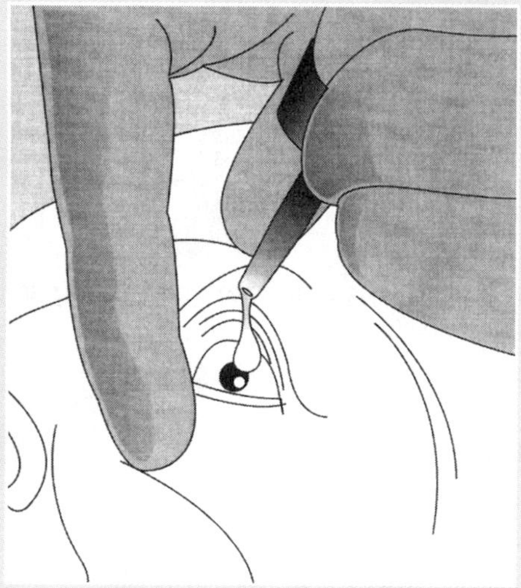

Instilling eyedrops.

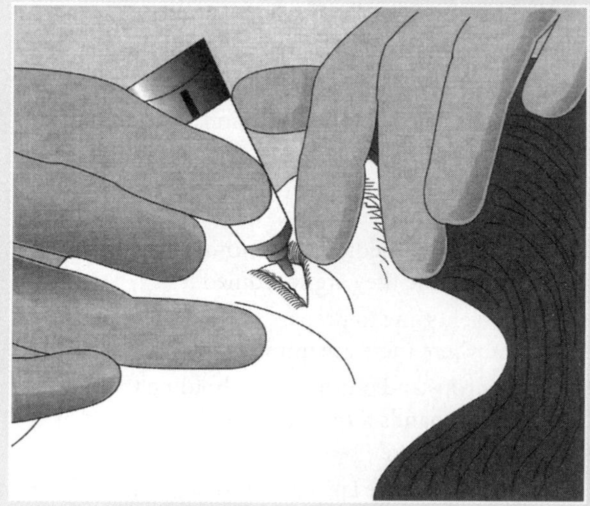

Instilling eye ointment.

Suggested Action	Reason for Action
Instruct the patient to close the eyelids gently and then blink several times.	Distributes the drug
Wipe the eyes with a clean tissue.	Removes excess drug and promotes comfort

Evaluation

- The five rights are upheld.
- The tip of the container remains uncontaminated.
- Sufficient drug is distributed within the eye.

Document

- Assessment data
- Medication administration on the MAR

SAMPLE DOCUMENTATION

Date and Time Prescribed eye medication instilled into L. eye before cataract surgery (see MAR). Conjunctiva appears pink and intact. Lens is opaque. Eyelashes have been clipped.

_______________________________ SIGNATURE, TITLE

CRITICAL THINKING

- Define the abbreviations O.S., O.D., O.U.
- Discuss actions the nurse should take if the tip of the ophthalmic medication container becomes contaminated.

SKILL 33-2

ADMINISTERING NASAL MEDICATIONS

Suggested Action	Reason for Action
Assessment	
Compare the medication administration record (MAR) with the written medical order.	Prevents medication errors
Review the patient's drug, allergy, and medical history.	Avoids potential complications
Consult a current drug reference concerning the drug's action, side effects, contraindications, and administration information.	Ensures appropriate administration based on a thorough knowledge of the drug
Planning	
Plan to administer medications within a half-hour to an hour of the time they are scheduled.	Demonstrates timely administration and compliance with the medical order
Allow sufficient time to prepare the medications in a location where there are minimal distractions.	Promotes safe preparation of drugs
Read and compare the label on the drug with the MAR at least three times—before, during, and after preparing the drug.	Ensures that the *right drug* is given at the *right time* by the *right route*
Implementation	
Wash your hands.	Removes colonizing microorganisms
Identify the patient by checking the wristband or asking the patient's name.	Ensures that medications are given to the *right patient*
Help the patient to a sitting position with his or her head tilted backward, or to the side if the drug needs to reach one or the other sinuses.	Facilitates depositing the drug where its effect is desired
If the patient cannot sit, place a rolled towel or pillow beneath the neck.	Provides support and aids in positioning
Remove the cap from liquid medication, to which a dropper is usually attached.	Provides a means for administering the drug
Aim the tip of the dropper toward the nasal passage and squeeze the rubber portion of the cap to administer the number of drops prescribed.	Deposits the drug within the nose rather than into the throat and ensures administering the *right dose*

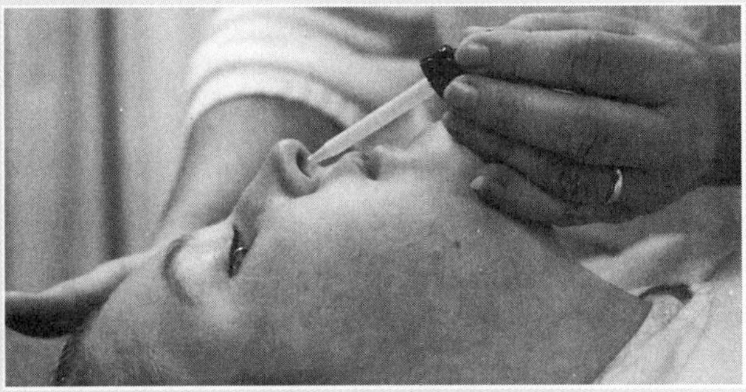

Instilling nasal medication. (Courtesy of Ken Timby.)

continued

SKILL 33-2

ADMINISTERING NASAL MEDICATIONS *Continued*

Suggested Action	Reason for Action
Instruct the patient to breathe through the mouth as the drops are instilled.	Prevents inhaling large droplets
If the drug is in a spray form, place the tip of the container just inside the nostril.	Confines the spray within the nasal passage
Occlude the opposite nostril.	Administers medication to one and then the other nasal passage
Instruct the patient to inhale as the container is squeezed.	Distributes the aerosol
Repeat in the opposite nostril.	Deposits the drug bilaterally for maximum effect
Advise the patient to remain in position for approximately 5 minutes.	Promotes local absorption
Recap the container and replace where medications are stored.	Supports principles of asepsis and demonstrates responsibility for the patient's property

Evaluation

- The five rights are upheld.
- Sufficient drug is distributed within the nose.
- Patient reports a decrease in nasal congestion.

Document

- Assessment data
- Medication administration on the MAR

SAMPLE DOCUMENTATION

Date and Time Indicates nasal passages are congested. Observed to be breathing through the mouth. Nasal medication administered (see MAR). States symptoms are relieved.

____ SIGNATURE, TITLE

CRITICAL THINKING

- What would you tell a person who uses a nasal decongestant more often than the label recommends?

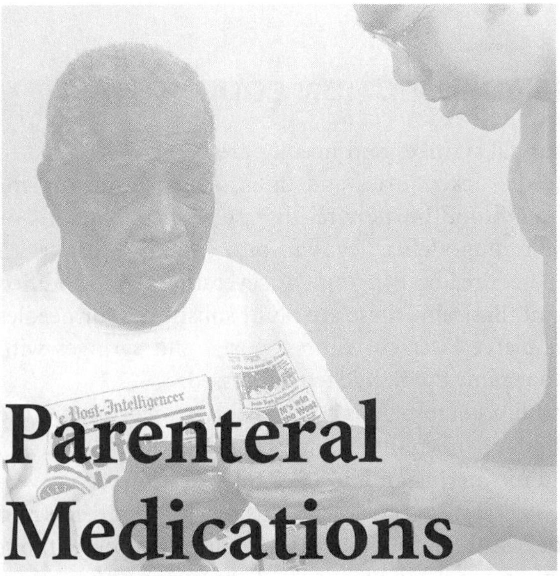

CHAPTER 34

Parenteral Medications

CHAPTER OUTLINE

NURSING GUIDELINES

SKILLS

NURSING CARE PLAN

KEY TERMS

ampule
barrel
deltoid site
dorsogluteal site
gauge
induration
insulin syringe
intradermal injection
intramuscular injection
intravenous injection
lipoatrophy
lipohypertrophy
parenteral route
plunger
prefilled cartridge
reconstitution
rectus femoris site
scoop method
shaft
subcutaneous injection
tip
tuberculin syringe
vastus lateralis site
ventrogluteal site
vial
wheal
Z-track technique

LEARNING OBJECTIVES

An understanding of the content within this chapter will be evidenced by the student's ability to:

- Name three parts of a syringe.
- List five factors to consider when selecting a syringe and needle.
- Explain the rationale for redesigning conventional syringes and needles.
- Name three ways parenteral drugs are prepared by pharmaceutical companies.
- Discuss an appropriate action to take before combining two drugs in a single syringe.
- List four injection routes.
- Identify common injection sites for an intradermal, subcutaneous, and intramuscular injection.
- Name a type of syringe that is commonly used to administer an intradermal, subcutaneous, and intramuscular injection.
- Describe the angle of entry for an intradermal, subcutaneous, and intramuscular injection.
- Discuss why most insulin combinations must be administered within 15 minutes of being mixed.
- Describe two techniques for preventing bruising when administering heparin subcutaneously.

The **parenteral route** (route of drug administration other than oral or through the gastrointestinal tract) commonly is used to refer to medications given by injection. This chapter discusses the techniques for administering injections. Preparation and administration follow the principles of asepsis and infection control.

Parenteral Administration Equipment

The major equipment used for parenteral drug administration consists of a syringe and a needle. Numerous types of syringes and needles are available.

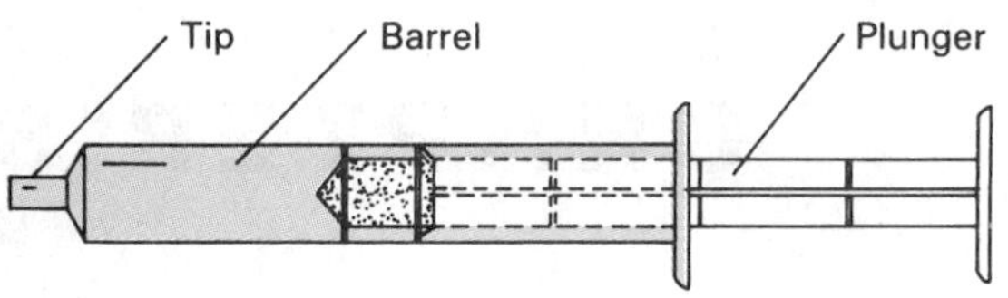

FIGURE 34–1. Parts of a syringe.

SYRINGES

All syringes contain a **barrel** (part of the syringe that holds the medication), a **plunger** (part of the syringe within the barrel that moves back and forth to withdraw and instill the medication), and a **tip** (part of the syringe to which the needle is attached; Fig. 34-1). Syringes are calibrated in milliliters (mL) or cubic centimeters (cc), units (U), and in some cases minims (m). When drugs are administered parenterally, syringes that hold 1 mL, or its equivalent in units, and up to 3 to 5 mL are most commonly used.

NEEDLES

Needles are supplied in various lengths and gauges. The **shaft** (length of the needle) depends on the depth to which the medication will be instilled. Needle lengths vary from approximately 0.5 to 2.5 inches. The tip of the shaft is beveled, or slanted, to pierce the skin more easily (see Chap. 15, Skill 15-3, Starting an Intravenous Infusion).

The needle **gauge** (diameter) refers to the width of the needle. For most injections, 18- to 27-gauge needles are used; the smaller the number, the larger the diameter. For example, an 18-gauge needle is wider than a 27-gauge needle. A wider diameter provides a larger lumen, or opening, through which drugs are administered into the tissue.

Several factors are considered when selecting a syringe and needle, including:

- Type of medication
- Depth of tissue
- Volume of prescribed drug
- Viscosity of the drug
- Size of the patient

Table 34-1 lists common sizes of syringes and needles used for various types of injections.

MODIFIED INJECTION EQUIPMENT

Conventional syringes and needles are being redesigned to avoid needlestick injuries and thus to reduce the risk for acquiring a blood-borne viral disease such as hepatitis or acquired immunodeficiency syndrome (AIDS). Most health agencies are already using one or several types of modified equipment. Basically, these are blunt substitutes for needles that can pierce laser-cut rubber ports, and syringes with shields that allow the needle to be recessed.

If modified equipment is not available, two techniques are used with standard equipment to prevent needlestick injuries. Before administering an injection, the protective cap covering a needle can be replaced by using the **scoop method** (technique of threading the needle within the cap without touching the cap itself; Fig. 34-2). After giving an injection, the needle is left uncapped and deposited in the nearest biohazard container, which is usually at the patient's bedside.

Should an accidental injury occur, health care workers should follow these recommendations:

- Report the injury to a supervisor.
- Document the injury in writing.
- Identify the patient, if possible.
- Obtain human immunodeficiency virus and hepatitis B virus patient status results, if it is legal to do so.
- Obtain counseling on the potential for infection.
- Receive the most appropriate postexposure prophylaxis.
- Be tested for the presence of antibodies at appropriate intervals.
- Monitor for potential symptoms and obtain medical follow-up.

Drug Preparation

Drug preparation involves withdrawing medication from an ampule or vial, or assembling a prefilled cartridge (Fig. 34-3).

AMPULES

An **ampule** (sealed glass drug container) must be broken to withdraw the medication.

TABLE 34–1. **Common Sizes of Syringes and Needles**

Type of Injection	Size of Syringe	Size of Needle
Intradermal (tuberculin)	1 mL calibrated or 0.01 mL or in minims	25-, 26-, or 27-gauge, ½- to ⅝-inch
Subcutaneous	1, 2, 2.5, or 3 mL calibrated in 0.1 mL	23-, 25-, or 26-gauge, ½- or ⅝-inch
Insulin, given subcutaneously	1 mL calibrated in units	25-, 26-, or 27-gauge, ½- or ⅝-inch
Intramuscular	3 or 5 mL calibrated in 0.2 mL	20-, 21-, 22-, or 23-gauge, 1½- or 2-inch

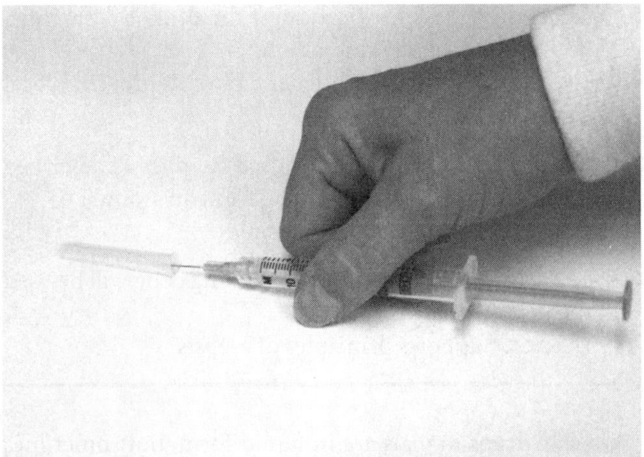

FIGURE 34–2. Scoop method for covering a needle. (Courtesy of Ken Timby.)

Nursing Guidelines For

Withdrawing Medication From an Ampule

- Select an appropriate syringe and needle.
  RATIONALE: Ensures appropriate drug administration
- Tap the top of the ampule.
  RATIONALE: Distributes all the medication to the lower portion of the ampule
- Protect your thumb and fingers with a gauze square or alcohol swab.
  RATIONALE: Reduces the potential for injury
- Snap the neck of the ampule away from your body.
  RATIONALE: Avoids accidental injury
- Insert the needle into the ampule. Avoid touching the outside of the ampule.
  RATIONALE: Ensures sterility of the needle

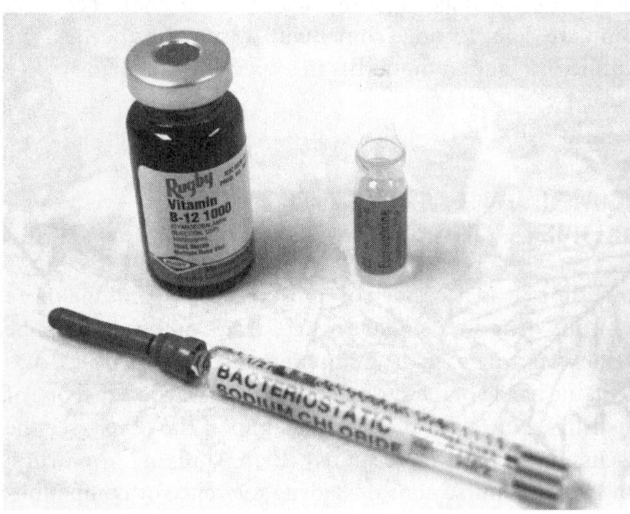

FIGURE 34–3. Vial, ampule, and prefilled cartridge. (Courtesy of Ken Timby.)

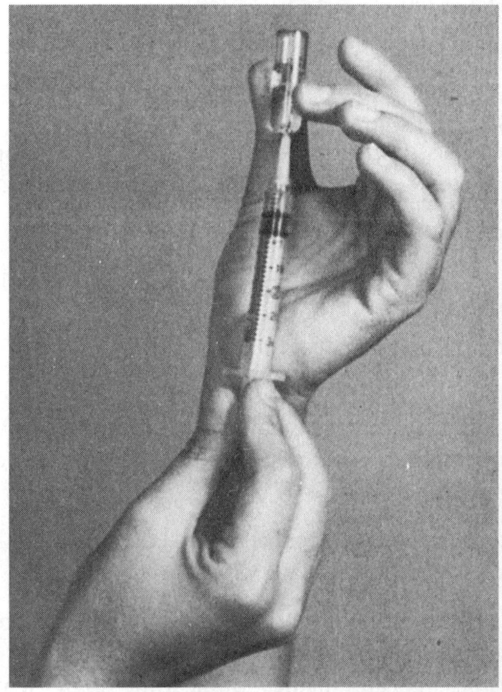

FIGURE 34–4. Withdrawing drug from an ampule.

- Invert the ampule (Fig. 34-4).
  RATIONALE: Facilitates withdrawing medication
- Pull back on the plunger.
  RATIONALE: Fills the syringe
- Remove the needle from the ampule when a sufficient volume has been withdrawn.
  RATIONALE: Prepares for drug administration
- Tap the barrel of the syringe near the hub.
  RATIONALE: Moves air toward the needle
- Push carefully on the plunger.
  RATIONALE: Expels air or excess medication
- Scoop the needle within its protective cap, or extend a guard that recesses the needle.
  RATIONALE: Reduces the risk of a needlestick injury
- Empty the unused portion of medication from the syringe.
  RATIONALE: Prevents illegal drug use
- Discard the glass ampule in a puncture-resistant container.
  RATIONALE: Prevents accidental injury

VIALS

A **vial** (glass or plastic container of parenteral medication with a self-sealing rubber stopper) must be pierced with a needle or a needleless adapter to remove medication. The amount of drug in a vial may be enough for one or several doses. Any unused drug is dated before it is stored for future use.

Nursing Guidelines For

Withdrawing Medication From a Vial

- ☑ Select an appropriate syringe and needle.
  RATIONALE: Ensures appropriate drug administration
- ☑ Remove the metal cover from the rubber stopper.
  RATIONALE: Facilitates inserting the needle or adapter
- ☑ Clean a preopened vial by swabbing it with an alcohol swab.
  RATIONALE: Removes colonizing microorganisms
- ☑ Fill the syringe with a volume of air equal to the volume that will be withdrawn from the vial.
  RATIONALE: Provides a means for increasing pressure within the vial
- ☑ Pierce the rubber stopper with the needle and instill the air.
  RATIONALE: Facilitates drug withdrawal
- ☑ Invert the vial, hold, and brace it while pulling on the plunger (Fig. 34-5).
  RATIONALE: Locates medication near the tip of the needle to facilitate its withdrawal
- ☑ Remove the needle when the desired volume has entered the barrel of the syringe.
  RATIONALE: Leaves remaining drug for additional administrations
- ☑ If the medication is a controlled substance such as a narcotic, aspirate the entire contents from the vial.
  RATIONALE: Prevents illegal drug use
- ☑ Discard any excess medication; if the drug is a narcotic, have someone witness this action.
  RATIONALE: Complies with federal laws to prevent illegal drug use
- ☑ Cover the needle, and care for used supplies as described in the guidelines for withdrawing from an ampule.
  RATIONALE: Follows similar principles
- ☑ Date and initial the vial if the remaining drug will be used in the near future.
  RATIONALE: Supports principles of asepsis

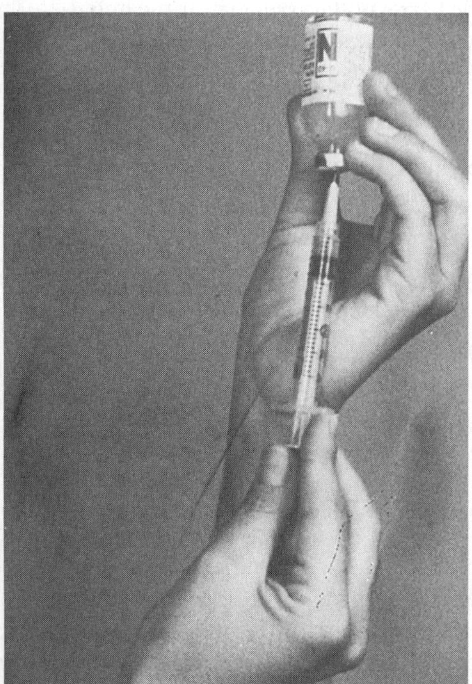

FIGURE 34–5. Withdrawing drug from a vial.

Usually drugs in vials are in liquid form, but sometimes they are supplied as powders that must be dissolved. **Reconstitution** (process of adding liquid, known as diluent, to a powdered substance) is done before administering the drug parenterally. Common diluents for injectable drugs are sterile water or sterile normal saline. Reconstituting a drug just before it is needed ensures that the drug's potency is at its maximum. When reconstitution is necessary, the drug label lists the following:

- Type of diluent to add
- Amount of diluent to use
- Dosage per volume after reconstitution
- Directions for storing the drug

If the medication will be used for more than one administration, the preparer writes the date and time on the vial label and initials it. In some cases, when the directions provide several options in diluent volumes, the amount added is also written on the vial.

PREFILLED CARTRIDGES

A **prefilled cartridge** (sealed glass cylinder of parenteral medication) is filled with medication by a pharmaceutical company. The cartridge comes with an attached needle. The cylinder is made so that it fits in a specially designed syringe (Fig. 34-6).

COMBINING MEDICATIONS IN ONE SYRINGE

Sometimes it is necessary or appropriate to combine more than one drug in a single syringe. Exact amounts must be withdrawn from each drug container, because once the drugs are in the barrel of the syringe, there is no way to expel one of the drugs without also expelling some of the other (see the discussion on mixing insulins). Before mixing any drugs, however, the nurse consults a drug reference or compatibility chart because some drugs may interact chemically when combined. The chemical reaction often causes a precipitate to form.

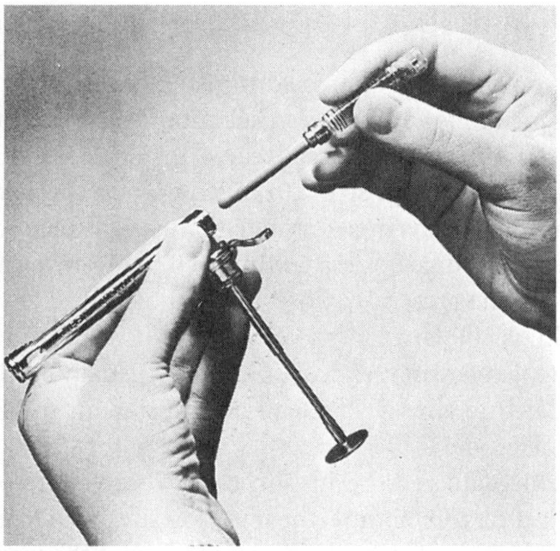

FIGURE 34–6. Inserting a prefilled cartridge.

Injection Routes

There are four injection routes for parenteral administration: **intradermal injections** (between the layers of the skin), **subcutaneous injections** (beneath the skin but above the muscle), **intramuscular injections** (in muscle tissue), and **intravenous injections** (instilled into veins; Fig. 34-7). Each site requires a slightly different injection technique. Intravenous medication administration is discussed in Chapter 35.

INTRADERMAL INJECTIONS

Intradermal injections are commonly used for diagnostic purposes. Examples include tuberculin tests and allergy testing. Small volumes, usually 0.01 to 0.05 mL, are injected because of the small tissue space.

Injection Sites

A common site for an intradermal injection is the inner aspect of the forearm. Other areas that may be used are the back and upper chest.

Injection Equipment

A **tuberculin syringe** (syringe that holds 1 mL of fluid and is calibrated in 0.01-mL increments; Fig. 34-8) is used to administer intradermal injections. A 25- to 27-gauge needle measuring a half-inch in length is commonly used when administering an intradermal injection.

Injection Technique

When giving an intradermal injection, the medication is instilled shallowly (Skill 34-1).

SUBCUTANEOUS INJECTIONS

A subcutaneous injection is administered more deeply than an intradermal injection. Medication is instilled between the skin and muscle and absorbed fairly rapidly: the medication usually begins acting within a half-hour of administration. The volume of a subcutaneous injection is usually up to 1 mL. The subcutaneous route is commonly used to administer insulin and heparin.

Injection Sites

The sites for giving a subcutaneous injection include the upper arm, thigh, abdomen, and back (Fig. 34-9).

Injection Equipment

The equipment used for a subcutaneous injection may depend on the type of medication prescribed. Insulin is prepared in an insulin syringe (see section on administering insulin). Heparin may be prepared in a tuberculin syringe, or it may be supplied in a prefilled cartridge. A 25-gauge needle is most often used because medications administered by the subcutaneous route usually are not viscous. Needle lengths may vary from 1/2 to 5/8 inch.

Injection Technique

To reach subcutaneous tissue in a heavy person, a half-inch needle is inserted at a 90° angle. For thin or average size patients, the

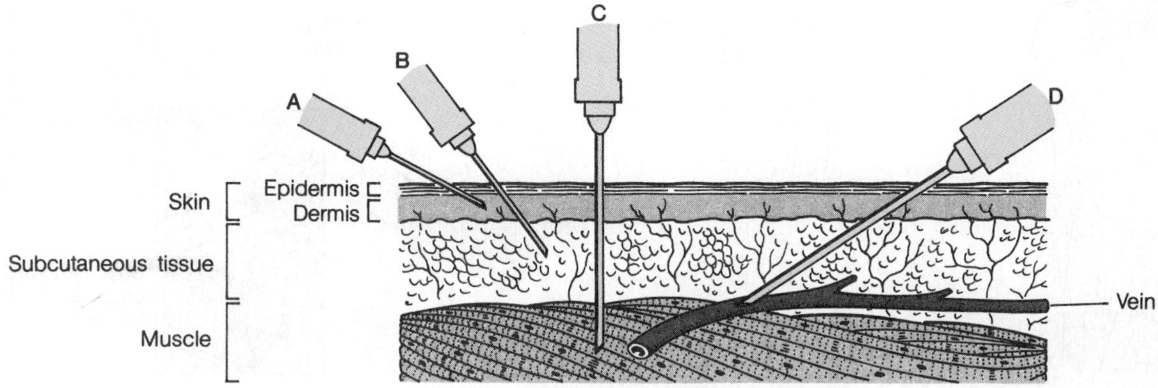

FIGURE 34–7. Injection routes. (*A*) Intradermal, (*B*) subcutaneous, (*C*) intramuscular, (*D*) intravenous. (Scherer JC: Introductory clinical pharmacology, 5th ed, p 15. Philadelphia, JB Lippincott, 1996)

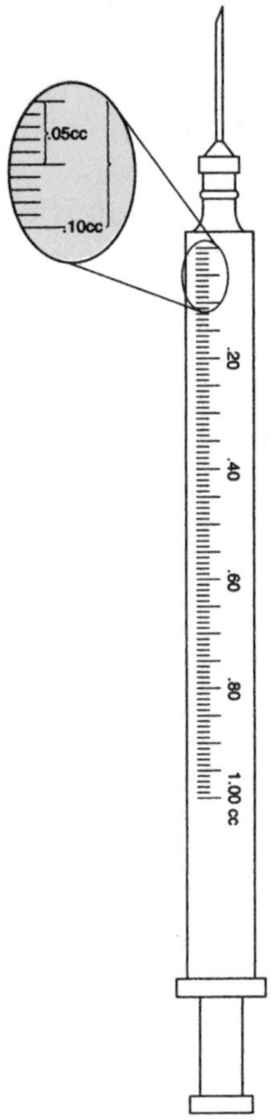

FIGURE 34–8. A tuberculin syringe.

needle is inserted at a 45° angle (Fig. 34-10). Skill 34-2 describes the technique for administering a subcutaneous injection.

In some situations the tissue is bunched between the thumb and fingers or stretched taut before administering the injection. The technique usually depends on the size of the patient. For thin patients and most children and infants, bunching is preferred.

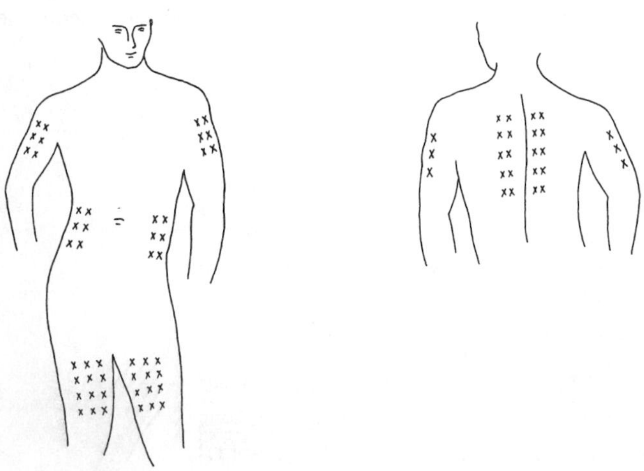

FIGURE 34–9. Subcutaneous injection sites.

Administering Insulin

Insulin is a hormone that is administered only by injection. Usually insulin is administered subcutaneously, but it can be administered intravenously. Because insulin is supplied and prescribed in a dosage strength called units, a special syringe called an **insulin syringe** (syringe that is calibrated in units) is used. The syringe holds a volume of 0.5 to 1 mL and is used to measure the prescribed dose. The standard dosage strength of insulin is 100 U/mL. Typically, a low-dose insulin syringe is used to deliver smaller doses of insulin, usually 50 U or less. A standard insulin syringe can administer up to 100 U of insulin (Fig. 34-11).

Patients who require insulin often receive one or more daily injections. Over time, the injection sites tend to undergo changes that interfere with the absorption of the insulin. To avoid **lipoatrophy** (breakdown of subcutaneous fat at the site of repeated insulin injections) and **lipohypertrophy** (buildup of subcutaneous fat at the site of repeated insulin injections), the sites are rotated each time an injection is administered.

Preparing Insulin

Types of insulin vary in their onset, peak effect, and duration of action. The nurse must read the vial labels carefully because they look similar to one another.

Some preparations of insulin contain an additive that delays its absorption. Insulin and the additive tend to separate on standing. Therefore, when preparing other than regular insulin, the vial is rotated between the palms to redistribute the two before the insulin is withdrawn.

Mixing Insulins

When mixed together, insulins tend to bind and become equilibrated. This means that each one's unique characteris-

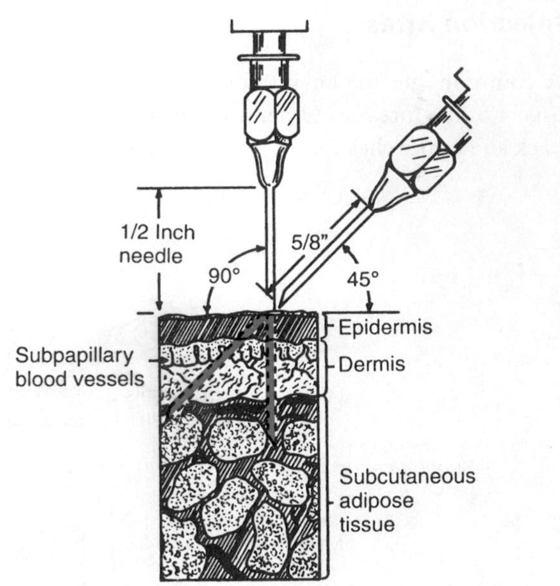

FIGURE 34–10. Angles and needle lengths for subcutaneous injections.

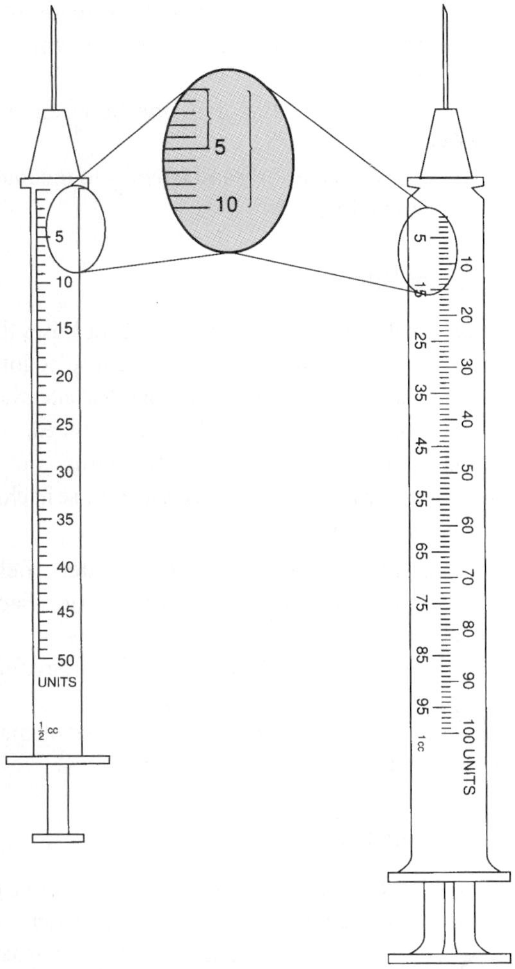

FIGURE 34–11. Low-dose and standard insulin syringes.

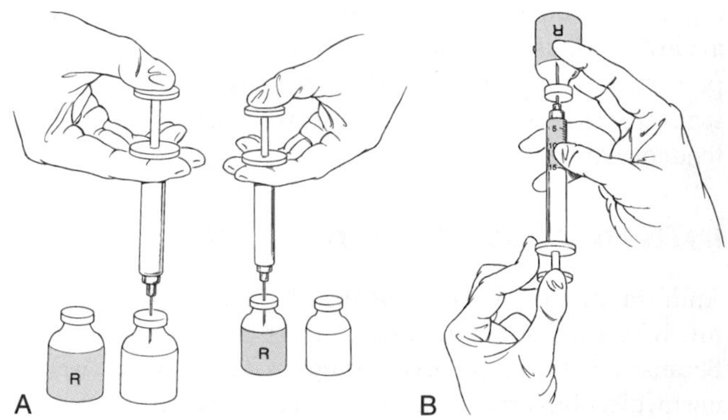

FIGURE 34–12. Mixing insulin. (*A*) Instilling air into vial with additive insulin. (*B*) Instilling air, then withdrawing from additive-free insulin vial.

tics are offset by the other. For this reason, most types of insulin are combined just before they are administered. When injected within 15 minutes of being combined, they act as if they had been injected separately. Regular insulin, which is additive-free, often is combined with an intermediate-acting insulin such as Humulin N.

Nursing Guidelines For
Mixing Insulins

☑ Roll the vial of insulin containing an additive between the palms.
RATIONALE: Mixes the insulin without damaging the protein molecules

☑ Cleanse the rubber stoppers of both vials of insulin.
RATIONALE: Removes colonizing microorganisms

☑ Instill an amount of air equal to the volume that will be withdrawn from the vial containing the insulin with the additive. Do not insert the needle into the insulin itself (Fig. 34-12*A*).
RATIONALE: Avoids coating the needle

☑ Withdraw the needle and use the same syringe to repeat the above step, but this time invert and withdraw the prescribed number of additive-free insulin units (see Fig. 34-12*B*).
RATIONALE: Prepares the partial dose

☑ Ask another nurse to check the label on the insulin and the number of units in the syringe.
RATIONALE: Prevents a medication error

☑ Swab the rubber stopper of the other vial and pierce it with the needle of the partially filled syringe.
RATIONALE: Facilitates withdrawing the other type of insulin

☑ Withdraw the specified number of units from the vial containing the insulin with the additive.
RATIONALE: Prepares the full prescribed dose

☑ Ask another nurse to check the label on the insulin and the number of units in the syringe.
RATIONALE: Prevents a medication error

☑ Administer within 15 minutes of mixing.
RATIONALE: Avoids equilibration

Administering Heparin

Heparin is an anticoagulant drug—that is, it prolongs the time it takes for blood to clot. Heparin is frequently administered subcutaneously as well as intravenously. The unique characteristics of the drug require special techniques when using the subcutaneous route for administration.

Heparin is supplied in multiple-dose vials or prefilled cartridges. The dosages are measured in tenths and hundredths of a milliliter. These very small volumes require a tuberculin syringe to ensure accuracy. The needle is removed after withdrawal of the drug from a multidose vial and replaced with another before administration.

Certain modifications are necessary to prevent bruising in the area of the injection. The needle is changed before injecting the patient. The sites are rotated with each injection to avoid a previous area where there has been local bleeding. The plunger is not aspirated once the needle is in place, and massaging the site is contraindicated because this can increase the tendency for local bleeding.

INTRAMUSCULAR INJECTIONS

An intramuscular injection is the administration of up to 3 mL of medication into one muscle or a muscle group. Because there are few nerve endings in deep muscles, irritating medications are commonly given intramuscularly. Except for medications injected directly into the bloodstream, absorption from an intramuscular injection occurs more rapidly than from the other parenteral routes.

Injection Sites

There are five common injection sites, named for the muscles into which the medications are injected: dorsogluteal, ventrogluteal, vastus lateralis, rectus femoris, and deltoid.

Dorsogluteal Site

The **dorsogluteal site** (injection area in the upper outer quadrant of the buttocks) is a common location for intramuscular injections. The primary muscle in this site is the gluteus maximus, which is large and therefore can hold a fair amount of injected medication with minimal postinjection discomfort. This site is avoided in patients younger than 3 years of age because their muscle is not sufficiently developed.

If the site is not identified correctly, damage to the sciatic nerve with subsequent paralysis of the leg can result. The nurse does the following to locate the appropriate landmarks (Fig. 34-13):

- Divide the buttock into four imaginary quadrants.
- Palpate the posterior iliac spine and the greater trochanter.
- Draw an imaginary diagonal line between the two landmarks.
- Insert the needle superiorly and laterally to the midpoint of the diagonal line.

Ventrogluteal Site

The **ventrogluteal site** (injection area in the hip) uses the gluteus medius and gluteus minimus muscles for injection. This site has several advantages over the dorsogluteal site: there are no large nerves or blood vessels in the injection area, and it is usually less fatty and cleaner because fecal contamination is rare at this site. The ventrogluteal site is also safe for use in children.

To locate the ventrogluteal site:

- Place the palm of the hand on the greater trochanter and the index finger on the anterior superior iliac spine (Fig. 34-14).
- Move the middle finger away from the index finger as far as possible along the iliac crest.
- Inject into the center of the triangle formed by the index finger, middle finger, and iliac crest.

Vastus Lateralis Site

The **vastus lateralis site** (injection area in the outer thigh) uses the vastus lateralis muscle, one of the muscles in the quadriceps group. Large nerves and blood vessels usually are absent in this area, which makes it safer. It is a particularly desirable site for administering injections to infants and small children and patients who are thin or debilitated, with poorly developed gluteal muscles.

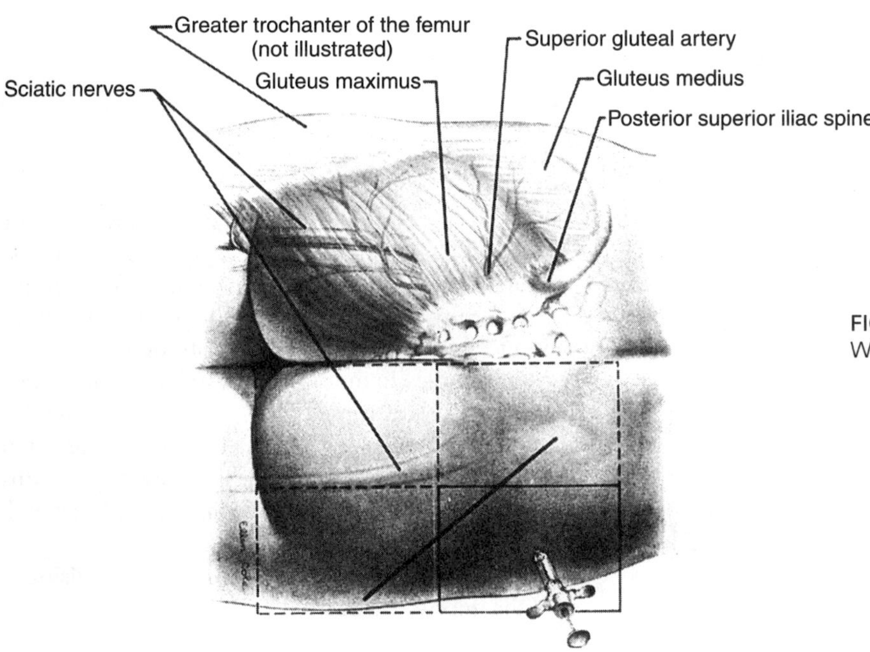

FIGURE 34–13. Dorsogluteal site. (Courtesy of Wyeth Laboratories, Philadelphia, PA.)

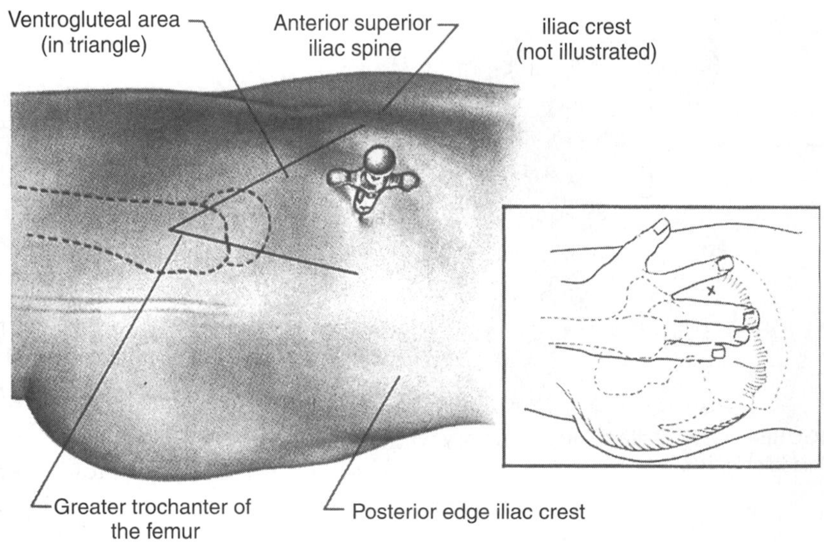

FIGURE 34–14. Ventrogluteal site. (Courtesy of Wyeth Laboratories, Philadelphia, PA.)

The vastus lateralis site is located by placing one hand just below the greater trochanter at the top of the thigh. The needle is then inserted into the lateral area of the thigh (Fig. 34-15).

Rectus Femoris Site

The **rectus femoris site** (injection area in the anterior aspect of the thigh) is the preferred injection site for infants. An injection in this site is placed in the middle third of the thigh, with the patient in a sitting or supine position (Fig. 34-16).

Deltoid Site

The **deltoid site** (injection area in the lateral aspect of the upper arm; Fig. 34-17) is the least-used intramuscular injection site because it is a smaller muscle than the others. The site is used only for adults because the muscle is not sufficiently developed in infants and children. Because of its small capacity, intramuscular injections into this site are limited to 1 mL of solution.

There is a risk of damaging the radial nerve and artery if the deltoid site is not well identified. To use this site safely:

- Have the patient lie down, sit, or stand with the shoulder well exposed.
- Palpate the lower edge of the acromion process.
- Draw an imaginary line at the axilla.
- Inject in the area between these two landmarks.

Injection Equipment

Generally, 3- to 5-mL syringes are used to administer medications by the intramuscular route. A 22-gauge needle that is 1.5 to 2 inches long usually is adequate for depositing medication in most sites.

Injection Technique

When administering intramuscular injections, a 90° angle is used for piercing the skin (Skill 34-3). Drugs that may be irri-

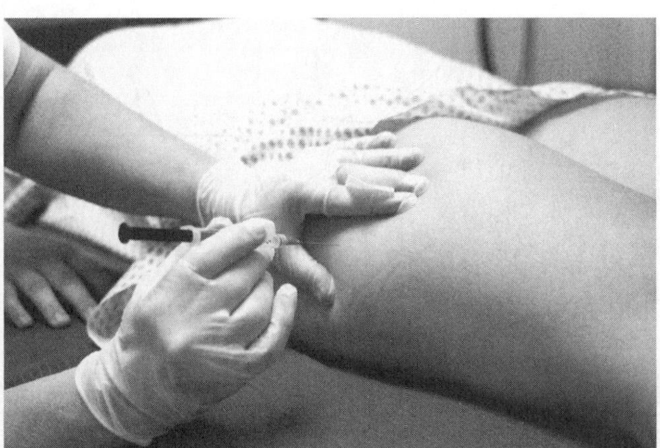

FIGURE 34–15. Vastus lateralis injection site. (Courtesy of Ken Timby.)

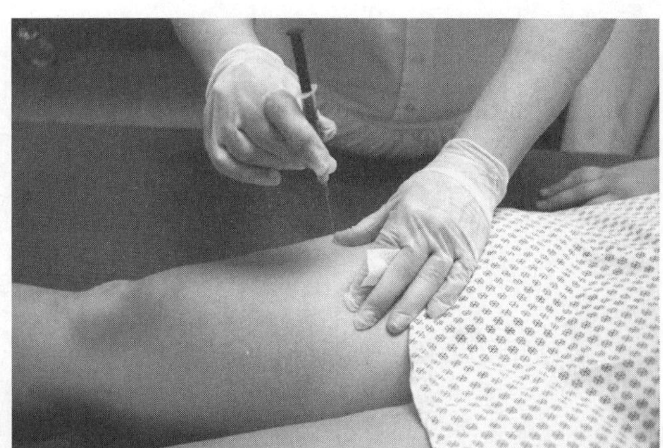

FIGURE 34–16. Rectus femoris injection site. (Courtesy of Ken Timby.)

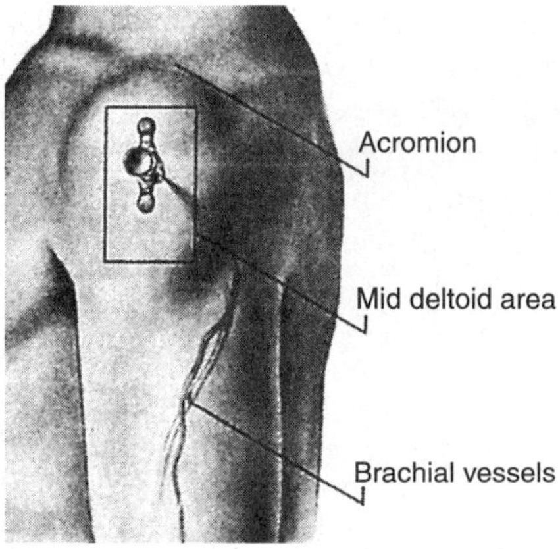

FIGURE 34–17. Deltoid site. (Courtesy of Wyeth Laboratories, Philadelphia, PA.)

tating to the upper levels of tissue may be administered by the **Z-track technique** (technique for manipulating the tissue to seal medication, especially an irritant, in the muscle). Sometimes called the zig-zag technique, the maneuver resembles the letter "Z."

Nursing Guidelines For

Giving an Injection by Z-Track Technique

- ☑ Fill the syringe with the prepared drug, then change the needle.
  RATIONALE: Prevents tissue contact with the irritating drug
- ☑ Attach a needle that is at least 1.5 to 2 inches long.
  RATIONALE: Helps deposit the drug deep within the muscle
- ☑ Add a 0.2-mL bubble of air in the syringe.
  RATIONALE: Flushes all the medication from the syringe during the injection
- ☑ Select a large muscular injection site, such as the ventrogluteal site.
  RATIONALE: Provides a location with a large capacity where the drug can be deposited and absorbed
- ☑ Wash your hands and don gloves.
  RATIONALE: Reduces the transmission of microorganisms
- ☑ Use the side of the hand to pull the tissue laterally about 1 inch (2.5 cm) until it is taut (Fig. 34-18*A*).
  RATIONALE: Creates the mechanism for sealing the drug within the muscle
- ☑ Insert the needle at a 90° angle while continuing to hold the tissue laterally.
  RATIONALE: Directs the tip of the needle well within the muscle
- ☑ Steady the barrel of the syringe with the fingers and use the thumb to manipulate the plunger (see Fig. 34-18*B*).
  RATIONALE: Avoids releasing the tissue held taut by the nondominant hand
- ☑ Aspirate for a blood return.
  RATIONALE: Determines whether the needle is in a blood vessel
- ☑ Instill the medication by depressing the plunger with the thumb.
  RATIONALE: Deposits the medication into the muscle
- ☑ Wait 10 seconds with the needle still in place and the skin still held taut.
  RATIONALE: Provides time for the medication to be distributed in a larger area
- ☑ Withdraw the needle and immediately release the taut skin.
  RATIONALE: Creates a diagonal path that prevents leaking into the subcutaneous and dermal layers of tissue (see Fig. 34-18*C*).
- ☑ Apply pressure, but do not massage the site.
  RATIONALE: Ensures that the medication remains sealed
- ☑ Discard the syringe without recapping the needle.
  RATIONALE: Reduces the potential for needlestick injury

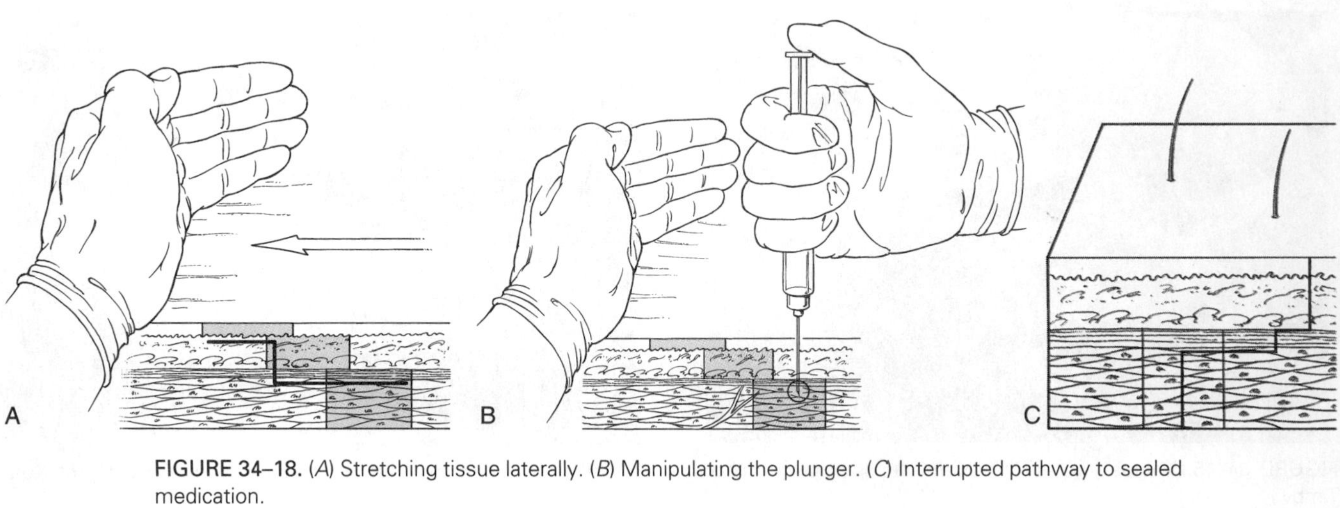

FIGURE 34–18. (*A*) Stretching tissue laterally. (*B*) Manipulating the plunger. (*C*) Interrupted pathway to sealed medication.

☑ Remove gloves and wash your hands.
RATIONALE: Reduces the transmission of microorganisms

☑ Document the medication administration.
RATIONALE: Maintains a current record of patient care

Any intramuscular injection can be given by the Z-track technique. Patients report slightly less pain during and the next day after a Z-track injection compared with the usual intramuscular injection technique.

Reducing Injection Discomfort

All injections cause discomfort, some more than others. A few products are available that produce anesthesia when applied to the skin or mucous membranes. One example is EMLA (eutectic mixture of local anesthetic), which reduces or eliminates the local discomfort of invasive procedures in which the skin is pierced. However, it can take 60 to 120 minutes after application for EMLA cream to take effect. Because these time constraints make EMLA impractical, the nurse can use the following alternative techniques to reduce the discomfort associated with injections:

- Use the smallest-gauge needle that is appropriate.
- Change the needle before administering a drug that is irritating to tissue.
- Select a site that is free of irritation.
- Rotate injection sites.
- Numb the skin with an ice pack before the injection.
- Insert and withdraw the needle without hesitation.
- Instill the medication slowly and steadily.
- Use the Z-track method for intramuscular injections.
- Apply pressure to the site during needle withdrawal.
- Massage the site afterward.

The patient also can assist in minimizing the pain associated with injections. Instructions commonly focus on positioning and relaxation techniques.

Patient Teaching Guidelines For
Reducing Injection Discomfort

Teach the patient to do the following:
- Lie prone and point the toes inward when receiving an injection into the dorsogluteal site.
- Perform deep breathing and other relaxation techniques before receiving an injection.
- Avoid watching when the injection is given.
- Ambulate or move the extremity where the injection was given as much as possible.

Nursing Implications

Nurses who administer parenteral medications may identify nursing diagnoses such as:
- Pain
- Anxiety
- Fear
- Risk for trauma
- Knowledge deficit
- Ineffective management of therapeutic regimen: individuals

The nursing care plan demonstrates the nursing process for a patient with the nursing diagnosis Ineffective management of therapeutic regimen: individuals, defined in the NANDA taxonomy (1999) as "a pattern of regulating and integrating into daily living a program for treatment of illness and the sequelae of illness that is unsatisfactory for meeting specific health goals."

Nursing Care Plan
Ineffective Management of Therapeutic Regimen: Individuals

Assessment

Subjective Data
States, "I don't know what happened. I gave myself my insulin and then I started cleaning the house. All of a sudden I fainted."

Objective Data
70-year-old newly diagnosed diabetic woman discharged 2 days earlier. Brought by ambulance to the Emergency Department after having been found unconscious at home by spouse. Blood sugar was 55 mg/dL on admission; current blood sugar is 85 mg per glucometer.

continued

Nursing Care Plan: *Ineffective Management of Therapeutic Regimen: Individuals* Continued

Diagnosis

Ineffective management of therapeutic regimen, individuals related to misunderstanding of how to balance insulin and dietary needs.

Plan

Goal

The patient will describe the need to eat food within ½ to 1 hour of insulin administration and ways to raise blood sugar if symptoms reappear.

Orders: 5/28

1. Request consult with dietitian.
2. Review onset, peak, and duration of Humulin N.
3. Review the signs and symptoms of low blood sugar.
4. Suggest ways of raising blood sugar quickly.
5. Have patient demonstrate use of glucometer and self-administration of insulin before discharge. ______ J. FULCHER, RN

Implementation (Documentation)

5/28 1345 Consult request sent to dietary department. Reviewed Humulin N onset at 1 to 1½ hours after eating, peak in 4 to 12 hours, and duration of 18 to 28 hours. Explained the meaning of terms. ______ K. DAMON, LPN

Evaluation (Documentation)

5/28 1800 Could explain purpose for eating within the onset time, but could not identify the time of peak and duration of action. Information repeated. ______ K. DAMON, LPN

FOCUS ON OLDER ADULTS

- Because older adults have less subcutaneous fat, it is best to bunch the tissue when administering an intramuscular injection to avoid striking the bone.
- Older adults with diabetes often have visual problems interfering with their ability to self-administer insulin. It is appropriate to collaborate with the prescribing practitioner on teaching patients who are visually impaired how to use a loading gauge that prevents filling a syringe with more than the prescribed dose. Sight Centers are a good resource for obtaining assistive devices to facilitate self-administration of insulin.
- Older adults who are learning to administer insulin may benefit from a referral for skilled nursing or diabetic health education after discharge. In many cases, the patient's health insurance company covers these services.
- Older adults who can administer insulin injections but cannot fill their own syringes may use pre-filled syringes as long as they roll the syringe to mix the solution before administering the injection.
- Older adults tend to experience more adverse effects from drugs administered parenterally because their ability to absorb and metabolize the drugs may be compromised by age-related changes and the possible existence of chronic diseases. Thus, older adults may require lower doses of parenteral medications.
- Injections into sites involving limbs that are paralyzed, inactive, or affected by poor circulation are to be avoided. The deltoid site may be best for older adults with impaired mobility.
- Dementia and musculoskeletal deformities such as contractures or those associated with arthritis often complicate the techniques for positioning older adults when selecting and identifying site landmarks appropriately. A second person's assistance is helpful when giving an injection to a person who has difficulty maintaining the required position for the injection. The second person can help with positioning and also offer comfort and distraction.
- When an older adult has a change in mental status or behavior coinciding with the administration of a new drug, the possibility of an adverse drug effect must be considered.

KEY CONCEPTS

- Three parts of a syringe are the barrel, plunger, and tip.
- When selecting a syringe and needle, the following factors are considered: type of medication, depth of tissue, volume of prescribed drug, viscosity of the drug, and size of the patient.
- Conventional syringes and needles are being redesigned to reduce the potential for needlestick injuries and the transmission of blood-borne pathogens.
- Pharmaceutical companies supply drugs for parenteral administration in ampules, vials, and prefilled cartridges.
- Before combining two drugs in a single syringe, it is important to consult a drug reference or a compatibility chart to determine whether a chemical interaction may occur.
- There are four parenteral injection routes: intradermal, subcutaneous, intramuscular, and intravenous.
- A common site for an intradermal injection is the inner forearm; subcutaneous injections are commonly given in the thigh, arm, or abdomen; intramuscular injections are given in the buttocks, hip, thigh, or arm.
- An intradermal injection is commonly given with a tuberculin syringe. Insulin is administered subcutaneously with an insulin syringe. Intramuscular injections are usually given with a syringe that holds a volume of 3 mL.
- For an intradermal injection, the needle is inserted at a 10° to 15° angle. For a subcutaneous injection, a 45° to 90° angle is used. For an intramuscular injection, a 90° angle is used.
- When two insulins are combined, they must be administered within 15 minutes to avoid equilibration (the loss of each insulin's unique characteristics).
- To prevent bruising when heparin is administered, the nurse avoids aspirating with the plunger and massaging the site afterward.
- Five sites used for administering intramuscular injections are the dorsogluteal site, the ventrogluteal site, the vastus lateralis site, the rectus femoris site, and the deltoid site.
- Intramuscular injections are given by Z-track technique to seal irritating substances in the muscle and to reduce discomfort after an injection.

CRITICAL THINKING EXERCISES

- Discuss the differences between administering injections by the intradermal, subcutaneous, and intramuscular routes.
- Discuss how an intramuscular injection would be different if given to a 3-year-old versus a 33-year-old.
- You are to administer an intramuscular injection to a 76-year-old patient. Discuss the factors you will consider before choosing your equipment and injection site.

SUGGESTED READINGS

Bodzin B. The needle-phobic patient with diabetes. Home Healthcare Nurse 1996;14(5):378–380.

Capriotti T. A new form of heparin is changing treatment of thrombotic disorders. MedSurg Nursing 1998;7(2):106–109.

Fleming DR. Challenging traditional insulin injection practices. American Journal of Nursing 1999;99(2):72–74.

Hadley SA, Chang M, Rogers K. Effect of syringe size on bruising following subcutaneous heparin injection. American Journal of Critical Care 1996; 5(4):271–276.

Hayes C. Injection technique. Nursing Times 1998;94(42):insert, 2p.

Heparin injections: Change is needed. Nursing 1998;28(7):12.

Insulin administration. Diabetes Care 1999;22(Suppl 1):S83–S86.

Jordan LS. Using the Dummy Tummy to teach insulin injection. Diabetes Educator 1996;22(3):245–246.

Knight J. Inserting an insulin catheter: Paving the way for multiple injections. Nursing 1998;28(2):58–60.

Maason V. Challenging tradition. American Journal of Nursing 1999;99(7):14.

McConnell EA. Administering intradermal injections. Nursing 1996;26(2):18.

NANDA nursing diagnoses: Definitions and classification, 1999–2000. Philadelphia, NANDA, 1999.

Rausch M. Update on insulin administration. American Journal of Nursing 1998;98(7):55.

Springs MH, Mulryan K, Fleming D. Shake, rattle, or roll? American Journal of Nursing 1999;99(7):14–17.

Turcios NL. Tuberculosis in children: Skin testing and screening. Journal of Respiratory Diseases 1997;18(7):674–683.

Workman B. Safe injection techniques. Nursing Standard 1999;13(39):47–54.

SKILL 34–1

ADMINISTERING INTRADERMAL INJECTIONS

Suggested Action	Reason for Action
Assessment	
Check the medical orders.	Collaborates nursing activities with medical treatment
Compare the medication administration record (MAR) with the written medical order.	Ensures accuracy
Read and compare the label on the drug with the MAR at least three times—before, during, and after preparing the drug.	Prevents errors
Check for any documented allergies to food or drugs.	Ensures safety
Determine how much the patient understands about the purpose and technique for administering the injection.	Provides an opportunity for health teaching
Planning	
Prepare to administer the injection according to the schedule prescribed.	Complies with medical orders
Obtain clean gloves, tuberculin syringe, appropriate needle, and alcohol swabs.	Facilitates drug preparation and administration
Prepare the syringe with the medication.	Fills the syringe with the appropriate volume
Implementation	
Wash your hands and don gloves.	Reduces the transmission of microorganisms
Read the name on the patient's identification band.	Prevents errors
Pull the privacy curtain.	Demonstrates respect for the patient's dignity
Select an area on the inner aspect of the forearm, about a hand's breadth above the patient's wrist.	Provides a convenient and easy location for accessing intradermal tissue
Cleanse the area with an alcohol swab using a circular motion outward from the site where the needle will pierce the skin.	Removes microorganisms following principles of asepsis
Allow the skin to dry.	Reduces tissue irritation
Hold the patient's arm and stretch the skin taut.	Helps control the placement of the needle
Hold the syringe almost parallel to the skin at a 10° to 15° angle with the bevel pointing upward. Then insert the needle about ⅛ inch.	Facilitates delivering the drug between the layers of the skin. Advances the needle to the desired depth.
Push the plunger of the syringe and watch for a small wheal (elevated circle) to appear.	Verifies that the drug has been injected correctly
Withdraw the needle at the same angle at which it was inserted.	Minimizes tissue trauma and discomfort
Do not massage the area after removing the needle.	Prevents interfering with test results
Deposit the uncapped needle and syringe in a puncture-resistant container.	Prevents injury
Remove your gloves and wash your hands	Reduces the risk for transmission of microorganisms
Observe the patient's condition for at least the first half-hour after performing an allergy test.	Ensures that emergency treatment can be quickly administered
Observe the area for signs of a local reaction at standard intervals, such as at 24 and 48 hours after the injection.	Determines the extent to which the patient responds to the injected substance

continued

SKILL 34–1

ADMINISTERING INTRADERMAL INJECTIONS *Continued*

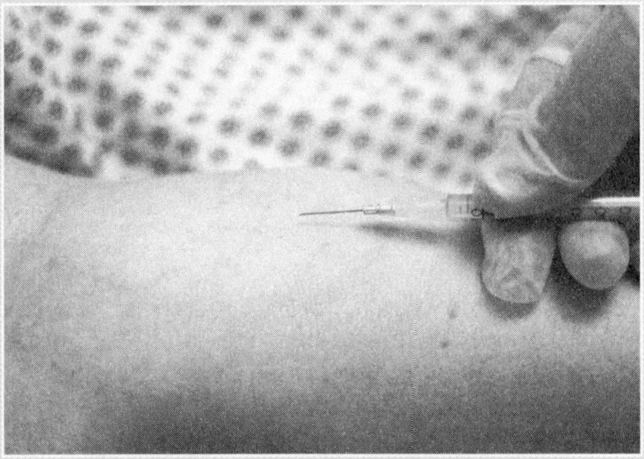

Entering the skin. (Courtesy of Ken Timby.)

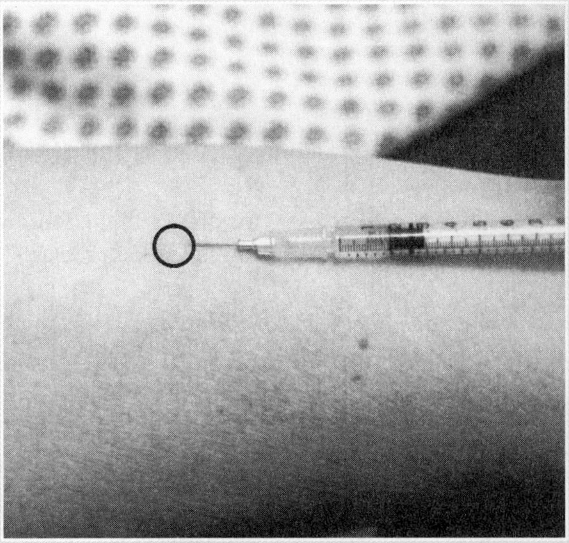

Forming a wheal. (Courtesy of Ken Timby.)

Evaluation

- Injection is administered.
- Patient remains free of any untoward effects.

Document

- The date, time, drug, dose, route, and specific site
- Response of the patient

SAMPLE DOCUMENTATION

Date and Time Tuberculin skin test administered intradermally in L. forearm with no immediate untoward effects. Instructed to return in 48 hours for inspection of site.

_______________________________ SIGNATURE, TITLE

CRITICAL THINKING

- Explain how you would modify this injection technique if the patient was a young child.
- What would you do if the patient begins to show signs of an allergic reaction to the agent given intradermally?

SKILL 34–2

ADMINISTERING SUBCUTANEOUS INJECTIONS

Suggested Action	Reason for Action
Assessment	
Check the medical orders.	Collaborates nursing activities with medical treatment
Compare the medication administration record (MAR) with the written medical order.	Ensures accuracy
Read and compare the label on the drug with the MAR at least three times—before, during, and after preparing the drug.	Prevents errors
Check for any documented allergies to food or drugs.	Ensures safety
Determine where the last injection was given to ensure site rotation.	Prevents tissue injury
Determine how much the patient understands about the purpose and technique for administering the injection.	Provides an opportunity for health teaching
Inspect the potential injection site for signs of bruising, swelling, redness, warmth, or tenderness.	Indicates injured tissue areas to be avoided
Planning	
Prepare to administer the injection according to the schedule prescribed.	Complies with medical orders
Obtain clean gloves, appropriate syringe and needle, and alcohol swabs.	Facilitates drug preparation and administration
Prepare the syringe with the medication.	Fills the syringe with the appropriate volume
Add 0.1 to 0.2 mL of air to the syringe.	Flushes all of the medication from the syringe at the time of the injection
Implementation	
Wash your hands and don gloves.	Reduces the transmission of microorganisms
Read the name on the patient's identification band.	Prevents errors
Pull the privacy curtain.	Demonstrates respect for the patient's dignity
Select and prepare an appropriate site by cleansing it with an alcohol swab.	Removes colonizing microorganisms
Allow the skin to dry.	Reduces tissue irritation
Bunch the skin at the site or spread it taut.	Facilitates placement in the subcutaneous level of tissue according to the patient's body composition and amount of adipose tissue
Pierce the skin at a 45° or 90° angle of entry.	Facilitates placement in the subcutaneous level of tissue according to the length of the needle being used
Release the tissue once the needle is inserted and use the hand to support the syringe at its hub.	Steadies the syringe
Pull back gently on the plunger* with a free hand and observe for blood in the barrel.	Determines if the needle lies in a blood vessel
Inject the medication by pushing on the plunger if there is no blood after aspiration.	Ensures subcutaneous administration
Withdraw the needle quickly while applying pressure against the medication site.	Controls bleeding
Massage the site, unless contraindicated.	Promotes absorption and relieves discomfort

continued

SKILL 34-2

ADMINISTERING SUBCUTANEOUS INJECTIONS *Continued*

Suggested Action	Reason for Action
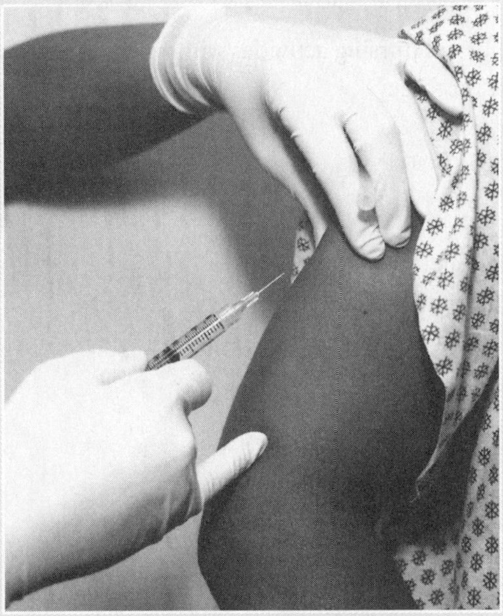 Entering the tissue at a 45° angle. (Courtesy of Ken Timby.)	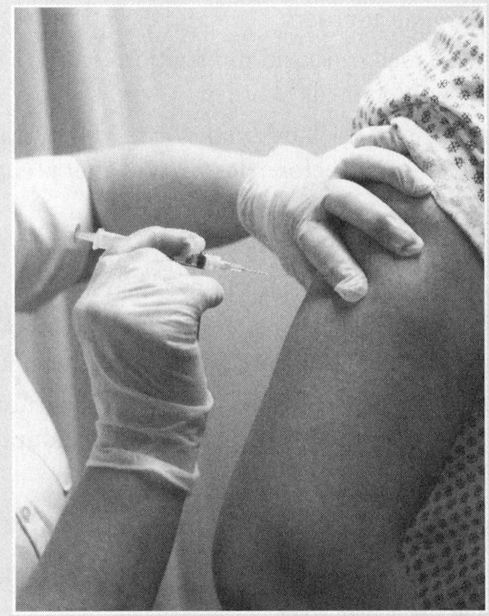 Entering the tissue at a 90° angle. (Courtesy of Ken Timby.)
Deposit the uncapped needle and syringe in a puncture-resistant container.	Prevents injury
Remove your gloves and wash your hands.	Reduces the transmission of microorganisms
Assess the patient's condition at least 30 minutes after giving the injection.	Aids in evaluating the drug's effectiveness

Evaluation

- Injection is administered.
- Patient experiences no untoward effects.

Document

- The date, time, drug, dose, route, and specific site
- Site assessment data
- Response of the patient

SAMPLE DOCUMENTATION[†]

Date and Time 25 U of regular insulin administered into L. upper arm. Site appears free of redness, swelling, warmth, tenderness, and bruising. Alert and oriented one half-hour after injection.

________________________________ Signature, Title

CRITICAL THINKING

- Besides documenting the site of a subcutaneous injection, discuss additional techniques for ensuring that sites are rotated with each subsequent injection.
- Compare and contrast the injection techniques for administering insulin and heparin.

* Skip this step if administering heparin.

† The administration of drugs is usually documented on the MAR.

SKILL 34-3

ADMINISTERING INTRAMUSCULAR INJECTIONS

Suggested Action	Reason for Action
Assessment	
Check the medical orders.	Collaborates nursing activities with medical treatment
Compare the medication administration record (MAR) with the written medical order.	Ensures accuracy
Read and compare the label on the drug with the MAR at least three times—before, during, and after preparing the drug.	Prevents errors
Check for any documented drug allergies.	Ensures safety
Determine where the last injection was given.	Prevents tissue injury
Determine how much the patient understands about the purpose and technique for administering the injection.	Provides an opportunity for health teaching
Inspect the potential injection site for signs of bruising, swelling, redness, warmth, tenderness, or **induration** (hardness).	Indicates tissue injury
Planning	
Prepare to administer the injection according to the schedule prescribed.	Complies with medical orders
Obtain clean gloves, appropriate syringe and needle, and alcohol swabs.	Facilitates drug preparation and administration
Prepare the syringe with the medication.	Fills the syringe with the appropriate volume
Add 0.2 mL of air to the syringe.	Flushes all of the medication from the syringe at the time of the injection
Implementation	
Wash your hands and don gloves.	Reduces the transmission of microorganisms
Read the name on the patient's identification band.	Prevents errors
Pull the privacy curtain.	Demonstrates respect for the patient's dignity
Select and prepare an appropriate site by cleansing it with an alcohol swab.	Removes colonizing microorganisms
Allow the skin to dry.	Reduces tissue irritation
Spread the tissue taut.	Facilitates placement in the muscle
Hold the syringe like a dart and pierce the skin at a 90° angle.	Reduces discomfort
Steady the syringe and aspirate to observe for blood.	Determines if the needle is in a blood vessel
Instill the drug if no blood is apparent.	Deposits the drug into the muscle
Withdraw the needle quickly at the same angle it was inserted while applying pressure against the site.	Reduces discomfort and controls bleeding
Massage the injection site with the alcohol swab, unless contraindicated.	Distributes the medication and reduces discomfort
Deposit the uncapped needle and syringe in a puncture-resistant container.	Prevents injury
Remove your gloves and wash your hands.	Reduces the transmission of microorganisms
Assess the patient's condition at least 30 minutes after giving the injection.	Aids in evaluating the drug's effectiveness

continued

SKILL 34–3

ADMINISTERING INTRAMUSCULAR INJECTIONS *Continued*

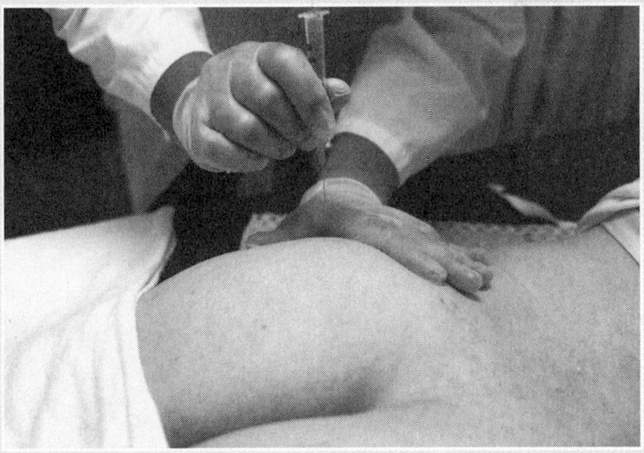

Holding syringe like a dart. (Courtesy of Ken Timby.)

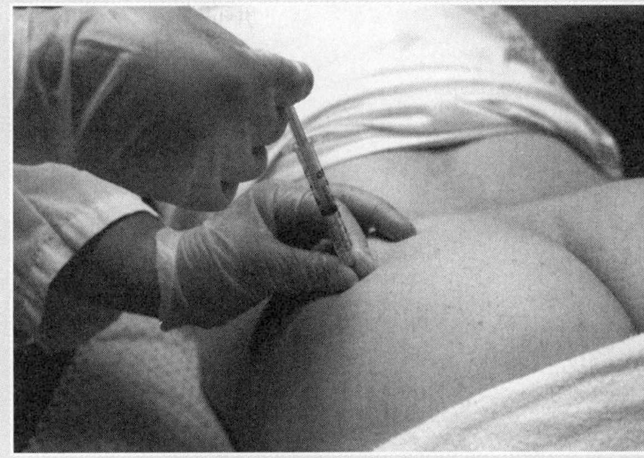

Aspirating for blood. (Courtesy of Ken Timby.)

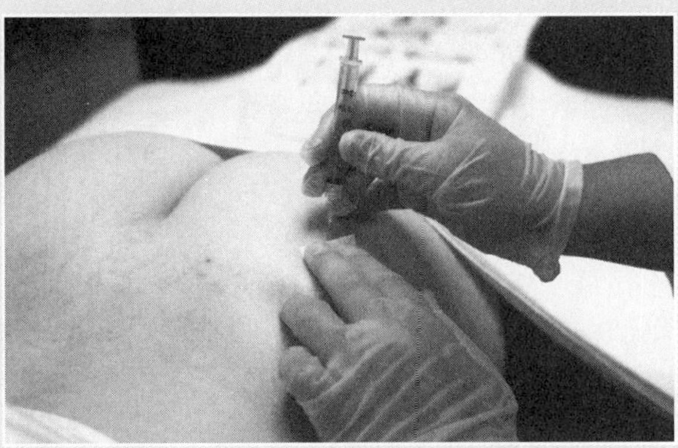

Withdrawing the needle. (Courtesy of Ken Timby.)

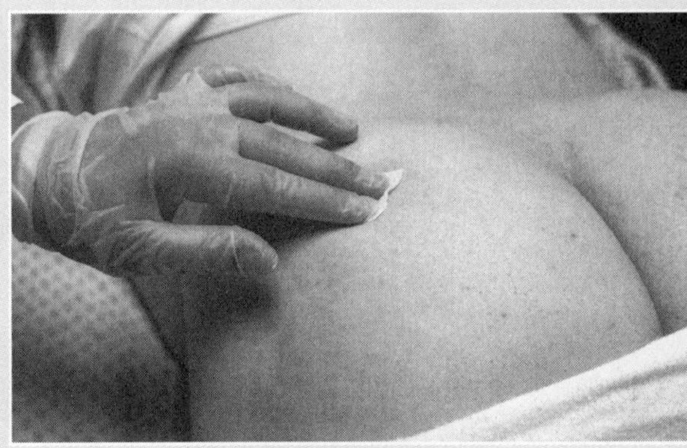

Massaging the site. (Courtesy of Ken Timby.)

Evaluation

- Injection is administered.
- Patient experiences no untoward effects.

Document

- The date, time, drug, dose, route, and specific site
- Site assessment data
- Response of the patient

SAMPLE DOCUMENTATION*

Date and Time Demerol 50 mg given IM into R. ventrogluteal site for pain rated as #8 on a scale of 0–10. No signs of irritation at the site. Rates pain at #5, 30 min. after injection.

______________________________ SIGNATURE, TITLE

CRITICAL THINKING

- Discuss the consequences that could occur if parenteral medication intended for the intramuscular route is instilled into a blood vessel.
- What consequences could occur if an intramuscular injection site is not identified accurately?

* The administration of drugs is usually documented on the MAR; prn drugs may be documented both in the nurse's notes and the MAR.

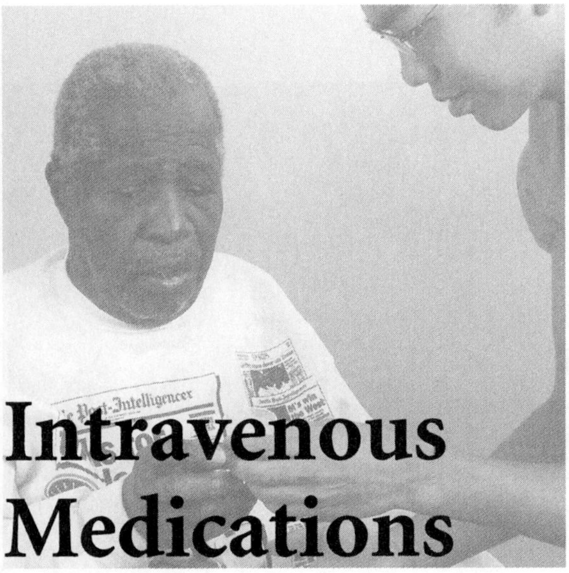

Intravenous Medications

CHAPTER 35

CHAPTER OUTLINE

Intravenous Medication Administration
Central Venous Catheters
Nursing Implications

NURSING GUIDELINES

ADMINISTERING MEDICATIONS THROUGH AN INTRAVENOUS PORT
ADMINISTERING MEDICATIONS THROUGH A LOCK
USING A CENTRAL VENOUS CATHETER

SKILLS

SKILL 35-1: ADMINISTERING INTRAVENOUS MEDICATION BY CONTINUOUS INFUSION
SKILL 35-2: ADMINISTERING AN INTERMITTENT SECONDARY INFUSION
SKILL 35-3: USING A VOLUME-CONTROL SET

NURSING CARE PLAN

ALTERED PROTECTION

KEY TERMS

antineoplastic drugs	intravenous route
bolus administration	port
central venous catheter	secondary infusion
continuous infusion	volume-control set
intermittent infusion	

LEARNING OBJECTIVES

An understanding of the content within this chapter will be evidenced by the student's ability to:

- Name two types of veins into which intravenous medications are administered.
- Describe at least three appropriate situations for administering intravenous medications.
- Name two ways intravenous medications are administered.
- Describe one method for giving bolus administrations of intravenous medications.
- Describe two methods for administering medicated solutions intermittently.
- Explain the technique for administering a piggyback infusion.
- Discuss two purposes for using a volume-control set.
- Describe a central venous catheter.
- Name three types of central venous catheters.
- Discuss two techniques for protecting oneself when administering antineoplastic drugs.

Administering intravenous solutions, which is discussed in Chapter 15, is considered a form of intravenous medication administration. The focus of this chapter, however, is on the methods for administering intravenous drugs, not fluid replacement solutions, and the techniques for using various venous access devices.

The **intravenous (IV) route** (drug administration via peripheral and central veins) provides an immediate effect. Consequently, this is the most dangerous route for drug administration. Drugs administered in this manner cannot be retrieved once they have been given. For this reason, only specially qualified nurses are permitted to administer IV medications. Even those who are responsible for IV medication administration must use extreme caution in preparation and instillation.

Intravenous Medication Administration

Despite its risks, IV administration, given either continuously or intermittently, is the route chosen when:

- A quick response is needed during an emergency.

- Patients have disorders that affect the absorption or metabolism of drugs (for instance, a seriously burned patient).
- Blood levels of drugs need to be maintained at a consistent therapeutic level, such as when treating infections caused by drug-resistant pathogens or when providing postoperative pain relief.
- It is in the patient's interest to avoid the discomfort of repeated intramuscular injections.
- A mechanism is needed to administer drug therapy over a prolonged period of time, as in patients with cancer.

CONTINUOUS ADMINISTRATION

A **continuous infusion** (instillation of a parenteral drug during a period of several hours), also called a continuous drip, involves adding medication to a large volume (500–1,000 mL) of IV solution (Skill 35-1). Drugs may be added to a new container of IV solution or to an existing infusion if there is a sufficient volume to dilute the drug.

After the medication has been added, the solution is administered by gravity infusion or more commonly with an electronic infusion device such as a controller or pump (see Chap. 15).

INTERMITTENT ADMINISTRATION

An **intermittent infusion** (parenteral administration of medication in a relatively short period) is instilled in a matter of minutes or up to 1 hour. There are three ways in which intermittent infusions are administered: bolus administrations, secondary administrations, and those in which a volume-control set is used.

Bolus Administration

The term *bolus* refers to a substance given all at one time. A **bolus administration** (undiluted medication given quickly into a vein) is sometimes described as a drug given by IV push. Although the term "push" is used, the medication is administered at the rate specified in a drug reference or at a rate of 1 mL (cc) per minute if no information is available.

Bolus administrations are given in one of two ways: through a port in an existing IV line or through a medication lock (see Chap. 15).

Using an IV Port

A **port** (sealed opening) extends from the IV tubing (Fig. 35-1). The seal is made of latex or another substance that can be pierced with a needle or needleless adapter.

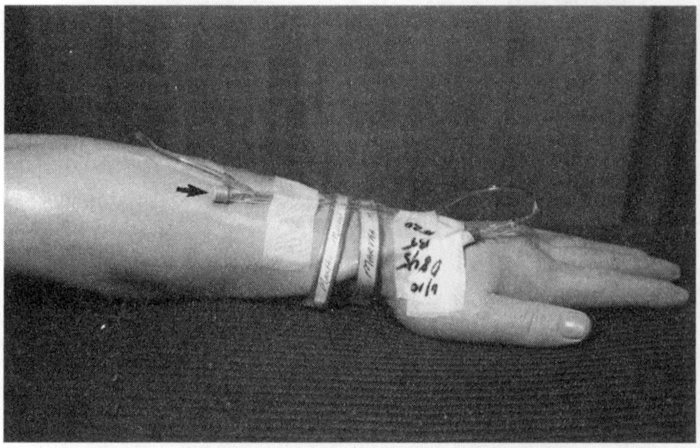

FIGURE 35–1. An intravenous port. (Courtesy of Ken Timby.)

Nursing Guidelines For

Administering Medications Through an Intravenous Port

- ☑ Prepare the medication in a syringe.
  RATIONALE: Provides a means for accessing the port
- ☑ Locate the port nearest the IV insertion site.
  RATIONALE: Provides the most rapid placement of medication in the circulatory system
- ☑ Swab the port with an alcohol sponge.
  RATIONALE: Removes colonizing microorganisms
- ☑ Pierce the port with the needle or needleless adapter.
  RATIONALE: Provides access to inside the tubing
- ☑ Pinch the tubing above the access port.
  RATIONALE: Temporarily stops the flow of IV fluid
- ☑ Pull back on the plunger of the syringe.
  RATIONALE: Creates negative pressure
- ☑ Observe for blood in the tubing near the IV catheter or insertion device.
  RATIONALE: Validates that the IV catheter is in the vein
- ☑ Gently instill a few tenths of a milliliter of medication (Fig. 35-2).
  RATIONALE: Initiates the bolus administration
- ☑ Release the tubing.
  RATIONALE: Allows some IV fluid to flow
- ☑ Continue the pattern of pinching the tubing, instilling a small amount of drug, and releasing the tubing until the medication has been administered over the specified period of time.
  RATIONALE: Delivers the drug gradually; keeps the catheter or venous insertion device patent when medication is not being instilled. Pinching the tubing while instilling drug ensures that the drug is administered to the patient rather than backfilling the tubing.

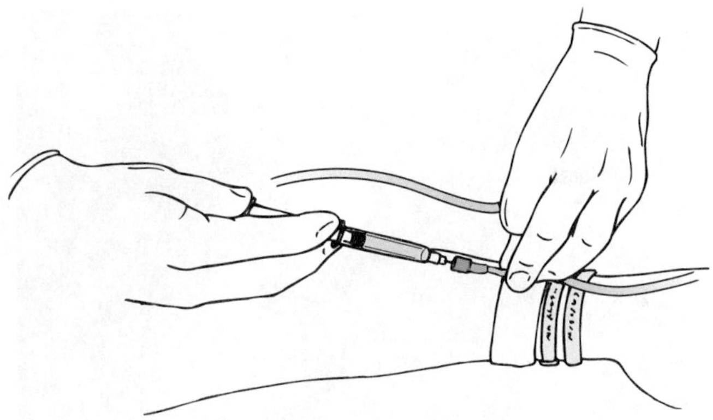

FIGURE 35–2. Instilling medication.

Because the entire dose is administered quickly, bolus administration has the greatest potential for causing life-threatening changes should a drug reaction occur. If the patient's condition changes for any reason, the administration is immediately ceased and emergency measures are taken to protect the patient's safety.

Using a Medication Lock

A medication lock is also called a saline or heparin lock or an intermittent infusion device. The insertion and technique for maintaining the patency of a medication lock are described in Chapter 15.

Briefly, a medication lock is a plug that, when inserted into the end of an IV catheter, allows instant access to the venous system. One of its best features is that it eliminates the need for a continuous, and sometimes unnecessary, administration of IV fluid.

Instilling IV medication through a lock is similar to the routine for keeping it patent (see Skill 15-6, Chap. 15). The technique varies depending on whether it is the agency's policy to maintain patency with saline or heparin. The trend is to use saline.

Nurses use the mnemonic "SAS" or "SASH" as a guide to the steps involved in administering IV medication into a lock. SAS stands for Saline—Administer drug—Saline; SASH refers to Saline—Administer drug—Saline—Heparin.

Nursing Guidelines For

Administering Medications Through a Lock

- ☑ Prepare three syringes, two with at least 1 mL of sterile normal saline and one with the prescribed medication.
  RATIONALE: Facilitates flushing the lock before and after medication administration
- ☑ Prepare a fourth syringe with heparin (10 units/mL), if it is the policy of the agency to use it.
  RATIONALE: Maintains patency by interfering with clot formation
- ☑ Label all the syringes in some way, such as attaching a piece of tape with the letters "S" and "H."
  RATIONALE: Identifies contents of syringes
- ☑ Check the identity of the patient.
  RATIONALE: Prevents medication errors
- ☑ Wipe the medication port with an alcohol swab.
  RATIONALE: Removes colonizing microorganisms
- ☑ Insert the needle or needleless device from the syringe containing saline through the "bull's eye" of the rubber seal on the medication lock (Fig. 35-3).
  RATIONALE: Provides the least resistance when introducing the needle
- ☑ Hold the lock and pull back on the plunger of the syringe.
  RATIONALE: Stabilizes the lock while aspirating for blood
- ☑ Observe for blood in the barrel of the syringe.
  RATIONALE: Verifies that the lock is still patent and in the vein (depending on the gauge of the needle, blood return may not always be observed)
- ☑ Instill the saline (the first "S" in the mnemonic).
  RATIONALE: Clears the lock and venous access device
- ☑ Remove the syringe when empty, wipe the tip of the lock, and insert the syringe containing the drug.
  RATIONALE: Facilitates administering the medication
- ☑ Gently and gradually administer the medication over the specified time period (the letter "A" in the mnemonic).
  RATIONALE: Ensures safety when recommendations from an authoritative source are followed
- ☑ Remove the syringe when it is empty, wipe the lock again, insert the second syringe with saline, and instill the fluid (the second "S" in the mnemonic).
  RATIONALE: Pushes the medication that remains in the lock into the venous system and fills the lock with saline

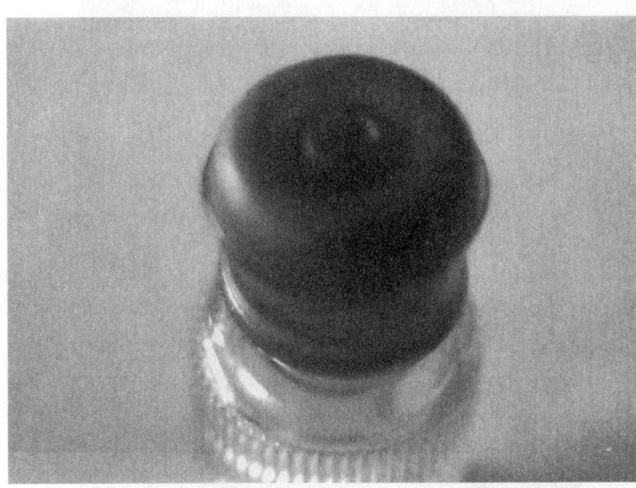

FIGURE 35–3. Bull's eye on a medication lock. (Courtesy of Ken Timby.)

☑ Begin to withdraw the syringe while instilling the last of the fluid in the syringe.
RATIONALE: Prevents drawing blood, which may clot, into the lumen of the IV catheter, and ensures future patency

☑ Wipe, insert, and instill the heparin, if that is agency policy, using the same technique for withdrawal (the "H" in the mnemonic).
RATIONALE: Maintains patency using an anticoagulant

☑ Deposit all uncapped syringes in the nearest puncture-resistant biohazard container.
RATIONALE: Prevents needlestick injuries

To maintain patency, medication locks are usually flushed every 8 hours with saline or heparin. The flushing technique is the same, except only one syringe of flush solution is required. Medication locks are changed when the IV site is changed, or at least every 72 hours. If patency cannot be verified by obtaining a blood return, and if there is resistance when administering the flush solution, the IV catheter is removed, the site is changed, and the lock is replaced.

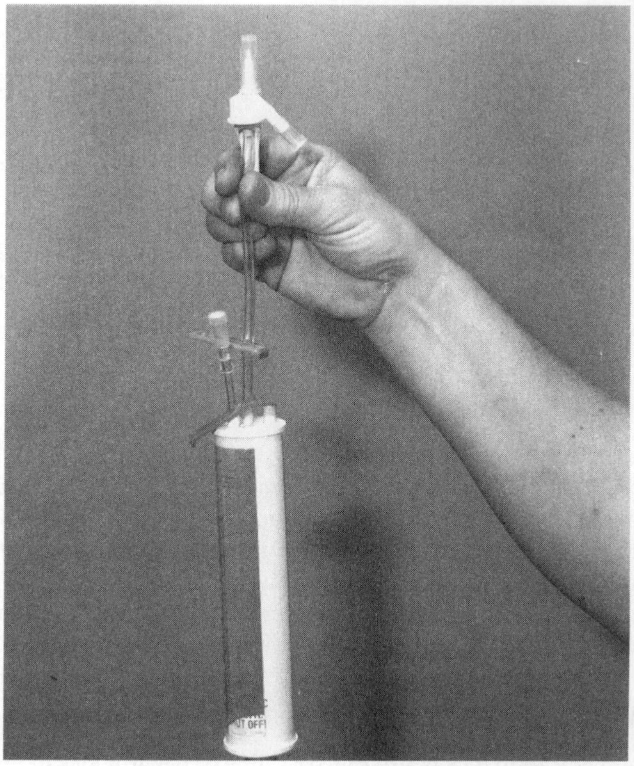

FIGURE 35–5. Volume-control set. (Courtesy of Ken Timby.)

Secondary Infusions

A **secondary infusion** (administration of a parenteral drug that has been diluted in a small volume of IV solution, usually 50–100 mL, over a period of 30 to 60 minutes) also is called a piggyback infusion because it is administered in tandem with a primary IV solution (Fig. 35-4). Both names are misnomers when the small volume of medicated solution is administered through a medication lock or the port of a central venous catheter (discussed below). When administered in this way, the medications are actually independent of a primary infusion. There are also instances when small volumes of medicated solution are given simultaneously with a primary infusion. This method involves using certain types of electronic infusion devices. Skill 35-2 describes how secondary infusions are administered by gravity in tandem with a currently infusing primary solution.

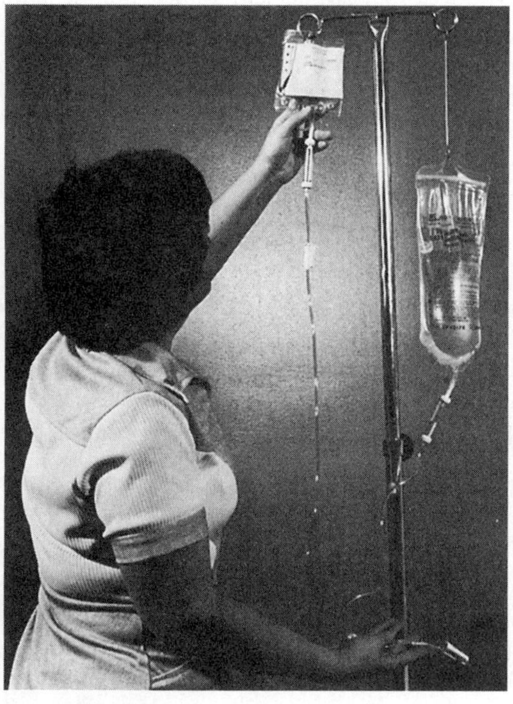

FIGURE 35–4. Piggyback arrangement.

Volume-Control Set

A **volume-control set** (chamber in IV tubing that holds a portion of the solution from a larger container; Fig. 35-5) is known by various commercial names such as Volutrol, Soluset, and Buretrol. A volume-control set is used for two purposes: to administer IV medication in a small volume of solution at intermittent intervals, and to avoid overloading the circulatory system. The volume-control set essentially substitutes for the separate secondary container of solution, therefore eliminating the need for additional fluid.

When caring for patients who are at risk for or who manifest signs of fluid excess, it may be appropriate to consult the physician and pharmacy department about using a volume-control set to administer intermittent IV medications (Skill 35-3).

Central Venous Catheters

A **central venous catheter** (CVC; venous access device that extends to the vena cava or right atrium) provides a means of administering parenteral medication in a large volume of blood. A CVC is used when:

- Patients require long-term IV fluid or medication administration.
- IV medications are irritating to peripheral veins.
- It is difficult to insert or maintain a peripherally inserted catheter.

CVCs have single or multiple lumens (Fig. 35-6). With multiple lumens, incompatible substances or more than one solution or drug can be given simultaneously. Each infuses through a separate channel and exits the catheter at a different location near the heart. Thus, the drugs or solutions never interact with one another. When a lumen is used only intermittently, it is capped with a medication lock. The unused lumen is kept patent by scheduled flushes with normal saline or heparin. There are three types of CVCs: percutaneous, tunneled, and implanted.

PERCUTANEOUS CATHETERS

A percutaneous catheter is inserted through the skin in a peripheral vein (for instance, the jugular or subclavian vein; see Chap. 15). This type of catheter is used when patients require short-term fluid or medication therapy, lasting a few days or weeks. Most are inserted by a physician and then sutured to the skin.

TUNNELED CATHETERS

Tunneled catheters are inserted into a central vein, with part of the catheter secured in the subcutaneous tissue. The end of the catheter exits from the skin lateral to the xiphoid process (Fig. 35-7). Tunneled catheters are used when patients require extended therapy. Tunneling helps stabilize the catheter and also reduces the potential for infection because an internal cuff acts as a barrier against migrating microorganisms. Some examples of tunneled catheters are the Hickman, Broviac, and Groshong catheters.

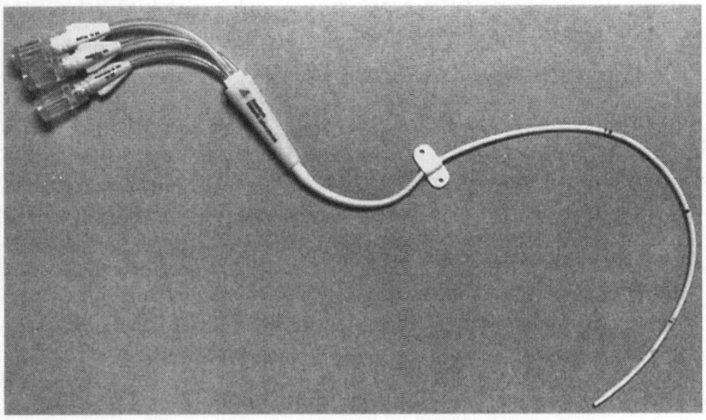

FIGURE 35–6. A triple-lumen central venous catheter. (Courtesy of Ken Timby.)

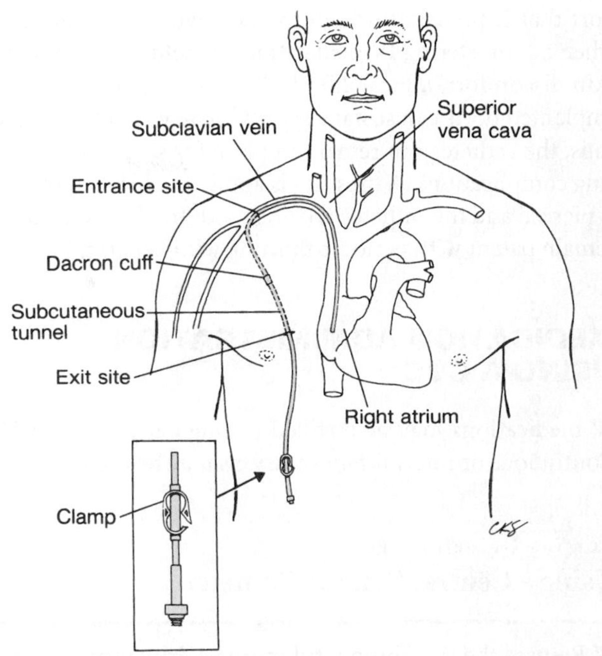

FIGURE 35–7. A tunneled catheter. (Ellis JR, Nowlis EA, Bentz PM: Modules for basic nursing skills, 6th ed. Philadelphia, Lippincott-Raven 1996.)

IMPLANTED CATHETERS

An implanted catheter (for example, the Porta-Cath) is sealed beneath the skin (Fig. 35-8). It provides the greatest protection against infection. Implanted catheters have a self-sealing

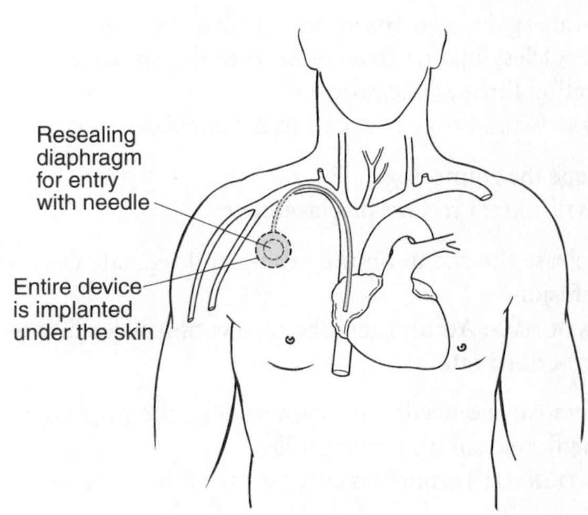

FIGURE 35–8. Placement of an implanted catheter. (Ellis JR, Nowlis EA, Bentz PM: Modules for basic nursing skills, 6th ed. Philadelphia, Lippincott-Raven, 1996.)

port that is pierced through the skin with a special needle when administering IV medications or solutions. To reduce skin discomfort, a local anesthetic is first applied topically. Implanted ports can sustain approximately 2,000 punctures; thus, the catheter can remain in place for several years, barring complications. A dressing is applied only when the port is pierced and the catheter is being used. Implanted catheters remain patent with periodic flushing with heparin.

MEDICATION ADMINISTRATION USING A CVC

IV medications may be instilled through any type of CVC. Continuous or intermittent infusions may be used.

Nursing Guidelines For

Using a Central Venous Catheter

- ☑ Prepare the IV solution, tubing, and drug using the steps for administering a continuous or secondary infusion.
  RATIONALE: Involves similar preparation principles
- ☑ Prepare a syringe with 3 to 5 mL of sterile normal saline solution.
  RATIONALE: Facilitates clearing the catheter of heparin if used to maintain patency
- ☑ Release the clamp, if there is one, on the exposed section of the catheter.
  RATIONALE: Facilitates flushing the catheter
- ☑ Swab the sealed port at the end of the catheter with alcohol.
  RATIONALE: Removes colonizing microorganisms
- ☑ Pierce the port with the syringe containing the saline and instill the flush solution (Fig. 35-9).
  RATIONALE: Clears the catheter of previous flush solution
- ☑ Swab again, and insert the needle, recessed needle, or needleless adapter that connects to the prepared IV medication through the port.
  RATIONALE: Provides access to the circulatory system
- ☑ Tape the connection.
  RATIONALE: Prevents displacement
- ☑ Release the clamp on the tubing and regulate the rate of infusion.
  RATIONALE: Administers the medication according to the prescribed rate
- ☑ Remove the needle or adapter from the port when the medicated solution has instilled.
  RATIONALE: Terminates current use of the catheter
- ☑ Flush the catheter with saline or heparin according to agency protocol.
  RATIONALE: Maintains catheter patency

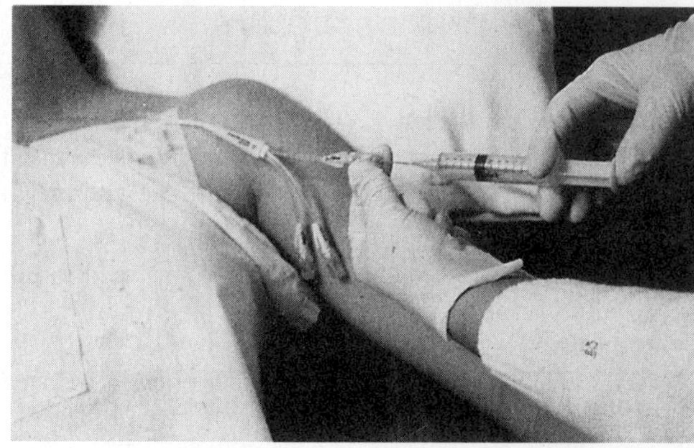

FIGURE 35–9. Flushing the lumen. (Courtesy of Ken Timby.)

- ☑ Reclamp the catheter.
  RATIONALE: Prevents complications such as air embolism (see Chap. 15)

Administering Antineoplastic Drugs

Antineoplastic drugs (medications used to destroy or slow the growth of malignant cells) are also commonly referred to as chemotherapy or just "chemo." CVCs are often used to administer antineoplastic drugs to patients with cancer.

Antineoplastic agents are toxic to both normal and abnormal cells. These drugs can even cause adverse effects in the pharmacists who mix them and the nurses who administer them. Antineoplastic drugs can be absorbed by caregivers through skin contact, inhalation of tiny fluid droplets or dust particles on which the droplets fall, or oral absorption of drug residue during hand-to-mouth contact. When transferred to the caregiver, these drugs can cause headaches, nausea, dizziness, and burning or itching of the skin. Long-term exposure can lead to changes in fast-growing body cells, including the sperm, ova, or fetal tissue. It is important, therefore, that nurses use safety measures when administering these drugs and avoid exposure and contact with hazardous materials.

In most cases, these drugs are reconstituted or diluted with sterile IV solutions in the pharmacy. The pharmacist wears protective clothing when preparing the drugs under a vertical flow containment hood or biologic safety cabinet (Fig. 35-10). The pharmacist usually attaches a special label to warn nurses to take special precautions during drug administration.

Common recommendations for avoiding self-contamination with antineoplastic drugs include the following:

- Cover the drug preparation area with a disposable paper pad, which will absorb a small drug spill.
- Wear a long-sleeved, cuffed, low-permeability gown with a closed front.
- Wear one or two pairs of surgical latex, *nonpowdered* gloves to reduce the potential for skin contact and inhalation of drug powder.

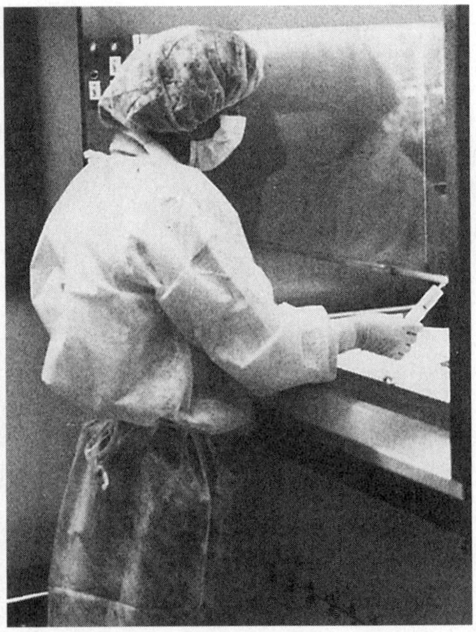

FIGURE 35–10. Pharmacy preparation of antineoplastic drugs. (Courtesy of Ken Timby.)

- Cover the cuffs of the gown with the cuffs of the gloves.
- Wear a mask or respirator and goggles if there is a potential for aerosolization or drug splash.
- Pour 70% alcohol over any drug spill to inactivate the drug.
- Clean the spill area with detergent and water at least three times and then rinse with clean water.
- Dispose of all substances that contain drug material in a biohazard container.
- Perform scrupulous handwashing.

Nursing Implications

Although the administration of all parenteral drugs involves specialized skills, the administration of IV medications in general and antineoplastic drugs in particular requires extreme caution. The following nursing diagnoses may be identified:

- Anxiety
- Fear
- Risk for injury
- Risk for infection
- Fluid volume excess
- Altered protection

The nursing care plan demonstrates the nursing process as it applies to a patient with the nursing diagnosis of Altered protection, defined in the 1999 NANDA taxonomy as "the state in which an individual experiences a decrease in the ability to guard the self from internal or external threats such as illness or injury." This diagnosis may be associated with the undesirable consequences of antineoplastic medication therapy; an example might be deficient immunity or a decreased ability to control bleeding.

Nursing Care Plan

Altered Protection

Assessment

Subjective Data

States, "I haven't been eating much. It's difficult to swallow; as a result I'm losing weight and feeling very weak."

Objective Data

26-year-old man admitted with enlarged cervical and axillary lymph nodes. Medical diagnosis is Hodgkin's lymphoma. Has had a Hickman central venous catheter inserted for chemotherapy. Complete blood count from 2 weeks ago reveals thrombocytopenia.

Diagnosis

Altered protection related to debilitated state and tendency to bleed secondary to chemotherapy

Plan

Goal

Blood loss will be minimal as evidenced by normal red blood cell count and negative occult blood tests on urine and stool throughout hospital stay.

Orders: 2/10

1. Obtain all blood samples from central line.
2. Monitor platelet count and hold chemotherapy if count is <100,000 until physician is consulted.

continued

Nursing Care Plan — *Altered Protection* Continued

3. Assess skin for bruising and catheter site for bleeding, and test urine and stool for occult blood q day.
4. Avoid aspirin or products containing salicylates.
5. Use a soft-bristle toothbrush or swabs for mouth care.
6. Substitute oral forms of medications rather than IM whenever possible.
7. If injections must be given, apply pressure for at least 3 minutes to control bleeding.

N. HURDER, RN

Implementation (Documentation)

2/10 1300 Blood for CBC and chemistry profile obtained from central venous catheter. Catheter flushed after blood draw. Results of blood tests unavailable at this time.

A. VALERIONI, LPN

Evaluation (Documentation)

2/10 1300 Skin is intact except at catheter insertion site. No evidence of bleeding from site. No bruises noted on skin. Urine and stool test negative for occult blood. Has not taken any over-the-counter aspirin products in the last 2 weeks. Soft-bristle toothbrush used for mouth care. No evidence of active bleeding from gums after mouth care. Not currently scheduled for injectable medications except those that will infuse through the central line.

A. VALERIONI, LPN

FOCUS ON OLDER ADULTS

- Older adults are the largest age group of patients cared for in acute and long-term health care agencies. Therefore, it is quite common for them to be recipients of IV medications. Increasing emphasis on early discharges may require teaching older adults how to flush venous access equipment such as medication locks on peripheral and central venous catheters, because some patients are discharged and then resume treatment on an out-patient basis. Problems with manual dexterity and vision, for example, may require repeated additional instructions and practice. A referral for skilled nursing care after discharge is appropriate.
- Older adults require frequent and comprehensive assessment before and after IV medication administration because they are more likely to manifest adverse reactions due to age-related changes.
- The veins of older adults tend to be quite fragile. Insertion of a percutaneous central venous line is often better than risking the trauma of repeated attempts at restarting or changing peripheral IV sites.
- To avoid the hazards of infiltrating tissue with medications delivered intravenously, it is appropriate to collaborate with the prescribing practitioner on the possibility of administering the same drug by another route.
- Explaining the purpose for each drug administered, especially by the IV route, is important because older adults often are reluctant to ask questions of health care professionals.
- A portion of many drugs is bound to protein in the blood. The portion not bound is called "free drug," the physiologically active form. Older adults tend to have more free drug in proportion to bound drug because of diminished protein components in their blood. Since the drug is being administered directly into the bloodstream, they are at greater risk for experiencing adverse drug effects with highly protein-bound drugs, for example, warfarin and sulfonamides.
- Older adults tend to metabolize and excrete drugs at a slower rate. This factor may predispose them to toxic effects from the accumulation of medications. This toxicity may occur more rapidly when the drug is administered IV. Adjustments may be needed in the amount or frequency of dosing.
- Health insurance coverage of IV medications is highly variable and may change depending on the setting. Older adults may need assistance in checking with their insurance company about coverage of IV medications, especially in long-term care settings.
- Older adults with dementia often experience more confusion and disorientation with an acute illness. They need extra vigilance to ensure safe administration of IV medications and maintenance of the IV insertion site. Family members or paid companion services are helpful in providing close observation in acute-care settings.

KEY CONCEPTS

- IV medications can be given into peripheral or central veins.
- The IV route is appropriate when a quick response is needed during an emergency, when patients have disorders that affect the absorption or metabolism of drugs, and when blood levels of drugs need to be maintained at a consistent therapeutic level.
- IV medications can be administered continuously or intermittently.
- Two methods for administering a bolus of IV medication are via a port on the IV tubing or a medication lock.
- IV medication solutions may be administered intermittently using secondary (piggyback) infusions or a volume-control set.
- A piggyback solution is a small volume of diluted medication that is connected to, and positioned higher than, the primary solution.
- A volume-control set is used to administer IV medication in a small volume of solution at intermittent intervals, to avoid overloading the circulatory system.
- A central venous catheter is a venous access device that extends to the vena cava or right atrium.
- There are three general types of central venous catheters: percutaneous, tunneled, and implanted.
- When administering antineoplastic drugs, the nurse should wear a cover gown, one or two pairs of gloves, and a disposable or respirator mask to protect against contact with or inhalation of the medication.

CRITICAL THINKING EXERCISES

- Discuss the advantages and disadvantages of giving IV medications to older adults.
- When preparing to administer an IV medication through an IV port or lock, you find no blood return on aspiration. Discuss the significance of this finding and what actions are appropriate.

SUGGESTED READINGS

Bagnall-Reeb H. Diagnosis of central venous access device occlusion: implications for nursing practice. Journal of Intravenous Nursing 1998; 21(55):S115–121.

Bean CA. High-tech homecare infusion therapies. Critical Care Nursing Clinics of North America 1998;10(3):287–303.

Boyne CG. Who's getting stuck, anyway? Nursing Management 1997; 28(10):20–23.

Buswell L, Beyea SC. Flushing protocols for tunneled central venous catheters: An integrative review of the literature. Online Journal of Knowledge Synthesis for Nursing 1998;5(3).

Cohen MR. Oral syringes and needleless systems: Bad connection. Nursing 1996;26(8):15.

Coppage D. A latex-free, needleless IV system. Surgical Services Management 1996;2(12):38–41.

Hunt ML Jr, Rapp RP. Intravenous medication errors. Journal of Intravenous Nursing 1996;19(3S):S9–S15.

Krzywda EA. Central venous access—catheters, technology, and physiology. MedSurg Nursing 1998;7(3):132–141.

Lawrence LW, Delclos GL, Felknor SA, et al. The effectiveness of a needleless intravenous connection system: An assessment by injury rate and user satisfaction. Infection Control and Hospital Epidemiology 1997;18(3): 175–182.

Lilley LL, Gaunci R. Using drug delivery devices. American Journal of Nursing 1996;96(10):14.

Medication administration series. Interactive Healthcare Newsletter 1997; 13(11/12):4.

NANDA nursing diagnoses: Definitions and classification, 1999–2000. Philadelphia, NANDA, 1999.

Orenstein R. The benefits and limitations of needle protectors and needleless intravenous systems. Journal of Intravenous Nursing 1999;22(3): 122–128.

Possanza CP. Special delivery: Using a syringe pump to administer IV drugs. Nursing 1997;27(9):43–45.

Preparing IV solutions: Shaken, not stirred. Nursing 1997;27(2):29.

Quick reference guide: Central venous lines. Nursing Standard 1999; 13(42):2p.

Sansivero GE. Venous anatomy and physiology: Considerations for vascular access device placement and function. Journal of Intravenous Nursing 1998;21(55):S107–S114.

Wenzel RP, Edmond MB. The evolving technology of venous access. New England Journal of Medicine 1999;340(1):48–50.

SKILL 35-1

ADMINISTERING INTRAVENOUS MEDICATION BY CONTINUOUS INFUSION

Suggested Action	Reason for Action
Assessment	
Check the medical orders.	Collaborates nursing activities with medical treatment
Compare the medication administration record (MAR) with the written medical order.	Ensures accuracy
Read the label on the drug and compare it with the MAR.	Prevents errors
Make sure the drug label indicates that it is for IV use.	Prevents patient injury
Check for any documented drug allergies.	Ensures safety

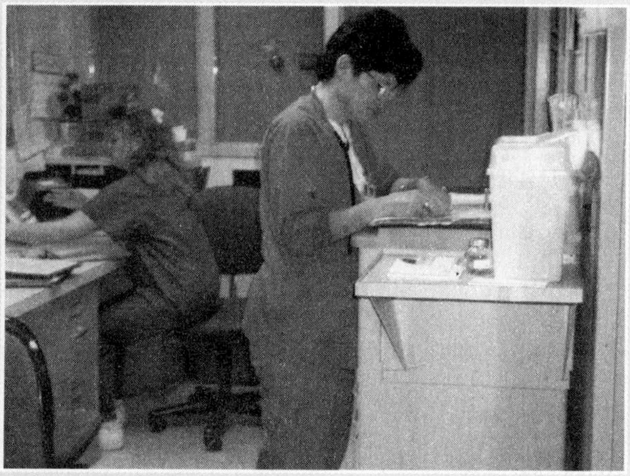

Checking the MAR. (Courtesy of Ken Timby.)

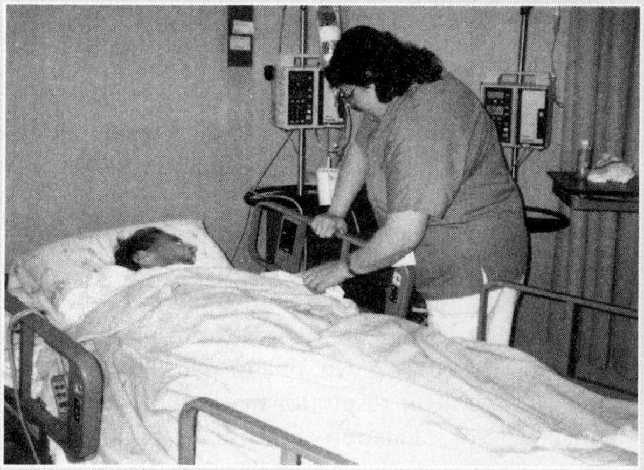

Assessing the infusion site. (Courtesy of Ken Timby.)

Suggested Action	Reason for Action
Review the drug action and side effects.	Promotes safe patient care
Consult a compatibility chart or drug reference.	Determines if the solution and drug are known to interact when mixed
Determine how much the patient understands about the purpose and technique for administering the medication.	Provides an opportunity for health teaching
Perform assessments that will provide a basis for evaluating the drug's effectiveness.	Provides a baseline for future comparisons
Inspect the current infusion site for swelling, redness, and tenderness.	Determines if a site change is needed
Planning	
Prepare the medication, taking care to read the medication label at least three times.	Avoids medication errors
Have a second nurse double-check your drug calculations.	Ensures accuracy
Implementation	
Wash your hands.	Reduces the transmission of microorganisms
Check the patient's identification band.	Prevents a medication error
Clamp or stop the current infusion of fluid.	Prevents administering a concentrated amount of medication while it is being added to the solution
Swab the appropriate port on the container of IV fluid.	Removes colonizing microorganisms

continued

SKILL 35–1

ADMINISTERING INTRAVENOUS MEDICATION BY CONTINUOUS INFUSION *Continued*

Suggested Action	Reason for Action
Instill the medication through the port into the full container of infusing fluid.	Promotes dilution of concentrated additive

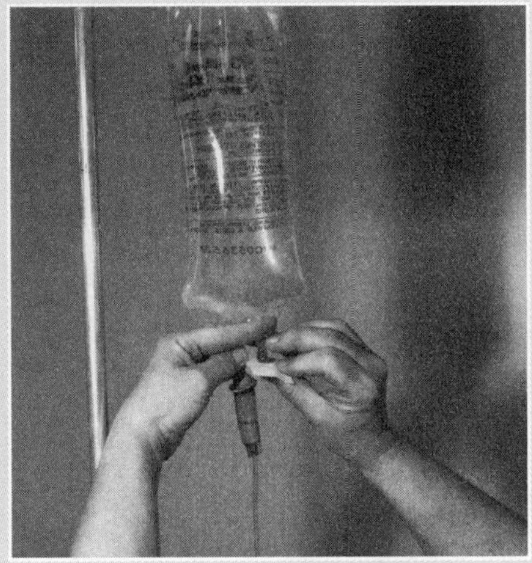

Swabbing the port on the container. (Courtesy of Ken Timby.)

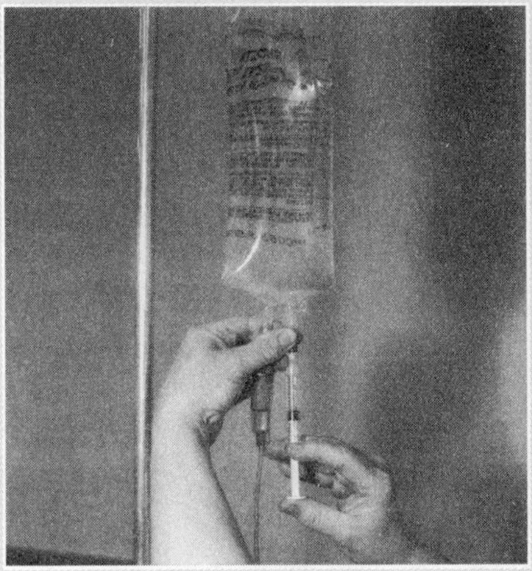

Instilling medication. (Courtesy of Ken Timby.)

Suggested Action	Reason for Action
Lower the bag and gently rotate it back and forth.	Distributes the medication equally throughout the fluid
Suspend the solution and release the clamp.	Facilitates infusion
Regulate the rate of flow by using the roller clamp or programming the rate on the electronic infusion device.	Promotes continuous infusion at prescribed rate

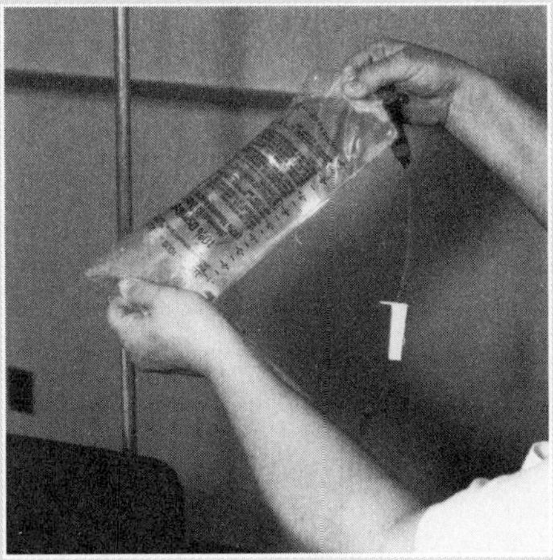

Rotating the container. (Courtesy of Ken Timby.)

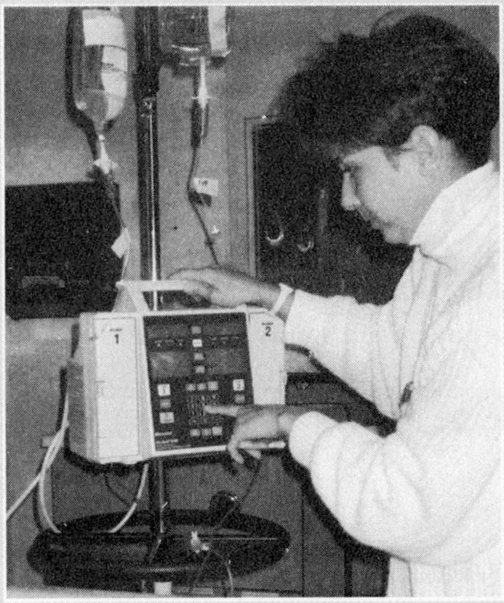

Programming the rate. (Courtesy of Ken Timby.)

Suggested Action	Reason for Action
Attach a label to the container of fluid identifying the drug, its dose, time it was added, and your initials.	Provides information for others and demonstrates accountability for nursing actions
Record the medication administration in the MAR.	Documents nursing care; avoids medication errors
Check the patient and the progress of the infusion at least hourly.	Promotes early intervention for complications

continued

SKILL 35–1

ADMINISTERING INTRAVENOUS MEDICATION BY CONTINUOUS INFUSION *Continued*

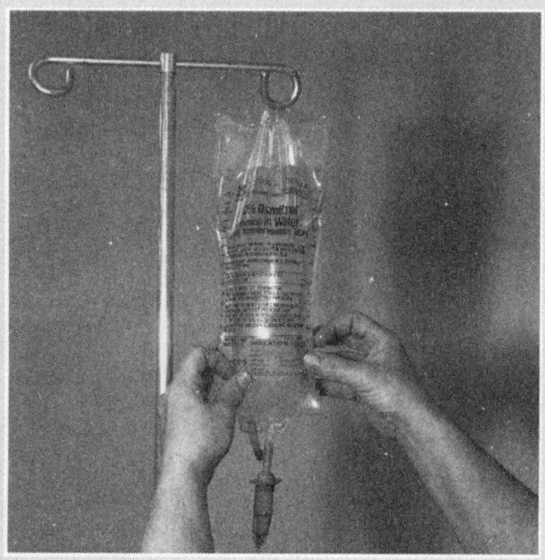

Attaching the label. (Courtesy of Ken Timby.)

Evaluation

- Medication instills at prescribed rate.
- Patient remains free of any adverse effects.

Document

- Patient and site assessment data
- The date, time, drug, dose, and initials
- Solution to which drug has been added
- Response of the patient

SAMPLE DOCUMENTATION*

Date and Time IV infusing in L. forearm. No tenderness, swelling, or redness observed. KCl 20 mEq added to 1,000 mL of D5/W. IV infusing at 125 mL/hr. Heart rate is regular and ranges between 65 and 75 bpm. ________________________ SIGNATURE, TITLE

CRITICAL THINKING

- Discuss potential advantages of administering IV medication by a continuous infusion.

* The administration of drugs is usually documented on the MAR.

SKILL 35-2

ADMINISTERING AN INTERMITTENT SECONDARY INFUSION

Suggested Action	Reason for Action
Assessment	
Check the medical orders.	Collaborates nursing activities with medical treatment
Compare the medication administration record (MAR) with the written medical order.	Ensures accuracy
Read the label on the medicated solution and compare with the MAR.	Prevents errors
Check for any documented drug allergies.	Ensures safety
Inspect the current infusion site for swelling, redness, and tenderness.	Determines if a site change is needed
Review the drug action and side effects.	Promotes safe patient care
Consult a compatibility chart or drug reference.	Determines if the drug in the secondary solution may interact when mixed with the solution in the primary tubing
Determine how much the patient understands about the purpose and technique for administering the medication.	Provides an opportunity for health teaching
Perform assessments that will provide a basis for evaluating the drug's effectiveness.	Provides a baseline for future comparisons
Planning	
Plan to administer the secondary infusion within 30 to 60 minutes of the scheduled time for drug administration established by the agency.	Complies with agency policy
Remove a refrigerated secondary solution at least 30 minutes before administration.	Warms the solution slightly to promote comfort during instillation
Check the drop factor on the package of secondary (short) IV tubing and calculate the rate for infusion (see Chap. 15).	Ensures that the secondary infusion will be instilled within the specified time
Have a second nurse double-check your calculations for the rate of infusion.	Ensures accuracy
Attach the tubing to the solution (see Skill 15-2), fill the drip chamber, and purge air from the tubing.	Prepares the medicated solution for administration
Attach a needle, recessed needle, or needleless adapter.	Facilitates piercing the port while minimizing the risk for needlestick injury
Implementation	
Wash your hands.	Reduces the transmission of microorganisms
Check the identity of the patient.	Prevents medication errors
Hang the secondary solution on the IV pole or standard.	Prepares the solution for administration
Lower the container of primary solution approximately 10 inches (25 cm) below the height of the secondary solution using a plastic or metal hanger.	Positions the secondary solution to instill under greater hydrostatic pressure
Wipe the *uppermost port* on the primary tubing with an alcohol swab.	Removes colonized microorganisms

continued

SKILL 35–2

ADMINISTERING AN INTERMITTENT SECONDARY INFUSION *Continued*

Suggested Action	Reason for Action
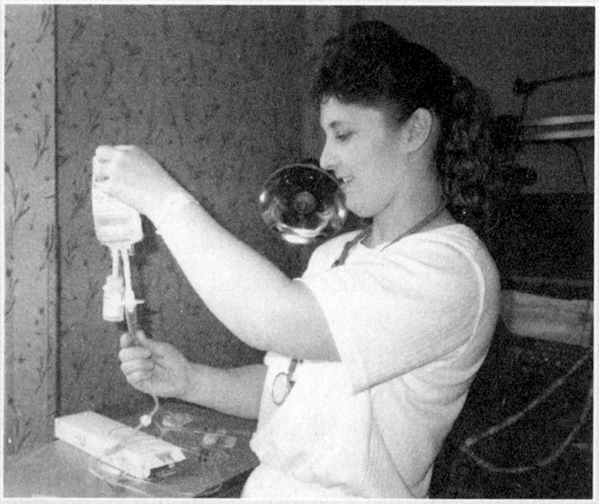 Preparing secondary infusion equipment. (Courtesy of Ken Timby.)	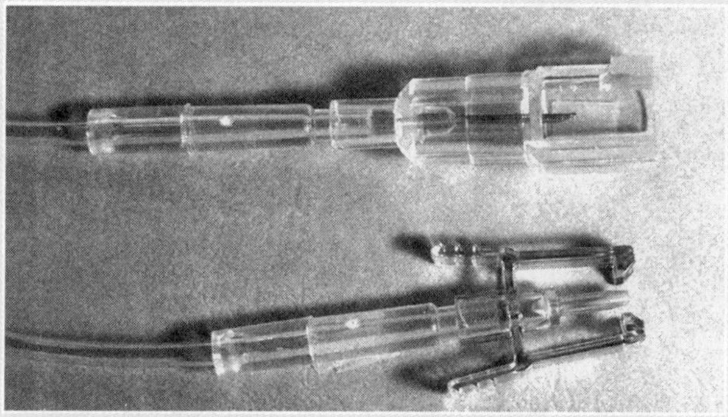 Recessed needle and needleless adapters. (Courtesy of Ken Timby.)
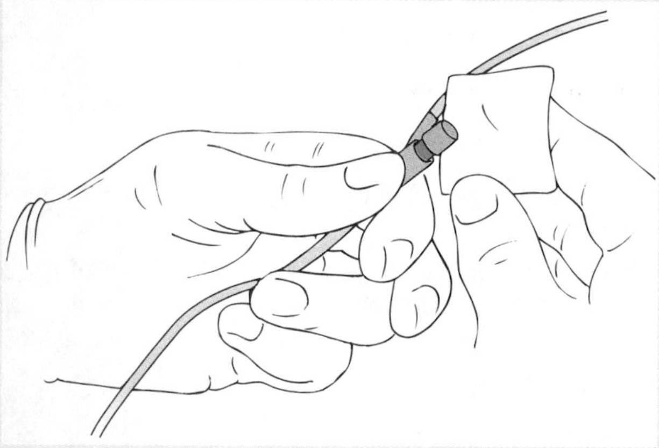 Swabbing the port. (Courtesy of Ken Timby.)	
Insert the needle or modified adapter within the port.	Provides access to the venous system
Tape the connection.	Prevents separation from the port
Release the roller clamp on the secondary solution.	Initiates the infusion
Regulate the rate of flow by counting the drip rate and adjusting the roller clamp.	Establishes the maintenance rate of flow to instill the solution in the time specified
Clamp the tubing when the solution has instilled.	Prevents backfilling with the primary solution
Rehang the primary container of solution and readjust the rate of flow.	Continues fluid replacement therapy at its appropriate rate
Leave the secondary tubing in place within the port if another secondary infusion of the same medication is scheduled again within the next 24 to 72 hours.	Controls health care costs without jeopardizing patient safety; different tubing, however, is used if other drugs are administered as secondary infusions

continued

SKILL 35-2

ADMINISTERING AN INTERMITTENT SECONDARY INFUSION *Continued*

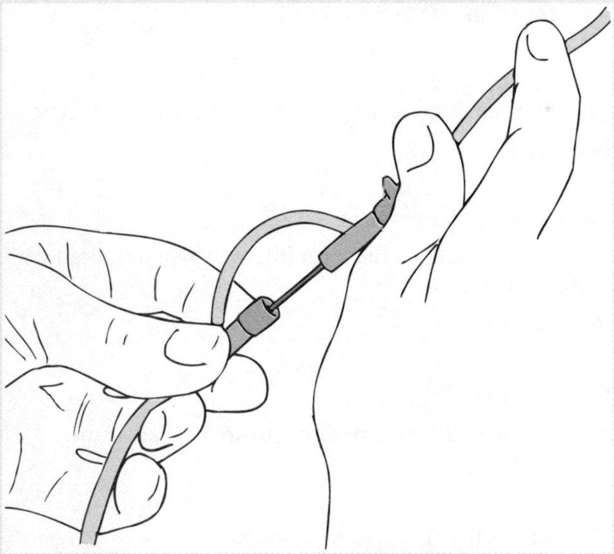

Inserting the needle. (Courtesy of Ken Timby.)

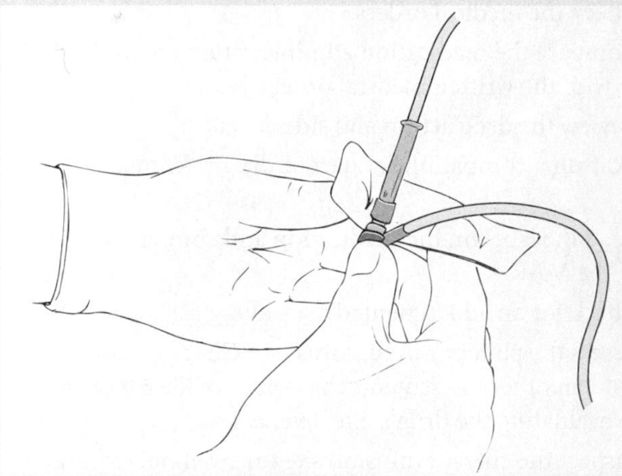

Taping the connection. (Courtesy of Ken Timby.)

Evaluation

- Secondary infusion instills at prescribed rate.
- Patient remains free of any adverse effects.

Document

- Patient and site assessment data
- The date, time, drug, dose, and initials
- Response of the patient

SAMPLE DOCUMENTATION*

Date and Time IV infusing in L. forearm. No tenderness, swelling, or redness observed. Vancomycin 1 g administered in 100 mL of NSS as a secondary infusion over 60 minutes without signs of a reaction. ________________ SIGNATURE, TITLE

CRITICAL THINKING

- Besides using a drug reference, who or what might you consult to determine the compatibility of two drugs that will infuse through the same IV tubing?

* The administration of drugs is usually documented on the MAR.

SKILL 35-3

USING A VOLUME-CONTROL SET

Suggested Action	Reason for Action
Assessment	
Check the medical orders.	Collaborates nursing activities with medical treatment
Compare the medication administration record (MAR) with the written medical order.	Ensures accuracy
Review the drug action and side effects.	Promotes safe patient care
Consult a compatibility chart or drug reference.	Determines if the medication interacts when diluted with the IV solution
Read the label on the medication and compare it with the MAR.	Prevents errors
Check for any documented drug allergies.	Ensures safety
Assess the patient's fluid status (see Chap. 15) and perform other assessments that will provide a basis for evaluating the drug's effectiveness.	Provides a baseline for making future comparisons
Inspect the current infusion site for swelling, redness, and tenderness.	Determines if a site change is needed
Determine how much the patient understands about the purpose and technique for administering the medication.	Provides an opportunity for health teaching
Planning	
Plan to administer the medication within 30 to 60 minutes of the scheduled time for drug administration established by the agency.	Complies with agency policy
Obtain a volume-control set.	Provides the means for instilling an intermittent infusion
Determine the drop factor on the volume-control set and calculate the rate of infusion.	Differs, in some instances, from the drop size on IV tubing
Have a second nurse double-check your calculations for the rate of infusion.	Ensures accuracy
Implementation	
Wash your hands and don gloves.	Reduces the transmission of microorganisms
Close all the clamps on the volume-control set and insert the spike into the IV solution.	Prepares the equipment for medication administration
Seal the air vent located to the side of the spike on the volume-control set if the solution is in a plastic bag; if the container is glass, leave the air vent open.	Facilitates the administration of fluid from collapsible or noncollapsible containers
Release the clamp above the fluid chamber.	Permits fluid to enter the calibrated container
Fill the calibrated chamber with approximately 30 mL of IV solution and retighten the clamp.	Provides a small volume with which to fill the drip chamber and purge air from the distal tubing
Squeeze and release the drip chamber until it is half full.	Fills the drip chamber with fluid
Note: *For volume-control sets with a membrane filter, the clamp below the drip chamber must be open when the drip chamber is filled or the set will be damaged.*	

continued

SKILL 35-3

USING A VOLUME-CONTROL SET *Continued*

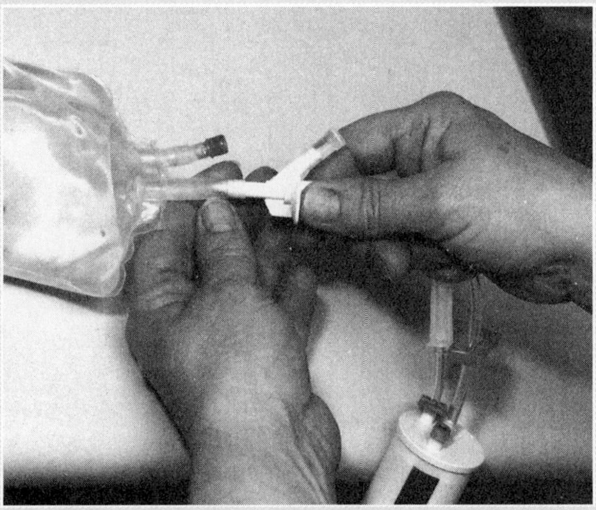

Inserting the spike. (Courtesy of Ken Timby.)

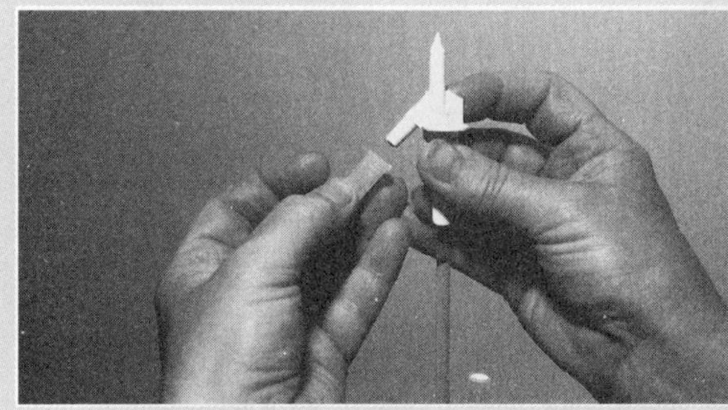

Capping the air vent. (Courtesy of Ken Timby.)

Suggested Action	Reason for Action
Open the lower clamp until the tubing is filled with fluid; then reclamp.	Purges air from the tubing
Open the clamp above the calibrated container, fill the chamber with the desired volume of fluid, and reclamp.	Provides diluent for the medication
Swab the injection port on the calibrated container.	Removes colonizing microorganisms
Instill the prepared medication.	Prepares the drug for administration

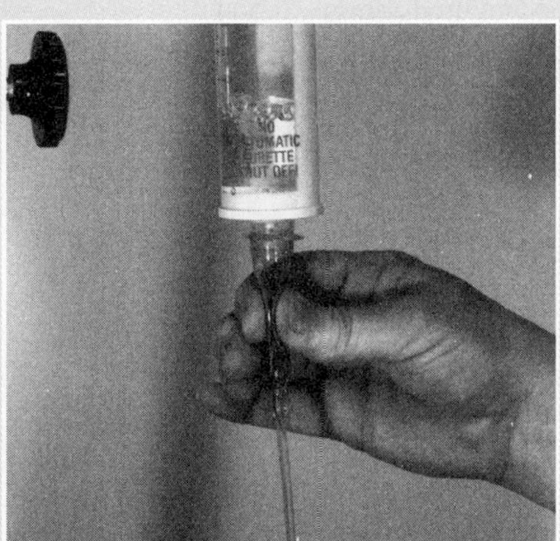

Squeezing the drip chamber. (Courtesy of Ken Timby.)

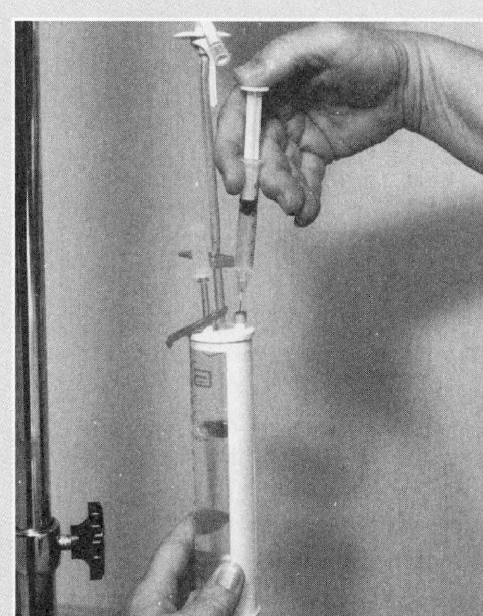

Instilling medication. (Courtesy of Ken Timby.)

continued

SKILL 35-3

USING A VOLUME-CONTROL SET *Continued*

Suggested Action	Reason for Action
Rotate the fluid chamber back and forth.	Mixes the drug throughout the fluid
Connect the tubing to the patient's IV catheter.	Completes the circuit for administering IV medication
Release the lower clamp and regulate the drip rate.	Continues the administration of fluid replacement
Add a label to the fluid chamber identifying the name of the drug, dose, time it was added, and your initials.	Provides information for other health professionals

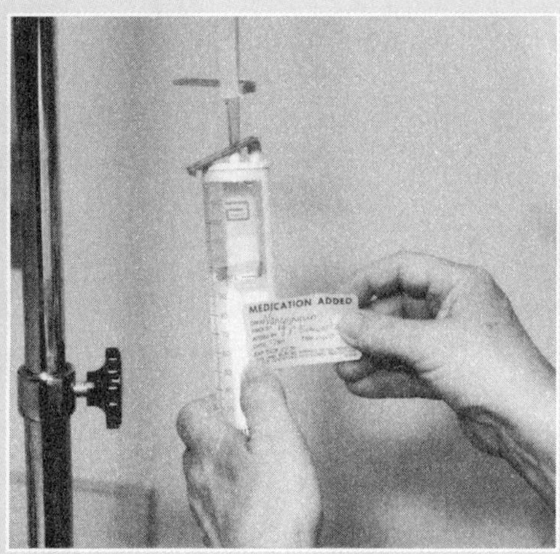

Attaching a drug label. (Courtesy of Ken Timby.)

Suggested Action	Reason for Action
Return before the time the medication is due to finish instilling.	Facilitates further fluid therapy
Release the upper clamp when the fluid chamber is empty and refill it with the next hour's worth of fluid.	Continues the administration of fluid replacement
Readjust the rate, if necessary.	Accommodates for differences between the rates for medication and fluid administration
Remove the drug label from the fluid chamber.	No longer applies after the medication is instilled

Evaluation

- Medicated solution instills within the specified period of time.
- Patient experiences no adverse effects.

Document

- Patient and site assessment data
- The date, time, drug, dose, and initials
- Solution to which drug has been added
- Response of the patient

continued

SKILL 35-3

USING A VOLUME-CONTROL SET *Continued*

SAMPLE DOCUMENTATION*

Date and Time Azactam 1 g added to 100 mL of D5/W within volume-control chamber and instilled IV over 60 min. Site is not irritated, tender, or swollen. Lungs sound clear. 100 mL urine output in the past hour. ______________________ SIGNATURE, TITLE

CRITICAL THINKING

- Explain why you would use a volume-control set to administer IV medications to a small child.

* The administration of drugs is usually documented on the MAR.

UNIT ELEVEN

INTERVENING IN EMERGENCY SITUATIONS

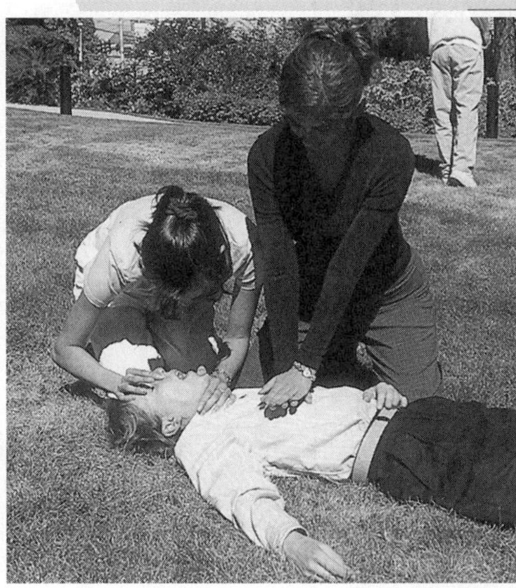

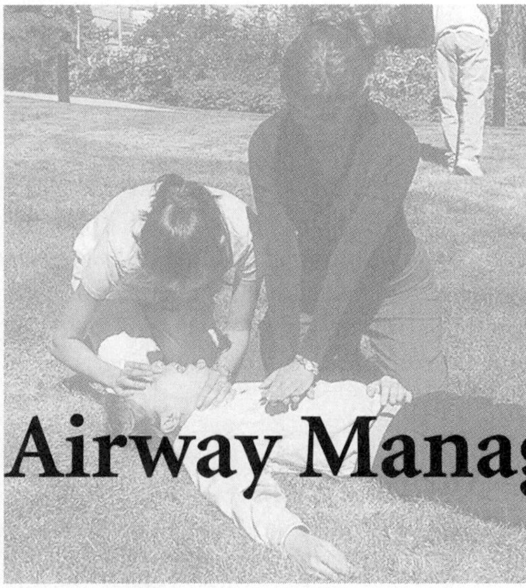

CHAPTER 36

Airway Management

CHAPTER OUTLINE

NURSING GUIDELINES

COLLECTING A SPUTUM SPECIMEN
INSERTING AN ORAL AIRWAY

SKILLS

SKILL 36-1: SUCTIONING THE AIRWAY
SKILL 36-2: PROVIDING TRACHEOSTOMY CARE

NURSING CARE PLAN

INEFFECTIVE AIRWAY CLEARANCE

KEY TERMS

airway	oropharyngeal suctioning
airway management	percussion
chest physiotherapy	postural drainage
inhalation therapy	sputum
mucus	suctioning
nasopharyngeal suctioning	tracheostomy
nasotracheal suctioning	tracheostomy care
oral airway	tracheostomy tube
oral suctioning	vibration

LEARNING OBJECTIVES

An understanding of the content within this chapter will be evidenced by the student's ability to:

- Identify the structural components of the airway.
- Describe the function of the airway.
- Discuss three natural mechanisms that protect the airway.
- Describe what airway management includes.
- Name two techniques for liquefying respiratory secretions.
- Explain the three techniques of chest physiotherapy.
- Describe at least three types of suctioning techniques that are used to clear secretions from the airway.
- Discuss two indications for inserting an artificial airway.
- Name two examples of artificial airways.
- Identify three components of tracheostomy care.

The primary function of the respiratory system is to permit ventilation for appropriate exchange of oxygen and carbon dioxide at the cellular level (see Chap. 20). Adequate ventilation, however, depends on clear air passages from the nose to the alveoli. This chapter focuses on the nursing skills that help ensure that the structures of the airway remain open and clear.

The Airway

The **airway** (collective system of tubes in the upper and lower respiratory tract) is the path through which gases travel during their passage to and from the alveoli (Fig. 36-1). The upper airway consists of the nose and pharynx, which is subdivided into the nasopharynx, oropharynx, and laryngopharynx. The lower airway is made up of the trachea, bronchi, and bronchioles. Additional structures and mechanisms keep the airway open and protect it from a wide variety of inhaled substances.

The main structures that protect the airway are the epiglottis, tracheal cartilage, mucous membrane, and cilia. The epiglottis is a protrusion of flexible cartilage located above the larynx. It acts as a lid that closes during swallowing so that fluid and food are directed toward the esophagus rather than the respiratory tract. The rings of tracheal cartilage ensure that the trachea, the portion of the airway beneath the larynx, remains open.

The respiratory passages are lined with mucous membrane, a type of tissue from which mucus is secreted. The

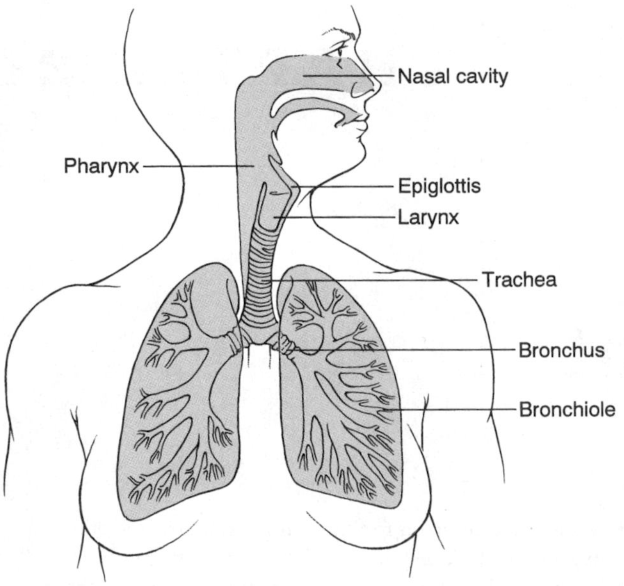

FIGURE 36–1. The airway and related structures.

sticky mucus traps particulate matter. In the nose, the debris can be cleared by sneezing or blowing. Debris that collects in the lower airway is beaten upward on hair-like projections called cilia (Fig. 36-2). **Sputum** (mucus raised to the level of the upper airways) is cleared from the upper airway by coughing, expectoration, or swallowing.

Among the factors that may jeopardize the patency of the airway are:

- Increased volume of mucus
- Thick mucus
- Fatigue or weakness
- Decreased level of consciousness
- Ineffective cough
- Impaired airway

Consequently, the nurse may need to assist patients with measures that support or replace their own natural efforts.

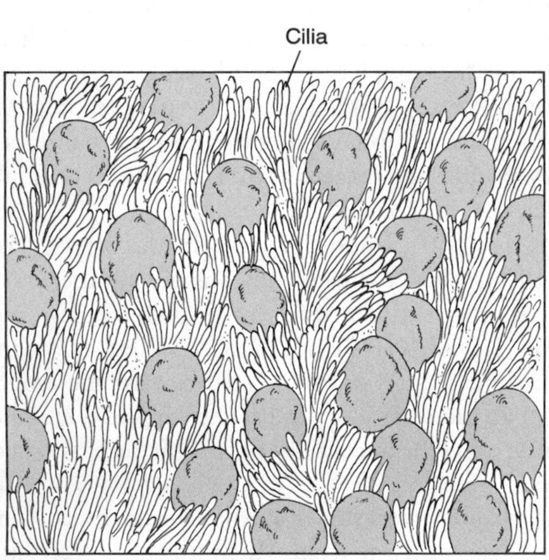

FIGURE 36–2. Cilia and mucus-producing cells.

Airway Management

Airway management (skills that maintain natural or artificial airways for compromised patients) is an essential nursing skill. The natural airway is most often maintained by keeping respiratory secretions liquefied, promoting their mobilization and expectoration with chest physiotherapy, or mechanically clearing mucus from the airway by suctioning.

LIQUEFYING SECRETIONS

Mucus (mixture of mucin, white blood cells, electrolytes, cells that have been shed through the natural process of tissue replacement, and water) is continuously produced. The volume of water affects the *viscosity,* or thickness, of the mucus.

Adequate hydration is important for keeping the mucus at a consistency that promotes expectoration (see Chap. 15). Hydration, the process of providing adequate fluid intake, tends to keep the mucous membranes moist and the mucus thin.

In addition, nurses may assist with **inhalation therapy** (respiratory treatments that provide a mixture of oxygen, humidification, and aerosolized medications directly to the lungs). The aerosol is delivered through a mask or hand-held mouthpiece (Fig. 36-3). Aerosol therapy improves breathing, encourages spontaneous coughing, and helps patients raise sputum for diagnostic purposes.

Nursing Guidelines For

Collecting a Sputum Specimen

☑ Plan to collect a sputum specimen just after the patient awakens or after an aerosol treatment.

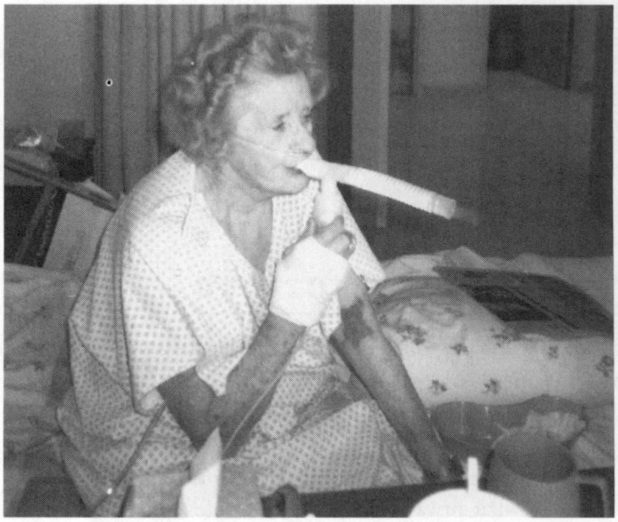

FIGURE 36–3. Aerosol therapy. (Courtesy of Ken Timby.)

RATIONALE: Allows collection at a time when there is more mucus available or it is in a thinner state

- Obtain a sterile sputum specimen cup.
  RATIONALE: Prevents contamination of the specimen
- Encourage the patient to rinse the mouth with tap water.
  RATIONALE: Removes some microorganisms and food residue from the mouth
- Explain that the desired specimen should be from deep within the respiratory passages, not saliva from within the mouth.
  RATIONALE: Avoids inconclusive or invalid test results
- Instruct the patient to take several deep breaths, attempt a forceful cough, and expectorate into the specimen container.
  RATIONALE: Helps mobilize secretions from the lower airway
- Collect at least a 1- to 3-mL (nearly a half-teaspoon) specimen.
  RATIONALE: Ensures a sufficient quantity for analysis
- Wear gloves and cover and enclose the specimen container in a clear plastic bag.
  RATIONALE: Reduces the potential for the transmission of microorganisms
- Offer oral hygiene.
  RATIONALE: Promotes comfort and well-being
- Attach a label and laboratory request form to the specimen.
  RATIONALE: Ensures correct specimen identification and test procedure
- Take the specimen to the laboratory immediately.
  RATIONALE: Allows prompt and accurate analysis of the specimen

MOBILIZING SECRETIONS

To mobilize secretions, **chest physiotherapy** (techniques for mobilizing secretions from distal airways using postural drainage, percussion, and vibration) is often used. It is usually indicated for patients with chronic respiratory diseases who have difficulty coughing or raising thick mucus.

Postural Drainage

Postural drainage (positioning technique that promotes gravity drainage from various lobes or segments of the lungs; Fig. 36-4) aids in mobilizing secretions. Its effectiveness is enhanced when it is combined with the two other techniques of chest physiotherapy, percussion and vibration. In most hospitals, respiratory therapists are responsible for postural drainage. In long-term care facilities and home health care, however, nurses may teach the patient and family to perform this technique.

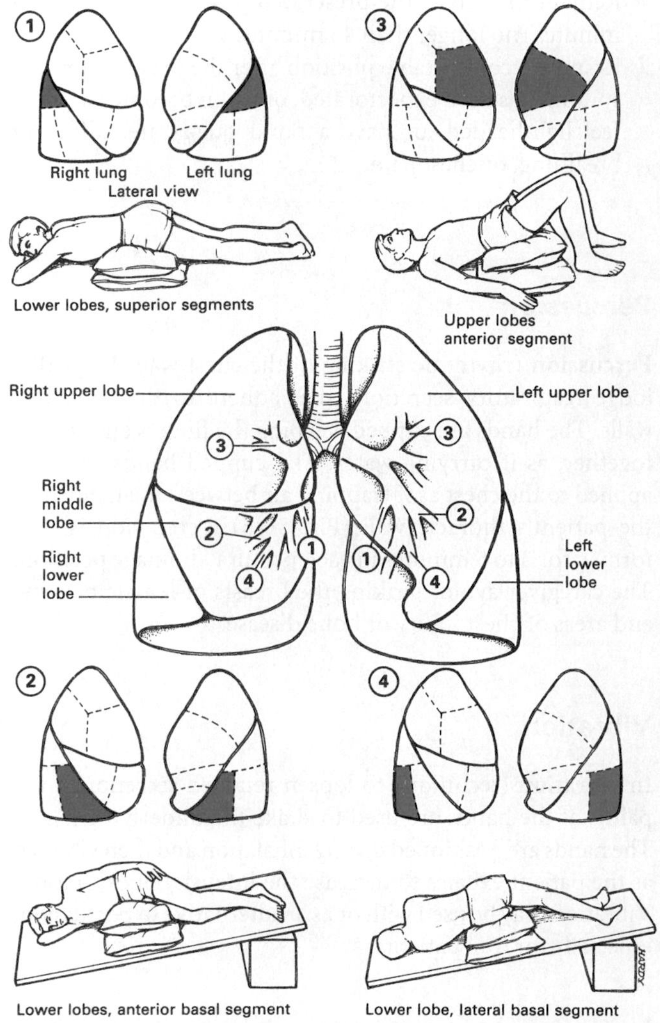

FIGURE 36–4. Lung segments and corresponding postural drainage positions. (Rosdahl C: Textbook of basic nursing, 7th ed, p 1201. Philadelphia, Lippincott Williams & Wilkins, 1999.)

Patient Teaching Guidelines For
Performing Postural Drainage

Teach the patient to do the following:

- Plan to perform postural drainage two to four times each day—for instance, before meals and at bedtime.
- Administer inhaled medications that have been prescribed (see Chap. 33) before performing postural drainage.
- Have paper tissues and a waterproof container nearby for collecting expectorated sputum.
- Position yourself to drain the appropriate areas of the lungs.
- Cough and expectorate the secretions that drain into the upper airway.

- Remain in each of the prescribed positions for 15 to 30 minutes (no longer than 45 minutes).
- Resume a comfortable position after the usual volume of sputum has been expectorated, or if you become fatigued, feel lightheaded, or have a rapid pulse rate, difficulty breathing, or chest pain.

Percussion

Percussion (rhythmic striking of the chest wall) helps dislodge respiratory secretions that adhere to the bronchial walls. The hands are cupped, keeping the fingers and thumb together, as if carrying water. The cupped hands are then applied to the chest as if trapping air between the hands and the patient's thoracic wall (Fig. 36-5). Percussion is performed for 3 to 5 minutes in each postural drainage position. The caregiver avoids striking the breasts of female patients and areas of chest injury or bone disease.

Vibration

In **vibration** (technique to loosen retained secretions), the palms of the hands are used to shake the underlying tissue. The hands are positioned during inhalation and then vibrated as the patient exhales to increase the intensity of expiration. Vibration may be used with or as an alternative to percussion, especially for frail patients.

SUCTIONING SECRETIONS

Suctioning (technique for removing liquid secretions with a catheter) uses negative (vacuum) pressure. The amount of negative pressure varies depending on the patient and the type of suction equipment (Table 36-1). In some cases, the upper airway, the lower airway, or both are suctioned. The airway is suctioned from the nose or mouth (Skill 36-1).

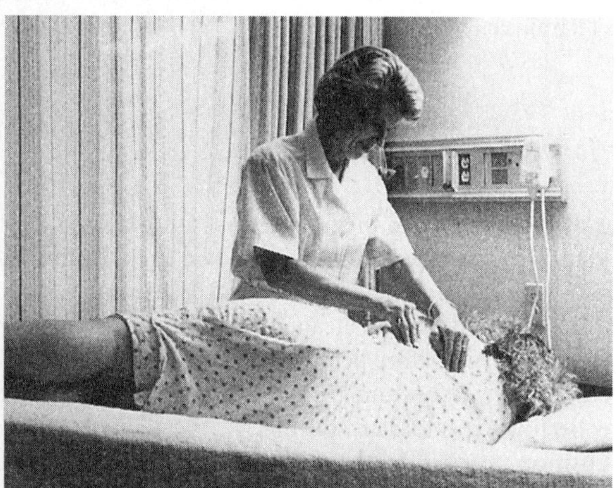

FIGURE 36–5. Performing percussion. (Courtesy of Ken Timby.)

TABLE 36–1. **Variations in Suction Pressure**

Age	Wall Suction	Portable Suction Machine
Adults	100–140 mm Hg	10–15 mm Hg
Children	95–100 mm Hg	5–10 mm Hg
Infants	50–95 mm Hg	2–5 mm Hg

Nasopharyngeal suctioning (removing secretions from the throat through a nasally inserted catheter) is more common than **nasotracheal suctioning** (removal of secretions from the distal airways through a nasally inserted catheter). A nasopharyngeal airway, sometimes called a trumpet (Fig. 36-6), can be used to protect the nostril if frequent suctioning is necessary.

An alternative method is **oropharyngeal suctioning** (removal of secretions from the throat through a catheter inserted through the mouth). **Oral suctioning** (removal of secretions from the mouth) is performed with a suctioning device called a Yankeur-tip or tonsil-tip catheter (Fig. 36-7).

Artificial Airways

If patients are at risk for an airway obstruction or long-term mechanical ventilation is necessary, an artificial airway may be used. Two common types of artificial airways are an oral airway and a tracheostomy tube.

ORAL AIRWAY

An **oral airway** (curved device that keeps the tongue positioned forward within the mouth) is most commonly used in patients who are unconscious and cannot protect their own airway, such as those recovering from general anesthesia or a seizure. It prevents the relaxed tongue from obstructing the upper airway.

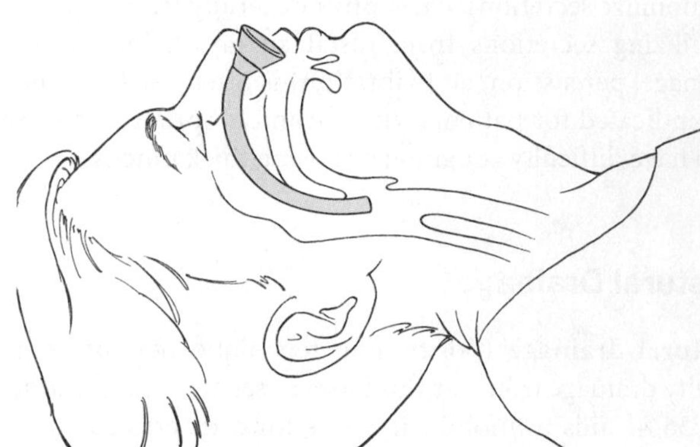

FIGURE 36–6. Placement of a nasopharyngeal trumpet.

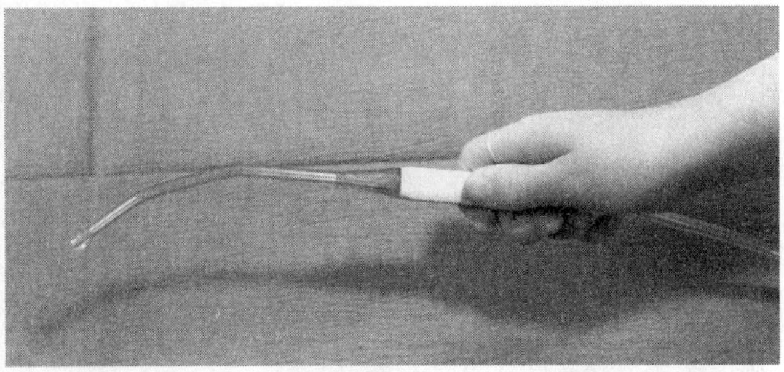

FIGURE 36–7. Yankeur-tip suction device for oral suctioning. (Courtesy of Ken Timby.)

Oral airways are usually used for a brief period and are inserted by nurses.

Nursing Guidelines For

Inserting an Oral Airway

- ☑ Gather the following supplies: various sizes of oral airways (most adults can accommodate an 80-mm airway), gloves, tongue blade, and suction equipment.
  RATIONALE: Promotes organization and efficient time management
- ☑ Place the airway on the outside of the cheek so that the front is parallel with the front teeth. Note whether the back of the airway reaches the angle of the jaw.
  RATIONALE: Determines the appropriate size to use (if the airway is too short, it will be ineffective; if it is too long, it will depress the epiglottis, increasing the risk of an airway obstruction)
- ☑ Wash your hands and don clean gloves.
  RATIONALE: Reduces the transmission of microorganisms
- ☑ Explain the procedure to the patient.
  RATIONALE: Provides information that some unconscious patients may comprehend, even though they may not respond verbally
- ☑ Perform oral suctioning if necessary.
  RATIONALE: Clears saliva from the mouth and prevents aspiration
- ☑ Place the patient in a supine position with the neck hyperextended, unless contraindicated.
  RATIONALE: Opens the airway and facilitates insertion
- ☑ Open the patient's mouth using a gloved finger and thumb or a tongue blade.
  RATIONALE: Prevents injury to the teeth during insertion
- ☑ Hold the airway so that the curved tip points upward toward the roof of the mouth (Fig. 36-8*A*) or toward the side of the cheek. Insert it about halfway.
  RATIONALE: Prevents pushing the tongue into the pharynx during insertion

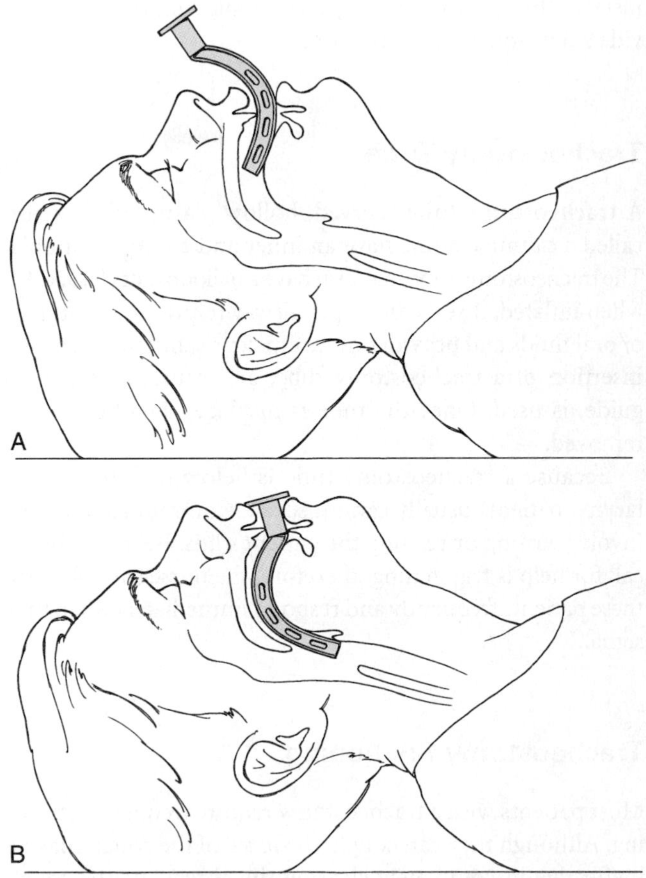

FIGURE 36–8. Oral airway insertion. (*A*) Initial insertion position. (*B*) Final position after rotation.

- ☑ Rotate the airway over the top of the tongue and continue inserting it until the front flange is flush with lips (see Fig. 36-8*B*).
  RATIONALE: Ensures that the artificial airway follows the natural curve of the upper airway
- ☑ Assess breathing.
  RATIONALE: Indicates that the natural airway is patent
- ☑ Remove the airway every 4 hours, provide oral hygiene, and clean and reinsert the airway.
  RATIONALE: Removes transient bacteria; promotes integrity of the oral mucosa

As the patient's level of consciousness improves, many patients extubate themselves independently.

TRACHEOSTOMY

Patients who are less stable, who have an upper airway obstruction, or who require prolonged ventilation and oxygenation are more likely to be candidates for a **tracheostomy** (surgically created opening into the trachea). A tube is inserted through the opening to maintain the airway and provide a new route for ventilation.

Tracheostomy Tube

A **tracheostomy tube** (curved, hollow plastic tube) is also called a cannula. Some have an inner and an outer cannula. The tracheostomy tube may also have a balloon cuff (Fig. 36-9); when inflated, it seals the upper airway to prevent aspiration of oral fluids and provides more efficient ventilation. During insertion of a tracheostomy tube, an obturator, a curved guide, is used. Once the tube is in place, the obturator is removed.

Because a tracheostomy tube is below the level of the larynx, patients usually cannot speak. Communication may involve writing or reading the patient's lips. Being unable to call for help is frightening; therefore, the nurse should check these patients frequently and respond immediately when they signal.

Tracheostomy Suctioning

Most patients with a tracheostomy require frequent suctioning. Although they can cough, the force of the cough may be ineffective in completely clearing the airway, or the cough may be inadequate to clear the volume of respiratory secretions. Therefore, suctioning is necessary when secretions are copious.

Tracheostomy suctioning is similar to nasotracheal suctioning, except that the catheter is inserted through the tracheostomy tube rather than the nose (Fig. 36-10). The catheter is also inserted a shorter distance because the tube lies in the trachea. The catheter is inserted approximately 4 to 5 inches (10–12.5 cm), or until resistance is felt. The resistance is caused by contact between the catheter tip and the carina, the ridge at the lower end of the tracheal cartilage where the main bronchi are located. The catheter is then raised about a half-inch (1.25 cm), and suction is applied.

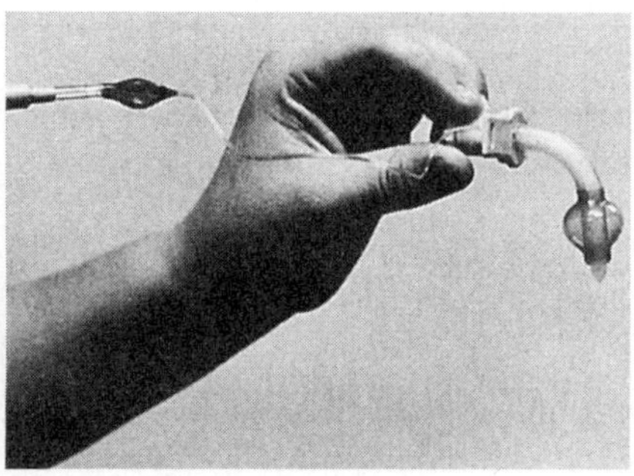

FIGURE 36–9. A cuffed tracheostomy tube. (Courtesy of Ken Timby.)

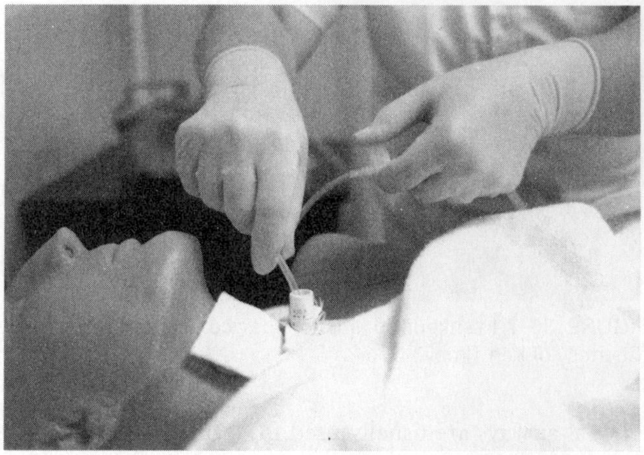

FIGURE 36–10. Suctioning through a tracheostomy tube. (Courtesy of Ken Timby.)

Tracheostomy Care

Tracheostomy care (cleaning the skin around the stoma, changing the dressing, and cleaning the inner cannula) is described in Skill 36-2. Tracheostomy care is performed at least every 8 hours or as often as needed to keep the secretions from becoming dried, thus narrowing or occluding the airway. Tracheal suctioning may be performed separately from or at the same time as tracheostomy care.

Nursing Implications

Maintaining an open and patent airway is a priority for nursing care. Lack of oxygen for more than 4 to 6 minutes can result in death or permanent brain damage. Therefore, it is essential to identify nursing diagnoses that apply to respiratory problems and to plan care accordingly for patients at risk. Some possible nursing diagnoses include:

- Ineffective airway clearance
- Impaired gas exchange
- Risk for infection
- Inability to sustain spontaneous ventilation
- Anxiety
- Knowledge deficit

The nursing care plan shows how the nursing process applies to a patient with the nursing diagnosis of Ineffective airway clearance, defined in the 1999 NANDA taxonomy as "the inability to clear secretions or obstructions from the respiratory tract to maintain a clear airway."

Nursing Care Plan

Ineffective Airway Clearance

Assessment

Subjective Data

States, "I've had such a hard time breathing this past week. I stayed home from work. Most of the time I slept in my recliner chair. I couldn't even eat or drink much."

Objective Data

48-year-old man with a history of smoking 2 packs of cigarettes per day admitted with possible bacterial pneumonia. T—101° (oral) P—100. Breathing is rapid (30/min) and shallow. Uses accessory muscles and demonstrates nasal flaring. Bronchial breath sounds and inspiratory gurgles heard in distal R. upper lobe both anteriorly and posteriorly; all other areas of lungs sound clear. Has a persistent cough but does not raise sputum. Skin is hot and dry. Urine is a dark, concentrated amber color.

Diagnosis

Ineffective airway clearance related to weak cough and retained secretions

Plan

Goal

The patient's lungs will sound clear throughout by 12/4.

Orders: 12/1

1. Auscultate lungs q shift, and before and after coughing or other respiratory therapy.
2. Elevate head of bed at all times.
3. Maintain 2,000–3,000 mL fluid intake of patient's choice (avoid milk) for 24 hours.
4. Instruct to take 3 deep breaths in through nose and out mouth, lean forward, and cough forcefully. Repeat q 1–2 hr while awake.
5. Perform oral/pharyngeal suctioning if secretions are loosened but not expectorated.

__________ L. HOWARD, RN

Implementation (Documentation)

12/1 0730 Continues to demonstrate effort at breathing. Sitting upright, nostrils flare, and physical activity is limited. Lungs clear except for inspiratory gurgles in RUL. Receiving 36% O_2 per nasal cannula at 4 L/min. IV of 1,000 mL of 5% D/W c̄ 800 mg of aminophyllin infusing at 30 mL per hour through infusion pump. Respiratory department contacted concerning new order for aerosol therapy. Instructed on deep breathing and coughing technique.

__________ A. SANTINI, LPN

Evaluation (Documentation)

0800 Breathing and coughing performed 3 times with no change in lung assessments. Able to drink a pot (240 mL) of hot tea with sugar and lemon.

__________ A. SANTINI, LPN

1000 Able to raise a small amount of tenacious, purulent sputum after breathing and coughing and aerosol therapy. Specimen sent to laboratory for culture and sensitivity. Lung sounds remain unchanged. __________ A. SANTINI, LPN

FOCUS ON OLDER ADULTS

- The muscular structures of the larynx tend to atrophy with age, which can affect the ability to clear the airway.
- Usually the bases of the older adult's lungs receive less ventilation, contributing to the retention of secretions and compromised ventilation. The respiratory cilia become less efficient with age, predisposing older adults to a high incidence of pneumonia.
- Diminished strength of accessory muscles for respiration, increased rigidity of the chest wall, and diminished cough reflex make it difficult for older adults to cough productively and effectively.
- Conditions affecting the respiratory system are among the most common life-threatening disorders experienced by older adults. The severity of chronic pulmonary diseases increases with age.
- Many older adults with pathologic pulmonary changes have a history of cigarette smoking since their youth, working in occupations where they inhaled pollutants that affected their lungs, or living a greater part of their lives in industrial areas known for their toxic emissions.
- Inquiring about their current history of coughing, determining how long the cough has been present, and observing and describing any sputum being raised are important when assessing older adults.
- Persistent, dry coughing consumes energy and causes fatigue in older adults if not relieved promptly.
- Deep-breathing exercises improve the older adult's ability to eliminate secretions from the respiratory tract. Maintenance of adequate hydration is important to facilitate elimination of respiratory secretions.
- The production of respiratory secretions is influenced by weather, such as high humidity or damp conditions.
- Older adults with difficulty swallowing (dysphagia), often associated with strokes or middle and later stages of dementia, are more vulnerable to aspiration pneumonia. Evaluation of dysphagia is important so that appropriate interventions are implemented to prevent aspiration.
- Older adults are at a higher risk for developing cardiac dysrhythmias when being suctioned because many have preexisting hypoxemia due to illnesses and age-related changes in ventilation.

KEY CONCEPTS

- The airway is the collective system of tubes in the upper and lower respiratory tract through which gases travel during their passage to and from the alveoli.
- The airway is composed of the nose, pharynx, trachea, bronchi, and bronchioles.
- The airway is protected by the epiglottis, which seals the airway when swallowing food and fluids; the rings of tracheal cartilage, which keep the trachea from collapsing; the mucous membrane, which traps particulate matter; and the cilia, which beat debris upward in the airway so it can be coughed, expectorated, or swallowed.
- Airway management refers to skills used to maintain natural or artificial airways for compromised patients. It includes measures for liquefying secretions, mobilizing secretions to promote their expectoration with chest physiotherapy, or mechanically clearing mucus from the airway by suctioning.
- When suctioning the airway, one of several approaches is used, such as nasopharyngeal, nasotracheal, oropharyngeal, oral, and tracheal suctioning.
- Artificial airways are used in patients at risk for an airway obstruction or those in whom long-term mechanical ventilation is necessary.
- Two examples of artificial airways are an oral airway and a tracheostomy tube.
- Tracheostomy care includes cleaning the skin around the stoma, changing the dressing, and cleaning the inner cannula.

CRITICAL THINKING EXERCISES

- Some patients with a tracheostomy learn to suction themselves. Develop a plan for teaching this procedure that would promote independence yet avoid overwhelming the patient.
- Discuss ways to relieve the anxiety of a patient with a tracheostomy who needs frequent suctioning but fears he or she will be unable to obtain assistance when needed.

SUGGESTED READINGS

Calianno C. Nosocomial pneumonia: repelling a deadly invader. Nursing 1996;26(5):34–39.

Carr J, Pryor JA, Hodson ME. Self chest clapping: Patients' views and the effects on oxygen saturation. Physiotherapy 1995;81(12):753–757.

Carroll P. Closing in on safer suctioning. RN 1998;61(5):22–26.

Ciesla ND. Chest physical therapy for patients in the intensive care unit. Physical Therapy 1996;76(6):609–625.

Druding MC. Re-examining the practice of normal saline instillation prior to suctioning. MedSurg Nursing 1997;6(4):209–212.

Glass C, Grap M. Ten tips for safer suctioning. American Journal of Nursing 1995;95(5):51–53.

Hardy KA. A review of airway clearance: New techniques, indications, and recommendations. Respiratory Care 1994;39:440–452.

Hatfield BO. Cost-effective trach teaching. RN 1997;60(3):48–49.

Hess DR. Managing the artificial airway. Respiratory Care 1999;44(7):759–776.

Inwood H, Cull C. Advanced airway management. Professional Nurse 1998;13(8):509–513.

NANDA nursing diagnoses: Definitions and classification, 1999–2000. Philadelphia, NANDA, 1999.

O'Hanlon-Nichols T. Basic assessment series. The adult pulmonary system. American Journal of Nursing 1998;98(2):38–45.

Orringer MK. The effects of tracheostomy tube placement on communication and swallowing. Respiratory Care 1999;44(7):845–855.

Reibel JF. Tracheotomy/tracheostomy. Respiratory Care 1999;44(7):820–827.

Shelton BK. Mounting an offense against lobar pneumonia. Nursing 1998; 28(12):42–47.

Somerson SJ, Husted CW, Somerson SW, et al. Mastering emergency airway management. American Journal of Nursing 1996;96(5):Nurse Pract. Extra Ed: 24–31.

Stauffer JL. Complications of endotracheal intubation and tracheotomy. Respiratory Care 1999;44(7):828.

St. John RE. Airway management. Critical Care Nursing 1999;19(4):79–83.

Stott S, Webster N. Nosocomial pneumonia. Care of the Critically Ill 1997; 13:139–144.

SKILL 36–1

SUCTIONING THE AIRWAY

Suggested Action	Reason for Action
Assessment	
Assess the patient's lung sounds, respiratory effort, and oxygen saturation level.	Determines the need for suctioning
Determine how much the patient understands about suctioning the airway.	Provides an opportunity for health teaching
Inspect the nose to determine which nostril is more patent.	Eases insertion of the catheter
Planning	
Obtain a suction kit. Equipment may vary, but all contain a basin and one or two sterile gloves. Some kits may also contain a sterile suction catheter.	Promotes organization and efficient time management
Select a catheter size, if one is not included, that will not occlude the diameter of the nostril; usually a 12 to 18F catheter is appropriate for an adult.	Promotes comfort and reduces the potential for injury
Obtain a flask of sterile normal saline and a suction machine, if a wall outlet is unavailable.	Provides items that are not prepackaged
Attach the suction canister to the wall outlet or plug a portable suction machine into an electrical outlet.	Provides a source for negative pressure
Connect the suction tubing to the canister.	Provides a means for connecting the canister to the suction catheter
Turn on the suction machine, occlude the suction tubing, and adjust the pressure gauge to the desired amount.	Ensures safe pressure during suctioning
Open the container of saline.	Reduces the risk for contamination later
Implementation	
Pull the privacy curtains.	Demonstrates respect for the patient's dignity
Elevate the head of the bed unless contraindicated.	Aids ventilation
Preoxygenate the patient for 1 to 2 minutes until the SpO_2 is maintained at 95% to 100%.	Reduces the risk of causing hypoxemia
Wash your hands.	Reduces the transmission of microorganisms
Open the suction kit without contaminating the contents.	Follows principles of asepsis
Don sterile glove(s). If only one is provided, don a clean glove on the nondominant hand and then don the sterile glove on the dominant hand.	Prevents the transmission of microorganisms
Pour sterile normal saline into the basin with your nondominant hand.	Prepares solution for wetting and rinsing the suction catheter
Consider the nondominant hand contaminated.	Follows principles of asepsis
Pick up the suction catheter with your sterile (dominant) hand and connect it to the suction tubing.	Completes the circuit for applying suction
Place the catheter tip in the saline and occlude the vent.	Wets the outer and inner surfaces of the catheter; reduces friction and facilitates insertion
Insert the catheter without applying suction along the floor of the nose or the side of the mouth.	Reduces the potential for sneezing or gagging

continued

SKILL 36–1

SUCTIONING THE AIRWAY *Continued*

Suggested Action	Reason for Action

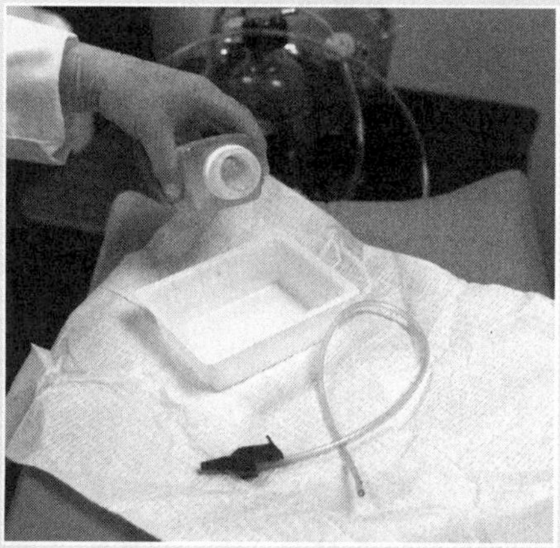

Pouring sterile saline. (Courtesy of Ken Timby.)

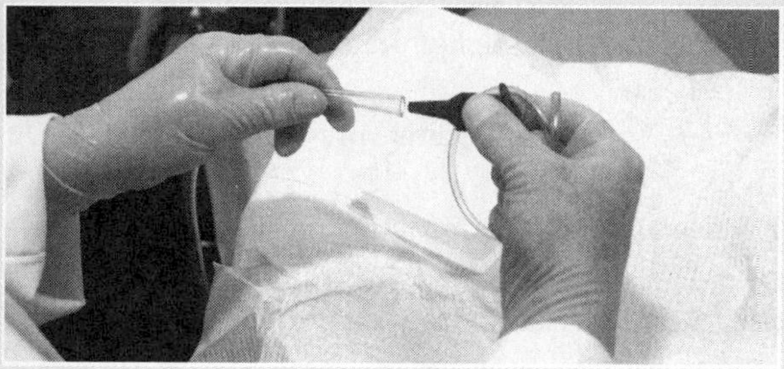

Connecting the catheter. (Courtesy of Ken Timby.)

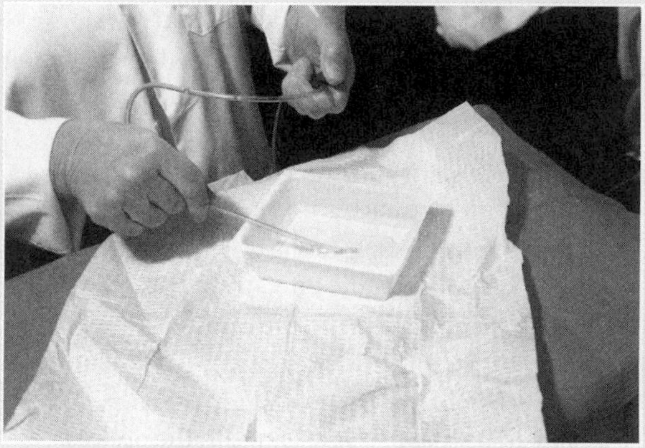

Wetting the catheter. (Courtesy of Ken Timby.)

Suggested Action	Reason for Action
Advance the catheter to a depth of 5 to 6 inches (12.5–15 cm) in the nose or 3 to 4 inches (7.5–10 cm) in the mouth.	Places the distal tip in the pharynx

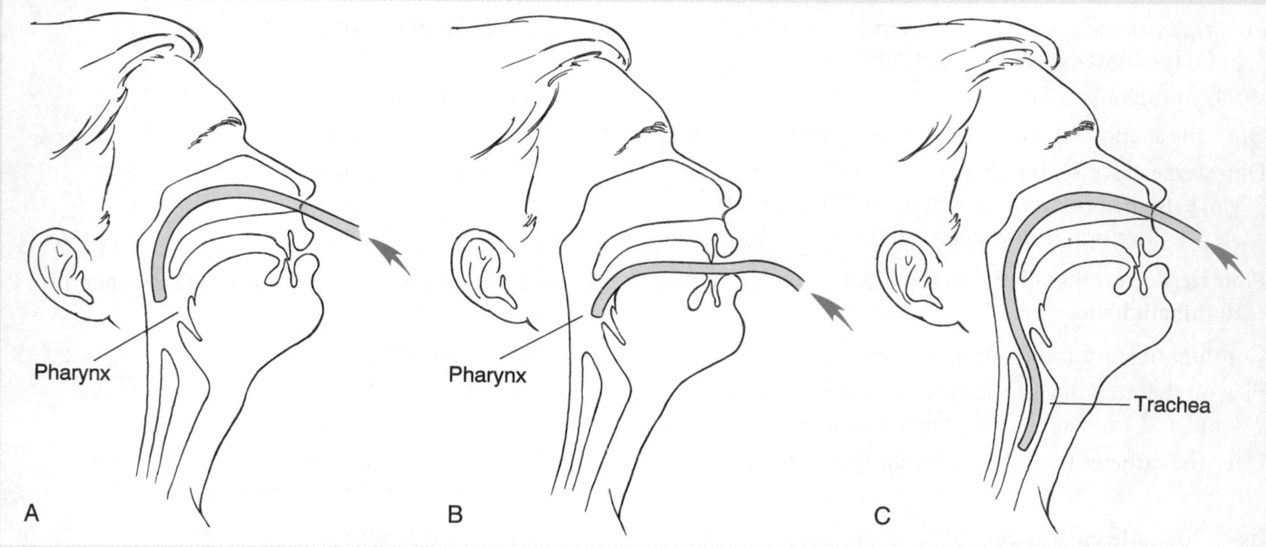

Catheter placement: (*A*) nasopharyngeal, (*B*) oropharyngeal, and (*C*) nasotracheal.

continued

SKILL 36–1

SUCTIONING THE AIRWAY *Continued*

Suggested Action	Reason for Action
For tracheal suctioning, wait until the patient takes a breath and advance the tubing 8 to 10 inches (20–25 cm).	Eases insertion below the larynx
Encourage the patient to cough if it does not occur spontaneously.	Breaks up mucus and raises secretions
Occlude the air vent and rotate the catheter as it is withdrawn.	Maximizes effectiveness of suctioning
Complete the process in no more than 15 seconds from the time of insertion of the catheter to its removal, occluding the vent no longer than 10 seconds.	Prevents hypoxemia
Rinse the secretions from the catheter by inserting the tip in the basin of saline and applying suction.	Flushes the mucus from the inner lumen
Provide a 2- to 3-minute period of rest while the patient continues to breathe oxygen.	Reoxygenates the blood
Suction again if necessary.	Bases decision on individual assessment data
Remove the gloves to enclose the suction catheter in an inverted glove.	Encloses the soiled catheter, reducing transmission of microorganisms

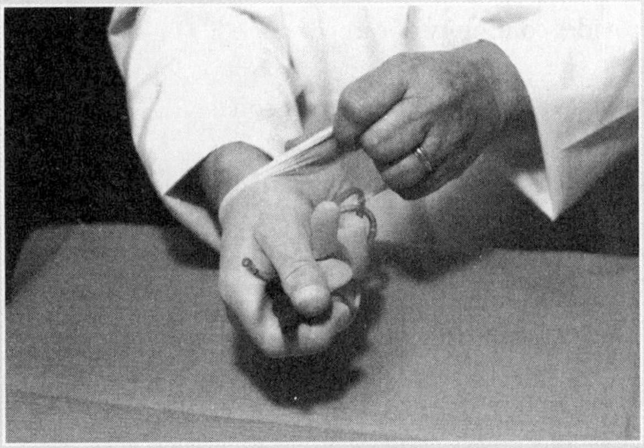

Enclosing the catheter. (Courtesy of Ken Timby.)

Suggested Action	Reason for Action
Discard suction kit, catheter, and gloves in a lined waste receptacle.	Follows principles of asepsis

Evaluation

- The airway is cleared of secretions.
- The SpO_2 level remains at 95% or more.
- Patient demonstrates breathing that requires less effort.

Document

- Preassessment data
- Type of suctioning performed
- Appearance of secretions
- Patient's response

continued

SKILL 36–1

SUCTIONING THE AIRWAY *Continued*

SAMPLE DOCUMENTATION

Date and Time Respirations are moist and noisy. SpO_2 shows a drop from 95% to 93% during last 15 minutes. Coughing effort is weak and ineffective. Raised to a high Fowler's position and oxygenated at 4 L per nasal cannula. Tracheal suctioning performed and reoxygenated. Lungs sound clear at this time. Pulse oximeter indicates SpO_2 at 95% at this time.

______________________________ SIGNATURE, TITLE

CRITICAL THINKING

- Besides an SpO_2 of less than 90%, what signs or symptoms are manifested by a person who is hypoxic?

SKILL 36–2

PROVIDING TRACHEOSTOMY CARE

Suggested Action	Reason for Action
Assessment	
Check the nursing care plan to determine the schedule for providing tracheostomy care.	Provides continuity of care
Review the patient's record for documentation concerning previous tracheostomy care.	Provides a data base for comparison
Assess the condition of the dressing and the skin around the tracheostomy tube.	Determines need for skin care and dressing change
Determine the patient's understanding of tracheostomy care.	Provides an opportunity for health teaching
Planning	
Consult with the patient on an appropriate time for performing tracheostomy care if only routine care is needed.	Demonstrates respect for the patient's right to participate in decisions.
Obtain a tracheostomy care kit, which usually includes sterile gloves, two basins, a drape, gauze squares, pipe cleaners, cotton-tipped applicators, forceps, stomal dressing, and twill ties.	Promotes organization and efficient time management
Obtain a container of hydrogen peroxide and a flask of normal saline. Remove the cap from each container.	Provides items that are not prepackaged and prevents contamination of one gloved hand later in the procedure
Implementation	
Wash your hands.	Removes colonizing microorganisms
Raise the bed to an appropriate height.	Prevents back strain
Place the patient in a supine or low Fowler's position.	Facilitates access to the tracheostomy tube
Don a clean glove and remove the soiled stomal dressing and discard it, glove and all, in a lined waste receptacle.	Follows principles of asepsis

continued

SKILL 36–2

PROVIDING TRACHEOSTOMY CARE *Continued*

Suggested Action	Reason for Action
Wash your hands again.	Reduces the transmission of microorganisms
Open the tracheostomy kit, taking care not to contaminate its contents.	Provides access to supplies and maintains their sterility
Don sterile gloves, one of which—usually the one on the dominant hand—must remain sterile.	Prevents transferring microorganisms to the lower airway
Lip the containers of solution and add sterile normal saline to one basin and sterile hydrogen peroxide to the other.	Follows principles of asepsis; the hand used to pour the liquids is now considered contaminated

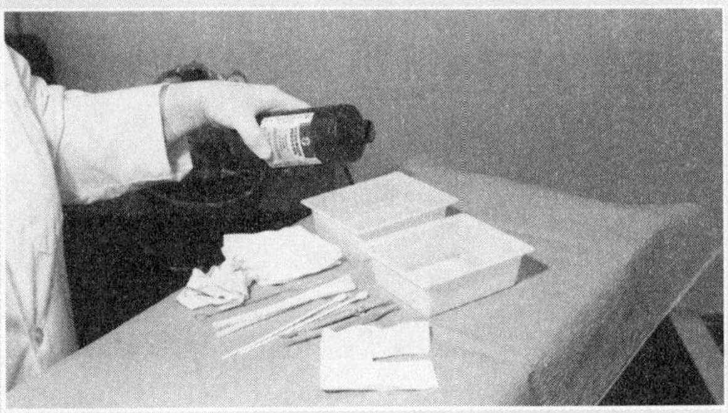

Adding cleaning solutions. (Courtesy of Ken Timby.)

Suggested Action	Reason for Action
Unlock the inner cannula (using the contaminated hand) by turning it counterclockwise and deposit it in the basin of hydrogen peroxide.	Loosens protein secretions and reduces the numbers of colonizing microorganisms
Clean the inside and outside of the cannula with pipe cleaners.	Removes gross debris

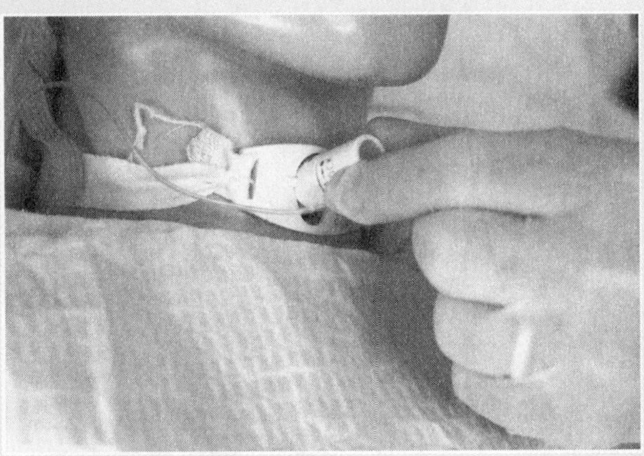

Removing the inner cannula. (Courtesy of Ken Timby.)

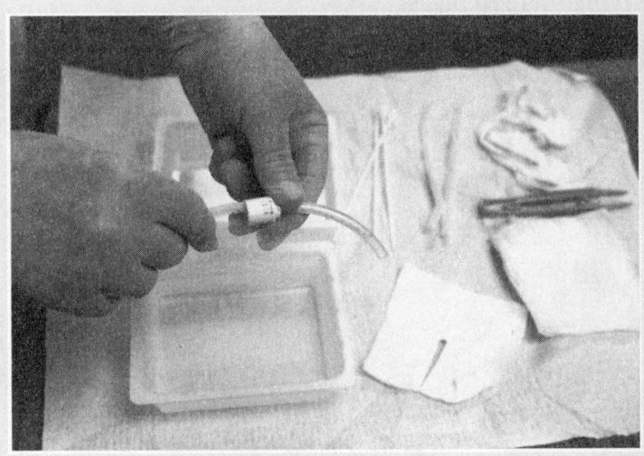

Cleaning the inner cannula. (Courtesy of Ken Timby.)

Suggested Action	Reason for Action
Deposit contaminated supplies in a lined or waterproof waste receptacle.	Reduces the potential for contaminating sterile supplies
Rinse the cleaned cannula in the basin of normal saline.	Removes remnants of hydrogen peroxide
Tap the rinsed cannula against the edge of the basin and wipe the excess solution with a gauze square.	Removes large droplets of fluid

continued

SKILL 36–2

PROVIDING TRACHEOSTOMY CARE *Continued*

Suggested Action	Reason for Action
Replace the inner cannula and turn it clockwise within the outer cannula.	Secures the inner cannula
Clean around the stoma with an applicator moistened with peroxide. Never go back over an area once it has been cleaned.	Removes secretions and colonizing microorganisms from the tracheal opening

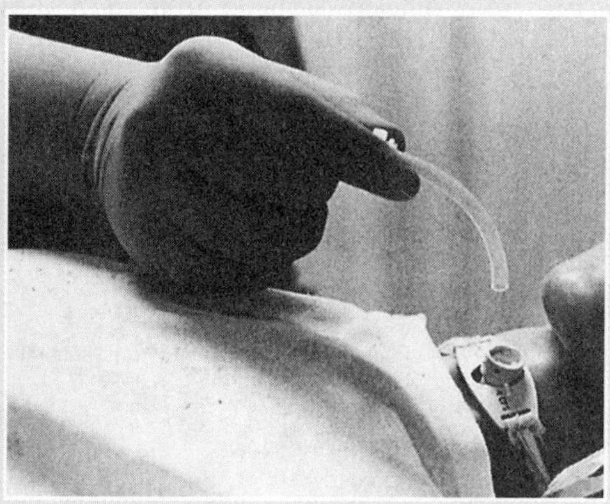

Replacing the inner cannula.

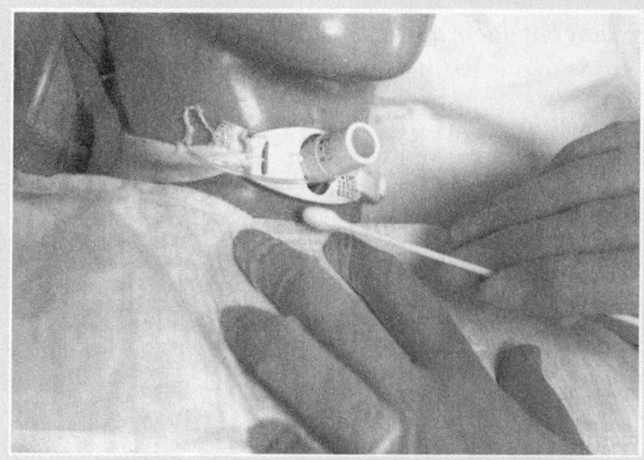

Cleaning the stoma. (Courtesy of Ken Timby.)

Suggested Action	Reason for Action
Wipe the same area in the same manner with another applicator moistened with saline.	Removes the hydrogen peroxide from the skin
Place the sterile stomal dressing around the tracheostomy tube.	Absorbs secretions and keeps the stomal area clean
Change the tracheostomy ties by threading them through the slits on the flange of the tracheostomy tube and tying them in place.	Holds the tracheostomy tube in place

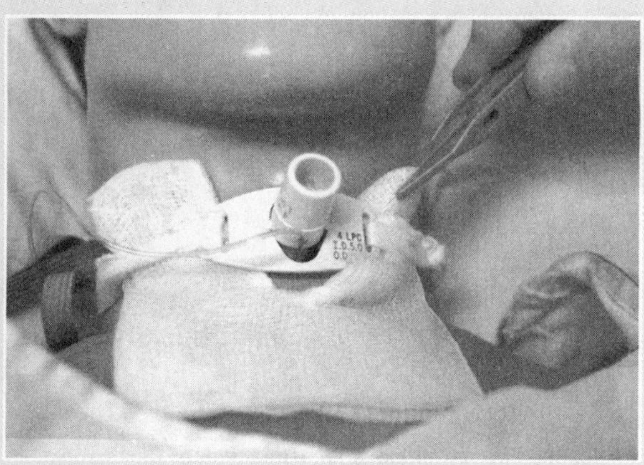

Applying the stomal dressing. (Courtesy of Ken Timby.)

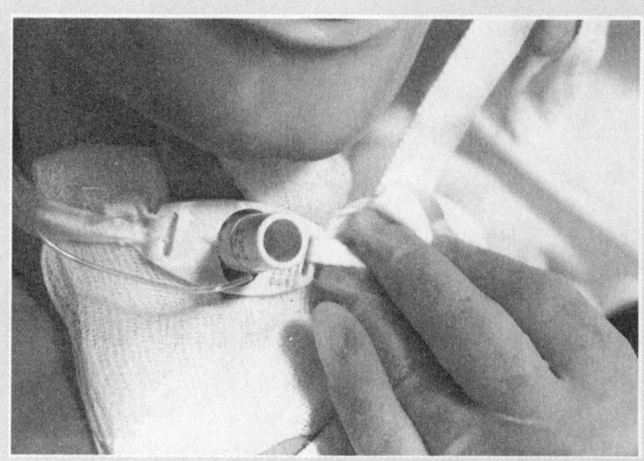

Securing the tracheostomy ties. (Courtesy of Ken Timby.)

Suggested Action	Reason for Action
Wait to remove the previous ties until after the new ones are secure, if working alone. Otherwise have an assistant stabilize the tracheostomy tube while the soiled ones are cut and the new ones are applied.	Prevents accidental extubation

continued

SKILL 36–2

PROVIDING TRACHEOSTOMY CARE *Continued*

Suggested Action	Reason for Action
Tie the two ends snugly, but not tightly, at the side of the neck.	Prevents skin impairment
Discard all soiled supplies, remove your gloves, and wash your hands.	Follows principles of asepsis
Return the patient to a position of comfort and safety.	Demonstrates concern for the patient's well-being

Evaluation

- The tracheostomy tube remains patent.
- The stomal opening is clean, without evidence of infection.
- The dressing is clean and dry.
- The neck skin is intact.

Document

- Preassessment data
- Procedure as it was performed
- Appearance of skin and secretions
- Response of the patient

SAMPLE DOCUMENTATION

Date and Time Respirations are quiet and effortless. Routine tracheostomy care provided. Moderate amount of clear mucus removed from inner cannula during cleaning. Stomal skin is pink but there is no redness, tenderness, swelling, or purulent drainage. Neck skin is intact; skin color is comparable to surrounding areas. ____________________ SIGNATURE, TITLE

CRITICAL THINKING

- Discuss methods of communicating with a patient who has a tracheostomy.
- Discuss the psychological effects of being unable to speak and having an artificial airway.

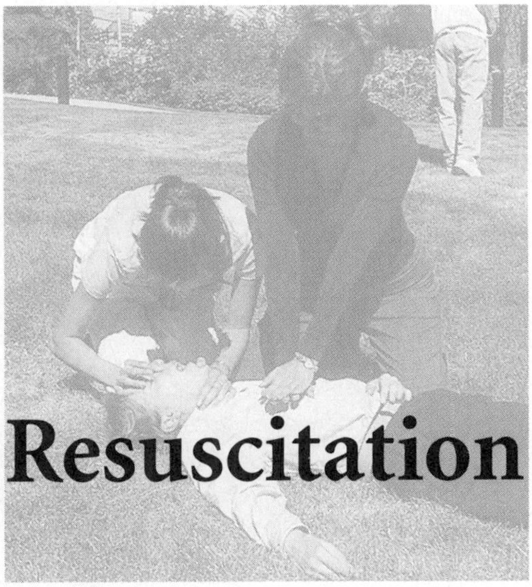

Resuscitation

CHAPTER 37

CHAPTER OUTLINE

SKILLS

NURSING CARE PLAN

KEY TERMS

automated external defibrillator
cardiopulmonary resuscitation
code
finger sweep
head tilt/chin lift technique
Heimlich maneuver
jaw-thrust maneuver
recovery position
rescue breathing
subdiaphragmatic thrust

LEARNING OBJECTIVES

An understanding of the content within this chapter will be evidenced by the student's ability to:

- Explain why an airway obstruction is life-threatening.
- Give at least three signs of an airway obstruction.
- Describe two appropriate actions if a patient has a partial airway obstruction.
- Explain the purpose of the Heimlich maneuver.
- Describe the circumstances for using subdiaphragmatic thrusts and chest thrusts.
- Discuss the technique used to dislodge an object from an infant's airway.
- Define cardiopulmonary resuscitation.
- Explain the ABCs of resuscitation.
- Name two techniques for opening the airway.
- List three ways to administer rescue breathing.
- Describe the purpose of chest compression.
- Identify the maximum time allowed for interrupting cardiopulmonary resuscitation.
- Name at least three criteria used in the decision to discontinue resuscitation efforts.

Nurses are often the first to respond to pulmonary or cardiac emergencies. This chapter reviews the most recent guidelines from the Emergency Cardiac Care Committee and Subcommittees of the American Heart Association for performing basic life support techniques.

Airway Obstruction

The upper airway, an area that includes the pharynx and trachea, can become occluded for various reasons. Sometimes the airway swells because of injury; an artificial airway may be needed to promote and sustain breathing (see Chap. 36). The airway may become mechanically obstructed with a bolus of food or some other foreign object. When the airway becomes obstructed, air exchange and subsequent oxygenation of cells and tissue become compromised. If an airway obstruction is not relieved, the victim will lose consciousness and eventually die.

IDENTIFYING SIGNS OF AIRWAY OBSTRUCTION

The signs of airway obstruction are similar to those of a heart attack, but there are differences. If distress occurs while the person is eating, airway obstruction is likely. The victim grasps the throat with the hands (Fig. 37-1) and makes aggressive efforts to cough and breathe. He or she makes a high-pitched sound while inhaling and turns pale and then blue.

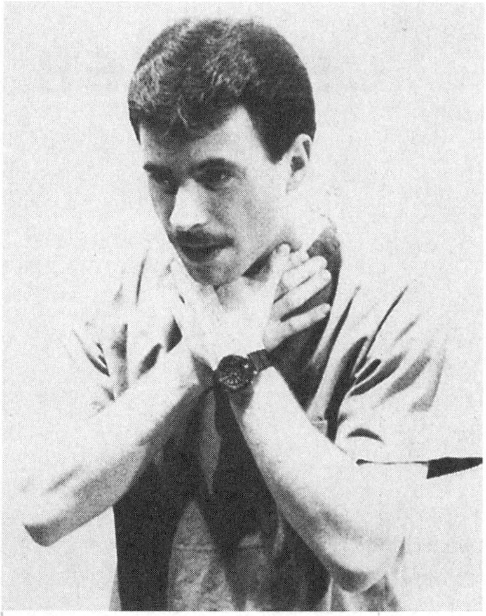

FIGURE 37–1. Universal sign for choking.

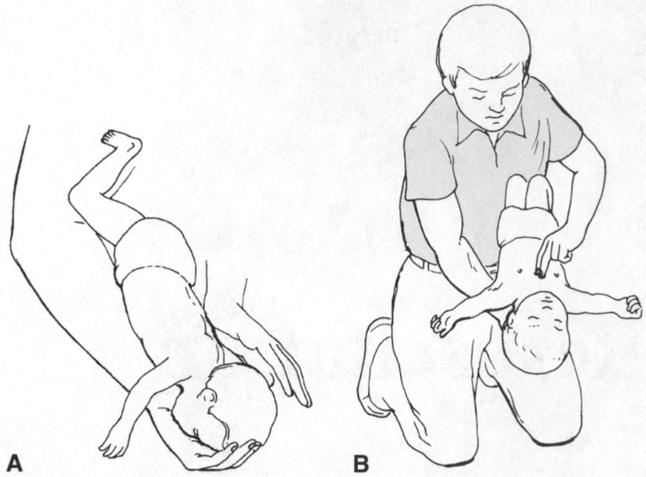

FIGURE 37–2. Assisting an infant with an obstruction. (*A*) Giving back blows. (*B*) Delivering chest thrusts.

RELIEVING AN OBSTRUCTION

If the victim can speak or cough, some air is being exchanged, indicating only a partial obstruction. No additional resuscitation efforts, other than encouraging and supporting the victim, are needed.

If the victim's efforts to relieve the partial obstruction are unsuccessful or if the situation worsens, it is appropriate to activate the emergency medical system. In the hospital, this is done by calling a **code** (summoning personnel trained in advanced life support techniques). In the community, assistance is obtained by dialing 911 or another emergency number.

If the obstruction becomes complete, immediate action is taken to dislodge the obstruction, as outlined in Skill 37-1. The **Heimlich maneuver** (method for relieving a mechanical airway obstruction) involves the use of **subdiaphragmatic thrusts** (pressure to the abdomen) or chest thrusts. Depending on the victim's age, there are differences in the way these are performed.

Adults and children older than 1 year are given five abdominal subdiaphragmatic thrusts to increase the intrathoracic pressure, equivalent to a cough. For obese adults or women in advanced pregnancy, five chest thrusts are given.

Because infants cannot talk or make a universal choking sign, the ability to cry is the best evidence of a partial obstruction. The infant is supported over the rescuer's forearm. With the baby in a prone position with the head held downward, the rescuer administers five back blows between the shoulder blades with the heel of one hand (Fig. 37-2*A*). If the infant is positioned supine, five chest thrusts are given with two fingers to the middle of the breastbone at about the level of the nipples (see Fig. 37-2*B*).

Cardiopulmonary Resuscitation

If the cause of distress is something other than an airway obstruction, other efforts are required. **Cardiopulmonary resuscitation** (CPR; techniques used to restore breathing and circulation) is performed once a quick assessment determines that the victim is unresponsive and is not breathing (Skill 37-2).

PERFORMING AN INITIAL ASSESSMENT

The initial assessment involves determining the victim's responsiveness by shaking the victim and shouting his or her name. If the victim is unresponsive and older than 8 years of age, the next step is to activate the emergency medical system before attempting resuscitation. The exception to this rule involves pediatric emergencies; in that case, resuscitation is attempted for a full minute before seeking emergency assistance.

OBTAINING ASSISTANCE

The sooner advanced life support measures are administered, the more likely it is that the victim will survive. If there is another person present, the task of obtaining assistance may be delegated. The following information should be given:

- The address (or room number) where assistance is needed
- The telephone number (or nursing unit) where the call is being made
- A description of the situation
- The current condition of the victim
- What actions have been taken

PERFORMING ABCS

The ABCs stand for **A**irway, **B**reathing, and **C**irculation, the steps involved in CPR.

Opening the Airway

Opening the airway may be all that is necessary to restore ventilation. The victim is positioned supine on a firm surface, taking care not to twist the spine in case there is unidentified trauma. In the absence of head or neck trauma, the **head tilt/chin lift technique** (method of choice for opening the airway; Fig. 37-3*A*) or the **jaw-thrust maneuver** (alternative method for opening the airway by grasping the lower jaw and lifting it while tilting the head backward) is used (Fig. 37-3*B*). If there is foreign material within the mouth, it is removed.

Once the airway is opened, the victim is assessed for spontaneous breathing. The rescuer observes for rising and falling of the chest and listens and feels for air escaping from the nose or mouth.

A breathing victim is then placed in the **recovery position** (side-lying position that helps to maintain an open airway and prevent aspiration of liquids). If breathing is not restored, the victim is kept supine and rescue breathing is attempted.

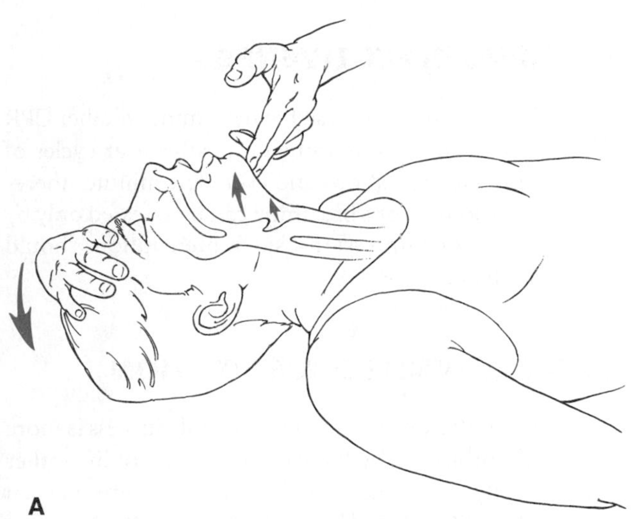

A

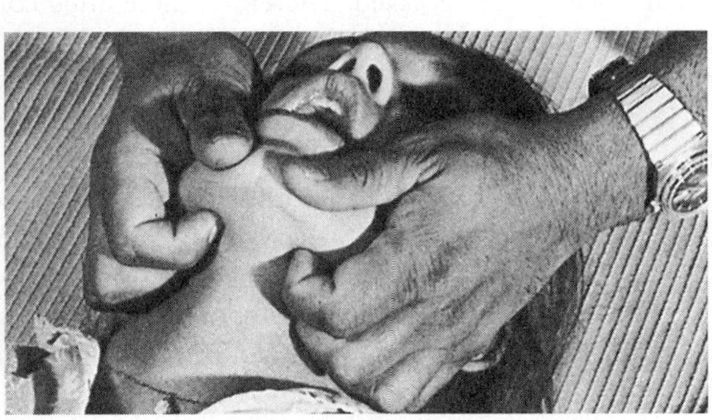

B

FIGURE 37–3. Techniques to open the airway. (*A*) Head tilt–chin lift technique. (*B*) Jaw-thrust technique.

Performing Rescue Breathing

Rescue breathing (process of ventilating the lungs) is done through the victim's mouth, nose, or stoma. A one-way valve mask or other protective face shield is used if available. These devices theoretically reduce the potential for acquiring infectious diseases such as hepatitis and AIDS, but lack of a barrier device should not interfere with attempting rescue breathing.

Mouth-to-Mouth Breathing

In mouth-to-mouth breathing, the victim's nose is sealed, the rescuer's mouth covers the victim's mouth, and the rescuer blows air into the victim. An open airway is maintained. Initially, two quick breaths are given before checking the victim's pulse. Rescue breathing resumes at a rate of 10 to 12 breaths per minute for adult victims.

Mouth-to-Nose Breathing

In mouth-to-nose breathing, an alternative method of providing rescue breathing, the mouth is sealed and the breaths are delivered through the nose. Mouth-to-nose breathing is provided when the victim is an infant or small child or when mouth-to-mouth breathing is impossible or unsuccessful.

Regardless of which method of rescue breathing is used, each breath is delivered (for an adult) over 1.5 to 2 seconds. This rate reduces the potential for distending the esophagus and stomach, which may promote regurgitation and aspiration.

Mouth-to-Stoma Breathing

Patients with a laryngectomy can be given rescue breathing by sealing the rescuer's mouth over the stoma. Because the upper airway is essentially a blind pathway, the nose does not require sealing.

For patients with a tracheostomy tube, rescue breathing may be given through the tube with the mouth or a one-way valve mask. If the tracheostomy tube does not have an inflated cuff, the nose must be sealed.

Promoting Circulation

To determine whether circulation requires support, the rescuer must determine whether the victim has a pulse. For an adult, this assessment is performed by compressing the carotid artery to the side of the trachea with two fingers (Fig. 37-4). The carotid artery is the most accessible site, but the femoral artery in the groin can also be used for assessment. The brachial artery in the upper arm is assessed when the victim is an infant. If the victim is pulseless, chest compressions are indicated.

Circulation is promoted by compressing the chest. Chest compressions circulate blood in one of two ways. Squeezing

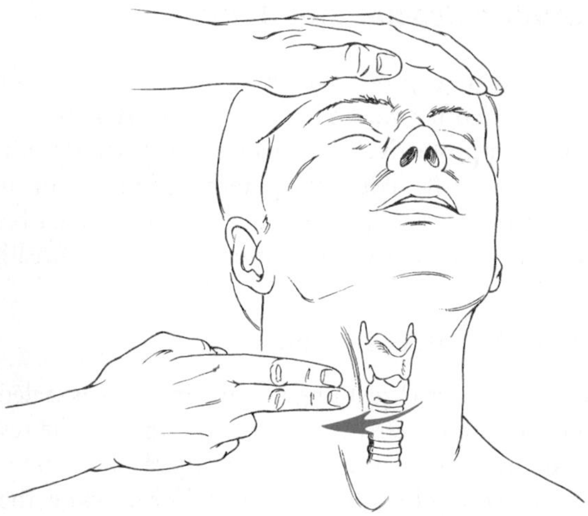

FIGURE 37–4. Assessing the carotid artery.

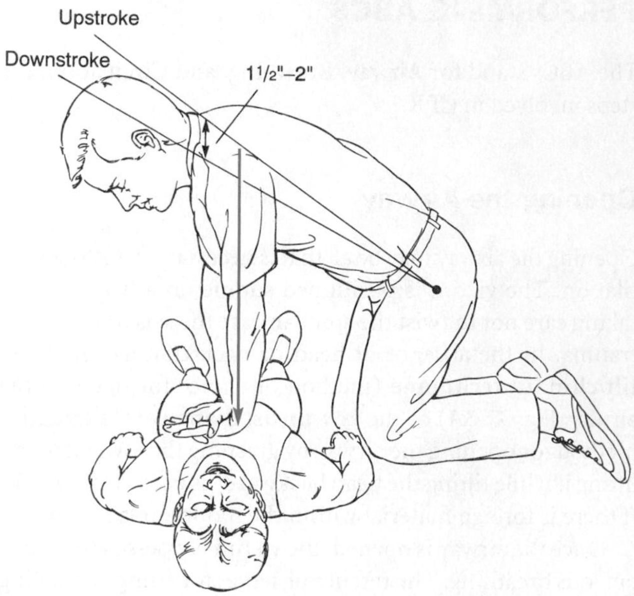

FIGURE 37–5. Correct hand and body position.

the heart between the sternum and the vertebrae increases the pressure in the ventricles; this is thought to push blood into the pulmonary arteries and aorta. Chest compressions are also thought to increase the pressure in blood vessels in the thorax, promoting systemic blood flow.

To be effective, cardiac compressions must be delivered at a rate of 80 to 100 times a minute for adult victims. For a one-person rescue, 15 chest compressions are given followed by two rescue breaths, or a ratio of 15:2. For a team of two persons, the ratio is five compressions to one breath, or 5:1.

The compression is given with sufficient force to cause a pulsation in the carotid artery. This may not occur unless the chest is depressed at least 1.5 to 2 inches. Assessment of carotid pulsation requires the assistance of a second rescuer.

The hands and body must be placed correctly. The heel of one hand is placed over the lower half of the sternum but above the xiphoid process. The other hand is placed on top, with the fingers interlocked or extended. The rescuer's body is positioned over the hands so that a straight-down motion is delivered with each compression (Fig. 37-5). The hands remain in contact with the chest, and the elbows are kept locked to avoid rocking back and forth over the victim.

Table 37-1 lists the variations that are made in rescue breathing and chest compressions to accommodate the anatomic differences and physiologic needs of various age groups.

Once CPR is initiated, it is not interrupted for more than 7 seconds except when:

- There is a pulse and the victim resumes breathing.
- The rescuer becomes exhausted.
- The victim's condition deteriorates despite the resuscitation efforts.
- There is written evidence that resuscitation is contrary to the victim's wishes.
- Advanced cardiac life support measures are administered, such as an automated external defibrillator.

An **automated external defibrillator** (device that delivers an electrical charge to the heart) is used when the heart is not beating effectively. Use of this equipment is not one of the techniques for basic life support.

ASSESSING EFFECTIVENESS

Periodically, the victim is assessed to determine whether CPR is effective. Assessment should be done after four cycles of compressions and ventilations and every few minutes thereafter. Signs of spontaneous breathing can be assessed only by interrupting chest compressions; such interruptions should last no more than 5 seconds.

DISCONTINUING RESUSCITATION

Not every resuscitation attempt is successful. Success is more appropriately measured by the victim's quality of life rather than its quantity. Severe neurologic deficits often result even when a victim's life is saved. Therefore, there often comes a time when a decision must be made to discontinue both basic and advanced life support efforts.

Because there are no clear-cut guidelines for suspending resuscitation, resuscitation efforts may extend for long periods in an attempt to save the victim. The decision to stop is a medical judgment made by the physician leading the code.

The decision to stop resuscitation efforts often is based on the time that elapsed before resuscitation began, the length of time that resuscitation has continued without any change in the victim's condition, the age and diagnosis of the victim, and objective data such as arterial blood gas results and electrolyte studies. Regardless of the basis for the decision, it is

TABLE 37–1. **Differences in Cardiopulmonary Resuscitation Among Infants, Children and Adults**

Technique	Infant (≤1 year of age)	Child (1–8 years of age)	Adult (≥8 years of age)
Rescue breaths			
Initial	2 breaths	2 breaths	2 breaths
Subsequent breaths	1 every 3 seconds	1 every 3 seconds	1 every 5 seconds
Rate	20/minute	20/minute	10–12/minute
Duration	1–1½ seconds	1–1½ seconds	1–1½ seconds
Compressions			
Location	In the midline, one fingerwidth below the nipples	Two fingerwidths above the tip of the sternum	Two fingerwidths above the tip of the sternum
Hand use	Two or three fingers	Heel of one hand	Two hands
Rate	At least 100/minute	100/min	80–100/min
Depth	½–1 in	1–1½ in	1½–2 in or more

not made lightly, and those involved in an unsuccessful code need the support of their colleagues.

Nursing Implications

Nurses have several responsibilities associated with resuscitation. They must learn to perform basic cardiac life support measures and maintain their certification to do so. If these skills are not used or refreshed at least every 2 years, they may be less than adequate. Nurses must support and participate in efforts to teach lay people, both adults and children, how to perform CPR. In most successful resuscitations, CPR was started early. Nurses should discuss advance directives (see Chap. 3) with patients. Honoring the patient's right to participate in the decision-making process is important.

The following nursing diagnoses may be relevant in a resuscitation situation:

- Ineffective airway clearance
- Inability to sustain spontaneous ventilation
- Impaired gas exchange
- Decreased cardiac output
- Impaired cardiopulmonary tissue perfusion
- Impaired cerebral tissue perfusion
- Impaired renal tissue perfusion
- Decisional conflict

The nursing care plan shows how the steps in the nursing process are used for a patient with a nursing diagnosis of Inability to sustain spontaneous ventilation, defined in the NANDA taxonomy (1999) as "a state in which the response pattern of decreased energy reserves results in an individual's inability to maintain breathing adequate to support life."

Nursing Care Plan

Inability to Sustain Spontaneous Ventilation

Assessment

Subjective Data

States, "It has been more and more difficult for me to breathe. My doctor told me that's the usual outcome from this disease."

Objective Data

34-year-old man with a history of amyotrophic lateral sclerosis (Lou Gehrig's disease) diagnosed 18 months ago. Admitted after being resuscitated by paramedics who responded to the family's 911 call for assistance. Currently has shallow respirations of 32 per min. SpO_2 is 80% with oxygen at 6 L per Venturi mask. Demonstrates difficulty talking and swallowing.

continued

Nursing Care Plan

Inability to Sustain Spontaneous Ventilation Continued

Diagnosis

Inability to sustain spontaneous ventilation related to progressive respiratory muscle weakness

Plan

Goal

The patient will receive assisted ventilation when SpO_2 falls below 60% or the PaO_2 is less than 50 mm Hg.

Orders: 9/18

1. Monitor SpO_2 with pulse oximeter at all times.
2. Place in Fowler's position.
3. Administer oxygen at 45% using Venturi mask.
4. Replace Venturi mask with a nonrebreather mask if SpO_2 falls below 60%.
5. Obtain arterial blood gas when SpO_2 is sustained at 60% for more than 10 minutes.
6. Perform CPR if respiratory and/or cardiac arrest occurs.
7. Withhold advanced cardiac life support per advance directive.

____________________ J. MANGOLD, RN

Implementation (Documentation)

9/18 1345 In Fowler's position. Monitored with pulse oximeter. Oxygen administered at 45% via Venturi mask. __________ S. OWENS, LPN

Evaluation (Documentation)

9/18 1500 SpO_2 ranges from 80% to 84%. Heart rate is 120 bpm. Alert and oriented. __________ S. OWENS, LPN

FOCUS ON OLDER ADULTS

- The resuscitation status of each patient must be documented somewhere within the record. If no information is documented, CPR is administered in any life-threatening situation, regardless of the patient's age. Some older adults fear that if they specify that they do not wish to be resuscitated, they will receive less-than-appropriate care and treatment of their illness.
- If possible, an older adult's advance directive should specify exactly the type of resuscitation that is allowed. For example, some may approve of emergency drugs but refuse to allow mechanical ventilation.
- Older adults may need very simple descriptions of various treatments and measures for resuscitation addressed in advance directives. Involving family caregivers, particularly those who are designated as having power of attorney, is important during any discussions of advance directives.
- When possible, it is important to allow older adults several days to think about advance directives before signing legal documents. They may benefit from consulting trusted members of their religious affiliation or trusted medical authorities. Also, discussing the implications of advance directives as they apply to various settings is important. For example, if a person at home has advance directives prohibiting resuscitation, family members and caregivers need to understand that it may not be appropriate to call 911 in some circumstances.
- Advance directives are to be reviewed periodically (at least annually and whenever there is a major change in the older adult's health status) and updated according to the current situation and living arrangement. For example, if an older adult is in a long-term care institutional setting, the staff needs specific directives about when to send him or her to an emergency room. Similarly, in home care situations, caregivers need very specific guidelines about what course of action to take under various circumstances.
- Older adults need to be informed that they may change their mind about their advance directives and instructions for resuscitation at any time. All changes must be communicated to the physician.
- When performing CPR, older adults are at a greater risk for fractured ribs because of the increased likelihood of osteoporosis.
- Some older adult patients with a history of chronic, life-threatening dysrhythmias that are unresponsive to drug therapy require an automatic cardiac defibrillator surgically inserted within their chest. The device senses the dysrhythmia and almost instantaneously delivers an electrical current to restore normal heart rhythm.
- Older adults who take daily doses of aspirin or other anticoagulant drugs are more apt to bleed internally when chest compressions are delivered.

KEY CONCEPTS

- An airway obstruction is potentially life-threatening because it interferes with ventilation and subsequently deprives cells and tissues of oxygen.
- An airway obstruction may be suspected when a person grasps the throat with the hands, makes an aggressive effort to cough and breathe, and produces a high-pitched sound while inhaling.
- When a partial airway obstruction occurs, encourage and support the victim's efforts to clear the obstruction independently, and prepare to call for emergency assistance if the victim's condition worsens.
- The Heimlich maneuver is the technique used to relieve a complete airway obstruction by performing a series of subdiaphragmatic thrusts or chest thrusts.
- Subdiaphragmatic thrusts are appropriate for almost all adults and children beyond infancy. Chest thrusts are used for obese adults and women with an advanced pregnancy.
- To dislodge an object from an infant's airway, a series of back blows is delivered, followed by a series of chest thrusts.
- CPR refers to the techniques used to restore breathing and circulation.
- The ABCs of resuscitation involve opening the airway and assessing and initiating breathing and circulation.
- The airway can be safely opened under most circumstances by using the head tilt/chin lift technique or the jaw-thrust maneuver.
- Rescue breathing is administered mouth-to-mouth, mouth-to-nose, or mouth-to-stoma.
- Chest compressions are used to circulate blood systemically.
- Once CPR is begun, it is never interrupted for more than 7 seconds (except in certain circumstances, such as when advanced electronic equipment is used).
- The decision to stop resuscitation efforts often is based on the time that elapsed before resuscitation began, the length of time that resuscitation has continued without any change in the victim's condition, and the age and diagnosis of the victim.

CRITICAL THINKING EXERCISES

- Arrange the following resuscitation steps in the sequence in which they are performed: administer 15 compressions; open the airway; activate the emergency medical system; check the carotid pulse; shake and shout; give two rescue breaths; tilt the head and lift the chin; look, listen, and feel for air.
- Discuss the possible consequences, positive and negative, of resuscitating a patient who has a written advance directive to the contrary.

SUGGESTED READINGS

Brennan RT, Braslow A. Skill mastery in public CPR classes. American Journal of Emergency Medicine 1998;16(7):653–657.

Buchanan SF. CPR directives: Part I, issues of concern. Clinical Geriatrics 1998;6(8):61–62.

Cardiopulmonary resuscitation. Nursing Standard 1999;13(30):insert, 2p.

CPR: Don't let gift of life be stolen by threat of infection. Hospital Infection Control 1999;26(4):Health Infec. Prev.: 1–4.

Devlin M. An evaluative study of the basic life support skills of nurses in an independent hospital. Journal of Clinical Nursing 1999;8(2):201–205.

Emergency Cardiac Care Committee and Subcommittees, American Heart Association. Guidelines for cardiopulmonary resuscitation and emergency cardiac care: Part II. Adult basic life support. Journal of the American Medical Association 1992;28(268):2184–2198.

Emergency Cardiac Care Committee and Subcommittees, American Heart Association. Guidelines for cardiopulmonary resuscitation and emergency cardiac care: Part V. Pediatric basic life support. Journal of the American Medical Association 1992;28(268):2251–2261.

Hadfield-Law L. Do relatives have a place in the resuscitation room? Care of the Critically Ill 1999;15(1):19–22.

Jevon P. Choose life . . . the key resuscitation skills. Nursing Times 1998; 94(48):24–26.

Mattern MF. Who prepares the nurse for preventing codes? Clinical Nurse Specialist 1999;13(3):145–146.

NANDA nursing diagnoses: Definitions and classification, 1999–2000. Philadelphia, NANDA, 1999.

Reece C, Fillion D. Pregnant code blue. American Journal of Maternal/Child Nursing 1999;24(1):53.

Rich K. Inhospital cardiac arrest: Pre-event variables and nursing response. Clinical Nurse Specialist 1999;13(3):147–156.

Safor P, Bircher N, Pretto E Jr, et al. Reappraisal of mouth-to-mouth ventilation. Annals of Emergency Medicine 1998;31(5):653–654.

Schueler A, Moser DK. The code nurse coordinator. American Journal of Nursing 1999;99(5, Suppl):48–52.

SKILL 37-1

RELIEVING AN AIRWAY OBSTRUCTION

Suggested Action	Reason for Action
Assessment	
Ask the victim who is still conscious if he or she is choking.	Identifies the nature of the problem
Look for the universal sign for choking.	Provides information nonverbally
Determine if the victim can speak.	Indicates whether the obstruction is partial or complete
Planning	
Call for immediate respiratory assistance, or if the crisis happens in the community, dial 911 or another emergency number.	Communicates that there is an emergency situation
Prepare to respond if the obstruction becomes complete or the situation becomes worse.	Demonstrates anticipation of performing life-saving measures
Implementation	
Stand behind the victim and lean the head lower than the chest.	Increases intrathoracic pressure and uses gravity to best advantage
If the victim is in a chair, grasp the person about the abdomen from behind.	Facilitates resuscitation
Place the fist of one hand with the thumb facing inward in the middle of the victim's abdomen, above the navel, and grasp it with the other hand.	Reduces the potential for injury to internal organs

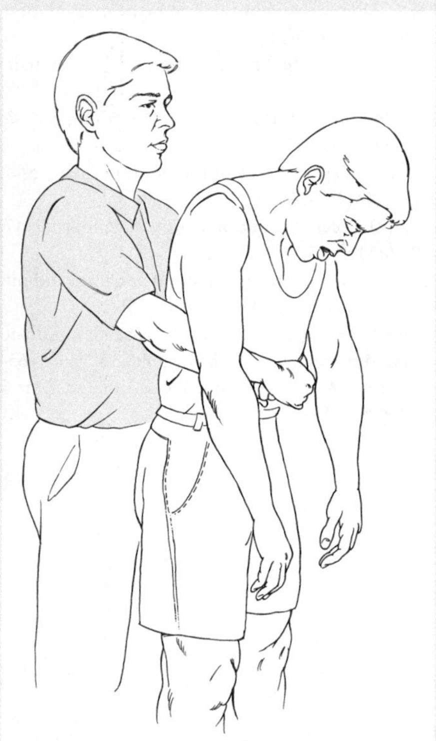

Giving subdiaphragmatic thrusts.

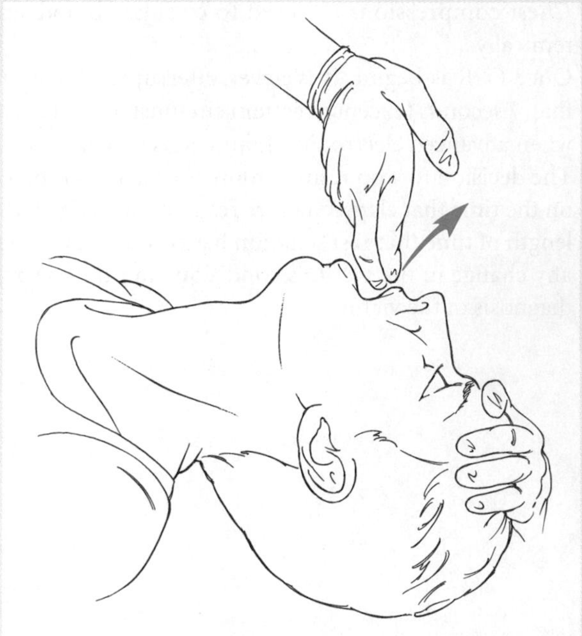

Performing a finger sweep.

continued

SKILL 37–1

RELIEVING AN AIRWAY OBSTRUCTION *Continued*

Suggested Action	Reason for Action
Lay an unconscious victim supine on the floor and perform a **finger sweep** (inserting the index finger along the inside of the cheek and deeply into the throat to the base of the tongue). Use a hooking motion to remove the substance.	Aids in removing the obstruction and facilitates resuscitation. Is performed only if the victim is unconscious.

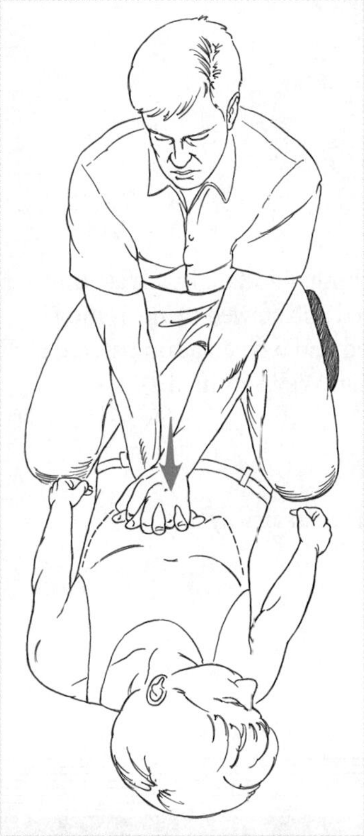

Assisting an unconscious victim.

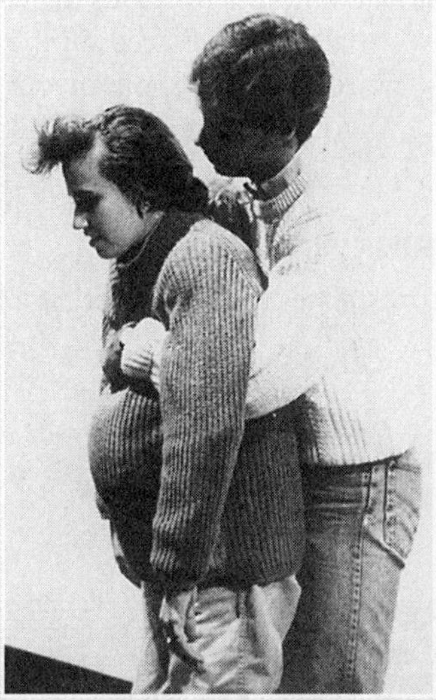

Chest thrusts.

Suggested Action	Reason for Action
For an unconscious victim, place the hands in midline above the navel with the heel of one hand above the other and the fingers interlocked.	Provides an alternative for hand positioning when the victim cannot be grasped
Deliver up to five forceful thrusts to the abdomen, one after the other.	Simulates the force of coughing
For a pregnant or obese victim, administer chest thrusts after positioning the fists in the middle of the victim's breastbone.	Provides an alternative when it is impossible to encircle the victim's abdomen
Reassess a conscious victim after each of the five thrusts, and repeat until the obstruction is relieved or the victim loses consciousness.	Provides continued safe and effective resuscitation efforts
Proceed to perform a finger sweep when the victim loses consciousness.	Aids in clearing the airway
Continue performing a series of five abdominal thrusts followed by finger sweeps until exhausted or until emergency assistance arrives.	Provides continuous resuscitation efforts

continued

SKILL 37-1

RELIEVING AN AIRWAY OBSTRUCTION *Continued*

Evaluation

- Victim clears the airway independently.
- Thrusts or finger sweeps dislodge obstructing substance.
- Resuscitation efforts are sustained until personnel with advanced life support skills can assist.

Document

- Time of discovery
- Assessment data
- Resuscitation efforts performed
- Time when request for assistance was made
- Outcome of resuscitation

SAMPLE DOCUMENTATION

Date and Time Found unconscious in chair @ 0745. No evidence of breathing. Food on breakfast tray partially eaten. Placed supine on floor. Finger sweep performed and stewed prune removed from throat. Spontaneous breathing resumed. Lifted to bed and oxygen administered at 8 L with a simple mask. Conscious and oriented at this time. Dr. Wells notified.

____ SIGNATURE, TITLE

CRITICAL THINKING

- Discuss circumstances in which there is a high risk for developing a mechanical airway obstruction.

SKILL 37-2

PERFORMING BASIC CARDIOPULMONARY RESUSCITATION

Suggested Action	Reason for Action
Assessment	
Shake patient and shout name.	Determines responsiveness
Planning	
Plan to administer CPR after calling for assistance.	Promotes successful outcome
Implementation	
Open the airway.	Facilitates spontaneous breathing
Look, listen, and feel for air.	Indicates the need to provide rescue breathing if no air is detected
Seal the nose and give two quick breaths lasting 1½ to 2 seconds through the patient's mouth, if there is no spontaneous breathing.	Initiates ventilations

continued

SKILL 37–2

PERFORMING BASIC CARDIOPULMONARY RESUSCITATION *Continued*

Suggested Action	Reason for Action
Use a face shield, if there is one available, or a one-way valve mask.	Reduces the potential for acquiring an infectious disease

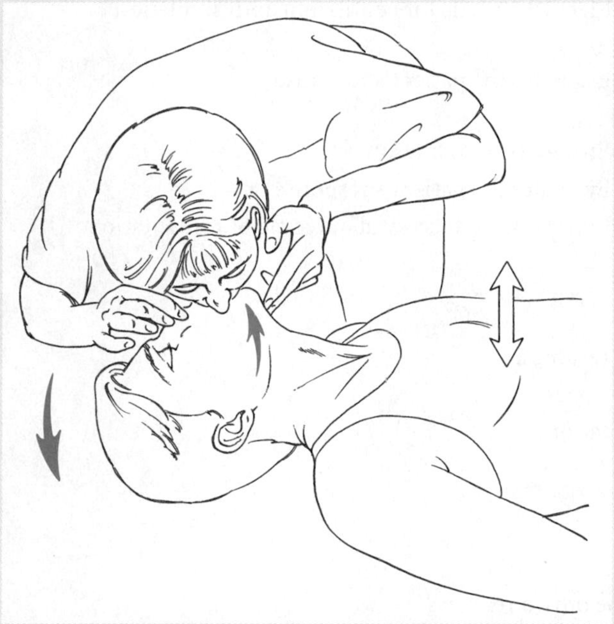

Mouth-to-mouth rescue breathing.

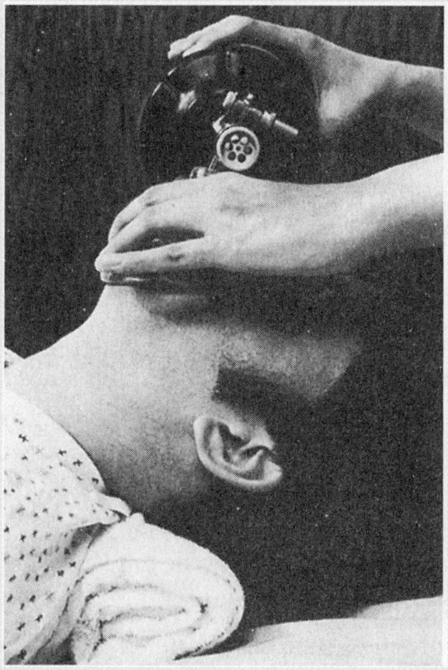

Using a one-way valve mask.

Suggested Action	Reason for Action
Reposition the head and reattempt ventilation if breathing is met with resistance or the chest does not rise.	Indicates narrowed or obstructed airway
Perform a finger sweep if the ventilation continues to be unsuccessful. Attempt the Heimlich maneuver.	Promotes relief of mechanical airway obstruction
Place in the recovery position if breathing resumes.	Prevents respiratory complications
Check for a pulse.	Determines the need for chest compressions
Place a backboard beneath the pulseless patient.	Promotes the efficiency of chest compressions
Position hands and body over the patient's chest.	Facilitates administering chest compressions

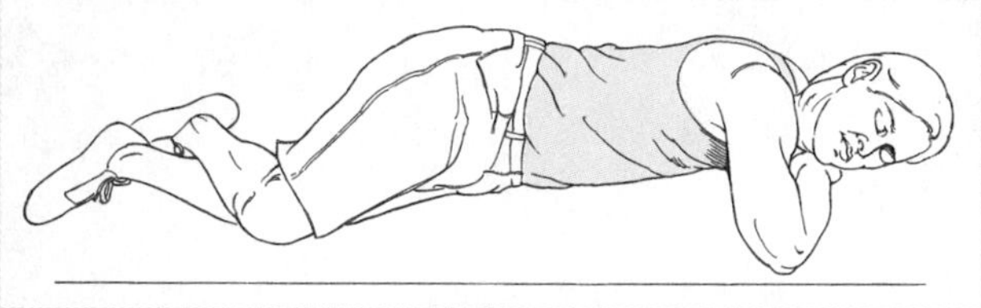

Recovery position.

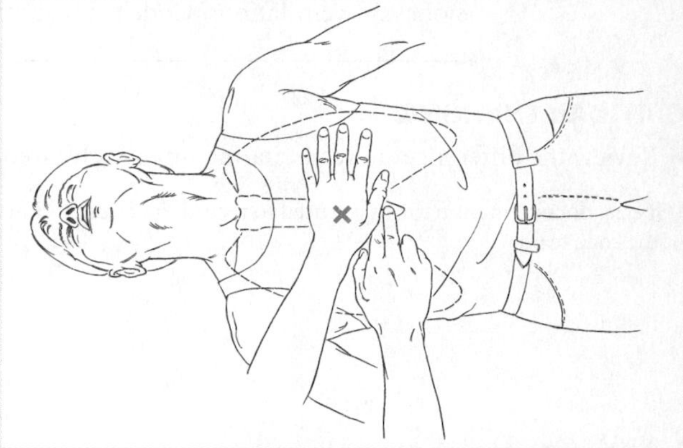

Location for chest compressions.

continued

SKILL 37-2

PERFORMING BASIC CARDIOPULMONARY RESUSCITATION *Continued*

Suggested Action	Reason for Action
Administer 15 compressions.	Circulates blood through the heart to the systemic circulation
Give two rescue breaths after each set of 15 chest compressions.	Meets the needs for ventilation and circulation
Reassess the patient after four cycles of chest compressions and ventilations.	Evaluates the patient's response
Continue CPR in the absence of breathing and pulse.	Promotes resuscitation
Reassess every few minutes.	Evaluates the patient's response
Assist code team with defibrillation, intubation, and administration of emergency drugs.	Enhances the successful outcome of resuscitation

Evaluation

- Spontaneous breathing occurs; circulation is maintained or resumes.
- Ventilation is assisted and defibrillation restores heart beat.
- Patient exhibits no response or improvement during resuscitation.

Document

- Time patient is discovered to be unresponsive
- Time the code is called
- Length of time CPR is administered, and if performed by one or two rescuers
- Time the code team arrives
- Methods used to restore ventilation and heart rate, including names of drugs, dose, route, and time given
- Names and results of laboratory tests to determine physiologic progress
- Response of the patient
- Time resuscitation is terminated

SAMPLE DOCUMENTATION*

Date and Time Unresponsive to shaking and shouting. Code called @ 1830. No breathing with opening of airway. Two rescue breaths given. No carotid pulse palpated. Backboard placed beneath patient. Cardiac compressions administered. No response after four cycles of compressions and ventilations. Code team arrived @ 1840. See resuscitation documentation form.

______________________________ SIGNATURE, TITLE

CRITICAL THINKING

- Review the differences in resuscitating infants, children, and adults.

* Special documentation forms are used to record the resuscitation activities of the code team.

UNIT TWELVE

CARING FOR THE TERMINALLY ILL

CHAPTER 38:
Death and Dying

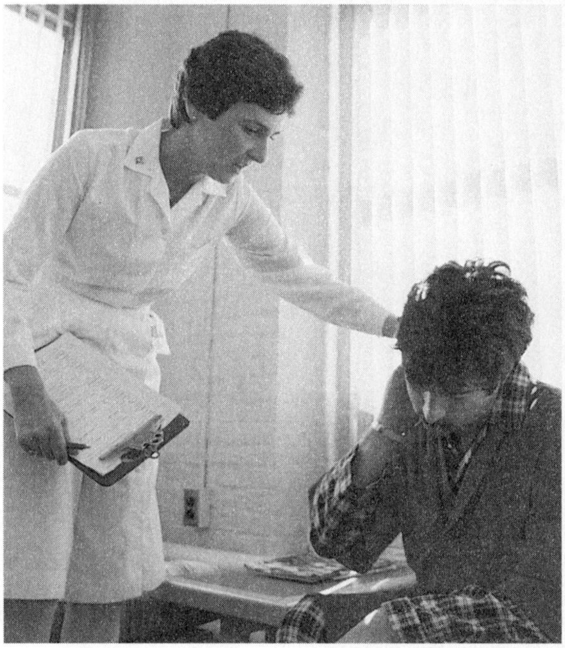

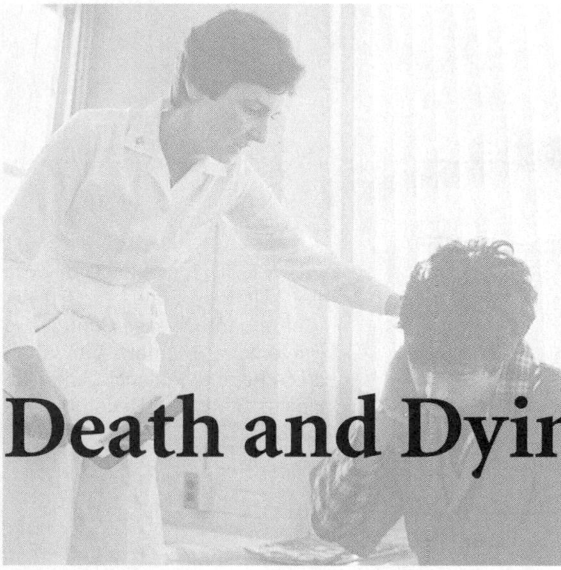

Death and Dying

CHAPTER 38

CHAPTER OUTLINE

Terminal Illness and Care
Grieving
Nursing Implications

NURSING GUIDELINES

HELPING DYING PATIENTS COPE
SUMMONING THE FAMILY OF A DYING PATIENT

SKILLS

SKILL 38-1: PERFORMING POSTMORTEM CARE

NURSING CARE PLAN

HOPELESSNESS

KEY TERMS

acceptance
anger
anticipatory grieving
autopsy
bargaining
coroner
death certificate
denial
depression
dying with dignity
grief response
grief work
grieving
hospice
morgue
mortician
multiple organ failure
paranormal experiences
pathologic grief
persistent vegetative state
postmortem care
respite care
shroud
terminal illness

LEARNING OBJECTIVES

An understanding of the content within this chapter will be evidenced by the student's ability to:

- Define terminal illness.
- Name five stages of dying.
- Describe two methods for promoting acceptance.
- Define respite care.
- Discuss the philosophy of hospice care.
- List at least five aspects of care addressed when providing terminal care.
- Name at least five signs of multiple organ failure.
- Explain why a discussion of organ donation must take place as expeditiously as possible.
- Name three components of postmortem care.
- Discuss the benefit of grieving.
- Describe one sign that a person's grief is becoming resolved.

Life expectancy continues to lengthen year by year (Fig. 38-1), but death is still a certainty. The only unknowns are when, where, and how it will occur. Nurses and other health personnel are probably involved more than any other group with people who experience impending death. This chapter deals with the grieving experience and aspects of caring for terminally ill patients.

Terminal Illness and Care

A **terminal illness** (condition from which recovery is beyond reasonable expectation) is devastating news. On learning that death is soon to come, patients tend to go through several stages as they process the information.

STAGES OF DYING

Dr. Elisabeth Kübler-Ross, an authority on dying, has described stages through which many terminally ill patients progress: denial, anger, bargaining, depression, and acceptance (Table 38-1).

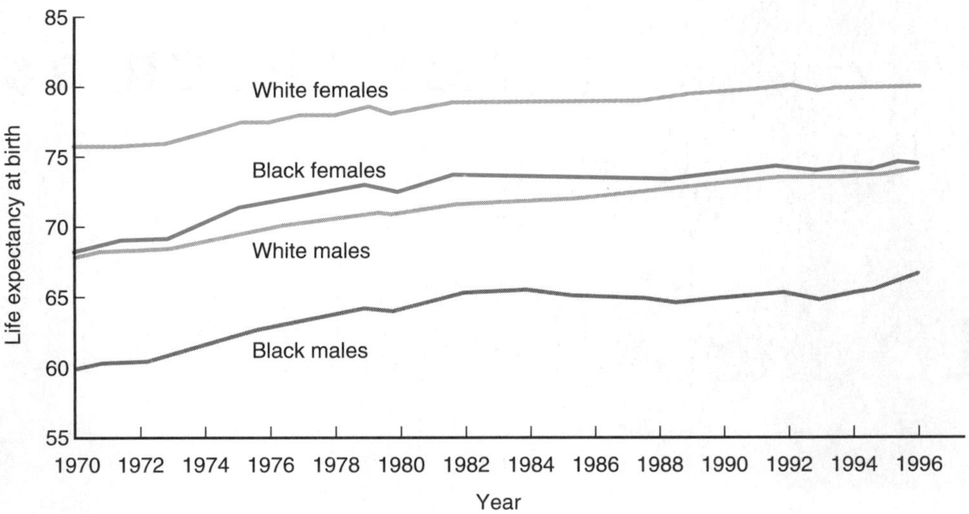

FIGURE 38–1. Life expectancy in the United States, 1970–96. (Centers for Disease Control and Prevention, Monthly Vital Statistics Report. National Center for Health Statistics, December 24, 1998;47:13)

Denial

Denial (psychological defense mechanism in which a person refuses to believe that certain information is true) helps people cope initially. Terminally ill patients may first refuse to believe that their diagnosis is accurate. They may speculate that the test results are wrong or that their reports have been mixed up with those of another.

Anger

Anger (emotional response to feeling victimized) occurs because there is no way to retaliate against fate. Patients often displace their anger onto nurses, the physician, the family, and even God. Anger may be expressed in less-than-obvious ways—for example, by complaining about care or overreacting to even the slightest aggravation.

Bargaining

Bargaining (psychological mechanism for delaying the inevitable) involves a process of negotiation, usually with God or some other higher power. Usually, the dying patient is willing to accept death but wants to extend his or her life temporarily until some significant event takes place (for instance, a son's or daughter's wedding).

TABLE 38–1. **Stages of Dying**

Stage	Typical Emotional Response	Typical Comment
First stage	Denial	"No, not me"
Second stage	Anger	"Why me?"
Third stage	Bargaining	"Yes, me, but if only. . . ."
Fourth stage	Depression	"Yes, me."
Fifth stage	Acceptance	"I am ready."

Depression

Depression (sad mood) indicates the dying patient's realization that death will come sooner, rather than later, than anticipated. The sad mood is a result of dealing with potential losses.

Acceptance

Acceptance (attitude of complacency) occurs after the patient has dealt with his or her losses and completed unfinished business. Kübler-Ross describes unfinished business in two ways. Literally, it refers to completing legal and financial matters to provide the best security for survivors. However, it also refers to social and spiritual matters, such as making peace with God and saying goodbye to loved ones. It is as important for dying patients as it is for their families to say, "Thank you for . . ." and "I'm sorry for . . ."

When all the loose ends are tied up, dying patients feel prepared to die. Some even happily anticipate death, viewing it as a bridge to a better dimension.

PROMOTING ACCEPTANCE

Nurses can help the patient pass from one stage to another by being available for emotional support and by supporting the patient's choices concerning terminal care.

Emotional Support

Patients who are dying require emotional support perhaps more than at any other time. Sometimes the dying patient simply wants an opportunity to vent feelings and verbally work through emotions. Nurses can act as a nonjudgmental sounding board.

Nursing Guidelines For

Helping Dying Patients Cope

- ☑ Accept the patient's behavior, no matter what it is.
  RATIONALE: Demonstrates respect for individuality
- ☑ Provide opportunities for the patient to express feelings freely.
  RATIONALE: Demonstrates attention to meeting individual needs
- ☑ Try to understand the patient's feelings.
  RATIONALE: Reinforces that each person is unique
- ☑ Use statements with broad openings such as, "It must be difficult for you" and "Do you want to talk about it?"
  RATIONALE: Encourages communication and allows the patient to choose the topic or manner of response

Besides being available for conversation, nurses provide emotional support to dying patients by acknowledging them as unique and worthwhile people. **Dying with dignity** (process in which dying patients are cared for with an attitude of respect, no matter what their emotional, physical, or cognitive state) addresses concepts stated in the Dying Patient's Bill of Rights (Display 38-1).

DISPLAY 38–1

The Dying Person's Bill of Rights

I have the right to be treated as a living human being until I die.
I have the right to maintain a sense of hopefulness, however changing its focus may be.
I have the right to be cared for by those who can maintain a sense of hopefulness, however changing this might be.
I have the right to express my feelings and emotions about my approaching death in my own way.
I have the right to participate in decisions concerning my care.
I have the right to expect continuing medical and nursing attention even though "cure" goals must be changed to "comfort" goals.
I have the right not to die alone.
I have the right to be free from pain.
I have the right to have my questions answered honestly.
I have the right not to be deceived.
I have the right to have help from and for my family in accepting my death.
I have the right to die in peace and dignity.
I have the right to retain my individuality and not be judged for my decisions which may be contrary to beliefs of others.
I have the right to discuss and enlarge my religious and/or spiritual experiences, whatever these may mean to others.
I have the right to expect that the sanctity of the human body will be respected after death.
I have the right to be cared for by caring, sensitive, knowledgeable people who will attempt to understand my needs and will be able to gain some satisfaction in helping me face my death.

From Barbus AJ. The Dying Person's Bill of Rights, © 1975, American Journal of Nursing Company. Reprinted with permission from the American Journal of Nursing January 1975; 75:99.

Arrangements for Care

Respect for the rights of dying patients includes helping them choose how and where they want to be cared for. Patients may find it comforting to prepare an advance directive (see Chap. 3). Many also appreciate learning about the options available for where they may receive care. In general, patients have four choices: home care, hospice care (which may be the same as home care), residential care, and acute care.

Home Care

Many patients with a terminal illness remain at home (Fig. 38-2). They may travel to and from a hospital or clinic for brief periods of treatment, tests, and medical evaluations. Nurses may help coordinate community services, secure home equipment, and arrange for home nursing visits.

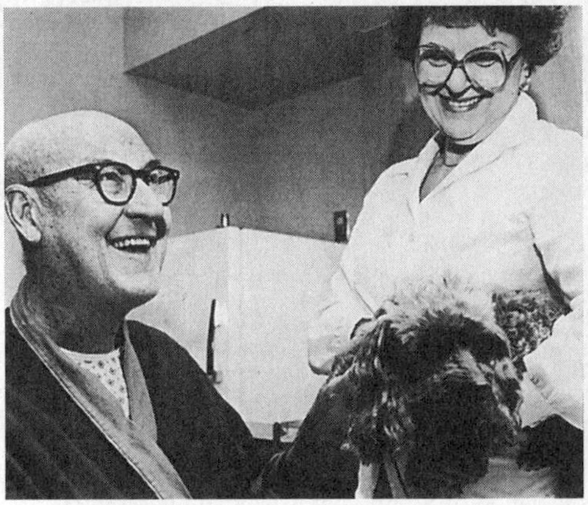

FIGURE 38–2. Home care.

Because the major burden of home care often falls on a spouse, family member, or significant other, nurses who care for home-bound patients periodically assess the toll this burden takes. The focus of support may shift back and forth from the patient to the caregiver. **Respite care** (relief for the caregiver by a surrogate) is important because it gives the caregiver an opportunity to enjoy brief periods away from home.

Hospice Care

A **hospice** (facility for or concept addressing the care of terminally ill patients) originally was a place of refuge for travelers. The hospice movement in the United States is modeled after facilities established by Dr. Cicely Saunders in England in the late 1960s. Whether the hospice is a building or a service that is provided in homes, hospice care involves helping patients live their final days in comfort and with dignity and meaning in a caring environment (Fig. 38-3).

In general, only patients who have 6 months or less to live are accepted for hospice care in the United States. Most are cared for in their own homes. The family's care is supported by a multidisciplinary team of hospice professionals and volunteers.

Hospice organizations also provide support programs for family members and significant others. Individual and group counseling is offered both during and after the patient's death to help survivors cope with their grief.

Residential Care

Residential care, a form of intermediate care, is provided in nursing homes or long-term care facilities, where the level of care is usually subacute. These facilities provide around-the-clock nursing care for patients who cannot live independently (Fig. 38-4). Family members have the peace of mind of knowing that their loved one is being cared for, and they enjoy the opportunity to visit as much as possible.

Residential care is costly. Once patients have exhausted their savings, their expenses may be paid by programs such as Medicaid.

Acute Care

Acute care, with its sophisticated technology and labor-intensive care, is needed if the patient's condition is unstable. It is the most expensive form of care. Bills for acute care provided in the hours, days, or weeks before a patient's death can be significant.

PROVIDING TERMINAL CARE

Throughout the terminal illness and immediately before death, the nurse meets the patient's basic physical needs for hydration, nourishment, elimination, hygiene, positioning, and comfort. Many of the skills described throughout this text are implemented to meet the multiple problems experienced by dying patients.

Hydration

Hydration involves the maintenance of an adequate fluid volume. If the swallowing reflex is present, water and other beverages are offered at frequent intervals. As swallowing becomes impaired, there is the risk for aspiration, followed by pneumonia. Sucking is one of the last reflexes to disappear as death approaches. Therefore, a moist cloth or wrapped ice cubes can be provided for the patient to suck. Eventually, intravenous fluids may be needed.

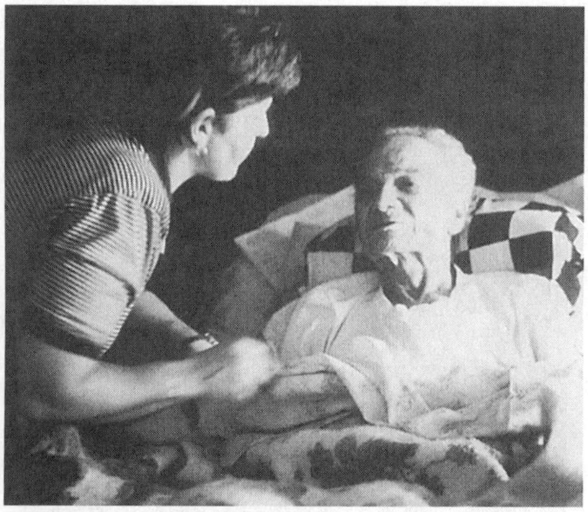

FIGURE 38-3. A hospice patient and nurse. (Courtesy of Visiting Nurse Association of Southwest Michigan.) (Timby BK, Scherer JC, Smith NE. Introductory medical-surgical nursing, 7th ed, p 282. Philadelphia, Lippincott Williams & Wilkins, 1999)

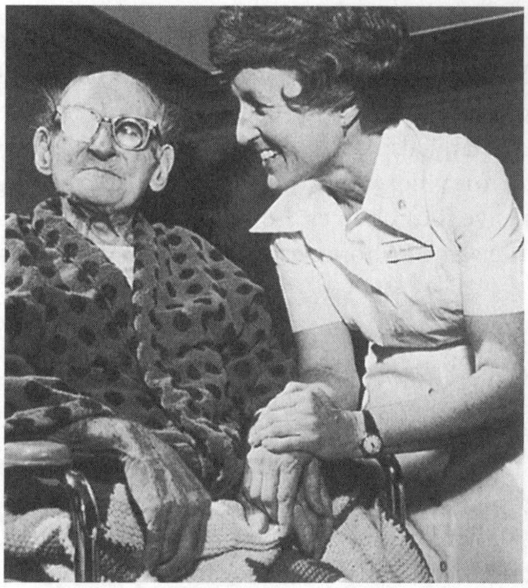

FIGURE 38-4. Residential care.

Nourishment

Some terminally ill patients have little interest in eating. The effort may be too exhausting, or nausea and vomiting may result in inadequate consumption of food. Poor nutrition leads to weakness, infection, and other complications, such as pressure sores. Consequently, tube feedings or total parenteral nutrition may be needed to maintain nutritional and fluid intake.

Elimination

Some terminally ill patients are incontinent of urine and stool; others may experience urinary retention and constipation. These are all uncomfortable. Cleansing enemas or suppositories may be ordered. Catheterization may also become necessary. Skin care becomes particularly important in an incontinent patient because urine and stool, if left in contact with the skin, contribute to skin breakdown and produce foul odors.

Hygiene

The dignity of patients is largely the result of their personal appearance. Therefore, dying patients are kept clean, well groomed, and free of unpleasant odors.

Mouth care may be necessary at more frequent intervals. Mucus that cannot be swallowed or expectorated is removed. The mouth is wiped with gauze or suctioned. Using a lateral position helps keep the mouth and throat free of accumulating secretions. The lips may need periodic lubrication because they may become dried from mouth breathing or the administration of oxygen.

Positioning

Even though the lateral position helps prevent choking and aspiration, the patient's position is changed at least every 2 hours, as for any other patient, to promote comfort and circulation.

Comfort

Relieving pain may be the most challenging problem in caring for dying patients. The goal is to keep the patient free from pain but not to dull consciousness or inhibit the ability to communicate.

Most patients are given nonnarcotics initially; later, the drug order may be changed to a narcotic. The route may also change from oral to parenteral, with the drug given on a routine schedule. Giving pain medication regularly, such as every 4 hours, rather than on an as-needed basis, maintains a consistent level of pain relief. The dosage will probably need to be increased because of drug tolerance (see Chap. 19). The possibility of addiction, however, does not stand in the way of pain control. Although tolerance develops to the pain-relieving property of the drug, tolerance to the drug's other actions does not appear as quickly. Therefore, respirations may become depressed and constipation may be more common with regular use of narcotic drugs.

Family Involvement

Family members may appreciate helping with the patient's care because they often feel helpless and welcome an opportunity to assist. However, they should not be burdened with major responsibilities. Involvement tends to maintain a family bond and helps survivors cope with their grief in the future (Fig. 38-5).

APPROACHING DEATH

As death nears, the patient exhibits signs indicating a decrease and then ultimately a cessation of function. As these signs appear, the family is informed that death is near.

Multiple Organ Failure

The signs of approaching death are the result of **multiple organ failure** (condition in which two or more organ systems gradually cease to function), which is directly related to the quality of cellular oxygenation. When the supply of oxygen falls below what cells need, cells, followed by tissues and organs, begin to die. The cardiovascular, pulmonary, hepatic, and renal systems are most vulnerable to failure.

As the cells die, their intracellular chemicals are released. The preexisting hypoxia is then complicated by a localized

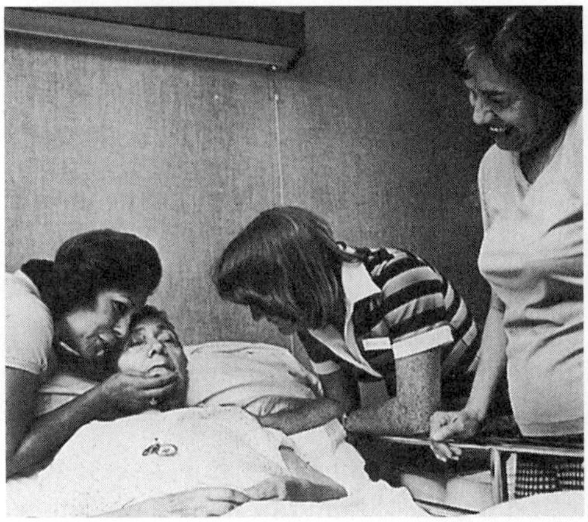

FIGURE 38–5. Family involvement.

TABLE 38–2. **Signs of Multiple Organ Failure**

Organ	Signs
Heart	• Hypotension • Irregular, weak, rapid pulse • Cold, clammy, mottled skin
Liver	• Internal bleeding • Edema • Jaundice • Impaired digestion, distention, anorexia, nausea, vomiting
Lungs	• Dyspnea • Accumulation of fluid ("death rattle")
Kidneys	• Oliguria • Anuria • Pruritus (itching skin)
Brain	• Fever • Confusion and disorientation • Hypoesthesia (reduced sensation) • Hyporeflexia (reduced reflexes) • Stupor • Coma

and then generalized inflammatory response (see Chap. 28) that causes the signs of multiple organ failure, heralding approaching death (Table 38-2). This process may take place gradually over a period of hours or days.

Family Notification

As the signs of approaching death appear, it is important to make the family aware that the end is near. The physician is informed first, however. If the death has already occurred, the physician is responsible for contacting the family and releasing that information. Sometimes the news is delayed until the family can be approached in person to avoid precipitating acts such as suicide or contributing to a traffic accident.

Nursing Guidelines For

Summoning the Family of a Dying Patient

☑ Plan to notify the family in a timely manner.
RATIONALE: Allows the family to be with the dying patient at the time of death

☑ Check the patient's medical record for the next of kin or a responsible party.
RATIONALE: Ensures notifying a person significantly involved in the patient's well-being

☑ Identify yourself by name, title, and location.
RATIONALE: Provides more personal communication

☑ Ask for the family member by name.
RATIONALE: Ensures communication of the information to the appropriate person

☑ Speak in a calm and controlled voice.
RATIONALE: Communicates a serious and competent demeanor

☑ Use short sentences to provide small bits of information.
RATIONALE: Helps the listener process and comprehend the news

☑ Explain that the patient's condition is deteriorating.
RATIONALE: Clarifies the purpose for the call

☑ Pause after giving the most important information.
RATIONALE: Allows the family member to respond

☑ Give brief answers to questions. Emphasize the level of care that is being given.
RATIONALE: Reinforces that the patient is receiving appropriate care

☑ Urge the family members to come as soon as possible.
RATIONALE: Ensures that the people most important to the patient are there at the time of death

☑ Document the time, the person to whom the information was communicated, and the message.
RATIONALE: Provides a permanent record of the communication

Meeting Relatives

To promote a smooth transition, relatives of the dying patient are met by the nurse who informed them. If that is not possible, another support person is designated.

On arrival, the family members are shown to a private room or area or are taken directly to the patient's bedside, depending on their wishes. Privacy allows people the freedom to express their feelings without social inhibitions. People have different ways of expressing grief: some may weep and sob uncontrollably, but those who do not may have sorrow that is just as genuine.

Discussing Organ Donation

Virtually anyone, from the very young to the elderly, may be an organ donor. If the donor is younger than 18 years, he or she must sign a donor card, along with the parents or legal guardian. Age requirements are determined on an individual basis (Table 38-3).

Some patients have the foresight to communicate whether they are interested in organ donation; others have not. In either case, if the dying or dead patient meets the donation criteria, the possibility of harvesting organs after death is discussed with the next of kin. This is done delicately because family members are under extreme duress when dealing with the death of a loved one. Typically, the facility's transplant coordinator is involved.

This matter cannot be delayed; some organs, such as the heart and lungs, must be harvested within a few hours to

TABLE 38–3. **Age Criteria for Organ Donation**

Organ	Age Range
Kidney	6 months–55 years
Liver	<50 years
Heart	<40 years
Pancreas	2–50 years
Corneas	Any age
Skin	15–74 years

Guidelines established by the Organ Procurement Agency of Michigan, Ann Arbor, MI.

ensure a successful transplant. To protect the health care facility from any legal consequences, permission is always obtained in writing (Fig. 38-6).

CONFIRMING DEATH

Death is determined on the basis that breathing and circulation have ceased. In most cases, when these criteria are met, there is no question that the patient is dead. Legally, a physician is responsible for pronouncing the patient dead, but in a few states nurses are authorized to do so.

Brain Death

Sometimes there are situations involving irreversible brain damage in which breathing can be sustained with a mechanical ventilator and circulation continues reflexively. The person is "brain dead," and continued life support may only sustain a **persistent vegetative state** (condition in which there is no cognitive function or capacity to experience emotions).

Consequently, brain function is now considered the most incontestable criterion for establishing whether a person is dead or alive. To ensure that brain activity is consistently and accurately assessed, the following standards are used as guidelines. Irreversible brain death is considered to be present if, in the absence of hypothermia or central nervous system depressants, there is:

- Unreceptiveness and unresponsiveness to even intense painful stimuli
- No movement or spontaneous respiration after 3 minutes of disconnection from a mechanical ventilator
- Complete absence of central and deep tendon reflexes
- Flat electroencephalogram for at least 10 minutes
- No change in response on a second assessment 24 hours later

Once death has been confirmed, the physician issues a death certificate and obtains written permission for an autopsy, if one is desirable.

Death Certificate

A **death certificate** (legal document attesting to the fact that the person named on the form has been found to be dead) also indicates the presumptive cause of the person's death. Death certificates are sent to local health departments, which use the information to compile mortality statistics. The statistics are important in identifying trends, needs, and problems in the fields of health and medicine.

The **mortician** (person who prepares the body for burial or cremation) is responsible for filing the death certificate with the proper authorities. The death certificate also carries the mortician's signature and, in some states, his or her license number.

Permission for Autopsy

An **autopsy** (examination of the organs and tissues of a human body after death) is not necessary after all deaths, but it is useful for determining more conclusively the cause of death. The findings may affect the medical care of blood relatives who may be at risk for a similar disorder, or the results may contribute to medical science. It is usually the physician's responsibility to obtain permission for an autopsy.

A **coroner** (person legally designated to investigate deaths that may not be the result of natural causes) has the right to order an autopsy. The coroner, who may or may not be a physician, does not need permission from the next of kin to do so. In general, a coroner orders an autopsy if the death involved a crime, was of a suspicious nature, or occurred without any prior medical consultation.

PERFORMING POSTMORTEM CARE

Postmortem care (care of the body after death) involves cleaning and preparing the body to enhance its appearance during viewing at the funeral home, ensuring proper identification, and releasing the body to mortuary personnel (Skill 38-1).

Grieving

Grieving (process of feeling acute sorrow over a loss) is a painful experience, but it helps the survivor resolve the loss. Some experience **anticipatory grieving** (grieving that begins before the loss occurs). The longer people have to anticipate a loss, the more quickly they eventually resolve it. **Grief work** (activities involved in grieving) includes participating in the burial rituals common in the culture. Although the rituals may differ, the **grief response** (psychological and physical phenomena experienced by those who are grieving) is universal.

Organ Procurement Agency of Michigan

Subsidiary Of
TRANSPLANTATION SOCIETY OF MICHIGAN
2203 Platt Road, Ann Arbor, Michigan 48104
(313) 973-1577

1-800-482-4881 Detroit—464-7988

ANATOMICAL GIFT DONATION STATEMENT

I understand that in the present state of medical practice, several organs and tissues are being removed from persons who have died unexpectedly, and are being used for transplantation to living persons or for medical or scientific research. I understand that organs are removed after my relative has died, and before the organs suffer any damage, (usually within eight [8] hours) and that this gift authorizes all examinations of the body which are necessary to assure the medical acceptability of the gift.

I appreciate the benefits that come from organ donation and also understand the criteria used in determining death in the case of decedent. I am the surviving:

(1) _____ Spouse
(2) _____ Adult son or daughter
(3) _____ Mother or Father
(4) _____ Adult brother or sister
(5) _____ Guardian of the patient at the time of death
(6) _____ Other person authorized or obligated to dispose of the body

____
Relationship

Relatives or persons in a class before my class are not available to sign this form (or have already signed such a form). I have no knowledge that during his or her lifetime the decedent, ____________________, was opposed to or said things against making an anatomical gift or organ donation such as the one described below. I do not know of any relative or person in a class before mine who is opposed to this gift, nor do I know of any person in the same class as myself who is opposed to this gift.

I hereby make the following anatomical gift from the body of ____________________:

( ) Any needed organs or parts, or
( ) Only the following organs or parts:

____
(Please specify the organ(s) or part(s)

The specified organ(s) and/or part(s) may be used for any of the purposes allowed by law, i.e. transplantation, therapy, medical research and education.

WITNESSES:

____________________ ____________________
Name

____________________ ____________________
Relation

____
Date

FIGURE 38–6. Organ procurement form.

Psychological reactions are commonly identified as the stages of grief:

- Shock and disbelief: refusal to accept that a loved one is about to die or has died
- Developing awareness: physical and emotional responses such as feeling sick, sad, empty, or angry
- Restitution period: recognition of the loss
- Idealization: exaggeration of the good qualities of the deceased

Some survivors have **paranormal experiences** (experiences outside scientific explanation), such as seeing, hearing, or feeling the continued presence of the deceased.

Physical symptoms are felt more acutely immediately after the death of a loved one. Some people who are grieving report symptoms such as anorexia, tightness in the chest and throat, difficulty breathing, lack of strength, and sleep disturbances. No identifiable pathologic state other than grief can explain these symptoms.

PATHOLOGIC GRIEF

Pathologic grief (condition in which a person cannot accept someone's death) also is called dysfunctional grief. Sometimes pathologic grief is manifested by bizarre or morbid behavior. For example, the survivor may keep the deceased's possessions exactly as they were at the time of death. Others may attempt to contact the deceased through seances. In rare instances, a survivor may keep a corpse in the home for an extended period after death.

RESOLUTION OF GRIEF

Mourning takes longer for some than for others. One sign that grief is becoming resolved is a person's ability to talk about the dead person without becoming emotionally overwhelmed. Another sign is that the grieving person describes the good and bad qualities of the deceased.

Nursing Implications

Nurses who care for dying patients, their family members, and their friends may identify many different nursing diagnoses, including:

- Pain
- Fear
- Spiritual distress
- Social isolation
- Altered role performance
- Altered family processes
- Ineffective individual coping
- Ineffective family coping
- Decisional conflict
- Hopelessness
- Powerlessness
- Dysfunctional grieving
- Anticipatory grieving
- Caregiver role strain
- Death anxiety
- Chronic sorrow

The nursing care plan applies the nursing process to the care of a patient with a diagnosis of Hopelessness, defined in NANDA's 1999 taxonomy as "a subjective state in which an individual sees limited or no alternatives or personal choices available and is unable to mobilize energy on (his) own behalf." Lynda Carpenito (1999) further explains, "Hopelessness differs from powerlessness in that a hopeless person sees no solution to his problem and/or way to achieve what is desired, even it he has control of his life. A powerless person, on the other hand, may see an alternative or answer to the problem, yet be unable to do anything about it because of lack of control and resources."

Nursing Care Plan

Hopelessness

Assessment

Subjective Data

States, "It doesn't matter what's done or not done anymore. One of these days you won't be able to stop the infections."

Objective Data

26-year-old man about to be discharged from acute care hospital after successful treatment of *Pneumocystis* pneumonia secondary to HIV infection. During interview patient made little eye contact; stared out window. Will be followed up with home health care. Significant other expressed, "I'm afraid he'll just stop eating and taking his medications."

continued

Nursing Care Plan — Hopelessness *Continued*

Diagnosis
Hopelessness related to eventual terminal outcome of illness

Plan

Goal

The patient will identify one future-related goal and participate in one goal-directed activity by time of discharge.

Orders: 1/14

1. Reinforce at appropriate times that although his illness is terminal, his current health status is stable.
2. After periodic physical examinations, verbalize normal as well as abnormal findings.
3. Present positive realistic choices.
4. Explore with patient the goals he hoped to accomplish before his illness.
5. Ask patient to identify goals he could achieve in the next year.
6. Encourage patient to develop a daily schedule and set aside time for working toward at least one goal. ______________________ E. HILLYARD, RN

Implementation (Documentation)

1/15 0800 Head-to-toe assessment performed. Lungs sound clear and heart rate is normal at 78 beats/min. Skin is intact. Discussed that there has been a ½ lb. weight loss since yesterday. Indicated that date of discharge remains unchanged. Offered one can of Ensure as dietary supplement. Encouraged to perform oral hygiene and use Mycostatin mouthwash to prevent yeast infection. ______________________ T. ROMIG, LPN

Evaluation (Documentation)

0830 Stated, "I think mouth care and anything else is futile. What a time for me to get sick. I'm a writer . . . or should I say, I was a writer. A publisher was interested in an idea I had, but it's past the deadline I was given." Encouraged to contact the publisher by phone before being discharged tomorrow. ______________________ T. ROMIG, LPN

FOCUS ON OLDER ADULTS

- Research has shown that some survivors develop life-threatening illnesses and die within 6 months of having experienced the death of a spouse. Allowing and encouraging older adults who have experienced the death of a close friend or family member to express their feelings associated with grieving is important. Referrals for individual counseling or grief support groups are appropriate.
- Older adults may read obituaries and death notices in the newspaper as a daily activity. Although families may view this activity as a morbid preoccupation, it may be an effective way of learning about what is happening to friends. It also may be an effective coping mechanism in helping older people develop a peaceful and accepting attitude toward death.
- Death is a very individualized experience, highly influenced by prior life experiences and one's level of personal development. Many older adults are realistically aware of their pending and inevitable death. Often they are relieved when health care providers are comfortable discussing this with them. Older adults may benefit from counseling with regard to their own death and dying, especially if they are cognitively aware and have a history of accepting help in coping with challenging issues.
- Hospice care should be considered for older adults who meet the medical criteria of having 6 months or less to live. Even older adults with chronic illnesses, such as dementia, and family may benefit from the hospice approach to care and available support services. Often families and older adults are relieved when the topic of hospice care is discussed so they can be involved in choices about the type of care they receive.
- Older adults, including those who are dying, must be included in as many aspects of their care as possible. The emphasis is on maintaining self-esteem and personal dignity.
- Older adults, and others as well, may feel their dignity is threatened by the use of machines and equipment designed to maintain life support.
- Many older adults are preparing advance directives concerning their health care and identifying a durable power of attorney at the same time they prepare a will. These advance directives must be reviewed and updated periodically and accessible to all those involved in the care of the person.
- Evaluation for the use of antidepressants and other therapies for older adults who are seriously depressed often is appropriate.
- Older adults have the highest rate of suicide, as well as the highest rate of completed suicides in proportion to unsuccessful attempts (Miller, 1999). Health care professionals need to assess suicide risk in older adults and implement appropriate precautions.

KEY CONCEPTS

- A terminal illness is one from which recovery is beyond reasonable expectation.
- The five stages of dying, as described by Dr. Elisabeth Kübler-Ross, are denial, anger, bargaining, depression, and acceptance.
- Acceptance can be promoted by providing emotional support to dying patients and helping them to arrange their care.
- Respite care provides relief for the caregiver.
- Hospice care involves helping patients live their final days in comfort and with dignity and meaning in a caring environment.
- Some aspects of care addressed when providing terminal care are hydration, nourishment, elimination, hygiene, positioning, and comfort.
- Many terminal illnesses result in death from multiple organ failure. Signs of multiple organ failure include hypotension, rapid heart rate, difficulty breathing, cold and mottled skin, and decreased urinary output.
- When the criteria for organ donation are met, permission for organ removal must be obtained in a timely manner to ensure a successful transplant.
- Criteria used to confirm that a patient has died include cessation of breathing and heart beat and absence of brain function.
- Postmortem care involves cleaning the body, ensuring proper identification, and releasing the body to mortuary personnel.
- Although grieving is a painful experience, it promotes resolution of the loss.
- One sign that a person's grief is becoming resolved is that the person can talk about the deceased person without becoming emotionally overwhelmed.

CRITICAL THINKING EXERCISES

- Does being maintained on life support equipment contradict the right to die in peace and dignity (see the Dying Person's Bill of Rights)?
- Select a right from the Dying Person's Bill of Rights and explain how it might be violated. How can this right be protected?

SUGGESTED READINGS

Akins SD. Vital signs. Teaching and grieving. American Journal of Nursing 1999;99(8):88.

Barbus AJ. The Dying Person's Bill of Rights. American Journal of Nursing 1975;75:99.

Baumrucker S. Science, hospice, and terminal dehydration. American Journal of Hospice and Palliative Care 1999;16(3):502–503.

Carpenito LJ. Nursing diagnosis: Application to clinical practice (8th ed). Philadelphia, Lippincott Williams & Wilkins, 1999.

Centers for Disease Control and Prevention. Monthly vital statistics report. National Center for Health Statistics, December 24, 1998;47:13.

Clayville L. When donor families and organ recipients meet. Journal of Transplant Coordination 1999;9(2):81–86.

deMontigny F, Beaudet L, Dumas L. A baby has died: The impact of perinatal loss on family social networks. Journal of Obstetric, Gynecologic, and Neonatal Nursing 1999;28(2):151–156.

Donnelly GF. Loss, death and grieving. Holistic Nursing Practice 1998; 23(1):v.

Enck RE. Pain control at the end-of-life. American Journal of Hospice and Palliative Care 1999;16(4):564–565.

Ferrell BR, Borneman T. Pain and suffering at the end of life for older patients and their families. Generations 1999;23(1):12–17.

Helping a grieving widower. Nursing 1999;29(8):64hh6.

Jarrett N, Payne S, Turner P, et al. "Someone to talk to" and "pain control": What people expect from a specialist palliative care team. Palliative Medicine 1999;13(2):139–144.

Kübler-Ross E. On death and dying. New York, Macmillan, 1969.

Mezey M, Miller LL, Linton-Nelson L. Caring for caregivers of frail elders at the end of life. Generations 1999;23(1):44–51.

Miller CA. Nursing care of older adults (3rd ed). Philadelphia, Lippincott Williams & Wilkins, 1999.

NANDA nursing diagnoses: Definitions and classification, 1999–2000. Philadelphia, NANDA, 1999.

Nemeth LL. If a facility's policy conflicts with your duty to provide care. RN 1999;62(8):68.

Pupolo AL. Gaining confidence to talk about end-of-life care. Nursing 1999; 29(7):49–51.

Quinn S. Helping the grieving process: A nurse's story. Nursing Times 1999;95(4):52–53.

Singer PA, Martin DK, Kelner M. Quality-of-life care: Patients' perspectives. Journal of the American Medical Association 1999;281(2):163–168.

Smith-Stoner M, Frost AL. How to build your "hope skills." Nursing 1999;29(9):24.

Thorns AR, Ellershaw JE. A survey of nursing and medical staff views on the use of CPR in the hospice. Palliative Medicine 1999;13(3):225–232.

Tilden VP. Ethics perspectives on end-of-life care. Nursing Outlook 1999; 47(4):162–167.

Ufema J. Insights on death and dying. Visitation policy: Surrounded by kith and kin. Nursing 1999;29(9):24.

Wink P. Addressing end-of-life issues: Spirituality and inner life. Generations 1999;23(1):75–80.

Zilberfein F. Coping with death: Anticipatory grief and bereavement. Generations 1999;23(1):69–74.

SKILL 38-1

PERFORMING POSTMORTEM CARE

Suggested Action	Reason for Action
Assessment	
Determine that the patient is dead by assessing breathing and circulation.	Confirms that the patient is lifeless in all but cases in which life support equipment is used
Determine if the physician and family have been notified.	Establishes the chain of communication
Notify the nursing supervisor and switchboard of the patient's death.	Makes others aware of a change in the status of the patient
Check the medical record for the name of the mortuary where the body will be taken.	Facilitates collaboration
Planning	
Contact the mortuary and inform them that the family has chosen them to manage the burial.	Communicates a need for services
Ask when mortuary personnel may be expected to arrive.	Facilitates efficient time management
Contact any individuals involved in organ procurement.	Promotes timely harvesting of organs
Obtain a postmortem kit or supplies for cleaning, wrapping, and identifying the body.	Promotes organization
Implementation	
Pull the curtains about the bed.	Ensures privacy
Don gloves.	Adheres to standard precautions
Place the body supine with the arms extended at the side or folded over the abdomen.	Prevents skin discoloration in areas that will be visible in a casket
Remove all medical equipment* such as an intravenous catheter, urinary catheter, and dressings.	Eliminates unnecessary equipment
Remove hairpins or clips.	Prevents accidental trauma about the face
Close the eyelids.	Ensures that they will close when the body is prepared
Replace or keep dentures in the mouth.	Maintains the natural contour of the face
Place a small rolled towel beneath the chin to close the mouth.	Promotes a natural appearance
Cleanse secretions and drainage from the skin.	Ensures delivery of a hygienic body
Apply one or more disposable pads between the legs and under the buttocks.	Absorbs stool or urine should they escape
Attach an identification tag to the ankle or wrist; pad the wrist first if it is used.	Facilitates accurate identification of the body; prevents damage to tissue that will be visible
Wrap the body in a paper **shroud** (covering for the body) and cover the body with a sheet.	Demonstrates respect for the dignity of the deceased person
Tidy the bedside area and dispose of soiled equipment.	Follows principles of medical asepsis
Remove gloves and wash your hands.	Removes colonizing microorganisms
Leave the room and close the door, or transport the body to the **morgue** (area where dead bodies are temporarily held or examined).	Provides a temporary location for the body until mortuary personnel arrive

continued

SKILL 38–1

PERFORMING POSTMORTEM CARE *Continued*

Suggested Action	Reason For Action

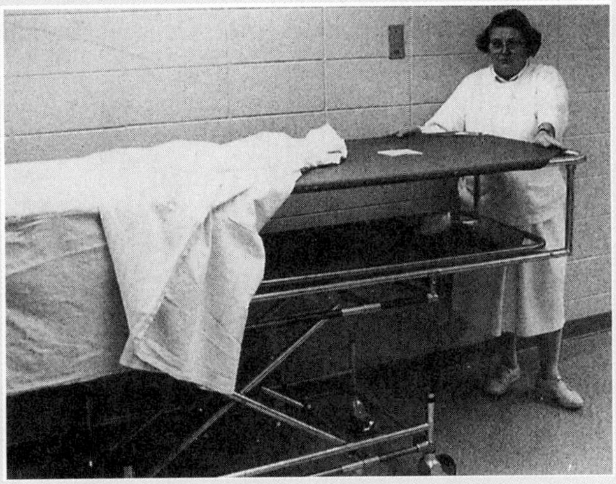

A morgue cart.

Suggested Action	Reason For Action
Make an inventory of valuables and send them to an administrative office, where they are placed in a safe.	Ensures safekeeping and accountability for valuables until they can be claimed by a family member
Notify housekeeping after the body is removed from the room.	Facilitates cleaning and preparation for another admission

Evaluation

- The body is cleaned and prepared appropriately.
- The body is transferred to mortuary personnel.

Document

- Assessments that indicate the patient is dead
- Time of death
- People notified of death
- Care of the body
- Time body is transported to the morgue or transferred to mortuary personnel

SAMPLE DOCUMENTATION

Date and Time No breathing noted and no pulse @ 1400. Dr. Williams notified @ 1415. Dr. Williams pronounced death and called patient's wife. Foster's Funeral Home notified. Mortuary personnel unavailable until 1800. Postmortem care provided. Body transported to morgue after wife and children departed. ________________________ SIGNATURE, TITLE

CRITICAL THINKING

- Discuss nursing activities that demonstrate dignity and respect for the body.

* Except in coroner's cases.

Glossary of Key Terms

Acceptance: attitude of complacency; last stage of dying, according to Dr. Kübler-Ross
Accommodation: pupil constriction when looking at a object close by and dilation when looking at an object in the distance
Active exercise: therapeutic activity performed independently
Active listening: demonstrating full attention to what is being said, hearing both the content being communicated and the unspoken message
Active transport: process of chemical distribution that requires an energy source
Actual diagnosis: problem that currently exists
Acultural nursing care: care that lacks concern for cultural differences
Acupressure: technique that involves tissue compression to reduce pain
Acupuncture: pain-management technique in which long, thin needles are inserted into the skin
Acute illness: one that comes on suddenly and lasts a short time
Acute pain: discomfort that is of short duration
Adaptation: manner in which an organism responds to change
Adjuvants: drugs that assist in accomplishing the desired effect of a primary drug
Administrative laws: legal provisions through which federal, state, and local agencies maintain self-regulation
Admission: entering a health care agency for nursing care and medical or surgical treatment
Advance directive: written statement identifying a competent person's wishes concerning terminal care
Advanced practice: specialized areas of nursing expertise, such as nurse practitioner and nurse midwifery
Aerobic bacteria: microorganisms that require oxygen to live
Aerobic exercise: rhythmically moving all parts of the body at a moderate to slow speed without hindering the ability to breathe
Aerosol: mist
Afebrile: absence of a fever
Affective domain: learning by appealing to a person's feelings, beliefs, or values
Affective touch: touching that demonstrates concern or affection
African Americans: those whose ancestral origin is Africa
Afterload: force against which the heart pumps when ejecting blood
Airborne precautions: measures that reduce the risk of transmitting airborne infectious agents
Air embolism: bubble of air in the vascular system
Airway: collective system of tubes in the upper and lower respiratory tract
Airway management: skills that maintain the patency of natural or artificial airways
Alignment: proper relation of one part to another
Allocation of scarce resources: process of deciding how to distribute limited life-saving equipment or procedures
Alternative medical therapy: treatment outside the mainstream of traditional medicine
Ambulatory electrocardiogram: continuous recording of heart rate and rhythm during normal activity
Ampule: sealed glass container for a drug
Anaerobic bacteria: microorganisms that exist without oxygen
Analgesic: pain-relieving drug
Anal sphincters: ring-shaped bands of muscles in the anus
Anatomic position: standing with arms at the sides and palms forward
Androgogy: principles of teaching adult learners
Anecdotal record: personal, handwritten account of an incident
Anesthesiologist: physician who administers chemical agents that temporarily eliminate sensation and pain
Anesthetist: nurse specialist who administers anesthesia under the direction of a physician
Anger: emotional response to feeling victimized
Anglo-Americans: those who trace their ancestry to the United Kingdom or Western Europe
Anions: electrolytes with a negative charge

Ankylosis: permanent loss of joint movement
Anorexia: loss of appetite
Anthropometric data: measurements of body size and composition
Anticipatory grieving: grieving that begins before a loss actually occurs
Antiembolism stockings: elastic stockings
Antimicrobial agents: chemicals that limit the number of infectious microorganisms by destroying them or suppressing their growth
Antineoplastic drugs: medications used to destroy or slow the growth of malignant cells
Antipyretics: drugs that reduce fever
Antiseptics: chemicals such as alcohol that inhibit the growth of, but do not kill, microorganisms
Anuria: absence of urine, or up to a 100-mL volume in 24 hours
Apical heart rate: number of ventricular contractions per minute
Apical-radial rate: number of sounds heard at the heart's apex and the rate of the radial pulse during the same period
Apnea: absence of breathing
Appliance: collection bag over a stoma
Aquathermia pad: electrical heating or cooling device
Arrhythmia: irregular pattern of heart beats
Art: ability to perform an act skillfully
Arterial blood gas: laboratory test using blood from an artery
Asepsis: practices that decrease or eliminate infectious agents, their reservoirs, and vehicles for transmission
Aseptic techniques: measures that reduce or eliminate microorganisms
Asian Americans: those who come from China, Japan, Korea, the Philippines, Thailand, Indochina, and Vietnam
Asphyxiation: inability to breathe
Assault: act in which there is a threat or attempt to do bodily harm
Assessment: systematic collection of information
Assessment skills: acts that involve collecting data
Atelectasis: airless, collapsed lung areas
Audiometry: measurement of hearing acuity at various sound frequencies
Auditors: inspectors who examine patient records
Auscultation: listening to body sounds
Auscultatory gap: period during which sound disappears then reappears when taking a blood pressure measurement
Autologous transfusion: self-donated blood
Automated external defibrillator: device that delivers an electrical charge to the heart
Automated monitoring devices: equipment that allows the simultaneous collection of multiple vital sign data
Autopsy: postmortem examination
Bag bath: technique for bathing that involves the use of 8 to 10 premoistened, warmed, disposable cloths contained in a plastic bag
Balance: steady position
Bandage: strip or roll of cloth
Bargaining: psychological mechanism for delaying the inevitable
Barrel: part of a syringe that holds the medication
Base of support: area on which an object rests
Basic care facility: agency that provides extended custodial care
Battery: unauthorized physical contact
Bed bath: washing with a basin of water at the bedside
Bed board: rigid structure placed under a mattress
Bedpan: seat-like container for elimination
Beliefs: concepts that a person holds to be true
Bilingual: able to speak a second language
Binder: type of bandage
Biofeedback: technique in which the patient learns to control or alter a physiologic phenomenon
Biologic defense mechanisms: methods that prevent microorganisms from causing an infectious disorder
Bivalved cast: cast that is cut in two lengthwise pieces
Blood pressure: force exerted by blood in the arteries
Board of nursing: regulatory agency that manages the provisions of a state's nurse practice act
Body cast: form of a cylinder cast that encircles the trunk of the body instead of an extremity
Body composition: amount of body tissue that is lean versus fat
Body-mass index: numeric data used to compare a person's size in relation to norms for the adult population
Body mechanics: efficient use of the musculoskeletal system
Body systems approach: collection of data according to the functional systems of the body
Bolus administration: undiluted medication given fairly quickly in a vein
Bolus dose: larger dose of a drug administered initially or when pain is intense
Bolus feeding: instillation of liquid nourishment four to six times a day in less than 30 minutes
Brace: custom-made or custom-fitted device designed to support weakened structures
Bradypnea: slower-than-normal respiratory rate at rest
Bridge: dental device that replaces one or several teeth
Bruxism: grinding of the teeth
Buccal application: drug placement against the mucous membranes of the inner cheek
Cachexia: general wasting of body tissue
Calorie: amount of heat that raises the temperature of 1 gram of water 1°C
Capillary action: movement of a liquid at the point of contact with a solid
Capillary refill time: amount of time it takes blood to resume flowing in the base of the nail beds
Capitation: strategy for controlling health care costs by paying a fixed amount per member
Carbohydrates: nutrients that contain molecules of carbon, hydrogen, and oxygen

Cardiac ischemia: impaired blood flow to the heart
Cardiac output: volume of blood ejected from the left ventricle per minute
Cardiopulmonary resuscitation: techniques used to restore breathing and circulation for lifeless victims
Caries: tooth cavities
Caring skills: nursing interventions that restore or maintain a person's health
Case method: pattern in which one nurse manages a patient's care for a designated period
Cast: rigid mold around a body part
Cataplexy: sudden loss of muscle tone, triggered by an emotional change such as laughing or anger
Catheter care: hygiene measures used to keep the meatus and adjacent area of the catheter clean
Catheter irrigation: flushing the lumen of a catheter
Catheterization: act of applying or inserting a hollow tube
Cations: electrolytes with a positive charge
Cellulose: undigestible fiber in the stems, skin, and leaves of fruits and vegetables
Center of gravity: point at which the mass of an object is centered
Centigrade scale: scale that uses 0°C as the temperature at which water freezes and 100°C as the point at which it boils
Central venous catheter: venous access device that extends to the vena cava
Cerumen: ear wax
Cervical collar: foam or rigid splint around the neck
Chain of infection: sequence that enables the spread of disease-producing microorganisms
Change of shift report: discussion between a nurse from the shift that is ending and personnel coming on duty
Chart: binder or folder that enables the orderly collection, storage, and safekeeping of a patient's medical records
Charting: process of writing information
Charting by exception: documentation method in which only abnormal assessment findings or care that deviates from the standard is charted
Checklist: form of documentation in which the nurse indicates with a check mark or initials that routine care has been performed
Chest physiotherapy: techniques for mobilizing pulmonary secretions
Chronic illness: one that comes on slowly and lasts a long time
Chronic pain: discomfort that lasts longer than 6 months
Circadian rhythm: phenomena that cycle on a 24-hour basis
Circulatory overload: severely compromised heart function
Civil laws: statutes that protect the personal freedoms and rights of individuals
Clean-catch specimen: voided sample of urine that is considered sterile
Climate control: mechanisms for maintaining temperature, humidity, and ventilation
Clinical pathways: standardized multidisciplinary plans for a specific diagnosis or procedure that identify specific aspects of care to be performed during a designated length of stay
Clinical résumé: summary of previous care
Clinical thermometers: instruments used to measure body temperature
Closed drainage system: device used to collect urine from a catheter
Closed wound: one in which there is no opening in the skin or mucous membrane
Code: summoning personnel to administer advanced life support techniques
Code of ethics: statements describing ideal behavior
Cognitive domain: style of processing information by listening or reading facts and descriptions
Cold spot: area with little or no radionuclide concentration
Collaborative problem: physiologic complication whose treatment requires both nurse- and physician-prescribed interventions
Collagen: protein substance that is tough and inelastic
Colloidal osmotic pressure: force for attracting water
Colloids: undissolved protein substances
Colloid solutions: water and molecules of suspended substances, such as blood cells, and blood products such as albumin
Colonization: condition in which microorganisms are present but the host manifests no signs or symptoms of infection
Colostomy: opening to some portion of the colon
Comfort: state in which a person is relieved of distress
Comforting skills: interventions that provide stability and security during a health crisis
Commode: portable chair used for elimination
Common law: decisions based on prior cases of a similar nature
Communicable diseases: infectious diseases that can be transmitted to other people
Communication: exchange of information
Community-acquired infections: infectious diseases that can be transmitted to other people
Complete proteins: those that contain all the essential amino acids
Compresses: moist cloths that may be warm or cool
Compression: pressure
Computed tomography: form of roentgenography that shows planes of tissue
Computerized charting: documenting patient information electronically
Concurrent disinfection: measures that keep the patient environment clean on a daily basis
Confidentiality: safeguarding a patient's health information from public disclosure
Congenital disorders: disorders present at birth that result from faulty embryonic development
Consensual response: brisk, equal, and simultaneous constriction of both pupils when one eye and then the other is stimulated with light

Constipation: condition in which dry, hard stool is difficult to pass
Contact precautions: measures used to block the transmission of pathogens by direct or indirect contact
Contagious diseases: infectious diseases that can be transmitted to other people
Continence training: process of restoring control of urination
Continent ostomy: surgically created opening in which liquid stool or urine is removed by siphoning
Continuity of care: uninterrupted patient care despite the change in caregivers
Continuous feeding: instillation of liquid nutrition without interruption
Continuous infusion: instillation of a parenteral drug over several hours
Continuous irrigation: ongoing instillation of solution
Continuous quality improvement: process of promoting care that reflects established agency standards
Continuous passive motion machine: electrical device that exercises joints
Contractures: permanently shortened muscles that resist stretching
Contrast medium: substance that adds density to a body organ or cavity, such as barium sulfate or iodine
Controlled substances: drugs whose prescription and dispensing are regulated by federal law because they have the potential for abuse
Coping mechanisms: unconscious tactics used to protect the psyche
Coping strategies: stress-reduction activities selected on a conscious level
Cordotomy: surgical interruption of pain pathways in the spinal cord
Core temperature: warmth at the center of the body
Coroner: person legally designated to investigate deaths that may not be the result of natural causes
Counseling skills: interventions that include communicating with patients, actively listening to the exchange of information, offering pertinent health teaching, and providing emotional support
CPAP mask: device that maintains positive pressure in the airway throughout the respiratory cycle
Credé maneuver: act of bending forward and applying hand pressure over the bladder to stimulate urination
Criminal laws: penal codes that protect citizens from persons who are a threat to the public good
Critical thinking: process of objective reasoning; analyzing facts to reach a valid conclusion
Cross-trained: ability to assume a nonnursing job position, depending on the census or levels of patient acuity on any given day
Crystalloid solution: water and other uniformly dissolved crystals, such as salt and sugar
Cultural shock: bewilderment over behavior that is culturally atypical
Culturally sensitive nursing care: care that respects and is compatible with each patient's culture
Culture: (1) values, beliefs, and practices of a particular group; (2) incubation of microorganisms
Cutaneous application: drug administration by rubbing medication into or placing it in contact with the skin
Cutaneous pain: discomfort that originates at the skin level
Cutaneous triggering: the act of lightly massaging or tapping the skin above the pubic area to stimulate urination
Cuticles: thin edge of skin at the base of the nail
Cyclic feeding: continuous instillation of liquid nourishment for 8 to 12 hours
Cylinder cast: rigid mold that encircles an arm or leg
Data base assessment: initial information about the patient's physical, emotional, social, and spiritual health
Death certificate: legal document confirming a person's death
Débridement: removal of dead tissue
Decompression: removal of gas and secretions from the stomach or bowel
Defamation: an act in which untrue information harms a person's reputation
Defecation: bowel elimination
Defendant: person charged with violating the law
Dehydration: fluid deficit in both extracellular and intracellular compartments
Deltoid site: injection area in the lateral upper arm
Denial: psychological defense mechanism in which a person refuses to believe that certain information is true
Dentures: artificial teeth
Deontology: ethical study based on duty or moral obligations
Depression: sad mood
Diagnosis: identification of health-related problems
Diagnostic examination: procedure that involves physical inspection of body structures and evidence of their function
Diaphragmatic breathing: breathing that promotes the use of the diaphragm rather than upper chest muscles
Diarrhea: urgent passage of watery stools
Diastolic pressure: pressure in the arterial system when the heart relaxes and fills with blood
Diet history: assessment technique used to obtain facts about a person's eating habits and factors that affect nutrition
Directed donors: relatives and friends who donate blood for a patient
Discharge: termination of care from a health care agency
Discharge instructions: directions for managing self-care and medical follow-up
Discharge planning: managing transitional needs and ensuring continuity
Disinfectants: chemicals that destroy active microorganisms but not spores
Distraction: intentional diversion of attention
Disuse syndrome: signs and symptoms that result from inactivity
Documenting: process of writing information

Doppler stethoscope: device that helps detect sounds created by the velocity of blood moving through a blood vessel
Dorsal recumbent position: reclining posture with the knees bent, hips rotated outward, and feet flat
Dorsogluteal site: injection area in the upper outer quadrant of the buttocks
Dose: amount of drug
Double-bagging: infection control measure in which one bag of contaminated items, such as trash or laundry, is placed within another
Douche: procedure for cleansing the vaginal canal
Drain: tube that provides a means for removing blood and drainage from a wound
Drape: sheet of soft cloth or paper
Drawdown effect: cooling of the ear when it comes in contact with a thermometer probe
Dressing: cover over a wound
Drop factor: number of drops per milliliter in intravenous tubing
Droplet precautions: measures that block pathogens in moist droplets larger than 5 microns
Drowning: situation in which fluid occupies the airway and interferes with ventilation
Drug tolerance: diminished effect of a drug at its usual dosage range
Dumping syndrome: cluster of symptoms resulting from the rapid deposition of calorie-dense nourishment into the small intestine
Dying with dignity: treating a terminally ill person with respect regardless of his or her emotional, physical, or cognitive state
Dyspnea: difficult or labored breathing
Dysrhythmia: irregular pattern of heart beats
Dysuria: difficult or uncomfortable voiding
Echography: soft tissue examination that uses sound waves in ranges beyond human hearing
Edema: excessive fluid in tissue
Electrical shock: discharge of electricity through the body
Electrocardiography: examination of the electrical activity in the heart
Electrochemical neutrality: balance of cations with anions
Electroencephalography: examination of the energy emitted by the brain
Electrolytes: chemical compounds, such as sodium and chloride, that are dissolved, absorbed, and distributed in body fluid and possess an electrical charge
Electromyography: examination of the energy produced by stimulated muscles
Emaciation: excessive leanness
Emboli: moving clots
Emesis: substance that is vomited
Empathy: intuitive awareness of what the patient is experiencing
Emulsion: mixture of two liquids, one of which is insoluble in the other
Endogenous opioids: naturally produced morphine-like chemicals
Endoscopy: visual examination of internal structures
Enema: introduction of a solution into the rectum
Energy: capacity to do work
Enteral nutrition: nourishment provided via the stomach or small intestine rather than the oral route
Enteric-coated tablet: tablet covered with a substance that does not dissolve until it is past the stomach
Environmental hazards: potentially dangerous conditions in the physical surroundings
Environmental psychologists: specialists who study how the environment affects behavior
Equianalgesic dose: oral dose that provides the same level of pain relief as a parenteral dose
Ergonomics: field of engineering science devoted to promoting comfort, performance, and health in the workplace
Eructation: belching
Essential amino acids: protein components that must be obtained from food because they cannot be synthesized by the body
Ethical dilemma: choice between two undesirable alternatives
Ethics: moral or philosophical principles
Ethnicity: bond or kinship a person feels with his or her country of birth or place of ancestral origin
Ethnocentrism: belief that one's own ethnicity is superior to all others
Evaluation: process of determining whether a goal has been reached
Exacerbation: reactivation of a disorder, or one that reverts from a chronic to an acute state
Excoriation: chemical skin injury
Exercise: purposeful physical activity
Exit route: means by which microorganisms escape from their original reservoir
Expiration: exhalation; breathing out
Extended care: services that meet the health needs of patients who no longer require acute hospital care
Extended care facility: health care agency that provides long-term care
External catheter: urine collecting device applied to the skin
External fixator: metal device inserted into and through one or more bones
Extracellular fluid: fluid outside cells
Extraocular movements: eye movements controlled by several pairs of eye muscles
Face tent: device that provides oxygen in an area around the nose and mouth
Facilitated diffusion: process in which certain dissolved substances require the assistance of a carrier molecule to pass from one side of a semipermeable membrane to the other
Fahrenheit scale: scale that uses 32°F as the temperature at which water freezes and 212°F as the point at which it boils
False imprisonment: interference with a person's freedom to move about at will without legal authority to do so

Fats: nutrients that contain molecules composed of glycerol and fatty acids called glycerides
Fat-soluble vitamins: those carried and stored in fat; vitamins A, D, E, and K
Febrile: elevated body temperature
Fecal impaction: condition in which it is impossible to pass feces voluntarily
Fecal incontinence: inability to control the elimination of stool
Feces: stool
Feedback loop: mechanism by which hormone production is turned off and on
Felony: serious criminal offense
Fenestrated drape: one with an open circle in its center
Fever: body temperature that exceeds 99.3°F (37.4°C)
Filtration: process that regulates the movement of water and substances from a compartment where the pressure is higher to one where the pressure is lower
Finger sweep: insertion of the index finger into the mouth along the inside of the cheek and deeply into the throat to the base of the tongue
Fire plan: procedure followed if there is a fire
First-intention healing: reparative process when wound edges are directly next to one another
Fitness: capacity to exercise
Fitness exercise: physical activity performed by healthy adults
Flatulence: accumulation of intestinal gas
Flatus: gas that is formed in the intestine and released from the rectum
Flowmeter: gauge used to regulate the number of liters of oxygen delivered to the patient
Flow sheet: form of documentation that contains sections for recording frequently repeated assessment data
Fluid imbalance: condition in which the body's water is not in the proper volume or location in the body
Fluoroscopy: form of radiography in which an image is displayed in real time
Focus assessment: information that provides more details about specific problems
Focus charting: modified form of SOAP charting
Folk medicine: health practices unique to a particular group of people
Food pyramid: guide for promoting the healthy intake of food
Foot drop: permanent dysfunctional position caused by shortening of the calf muscles and lengthening of the opposing muscles on the anterior leg
Forced coughing: coughing that is purposely produced
Fowler's position: upright seated position
Fraction of inspired oxygen: portion of oxygen in relation to total inspired gas
Frenulum: structure that attaches the undersurface of the tongue to the fleshy portion of the mouth
Frequency: need to urinate often
Functional brace: brace that provides stability for a joint
Functionally illiterate: possessing minimal literacy skills
Functional mobility: alignment that maintains the potential for movement and ambulation
Functional nursing: pattern in which each nurse on a unit is assigned specific tasks
Functional position: position that promotes continued use and mobility
Gastric reflux: reverse flow of gastric contents
Gastric residual: volume of liquid remaining in the stomach
Gastrocolic reflex: increased peristaltic activity
Gastrostomy tube, G-tube: transabdominal tube located in the stomach
Gate-control theory: belief about how pain is transmitted and blocked
Gauge: diameter
Gavage: provision of nourishment
General adaptation syndrome: collective physiologic processes that occur in response to a stressor
Generic name: chemical drug name that is not protected by a manufacturer's trademark
Gerogogy: techniques that enhance learning among older adults
Glucometer: instrument that measures the amount of glucose in capillary blood
Gingivitis: inflammation of the gums
Goal: expected or desired outcome
Good Samaritan laws: legal immunity for passersby who provide emergency first aid to accident victims
Gram staining: process of adding a dye to a microscopic specimen
Granulation tissue: combination of new blood vessels, fibroblasts, and epithelial cells
Gravity: force that pulls objects toward the center of the earth
Grief response: psychological and physical phenomena experienced by those who are grieving
Grief work: activities involved in grieving
Grieving: process of feeling acute sorrow over a loss
Hand antisepsis: removal and destruction of transient microorganisms from the hands
Handwashing: aseptic practice that involves scrubbing the hands with plain soap or detergent, water, and friction
Head tilt/chin lift technique: preferred method for opening the airway
Head-to-toe approach: gathering data from the top of the body to the feet
Health: state of complete physical, mental, and social well-being; not merely the absence of disease or infirmity
Health care system: network of available health services
Hearing acuity: ability to hear and discriminate sound
Heimlich maneuver: method for removing a mechanical airway obstruction
Hereditary condition: disorder acquired from the genetic codes of one or both parents
Holism: philosophical concept of interrelatedness
Home health care: health care provided in the home by an employee of a home health agency

Homeostasis: relatively stable state of physiologic equilibrium
Hospice: facility for or concept addressing the care of terminally ill patients
Hot spot: area where radionuclide is intensely concentrated
Human needs: factors that motivate behavior
Humidifier: device that produces small water droplets
Humidity: amount of moisture in the air
Hydrostatic pressure: pressure exerted against a membrane
Hydrotherapy: therapeutic use of water
Hygiene: practices that promote health through personal cleanliness
Hyperbaric oxygen therapy: delivery of 100% oxygen at three times the normal atmospheric pressure in an airtight chamber
Hypercarbia: excessive levels of carbon dioxide in the blood
Hypersomnia: sleep disorder characterized by feeling sleepy despite getting a normal amount of sleep
Hypersomnolence: excessive sleeping
Hypertension: high blood pressure
Hyperthermia: excessively high core temperature
Hypertonic solution: solution that is more concentrated than body fluid
Hyperventilation: rapid or deep breathing, or both
Hypervolemia: higher-than-normal volume of water in the intravascular fluid compartment
Hypnogogic hallucinations: dream-like auditory or visual experiences while dozing or falling asleep
Hypnosis: therapeutic technique in which a person enters a trance-like state
Hypnotic: agent that produces sleep
Hypoalbuminemia: deficit of albumin in the blood
Hypopnea: hypoventilation
Hypotension: low blood pressure
Hypothalamus: temperature-regulating structure in the brain
Hypothermia: core body temperature less than 95°F (35°C)
Hypotonic solution: one that contains fewer dissolved substances than normally found in plasma
Hypoventilation: diminished breathing
Hypovolemia: low volume in the extracellular fluid compartments
Hypoxemia: insufficient oxygen in arterial blood
Hypoxia: inadequate oxygen at the cellular level
Idiopathic illness: one whose cause is unexplained
Ileostomy: surgically created opening to the ileum
Illiterate: unable to read or write
Illness: state of discomfort
Imagery: using the mind to visualize an experience
Immobilizer: commercial splint made from cloth and foam
Implementation: carrying out the plan of care
Incentive spirometry: technique for deep breathing using a calibrated device
Incident report: written account of an unusual event involving a client, employee, or visitor that has the potential for being injurious
Incomplete proteins: those that contain some, but not all, of the essential amino acids
Incontinence: inability to control either urinary or bowel elimination
Individual supply: single container of drugs with several days' worth of doses
Induration: area of hardness
Infection: condition that results when microorganisms cause injury to a host
Infection control precautions: physical measures designed to curtail the spread of infectious diseases
Infectious diseases: diseases spread from one person to another
Inflammation: physiologic defense that occurs immediately after tissue injury
Inflatable splint: immobilizing device that becomes rigid when filled with air
Infiltration: escape of intravenous fluid into the tissue
Informed consent: permission a person gives after having the risks, benefits, and alternatives explained
Infusion pump: device that uses pressure to infuse solutions
Inhalant route: drug administration into the lower airways
Inhalation therapy: respiratory treatments that provide a mixture of oxygen, humidification, and aerosolized medication
Inhaler: hand-held device for delivering medication to the respiratory passages
Inpatient surgery: operative procedures performed on patients who are admitted to the hospital and are expected to remain for a period of time
Insomnia: sleep disorder involving early awakening or difficulty falling asleep or staying asleep
Inspection: purposeful observation
Inspiration: inhalation; breathing in
Insulin syringe: syringe that is calibrated in units and holds a volume of 0.5 to 1 mL of medication
Intake and output: record of a patient's fluid intake and fluid loss over a 24-hour period
Intentional tort: lawsuit in which a plaintiff charges that the defendant committed a deliberately aggressive act
Intermediate care facility: agency that provides health-related care and services to people who, because of their mental or physical condition, require institutional care but not 24-hour nursing care
Intermittent feeding: gradual instillation of liquid nourishment four to six times a day
Intermittent infusion: parenteral administration of medication over a relatively short period
Intermittent venous access device: sealed chamber that provides a means for administering intravenous medications or solutions on a periodic basis
Interstitial fluid: fluid in the tissue space between and around cells
Intestinal decompression: removal of gas and intestinal contents
Intimate space: distance within 6 inches
Intracellular fluid: fluid inside cells

Intractable pain: pain unresponsive to methods of pain management

Intradermal injection: parenteral drug administration between the layers of the skin

Intramuscular injection: parenteral drug administration into muscle

Intraoperative period: time during which the patient undergoes surgery

Intraspinal analgesia: method of relieving pain by instilling a narcotic or local anesthetic via a catheter into the subarachnoid or epidural space of the spinal cord

Intravascular fluid: watery plasma, or serum, portion of blood

Intravenous fluids: solutions infused into a patient's vein

Intravenous injection: parenteral drug administration into a vein

Introductory phase: period of getting acquainted

Intubation: placement of a tube into a structure of the body

Inunction: medication incorporated into an agent such as an ointment, oil, lotion, or cream

Invasion of privacy: failure to leave people and their property alone

Ions: substances that carry either a positive or negative electrical charge

Irrigation: technique for flushing debris

Isometric exercise: stationary exercises that are generally performed against a resistive force

Isotonic exercise: activity that involves movement and work

Isotonic solution: solution that contains the same concentration of dissolved substances as normally found in plasma

Jaeger chart: visual assessment tool with small print

Jaw-thrust maneuver: alternative method for opening the airway

Jejunostomy tube; J-tube: transabdominal tube that leads to the jejunum of the small intestine

Jet lag: emotional and physical changes experienced when arriving in a different time zone

Kardex: quick reference for current information about the patient and the patient's care

Kilocalories: 1,000 calories, or the amount of heat that raises the temperature of 1 kilogram of water 1°C

Kinesics: body language

Knee-chest position: position in which the patient rests on the knees and chest

Korotkoff sounds: sounds that result from the vibrations of blood in the arterial wall or changes in blood flow

Laboratory test: procedure that involves the examination of body fluids or specimens

Lateral oblique position: variation of a side-lying position

Lateral position: side-lying position

Latex-safe environment: room stocked with latex-free equipment and wiped clean of glove powder

Latex sensitivity: allergic response to the proteins in latex

Latinos: those who trace their ethnic origin to South America

Lavage: wash out; remove poisonous substances

Laws: rules of conduct established and enforced by the government of a society

Leukocytes: white blood cells

Leukocytosis: increased production of white blood cells

Liability insurance: contract between a person or corporation and a company who is willing to provide legal services and financial assistance when the policyholder is involved in a malpractice lawsuit

Libel: damaging statement that is written and read by others

Line of gravity: imaginary vertical line that passes through the center of gravity

Lipoatrophy: breakdown of subcutaneous fat at the site of repeated insulin injections

Lipohypertrophy: buildup of subcutaneous fat at insulin injection sites

Lipoproteins: combinations of fats and proteins

Liquid oxygen unit: device that converts cooled liquid oxygen to a gas by passing it through heated coils

Literacy: ability to read and write

Lithotomy position: reclining posture with the feet in metal supports called stirrups

Loading dose: larger dose of a drug administered initially or when pain is intense

Long-term goals: desirable outcomes that take weeks or months to accomplish

Lumbar puncture: procedure that involves insertion of a needle between lumbar vertebrae in the spine but below the spinal cord itself

Lumen: channel

Macrophages: white blood cells that consume cellular debris

Macroshock: harmless distribution of low-amperage electricity over a large area of the body

Magnetic resonance imaging: technique for producing an image by using atoms subjected to a strong electromagnetic field

Malingerer: someone who pretends to be sick or in pain

Malnutrition: condition resulting from a lack of proper nutrients in the diet

Malpractice: professional negligence

Managed care practices: cost-containment strategies used to plan and coordinate a patient's care to avoid delays, unnecessary services, or overuse of expensive resources

Manual traction: pulling on the body using a person's hands and muscular strength

Mattress overlays: layers of foam or other devices placed on top of the mattress

Maximum heart rate: highest limit for heart rate during exercise

Medical asepsis: practices that confine or reduce the numbers of microorganisms

Medical records: written collection of information about a person's health problems, the care provided by health practitioners, and the progress of the patient

Medication: chemical substance that changes body function
Medication administration record: agency form used to document drug administration
Medication order: name and directions for giving a drug
Meditation: concentrating on a word or idea that promotes tranquility
Megadoses: amounts exceeding those considered adequate for health
Melatonin: hormone that induces drowsiness and sleep
Mental status assessment: technique for determining the level of a patient's cognitive functioning
Metabolic energy equivalent: measure of energy and oxygen consumption during exercise
Metabolic rate: use of calories for sustaining body functions
Metered-dose inhaler: canister that contains medication under pressure
Microabrasions: tiny cuts that provide an entrance for microorganisms
Microorganisms: living animals or plants visible only with a microscope
Microshock: low-voltage but high-amperage electricity
Microsleep: Unintentional sleep lasting 20 to 30 seconds
Midarm circumference: measurement used to assess skeletal muscle mass
Military time: time based on a 24-hour clock
Minerals: noncaloric substances in food that are essential to all cells
Misdemeanor: minor criminal offense
Mode of transmission: manner in which infectious microorganisms move to another location
Modified standing position: position in which the upper half of the body is leaning forward
Molded splint: orthotic device made of rigid material
Montgomery straps: strips of tape with eyelets
Morbidity: incidence of a specific disease, disorder, or injury
Morgue: area where dead bodies are temporarily held or examined
Mortality: incidence of deaths
Mortician: person who prepares the body for burial or cremation
Mucus: substance that keeps mucous membranes moist
Multicultural diversity: unique characteristics of ethnic groups
Multiple organ failure: condition in which two or more organ systems gradually cease to function
Multiple sleep latency test: assessment of daytime sleepiness
Muscle spasms: sudden, forceful, involuntary muscle contractions
Narcolepsy: sleep disorder characterized by the sudden onset of daytime sleep, a short NREM period before the first REM phase, and pathologic manifestations of REM sleep
Narrative charting: style of documentation generally used in source-oriented records
Nasal cannula: hollow tube with prongs that are placed into the patient's nostrils for delivering oxygen
Nasal catheter: tube for delivering oxygen that is inserted through the nose into the posterior nasal pharynx
Nasogastric tube: tube that is placed in the nose and advanced to the stomach
Nasointestinal tube: tube that is inserted through the nose for distal placement below the stomach
Nasopharyngeal suctioning: removal of secretions from the throat through a nasally inserted catheter
Nasotracheal suctioning: removal of secretions from the trachea through a nasally inserted catheter
Native Americans: Indian nations found in North America, including the Eskimos and Aleuts
Nausea: feeling that usually precedes vomiting
Necrotic tissue: nonliving tissue
Needleless systems: intravenous tubing that eliminates the need for access needles
Negligence: harm that results because a person did not act reasonably
Neuropathic pain: pain with atypical characteristics
Neurotransmitters: chemical messengers synthesized in the neurons
Neutral position: limb that is turned neither toward nor away from the body's midline
NEX measurement: distance from the nose to the earlobe to the xiphoid process
Nociceptors: nerve receptors that transmit pain impulses
Nocturia: nighttime urination
Nocturnal enuresis: bedwetting
Nocturnal polysomnography: technique used to obtain physiologic data during nighttime sleep
Nonelectrolytes: chemical compounds that remain bound together when dissolved in solution
Nonessential amino acids: protein components manufactured in the body
Nonopioids: nonnarcotic drugs
Nonpathogens: harmless and beneficial microorganisms
Nonrebreather mask: oxygen delivery device in which all the exhaled air leaves the mask rather than partially entering the reservoir bag
Nonverbal communication: exchange of information without using words
Normal flora: microorganisms that reside in and on humans
Nosocomial infections: infections acquired while a person is being cared for in a hospital or other health care agency
Nuclear medicine department: unit responsible for radionuclide imaging
Nurse-managed care: pattern in which a nurse manager plans the nursing care of patients based on their illness or medical diagnosis
Nurse practice act: statute that legally defines the unique role of the nurse and differentiates it from that of other health care practitioners, such as physicians
Nursing care plan: written list of the patient's problems, goals, and nursing orders for patient care

Nursing diagnosis: health problem that can be prevented, reduced, or resolved through independent nursing measures
Nursing orders: directions for a patient's care
Nursing process: organized sequence of problem-solving steps: assessment, diagnosis, planning, implementation, and evaluation
Nursing skills: activities unique to the practice of nursing
Nursing team: personnel who care for patients directly
Nursing theory: proposal on what is involved in the process of nursing
Nutrition: process by which the body uses food
Obesity: condition in which a person's body-mass index exceeds $30/m^2$ or the triceps skinfold measurement exceeds 15 mm
Objective data: facts that are observable and measurable
Occupied bed: changing linen while the patient remains in bed
Offsets: predictive mathematical conversions
Oliguria: urine output of less than 400 mL per 24 hours
Open wound: wound in which the surface of the skin or mucous membrane is no longer intact
Ophthalmic application: method of applying drugs onto the mucous membrane of one or both eyes
Ophthalmologist: medical doctor who treats eye disorders
Opioids: narcotic drugs; synthetic narcotics
Opportunistic infections: disorders caused by nonpathogens that occur in people with compromised health
Optometrist: person who prescribes corrective lenses
Oral airway: curved device that keeps the tongue positioned forward within the mouth
Oral hygiene: practices used to clean the mouth, especially the teeth
Oral route: drug administration by swallowing or instillation through an enteral tube
Oral suctioning: removal of secretions from the mouth
Orientation: helping a person become familiar with a new environment
Orogastric tube: tube that is inserted from the mouth into the stomach
Oropharyngeal suctioning: removal of secretions from the throat through a catheter inserted through the mouth
Orthopnea: breathing that is facilitated by sitting up or standing
Orthopneic position: seated position with the arms supported on pillows or the arm rests of a chair
Orthoses: orthopedic devices that support or align a body part and prevent or correct deformities
Orthostatic hypotension: sudden but temporary drop in blood pressure when rising from a reclining position
Osmosis: process that regulates the distribution of water
Ostomate: person with an ostomy
Ostomy: surgically created opening
Otic application: drug instillation in the outer ear
Outpatients: persons who receive health care in a hospital department but return home in less than 24 hours
Outpatient surgery: operative procedures from which patients recover and return home on the same day
Over-the-counter medication: nonprescription drug
Oxygen concentrator: machine that collects and concentrates oxygen from room air and stores it for patient use
Oxygen tent: clear plastic enclosure that provides cooled, humidified oxygen
Oxygen therapy: therapeutic intervention for administering more oxygen than exists in the atmosphere
Oxygen toxicity: lung damage that develops when oxygen concentrations of more than 50% are administered for longer than 48 to 72 hours
Pack: commercial device for applying moist heat
Pain: unpleasant sensation usually associated with disease or injury
Pain management: techniques for preventing, reducing, or relieving pain
Pain perception: conscious experience of discomfort
Pain threshold: point at which sufficient pain-transmitting neurochemicals reach the brain to cause awareness of discomfort
Pain tolerance: amount of pain a person endures once the pain threshold is surpassed
Palpation: lightly touching the body or applying pressure
Palpitation: awareness of one's own heart contraction without having to feel the pulse
Pap test: screening test that detects abnormal cervical cells, the status of reproductive hormone activity, or the presence of normal or infectious microorganisms in the uterus or vagina
Paracentesis: procedure for withdrawing fluid from the abdominal cavity
Paralanguage: vocal sounds that are not actually words
Paranormal experiences: those outside scientific explanation
Parasomnias: conditions associated with activities that cause arousal or partial arousal, usually during transitions in NREM periods of sleep
Parenteral nutrition: nutrients, such as proteins, carbohydrate, fat, vitamins, minerals, and trace elements, that are administered intravenously
Parenteral route: route of drug administration other than oral or through the gastrointestinal tract; administration by injection
Partial bath: washing only the areas of the body that are subject to the greatest soiling or that are sources of body odor
Partial rebreather mask: oxygen delivery device through which a patient inhales a mixture of atmospheric air, oxygen from its source, and oxygen contained in a reservoir bag
Passive diffusion: physiologic process in which dissolved substances, such as electrolytes and gases, move from an

area of higher concentration to one of lower concentration through a semipermeable membrane

Passive exercise: therapeutic activity performed with assistance

Paste: vehicle that contains a drug in a viscous base

Pathogens: microorganisms that cause illness

Pathologic grief: condition in which a person cannot accept someone's death

Patient-controlled analgesia: intervention that allows patients to self-administer pain medication

Pedagogy: science of teaching children or those who have comparable cognitive ability

Pelvic examination: physical inspection of the vagina and cervix, with palpation of the uterus and ovaries

Percussion: (1) striking or tapping a part of the body; (2) type of chest physiotherapy performed by rhythmically striking the chest wall

Percutaneous electrical nerve stimulation: pain management technique involving a combination of acupuncture needles and transcutaneous electrical nerve stimulation

Percutaneous endoscopic gastrostomy (PEG) tube: transabdominal tube inserted into the stomach under endoscopic guidance

Percutaneous endoscopic jejunostomy (PEJ) tube: tube that is passed through a PEG tube into the jejunum

Perineal care: techniques used for cleansing the perineum

Periodontal disease: condition that results in destruction of the tooth-supporting structures and jawbone

Perioperative care: care that patients receive before, during, and after surgery

Peripheral parenteral nutrition: isotonic or hypotonic intravenous nutrient solution instilled in a vein distant from the heart

Peristalsis: rhythmic contractions of smooth muscle

Peristomal skin: skin around a stoma

Persistent vegetative state: condition in which there is no cognitive function or capacity to experience emotions

Personal protective equipment: garments that block the transfer of pathogens from one person, place, or object to oneself or others

Personal space: distance of 6 inches to 4 feet

Petals: strips of adhesive used to eliminate rough cast edges

Phagocytosis: process in which white blood cells consume cellular debris

Phlebitis: inflammation of a vein

Photoperiod: number of daylight hours

Phototherapy: technique for suppressing melatonin by stimulating light receptors in the eye

Physical assessment: systematic examination of body structures

PIE charting: method of recording the patient's progress under the headings of problem, intervention, and evaluation

Placebo: inactive substance

Plaintiff: person claiming injury

Planning: process of prioritizing nursing diagnoses and collaborative problems, identifying measurable goals or outcomes, selecting appropriate interventions, and documenting the plan for care

Plaque: substance composed of mucin and other gritty substances that becomes deposited on teeth

Plume: vaporized tissue, carbon, and water released during laser surgery

Plunger: part of a syringe inside the barrel that moves back and forth to withdraw and instill medication

Pneumatic compression device: machine that promotes circulation of venous blood and the movement of excess fluid into the lymphatic vessels

Pneumonia: lung infection

Podiatrist: person with special training in caring for feet

Poisoning: injury caused by the ingestion, inhalation, or absorption of a toxic substance

Polypharmacy: administration of multiple drugs to the same person

Polyuria: larger-than-normal urinary volume

Port of entry: site where microorganisms find their way onto or into a host

Port: sealed opening

Positron emission tomography: radionuclide scanning with the layered analysis of tomography

Possible diagnosis: problem that may be present, but more information is needed to rule out or confirm its existence

Postanesthesia care unit: area in the surgical department where patients are intensively monitored

Postmortem care: care of the body after death

Postoperative care: nursing care after surgery

Postoperative period: interval that begins after surgery is completed

Postural drainage: positioning technique that facilitates drainage of secretions from the lungs

Postural hypotension: sudden but temporary drop in blood pressure when rising from a reclining position

Posture: position of the body, or the way in which it is held

Potential diagnosis: problem a patient is at risk for developing

Prefilled cartridge: sealed glass cylinder of parenteral medication with a preattached needle

Preload: volume of blood that fills the heart and stretches the heart muscle fibers during its resting phase

Preoperative checklist: form that identifies the status of essential presurgical activities

Preoperative period: time that starts when the patient is informed that surgery is necessary and ends when he or she is transported to the operating room

Primary care: the first health care worker or agency to assess a person with a health need

Primary illness: one that develops independently of any other disease

Primary nursing: pattern in which the admitting nurse assumes responsibility for planning patient care and evaluating the progress of the patient

Problem-oriented records: records organized according to the patient's health problems
Progressive care units: units for patients who were once in critical condition but have recovered sufficiently to require less intensive nursing care
Progressive relaxation: therapeutic exercise in which a person actively contracts and then relaxes muscle groups
Projectile vomiting: vomiting that occurs with great force
Proliferation: period during which new cells fill and seal a wound
Prone position: position in which the patient lies on the abdomen
Prophylactic brace: brace used to prevent or reduce the severity of a joint injury
Protein: nutrient composed of amino acids, chemical compounds made up of nitrogen, carbon, hydrogen, and oxygen
Protein complementation: combining plant sources of protein
Proxemics: relation of space to communication
Psychomotor domain: learning by doing
Public space: distance of 12 or more feet
Pulmonary embolism: blood clot that travels to the lung
Pulse: wave-like sensation that can be palpated in a peripheral artery
Pulse deficit: difference between the apical and radial pulse rates
Pulse oximetry: noninvasive, transcutaneous technique for periodically or continuously monitoring the oxygen saturation of blood
Pulse pressure: difference between systolic and diastolic blood pressure measurements
Pulse rate: number of peripheral arterial pulsations palpated in a minute
Pulse rhythm: pattern of the pulsations and pauses between them
Pulse volume: quality of the pulsations that are felt
Pursed-lip breathing: form of controlled ventilation in which the expiration phase of breathing is consciously prolonged
Purulent drainage: white- or green-tinged fluid
Pyrexia: fever
Quality assurance: process of promoting care that reflects established agency standards
Race: biologic variations
Radiography: diagnostic procedures that use x-rays
Radionuclides: elements whose molecular structures are altered to produce radiation
Range-of-motion exercises: therapeutic activity in which joints are moved
Receiving room: presurgical holding area
Reciprocity: licensure based on evidence of having met licensing criteria in another state
Reconstitution: process of adding liquid to a powdered substance
Recording: process of writing information
Recovery index: guide for determining a person's fitness level
Recovery position: side-lying position that helps to maintain an open airway and prevent aspiration of liquids
Rectus femoris site: injection area in the anterior thigh
Referral: process of sending someone to another person or agency for special services
Referred pain: discomfort perceived in an area of the body away from the site of origin
Regeneration: cell duplication
Regurgitation: bringing stomach contents to the throat and mouth without the effort of vomiting
Rehabilitative brace: brace that allows protected motion of an injured joint that has been treated surgically
Relationship: association between two people
Relative humidity: ratio between the amount of moisture in the air and the greatest amount of water vapor the air can hold at a given temperature
Relaxation: technique for releasing muscle tension and quieting the mind
Remission: disappearance of signs and symptoms associated with a particular disease
Remodeling: period during which a wound undergoes changes and maturation
Repetitive strain injuries: disorders that result from cumulative trauma to musculoskeletal structures
Rescue breathing: process of ventilating a nonbreathing victim's lungs
Resident microorganisms: generally nonpathogens that are constantly present on the skin
Residual urine: urine that remains in the bladder after voiding
Resolution: process by which damaged cells recover and reestablish their normal function
Respiration: exchange of oxygen and carbon dioxide
Respiratory rate: number of ventilations per minute
Respite care: relief for a caregiver
Rest: waking state characterized by reduced activity and reduced mental stimulation
Restless legs syndrome: movement typically in the legs, but occasionally in the arms or other body parts, to relieve disturbing skin sensations
Restraint alternatives: protective or adaptive devices that promote patient safety and postural support, but which the patient can release independently
Restraints: devices or chemicals that restrict movement or access to one's body
Retching: act of vomiting without producing vomitus
Retention catheter: urinary tube that is left in place for a period of time
Retention enema: solution held in the large intestine
Rhizotomy: surgical sectioning of a nerve root close to the spinal cord
Rinne test: assessment technique for comparing air versus bone conduction of sound

Roentgenography: general term for procedures that use x-rays
Rounds: visit to patients on an individual basis or as a group
Safety: measures that prevent accidents or unintentional injuries
Saturated fats: lipids that contain as much hydrogen as their molecular structure can hold
Scar formation: replacement of damaged cells with fibrous tissue
Science: body of knowledge unique to a particular subject
Scoop method: technique for threading the needle of a syringe into the cap without touching the cap itself
Scored tablet: tablet with a groove in its center
Secondary care: health services to which primary caregivers refer patients for consultation and additional testing
Secondary illness: disorder that develops from a preexisting condition
Secondary infusion: administration of a diluted intravenous drug at the same time a solution is infusing, or intermittently with an infusing solution
Second-intention healing: reparative process when wound edges are widely separated
Sedatives: drugs that produce a relaxing and calming effect
Sequela: consequences of a disease or its treatment
Serous drainage: leaking plasma
Sepsis: potentially fatal systemic infection
Set point: optimal body temperature
Shaft: long portion of a needle
Shearing: force exerted against the surface and layers of the skin as tissues slide in opposite but parallel directions
Shell temperature: warmth at the skin surface
Short-term goals: outcomes that can be met in a few days to a week
Shroud: covering for a dead body
Signs: objective data; information that is observable and measurable
Silence: intentionally withholding verbal comments
Simple mask: device for administering oxygen that fits over the nose and mouth
Sims' position: lying on the left side with the chest leaning forward, the right knee bent toward the head, the right arm forward, and the left arm extended behind the body
Sitz bath: soak of the perianal area
Skeletal traction: pull exerted directly on the skeletal system by attaching wires, pins, or tongs into or through a bone
Skilled nursing facility: nursing home that provides 24-hour nursing care under the direction of a registered nurse
Skin patches: drugs that are bonded to an adhesive bandage
Skin tear: shallow break in the skin
Skin traction: pulling effect on the skeletal system by applying devices to the skin
Slander: character attack that is uttered in the presence of others
Sleep: state of arousable unconsciousness
Sleep apnea/hypopnea syndrome: sleep disorder in which the sleeper stops breathing or the breathing slows for 10 seconds or longer, five or more times per hour
Sleep diary: daily account of sleeping and waking activities
Sleep paralysis: inability to move for a few minutes just before falling asleep or awakening
Sleep rituals: habitual activities performed before retiring
Sleep-wake cycle disturbance: condition that results from a sleep schedule that involves daytime sleeping
Sling: cloth device used to elevate, cradle, and support parts of the body
Smelling acuity: ability to smell and identify odors
Snellen eye chart: tool for assessing far vision
Soak: procedure in which a part of the body is submerged in fluid
SOAP charting: documentation style more likely to be used in a problem-oriented record
Social space: distance of 4 to 12 feet
Somatic pain: discomfort generated from deeper connective tissue
Somnambulism: sleep-walking
Sordes: dried crusts around the mouth containing mucus, microorganisms, and epithelial cells shed from the oral mucous membrane
Source-oriented records: records organized according to the source of information
Spacer: chamber that is attached to an inhaler
Specimens: samples of tissue or body fluids
Speculum: metal or plastic instrument for widening the vagina or other body cavity
Sphygmomanometer: device for measuring blood pressure
Spica cast: rigid mold that encircles one or both arms or legs and the chest or trunk
Spinal tap: procedure that involves insertion of a needle between lumbar vertebrae in the spine but below the spinal cord itself
Splint: device that immobilizes and protects an injured part of the body
Spore: temporarily inactive microbial life form
Sputum: mucus raised to the level of the upper airways
Standard precautions: measures for reducing the risk of microorganism transmission from both recognized and unrecognized sources of infection
Standards for care: policies that ensure quality patient care
Staples: wide metal clips
Stasis: lack of movement
Statute of limitations: designated amount of time within which a person can file a lawsuit
Statutory laws: laws enacted by federal, state, or local legislatures
Stent: tube that keeps a channel open
Stepdown units: units for patients who were once in critical condition but have recovered sufficiently to require less intensive nursing care

Step test: submaximal fitness test involving a timed stepping activity
Stereotypes: fixed attitudes about all people who share a common characteristic
Sterile field: work area free of microorganisms
Sterile technique: practices that avoid contaminating microbe-free items
Sterilization: physical and chemical techniques that destroy all microorganisms, including spores
Stertorous breathing: noisy ventilation
Stethoscope: instrument that carries sound to the ears
Stimulants: drugs that excite structures in the brain
Stock supply: drugs kept in a nursing unit for use in an emergency
Stoma: entrance to a surgically created opening
Straight catheter: urine drainage tube that is inserted but not left in place
Stress: physiologic and behavioral reactions that occur in response to disequilibrium
Stress electrocardiogram: test of electrical conduction through the heart during maximal activity
Stressors: changes that have the potential for disturbing equilibrium
Stridor: harsh, high-pitched sound heard on inspiration when there is laryngeal obstruction
Stylet: metal guidewire
Subcultures: unique cultural groups that coexist within the dominant culture
Subcutaneous injection: parenteral drug administration beneath the skin but above the muscle
Subjective data: information that only the patient feels and can describe
Sublingual application: placement of a drug under the tongue
Submaximal fitness test: exercise test that does not stress a person to exhaustion
Suctioning: technique for removing liquid secretions with a catheter
Suffering: emotional component of pain
Sump tube: one that contains a double lumen
Sundown syndrome: onset of disorientation as the sun sets
Sunrise syndrome: early-morning confusion
Supine position: position in which the person lies on the back
Suppository: medicated oval or cone-shaped mass
Surfactant: lipoprotein produced by cells in the alveoli that promotes elasticity of the lungs and enhances gas diffusion
Surgical asepsis: measures that render supplies and equipment totally free of microorganisms
Surgical waiting area: room where family and friends await information about the surgical patient
Susceptible host: one whose biologic defense mechanisms are weakened in some way
Sustained release: drug that dissolves at timed intervals
Sutures: knotted ties that hold an incision together
Symptoms: subjective data; that which only the patient can identify
Sympathy: feeling as emotionally distraught as the patient
Syndrome diagnosis: cluster of problems that are present due to an event or situation
Systolic pressure: pressure in the arterial system when the heart contracts
Tachycardia: heart rate between 100 and 150 beats per minute (bpm) at rest
Tachypnea: rapid respiratory rate
Tamponade: pressure
Target heart rate: goal for heart rate during exercise
Tartar: hardened plaque
Task-oriented touch: personal contact that is required when performing nursing procedures
Team nursing: pattern in which nursing personnel divide the patients into groups and complete their care together
Teleology: ethical theory based on final outcomes
Temperature translation: conversion of tympanic temperature into an oral, rectal, or core temperature
Tension pneumothorax: extreme air pressure in the lung when there is no avenue for its escape
Terminal disinfection: measures used to clean the patient environment after discharge
Terminal illness: illness with no potential for cure
Terminating phase: ending of a nurse–patient relationship when there is mutual agreement that the patient's immediate health problems have improved
Tertiary care: health services provided at hospitals or medical centers that offer specialists and complex technology
Theory: opinion, belief, or view that explains a process
Therapeutic baths: baths performed for other than hygiene purposes
Therapeutic exercise: activity performed by people with health risks or those being treated for a health problem
Therapeutic verbal communication: using words and gestures to accomplish a particular objective
Thermal burn: skin injury caused by flames, hot liquids, or steam
Thermister: temperature sensor
Thermoregulation: ability to maintain stable body temperature
Third-intention healing: reparative process when a wound is widely separated and later brought together with some type of closure material
Third-spacing: movement of intravascular fluid to nonvascular fluid compartments, where it becomes trapped and useless
Thrombus: stationary blood clot
Tidaling: rhythmic rise and fall of water in a chest tube drainage system
Tip: part of a syringe to which the needle is attached

Topical route: drug administration to the skin or mucous membranes

Tort: litigation in which one person asserts that an injury, which may be physical, emotional, or financial, occurred as a consequence of another's actions or failure to act

Total parenteral nutrition: hypertonic solution of nutrients designed to meet almost all the caloric and nutritional needs of patients

Total quality improvement: process of promoting care that reflects established agency standards

Touch: tactile stimulus produced by making personal contact with another person or an object

Towel bath: technique for bathing in which a single large towel is used to cover and wash a patient

T-piece: device that fits securely onto a tracheostomy tube or endotracheal tube

Tracheostomy: surgically created opening into the trachea

Tracheostomy care: hygiene and maintenance of a tracheostomy and tracheostomy tube

Tracheostomy collar: device that delivers oxygen near an artificial opening in the neck

Tracheostomy tube: curved, hollow plastic tube in the trachea

Traction: pulling on a part of the skeletal system

Traction splint: metal device that immobilizes and pulls on muscles that are in a state of contraction

Trade name: name used by the pharmaceutical company for the drug it sells

Traditional time: time based on two 12-hour revolutions on a clock

Training effect: heart rate and consequently pulse rate become consistently lower than average with regular exercise

Tranquilizers: drugs that produce a relaxing and calming effect

Transabdominal tube: tube placed through the abdominal wall

Transcultural nursing: providing nursing care in the context of another's culture

Transcutaneous electrical nerve stimulation: medically prescribed pain management technique that delivers bursts of electricity to the skin and underlying nerves

Transdermal application: method of applying a drug on the skin and allowing it to become passively absorbed

Transducer: instrument that receives and transmits biophysical energy

Transfer: (1) discharging a patient from one unit or agency and immediately admitting him or her to another; (2) moving a patient from place to place

Transfer summary: written review of the patient's previous care

Transient microorganisms: pathogens picked up during brief contact with contaminated reservoirs

Transmission-based precautions: measures for controlling the spread of infectious agents from patients known to be or suspected of being infected with highly transmissable or epidemiologically important pathogens

Transtracheal catheter: hollow tube inserted in the trachea to deliver oxygen

Trauma: injury

Truth telling: ethical principle proposing that all patients have the right to receive complete and accurate information

Tuberculin syringe: syringe that holds 1 mL of fluid and is calibrated in 0.01-mL increments

Turbo-inhaler: propeller-driven device used to instill medication into the airways

Turgor: resiliency of the skin

Twenty-four-hour specimen: collection of all the urine produced in a full 24-hour period

Ultrasonography: soft tissue examination that uses sound waves in ranges beyond human hearing

Unintentional tort: situation that results in an injury, although the person responsible did not mean to cause harm

Unit dose: self-contained packet that holds one tablet or capsule

Unoccupied bed: changing the linen when the bed is empty

Unsaturated fats: lipids that are missing some hydrogen

Urgency: strong feeling that urine must be eliminated quickly

Urinal: cylindrical container for collecting urine

Urinary diversion: procedure in which one or both ureters are surgically implanted elsewhere

Urinary elimination: process of releasing excess fluid and metabolic wastes

Urinary retention: condition in which urine is produced but is not released from the bladder

Urinary suppression: failure of the kidneys to produce sufficient urine

Urine: fluid in the bladder

Urostomy: urinary diversion that discharges urine from an opening on the abdomen

Valsalva maneuver: act of closing the glottis and contracting the pelvic and abdominal muscles to increase abdominal pressure

Values: ideals that a person believes are important

Vastus lateralis site: injection area in the outer thigh

Vegans: persons who rely exclusively on plant sources for protein

Vegetarians: persons who do not consume animal food sources

Venipuncture: accessing the venous system by piercing a vein with a needle

Ventilation: (1) movement of air in and out of the lungs; (2) movement of air in the environment

Ventrogluteal site: injection area in the hip

Venturi mask: oxygen delivery device that mixes a precise amount of oxygen and atmospheric air

Verbal communication: communication that uses words

Vial: glass or plastic container of parenteral medication with a self-sealing rubber stopper

Vibration: type of chest physiotherapy used to loosen retained secretions

Viral load: number of viral copies
Visceral pain: discomfort arising from internal organs
Visual acuity: ability to see both far and near
Visual field examination: assessment of peripheral vision and continuity in the visual field
Vital signs: body temperature, pulse rate, respiratory rate, and blood pressure
Vitamins: chemical substances that are necessary in minute amounts for normal growth, maintenance of health, and functioning of the body
Voided specimen: freshly urinated sample of urine
Voiding reflex: spontaneous relaxation of the urinary sphincter in response to physical stimulation
Volume-control set: chamber in intravenous tubing that holds a portion from a larger volume of intravenous solution
Volumetric controller: electronic infusion device that instills intravenous solutions by gravity
Vomiting: loss of stomach contents through the mouth
Vomitus: substance that is vomited
Walk-a-mile test: fitness test that measures the time it takes a person to walk a mile
Water-seal chest tube drainage: technique for evacuating air or blood from the pleural cavity
Water-soluble vitamins: vitamins present and carried in body water; B complex and vitamin C
Weber test: assessment technique for determining equality or disparity of bone-conducted sound
Wellness: full and balanced integration of all aspects of health
Wellness diagnosis: situation in which a healthy person obtains nursing assistance to maintain his or her health or perform at a higher level
Window: square cut from a cast
Wheal: elevated circle on the skin
Whistle-blowing: reporting incompetent or unethical practices
Whitecoat hypertension: condition in which the blood pressure is elevated when taken by a health care worker but is normal at other times
Working phase: period during which the nurse and patient plan the patient's care and put the plan into action
Wound: damaged skin or soft tissue
Z-track technique: injection method that prevents medication from leaking outside the muscle

APPENDIX A

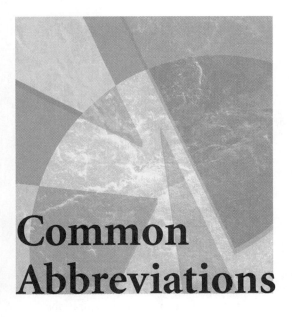

Common Abbreviations

Symbols

<	less than
≤	equal to or less than
>	more than
≥	equal to or more than
±	plus or minus
°	degree

Words

ADL	activities of daily living
AHCPR	Agency for Health Care Policy and Research
AIDS	acquired immune deficiency syndrome
ANA	American Nurses Association
AMA	against medical advice; or American Medical Association
BP	blood pressure
bpm	beats per minute
cal	calorie
CBC	complete blood count
CDC	Centers for Disease Control and Prevention
CHO	carbohydrate
CO_2	carbon dioxide
CPR	cardiopulmonary resuscitation
CT	computed tomography (also CAT)
CVC	central venous catheter
dL	deciliter (100 mL)
ECG	electrocardiogram (also EKG)
EEG	electroencephalogram
EMG	electromyography
EOMs	extraocular movements
g	gram
GI	gastrointestinal
HIV	human immunodeficiency virus
JCAHO	Joint Commission on Accreditation of Healthcare Organizations
I & O	intake and output
ICN	International Council of Nurses
IM	intramuscular
IV	intravenous
IVP	IV push
IVPB	IV piggyback
kcal	kilocalorie
kg	kilogram (1000 g)
L	liter
LPN	licensed practical nurse (also LVN, licensed vocational nurse)
MAR	medication administration record
mEq	milliequivalent
mg	milligram (one-thousandth g)
mL	milliliter (one-thousandth L)
mm Hg	millimeters of mercury
mph	miles per hour
MRI	magnetic resonance imaging
NANDA	North American Nursing Diagnosis Association
NAPNES	National Association for Practical Nurse Education and Service
NCLEX-PN	National Council Licensure Examination for Practical Nurses
NCLEX-RN	National Council Licensure Examination for Registered Nurses
NEX	nose, earlobe, xiphoid process
NKA	no known allergies
NLN	National League for Nursing
NPO	*nil per os,* nothing by mouth

NREM	nonrapid eye movement (sleep phase)
NSS	normal saline solution
NWB	nonweight bearing
O_2	oxygen
OTC	over the counter (eg, nonprescription)
PACU	postanesthesia care unit
$PaCO_2$	partial pressure of carbon dioxide; that which is dissolved in plasma
PaO_2	partial pressure of oxygen; that which is dissolved in plasma
PCA	patient-controlled analgesia
PEG	percutaneous endoscopic gastrostomy
PEJ	percutaneous endoscopic jejunostomy
PERRLA	pupils equally round and respond to light and accommodation
PET	positron emission tomography
pH	degree of acidity or alkalinity
PICC	peripherally inserted central catheter
PPN	peripheral parenteral nutrition
PWB	partial weight bearing
QA	quality assurance
RBC	red blood cell
REM	rapid eye movement (sleep phase)
RN	registered nurse
R/O	rule out; either confirm or eliminate
ROM	range of motion
SAD	seasonal affective disorder
SaO_2	oxygen saturation; percent of hemoglobin molecules saturated with oxygen
SNF	skilled nursing facility
SSE	soap suds enema
TPN	total parenteral nutrition
TPR	temperature, pulse, and respirations
WBC	white blood cell
WHO	World Health Organization

APPENDIX B

NANDA-Approved Nursing Diagnoses

This list represents the NANDA-approved nursing diagnoses for clinical use and testing (1999–2000).

Pattern 1: Exchanging

1.1.2.1	Altered Nutrition: More Than Body Requirements
1.1.2.2	Altered Nutrition: Less Than Body Requirements
1.2.2.3	Altered Nutrition: Risk for More Than Body Requirements
1.2.1.1	Risk for Infection
1.2.2.2	Hypothermia
1.2.2.3	Hyperthermia
1.2.2.4	Ineffective Thermoregulation
1.2.3.1	Dysreflexia
1.2.3.2	Risk for Autonomic Dysreflexia
1.3.1.1	Constipation
1.3.1.1.1	Perceived Constipation
1.3.1.2	Diarrhea
1.3.1.3	Bowel Incontinence
1.3.1.4	Risk for Constipation
1.3.2	Altered Urinary Elimination
1.3.2.1.1	Stress Incontinence
1.3.2.1.2	Reflex Urinary Incontinence
1.3.2.1.3	Urge Incontinence
1.3.2.1.4	Functional Urinary Incontinence
1.3.2.1.5	Total Incontinence
1.3.2.1.6	Risk for Urinary Urge Incontinence
1.3.2.2	Urinary Retention
1.4.1.1	Altered (Specify Type) Tissue Perfusion (Renal, cerebral, cardiopulmonary, gastrointestinal, peripheral)
1.4.1.2	Risk for Fluid-Volume Imbalance
1.4.1.2.1	Fluid Volume Excess*
1.4.1.2.2.1	Fluid Volume Deficit*
1.4.1.2.2.2	Risk for Fluid Volume Deficit
1.4.2.1	Decreased Cardiac Output*
1.5.1.1	Impaired Gas Exchange
1.5.1.2	Ineffective Airway Clearance
1.5.1.3	Ineffective Breathing Pattern*
1.5.1.3.1	Inability to Sustain Spontaneous Ventilation
1.5.1.3.2	Dysfunctional Ventilatory Weaning Response (DVWR)
1.6.1	Risk for Injury
1.6.1.1	Risk for Suffocation
1.6.1.2	Risk for Poisoning
1.6.1.3	Risk for Trauma
1.6.1.4	Risk for Aspiration
1.6.1.5	Risk for Disuse Syndrome
16.1.6	Latex Allergy
1.6.1.7	Risk for Latex Allergy
1.6.2	Altered Protection
1.6.2.1	Impaired Tissue Integrity
1.6.2.1.1	Altered Oral Mucous Membrane
1.6.2.1.2	Altered Dentition
1.6.2.1.2.1	Impaired Skin Integrity
1.6.2.1.2.2	Risk for Impaired Skin Integrity
1.7.1	Decreased Adaptive Capacity: Intracranial
1.8	Energy Field Disturbance

Pattern 2: Communication

2.1.1.1	Impaired Verbal Communication

Pattern 3: Relating

3.1.1.1	Impaired Social Interaction
3.1.2	Social Isolation
3.1.3	Risk for Loneliness
3.2.1	Altered Role Performance
3.2.1.1.1	Altered Parenting
3.2.1.1.2	Risk for Altered Parenting
3.2.1.1.2.1	Risk for Altered Parent/Infant/Child Attachment
3.2.1.2.1	Sexual Dysfunction
3.2.2	Altered Family Processes
3.2.2.1	Caregiver Role Strain
3.2.2.2	Risk for Caregiver Role Strain
3.2.2.3.1	Altered Family Process: Alcoholism
3.2.3.1	Parental Role Conflict
3.3	Altered Sexuality Patterns

Pattern 4: Valuing

4.1.1	Spiritual Distress (Distress of the Human Spirit)
4.1.2	Risk for Spiritual Distress
4.2	Potential for Enhanced Spiritual Well-Being

Pattern 5: Choosing

5.1.1.1	Ineffective Individual Coping*
5.1.1.1.1	Impaired Adjustment
5.1.1.1.2	Defensive Coping
5.1.1.1.3	Ineffective Denial
5.1.2.1.1	Ineffective Family Coping: Disabling*
5.1.2.1.2	Ineffective Family Coping: Compromised*
5.1.2.2	Family Coping: Potential for Growth
5.1.3.1	Potential for Enhanced Community Coping
5.1.3.2	Ineffective Community Coping
5.2.1	Ineffective Management of Therapeutic Regimen (Individuals)
5.2.1.1	Noncompliance (Specify)
5.2.2	Ineffective Management of Therapeutic Regimen: Families
5.2.3	Ineffective Management of Therapeutic Regimen: Community
5.2.4	Effective Management of Therapeutic Regimen: Individual
5.3.1.1	Decisional Conflict (Specify)
5.4	Health-Seeking Behaviors (Specify)

Pattern 6: Moving

6.1.1.1	Impaired Physical Mobility
6.1.1.1.1	Risk for Peripheral Neurovascular Dysfunction
6.1.1.1.2	Risk for Perioperative Positioning Injury
6.1.1.1.3	Impaired Walking
6.1.1.1.4	Impaired Wheelchair Mobility
6.1.1.1.5	Impaired Wheelchair Transferability
6.1.1.1.6	Impaired Bed Mobility
6.1.1.2	Activity Intolerance
6.1.1.2.1	Fatigue
6.1.1.3	Risk for Activity Intolerance
6.2.1	Sleep Pattern Disturbance
6.2.1.1	Sleep Deprivation
6.3.1.1	Diversional Activity Deficit
6.4.1.1	Impaired Home Maintenance Management
6.4.2	Altered Health Maintenance
6.4.2.1	Delayed Surgical Recovery
6.4.2.2	Adult Failure to Thrive
6.5.1	Feeding Self-Care Deficit
6.5.1.1	Impaired Swallowing
6.5.1.2	Ineffective Breastfeeding
6.5.1.2.1	Interrupted Breastfeeding
6.5.1.3	Effective Breastfeeding
6.5.1.4	Ineffective Infant Feeding Pattern
6.5.2	Bathing/Hygiene Self-Care Deficit
6.5.3	Dressing/Grooming Self-Care Deficit
6.5.4	Toileting Self-Care Deficit
6.6	Altered Growth and Development
6.6.1	Risk for Altered Development
6.6.2	Risk for Altered Growth
6.7	Relocation Stress Syndrome
6.8.1	Risk for Disorganized Infant Behavior
6.8.2	Disorganized Infant Behavior
6.8.3	Potential for Enhanced Organized Infant Behavior

Pattern 7: Perceiving

7.1.1	Body Image Disturbance
7.1.2	Self-Esteem Disturbance*
7.1.2.1	Chronic Low Self-Esteem*
7.1.2.2	Situational Low Self-Esteem*
7.1.3	Personal Identity Disturbance
7.2	Sensory/Perceptual Alterations (Specify) (Visual, auditory, kinesthetic, gustatory, tactile, olfactory)
7.2.1.1	Unilateral Neglect
7.3.1	Hopelessness
7.3.2	Powerlessness

Pattern 8: Knowing

8.1.1	Knowledge Deficit (Specify)*
8.2.1	Impaired Environmental Interpretation Syndrome
8.2.2	Acute Confusion
8.2.3	Chronic Confusion
8.3	Altered Thought Processes*
8.3.1	Impaired Memory

Pattern 9: Feeling

9.1.1	Pain*
9.1.1.1	Chronic Pain*
9.1.2	Nausea
9.2.1.1	Dysfunctional Grieving*
9.2.1.2	Anticipatory Grieving*
9.2.1.3	Chronic Sorrow
9.2.2	Risk for Violence: Directed at Others*
9.2.2.1	Risk for Self-Mutilation
9.2.2.2	Risk for Violence: Self-Directed
9.2.3	Post-Trauma Response
9.2.3.1	Rape-Trauma Syndrome
9.2.3.1.1	Rape-Trauma Syndrome: Compound Reaction
9.2.3.1.2	Rape-Trauma Syndrome: Silent Reaction
9.2.4	Risk for Post-Trauma/Stress Syndrome
9.3.1	Anxiety
9.3.1.1	Death Anxiety
9.3.2	Fear

* Diagnoses revised by small work groups at the 1998 Biennial Conference on the Classification of Nursing Diagnoses.

INDEX

Note: Page numbers in *italics* indicate illustrations; those followed by t indicate tables; and those followed by d indicate display material.

A

B

E

N

O

Q

R

S

T

U

V

W

X

Y

Z

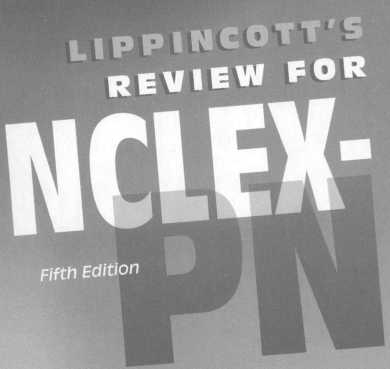